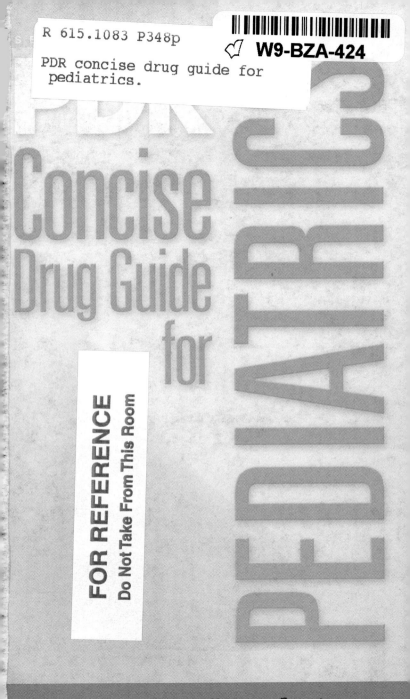

PDR
Concise
Drug Guide
for
PEDIATRICS

PDR® CONCISE DRUG GUIDE FOR PEDIATRICS

SECOND EDITION

Senior Director, Editorial & Publishing: Bette LaGow
Director, Clinical Services: Michael DeLuca, PharmD, MBA
Manager, Clinical Services: Nermin Shenouda, PharmD
Drug Information Specialists: Anila Patel, PharmD; Greg Tallis, RPh
Manager, Editorial Services: Lori Murray
Project Editors: Sabina Borza, Kathleen Engel
Associate Editor: Jennifer Reed
Contributing Editors: Mariam Gerges; Majid Kerolous, PharmD; Cathy Kim, PharmD; Katie Rodgers, RPh
Senior Director, Client Services: Stephanie Struble
Project Manager: John Castro
Manager, Production Purchasing: Thomas Westburgh
Manager, Art Department: Livio Udina
Electronic Publishing Designers: Deana DiVizio, Carrie Faeth
Production Associate: Joan K. Akerlind

Senior Director, Copy Sales: Bill Gaffney
Senior Product Manager: Richard Buchwald

PHYSICIANS' DESK REFERENCE

Executive Vice President, PDR: Thomas F. Rice
Vice President, Publishing & Operations: Valerie Berger
Vice President, Clinical Relations: Mukesh Mehta, RPh
Vice President: Product Management: Cy Caine
Vice President, Strategy & Business Development: Ray Zoeller
Vice President, Pharmaceutical Sales: Anthony Sorce
Vice President, Manufacturing & Vendor Management: Brian Holland

Officers of Thomson Reuters: *President & Chief Executive Officer, Healthcare:* Mike Boswood; *Senior Vice President & Chief Technology Officer:* Frank Licata; *Chief Strategy Officer:* Courtney Morris; *Executive Vice President, Payer Decision Support:* Jon Newpol; *Executive Vice President, Provider Markets:* Terry Cameron; *Executive Vice President, Marketing & Innovation:* Doug Schneider; *Senior Vice President, Finance:* Phil Buckingham; *Senior Vice President, Human Resources:* Pamela M. Bilash; *General Counsel:* Darren Pocsik

ISBN: 978-156363-717-9

Printed in the United States

CONTENTS

Miscellaneous

CDC Growth Charts

FOREWORD

There are many challenges facing the pediatrician in the new millennium. Children with complex diseases are living long and living well. Fiscal concerns and regulatory agencies impose seemingly unreasonable time constraints for care. There is a steady stream of new drugs on the market and there are new indications for familiar drugs. There is more direct pharmaceutical marketing to consumers than ever. Pediatricians and others concerned with the health of infants and children are called upon daily to make critical decisions regarding the best treatment regimen for their patients, which often includes choosing the best drug therapy for a particular disease. There are drug interactions to consider, dosages to remember and to adjust for chronic disease, potential side effects to consider, and more.

The *PDR® Concise Drug Guide for Pediatrics, 2nd Ed.*, was developed to help the pediatric and neonatal healthcare professional get accurate information quickly, easily, and without computer access. This guide provides concise yet comprehensive monographs on more than 800 drugs with FDA-approved pediatric indications, as well entries on more than 150 drugs used in the care of neonates. It is an ideal point-of-care reference.

Vaccines, antibiotics, allergy and asthma medications, treatments for acne and dermatitis—all of the most commonly prescribed drugs in the pediatric setting—are included here. Additionally, this book contains a number of helpful reference tables, including comparison charts of both Rx and OTC medications, an extensive antibiotic sensitivity chart, CDC vaccination recommendations, and drugs excreted in breast milk, just to name a few.

The *PDR® Concise Drug Guide for Pediatrics* should be in the library of all healthcare professionals in the specialties of pediatrics and neonatology. It should sit on the nurses' station of every pediatric hospital ward service. It should be available for home care professionals and school nurses, daycare workers, and teachers. In all venues where there are infants and children who may be on prescription medications, there should be a copy of the *PDR® Concise Drug Guide for Pediatrics*.

Madelyn Kahana, MD
Professor of Pediatrics and Anesthesia and Critical Care
Medical Director, Pediatric Intensive Care Unit
Program Director, Pediatric Residency Training Program
University of Chicago Comer Children's Hospital

HOW TO USE THIS BOOK

The *PDR® Concise Drug Guide for Pediatrics, 2nd Ed.* allows you to quickly locate important drug information so you can care for patients with confidence. With over 800 monographs providing current, organized information from *PDR®*, and more than 150 monographs from *NeoFax®*, this handy reference is the perfect companion for the busy healthcare professional involved in pediatric care.

This compact guide is divided into five discrete sections. The first section consists of over 800 concise drug monographs with FDA-approved pediatric indications. The information provided in these monographs is based on FDA-approved prescribing information. These monographs are organized alphabetically by brand name. When a brand is no longer available, the generic name is used. Monographs may consist of:

- Brand Name
- Generic Name
- Manufacturer
- FDA/DEA Schedule
- Black Box Warnings
- Therapeutic Class
- Indications
- Dosage (adults, pediatrics, special populations)
- How Supplied (dosage form/strength)
- Contraindications
- Warnings/Precautions
- Interactions
- Adverse Reactions
- Pregnancy Category/Breastfeeding Precautions
- Mechanism of Action
- Pharmacokinetics

The second section comprises more than 150 drug monographs with evidence-based uses for neonatal patients. These monographs are organized alphabetically by generic name. Monographs may consist of:

- Generic Name
- Dose and Administration
- Uses
- Monitoring
- Adverse Effects/Precautions
- Pharmacology
- Special Considerations/Preparation
- Selected References

An explanatory note about NeoFax antibiotic dosing charts

The antibiotic dosing charts reflect the fact that renal function and drug elimination are most strongly correlated with Postmenstrual Age ("PMA," which is equivalent to Gestational Age plus Postnatal Age). Postmenstrual Age is therefore used as the primary determinant of dosing interval, with Postnatal Age as a secondary qualifier.

Example: A baby born at 28 weeks gestation is now 21 days old. To determine the dosing interval for cefotaxime, first find the row on the chart containing the Postmenstrual Age of 31 weeks (30 to 36), and then the Postnatal Age of 21 days (>14) to arrive at a dosing interval of 8 hours.

The third section of this guide contains two indices—one with drugs indexed by both brand and generic name, and the other organized by therapeutic class.

In the middle of the book you'll find a Visual Identification Guide featuring hundreds of product images listed by brand name. This section helps you quickly verify the identity of many forms of medications, from tablets to oral solutions. Each product image contains both the generic and brand name, strength, and the name of its supplier. Other strengths and dosage forms may be available; please check FDA-approved prescribing information for a complete listing of all strengths and dosage forms.

The last section is an extensive collection of tables and key references to help healthcare professionals care for pediatric patients. Tables provided include drug comparisons (both Rx and OTC), recommended immunization schedules, growth charts, poison control centers, and much more. The drug comparison tables, which are organized alphabetically by class, may include:

- Brand/Generic Name
- How Supplied (dosage form/strength)
- Initial and Max Dosages
- Usual Dosage Range
- Indications

Important Information About Product Labeling

Entries in the *PDR® Concise Drug Guide for Pediatrics, 2nd Ed.* are drawn from either FDA-approved product labeling as published in *Physicians' Desk Reference®* or supplied by the manufacturer, or in the case of NeoFax, from reliable sources believed to be in accord with good medical practice. The PDR entries are compiled and updated on a regular basis by a staff of experienced pharmacists. While diligent efforts have been made to ensure the accuracy of each entry, it is essential to bear in mind that the information presented here is merely a synopsis of key points in the official labeling, and that the complete labeling contains additional precautionary information that may be of significance in specific cases. Similarly, please remember that only common and dangerous adverse reactions and interactions are included here, and that numerous less-prevalent adverse effects may be reported in the complete labeling. If an entry leaves any question unanswered, be sure to consult *Physicians' Desk Reference* or the manufacturer for additional information.

The function of the publisher is the compilation, organization, and distribution of this information. In organizing and presenting the material in the *PDR® Concise Drug Guide for Pediatrics, 2nd Ed.*, the publisher does not warrant or guarantee any of the products described, or perform any independent analysis in connection with any of the product information contained herein.

The *PDR® Concise Drug Guide for Pediatrics, 2nd Ed.* assumes no obligation to obtain and include any information in the PDR entries other than that provided by the manu-facturer. The publisher does not warrant, guarantee, or advocate the use of any product described herein. The publisher and editors do not assume, and expressly disclaim, any liability for error, omissions, or typographical errors in the information contained herein or for misuse of any of the products listed.

PDR® DRUG MONOGRAPH KEY[1, 2]

BRAND NAME
FDA/DEA Class*

generic (Manufacturer)

> **Black Box Warning:** A brief description of the black box warning(s) that appear in the beginning of the official FDA-approved labeling for the drug.

OTHER BRAND NAMES: Brand name drugs that have the same generic components as the monograph drug.

THERAPEUTIC CLASS: Based on the active ingredients and their mechanism of action.

INDICATIONS: Only includes FDA-approved indications.

DOSAGE: Dosages for adults, pediatrics, and/or special populations as indicated in the official FDA-approved labeling.

HOW SUPPLIED: Product description including strength, formulation, [package size], and scored tablet information.

CONTRAINDICATIONS: Details harmful conditions related to the use of the drug and disease states or patient populations in which use of the monograph drug should be avoided.

WARNINGS/PRECAUTIONS: Details harmful conditions related to the use of the drug and disease states or patient populations where caution is dictated.

ADVERSE REACTIONS: Denotes side effects and adverse reactions listed in the official FDA-approved labeling as occurring with greater frequency (generally at a rate of ≥3%) or deemed significant based on the clinical judgment of the editors. Other side effects may be included if deemed serious or life-threatening. For a complete list of adverse reactions, please refer to the official FDA-approved labeling.

INTERACTIONS: Includes the effects and implications of other drugs and food on the monograph drug based on official FDA-approved labeling.

PREGNANCY: Indicated pregnancy and breastfeeding precautions and, when available, the FDA pregnancy rating system category.[†]

MECHANISM OF ACTION: Includes pharmacologic drug class and a brief description, or proposed mechanism, of how the drug produces its therapeutic effect.

PHARMACOKINETICS: Brief description of the important parameters described in the FDA-approved labeling related to the absorption, distribution, metabolism, and elimination of the drug. The majority of parameters included are an average or the approximate values provided in the FDA-approved labeling. Only a select group of parameters are included. Refer to the full prescribing information for more detailed pharmacokinetics information.

- **Absorption:** The process by which the drug enters the bloodstream and becomes bioavailable. Absorption parameters may include time to peak plasma concentration (T_{max}), area under the curve (AUC), peak plasma concentration (C_{max}), and absolute bioavailability.

- **Distribution:** Parameters related to the dispersion and dissemination of the monograph drug through bodily fluids and tissues. Distribution parameters may include plasma protein binding and volume of distribution (V_d).

- **Metabolism:** Summary of the biotransformation or detoxification of the parent compound into metabolites. Associated enzymes and active metabolites are included if applicable.

- **Elimination:** The parameters associated with the removal of the drug from the body. Elimination parameters may include elimination/terminal half-life ($T_{1/2}$) and percentage eliminated through urine or feces.

[1] Drug monographs contain concise information. Not all fields described in the Drug Monograph Key are included in every monograph. For more detailed information, please see the full FDA-approved labeling information for the drug.

[2] To identify abbreviated terms used within monographs, refer to the Abbreviations, Acronyms, and Symbols table in the appendix on page A1.

*FDA/DEA CLASS

OTC:	Available over-the-counter.
RX:	Requires a prescription.
CII:	Controlled substance; high potential for abuse.
CIII:	Controlled substance; some potential for abuse.
CIV:	Controlled substance; low potential for abuse.
CV:	Controlled substance; subject to state and local regulation.

†FDA USE-IN-PREGNANCY RATINGS

The FDA use-in-pregnancy rating system weighs the degree to which available information has ruled out risk to the fetus against the drug's potential benefit to the patient. The ratings, and the interpretation, are as follows:

CATEGORY	INTERPRETATION
A	**CONTROLLED STUDIES SHOW NO RISK.** Adequate, well-controlled studies in pregnant women have failed to demonstrate a risk to the fetus in any trimester of pregnancy.
B	**NO EVIDENCE OF RISK IN HUMANS.** Adequate, well controlled studies in pregnant women have not shown increased risk of fetal abnormalities despite adverse findings in animals, or, in the absence of adequate human studies, animal studies show no fetal risk. The chance of fetal harm is remote, but remains a possibility.
C	**RISK CANNOT BE RULED OUT.** Adequate, well-controlled human studies are lacking, and animal studies have shown a risk to the fetus or are lacking as well. There is a chance of fetal harm if the drug is administered during pregnancy; but the potential benefits may outweigh the potential risk.
D	**POSITIVE EVIDENCE OF RISK.** Studies in humans, or investigational or post-marketing data, have demonstrated fetal risk. Nevertheless, potential benefits from the use of the drug may outweigh the potential risk. For example, the drug may be acceptable if needed in a life-threatening situation or serious disease for which safer drugs cannot be used or are ineffective.
X	**CONTRAINDICATED IN PREGNANCY.** Studies in animals or humans, or investigational or post-marketing reports, have demonstrated positive evidence of fetal abnormalities or risk which clearly outweighs any possible benefit to the patient.

NEOFAX® DRUG MONOGRAPH KEY[1, 2]

MONOGRAPH NAME

DOSE & ADMINISTRATION: Evidence-based dosage and administration information for neonates.

USES: Includes evidence-based indications.

MONITORING: Important monitoring parameters.

ADVERSE EFFECTS/PRECAUTIONS: Details harmful conditions and adverse reactions related to the use of the drug.

PHARMACOLOGY: Summary of the pharmacological characteristics of the drug.

SPECIAL CONSIDERATIONS/PREPARATION: Brief description of how to prepare the medicine for administration. Also highlights the drug's compatibilities and incompatibilities.

SELECTED REFERENCES: Citations for evidence-based information.

---

[1] Drug monographs contain concise information. Some monographs may not include all fields described in the Drug Monograph Key. For more detailed information, please see the full FDA-approved labeling information for the drug.

[2] To identify abbreviated terms used within monographs, refer to the Abbreviations, Acronyms, and Symbols table in the appendix on page A1.

PDR® Concise Drug Monographs

1-DAY
OTC
tioconazole (Personal Products Company)

THERAPEUTIC CLASS: Azole antifungal

INDICATIONS: Treatment of recurrent vaginal yeast infections.

DOSAGE: *Adults:* Insert contents of applicator intravaginally once hs.
Pediatrics: ≥12 yrs: Insert contents of applicator intravaginally once hs.

HOW SUPPLIED: Oint: 6.5% (4.6g)

WARNINGS/PRECAUTIONS: Do not use if abdominal pain, fever (>100°F), chills, nausea, vomiting, diarrhea, or foul smelling discharge. Avoid tampons, douches, spermicides, and other vaginal products. Do not rely on condoms or diaphragm to prevent STDs or pregnancy until 3 days after last use. Avoid vaginal intercourse.

ADVERSE REACTIONS: Vulvovaginal burning.

PREGNANCY: Safety in pregnancy and nursing not known.

ABELCET
RX
amphotericin B (lipid complex) (Enzon)

THERAPEUTIC CLASS: Polyene antifungal

INDICATIONS: Treatment of invasive fungal infections in patients refractory to or intolerant of conventional amphotericin B therapy.

DOSAGE: *Adults:* 5mg/kg IV at 2.5mg/kg/hr.
Pediatrics: ≥16 yrs: 5mg/kg IV at 2.5mg/kg/hr.

HOW SUPPLIED: Inj: 5mg/mL

WARNINGS/PRECAUTIONS: Anaphylaxis reported. D/C if respiratory distress occurs. Monitor SCr, LFTs, serum electrolytes, CBC during therapy.

ADVERSE REACTIONS: Chills, fever, increased SCr, multi-organ failure, NV, hypotension, respiratory failure, dyspnea, sepsis, diarrhea, headache, heart arrest, HTN, hypokalemia, infection, kidney failure, pain, thrombocytopenia.

INTERACTIONS: Antineoplastics may potentiate renal toxicity, bronchospasm, hypotension. Corticosteroids and corticotropin may potentiate hypokalemia predisposing patients to cardiac dysfunction. May potentiate digitalis toxicity. Increased risk of flucytosine toxicity. Acute pulmonary toxicity reported with leukocyte transfusions. Nephrotoxic drugs (eg, aminoglycosides, pentamidine) enhance potential for renal toxicity. Cyclosporine within several days of bone marrow ablation associated with nephrotoxicity. Hypokalemia effect may enhance curariform effect of skeletal muscle relaxants. May cause increased myelotoxicity and nephrotoxicity with concomitant zidovudine.

PREGNANCY: Category B, not for use in nursing.

MECHANISM OF ACTION: Acts by binding to sterols in cell membrane of susceptible fungi, with resultant change in membrane permeability.

PHARMACOKINETICS: **Absorption:** C_{max}=1.7mcg/mL, AUC=14mcg•h/mL. **Distribution:** V_d=131L/kg. **Elimination:** $T_{1/2}$=173.4 hrs.

ABILIFY
RX
aripiprazole (Bristol-Myers Squibb/Otsuka America)

> **Elderly patients with dementia-related psychosis treated with atypical antipsychotic drugs are at an increased risk of death; most appeared to be cardiovascular (eg, heart failure, sudden death) or infectious (eg, pneumonia) in nature. Aripiprazole is not approved for the treatment of patients with dementia-related psychosis. Children, adolescents, and young adults taking antidepressants for major depressive disorder and other psychiatric disorders are at increased risk of suicidal thinking and behavior.**

OTHER BRAND NAME: Abilify Discmelt (Bristol-Myers Squibb/Otsuka America)

THERAPEUTIC CLASS: Partial D_2/$5HT_{1A}$ agonist/$5HT_{2A}$ antagonist

INDICATIONS: (PO) Acute and maintenance treatment of schizophrenia in adults and adolescents aged 13-17 yrs. Acute and maintenance treatment of manic and mixed episodes associated with bipolar I disorder with or without psychotic features in adults and pediatrics aged 10-17 yrs. Adjunctive therapy to antidepressants for acute treatment of major depressive disorder (MDD) in adults. Adjunctive therapy to either lithium or valproate for the acute treatment of manic and mixed episodes associated with bipolar I disorder with or without psychotic features in adults and pediatrics aged 10-17 yrs. (Inj) Acute treatment of agitation associated with schizophrenia or bipolar disorder, manic or mixed, in adults.

DOSAGE: *Adults:* (PO) Schizophrenia: Initial/Target: 10-15mg qd. Titrate: Should not increase before 2 weeks. Max: 30mg/day. Bipolar Disorder (Monotherapy or Adjunct): Initial/Target: 15mg/day. Max: 30mg/day. MDD: Initial: 2-5mg/day. Titrate: May adjust dose at increments of ≤5mg/day at intervals ≥1 week. Range: 2-15mg/day. Max: 15mg/day. Periodically reassess need for maintenance therapy. Oral sol can be given on mg-per-mg basis up to 25mg. Patients receiving 30mg tabs should receive 25mg of oral sol. (Inj) Agitation: 9.75mg IM. Range: 5.25-15mg IM. Max: 30mg/day; initiate PO therapy as soon as possible. Concomitant Strong CYP3A4 Inhibitors (eg, ketoconazole, clarithromycin): Reduce usual aripiprazole dose by 50%. Concomitant CYP2D6 Inhibitors (eg, quinidine, fluoxetine, paroxetine): Reduce usual aripiprazole dose by 50%. Concomitant CYP3A4 Inducers (eg, carbamazepine): Double aripiprazole dose.
Pediatrics: Schizophrenia (13-17 yrs)/Bipolar Disorder (Monotherapy or Adjunct) (10-17 yrs): Initial: 2mg/day. Titrate: 5mg after 2 days. May adjust dose in 5mg/day increments. Recommended: 10mg/day. Max: 30mg/day. Periodically reassess need for maintenance therapy. Oral sol can be given on mg-per-mg basis up to 25mg. Patients receiving 30mg tabs should receive 25mg of oral sol. Concomitant Strong CYP3A4 Inhibitors (eg, ketoconazole, clarithromycin): Reduce usual aripiprazole dose by 50%. Concomitant CYP2D6 Inhibitors (eg, quinidine, fluoxetine, paroxetine): Reduce usual aripiprazole dose by 50%. Concomitant CYP3A4 Inducers (eg, carbamazepine): Double aripiprazole dose.

HOW SUPPLIED: Tab, Orally Disintegrating: (Discmelt) 10mg, 15mg; Tab: 2mg, 5mg, 10mg, 15mg, 20mg, 30mg; Sol: 1mg/mL (150mL); Inj: 7.5mg/mL

WARNINGS/PRECAUTIONS: May develop tardive dyskinesia, NMS. Monitor for hyperglycemia, worsening of glucose control with DM, FBG levels with diabetes risk. Increased incidence of cerebrovascular adverse events (stroke) in elderly dementia patients. Orthostatic hypotension reported; caution with cardiovascular disease, conditions predisposed to hypotension (eg, dehydration, hypovolemia). May lower seizure threshold. Potential for cognitive and motor impairment. May disrupt body's temperature regulation. Possible esophageal dysmotility and aspiration; caution in patients at risk for aspiration pneumonia. Observe vigilance in treating psychosis associated with Alzheimer's.

ADVERSE REACTIONS: Headache, asthenia, rash, blurred vision, rhinitis, cough, tremor, anxiety, insomnia, nausea, vomiting, lightheadedness, somnolence, constipation, akathisia, extrapyramidal disorder, somnolence, oropharyngeal spasm, grand mal seizure, jaundice, nasopharyngitis, dizziness.

INTERACTIONS: May potentiate effect of antihypertensives. Caution with anticholinergic agents, other centrally acting drugs. Avoid alcohol. CYP3A4 inducers (eg, carbamazepine) may lower blood levels. CYP3A4 inhibitors (eg, ketoconazole, itraconazole) or 2D6 inhibitors (eg, quinidine, fluoxetine, paroxetine) can increase blood levels.

PREGNANCY: Category C, not for use in nursing.

MECHANISM OF ACTION: Not established; proposed that efficacy is mediated through a combination of partial agonist activity at D_2 and $5-HT_{1A}$ receptors and antagonist activity at $5-HT_{2A}$ receptors.

PHARMACOKINETICS: Absorption: Absolute bioavailability 87% (PO), 100% (IM); T_{max}=3-5 hrs (PO), 1-3 hrs (IM). **Distribution:** V_d=404L or 4.9L/kg (PO), plasma protein binding 99% (PO). **Metabolism:** Hepatic via dehydrogenation, hydroxylation, and N-dealkylation. Dehydro-aripiprazole (active metabolite) CYP3A4 and 2D6 enzymes (PO). Not systemically evaluated (IM). **Elimination:** Urine (25%), feces (55%); $T_{1/2}$=75-146 hrs.

ABREVA OTC
docosanol (GlaxoSmithKline Consumer)

THERAPEUTIC CLASS: Antiviral

INDICATIONS: To treat cold sore/fever blisters on the face or lips.

DOSAGE: *Adults:* Apply to affected area on face or lips at 1st sign of cold sore/fever blister (tingle). Use 5x/day until healed.
Pediatrics: ≥12 yrs: Apply to affected area on face or lips at 1st sign of cold sore/fever blister (tingle). Use 5x/day until healed.

HOW SUPPLIED: Cre: 10% (2g)

WARNINGS/PRECAUTIONS: Avoid in or near eyes, and inside mouth. D/C if sore worsens or does not heal in 10 days.

PREGNANCY: Safety in pregnancy and nursing is not known.

MECHANISM OF ACTION: Antiviral; works on the cell membrane to inhibit the ability of the virus to fuse with the cell membrane.

ACCOLATE RX
zafirlukast (AstraZeneca)

THERAPEUTIC CLASS: Leukotriene receptor antagonist

INDICATIONS: Prophylaxis and chronic treatment of asthma.

DOSAGE: *Adults:* 20mg bid. Administer 1 hr ac or 2 hrs pc.
Pediatrics: ≥12 yrs: 20mg bid. 5-11 yrs: 10mg bid. Administer 1 hr ac or 2 hrs pc.

HOW SUPPLIED: Tab: 10mg, 20mg

WARNINGS/PRECAUTIONS: Not for treatment of acute asthma attacks. Bioavailability decreases with food. Hepatic dysfunction and systemic eosinophilia reported.

ADVERSE REACTIONS: Headache, infection, nausea, diarrhea, hypersensitivity reactions including angioedema.

INTERACTIONS: Potentiates warfarin. Caution with drugs metabolized by CYP2C9 (eg, tolbutamide, phenytoin, carbamazepine) or CYP3A4 (eg, dihydropyridine CCBs, cyclosporine, cisapride, astemizole). Increased levels with ASA. Decreased levels by erythromycin, theophylline. May increase theophylline levels.

PREGNANCY: Category B, not for use in nursing.

MECHANISM OF ACTION: Leukotriene receptor antagonist (LTRA); selective and competitive receptor antagonist of leukotriene D_4 and E_4 (LTD$_4$ and LTE$_4$), components of slow-reacting substance of anaphylaxis (SRSA); inhibits bronchoconstriction.

PHARMACOKINETICS: Absorption: Rapid. (Adult) C_{max}=326ng/mL; T_{max}=2 hrs; AUC=1137ng•h/mL. (7-11 yrs) C_{max}=601ng/mL; T_{max}=2.5 hrs; AUC=2027ng•h/mL. (5-6 yrs) C_{max}=756ng/mL; T_{max}=2.1 hrs; AUC=2458ng•h/mL. **Distribution:** V_d=approximately 70L; plasma protein binding (>99%). **Metabolism:** Liver, hydroxylation via CYP2C9. **Elimination:** $T_{1/2}$=10 hrs.

ACCUNEB RX
albuterol sulfate (Dey)

THERAPEUTIC CLASS: Beta$_2$ -agonist

INDICATIONS: Relief of bronchospasm with asthma.

DOSAGE: *Pediatrics:* 2-12 yrs: Initial: 0.63mg or 1.25mg tid-qid via nebulizer. 6-12 yrs with severe asthma, >40kg or 11-12 yrs: Initial: 1.25mg tid-qid.

HOW SUPPLIED: Sol: 1.25mg/3mL, 0.63mg/3mL (3mL, 25^s)

WARNINGS/PRECAUTIONS: Hypersensitivity reactions reported. Fatalities reported with excessive use. Caution with cardiovascular disorders, especially coronary insufficiency, arrhythmias and HTN. May need concomitant anti-inflammatory agents. Can produce paradoxical bronchospasm. Caution with DM. May cause hypokalemia.

ADVERSE REACTIONS: Asthma exacerbation, otitis media, allergic reaction, gastroenteritis, cold symptoms.

INTERACTIONS: Avoid other short-acting sympathomimetic bronchodilators and epinephrine. Extreme caution within 2 weeks of MAOI or TCA use. Monitor digoxin. ECG changes and/or hypokalemia with non-K$^+$-sparing diuretics may worsen. May be antagonized by β-blockers.

PREGNANCY: Category C, not for use in nursing.

MECHANISM OF ACTION: β$_2$ adrenergic agonist; stimulates adenyl cyclase, the enzyme that catalyzes the formation of ATP.

PHARMACOKINETICS: Absorption: (3mg): C_{max}=2.1ng/mL, T_{max}=0.5 hrs. **Elimination:** (4 mg): $T_{1/2}$=5-6 hrs.

ACCUTANE RX
isotretinoin (Roche Labs)

Not for use by females who are or may become pregnant, or if breastfeeding. Birth defects have been documented. Increased risk of spontaneous abortion, and premature births reported. Approved for marketing only under special restricted distribution program called iPLEDGE™. Must have 2 negative pregnancy tests. Repeat pregnancy test monthly. Use 2 forms of contraception at least 1 month prior, during, and 1 month following discontinuation. Must fill written prescriptions within 7 days; refills require new prescriptions. May dispense maximum of 1 month supply. Prescriber, dispensing pharmacy, and patient must be registered with iPLEDGE.

OTHER BRAND NAMES: Amnesteem (Genpharm) - Claravis (Barr) - Sotret (Ranbaxy)

THERAPEUTIC CLASS: Retinoid

INDICATIONS: Severe recalcitrant nodular acne unresponsive to conventional therapy, including systemic antibiotics.

DOSAGE: *Adults:* Initial/Usual: 0.5-1mg/kg/day given bid for 15-20 weeks. Max: 2mg/kg/day (for very serious cases). Adjust for side effects and disease response. May discontinue if nodule count reduced by >70% prior to completion. Repeat only if necessary after 2 months off drug. Take with food.
Pediatrics: ≥12 yrs: Initial/Usual: 0.5-1mg/kg/day given bid for 15-20 weeks. Max: 2mg/kg/day (for very serious cases). Adjust for side effects and disease response. May discontinue if nodule count reduced by >70% prior to completion. Repeat only if necessary after 2 months off drug. Take with food.

HOW SUPPLIED: Cap: 10mg, 20mg, 40mg

CONTRAINDICATIONS: Pregnancy, paraben sensitivity (preservative in gelatin cap).

WARNINGS/PRECAUTIONS: Acute pancreatitis, impaired hearing, anaphylactic reactions, inflammatory bowel disease, elevated TG and LFTs, hepatotoxicity, premature epiphyseal closure, and hyperostosis reported. May cause depression, psychosis, aggressive and/or violent behaviors, rarely suicidal ideation/attempts and suicide; may need further evaluation after discontinuation. May cause decreased night vision, and corneal opacities. Associated with pseudotumor cerebri. Check lipids before therapy, and then at intervals until response established (within 4 weeks). D/C if significant decrease in WBC, hearing or visual impairment, abdominal pain, rectal bleeding, or severe diarrhea occurs. Monitor LFTs before therapy, weekly or biweekly until response established. May develop musculoskeletal symptoms. Avoid prolonged UV rays or sunlight, and donating blood up to 1 month after discontinuing therapy. Caution with genetic predisposition for age-related osteoporosis, history of childhood osteoporosis, osteomalacia, other bone metabolism disorders (eg, anorexia nervosa). Spontaneous osteoporosis, osteopenia, bone fractures, and delayed fracture healing reported; caution in sports with repetitive impact. Use 2 forms of effective contraception for 1 month. Female patients of childbearing potential must fill and pick up the prescription within 7 days of the date of specimen collection for the pregnancy test. Must only be dispensed in no more than 30-day supply and with a Medication Guide.

ADVERSE REACTIONS: Cheilitis, dry skin and mucous membranes, conjunctivitis, blood dyscrasias, epistaxis, decreased HDL, elevated cholesterol and TG, elevated blood sugar, arthralgias, back pain, hearing/vision impairment, rash, photosensitivity reactions, psychiatric disorders, abnormal menses, cardiovascular disorders.

INTERACTIONS: Avoid vitamin A. Limit alcohol consumption. Aoid use with tetracyclines; increased incidence of pseudotumor cerebri. Pregnancy reported with oral and injectable/implantable contraceptives. Avoid St. John's wort; may cause breakthrough bleeding with oral contraceptives. Caution with drugs that cause drug-induced osteoporosis/osteomalacia and affect vitamin D metabolism (eg, corticosteroids, phenytoin).

PREGNANCY: Category X, not for use in nursing.

MECHANISM OF ACTION: Retinoid; MOA not established. Suspected to inhibit sebaceous gland function and keratinization.

PHARMACOKINETICS: Absorption: C_{max}=862ng/mL (fed), 301ng/mL (fasted); T_{max}=5.3 hrs (fed), 3.2 hrs (fasted); AUC=10,004ng•hr/mL (fed), 3703ng•hr/mL (fasted). **Distribution:** Plasma protein binding (99.9%). **Metabolism:** Liver via CYP2C8, 2C9, 3A4, and 2B6; 4-oxo-isotretinoin, retinoic acid, and 4-oxo-retinoic acid (active metabolites). **Elimination:** Urine, feces; $T_{1/2}$=21 hrs (isotretinoin), 24 hrs (4-oxo-isotretinoin).

ACETYLCYSTEINE   RX
acetylcysteine (Various)

THERAPEUTIC CLASS: Acetaminophen antidote/Mucolytic

INDICATIONS: Adjunctive mucolytic therapy in acute and chronic bronchopulmonary disease; pulmonary complications of cystic fibrosis and surgery; tracheostomy care; during anesthesia; post-traumatic chest conditions; atelectasis; diagnostic bronchial studies. Antidote for acute acetaminophen (APAP) toxicity.

DOSAGE: *Adults:* Antidote: Empty stomach by lavage or emesis before administration. Administer immediately, regardless of quantity, if APAP ingestion ≤24hrs. LD: 140mg/kg PO then 70mg/kg PO q4h for 17 doses starting 4 hrs after LD. D/C if predetoxification APAP level is in nontoxic range and overdose occurred at least 4 hrs before assay. Obtain 2nd plasma level if range is nontoxic and time of ingestion is unknown or <4 hrs. Mucolytic: Nebulization (face mask, mouth piece, tracheostomy): 1-10mL of 20% or 2-10mL of 10% q2-6h. Usual: 3-5mL of 20% or 6-10mL of 10% 3-4 times/day. Closed Tent or Croupette: Up to 300mL of 10% or 20%. Direct Instillation: 1-2 mL of 10% or 20% q1-4h. Percutaneous Intratracheal Catheter: 1-2mL of 20% or 2-4mL of 10% q1-4h. Diagnostic Bronchograms: Give before procedure. 2-3 doses of 1-2mL of 20% or 2-4mL of 10%. *Pediatrics:* Antidote: Empty stomach by lavage or emesis before administration. Administer immediately, regardless of quantity, if APAP ingestion ≤24hrs. LD: 140mg/kg PO then 70mg/kg PO q4h for 17 doses starting 4 hours after LD. D/C if predetoxification APAP level is in nontoxic range and overdose occurred at least 4 hrs before assay. Obtain 2nd plasma level if range is nontoxic and time of ingestion is unknown or <4 hrs. Mucolytic: Nebulization (face mask, mouth piece, tracheostomy): 1-10mL of 20% or 2-10mL of 10% q2-6h. Usual: 3-5mL of 20% or 6-10mL of 10% 3-4 times/day. Closed Tent or Croupette: Up to 300mL of 10% or 20%. Direct Instillation: 1-2 mL of 10% or 20% q1-4h. Percutaneous Intratracheal Catheter: 1-2mL of 20% or 2-4mL of 10% q1-4h. Diagnostic Procedures: Give before procedure. 2-3 doses of 1-2mL of 20% or 2-4mL of 10%.

HOW SUPPLIED: Sol: 10%, 20%

WARNINGS/PRECAUTIONS: (Oral) D/C if generalized urticaria or encephalopathy due to hepatic failure develops. May aggravate vomiting; evaluate with risk of gastric hemorrhage. (Inhalation) Monitor asthmatics. D/C if bronchospasm progresses.

ADVERSE REACTIONS: (Oral) N/V, other GI symptoms. (Inhalation) Stomatitis, NV, fever, rhinorrhea, drowsiness, clamminess, chest tightness, bronchoconstriction.

PREGNANCY: Category B, caution in nursing.

MECHANISM OF ACTION: N-acetyl derivative. Mucolytic: Opens disulfide linkages in mucus, thereby lowering viscosity. Antidote: Protects liver by maintaining or restoring glutathione levels, or by acting as alternate substrate for conjugation with, and thus detoxification of reactive metabolites, reducing extent of liver injury.

PHARMACOKINETICS: Metabolism: Deacetylation, oxidation.

ACIPHEX
rabeprazole sodium (Eisai/PRICARA)

RX

THERAPEUTIC CLASS: Proton pump inhibitor

INDICATIONS: Short-term treatment in the healing and symptomatic relief of erosive or ulcerative gastroesophageal reflux disease (GERD). Maintenance of healing and reduction in relapse rates of heartburn symptoms in patients with erosive or ulcerative GERD. Treatment of daytime and nighttime heartburn and other symptoms associated with GERD. Short-term treatment in the healing and symptomatic relief of duodenal ulcers (DU). In combination with amoxicillin and clarithromycin as a 3-drug regimen for the treatment of patients with H.pylori infection and DU disease (active or history within the past 5 yrs) to eradicate H.pylori and reduce the risk of DU recurrence. Long-term treatment of pathological hypersecretory conditions, including Zollinger-Ellison syndrome.

DOSAGE: *Adults:* Erosive/Ulcerative GERD: Healing: 20mg qd for 4-8 weeks. May repeat for 8 weeks if needed. Maint: 20mg qd. Symptomatic GERD: 20mg qd for 4 weeks. May repeat for 4 weeks if needed. DU: 20mg qd after morning meal for up to 4 weeks. May need additional therapy. H.pylori Triple Therapy: 20mg + clarithromycin 500mg + amoxicillin 1g, all bid (qam and qpm) with food for 7 days. Pathological Hypersecretory Conditions: Initial: 60mg qd. Titrate: Adjust according to need. Maint: Up to 100mg qd or 60mg bid. May treat up to 1 yr. Swallow tabs whole; do not chew, crush, or split.
Pediatrics: ≥12 yrs: Symptomatic GERD: 20mg qd for up to 8 weeks.

HOW SUPPLIED: Tab, Delayed-Release: 20mg

WARNINGS/PRECAUTIONS: Symptomatic response does not preclude the presence of gastric malignancy. Caution with severe hepatic impairment.

ADVERSE REACTIONS: Headache. Diarrhea and taste perversion with triple therapy.

INTERACTIONS: May alter absorption of pH-dependent drugs (eg, ketoconazole, digoxin). May inhibit cyclosporine metabolism. May increase digoxin plasma levels and decrease ketoconazole levels. Monitor PT/INR with warfarin. Increased rabeprazole and clarithromycin levels with triple therapy.

PREGNANCY: Category B, not for use in nursing.

MECHANISM OF ACTION: Proton pump inhibitor; suppresses gastric acid secretion by inhibiting the gastric (H^+, K^+)-ATPase enzyme at the secretory surface of the gastric parietal cell. Blocks the final step of gastric acid secretion.

PHARMACOKINETICS: Absorption: T_{max}=2-5 hrs; absolute bioavailability (52%). **Distribution:** Plasma protein binding (96.3%). **Metabolism:** Extensive. Liver via CYP3A4 to sulphone (primary metabolite) and CYP2C19 to desmethyl rabeprazole (primary metabolite). **Elimination:** Urine (90%), feces; $T_{1/2}$=1-2 hrs.

ACLOVATE
alclometasone dipropionate (GlaxoSmithKline)

RX

THERAPEUTIC CLASS: Corticosteroid

INDICATIONS: Relief of the inflammatory and pruritic manifestations of corticosteroid responsive dermatoses.

DOSAGE: *Adults:* Apply bid-tid. Reassess if no improvement after 2 weeks.
Pediatrics: ≥1 yr: Apply bid-tid. Reassess if no improvement after 2 weeks.

HOW SUPPLIED: Cre, Oint: 0.05% (15g, 45g, 60g)

WARNINGS/PRECAUTIONS: May produce reversible HPA axis suppression, manifestations of Cushing's syndrome, hyperglycemia, and glucosuria. Use appropriate antifungal or antibacterial agent with dermatological infections. Peds may be more susceptible to systemic toxicity. Avoid occlusive dressings. Avoid diaper area. Not for use in diaper dermatitis. D/C if irritation occurs. Caution in peds.

ADVERSE REACTIONS: Itching, burning, erythema, dryness, irritation, papular rash, folliculitis, acneiform eruptions, hypopigmentation, perioral dermatitis, allergic contact dermatitis, secondary infection, skin atrophy, striae.

PREGNANCY: Category C, caution in nursing.

MECHANISM OF ACTION: Corticosteroid; has anti-inflammatory, antipruritic, and vaso-constrictive properties. Anti-inflammatory mechanism not established. Suspected to act by the induction of phospholipase A_2 inhibitory proteins (lipocortins), which may control the biosynthesis of potent mediators of inflammation (eg, prostaglandins, leukotrienes) by inhibiting the release of their common precursor, arachidonic acid. Arachidonic acid is released from membrane phospholipids by phospholipase A_2.

PHARMACOKINETICS: Distribution: Systemically administered corticosteroids are found in breast milk.

AcтHIB   RX
haemophilus B conjugate (Sanofi Pasteur)

THERAPEUTIC CLASS: Vaccine

INDICATIONS: Solo or combined with DTP (Aventis Pasteur) for active immunization of children 2-18 months for prevention of invasive disease caused by *H.influenzae* type B and/or diphtheria, tetanus, and pertussis. Combined with Tripedia (TriHIBit) for active immunization of children 15-18 months for prevention of invasive disease caused by *H.influenzae* type B and diphtheria, tetanus, and pertussis.

DOSAGE: *Pediatrics:* Reconstituted with DTP or Saline: 0.5mL IM in deltoid or thigh at 2, 4, and 6 months old; 4th dose at 15-18 months; 5th dose at 4-6 yrs. Reconstituted with Tripedia (as 4th dose in series): 0.5mL IM in deltoid or thigh given at 15-18 months; 5th dose at 4-6 yrs. Previously Unvaccinated: 7-11 months old: 2 doses at 8 week intervals with a booster at 15-18 months. 12-14 months: 1 dose followed by a booster 2 months later.

HOW SUPPLIED: Inj: 10mcg

WARNINGS/PRECAUTIONS: Immunosuppressed patients may not obtain expected anti-body response. Have epinephrine injection (1:1000) available.

ADVERSE REACTIONS: Local: tenderness, erythema, induration. Systemic: fever, irritability, drowsiness, anorexia, nausea, diarrhea, vomiting.

INTERACTIONS: Immunosuppressive therapies may reduce effectiveness.

PREGNANCY: Category C, safety in nursing not known.

MECHANISM OF ACTION: Vaccine; bactericidal activity against *H.influenzae* type B, diphtheria, tetanus, and pertussis.

Acticin   RX
permethrin (Mylan Bertek)

THERAPEUTIC CLASS: Pyrethroid scabicidal agent

INDICATIONS: Treatment of scabies.

DOSAGE: *Adults:* Massage into skin from head to soles of feet. Wash off after 8-14 hrs. One treatment should be adequate. Retreat if living mites present after 14 days. *Pediatrics:* ≥2 months: Massage into skin from head (scalp, temples and forehead) to soles of feet. Wash off after 8-14 hrs. One treatment should be adequate. Retreat if living mites present after 14 days.

HOW SUPPLIED: Cre: 5% (60g)

CONTRAINDICATIONS: Allergy to synthetic pyrethroid or pyrethrin.

WARNINGS/PRECAUTIONS: May temporarily exacerbate infection (eg pruritus, edema, erythema). Avoid eyes. D/C if hypersensitivity occurs.

ADVERSE REACTIONS: Burning, stinging, pruritus, erythema, numbness, tingling, rash.

PREGNANCY: Category B, not for use in nursing.

MECHANISM OF ACTION: Pyrethroid scabicidal agent; acts on the nerve cell membrane to disrupt the sodium channel current by which the polarization of the membrane is regulated. Results in depolarization and paralysis of pests. Active against a broad range of pests including lice, ticks, fleas, mites, and other arthropods.

PHARMACOKINETICS: Metabolism: Liver via ester hydrolysis. **Excretion:** Urine.

ACTIQ
fentanyl citrate (Cephalon)

> May cause life-threatening hypoventilation in opioid non-tolerant patients. Only for cancer pain in opioid tolerant patients with malignancies. Keep out of reach of children and discard properly. Concomitant use with moderate and strong CYP3A4 inhibitors may cause fatal respiratory depression.

THERAPEUTIC CLASS: Opioid analgesic

INDICATIONS: Management of breakthrough cancer pain in patients with malignancies who are already receiving and are tolerant to opioid therapy.

DOSAGE: *Adults:* Initial: 0.2mg (consume over 15 min). Titrate: Redose 15 min after previous dose is completed. No more than 2 units per breakthrough pain episode. May increase to next highest available strength if several breakthrough episodes (1-2 days) require more than 1 unit per pain episode. Repeat titration for each new dose. Max: 4 units/day. Prescribe 6 units with each new titration. The lozenge should be sucked, not chewed, and consumed over 15 min.
Pediatrics: ≥16 yrs: Initial: 0.2mg (consume over 15 min). Titrate: Redose 15 min after previous dose is completed. No more than 2 units per breakthrough pain episode. May increase to next highest available strength if several breakthrough episodes (1-2 days) require more than 1 unit per pain episode. Repeat titration for each new dose. Max: 4 units/day. Prescribe 6 units with each new titration. The lozenge should be sucked, not chewed, and consumed over 15 min.

HOW SUPPLIED: Loz: 0.2mg, 0.4mg, 0.6mg, 0.8mg, 1.2mg, 1.6mg

CONTRAINDICATIONS: Opioid non-tolerant patients and management of acute or postoperative pain.

WARNINGS/PRECAUTIONS: Caution with COPD, hepatic or renal dysfunction. Risk of clinically significant hypoventilation. Extreme caution with evidence of increased ICP or impaired consciousness. Can produce morphine-like dependence. Increased risk of dental decay; ensure proper oral hygiene. Caution with bradyarrhythmias, liver or kidney dysfunction. Patients on concomitant CNS depressants must be monitored for a change in opioid effects. May impair mental and/or physical status.

ADVERSE REACTIONS: Respiratory depression, circulatory depression, headache, hypotension, shock, NV, constipation, dizziness, dyspnea, anxiety, somnolence.

INTERACTIONS: Concomitant use with other CNS depressants, including opioids, sedatives, hypnotics, general anesthetics, phenothiazines, tranquilizers, skeletal muscle relaxants, sedating antihistamines, potent inhibitors of CYP3A4 (eg, erythromycin, ketoconazole, itraconazole, ritonavir, troleandomycin, clarithromycin, nelfinavir and nefazodone) or moderate inhibitors (eg, amprenavir, aprepitant, diltiazem, erythromycin, fluconazole, fosamprenavir, and verapamil) and alcohol may result in increased plasma concentrations. Avoid grapefruit juice. Avoid within 14 days of MAOIs.

PREGNANCY: Category C, not for use in nursing.

MECHANISM OF ACTION: Narcotic agonist analgesic: Principle therapeutic effect is analgesia. Not established. A μ-opioid receptor agonist. Specific CNS opioid receptors for endogenous compounds have been identified throughout brain and spinal cord and play a role in analgesic effects.

PHARMACOKINETICS: Absorption: Rapidly absorbed from buccal mucosa; slow absorption of swallowed fentanyl from GI tract. Absolute bioavailability (50%); C_{max}= 0.39-2.51ng/mL; T_{max}=20-40 min. **Distribution:** V_d=4L/kg; plasma protein binding (80-85%). Rapidly distributed to brain, heart, lungs, kidneys, spleen; slowly to muscles and fat. Readily crosses placenta; found in breast milk. . **Metabolism:** Liver, via CYP3A4; intestinal mucosa; norfentanyl (metabolite). **Elimination:** Urine (major), feces; $T_{1/2}$=7 hrs.

ACULAR
ketorolac tromethamine (Allergan)

RX

THERAPEUTIC CLASS: NSAID

INDICATIONS: Ocular itching due to seasonal allergic conjunctivitis. Postoperative inflammation in cataract extraction.

DOSAGE: *Adults:* 1 drop qid. Post-op Inflammation: Begin 24 hrs post-op and continue for 2 weeks.
Pediatrics: ≥3 yrs: 1 drop qid. Post-op Inflammation: Begin 24 hrs post-op and continue for 2 weeks.

HOW SUPPLIED: Sol: 0.5% (3mL, 5mL, 10mL)

WARNINGS/PRECAUTIONS: May increase ocular tissue bleeding in conjunction with ocular surgery. Avoid use with contact lenses. D/C if corneal epithelium breakdown occurs. Caution in known bleeding tendencies, complicated ocular surgeries, corneal denervation, corneal epithelial defects, DM, ocular surface diseases (eg, dry eye syndrome), rheumatoid arthritis, or repeat ocular surgeries within a short period of time. Caution if used >24 hrs prior to surgery and use beyond 14 days post-surgery.

ADVERSE REACTIONS: Transient stinging/burning, superficial keratitis or infections, allergic reactions, ocular inflammation, corneal edema, iritis.

INTERACTIONS: Potential for cross-sensitivity to acetylsalicylic acid, phenylacetic acid derivatives, and other NSAIDs. Caution with agents that may prolong bleeding time. Increased potential for healing problems with topical steroids.

PREGNANCY: Category C, caution in nursing.

MECHANISM OF ACTION: NSAID; inhibits prostaglandin biosynthesis.

PHARMACOKINETICS: Absorption: C_{max} =95ng/mL; T_{max} =12hrs.

ADACEL
RX

diphtheria toxoid, reduced - pertussis vaccine acellular, adsorbed - tetanus toxoid (Sanofi Pasteur)

THERAPEUTIC CLASS: Vaccine

INDICATIONS: Active booster immunization against tetanus, diphtheria, and pertussis in persons 11-64 years of age.

DOSAGE: *Adults:* ≤64 yrs: 0.5mL IM (deltoid).
Pediatrics: ≥11 yrs: 0.5mL IM (deltoid).

HOW SUPPLIED: Inj: 0.5mL

CONTRAINDICATIONS: Encephalopathy not attributable to another identifiable cause within 7 days from initial vaccination. Progressive neurological disorder, uncontrolled epilepsy, or progressive encephalopathy.

WARNINGS/PRECAUTIONS: Evaluate risks/benefits of subsequent doses if temperature ≥105°F within 48 hrs not due to another identifiable cause; if collapse/shock occurs; persistent crying for ≥3 hrs within 48 hrs; and convulsions with or without fever within 3 days of vaccine. Continue with Td vaccine if pertussis must be withheld. Have epinephrine (1:1000) available. May not achieve expected immune response in immunosuppressed patients. Avoid injection into blood vessel. Should not be administered into the buttocks nor by the intradermal route.

ADVERSE REACTIONS: Injection site reactions, fever, headache, body aches, tiredness, chills, sore joints, nausea, lymph node swelling, diarrhea, and vomiting.

INTERACTIONS: Immunosuppressives (eg, irradiation, antimetabolites, alkylating agents, cytotoxic drugs, and corticosteroids) may reduce the immune response to vaccines.

PREGNANCY: Category C, caution in nursing

MECHANISM OF ACTION: Immunostimulant; elicits production of antibodies that may protect against tetanus, diphtheria, and pertussis.

ADDERALL
CII

amphetamine salt combo (Shire)

> High potential for abuse; avoid prolonged use. Misuse of amphetamine may cause sudden death and serious cardiovascular adverse events.

THERAPEUTIC CLASS: Sympathomimetic amine

INDICATIONS: Treatment of attention deficit disorder with hyperactivity (ADHD) and narcolepsy.

ADDERALL XR

DOSAGE: *Adults:* Narcolepsy: Initial: 10mg/day. Titrate: May increase by 10mg/day every week. Usual: 5-60mg/day. Give 1st dose upon awakening, and additional doses q4-6h.

Pediatrics: ADHD: 3-5 yrs: Initial: 2.5mg qd. Titrate: May increase by 2.5mg weekly. ≥6 yrs: 5mg qd-bid. May increase by 5mg weekly. Max (usual): 40mg/day. Narcolepsy: 6-12 yrs: Initial: 5mg/day. May increase by 5mg weekly. ≥12 yrs: Initial: 10mg/day. Titrate: May increase by 10mg/day every week. Usual: 5-60mg/day. Give 1st dose upon awakening, and additional doses q4-6h.

HOW SUPPLIED: Tab: 5mg*, 7.5mg*, 10mg*, 12.5mg*, 15mg*, 20mg*, 30mg* *scored

CONTRAINDICATIONS: Advanced arteriosclerosis, symptomatic cardiovascular disease, moderate to severe HTN, hyperthyroidism, glaucoma, agitated states, history of drug abuse, during or within 14 days of MAOI use.

WARNINGS/PRECAUTIONS: May exacerbate symptoms of behavior disturbance and thought disorder in psychotic patients. Caution when using stimulants to treat patients with comorbid bipolar disorder because of concern for possible induction of mixed/manic episode in such patients. Stimulants at usual doses can cause treatment emergent psychotic or manic symptoms (eg, hallucinations, delusional thinking, mania) in children and adolescents without prior history of psychotic illness. Aggressive behavior or hostility reported in clinical trials and the postmarketing experience of some medications indicated for the treatment of ADHD. Monitor growth in children. May lower convulsive threshold; d/c in presence of seizures. Visual disturbances reported with stimulant treatment. May exacerbate Tourette's syndrome and phonic or motor tics. Caution with HTN and monitor BP. Interrupt occasionally to determine if patient requires continued therapy. Sudden death reported in children with structural cardiac abnormalities; avoid use in children or adults with structural cardiac abnormalities.

ADVERSE REACTIONS: HTN, tachycardia, palpitations, CNS overstimulation, dry mouth, GI disorders, anorexia, impotence, urticaria, rash, angioedema, anaphylaxis, Stevens-Johnson syndrome.

INTERACTIONS: GI acidifying agents (guanethidine, reserpine, glutamic acid, etc) and urinary acidifying agents (ammonium chloride, etc) decrease efficacy. MAOIs may cause hypertensive crisis. Potentiated by GI and urinary alkalinizers, propoxyphene overdose. Potentiated effects of both agents with TCAs. May delay absorption of phenytoin, ethosuximide, phenobarbital. Potentiates meperidine, norepinephrine, phenobarbital, phenytoin. Antagonized by haloperidol, chlorpromazine, lithium. Antagonizes adrenergic blockers, antihistamines, antihypertensives, veratrum alkaloids (antihypertensive). Avoid co-administration with alkalinizing agents (eg, antacids).

PREGNANCY: Category C, not for use in nursing.

MECHANISM OF ACTION: CNS stimulant; thought to block reuptake of norepinephrine and dopamine into presynaptic neuron and increase release of these monoamines into extraneuronal space.

PHARMACOKINETICS: Absorption: T_{max}=approximately 3 hrs (fasted). **Metabolism**: CYP2D6 (oxidation): 4-hydroxy-amphetamine and norephedrine. **Elimination**: Urine, $T_{1/2}$=9.77-11 hrs (d-amphetamine), 11.5-13.8 hrs (l-amphetamine).

ADDERALL XR
amphetamine salt combo (Shire)

> High potential for abuse; avoid prolonged use. Misuse of amphetamine may cause sudden death and serious cardiovascular adverse events.

THERAPEUTIC CLASS: Sympathomimetic amine

INDICATIONS: Treatment of attention deficit hyperactivity disorder (ADHD).

DOSAGE: *Adults:* Initial: 20mg qam. Currently Using Adderall: Switch to Adderall XR at the same total daily dose, taken once daily. Titrate at weekly intervals as needed. Swallow cap whole or open cap and sprinkle contents on applesauce; do not chew beads.

Pediatrics: ≥6 yrs: Initial: 10mg qam. Titrate: May increase weekly by 5-10mg/day. Max: 30mg/day. 13 to 17 yrs: Initial: 10mg/day. Titrate: May increase to 20mg/day after one week. Currently Using Adderall: Switch to Adderall XR at the same total daily dose, taken once daily. Titrate at weekly intervals as needed. Swallow cap whole or open cap and sprinkle contents on applesauce; do not chew beads.

HOW SUPPLIED: Cap, Extended-Release: 5mg, 10mg, 15mg, 20mg, 25mg, 30mg

CONTRAINDICATIONS: Advanced arteriosclerosis, symptomatic cardiovascular disease, moderate to severe HTN, hyperthyroidism, glaucoma, agitated states, history of drug abuse, during or within 14 days of MAOI use.

WARNINGS/PRECAUTIONS: May exacerbate symptoms of behavior disturbance and thought disorder in psychotic patients. Caution when using stimulants to treat patients with comorbid bipolar disorder because of concern for possible induction of mixed/manic episode in such patients. Stimulants at usual doses can cause treatment emergent psychotic or manic symptoms (eg, hallucinations, delusional thinking, mania) in children and adolescents without prior history of psychotic illness. Aggressive behavior or hostility reported in clinical trials and postmarketing experience of some medications indicated for the treatment of ADHD. Monitor growth in children. May lower convulsive threshold; d/c in presence of seizures. Visual disturbances reported with stimulant treatment. May exacerbate Tourette's syndrome and phonic or motor tics. Caution with HTN and monitor BP. Interrupt occasionally to determine if patient requires continued therapy. Sudden death reported in children with structural cardiac abnormalities; avoid use in children or adults with structural cardiac abnormalities. May decrease appetite.

ADVERSE REACTIONS: Abdominal pain, asthenia, fever, infection, viral infection, loss of appetite, diarrhea, nausea, vomiting, emotional lability, insomnia, nervousness, weight loss, dry mouth, headache, urticaria, anaphylaxis.

INTERACTIONS: GI acidifying agents (guanethidine, reserpine, glutamic acid, etc) and urinary acidifying agents (ammonium chloride, etc) decrease efficacy. MAOIs may cause hypertensive crisis. Potentiated by GI and urinary alkalinizers, propoxyphene overdose. Potentiated effects of both agents with TCAs. May delay absorption of phenytoin, ethosuximide, phenobarbital. Potentiates meperidine, norepinephrine, phenobarbital, phenytoin. Antagonized by haloperidol, chlorpromazine, lithium. Antagonizes adrenergic blockers, antihistamines, antihypertensives, veratrum alkaloids (antihypertensive). Avoid coadministration of alkalinizing agents (eg, antacid).

PREGNANCY: Category C, not for use in nursing.

MECHANISM OF ACTION: CNS stimulant; thought to block reuptake of norepinephrine and dopamine into presynaptic neuron and increase release of these monoamines into extraneuronal space.

ADENOCARD

RX

adenosine (Astellas)

THERAPEUTIC CLASS: Endogenous nucleoside

INDICATIONS: Conversion of paroxysmal supraventricular tachycardia (including Wolff-Parkinson-White syndrome) to sinus rhythm (SR).

DOSAGE: *Adults:* 6mg rapid IV bolus infusion over 1-2 sec. If not converted to SR within 1-2 min, give 12mg rapid IV bolus; may give 2nd 12mg dose if needed. Max: 12mg/dose.
Pediatrics: <50kg: 0.05-0.1mg/kg rapid IV bolus. If not converted to SR within 1-2 min, give additional bolus doses incrementally increasing amount by 0.05-0.1mg/kg. Follow each bolus with a saline flush. Continue process until SR or a maximum single dose of 0.3mg/kg is used. ≥50kg: 6mg rapid IV bolus infusion over 1-2 sec. If not converted to SR within 1-2 min, give 12mg rapid IV bolus; may give 2nd 12mg dose if needed. Max: 12mg/dose.

HOW SUPPLIED: Inj: 3mg/mL (2mL, 4mL)

CONTRAINDICATIONS: 2nd- or 3rd-degree AV block (except with pacemaker), sinus node disease such as sick sinus syndrome or symptomatic bradycardia (except with pacemaker).

WARNINGS/PRECAUTIONS: May produce short-lasting heart block. Transient or prolonged asystole, respiratory alkalosis, ventricular fibrillation reported. Caution with obstructive lung disease not associated with bronchoconstriction (eg, emphysema, bronchitis). Avoid with bronchoconstriction/bronchospasm (eg, asthma). D/C if severe respiratory difficulties develop. New arrhythmias may appear on ECG at time of conversion. Caution in elderly.

ADVERSE REACTIONS: Facial flushing, dyspnea/SOB, chest pressure, nausea.

INTERACTIONS: Antagonized by methylxanthines (eg, theophylline, caffeine); may need larger adenosine dose. Potentiated by dipyridamole; use lower adenosine dose. Caution with digoxin, verapamil; ventricular fibrillation reported and potential for additive/ synergistic depressant effects on SA and AV nodes. Possible higher degrees of heart block with carbamazepine.

PREGNANCY: Category C, safety in nursing not known.

MECHANISM OF ACTION: Endogenous nucleoside; slows conduction time through A-V node, can interrupt reentry pathways through the A-V node, and can restore normal sinus rhythm in patients with paroxysmal supraventricular tachycardia associated with Wolff-Parkinson-White syndrome.

PHARMACOKINETICS: Metabolism: Rapid (intracellular), through phosphorylation and deamination. **Elimination:** $T_{1/2} < 10$ seconds.

ADIPEX-P
phentermine HCl (Gate)

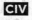

THERAPEUTIC CLASS: Anorectic sympathomimetic amine

INDICATIONS: Short-term adjunct for exogenous obesity if initial BMI $\geq 30 kg/m^2$ or $\geq 27 kg/m^2$ with other risk factors (eg, HTN, diabetes, hyperlipidemia).

DOSAGE: *Adults:* Usual: 37.5mg before breakfast or 1-2 hrs after breakfast. Alternate Schedule: 18.75mg qd-bid. Avoid late evening dosing.
Pediatrics: >16 yrs: Usual: 37.5mg before breakfast or 1-2 hrs after breakfast. Alternate Schedule: 18.75mg qd-bid. Avoid late evening dosing.

HOW SUPPLIED: Cap: 37.5mg; Tab: 37.5mg* *scored

CONTRAINDICATIONS: Advanced arteriosclerosis, cardiovascular disease, moderate to severe HTN, hyperthyroidism, glaucoma, agitated states, history of drug abuse, within 14 days of MAOI use.

WARNINGS/PRECAUTIONS: Only for short-term therapy. Primary pulmonary HTN and valvular heart disease reported. Abuse potential. Caution with mild HTN. Tolerance may develop.

ADVERSE REACTIONS: Primary pulmonary hypertension, regurgitant valvular heart disease, palpitation, tachycardia, BP elevation, CNS overstimulation, dry mouth, impotence, urticaria.

INTERACTIONS: May alter insulin requirements. Avoid alcohol and other weight loss products including SSRIs. Valvular heart disease and primary pulmonary hypertension reported with fenfluramine and dexfenfluramine. May decrease effects of guanethidine.

PREGNANCY: Category C, not for use in nursing.

MECHANISM OF ACTION: Anorectic sympathomimetic amine; not established as appetite suppressor; causes CNS stimulation and elevation of BP.

ADVAIR
fluticasone propionate - salmeterol xinafoate (GlaxoSmithKline)

RX

> Long-acting β_2-adrenergic agonists, such as salmeterol, may increase risk of asthma-related deaths. Use of diskus should be reserved for patients not adequately controlled on other medications or whose disease severity warrants initiation with 2 maintenance therapies.

THERAPEUTIC CLASS: Corticosteroid/beta$_2$ agonist

INDICATIONS: Long-term, maintenance treatment of asthma in patients ≥4 yrs. (250/50 only): Maintenance treatment of airflow obstruction in patients with COPD, including chronic bronchitis and/or emphysema; to reduce exacerbations of COPD in patients with history of exacerbations.

DOSAGE: *Adults:* Asthma: 1 inh q12h. Without Prior Inhaled Corticosteroid (CS) Therapy/Inadequate Control on Current Inhaled CS: Initial: 100/50 or 250/50 bid. Max: 500/50 bid. If no response within 2 weeks, may increase to higher strength. COPD: (250/50 only): 1 inh q12h. Rinse mouth after use.
Pediatrics: ≥12 yrs: Asthma: 1 inh q12h. Without Prior Inhaled Corticosteroid (CS)Therapy/Inadequate Control on Current Inhaled CS: Initial: 100/50 or 250/50 bid. Max: 500/50 bid. If no response within 2 weeks, may increase to higher strength. (100/50 only): 4-11 yrs: Symptomatic on Inhaled CS: 1 inh q12h. Rinse mouth after use.

HOW SUPPLIED: Disk (Inhalation): (Fluticasone-Salmeterol) (100/50) 0.1mg-0.05mg/inh, (250/50) 0.25mg-0.05mg/inh, (500/50) 0.5mg-0.05mg/inh (60 blisters)

CONTRAINDICATIONS: Status asthmaticus, other acute asthma or COPD episodes, and hypersensitivity to milk proteins.

WARNINGS/PRECAUTIONS: Deaths due to adrenal insufficiency have occurred with transfer from systemic corticosteroids to inhaled corticosteroids. Resume oral corticosteroids during stress or severe asthma attack. Observe for adrenal insufficiency, systemic corticosteroid withdrawal effects, hypercorticism, reduction in growth velocity (pediatrics). More susceptible to infection. Not for acute bronchospasm. D/C if bronchospasm occurs after dosing. Caution with TB; untreated systemic fungal, bacterial, viral, or parasitic infections; or ocular herpes simplex. *Candida* infection of mouth and pharynx, glaucoma, hypersensitivity reactions, increased IOP, cataracts reported. Monitor for increasing use of β_2 agonists. QTc interval prolongation reported with large doses. D/C if paradoxical bronchospasm occurs. Caution with cardiovascular or CNS disorders, convulsive disorders, thyrotoxicosis, DM, and keto-acidosis. May produce hypokalemia, hyperglycemia, and eosinophilic conditions.

ADVERSE REACTIONS: Upper respiratory tract inflammation, pharyngitis, sinusitis, cough, hoarseness, headaches, GI effects, musculoskeletal pain, palpitations.

INTERACTIONS: Extreme caution with TCAs or MAOIs during or within 14 days of use. Antagonized by β-blockers. Caution with non-potassium sparing diuretics; ECG changes, hypokalemia may develop. Concomitant use with strong CYP3A4 inhibitors (eg, ritonavir, atazanavir, indinavir, ketoconazole) is not recommended .

PREGNANCY: Category C, caution in nursing.

MECHANISM OF ACTION: Fluticasone: Corticosteroid with anti-inflammatory activity; inihibits multiple cell types (eg, mast cells, eosinophils, neutrophils, macrophages, lymphocytes) and mediators (eg, histamine, eicosanoids, leukotrienes and cytokines) involved in inflammation and asthmatic response. Salmeterol: Long-acting β_2-adrenergic agonist; stimulates intracellular adenyl cyclase, which catalyzes conversion of ATP to cAMP, producing relaxation of bronchial smooth muscle and inhibition of release of immediate hypersensitivity mediators from cells (eg, mast cells).

PHARMACOKINETICS: Absorption: Fluticasone: (Asthma, 500 bid) C_{max}=110pg/mL, (COPD, 250 bid) 53pg/mL. Salmeterol: C_{max}=167pg/mL, T_{max}=20 min. **Distribution:** Fluticasone: V_d=4.2L/kg; plasma protein binding (91%). Salmeterol: Plasma protein binding (96%). **Metabolism:** Fluticasone: Liver via CYP3A4. Salmeterol: Liver, via CYP3A4 to α-hydroxysalmeterol (metabolite). **Elimination:** Urine, feces; Fluticasone: $T_{1/2}$=7.8 hrs. Salmeterol: $T_{1/2}$=5.5 hrs.

Advair HFA
RX
fluticasone propionate - salmeterol xinafoate (GlaxoSmithKline)

> Long-acting β_2-adrenergic agonists, such as salmeterol, may increase risk of asthma-related deaths.

THERAPEUTIC CLASS: Corticosteroid/beta$_2$ agonist

INDICATIONS: For long-term, maintenance treatment of asthma.

DOSAGE: *Adults:* Asthma: 2 inh q12h. Without Prior Inhaled Corticosteroid (CS): Initial: 2 inh of 45/21 bid or 1 inh of 115/21 bid. Max: 2 inh of 230/21 bid. Current Inhaled CS: Beclomethasone: ≤160mcg/day use 2 inh of 45/21 bid, 320mcg/day use 2 inh of 115/21 bid, 640mcg/day use 2 inh of 230/21 bid. Budesonide: ≤400mcg/day use 2 inh of 45/21 bid, 800-1200mcg/day use 2 inh of 115/21 bid, 1600mcg/day use 2 inh of 230/21 bid. Flunisolide: ≤1000mcg/day use 2 inh of 45/21 bid, 1250-2000mcg/day use 2 inh of 115/21 bid. Flunisolide HFA: ≤320mcg/day use 2 inh of 45/21 bid, 640mcg/day use 2 inh of 115/21 bid. Fluticasone Aerosol: ≤176mcg/day use 2 inh of 45/21 bid, 440mcg/day use 2 inh of 115/21 bid, 660-880mcg/day use 2 inh of 230/21 bid. Fluticasone Powder: ≤200mcg/day use 2 inh of 45/21 bid, 500mcg/day use 2 inh of 115/21 bid, 1000mcg/day use 2 inh of 230/21 bid. Mometasone Powder: 220mcg/day use 2 inh of 45/21 bid, 440mcg/day use 2 inh of 115/21 bid, 880mcg/day use 2 inh of 230/21 bid. Triamcinolone: ≤1000mcg/day use 2 inh of 45/21 bid, 1100-1600mcg/day use 2 inh of 115/21 bid. If no response within 2 weeks, increase to higher strength.

Pediatrics: ≥12 yrs: Asthma: 2 inh q12h. Without Prior Inhaled Corticosteroid (CS): Initial: 2 inh of 45/21 bid or 1 inh of 115/21 bid. Max: 2 inh of 230-21 bid. Current Inhaled CS: Beclomethasone: ≤160mcg/day use 2 inh of 45/21 bid, 320mcg/day use 2 inh of 115/21 bid, 640mcg/day use 2 inh of 230/21 bid. Budesonide: ≤400mcg/day use 2 inh of 45/21 bid, 800-1200mcg/day use 2 inh of 115/21 bid, 1600mcg/day use 2 inh of 230/21 bid. Flunisolide: ≤1000mcg/day use 2 inh of 45/21 bid, 1250-2000mcg/day use 2 inh of 115/21 bid. Flunisolide HFA: ≤320mcg/day use 2 inh of 45/21 bid, 640mcg/day use 2 inh of 115/21 bid. Fluticasone Aerosol: ≤176mcg/day use 2 inh of 45/21 bid, 440mcg/day use 2 inh of 115/21 bid, 660-880mcg/day use 2 inh of 230/21 bid. Fluticasone Powder: ≤200mcg/day use 2 inh of 45/21 bid, 500mcg/day use 2 inh of 115/21 bid, 1000mcg/day use 2 inh of 230/21 bid. Mometasone powder: 220mcg/day use 2 inh of 45/21 bid, 440mcg/day use 2 inh of 115/21 bid, 880mcg/day use 2 inh of 230/21 bid. Triamcinolone: ≤1000mcg/day use 2 inh of 45/21 bid, 1100-1600mcg/day use 2 inh of 115/21 bid. If no response within 2 weeks, increase to higher strength.

HOW SUPPLIED: MDI: (Fluticasone-Salmeterol) (45/21) 0.045mg-0.021mg/inh, (115/21) 0.115mg-0.021mg/inh, (230/21) 0.230mg-0.021mg/inh (120 inhalations)

CONTRAINDICATIONS: Status asthmaticus or other acute asthma.

WARNINGS/PRECAUTIONS: See Contraindications. Deaths due to adrenal insufficiency have occurred with transfer from systemic corticosteroids to inhaled corticosteroids. Resume oral corticosteroids during stress or severe asthma attack. Observe for adrenal insufficiency, systemic corticosteroid withdrawal effects, hypercorticism, reduction in growth velocity (pediatrics). More susceptible to infection. Not for acute bronchospasm. D/C if bronchospasm occurs after dosing. Caution with TB; untreated systemic fungal, bacterial, viral, or parasitic infections; or ocular herpes simplex. *Candida* infection of mouth and pharynx, glaucoma, hypersensitivity reactions, increased IOP, cataracts reported. Monitor for increasing use of β_2 agonists. QTc interval prolongation reported with large doses. D/C if paradoxical bronchospasm occurs. Caution with cardiovascular disorders.

ADVERSE REACTIONS: Upper respiratory tract infection, throat irritation, upper respiratory tract inflammation, headaches, nausea, vomiting, musculoskeletal pain, menstruation symptoms.

INTERACTIONS: Extreme caution with TCAs or MAOIs during or within 14 days of use. Antagonized by β-blockers. Caution with non-potassium sparing diuretics; ECG changes, hypokalemia may develop. Potentiated by ketoconazole, other CYP3A4 inhibitors.

PREGNANCY: Category C, caution in nursing.

MECHANISM OF ACTION: Fluticasone: Corticosteroid with anti-inflammatory activity. Inihibits multiple cell types (eg, mast cells, eosinophils, neutrophils, macrophages, lymphocytes) and mediators (eg, histamine, eicosanoids, leukotrienes and cytokines) involved in inflammation and asthmatic response. Salmeterol: β_2-adrenergic agonist; stimulates intracellular adenyl cyclase, which catalyzes conversion of ATP to cAMP, producing relaxation of bronchial smooth muscle and inhibition of release of immediate hypersensitivity mediators from cells (eg, mast cells).

PHARMACOKINETICS: Absorption: Salmeterol: C_{max}=150pg/mL. **Distribution:** Fluticasone: V_d=4.2 L/kg; plasma protein binding (99%). Salmeterol: Plasma protein binding (96%). **Metabolism:** Fluticasone: Liver, via CYP3A4. Salmeterol: Extensive by hydroxylation. **Elimination:** Fluticasone: Feces (major), urine (<5%); $T_{1/2}$=7.8 hrs. Salmeterol: Feces (60%), urine (25%); $T_{1/2}$=5.5 hrs.

AEROBID
flunisolide (Forest)

RX

OTHER BRAND NAME: Aerobid-M (with menthol) (Forest)

THERAPEUTIC CLASS: Corticosteroid

INDICATIONS: Maintenance treatment of asthma as prophylactic therapy in patients ≥6 years and to reduce or eliminate the need for oral systemic corticosteroidal therapy.

DOSAGE: *Adults:* Initial: 2 inh bid. Max: 4 inh bid. Rinse mouth after use.
Pediatrics: 6-15 yrs: 2 inh bid. Rinse mouth after use.

HOW SUPPLIED: MDI: 0.25mg/inh (7g)

CONTRAINDICATIONS: Primary treatment of status asthmaticus or other acute asthma attacks.

WARNINGS/PRECAUTIONS: Deaths due to adrenal insufficiency have occurred with transfer from systemic corticosteroids to inhaled corticosteroids. Resume oral corticosteroids during stress or severe asthma attack. Observe for adrenal insufficiency, systemic corticosteroid withdrawal effects, and growth suppression (children). More susceptible to infections. Not for acute bronchospasm. D/C if bronchospasm occurs after dosing. Caution with tuberculosis of the respiratory tract; untreated systemic fungal, bacterial, viral, or parasitic infections; or ocular herpes simplex. *Candida* infection of the mouth and pharynx reported.

ADVERSE REACTIONS: Upper respiratory infection, diarrhea, stomach upset, cold symptoms, nasal congestion, headache, nausea, vomiting, sore throat, unpleasant taste.

PREGNANCY: Category C, caution with nursing.

MECHANISM OF ACTION: Corticosteroid; demonstrated marked anti-inflammatory and anti-allergic activity in test systems.

PHARMACOKINETICS: Metabolism: Liver (1st pass). Metabolite (6β-OH). **Elimination:** $T_{1/2}=1.8$ hrs.

AGRYLIN
anagrelide HCl (Shire)

RX

THERAPEUTIC CLASS: Platelet-reducing agent

INDICATIONS: Treatment of thrombocythemia secondary to myeloproliferative disorders.

DOSAGE: *Adults:* Initial: 0.5mg qid or 1mg bid for at least 1 week. Moderate Hepatic Impairment: Initial: 0.5mg qd for at least 1 week. Titrate: Increase by no more than 0.5mg/day per week. Max: 10mg/day or 2.5mg/dose. Adjust lowest effective dose to reduce and maintain platelets <600,000/mcL. Monitor platelets every 2 days during first week, then weekly thereafter until reach maintenance dose.
Pediatrics: Initial: 0.5mg qd. Titrate: Increase by no more than 0.5mg/day per week. Max: 10mg/day or 2.5mg/dose. Adjust to lowest effective dose to reduce and maintain platelets <600,000/mcL. Monitor platelets every 2 days during first week, then weekly thereafter until reach maintenance dose.

HOW SUPPLIED: Cap: 0.5mg, 1mg

CONTRAINDICATIONS: Severe hepatic impairment.

WARNINGS/PRECAUTIONS: Caution with heart disease, renal or hepatic dysfunction. Perform pre-treatment cardiovascular exam and monitor during treatment; may cause cardiovascular effects (eg, vasodilation, tachycardia, palpitations, CHF). Monitor closely for renal toxicity if creatinine ≥2mg/dL or hepatic toxicity if bilirubin, SGOT, or LFTs >1.5x ULN. Monitor blood counts, renal and hepatic function while platelets are lowered. Increase in platelets after therapy interruption. Reduce dose in moderate hepatic impairment.

ADVERSE REACTIONS: Headache, palpitations, asthenia, edema, GI effects, dizziness, pain, dyspnea, fever, chest pain, rash, tachycardia, malaise, pharyngitis, cough, paresthesia.

INTERACTIONS: Sucralfate may interfere with absorption. Exacerbated effects of products that inhibit cyclic AMP PDE III (inotropes: milrinone, enoximone, amrinone, olparinone, cilostazol).

PREGNANCY: Category C, not for use in nursing.

MECHANISM OF ACTION: Platelet-reducing agent; not established. Suspected to reduce platelet production resulting from a decrease in megakaryocyte hypermaturation. Inhibits cyclic AMP phosphodiesterase III (PDEIII). PDEIII inhibitors can also inhibit platelet aggregation.

PHARMACOKINETICS: Metabolism: Liver, CYP1A2 (partial). RL603 and 3-hydroxy anagrelide (major metabolites). **Elimination:** Urine; $T_{1/2}$=1.3 hrs.

AK-FLUOR RX
fluorescein sodium (Akorn)

THERAPEUTIC CLASS: Diagnostic dye

INDICATIONS: Indicated in diagnostic fluorescein angiography or angioscopy of the fundus and iris vasculature.

DOSAGE: *Adults:* Perform intradermal skin test before IV use if suspect potential allergy. Inject contents of ampule rapidly into antecubital vein. A syringe with fluorescein is attached to transparent tubing and a 25 gauge scalp vein needle for injection. Insert needle and draw patient's blood to hub of syringe so small air bubble separates patient's blood in tubing from fluorescein. With room lights on, inject blood back into vein while watching skin over needle tip. If needle extravasated, patient's blood will bulge skin; stop injection before injecting fluorescein. When certain there is no extravasation, turn room light off and complete fluorescein injection. Luminescence appears in retina and choroidal vessels in 9-14 seconds.
Pediatrics: Perform intradermal skin test before IV use if suspect potential allergy. Dose is 35mg/10lbs. Inject contents of ampule/vial rapidly into antecubital vein. A syringe with fluorescein is attached to transparent tubing and a 25 gauge scalp vein needle for injection. Insert needle and draw patient's blood to hub of syringe so small air bubble separates patient's blood in tubing from fluorescein. With room lights on, inject blood back into vein while watching skin over needle tip. If needle extravasated, patient's blood will bulge skin; stop injection before injecting fluorescein. When certain there is no extravasation, turn room light off and complete fluorescein injection. Luminescence appears in retina and choroidal vessels in 9-14 seconds.

HOW SUPPLIED: Inj: 10% (5mL), 25% (2mL)

WARNINGS/PRECAUTIONS: Avoid extravasation; severe local tissue damage can occur. Caution with history of allergy or bronchial asthma. Have emergency tray (eg, 0.1% epinephrine IV/IM, antihistamine, soluble steroid, IV aminophylline) and oxygen available. Avoid angiography in pregnancy, especially 1st trimester. Skin attains temporary yellowish discoloration and urine attains bright yellow color.

ADVERSE REACTIONS: Nausea, vomiting, headache, GI distress, syncope, hypotension, cardiac arrest, basilar artery ischemia, severe shock, convulsions, thrombophlebitis.

PREGNANCY: Safety in pregnancy not known, caution in nursing.

MECHANISM OF ACTION: A diagnostic dye; demacrates the vascular area under observation, distinguishing it from adjacent areas.

ALACOL DM RX
brompheniramine maleate - dextromethorphan HBr - phenylephrine HCl
(Ballay)

THERAPEUTIC CLASS: Antihistamine/antitussive/sympathomimetic

INDICATIONS: Relief of cough and upper respiratory symptoms including nasal congestion, associated with allergy or the common cold.

DOSAGE: *Adults:* 10mL q4h. Max: 6 doses/24 hrs.
Pediatrics: >12 yrs: 10mL q4h. 6-12 yrs: 5mL q4h. 2-6 yrs: 2.5mL q4h. Max: 6 doses/24 hrs.

HOW SUPPLIED: Syrup: (Brompheniramine-Dextromethorphan-Phenylephrine) 2mg-10mg-5mg/5mL

CONTRAINDICATIONS: Newborns, premature infants, nursing, severe HTN or CAD, with MAOIs, lower respiratory tract conditions including asthma.

WARNINGS/PRECAUTIONS: Caution with persistent or chronic cough (eg, associated with asthma, emphysema, smoking, excessive phlegm). Persistent cough may be a sign of a serious condition. May diminish mental alertness. May produce excitation in children. Caution with asthma, narrow-angle glaucoma, GI obstruction, urinary bladder neck obstruction, DM, HTN, heart and thyroid disease.

ADVERSE REACTIONS: Sedation, thickening of bronchial secretions, dizziness, dryness of mouth, nose, and throat.

INTERACTIONS: Additive effects with alcohol, CNS depressants (eg, hypnotics, sedatives, tranquilizers, anxiolytics). MAOIs may prolong/intensify anticholinergic effects of antihistamines and phenylephrine. May reduce effects of antihypertensives.

PREGNANCY: Category C, contraindicated in nursing.

MECHANISM OF ACTION: Brompheniramine: Histamine antagonist, specifically H_2-receptor-blocking agent belonging to the alkylamine class of antihistamines. Competes with histamine for receptor sites in effector cells. Phenylephrine: Sympathomimetic amine; acts as decongestant to respiratory tract mucus membranes. Dextromethorphan: Non-narcotic antitussive; acts in the medulla oblongata to elevate cough threshold.

PHARMACOKINETICS: Absorption: Brompheniramine: Well absorbed. T_{max}=5 hrs. **Metabolism:** Dextromethorphan: Rapid. **Elimination:** Brompheniramine: Urine. Phenylephrine: Urine; $T_{1/2}$=6-8 hrs. Dextromethorphan: Urine.

Alamast   RX
pemirolast potassium (Vistakon)

THERAPEUTIC CLASS: Mast cell stabilizer

INDICATIONS: Prevention of ocular itching due to allergic conjunctivitis.

DOSAGE: *Adults:* 1-2 drops in affected eye qid.
Pediatrics: ≥3 yrs: 1-2 drops in affected eye qid.

HOW SUPPLIED: Sol: 0.1% (10mL)

WARNINGS/PRECAUTIONS: May reinsert soft contact lens after 10 min, if eyes are not red. Contains lauralkonium chloride; may be absorbed by soft contact lens.

ADVERSE REACTIONS: Headache, rhinitis, cold/flu symptoms, ocular burning/discomfort, dry eye, foreign body sensation.

PREGNANCY: Category C, caution in nursing.

MECHANISM OF ACTION: Mast cell stabilizer; inhibits type I immediate hypersensitivity reaction, antigen-induced release of inflammatory mediators (eg, histamine, leukotriene C_4, D_4, E_4) from human mast cell; also inhibits the chemotaxis of eosinophils into ocular tissue, blocks the release of mediators from human eosinophils, and prevents calcium influx into mast cells upon antigen stimulation (not established).

PHARMACOKINETICS: Absorption: C_{max}=4.7ng/mL, T_{max}=0.42 hrs. **Elimination:** Urine (10-15% unchanged); $T_{1/2}$=4.5 hrs.

Albenza   RX
albendazole (GlaxoSmithKline)

THERAPEUTIC CLASS: Broad-spectrum anthelmintic

INDICATIONS: Treatment of parenchymal neurocysticercosis and cystic hydatid disease of the liver, lung, and peritoneum.

DOSAGE: *Adults:* Hydatid Disease: ≥60kg: 400mg bid. <60kg: 7.5mg/kg bid up to 800mg/day. Take with meals for 28 days, then 14 days drug-free, repeat for a total of 3 cycles. Neurocysticercosis: Same dose as Hydatid disease. Treat for 8-30 days.
Pediatrics: ≥6 yrs: Hydatid Disease: ≥60kg: 400mg bid. <60kg: 7.5mg/kg bid up to 800mg/day. Take with meals for 28 days, then 14 days drug-free, repeat for a total of 3 cycles. Neurocysticercosis: Same dose as Hydatid disease. Treat for 8-30 days.

HOW SUPPLIED: Tab: 200mg

WARNINGS/PRECAUTIONS: Monitor blood counts at the beginning of each 28-day cycle, and every 2 weeks during therapy; bone marrow suppression, aplastic anemia, and agranulocytosis have been reported. May continue if total WBC and absolute neutrophil count decrease are modest and do not progress. Not for use in pregnancy unless no other therapy is appropriate. Avoid pregnancy at least 1 month after discontinuing therapy. D/C immediately if become pregnant. Treatment for neurocysticercosis should include anticonvulsants and steroids. Examine for retinal lesions before therapy. Elevated LFTs reported. Can cause bone marrow suppression, aplastic anemia, and agranulocytosis in patients with and without underlying hepatic dysfunction.

ADVERSE REACTIONS: Abnormal LFTs, abdominal pain, NV, headache.

INTERACTIONS: Monitor theophylline levels during and after therapy. Increased levels with dexamethasone, praziquantel, and cimetidine.

PREGNANCY: Category C, caution in nursing.

MECHANISM OF ACTION: Broad-spectrum anthelmintic; exerts action by inhibitory effect on tubulin polymerization, which results in loss of cytoplasmic microtubules.

PHARMACOKINETICS: Absorption: GI tract (poorly absorbed); C_{max}=1.31mcg/mL; T_{max}=2-5 hrs. **Distribution:** Plasma protein binding (70%). **Metabolism:** Liver; metabolite: Albendazole sulfoxide (major metabolite). **Elimination:** Bile, urine (<1%); $T_{1/2}$=8-12 hrs.

ALBUTEROL   RX
albuterol sulfate (Various)

THERAPEUTIC CLASS: Beta$_2$-agonist

INDICATIONS: (Aerosol) Prevention and treatment of bronchospasm with reversible obstructive airway disease. Prevention of Exercise-Induced Bronchospasm (EIB). (Sol) Relief of bronchospasm with reversible obstructive airway disease and acute attacks of bronchospasm in patients ≥12 yrs. (Tab, Tab, Extended-Release) Relief of bronchospasm with reversible obstructive airway disease in patients ≥6 yrs. (Syrup) Relief of bronchospasm in patients ≥2 yrs with reversible obstructive airway disease.

DOSAGE: *Adults:* Bronchospasm: (Aerosol) 2 inh q4-6h or 1 inh q4h. (Repetabs) Initial: 4-8mg q12h. Max: 32mg/day. (Sol) 2.5mg tid-qid by nebulizer. (Syrup, Tabs) 2-4mg tid-qid. Max: 32mg/day (8mg qid). Elderly/β-Adrenergic Sensitivity: (Syrup, Tabs) Initial: 2mg tid-qid. Max: 8mg tid-qid. EIB: (Aerosol) 2 inh 15 min before activity.
Pediatrics: Bronchospasm: >14 yrs: (Syrup) Initial: 2-4mg tid-qid. Max: 8mg qid. ≥12 yrs: (Aerosol) 2 inh q4-6h or 1 inh q4h. (Sol) 2.5mg tid-qid by nebulizer. (Tabs) Initial: 2-4mg tid-qid. Max: 8mg qid. >12 yrs: (Repetabs) Initial: 4-8mg q12h. Max: 32mg/day. 6-14 yrs: (Syrup) Initial: 2mg tid-qid. Max: 24mg/day. 6-12 yrs: (Repetabs) Initial: 4mg q12h. Max: 24mg/day. (Tabs) Initial: 2mg tid-qid. Max: 24mg/day. 2-5 yrs: (Syrup) Initial: 0.1mg/kg tid (not to exceed 2mg tid). Titrate: May increase to 0.2mg/kg/day. Max: 4mg tid. EIB: ≥12 yrs: (Aerosol) 2 inh 15 min before activity.

HOW SUPPLIED: MDI: 0.09mg/inh (17g); Sol (neb): 0.083% (3mL, 25's), 0.5% (20mL); Syrup: 2mg/5mL; Tab: 2mg*, 4mg*; Tab, Extended-Release (Repetabs): 4mg *scored

WARNINGS/PRECAUTIONS: Hypersensitivity reactions reported. Monitor for worsening asthma. Fatalities reported with excessive use. Caution with cardiovascular disorders, especially coronary insufficiency, arrhythmias and HTN. May need concomitant corticosteroids. Can produce paradoxical bronchospasm. Caution with DM, hyperthyroidism, seizures. May cause transient hypokalemia.

ADVERSE REACTIONS: Tachycardia, increased BP, tremor, nervousness, dizziness, nausea/vomiting, palpitations, paradoxical bronchospasm, heartburn, rhinitis, respiratory tract infection.

INTERACTIONS: Avoid other sympathomimetic agents. Extreme caution with MAOIs and TCAs. Monitor digoxin. May worsen ECG changes and/or hypokalemia with nonpotassium-sparing diuretics. Antagonized by β-blockers.

PREGNANCY: Category C, not for use in nursing.

MECHANISM OF ACTION: β$_2$-adrenergic agonist; stimulates intracellular adenyl cyclase, which catalyzes conversion of ATP to cAMP to produce relaxation of bronchial smooth muscle and inhibition of release of mediators of immediate hypersensitivity from cells (mast cells).

PHARMACOKINETICS: Absorption: (Aerosol) T$_{max}$=2-4 hrs. (Syrup, Tab) Rapid. C$_{max}$=18ng/mL; T$_{max}$=2 hrs. **Elimination:** (Aerosol) Urine (28%); T$_{1/2}$=3.8 hrs. (Syrup, Tab) T$_{1/2}$=5 hrs.

ALCORTIN   RX
hydrocortisone - iodoquinol (Primus)

THERAPEUTIC CLASS: Corticosteroid/Anti-infective

INDICATIONS: "Possibly" Effective: Contact or atopic dermatitis, impetiginized eczema, nummular eczema, endogenous chronic infectious dermatitis, stasis dermatitis, pyoderma, nuchal eczema and chronic eczematoid otitis externa, acne urticata, localized or disseminated neurodermatitis, lichen simplex chronicus, anogenital pruritus (vulvae, scroti, ani), folliculitis, bacterial dermatoses, mycotic dermatoses such as tinea (capitis, cruris, corporis, pedis), monliasis, intertrigo.

DOSAGE: *Adults:* Apply to affected area(s) tid-qid.
Pediatrics: ≥12 yrs: Apply to affected area(s) tid-qid.

HOW SUPPLIED: Gel: (Hydrocortisone-Iodoquinol) 2%-1% (2g)

WARNINGS/PRECAUTIONS: For external use only. Avoid eyes. D/C if irritation develops. May stain skin, hair, or fabrics. Risk of systemic absorption with treatment of extensive areas or use of occlusive dressings. Increased risk of systemic absorption in children. Iodoquinol may interfere with thyroid tests. False-positive phenylketonuria test reported. Prolonged use may result in overgrowth of nonsusceptible organisms.

ADVERSE REACTIONS: Burning, itching, irritation, dryness, folliculitis, hypertrichosis, acneiform eruptions, hypopigmentation, perioral dermatitis, allergic dermatitis, skin maceration, secondary infection, skin atrophy, striae, miliaria.

PREGNANCY: Category C, caution in nursing.

MECHANISM OF ACTION: Corticosteroid/Anti-infective. Hydrocortisone: Corticosteroid; possesses anti-inflammatory, antipruritic, and vasoconstrictive properties. Anti-inflammatory effect unclear; however, there is a recognizable correlation between vasoconstrictor potency and therapeutic efficacy. Iodoquinol: Anti-infective; possesses both antifungal and antibacterial properties.

PHARMACOKINETICS: Absorption: Hydrocortisone: Absorbed from normal intact skin. Inflammation of skin increases absorption. **Metabolism:** Hydrocortisone: Liver and most body tissues. Tetrahydrocortisone and tetrahydrocortisol (metabolites). **Elimination:** Hydrocortisone: Urine (unchanged and glucuronides). Iodoquinol: Urine (3-5% glucuronide).

ALDARA   RX
imiquimod (Graceway)

THERAPEUTIC CLASS: Immune response modifier

INDICATIONS: Actinic keratoses on face or scalp in immunocompetent adults. External genital and perianal warts/condyloma acuminata. Biopsy-confirmed, primary superficial basal cell carcinoma (sBCC) in immunocompetent adults, with a maximum tumor diameter of 2cm, located on trunk (excluding anogenital skin), neck, or extremities (excluding hands and feet), only when surgical methods are medically less appropriate and follow-up can be assured.

DOSAGE: *Adults:* Use before bedtime. Actinic Keratosis: Usual: Apply 2x/week to defined area on face or scalp (but not both concurrently). Wash off after 8 hrs with soap and water. Max: 16 weeks. External Genital and Perianal Warts/Condyloma: Usual: Apply 3x/week. Wash off after 6-10 hrs with soap and water. Use until warts are clear. Max: 16 weeks. May suspend use for several days to manage local reactions. Do not occlude treatment area. sBCC: Apply 5x/week for 6 weeks. If tumor diameter is 0.5 to <1cm, use 4mm (10mg) of cream. If tumor is ≥1 to <1.5cm, use 5mm (25mg) of cream. If tumor is ≥1.5 to 2cm, use 7mm (40mg) of cream. Max diameter of tumor: ≤2cm. Treatment area should include a 1cm margin of skin around the tumor. Wash off after 8 hrs with soap and water.
Pediatrics: ≥12 yrs: External Genital and Perianal Warts/Condyloma: Usual: Apply

3x/week before bedtime. Wash off after 6-10 hrs with soap and water. Use until warts are clear. Max: 16 weeks. May suspend use for several days to manage local reactions. Do not occlude treatment area.

HOW SUPPLIED: Cre: 5% (12 pkts)

WARNINGS/PRECAUTIONS: Not for urethral, intra-vaginal, cervical, rectal, or intra-anal human papilloma viral disease. Avoid sexual contact while cream is on skin. May weaken condoms and diaphragms; avoid concurrent use. Avoid or minimize exposure to sunlight. May exacerbate inflammatory skin conditions. Avoid contact with eyes, lips, nostrils. Avoid after surgery or with sunburn until tissue is healed.

ADVERSE REACTIONS: Wart (erythema, erosion, flaking, edema) and application site reactions (bleeding, burning, itching, pain), flu-like symptoms, headache.

INTERACTIONS: Avoid topical drugs immediately after treatment of warts.

PREGNANCY: Category C, safety in nursing not known.

MECHANISM OF ACTION: Immune response modifier; not established. In basal cell carcinoma, suspected to increase infiltration of lymphocytes, dendritic cells, and macrophages in the tumor lesion. In external genital warts, suspected to induce mRNA encoding cytokines, including interferon-α at the treatment site.

PHARMACOKINETICS: Absorption: C_{max}=0.1ng/mL (12.5mg, face), 0.2ng/mL (25mg, scalp), 3.5ng/mL (75mg, hands/arms). **Distribution:** Excreted in breast milk. **Elimination:** Urine: Male (0.11%), female (2.41%).

ALEVE OTC
naproxen sodium (Bayer Healthcare)

THERAPEUTIC CLASS: NSAID

INDICATIONS: Relief of minor aches and pains. Reduction of fever.

DOSAGE: *Adults:* Initial: 1-2 tabs, then 1 tab q8-12h. Max: 660mg/24 hrs or 440mg/12 hrs. Elderly: >65 yrs: 1 tab q12h.
Pediatrics: ≥12 yrs: Initial: 1-2 tabs, then 1 tab q8-12h. Max: 660mg/24 hrs or 440mg/12 hrs.

HOW SUPPLIED: Tab: 220mg

WARNINGS/PRECAUTIONS: Avoid during last trimester of pregnancy. Do not use >10 days for pain or >3 days for fever.

INTERACTIONS: Increased risk of GI bleeding with alcohol.

PREGNANCY: Safety in pregnancy or nursing not known.

ALINIA RX
nitazoxanide (Romark)

THERAPEUTIC CLASS: Antiprotozoal agent

INDICATIONS: Treatment of diarrhea caused by *Cryptosporidium parvum* and *Giardia lamblia.*

DOSAGE: *Adults:* ≥12 yrs: *G.lamblia* Diarrhea: 500mg q12h for 3 days. Take with food.
Pediatrics: C.parvum/G.lamblia Diarrhea: 1-3 yrs: 100mg (5mL) q12h for 3 days. 4-11yrs: 200mg (10mL) q12h for 3 days. *G.lamblia* Diarrhea: ≥12 yrs: 500mg (1 tab or 25mL) q12h for 3 days. Take with food.

HOW SUPPLIED: Sus: 100mg/5mL (60mL); Tab: 500mg (60s, 3-Day Therapy Packs, 6s)

WARNINGS/PRECAUTIONS: Caution with hepatic and biliary disease, renal disease. Contains 1.48g sucrose/5mL. Safety and effectiveness have not been established in HIV positive or immunodeficient patients.

ADVERSE REACTIONS: Abdominal pain, diarrhea, headache, nausea.

INTERACTIONS: Highly protein bound; caution with other highly plasma protein-bound drugs with narrow therapeutic indices.

PREGNANCY: Category B; caution in nursing.

MECHANISM OF ACTION: Antiprotozoal agent; interferes with the pyruvate, ferredoxin oxidoreductase enzyme-dependent electron transfer reaction, which is essential to anaerobic energy metabolism.

PHARMACOKINETICS: Absorption: Tizoxanide: (Tab, 500mg) 12-17 yrs: C_{max}=9.1mcg/mL, T_{max}=4 hrs, AUC=39.5mcg•hr/mL; ≥18 yrs: C_{max}=10.6mcg/mL, T_{max}=3 hrs, AUC=41.9mcg•hr/mL. (Sus, 100mg) 1-3 yrs: C_{max}=3.11mcg/mL, T_{max}=3.5 hrs, AUC=11.7mcg•hr/mL; 4-11 yrs: C_{max}=3mcg/mL, T_{max}=2 hrs, AUC=13.5mcg•hr/mL. **Distribution**: Tizoxanide: Plasma protein binding (>99%). **Metabolism**: Hydrolysis, glucuronidation: Tizoxanide and tizoxanide glucuronide (active). **Elimination**: Urine (33%), bile and feces (66%). Refer to PI for complete kinetics information.

ALLEGRA
fexofenadine HCl (Sanofi-Aventis)
RX

THERAPEUTIC CLASS: H_1-antagonist

INDICATIONS: (ODT) 6-11 yrs; (Sus) 2-11 yrs: Relief of symptoms associated with seasonal allergic rhinitis in children. (ODT) 6-11 yrs; (Sus) 6 months-11 yrs: Treatment of uncomplicated skin manifestations of chronic idiopathic urticaria in children. (Tab) Relief of symptoms associated with seasonal allergic rhinitis and treatment of uncomplicated skin manifestations of chronic idiopathic urticaria in adults and children ≥6 yrs.

DOSAGE: *Adults:* Tab: Rhinitis/Urticaria: 60mg bid or 180mg qd. Renal Dysfunction: Initial: 60mg qd.
Pediatrics: Tab: ≥12 yrs: Rhinitis/Urticaria: 60mg bid or 180mg qd. Renal Dysfunction: Initial: 60mg qd. 6-11 yrs: Rhinitis/Urticaria: 30mg bid. Renal Dysfunction: Initial: 30mg qd. ODT: Rhinitis/Urticaria: 6-11 yrs: 30mg bid. Renal Dysfunction: 30mg qd. Sus: Rhinitis: 2-11 yrs: 30mg (5mL) bid. Renal Dysfunction: 30mg (5mL) qd. Urticaria: 2-11 yrs: 30mg (5mL) bid. Renal Dysfunction: 30mg (5mL) qd. 6 months to <2 yrs: 15mg (2.5mL) bid. Renal Dysfunction: 15mg (2.5mL) qd.

HOW SUPPLIED: Tab: 30mg, 60mg, 180mg; Tab, Orally Disintegrating: 30mg; Sus: 30mg/5mL

ADVERSE REACTIONS: Headache, cough, upper respiratory tract infection, back pain, fever, pain, otitis media, vomiting, diarrhea.

INTERACTIONS: Increased plasma levels with erythromycin or ketoconazole. Avoid concomitant aluminum- and magnesium-containing antacids. Fruit juices (eg, grapefruit, orange, and apple) may decrease levels.

PREGNANCY: Category C, caution in nursing.

MECHANISM OF ACTION: Antihistamine with selective peripheral H_1-receptor antagonist activity; prevents antigen-induced bronchospasm and histamine release from periotoneal mast cells.

PHARMACOKINETICS: Absorption: Rapid; (Cap, 120mg) T_{max}=2.6 hrs; (Cap, 60mg) C_{max}=131ng/mL; (Tab, 60mg) C_{max}=142ng/mL; (Tab, 180mg) C_{max}=494ng/mL; (Sus, 30mg) C_{max}=118.0ng/mL, T_{max}=1.0 hrs. **Distribution:** Plasma protein binding (60-70%). **Metabolism:** Liver (5%). **Elimination:** Urine (80%), feces (11%); $T_{1/2}$=14.4 hrs.

ALLEGRA-D
fexofenadine HCl - pseudoephedrine HCl (Sanofi-Aventis)
RX

THERAPEUTIC CLASS: H_1-antagonist/sympathomimetic amine

INDICATIONS: Relief of symptoms of seasonal allergic rhinitis.

DOSAGE: *Adults:* 60mg-120mg tab bid or 180mg-240mg tab qd without food. Renal Dysfunction: Initial: 60mg-120mg tab qd; avoid 180mg-240mg tab. Do not crush or chew.
Pediatrics: ≥12 yrs: 60mg-120mg tab bid or 180mg-240mg tab qd without food. Renal Dysfunction: Initial: 60mg-120mg tab qd; avoid 180mg-240mg tab. Do not crush or chew.

HOW SUPPLIED: Tab, Extended-Release: (Fexofenadine-Pseudoephedrine) (12-Hour) 60mg-120mg, (24-Hour) 180mg-240mg

CONTRAINDICATIONS: Narrow-angle glaucoma, urinary retention, severe HTN, severe CAD, within 14 days of MAOI therapy.

WARNINGS/PRECAUTIONS: Caution with HTN, DM, ischemic heart disease, increased IOP, hyperthyroidism, renal impairment, or prostatic hypertrophy. May produce CNS stimulation with convulsions or cardiovascular collapse with hypotension.

ADVERSE REACTIONS: Headache, insomnia, nausea, dry mouth, dyspepsia, throat irritation.

INTERACTIONS: Increased plasma levels with erythromycin or ketoconazole. Avoid MAOIs. Increased ectopic pacemaker activity can occur with digitalis. Caution with other sympathomimetic amines. Reduced effects of antihypertensive drugs which interfere with sympathetic activity (eg, methyldopa, mecamylamine, reserpine).

PREGNANCY: Category C, caution with nursing.

MECHANISM OF ACTION: H_1-receptor antagonist/sympathomimetic amine. Fexofenadine: Selective peripheral H_1-receptor antagonist; inhibits antigen-induced bronchospasm and histamine release from peritoneal mast cells. Pseudoephedrine: Exerts a decongestant action on the nasal mucosa.

PHARMACOKINETICS: Absorption: Fexofenadine: Rapidly absorbed; C_{max}=634ng/mL (single dose), 674ng/mL (multiple doses); T_{max}=1.8-2 hrs. Pseudoephedrine: C_{max}=394ng/mL (single dose), 495ng/mL (multiple doses); T_{max}=12 hrs. **Distribution:** Fexofenadine: Plasma protein binding (60-70%). Pseudoephedrine: V_d=2.6-3.5L/kg. **Metabolism:** Fexofenadine and pseudoephedrine: Hepatic (5% of fexofenadine; <1% of pseudoephedrine). **Elimination:** Fexofenadine: Feces (80%), urine (11%); $T_{1/2}$=14.6 hrs. Pseudoephedrine: $T_{1/2}$=7 hrs.

ALLERX

RX

chlorpheniramine maleate - methscopolamine nitrate - pseudoephedrine HCl
(Cornerstone)

THERAPEUTIC CLASS: Antihistamine/anticholinergic/decongestant

INDICATIONS: Temporary relief of symptoms associated with allergic rhinitis, vasomotor rhinitis, sinusitis, and the common cold.

DOSAGE: *Adults:* 1 AM Dose tab in morning and 1 PM Dose tab in evening. *Pediatrics:* ≥12 yrs: 1 AM Dose tab in morning and 1 PM Dose tab in evening.

HOW SUPPLIED: Tab, Extended-Release: (AM Dose) (Methscopolamine-Pseudoephedrine) 2.5mg-120mg; (PM Dose) (Chlorpheniramine-Methscopolamine) 8mg-2.5mg

CONTRAINDICATIONS: Severe HTN or CAD, MAOI use or within 14 days of discontinuation, nursing mothers taking MAOIs, narrow-angle glaucoma, urinary retention, peptic ulcer, during asthma attack.

WARNINGS/PRECAUTIONS: Caution with elderly, HTN, DM, ischemic heart disease, hyperthyroidism, prostatic hypertrophy, CVD, increased IOP. May produce CNS stimulation with convulsions or cardiovascular collapse with hypotension. Excitability reported especially in children.

ADVERSE REACTIONS: Drowsiness, lassitude, nausea, giddiness, dry mouth, blurred vision, cardiac palpitations, flushing, increased irritability.

INTERACTIONS: May enhance effects of TCAs, barbiturates, alcohol, other CNS depressants. May diminish antihypertensive effects of reserpine, veratrum alkaloids, methyldopa, mecamylamine. Increased sympathomimetic effect with β-blockers and MAOIs. Contraindicated with or within 14 days of discontinuing MAOIs. Hypotension potentiated with sildenafil or other organic nitrates; avoid concomitant use. Caution with hyperactivity to sympathomimetics.

PREGNANCY: Category C, not for use in nursing.

MECHANISM OF ACTION: Pseudoephedrine: Antihistamine decongestant; indirect-acting sympathomimetic amine that exerts decongestant action on the nasal mucosa. Chlorpheniramine: Alkylamine-type antihistamine. Methscopolamine: Anticholinergic; quaternary ammonium derivative of the anticholinergic scopolamine which possesses the peripheral actions of the belladonna alkaloids. Causes inhibition of salivary secretions, reduction in vol and total acid content of gastric secretion and inhibition of GI motility.

PHARMACOKINETICS: Absorption: Pseudoephedrine: Rapidly and almost completely absorbed by GIT. Methscopolamine: Poorly absorbed. **Distribution:** Methscopolamine:

Crosses blood-brain barrier. **Metabolism:** Pseudoephedrine: Liver via N-demethylation, parahydroxylation and oxidative deamination. **Elimination:** Pseudoephedrine: Urine (50-75% unchanged). Methscopolamine: Urine, bile, feces; $T_{1/2}$=4-6 hrs.

ALOCRIL   RX
nedocromil sodium (Allergan)

THERAPEUTIC CLASS: Mast cell stabilizer

INDICATIONS: Treatment of itching associated with allergic conjunctivitis.

DOSAGE: *Adults:* 1-2 drops bid. Continue throughout period of exposure.
Pediatrics: ≥3 yrs: 1-2 drops bid. Continue throughout period of exposure.

HOW SUPPLIED: Sol: 2% (5mL)

WARNINGS/PRECAUTIONS: Avoid wearing contacts while symptoms of allergic conjunctivitis persist.

ADVERSE REACTIONS: Headache, ocular burning, irritation, stinging, unpleasant taste, nasal congestion, asthma, conjunctivitis, eye redness, photophobia, rhinitis.

PREGNANCY: Category B, caution in nursing.

MECHANISM OF ACTION: Mast cell stabilizer; inhibits release of mediators from cells involved in hypersensitivity reactions, decreases chemotaxis and activation of eosinophils.

PHARMACOKINETICS: Absorption: Low systemic absorption. **Metabolism:** Not metabolized. **Elimination:** Urine (70% unchanged), feces (30%).

ALOMIDE   RX
lodoxamide tromethamine (Alcon)

THERAPEUTIC CLASS: Mast cell stabilizer

INDICATIONS: Ocular disorders including vernal keratoconjunctivitis, vernal conjunctivitis, and vernal keratitis.

DOSAGE: *Adults:* 1-2 drops qid for up to 3 months.
Pediatrics: >2 yrs: 1-2 drops qid for up to 3 months.

HOW SUPPLIED: Sol: 0.1% (10mL)

WARNINGS/PRECAUTIONS: Do not wear soft contacts during treatment. Transient burning and stinging upon instillation.

ADVERSE REACTIONS: Ocular pruritus, blurred vision, dry eye, tearing, discharge, hyperemia, crystalline deposits, foreign body sensation.

PREGNANCY: Category B, caution in nursing.

MECHANISM OF ACTION: Mast cell stabilizer; not established; suspected to inhibit the Type I immediate hypersensitivity reaction, decrease cutaneous vascular permeability associated with reagin or IgE and antigen-mediated reactions, and prevent calcium influx into mast cells upon stimulation.

PHARMACOKINETICS: Elimination: Urine; $T_{1/2}$=8.5 hrs.

ALOPRIM   RX
allopurinol sodium (Nabi)

THERAPEUTIC CLASS: Xanthine oxidase inhibitor

INDICATIONS: Management of elevated serum and urinary uric acid levels in patients with leukemia, lymphoma, and solid tumor malignancies receiving cancer therapy when oral therapy is not tolerated.

DOSAGE: *Adults:* Initial: 200-400mg/m^2/day IV as qd or in divided doses every 6, 8, or 12 hrs. Max: 600mg/day. CrCl 10-20mL/min: 200mg/day. CrCl 3-10mL/min: 100mg/day. CrCl <3mL/min: 100mg/day at extended intervals.
Pediatrics: Initial: 200mg/m^2/day IV as qd or in divided doses every 6, 8, or 12 hrs.

HOW SUPPLIED: Inj: 500mg

CONTRAINDICATIONS: Previous severe reaction to therapy.

WARNINGS/PRECAUTIONS: D/C at first appearance of hypersensitivity; increased risk in decreased renal function. Monitor LFTs during early stages of therapy in liver disease. Monitor renal function and uric acid levels; adjust dose if needed. Maintain sufficient fluid intake to yield a daily urinary output ≥2L. Drowsiness, hepatotoxicity, bone marrow suppression reported.

ADVERSE REACTIONS: Skin rash, eosinophilia, local injection site reaction, nausea, vomiting, diarrhea, renal failure/insufficiency.

INTERACTIONS: Decrease mercaptopurine and azathioprine dose to 1/3-1/4 of usual dose. Increased risk of skin rash with ampicillin, amoxicillin. Increased toxicity and risk of hypersensitivity with thiazide diuretics; monitor renal function. Caution with anticoagulants. Hypoglycemia reported with chlorpropamide. Enhanced myelosuppressive effects of cyclophosphamide, other cytotoxic agents. Increased cyclosporine levels. Increased urinary excretion of uric acid with uricosuric agents. Monitor PT with dicumarol.

PREGNANCY: Category C, caution in nursing.

MECHANISM OF ACTION: Xanthine oxidase inhibitor; reduces production of uric acid by inhibiting the biochemical reactions immediately preceding its formation.

PHARMACOKINETICS: Absorption: Absolute bioavailability (100%); C_{max}=1.58μg/mL (100mg), 5.12μg/mL (300mg); T_{max}=0.5 hrs; AUC=1.99 hr•μg/mL (100mg), 7.1 hr•μg/mL (300mg). **Metabolism:** Oxidative; oxypurinol (active metabolite). **Elimination:** Urine (12% unchanged); $T_{1/2}$=1 hr (parent), 24.1 hrs (oxypurinol).

ALPHAGAN P   RX
brimonidine tartrate (Allergan)

THERAPEUTIC CLASS: Selective alpha₂ agonist

INDICATIONS: Treatment of open-angle glaucoma and ocular hypertension.

DOSAGE: *Adults:* 1 drop tid, give q8h. Space dosing of other topical products that lower IOP by 5 min.
Pediatrics: ≥2 yrs: 1 drop tid, give q8h. Space dosing of other topical products that lower IOP by 5 min.

HOW SUPPLIED: Sol: 0.1% (5mL, 10mL, 15mL), 0.15% (5mL, 10mL, 15mL) (contains Purite)

CONTRAINDICATIONS: Concomitant MAOI therapy.

WARNINGS/PRECAUTIONS: Caution with severe CV disease, hepatic or renal dysfunction, depression, cerebral or coronary insufficiency, Raynaud's phenomenon, orthostatic hypotension, thromboangiitis obliterans. Wait 15 min before reinserting contacts with 0.2% solution. Monitor IOP.

ADVERSE REACTIONS: Oral dryness, ocular hyperemia, ocular pruritus, burning, stinging, ocular allergic reaction, blurred vision, foreign body sensation, fatigue, drowsiness, headache, conjunctival follicles.

INTERACTIONS: See Contraindications. May potentiate CNS depressants. May reduce BP; caution with β-blockers, antihypertensives, cardiac glycosides. Caution with TCAs. May be given with other topical products to lower IOP.

PREGNANCY: Category B, not for use in nursing.

MECHANISM OF ACTION: An α-2-adrenergic receptor agonist; reduces aqueous humor production and increases uveoscleral outflow.

PHARMACOKINETICS: Absorption: T_{max}=0.5-2.5 hrs. **Metabolism:** Liver (extensive). **Elimination:** Urine (74%).

ALTABAX   RX
retapamulin (GlaxoSmithKline)

THERAPEUTIC CLASS: Pleuromutilin antibacterial

INDICATIONS: Topical treatment of impetigo caused by susceptible strains of microorganisms, in patients ≥9 months.

DOSAGE: *Adults*: Apply thin layer (up to 100 cm^2 in total area) bid for 5 days. May cover with sterile bandage or gauze.
Pediatrics: ≥9 months: Apply thin layer (up to 2% total BSA) bid for 5 days. May cover with sterile bandage or gauze.

HOW SUPPLIED: Oint: 1% (5g, 10g, 15g)

WARNINGS/PRECAUTIONS: D/C if sensitization or irritation occurs. Not intended for oral, intranasal, ophthalmic or intravaginal use. May cause superinfection during therapy.

ADVERSE REACTIONS: Application site reactions.

INTERACTIONS: Coadministration with ketoconazole may increase levels.

PREGNANCY: Category B, caution in nursing.

MECHANISM OF ACTION: Pleuromutilin antibacterial; selectively inhibits bacterial protein synthesis by interacting at a site on the 50S subunit of the bacterial ribosome. The binding site involves ribosomal protein L3 and is in the region of the ribosomal P site and peptidyl transferase center. By binding to this site, peptidyl transfer is inhibited, P-site interactions are blocked, and the formation of normal active 50S ribosomal subunits is prevented.

PHARMACOKINETICS: Absorption: Low systemic exposure. Following application to 800cm^2 of intact skin: C_{max}=3.5ng/mL (multiple doses). Following application to 200cm^2 of abraded skin: C_{max}=11.7ng/mL (single dose), 9.0ng/mL (multiple doses). **Distribution:** Plasma protein binding (94%). **Metabolism:** Liver via CYP3A4 (mono-oxygenation, N-demethylation). **Elimination:** Not investigated.

ALVESCO
ciclesonide (Sepracor)

RX

THERAPEUTIC CLASS: Non-halogenated glucocorticoid

INDICATIONS: Maintenance treatment of asthma as prophylactic therapy in adult and adolescents ≥12 yrs.

DOSAGE: *Adults:* Previous Bronchodilator Alone: Initial: 80mcg bid. Max: 160mcg bid. Previous Inhaled Corticosteroid Therapy: Initial: 80mcg bid. Max: 320mcg bid. Previous Oral Corticosteroid Therapy: Initial: 320mcg bid. Max: 320mcg bid.
Pediatrics: ≥12 yrs: Previous Bronchodilator Alone:: Initial: 80mcg bid. Max: 160mcg bid. Previous Inhaled Corticosteroid Therapy: Initial: 80mcg bid. Max: 320mcg bid. Previous Oral Corticosteroid Therapy: : Initial: 320mcg bid. Max: 320mcg bid.

HOW SUPPLIED: MDI: 80mcg/actuation (60 actuations), 160mcg/actuation (60 or 120 actuations)

CONTRAINDICATIONS: Status asthmaticus or other acute episodes of asthma.

WARNINGS/PRECAUTIONS: *Candida albicans* infections of mouth and pharynx may occur; examine periodically and treat accordingly. Advise to rinse mouth after inhalation. Caution with active or quiescent TB infections, untreated local/systemic bacterial/fungal infections, systemic viral or parasitic infections, or ocular herpes simplex. Risk for more severe/fatal course of infections (eg, chickenpox, measles); avoid exposure in patients who have not had the disease or been properly immunized. Risk of adrenal insufficiency and withdrawal symptoms when replacing oral corticosteroids with inhaled corticosteroids; monitor closely. Taper dose if symptoms of hypercorticism and adrenal suppression occur. May cause growth velocity reduction in pediatrics. May decrease bone mineral density (BMD) with prolonged treatment; monitor and treat accordingly. Caution with history of glaucoma, increased IOP, and cataracts; monitor closely. Acute asthma episodes or bronchospasm may occur; d/c use and institute alternative treatment if occur.

ADVERSE REACTIONS: Headache, nasopharyngitis, sinusitis, pharyngolaryngeal pain, upper respiratory infection, arthralgia, nasal congestion, pain in extremity, back pain.

INTERACTIONS: Ketoconazole may increase levels of the pharmacologically active metabolite des-ciclesonide; co-administer with caution.

PREGNANCY: Category C, caution in nursing.

MECHANISM OF ACTION: Corticosteroid: exerts anti-inflammatory actions with affinity to glucocorticoid receptor that inhibits activities of multiple cell types (mast cells, eosinophils, basophils, lymphocytes, macrophages, and neutrophils) and mediators (histamine, eicosanoids, leukotrienes, and cytokines) involved in asthmatic response.

PHARMACOKINETICS: Absorption: Ciclesonide: Absolute bioavailability: 22%. Desciclesonide (active metabolite): 63%; C_{max}=1.02ng/mL in asthmatic patient. **Distribution:** Ciclesonide: V_d=2.9L/kg. Des-ciclesonide: V_d=12.1L/kg. **Metabolism:** Liver, via CYP3A4, CYP2D6 (hydrolysis); des-ciclesonide (active metabolite). **Elimination:** Feces (60%), urine (≤20%), and bile. $T_{1/2}$=ciclesonide (0.71 hrs), des-ciclesonide (6-7 hrs).

AmBisome   RX
amphotericin B (Astellas)

THERAPEUTIC CLASS: Polyene antifungal

INDICATIONS: Empirical therapy for presumed fungal infection in febrile, neutropenic patients. Treatment of *Aspergillus, Candida,* or *Cryptococcus* infections refractory to amphotericin B deoxycholate or where renal impairment or unacceptable toxicity precludes its use. Treatment of cryptococcal meningitis in HIV-infected patients. Treatment of visceral leishmaniasis.

DOSAGE: *Adults:* Empiric Therapy: 3mg/kg/day IV. Systemic Infections (*Aspergillus, Candida, Cryptococcus*): 3-5mg/kg/day IV. Cryptococcal Meningitis in HIV: 6mg/kg/day IV. Visceral Leishmaniasis: Immunocompetent: 3mg/kg/day IV on Days 1-5, 14, 21. May repeat course if needed. Immunocompromised: 4mg/kg/day IV on Days 1-5, 10, 17, 24, 31, 38.
Pediatrics: 1 month-16 yrs: Empirical Therapy: 3mg/kg/day IV. Systemic Infections (*Aspergillus, Candida, Cryptococcus*): 3-5mg/kg/day IV. Cryptococcal Meningitis in HIV: 6mg/kg/day IV. Visceral Leishmaniasis: Immunocompetent: 3mg/kg/day IV on Days 1-5, 14, 21. May repeat course if needed. Immunocompromised: 4mg/kg/day IV on Days 1-5, 10, 17, 24, 31, 38.

HOW SUPPLIED: Inj: 50mg

WARNINGS/PRECAUTIONS: If anaphylaxis occurs, d/c all further infusions. Significantly less toxic than amphotericin B deoxycholate. Monitor renal, hepatic, hematopoietic function and electrolytes (especially K^+, Mg^{++}).

ADVERSE REACTIONS: Chills, asthenia, back pain, pain, infection, chest pain, HTN, hypotension, tachycardia, GI hemorrhage, diarrhea, NV, hyperglycemia, hypokalemia, dyspnea.

INTERACTIONS: Concurrent use of antineoplastic agents may potentiate renal toxicity, bronchospasm, hypotension. Corticosteroids and corticotropin may potentiate hypokalemia. May potentiate digitalis toxicity. May increase flucytosine toxicity. Acute pulmonary toxicity with leukocyte transfusions reported. Nephrotoxic drugs enhance potential for renal toxicity. May enhance curariform effect of skeletal muscle relaxants due to hypokalemia. Imidazoles (eg, ketocoazole, miconazole, clotrimazole, fluconazole) may induce fungal resistance; caution with combination therapy especially in immunocompromised patients.

PREGNANCY: Category B, not for use in nursing.

MECHANISM OF ACTION: Antifungal agent; acts by binding to the sterol component of the cell membrane, which leads to changes in cell permeability and cell death in susceptible fungi. Also binds to the cholesterol component of the mammalian cell, leading to cytotoxicity.

PHARMACOKINETICS: Absorption: IV administration of variable doses resulted from different parameters. **Metabolism:** Not known.

AMCINONIDE   RX
amcinonide (Various)

THERAPEUTIC CLASS: Corticosteroid

INDICATIONS: Corticosteroid responsive dermatoses.

DOSAGE: *Adults:* Apply bid-tid depending on severity.
Pediatrics: Apply bid-tid depending on severity.

HOW SUPPLIED: Cre, Oint: 0.1% (15g, 30g, 60g); Lot: 0.1% (20mL, 60mL)

WARNINGS/PRECAUTIONS: Systemic absorption may produce reversible HPA axis suppression, manifestations of Cushing's syndrome, hyperglycemia, and glucosuria. D/C if irritation occurs. Use appropriate antifungal or antibacterial agent with dermatological infections. Pediatrics may be more susceptible to systemic toxicity. Caution when applied to large surface areas or with occlusive dressings.

ADVERSE REACTIONS: Itching, stinging, soreness, burning, irritation, folliculitis, hypertrichosis, hypopigmentation, perioral dermatitis, skin maceration, striae, miliaria, skin atrophy, secondary infection, contact dermatitis.

PREGNANCY: Category C, not for use in nursing.

MECHANISM OF ACTION: Corticosteroid: possesses anti-inflammatory, antipruritic and vasoconstrictive properties. Anti-inflammatory effects not established.

PHARMACOKINETICS: Absorption: Percutaneous; inflammation, other disease states, and use of occlusive dressings may increase absorption. **Distribution:** Systemically administered corticosteroids found in breast milk. **Metabolism:** Liver. **Elimination:** Renal, bile.

AMIDATE   RX
etomidate (Hospira)

THERAPEUTIC CLASS: General anesthetic

INDICATIONS: For induction of general anesthesia. For supplementation of subpotent anesthetic agents, such as nitrous oxide in oxygen, during maintenance of anesthesia for short operative procedures.

DOSAGE: *Adults:* 0.2-0.6mg/kg IV. Usual: 0.3mg/kg IV, over 30 to 60 seconds. *Pediatrics:* >10 yrs: 0.2-0.6mg/kg IV. Usual: 0.3mg/kg IV, over 30 to 60 seconds.

HOW SUPPLIED: Inj: 2mg/mL

WARNINGS/PRECAUTIONS: Not for prolonged infusion. Reduction of plasma cortisol and aldosterone concentrations have occurred; consider exogenous replacement during severely stressful conditions.

ADVERSE REACTIONS: Transient venous pain, transient skeletal muscle movements, including myoclonus, hyper/hypoventilation, apnea of short duration, hyper/hypotension, tachycardia, bradycardia.

PREGNANCY: Category C, caution in nursing.

MECHANISM OF ACTION: Hypnotic and general anesthetic.

PHARMACOKINETICS: Metabolism: Hydrolysis; carboxylic acid (metabolite). **Elimination:** Urine; $T_{1/2}$=75 mins.

AMIKACIN   RX
amikacin sulfate (Various)

> Potential for ototoxicity and nephrotoxicity. Neuromuscular blockade, respiratory blockade reported. Avoid potent diuretics and other neurotoxic, nephrotoxic, and ototoxic drugs.

THERAPEUTIC CLASS: Aminoglycoside

INDICATIONS: Short-term treatment of serious infections due to susceptible strains of gram-negative bacteria. Shown to be effective in bacterial septicemia; respiratory tract, bone/joint, CNS (including meningitis), skin and soft tissue, and intra-abdominal infections; burns and postoperative infections; complicated and recurrent urinary tract infections (UTI) due to susceptible strains of microorganisms.

DOSAGE: *Adults:* (IM/IV) 15mg/kg/day given q8h or q12h. Max: 15mg/kg/day. Heavier Wt Patients: Max: 1.5g/day. Recurrent Uncomplicated UTI: 250mg bid. Usual Duration: 7-10 days. D/C therapy if no response after 3-5 days. D/C if azotemia increases or if progressive decrease in urinary output occurs. Renal Impairment: Reduce dose. *Pediatrics:* 15mg/kg/day given q8h or q12h. Newborns: LD: 10mg/kg. Maint: 7.5mg/kg q12h. Usual Duration: 7-10 days. D/C therapy if no response after 3-5 days. D/C if azotemia increases or if progressive decrease in urinary output occurs. Renal Impairment: Reduce dose.

HOW SUPPLIED: Inj: 50mg/mL, 250mg/mL

CONTRAINDICATIONS: History of serious toxic reactions to aminoglycosides.

WARNINGS/PRECAUTIONS: May aggravate muscle weakness; caution with muscular disorders (eg, myasthenia gravis, parkinsonism). May cause fetal harm in pregnancy. Contains sodium metabisulfite, allergic reactions may occur especially in asthmatics. Maintain adequate hydration. Assess kidney function before therapy, then daily.

ADVERSE REACTIONS: Ototoxicity, neuromuscular blockage, nephrotoxicity, skin rash, drug fever, headache, paresthesia, tremor, nausea, arthralgia, anemia, hypotension.

INTERACTIONS: Increased nephrotoxicity with cephalosporins. Significant mutual inactivation may occur with β-lactams (eg, penicillin, cephalosporins). Cross-allergenicity between aminoglycosides. Avoid potent diuretics (eg, ethacrynic acid, furosemide), bacitracin, cisplatin, amphotericin B, paromomycin, polymyxin B, colistin, vancomycin, other aminoglycosides, and other neurotoxic, nephrotoxic and ototoxic drugs. Increased risk of neuromuscular blockade and respiratory paralysis with anesthetics, neuromuscular blockers, or massive transfusions of citrate-anticoagulated blood.

PREGNANCY: Category D, not for use in nursing.

MECHANISM OF ACTION: Semi-synthetic aminoglycoside antibiotic derived from kanamycin.

PHARMACOKINETICS: Absorption: Rapidly absorbed after IM administration. (IV) C_{max}=38mcg/mL. **Distribution**: V_d=24L; plasma protein binding (0-11%); crosses placenta. **Elimination**: Urine; $T_{1/2}$≥2 hr; (IM) 91.9% at 8 hrs, 98.2% at 24 hrs; (IV) 84% at 9 hrs, 94% at 24 hrs.

AMOXIL   RX
amoxicillin (GlaxoSmithKline)

THERAPEUTIC CLASS: Semisynthetic ampicillin derivative

INDICATIONS: Treatment of infections of the ear, nose, throat, genitourinary tract, skin and skin structure, lower respiratory tract (LRTI); acute, uncomplicated gonorrhea due to susceptible (β-lactamase negative) strains of microorganisms. Combination therapy for H.pylori eradication to reduce the risk of duodenal ulcer recurrence.

DOSAGE: Adults: Ear/Nose/Throat/SSSI/GU: (Mild/Moderate) 500mg q12h or 250mg q8h. (Severe) 875mg q12h or 500mg q8h. LRTI: 875mg q12h or 500mg q8h. Gonorrhea: 3g as single dose. H.pylori: (Dual Therapy) 1g + 30mg lansoprazole, both tid x 14 days. (Triple Therapy) 1g + 30mg lansoprazole + 500mg clarithromycin, all q12h x 14 days. (Amoxicillin) CrCl 10-30mL/min: 250-500mg q12h. CrCl <10mL/min: 250-500mg q24h. Hemodialysis: 250-500mg or 250mg q24h, additional dose during and at end of dialysis. Pediatrics: Neonates: ≤12 weeks: Max: 30mg/kg/day divided q12h. >3 months: Ear/Nose/Throat/SSSI/GU: (Mild/Moderate) 25mg/kg/day given q12h or 20mg/kg/day given q8h. (Severe): 45mg/kg/day given q12h or 40mg/kg/day given q8h. LRTI: 45mg/kg/day given q12h or 40mg/kg/day given q8h. Gonorrhea: (Prepubertal) 50mg/kg with 25mg/kg probenecid as single dose. (Not for <2yrs). >40kg: Dose as adult.

HOW SUPPLIED: Cap: 500mg; Sus: 50mg/mL (30mL), 200mg/5mL (50mL, 75mL, 100mL), 250mg/5mL (100mL, 150mL), 400mg/5mL (50mL, 75mL, 100mL); Tab: 500mg, 875mg; Tab, Chewable: 200mg, 400mg

WARNINGS/PRECAUTIONS: Serious, sometimes fatal, hypersensitivity reactions reported with PCN therapy. Clostridium difficile-associated diarrhea has been reported. Monitor renal, hepatic, and blood with prolonged use. The 200mg and 400mg chewable tabs contain phenylalanine.

ADVERSE REACTIONS: NV, diarrhea, pseudomembranous colitis, hypersensitivity reactions, blood dyscrasias, superinfection (prolonged use).

INTERACTIONS: Increased levels with probenecid. Chloramphenicol, macrolides, sulfonamides, tetracyclines may interfere with bactericidal effects. False (+) for urine glucose with Clinitest, Benedict's or Fehling's solution.

PREGNANCY: Category B, caution in nursing.

MECHANISM OF ACTION: Ampicillin analog; has broad-spectrum bactericidal activity against susceptible organisms during active multiplication; acts through inhibition of biosynthesis of cell-wall mucopeptide.

PHARMACOKINETICS: Absorption: Rapid. Cap (500mg): T_{max}=1-2 hrs. Tab (875mg): C_{max}=13.8mcg/mL, AUC=35.4mcg•hr/mL. Oral suspension (400mg): C_{max}=5.92mcg/mL, AUC=17.1mcg•hr/mL. Chewable tab (400mg): C_{max}=5.18mcg/mL, AUC=17.9mcg•hr/

mL. Oral suspension (125-250mg) T_{max}=1-2 hrs. **Distribution:** Plasma protein binding, (20%). Diffuses to spinal fluid and brain only if meninges inflamed. **Elimination:** Urine (unchanged); $T_{1/2}$=61.3 min.

AMPHOTEC   RX
amphotericin B cholesteryl sulfate (Three Rivers)

THERAPEUTIC CLASS: Polyene antifungal

INDICATIONS: Treatment of invasive aspergillosis in patients with renal impairment, unacceptable toxicity, or previous failure to amphotericin deoxycholate.

DOSAGE: *Adults:* Test Dose: Infuse small amount over 15-30 min. Treatment: 3-4mg/kg/day IV at 1mg/kg/hr.
Pediatrics: Test Dose: Infuse small amount over 15-30 min. Treatment: 3-4mg/kg/day IV at 1mg/kg/hr.

HOW SUPPLIED: Inj: 50mg, 100mg

WARNINGS/PRECAUTIONS: Anaphylaxis may occur. D/C if severe respiratory distress occurs. Acute reactions (eg, fever, shaking chills, hypotension, nausea, tachypnea) 1-3 hrs after starting infusion. Monitor renal/hepatic function, electrolytes, CBC, PT during therapy.

ADVERSE REACTIONS: Chills, fever, headache, hypotension, tachycardia, HTN, nausea, vomiting, thrombocytopenia, increased creatinine, hypokalemia, dyspnea, hypoxia.

INTERACTIONS: Antineoplastics may potentiate renal toxicity, bronchospasm, hypotension. Corticosteroids and corticotropin may potentiate hypokalemia. May increase flucytosine toxicity. Caution with imidazoles (eg, ketoconazole, clotrimazole, miconazole, fluconazole). Increased risk of renal toxicity with nephrotoxic drugs (eg, aminoglycosides, cyclosporine, pentamidine). May enhance curariform effect of skeletal muscle relaxants (eg, tubocurarine) or digitalis toxicity with hypokalemia.

PREGNANCY: Category B, not for use in nursing.

MECHANISM OF ACTION: Polyene antibiotic; binds to sterols (primarily ergosterol) in cell membranes of sensitive fungi, with subsequent leakage of intracellular contents and cell death. Also binds to cholesterol in mammalian cell membranes, which may account for human toxicity.

PHARMACOKINETICS: Administration: Variable doses resulted in altered parameters. **Absorption:** 3mg/kg/day: AUC=29µg/mL•hr, C_{max}=2.6µg/mL. 4mg/kg/day: AUC=36µg/mL•hr, C_{max}=2.9µg/mL. **Distribution:** 3mg/kg/day: V_d=3.8L/kg. 4mg/kg/day: V_d =4.1L/kg. **Metabolism:** Unknown. **Elimination:** 3mg/kg/day: $T_{1/2}$ =27.5 hrs. 4mg/kg/day: $T_{1/2}$ =28.2 hrs.

AMPICILLIN INJECTION   RX
ampicillin sodium (Various)

THERAPEUTIC CLASS: Semisynthetic penicillin derivative

INDICATIONS: Treatment of respiratory tract, urinary tract, and GI infections, bacterial meningitis, septicemia, and endocarditis caused by susceptible strains of microorganisms.

DOSAGE: *Adults:* IM/IV: Respiratory Tract/Soft Tissues: ≥40kg: 250-500mg q6h. <40kg: 25-50mg/kg/day given q6-8h. GI/GU: ≥40kg: 500mg q6h. <40kg: 50mg/kg/day given q6-8h. Urethritis (Caused by *N.gonorrhea* in Males): 500mg q8-12h for 2 doses; may retreat if needed. Bacterial Meningitis: 150-200mg/kg/day given q3-4h. Septicemia: 150-200mg/kg/day IV for 3 days, continue with IM q3-4h. Treatment of all infections should be continued for a minimum of 48-72 hrs after becoming asymptomatic. Minimum of 10 days treatment recommended for Group A β-hemolytic streptococci. *Pediatrics:* Bacterial Meningitis: 150-200mg/kg/day given q3-4h. Septicemia: 150-200mg/kg/day IV given q3-4h for 3 days, continue with IM q3-4h. Treatment of all infections should be continued for a minimum of 48-72 hrs after becoming asymptomatic. Minimum of 10 days treatment recommended for Group A β-hemolytic streptococci.

HOW SUPPLIED: Inj: 250mg, 500mg, 1g, 2g

WARNINGS/PRECAUTIONS: Serious, sometimes fatal, hypersensitivity reactions reported with PCN therapy. Caution with renal impairment. Cross-sensitivity with other β-lactams. May cause skin rash, especially in mononucleosis; avoid use. Pseudomembranous colitis reported. May result in overgrowth of nonsusceptible organisms.

ADVERSE REACTIONS: Headache, NV, oral and vaginal candidiasis, diarrhea, urticaria, allergic reactions, anaphylaxis, serum sickness-like reactions, exfoliative dermatitis.

INTERACTIONS: Potentiated by probenecid. May decrease effects of oral contraceptives. Allopurinol increases incidence of skin rash.

PREGNANCY: Category B, caution in nursing.

MECHANISM OF ACTION: Penicillin derivative; bactericidal against gram-positive and gram-negative organisms.

PHARMACOKINETICS: Distribution: Plasma protein binding (20%), found in breast milk. Penetrates to CSF and brain only if meninges are inflamed. **Elimination:** Urine (unchanged).

AMPICILLIN ORAL
ampicillin (Various)

RX

THERAPEUTIC CLASS: Semisynthetic penicillin derivative

INDICATIONS: Genitourinary tract (GU) infections, including gonorrhea, respiratory and GI tract infections, and meningitis.

DOSAGE: *Adults:* GI/GU: 500mg qid. Use larger doses in chronic or severe infections. Gonorrhea: 3.5g single dose with 1g probenecid. Respiratory: 250mg qid. Treat minimum 48-72 hrs after eradication. Treat minimum 10 days for hemolytic strains of strep. *Pediatrics:* >20kg: GI/GU: 500mg qid. Respiratory: 250mg qid. ≤20kg: GI/GU: 25mg/kg qid. Respiratory: 50mg/kg/day given tid-qid. Do not exceed adult doses. Use larger doses in chronic or severe infections. Treat minimum 48-72 hrs after eradication. Treat minimum 10 days for hemolytic strains of strep.

HOW SUPPLIED: Cap: 250mg, 500mg; Sus: 125mg/5mL, 250mg/5mL (100mL, 200mL)

CONTRAINDICATIONS: Infections caused by penicillinase-producing organisms.

WARNINGS/PRECAUTIONS: Possible cross-sensitivity with cephalosporins. Pseudomembranous colitis and anaphylatic reactions may occur.

ADVERSE REACTIONS: Stomatitis, NV, diarrhea, rash, SGOT elevation, blood dyscrasias, eosinophilia, thrombocytopenic purpura, hypersensitivity reactions, superinfection (prolonged use).

INTERACTIONS: Increased risk of rash with allopurinol. Bacteriostatic antibiotics (eg, chloramphenicol, erythromycins, sulfonamides or tetracyclines) may interfere with bactericidal activity. May decrease the effectiveness of oral contraceptives. Increased blood levels with probenecid.

PREGNANCY: Category B, not for use in nursing.

MECHANISM OF ACTION: Penicillin derivative; bactericidal against gram-positive and gram-negative organisms.

PHARMACOKINETICS: Absorption: Well-absorbed; (500mg Cap) C_{max}=3mcg/mL; (250mg Sus) C_{max}=2.3mcg/mL. **Distribution:** Plasma protein binding (20%). **Elimination:** Urine (unchanged).

ANAFRANIL
clomipramine HCl (Mallinckrodt)

RX

> Antidepressants increased the risk of suicidal thinking and behavior (suicidality) in short-term studies in children, adolescents, and young adults with Major Depressive Disorder (MDD) and other psychiatric disorders. Clomipramine is not approved for use in pediatric patients except for patients with OCD.

THERAPEUTIC CLASS: Tricyclic antidepressant

INDICATIONS: Treatment of OCD.

DOSAGE: *Adults:* Initial: 25mg/day with meals. Titrate: Increase within 2 weeks to 100mg/day. Increase further over several weeks. Max: 250mg/day. Maint: May give total daily dose at bedtime.

Pediatrics: >10 yrs: Initial: 25mg/day with meals. Titrate: Increase within 2 weeks to 3mg/kg or 100mg/day, whichever is smaller. Increase further over several weeks. Max: 3mg/kg/day or 200mg/day. Maint: May give total daily dose at bedtime.

HOW SUPPLIED: Cap: 25mg, 50mg, 75mg

CONTRAINDICATIONS: MAOI use within 14 days, acute recovery period following MI.

WARNINGS/PRECAUTIONS: Pooled analyses of short-term placebo-controlled trials of antidepressant drugs showed that these drugs increase the risk of suicidal thinking and behavior (suicidality) in children, adolescents, and young adults (ages 18-24) with major depressive disorder (MDD) and other psychiatric disorders. Increased risks with electroconvulsive therapy. D/C prior to elective surgery. Avoid abrupt withdrawal. Caution with seizure disorder, conditions predisposing to seizures (eg, brain damage, alcoholism), urinary retention, narrow-angle glaucoma, adrenal medulla tumors, increased IOP, hyperthyroidism, cardiovascular disorders, liver dysfunction, significant renal dysfunction. Monitor hepatic enzymes with liver dysfunction. Weight changes, sexual dysfunction, blood dyscrasias, elevated liver enzymes reported. Hypomania/mania reported with affective disorder. Psychosis reported with schizophrenia. All patients being treated with antidepressants for any indication should be monitored appropriately and observed closely for clinical worsening, suicidality, and unusual changes in behavior, especially during the initial few months of therapy or at times of dose changes.

ADVERSE REACTIONS: Dry mouth, constipation, nausea, dyspepsia, anorexia, weight gain, increased sweating, increased appetite, myoclonus, nervousness, libido change, dizziness, tremor, somnolence, impotence, visual changes.

INTERACTIONS: See Contraindications. Caution with anticholinergics, sympathomimetics, thyroid and CNS drugs. May block effects of clonidine, guanethidine. Increased levels with haloperidol, methylphenidate, highly protein bound drugs, CYP2D6 inhibitors (eg, quinidine, cimetidine, SSRIs) and enzyme substrates (eg, phenothiazines, propafenone, flecainide). At least 5 weeks must elapse before starting TCA therapy after fluoxetine discontinuation. Decreased levels with enzyme inducers (eg, barbiturates, phenytoin). Additive effects with CNS depressants, barbiturates, alcohol. NMS reported with neuroleptics. Increases phenobarbital and highly protein bound drugs (eg, warfarin, digoxin) plasma levels.

PREGNANCY: Category C, not for use in nursing.

MECHANISM OF ACTION: Dibenzazepine (TCA); unknown, capacity to inhibit reuptake of 5-HT.

PHARMACOKINETICS: Absorption: Administration of variable doses resulted in different parameters. **Distribution:** Plasma protein binding (97%); excreted in breast milk. **Metabolism:** Hepatic (biotransformation). Metabolite (desmethylclomipramine). **Elimination:** Biliary excretion. Clomipramine: $T_{1/2}$=32 hrs. Desmethylclomipramine: $T_{1/2}$=69 hrs.

ANALPRAM-HC
hydrocortisone acetate - pramoxine HCl (Ferndale)

RX

THERAPEUTIC CLASS: Corticosteroid/anesthetic

INDICATIONS: Corticosteroid responsive dermatoses of the anal region.

DOSAGE: *Adults:* Apply tid-qid. May use occlusive dressings in psoriasis or recalcitrant conditions. For cleansing anogenital area, spread lotion on cotton or tissue and wipe affected area.
Pediatrics: Apply tid-qid. May use occlusive dressings in psoriasis or recalcitrant conditions. For cleansing anogenital area, spread lotion on cotton or tissue and wipe affected area.

HOW SUPPLIED: Cre: (Hydrocortisone-Pramoxine) 1%-1%, 2.5%-1% (30g); Lot: 2.5%-1% (60mL)

WARNINGS/PRECAUTIONS: May produce reversible HPA axis suppression, manifestations of Cushing's syndrome, hyperglycemia, and glucosuria. D/C use if irritation occurs. Avoid eyes. Peds may be more susceptible to systemic toxicity. Use appropriate therapy with infections.

ADVERSE REACTIONS: Burning, itching, irritation, dryness, folliculitis, hypertrichosis, acneiform eruptions, hypopigmentation, perioral dermatitis, allergic contact dermatitis, secondary infection, skin maceration, skin atrophy, striae, miliaria.

PREGNANCY: Category C, caution in nursing.

MECHANISM OF ACTION: Unknown. Hydrocortisone: Suspected to act as anti-inflammatory, anti-pruritic, and vasoconstrictor. Pramoxine: Anesthetic agent, suspected to stabilize neuronal membrane of nerve endings.

PHARMACOKINETICS: Absorption: Absorbed from normal intact skin. **Distribution:** Plasma protein binding in varying degrees. **Metabolism:** Liver. **Elimination:** Kidney, bile (metabolites).

ANDRODERM
testosterone (Watson)

THERAPEUTIC CLASS: Androgen

INDICATIONS: Testosterone replacement therapy in males due to primary or secondary hypogonadism.

DOSAGE: *Adults:* Initial: 5mg/day. Maint: 2.5mg-7.5mg/day. Apply patch nightly to intact skin of back, abdomen, upper arm or thigh. Rotate sites; avoid same site for 7 days. Do not apply to scrotum or oily, damaged, irritated areas. May apply 2 patches at same time.
Pediatrics: ≥15 yrs: Initial: 5mg/day. Maint: 2.5mg-7.5mg/day. Apply patch nightly to intact skin of back, abdomen, upper arm or thigh. Rotate sites; avoid same site for 7 days. Do not apply to scrotum or oily, damaged, irritated areas. May apply 2 patches at same time.

HOW SUPPLIED: Patch: 2.5mg/24 hrs (60s), 5mg/24 hrs (30s)

CONTRAINDICATIONS: Breast or prostate cancer in men. Women.

WARNINGS/PRECAUTIONS: Prolonged use is associated with serious hepatic effects. Increased risk for prostatic hyperplasia/carcinoma in elderly. Risk of edema with pre-existing cardiac, renal, or hepatic disease; d/c if edema occurs. Risk of virilization of female sex partner. Monitor LFTs, Hgb, Hct, PSA, cholesterol, lipids.

ADVERSE REACTIONS: Gynecomastia, pruritus/erythema/vesicles/blister at application site, prostate abnormalities, headache, depression.

INTERACTIONS: May potentiate effects of anticoagulants, oxyphenbutazone. May decrease blood glucose and insulin requirements in diabetics. Pretreatment with ointments may reduce testosterone absorption.

PREGNANCY: Category X, not for use in nursing.

MECHANISM OF ACTION: Endogenous androgen; responsible for normal growth and development of male sex organs and for maintenance of secondary sex characteristics.

PHARMACOKINETICS: Absorption: C_{max}=753ng/dL, T_{max}=7.9 hrs. **Ditribution:** SHBG and albumin binding. **Metabolism:** Liver, estradiol, and DHT (major metabolite). **Elimination:** (IM) Urine=90% (glucuronide and sulfate conjugates), feces=6% (unconjugated); $T_{1/2}$=71 min.

ANECTINE   RX
succinylcholine chloride (Sandoz)

> **Rare reports of acute rhabdomyolysis with hyperkalemia followed by ventricular dysrhythmias, cardiac arrest, and death in children with undiagnosed skeletal muscle myopathy. Reserve in children for emergency intubation where securing airway is necessary.**

THERAPEUTIC CLASS: Skeletal muscle relaxant (depolarizing)

INDICATIONS: Adjunct to general anesthesia to facilitate tracheal intubation and to provide skeletal muscle relaxation during surgery or mechanical ventilation.

DOSAGE: *Adults:* Short Surgical Procedure: Average Dose: 0.6mg/kg IV. Range: 0.3-1.1mg/kg IV. Blockade develops in 1 min, may persist up to 2 min. Long Surgical Procedure: 2.5-4.3mg/min IV; or 0.3-1.1mg/kg initial IV inj, then 0.04-0.07mg/kg IV at

appropriate intervals. IM (if vein not accessible): Up to 3-4mg/kg IM. Max: 150mg/total dose. Effect observed in 2-3 min.
Pediatrics: Procedure to Secure Airway: Infants/Small Children: 2mg/kg IV. Older Children/Adolescents: 1mg/kg IV. IM (if vein not accessible): Infants/Older Children: Up to 3-4mg/kg IM. Max: 150mg/total dose. Effect observed in 2-3 min.

HOW SUPPLIED: Inj: 20mg/mL

CONTRAINDICATIONS: Personal or familial history of malignant hyperthermia, skeletal muscle myopathies. Acute phase of injury following major burns, multiple trauma, extensive skeletal muscle denervation, upper motor neuron injury.

WARNINGS/PRECAUTIONS: Avoid administration before unconsciousness has been induced. May induce arrhythmias or cardiac arrest in electrolyte abnormalities or massive digitalis toxicity. Caution with chronic abdominal infection, subarachnoid hemorrhage, conditions causing degeneration of central and peripheral nervous system, fractures, muscle spasms, reduced plasma cholinesterase activity, and acute phase of injury following major burns, multiple trauma, extensive skeletal muscle denervation, upper motor neuron injury. Malignant hyperthermia reported. Higher incidence of bradycardia progressing to asystole with 2nd dose. May increase IOP, intracranial or intragastric pressure. With prolonged therapy, Phase I block will progress to Phase II block associated with prolonged respiratory paralysis and weakness. Confirm Phase II block before therapy. Hypokalemia or hypocalcemia prolong neuromuscular blockade.

ADVERSE REACTIONS: Respiratory depression, cardiac arrest, malignant hyperthermia, arrhythmia, bradycardia, tachycardia, HTN, hypotension, hyperkalemia, increased IOP, muscle fasciculation, jaw rigidity, post-op muscle pains.

INTERACTIONS: Enhanced effects with promazine, oxytocin, certain non-penicillin antibiotics, β-blockers, procainamide, lidocaine, trimethaphan, lithium carbonate, magnesium salts, quinine, aprotinin, chloroquine, diethylether, isoflurane, desflurane, metoclopramide, terbutaline, and drugs that reduce plasma cholinesterase activity (eg, chronically administered oral contraceptives, glucocorticoids, certain MAOIs) or inhibit plasma cholinesterase. Increased risk of malignant hyperthermia with volatile anesthetics.

PREGNANCY: Category C, caution in nursing.

MECHANISM OF ACTION: Depolarizing skeletal muscle relaxant; combines with the cholinergic receptors of motor end plate to produce depolarization, and subsequent neuromuscular transmission inhibition.

PHARMACOKINETICS: Metabolism: Rapid; via plasma cholinesterases through hydrolysis to succinylmonocholine and to succinic and choline. **Elimination:** Urine 10% (unchanged).

ANTIVENIN   RX
black widow spider antivenin [lactrodectus mactans] (Merck)

THERAPEUTIC CLASS: Immunoglobulin

INDICATIONS: Treat symptoms due to black widow spider bites.

DOSAGE: *Adults:* 1 vial (2.5mL) IM, preferably given in anterolateral thigh. May repeat if necessary. Shock/Severe Cases: 1 vial (2.5mL) IV in 10-50mL saline solution over 15 min. *Pediatrics:* <12 yrs: 1 vial (2.5mL) IV in 10-50mL saline solution over 15 min.

HOW SUPPLIED: Inj: 6000 U

WARNINGS/PRECAUTIONS: Serum sickness/death could result from the use of horse serum in sensitive patients. Perform skin test prior to treatment. Observe for serum sickness for 8-12 days following treatment. Attempt desensitization only to save life.

ADVERSE REACTIONS: Anaphylaxis, serum sickness.

PREGNANCY: Category C, caution in nursing.

MECHANISM OF ACTION: Venom neutralizing globulin; not established.

ANTIVERT
meclizine HCl (Pfizer)

RX

THERAPEUTIC CLASS: Antihistamine

INDICATIONS: Management of nausea, vomiting and dizziness associated with motion sickness. Management of vertigo associated with diseases affecting the vestibular system.

DOSAGE: *Adults:* Motion Sickness: 25-50mg 1 hr prior to trip/departure, repeat q24h prn. Vertigo: 25-100mg/day in divided doses.
Pediatrics: ≥12 yrs: Motion Sickness: 25-50mg 1 hr prior to trip/departure, repeat q24h prn. Vertigo: 25-100mg/day in divided doses.

HOW SUPPLIED: Tab: 12.5mg, 25mg, 50mg* *scored

WARNINGS/PRECAUTIONS: Caution with asthma, glaucoma, prostatic hypertrophy.

ADVERSE REACTIONS: Drowsiness, dry mouth, blurred vision (rare).

INTERACTIONS: Avoid alcoholic beverages.

PREGNANCY: Category B, safety in nursing is not known.

MECHANISM OF ACTION: Antihistaminic agent; blocks vasodepressor response to histamine; slight blocking against acetylcholine.

ANUSOL-HC CREAM
hydrocortisone (Salix)

RX

OTHER BRAND NAMES: Proctocream HC (Schwarz Pharma) - Proctosol HC (NuCare) - Proctozone-HC (Rising)

THERAPEUTIC CLASS: Corticosteroid

INDICATIONS: Corticosteroid responsive dermatoses.

DOSAGE: *Adults:* Apply bid-qid. May use occlusive dressings for psoriasis or recalcitrant conditions; d/c dressings if infection develops.
Pediatrics: Apply bid-qid. May use occlusive dressings for psoriasis or recalcitrant conditions; d/c dressings if infection develops.

HOW SUPPLIED: Cre: 2.5% (30g)

WARNINGS/PRECAUTIONS: May cause reversible adrenal suppression, manifestations of Cushing's syndrome, hyperglycemia, glucosuria. Caution when applied to large surface areas or under occlusive dressings. Use appropriate therapy with infections. Pediatrics may be more susceptible to systemic toxicity. D/C if irritation occurs. Avoid eyes.

ADVERSE REACTIONS: Burning, itching, irritation, dryness, folliculitis, hypertrichosis, acneiform eruptions, hypopigmentation, perioral dermatitis, allergic contact dermatitis, maceration skin, secondary infection, skin atrophy, striae, miliaria.

PREGNANCY: Category C, caution in nursing.

MECHANISM OF ACTION: Topical corticosteroid, suspected to produce anti-inflammatory, antipruritic, and vasoconstrictive actions.

PHARMACOKINETICS: Absorption: Absorbed from normal intact skin. **Distribution:** Plasma protein binding in varying degrees. **Metabolism:** Liver. **Elimination:** Kidneys, bile (metabolites). $T_{1/2}$=8-12 hr.

ANZEMET
dolasetron mesylate (Sanofi-Aventis)

RX

THERAPEUTIC CLASS: 5-HT$_3$-antagonist

INDICATIONS: (Inj) Prevention of nausea/vomiting associated with emetogenic cancer chemotherapy including high-dose cisplatin. Prevention and treatment of post-op nausea/vomiting. (Tab) Prevention of nausea/vomiting associated with moderately emetogenic cancer chemotherapy and prevention of post-op nausea/vomiting.

DOSAGE: *Adults:* (Inj) Prevention of Chemotherapy Nausea/Vomiting: 1.8mg/kg IV single dose or 100mg IV 30 min before chemotherapy. Prevention/Treatment of Post-op Nausea/Vomiting: 12.5mg IV single dose 15 min before cessation of anesthesia or as soon as nausea/vomiting presents. (Tab) Prevention of Chemotherapy-Induced Nausea/Vomiting: 100mg PO within 1 hr before chemotherapy. Prevention of Postoperative Nausea/Vomiting: 100mg PO within 2 hrs before surgery.

Pediatrics: 2-16 yrs: (Inj) Prevention of Chemotherapy Nausea/Vomiting: 1.8mg/kg IV single dose 30 min before chemotherapy. Max: 100mg. May mix inj in apple or grape juice and take orally within 1 hr before chemotherapy. Prevention/Treatment of Post-op Nausea/Vomiting: 0.35mg/kg IV single dose 15 min before cessation of anesthesia or as soon as nausea/vomiting presents. Max: 12.5mg single dose. May mix 1.2mg/kg inj in apple or grape juice and take orally within 2 hrs before surgery. Max: 100mg/dose. (Tab) Prevention of Chemotherapy-Induced Nausea/Vomiting: 1.8mg/kg PO within 1 hr before chemotherapy. Max: 100mg. Prevention of Postoperative Nausea/Vomiting: 1.2mg/kg PO within 2 hrs before surgery. Max: 100mg.

HOW SUPPLIED: Inj: 20mg/mL; Tab: 50mg, 100mg

WARNINGS/PRECAUTIONS: Caution in patients with or who may develop cardiac conduction interval prolongation, especially those with congenital QT syndrome, hypokalemia and hypomagnesemia, Cross sensitivity may occur with other 5-HT$_3$ antagonists. Can cause ECG interval changes.

ADVERSE REACTIONS: Headache, diarrhea, fever, fatigue, dizziness, abnormal hepatic function, chills/shivering, urinary retention, abdominal pain, HTN, wide complex tachycardia or ventricular tachycardia, ventricular fibrillation.

INTERACTIONS: Increased risk of prolongation of cardiac conduction intervals with diuretics, antiarrhythmics, drugs that prolong QTc interval and cumulative high dose anthracycline therapy. Increased levels with cimetidine. Decreased levels with rifampin. Decreased clearance with IV atenolol.

PREGNANCY: Category B, caution in nursing.

MECHANISM OF ACTION: 5-HT$_3$ receptor antagonist.

PHARMACOKINETICS: Absorption: T_{max}=0.6 hr. **Distribution:** V_d=5.8L/Kg; plasma protein binding (77%). **Metabolism:** Complete. Via carbonyl reductase CYP2D6 and flavin monooxygenase through reduction, hydroxylation, and N-oxidation. **Elimination:** Urine 53% (unchanged), feces; $T_{1/2}$=7.3 hrs.

ARALEN   RX
chloroquine phosphate (Sanofi-Aventis)

THERAPEUTIC CLASS: Aminoquinolone

INDICATIONS: Treatment of extraintestinal amebiasis and acute attacks of malaria. Suppression of malaria.

DOSAGE: *Adults:* Malaria: Initial: 1g, then 500mg 6-8 hrs later, then 500mg qd for 2 consecutive days (total of 2.5g in 3 days). Suppression: 500mg on the same day each week. Start 2 weeks before exposure (double initial dose if <2 weeks before exposure) and continue for 8 weeks after return. Extraintestinal Amebiasis: 1g qd for 2 days, then 500mg qd for at least 2-3 weeks. Treatment usually combined with intestinal amebicide. *Pediatrics:* Malaria: Total dose of 25mg base/kg taken over 3 day, as follows: 1st Dose: 10mg base/kg (max 600mg base single dose). 2nd Dose: 5mg base/kg (300mg base single dose) 6 hrs after 1st dose. 3rd Dose: 5mg base/kg 18 hrs after 2nd dose. 4th Dose: 5mg base/kg 24 hrs after 3rd dose. Suppression: 5mg base/kg/week. Max: 300mg base/dose. Start 2 weeks before exposure (double initial dose if <2 weeks before exposure) and continue for 8 weeks after return.

HOW SUPPLIED: Tab: (Phosphate) 500mg (500mg tab=300mg base)

CONTRAINDICATIONS: Retinal or visual field changes.

WARNINGS/PRECAUTIONS: Caution with G6PD deficiency, pre-existing auditory damage, hepatic impairment, alcoholism, porphyria, psoriasis, elderly, and history of seizures. Monitor CBCs, vision, reflexes with prolonged use. D/C if visual or hematological disturbances, muscle weakness, hearing defects develop. Chloroquine resistance is widespread.

ADVERSE REACTIONS: Headache, pruritus, psychic stimulation, visual disturbances, pleomorphic skin eruptions, GI effects, convulsions, tinnitus, nerve type deafness.

INTERACTIONS: Caution with hepatotoxic drugs. Space dosing of antacids/kaolin by 4 hours. Increased levels with cimetidine; avoid concomitant use. Space dosing of ampicillin by at least 2 hours. May increase cyclosporine levels; monitor closely.

PREGNANCY: Avoid in pregnancy except for treatment of malaria if benefits outweigh risks. Not for use in nursing.

MECHANISM OF ACTION: Antimalarial aminoquinolone; unknown, suspected to inhibit certain enzymes, resulting from its interaction with DNA.

PHARMACOKINETICS: Absorption: Rapidly and completely absorbed (GIT). **Distribution:** Plasma protein binding (approximately 55%). Crosses placenta. **Metabolism:** Undergoes appreciable degradation. Desethylchloroquine (main metabolite). **Elimination:** Urine (unchanged).

ARANESP RX
darbepoetin alfa (Amgen)

> Increased mortality, serious cardiovascular/thromboembolic events, and tumor progression. Erythropoiesis-stimulating agents (ESAs) may increase risk for death and/or serious cardiovascular events when administered to a target Hgb >12g/dL. Use lowest level sufficient to avoid need for RBC transfusion. When ESAs are used preoperatively for reduction of allogenic RBC transfusions, a higher incidence of DVT was reported in patients not receiving prophylactic anticoagulation; darbepoetin alfa is not approved for this indication. ESAs shortened overall survival in patients with breast, head and neck, lymphoid, non-small cell lung, and cervical cancers when dosed to target Hgb ≥ 12 g/dL. Use only for treatment of anemia due to concomitant myelosuppressive chemotherapy. D/C following completion of chemotherapy.

THERAPEUTIC CLASS: Erythropoiesis stimulator

INDICATIONS: Treatment of anemia associated with chronic renal failure (CRF), and anemia in patients with non-myeloid malignancies due to chemotherapy.

DOSAGE: *Adults:* CRF: Initial: 0.45mcg/kg IV/SQ weekly. Titrate: Adjust to target Hgb <12g/dL. If Hgb increases >1g/dL in a 2-week period or is approaching 12g/dL, decrease dose by 25%. If Hgb continues to increase, hold dose until Hgb begins to decrease, and reinitiate at 25% below previous dose. Do not increase more than once monthly. Conversion from Epoetin Alfa: Base dose on weekly epoetin dose. Give once weekly if receiving epoetin 2-3x/week. Give every 2 weeks if receiving epoetin once weekly. (See PI for details). Malignancy: Initial: 2.25mcg/kg SQ weekly or 500mcg once every 3 weeks. Titrate: Increase to 4.5mcg/kg if Hgb increases <1g/dL after 6 weeks of therapy. If Hgb increases by >1g/dL in a 2-week period or if Hgb >12g/dL, decrease dose by 40%. If Hgb >13g/dL, hold dose until Hgb falls to 12g/dL and reinitiate at 40% below previous dose.
Pediatrics: ≥1 years: CRF: Conversion from Epoetin Alfa: Base dose on weekly epoetin dose. Give once weekly if receiving epoetin 2-3x/week. Give every 2 weeks if receiving epoetin once weekly. (See Full Prescribing Information for details).

HOW SUPPLIED: Inj: Syringe: 0.025mg/0.42mL, 0.04mg/0.4mL, 0.06mg/0.3mL, 0.1mg/0.5mL, 0.15mg/0.3mL, 0.2mg/0.4mL, 0.3mg/0.6mL, 0.5mg/mL; SDV: 0.025mg/mL, 0.04mg/mL, 0.06mg/mL, 0.1mg/mL, 0.15mg/0.75mL, 0.2mg/mL, 0.3mg/mL

CONTRAINDICATIONS: Uncontrolled HTN.

WARNINGS/PRECAUTIONS: Pure red cell aplasia and severe anemia (with or without other cytopenias) may occur. Due to increased Hgb, increased risk of cardiovascular events including death may occur. This includes MI, stroke, CHF, and hemodialysis vascular access thrombosis. Control BP before therapy. Seizures reported. Increased risk of thrombotic events. Evaluate etiology if lack/loss of response occurs. Permanently d/c if serious allergic reaction occurs. Monitor renal function, fluid, and electrolytes. Albumin solution carries risk of transmission of viral diseases. May need interval of 2-6 weeks between dose adjustment and response. Monitor Hgb weekly until stabilized and maintenance dose is established, and for at least 4 weeks after dosage change. Monitor iron status before and during therapy. Increases RBCs and decreases plasma volume. ESAs shortened time to tumor progression in patients with advanced head and neck cancer receiving radiation therapy.

ADVERSE REACTIONS: Thrombic events, infection, myalgia, HTN, hypotension, headache, diarrhea, fatigue, edema, nausea, vomiting, fever, dyspnea.

PREGNANCY: Category C, caution in nursing.

MECHANISM OF ACTION: Erythropoiesis stimulating protein; stimulates erythropoiesis (same mechanism as endogenous erythropoietin) in response to hypoxia by interacting with progenitor stem cells to increase RBC production.

PHARMACOKINETICS: Absorption: *Adults:* (SQ) Bioavailability (37%). (2.25mcg/kg; 6.75mcg/kg) T_{max}=90 hrs; 71 hrs. *Pediatrics:* Bioavailability (54%). **Elimination:** (IV, SQ): $T_{1/2}$=21 hrs; 74 hrs.

ARMOUR THYROID   RX
thyroid (Forest)

THERAPEUTIC CLASS: Thyroid replacement hormone

INDICATIONS: Treatment of hypothyroidism. As a pituitary TSH suppressant in the treatment or prevention of various types of euthyroid goiters. Diagnostic agent in suppression tests to differentiate suspected mild hyperthyroidism or thyroid gland autonomy. Management of thyroid cancer.

DOSAGE: *Adults:* Hypothyroidism; Initial: 30mg qd. Titrate: Increase by 15mg q2-3 weeks. Myxedema with Cardiovascular Disorder: 15mg qd. Maint: 60-120mg/day. Thyroid Cancer: Higher doses than replacement therapy are required. Myxedema Coma: Levothyroxine Sodium: Initial: 400mcg IV then 100-200mcg/day IV. Continue with oral therapy when stabilized. Thyroid Suppression: 1.56mg/kg/day for 7-10 days. Elderly: Initial: Use lower dose (eg, 15-30mg qd).
Pediatrics: Hypothyroidism: 0-6 months: 4.8-6mg/kg/day; 6-12 months: 3.6-4.8mg/kg/day; 1-5 yrs: 3-3.6mg/kg/day; 6-12 yrs: 2.4-3mg/kg/day; >12 yrs: 1.2-1.8mg/kg/day.

HOW SUPPLIED: Tab: 15mg, 30mg, 60mg, 90mg, 120mg, 180mg, 240mg, 300mg

CONTRAINDICATIONS: Untreated thyrotoxicosis; uncorrected adrenal cortical insufficiency.

WARNINGS/PRECAUTIONS: Do not use in the treatment of obesity; larger doses in euthyroid patients can cause serious or even life threatening toxicity. Caution with cardiovascular disease, DM, diabetes insipidus, elderly, and adrenal cortical insufficiency.

INTERACTIONS: May increase insulin or oral hypoglycemic requirements. Reduced absorption with cholestyramine and colestipol; space dosing by 4-5 hrs. Altered effect of oral anticoagulants; monitor PT/INR. Estrogens increase thyroxine-binding globulin; increase in thyroid dose may be needed. Serious or life-threatening side effects can occur with sympathomimetic amines. Androgens, corticosteroids, estrogens, iodine-containing preparations, and salicylates may interfere with thyroid lab tests.

PREGNANCY: Category A, caution in nursing.

MECHANISM OF ACTION: Thyroid hormone; not established, suspected to enhance oxygen consumption by most tissues of the body, increase the basal metabolic rate and metabolism of carbohydrates, lipids, and proteins.

PHARMACOKINETICS: Abosrption: (T_3) Completely absorbed; T_{max}=4 hrs; (T_4) partially absorbed. **Distribution:** Plasma protein binding (>99%), found in breast milk. **Metabolism:** Deiodination in liver, kidneys, other tissues.

ARRANON   RX
nelarabine (GlaxoSmithKline)

> Severe neurologic events reported; close monitoring is strongly recommended. Discontinue for neurologic events of NCI Common Toxicity Criteria ≥ grade 2.

THERAPEUTIC CLASS: Deoxyguanosine analogue

INDICATIONS: Treatment of T-cell acute lymphoblastic leukemia and T-cell lymphoblastic lymphoma in patients whose disease has not responded to or has relapsed following treatment with at least two chemotherapy regimens.

DOSAGE: *Adults:* 1500mg/m^2 IV over 2 hrs on days 1, 3, and 5 repeated every 21 days. CrCl <50ml/min: Insufficient data to support dose recommendation.
Pediatrics: 650mg/m^2/day IV over 1 hr daily for 5 consecutive days. Repeat every 21 days. CrCl <50ml/min: Insufficient data to support dose recommendation.

HOW SUPPLIED: Inj: 5mg/mL

WARNINGS/PRECAUTIONS: Leukopenia, thrombocytopenia, anemia, neutropenia/febrile neutropenia reported; regularly monitor CBC including platelets. Intravenous hydration recommended for management of hyperuricemia with risk of tumor lysis syndrome; may also consider allopurinol. Avoid administration of live vaccines. Closely monitor toxicities with severe renal impairment (eg, CrCl <30mL/min) and/or severe hepatic impairment (eg, bilirubin >3mg/dL); increased risk of adverse reactions.

ADVERSE REACTIONS: See Black Box Warning, Warnings/Precautions. *Pediatrics:* headache, increased transaminases, decreased blood potassium, decreased/increased blood albumin, vomiting. *Adults:* fatigue, nausea, diarrhea, vomiting, constipation, cough, dyspnea, dizziness, pyrexia, blurred vision.

PREGNANCY: Category D, not for use in nursing.

MECHANISM OF ACTION: Deoxyguanosine analogue; inhibits DNA synthesis, causing cell death.

PHARMACOKINETICS: Absorption: Nelarabine: C_{max}=5μg/mL; AUC=162μg•h/mL. ara-G: C_{max}=31.4μg/mL; AUC=4.4μg•h/mL. **Distribution:** Plasma protein binding (<25%). Nelarabine: (Adults) V_{ss}=197L/m^2; (Pediatrics) V_{ss}=213L/m^2. ara-G: (Adults) V_{ss}=50L/m^2; (Pediatrics) V_{ss}=33L/m^2. **Metabolism:** O-demethylation via adenosine deaminase. (Metabolite): Ara-G. **Elimination:** Kidneys (partial). Nelarabine: Urine (6.6%); $T_{1/2}$=30 min. ara-G: Urine (27%); $T_{1/2}$=3 hrs.

ASMANEX   RX
mometasone furoate (Schering)

THERAPEUTIC CLASS: Corticosteroid

INDICATIONS: Maintenance treatment of asthma as prophylactic therapy in patients ≥4 yrs.

DOSAGE: *Adults:* Previous Therapy with Bronchodilators Alone or Inhaled Corticosteroids: Initial: 220mcg qpm. Max: 440mcg qpm or 220mcg bid. Previous Therapy with Oral Corticosteroids: Initial: 440mcg bid. Max: 880mcg/day. Titrate to lowest effective dose once asthma stability achieved.
Pediatrics: ≥12 yrs: Previous Therapy with Bronchodilators Alone or Inhaled Corticosteroids (CS): Initial: 220mcg qpm. Max: 440mcg qpm or 220mcg bid. Previous Therapy with Oral CS: Initial: 440mcg bid. Max: 880mcg/day. 4-11 yrs: 110mcg qpm regardless of prior therapy. Titrate to lowest effective dose once asthma stability achieved.

HOW SUPPLIED: Twisthaler: 110mcg/inh, 220mcg/inh

CONTRAINDICATIONS: Primary treatment of status asthmaticus or other acute episodes of asthma where intensive measures are required.

WARNINGS/PRECAUTIONS: Deaths due to adrenal insufficiency have occurred with transfer from systemic corticosteroids to inhaled corticosteroids. Wean slowly from systemic corticosteroid therapy. Resume oral corticosteroids during stress or severe asthma attack. May unmask allergic conditions previously suppressed by systemic corticosteroid therapy. May increase susceptibility to infections. Not for rapid relief of bronchospasm or other acute episodes of asthma. D/C if bronchospasm occurs after dosing. Observe for systemic corticosteroid withdrawal effects, hypercorticism, reduced bone mineral density, and adrenal suppression; reduce dose slowly if needed. Decreased growth velocity may occur in pediatric patients. *Candida* infections in the mouth and pharynx reported. Caution with active or quiescent TB infection of respiratory tract; untreated systemic fungal, bacterial, viral, or parasitic infections; or ocular herpes simplex. Glaucoma, increased IOP, and cataracts reported.

ADVERSE REACTIONS: Headache, allergic rhinitis, pharyngitis, upper respiratory tract infection, sinusitis, oral candidiasis, dysmenorrhea, musculoskeletal pain, back pain, dyspepsia, myalgia, abdominal pain, nausea.

INTERACTIONS: Ketoconazole may increase plasma levels.

PREGNANCY: Category C, caution in nursing.

MECHANISM OF ACTION: Corticosteroid; shown to have inhibitory effects on multiple cell types (mast cells, eosinophils, neutrophils, macrophages, and lymphocytes) and mediators (histamine, eicosanoids, leukotrienes and cytokines), involved in inflammatory and asthmatic response.

PHARMACOKINETICS: Absorption: Absolute bioavailability (≤1%); C_{max}=94-114pcg/mL; T_{max}=1.0-2.5 hrs. **Distribution:** V_d=152L, plasma protein binding (98-99%). **Metabolism:** Liver, via CYP3A4. **Elimination:** $T_{1/2}$=5 hrs.

ASTELIN
azelastine HCl (MedPointe)

RX

THERAPEUTIC CLASS: Antihistamine

INDICATIONS: Treatemnt of the symptoms of seasonal allergic rhinitis and vasomotor rhinitis.

DOSAGE: *Adults:* 2 sprays per nostril bid.
Pediatrics: Seasonal Allergic/Vasomotor Rhinitis: ≥12 yrs: 2 sprays per nostril bid. Seasonal Allergic Rhinitis: 5-11 yrs: 1 spray per nostril bid.

HOW SUPPLIED: Spray: 137mcg/spray (30mg)

ADVERSE REACTIONS: Bitter taste, somnolence, weight increase, headache, nasal burning, pharyngitis, paroxysmal sneezing, dry mouth, nausea, atrial fibrillation, palpitations.

INTERACTIONS: Avoid alcohol or other CNS depressants; additive CNS impairment may occur. Increased azelastine levels with cimetidine.

PREGNANCY: Category C, caution in nursing.

MECHANISM OF ACTION: Phthalazinone derivative; inhibits histamine H_1 receptor activity.

PHARMACOKINETICS: Absorption: T_{max}=2-3 hrs. **Distribution:** Azelastine: Plasma protein binding (88%); Desmethylazelastine: V_d=14.5L/kg; plasma protein binding (97%).

ATGAM
lymphocyte immune globulin, anti-thymocyte globulin (Equine)
(Pharmacia & Upjohn)

RX

> **Administer by experienced physician in immunosuppressive therapy in facility equipped and staffed with adequate lab and supportive medical resources.**

THERAPEUTIC CLASS: Lymphocyte-selective immunosuppressant

INDICATIONS: Management of allograft rejection in renal transplantation. Treatment of moderate to severe aplastic anemia unsuitable for bone marrow transplantation.

DOSAGE: *Adults:* Renal Transplant: Delaying Rejection Onset: 15mg/kg/day for 14 days, then every other day for 14 days for total of 21 doses in 28 days. Give 1st dose 24 hrs before or after transplant. Rejection Treatment: 10-15mg/kg/day for 14 days. May give additional alternate day therapy up to total of 21 doses. May delay 1st dose until diagnosis of 1st rejection episode. Aplastic Anemia: 10-20mg/kg/day for 8-14 days. May give additional alternate day therapy up to total of 21 doses.
Pediatrics: Renal Transplant: Delaying Rejection Onset: 15mg/kg/day for 14 days, then every other day for 14 days for total of 21 doses in 28 days. Give 1st dose 24 hrs before or after transplant. Rejection Treatment: 10-15mg/kg/day for 14 days. May give additional alternate day therapy up to total of 21 doses. May delay 1st dose until diagnosis of 1st rejection episode. Aplastic Anemia: 10-20mg/kg/day for 8-14 days. May give additional alternate day therapy up to total of 21 doses.

HOW SUPPLIED: Inj: 50mg/mL (5mL)

CONTRAINDICATIONS: History of severe systemic reaction to this product or other equine gamma globulin agents.

WARNINGS/PRECAUTIONS: Potency of agent may vary from lot to lot. D/C if anaphylaxis (eg, respiratory distress, hypotension) occurs, or if severe and unremitting thrombocytopenia or leukopenia occur in renal transplant patients. Risk of infectious transmission due to equine and human blood components. Monitor for leukopenia, thrombocytopenia, or infection (eg, CMV). Decide whether or not to continue therapy based on clinical circumstances (eg, infection).

ADVERSE REACTIONS: Fever, chills, leukopenia, thrombocytopenia, rash, pruritus, urticaria, wheal, flare, arthralgia, headache, phlebitis, chest/back pain, diarrhea, vomiting, nausea, dyspnea, hypotension, night sweats, stomatitis.

INTERACTIONS: Previously masked reactions may appear with corticosteroid or immuno-suppressant dose reduction. Do not dilute with dextrose or use highly acidic infusions.

PREGNANCY: Category C, caution in nursing.

MECHANISM OF ACTION: Lymphocyte-selective immunosuppressant; reduces the number of circulating, thymus-dependent lymphocytes.

ATIVAN
lorazepam (Biovail)

THERAPEUTIC CLASS: Benzodiazepine

INDICATIONS: Management of anxiety disorders or for short-term relief of the symptoms of anxiety or anxiety associated with depressive symptoms.

DOSAGE: *Adults:* Initial: 2-3mg/day given bid-tid. Usual: 2-6mg/day in divided doses. Insomnia: 2-4mg qhs. Elderly/Debilitated: 1-2mg/day in divided doses.
Pediatrics: >12 yrs: Initial: 2-3mg/day given bid-tid. Usual: 2-6mg/day in divided doses. Insomnia: 2-4mg qhs.

HOW SUPPLIED: Tab: 0.5mg, 1mg*, 2mg* *scored

CONTRAINDICATIONS: Acute narrow-angle glaucoma.

WARNINGS/PRECAUTIONS: Avoid with primary depression or psychosis. Withdrawal symptoms with abrupt discontinuation. Careful supervision if addiction-prone. Caution in patients with compromised respiratory function. Caution with elderly, and renal or hepatic dysfunction. Monitor for GI disease with prolonged therapy. Periodic blood counts and LFTs with long-term therapy.

ADVERSE REACTIONS: Sedation, dizziness, weakness, unsteadiness, transient amnesia, memory impairment, visual disturbance, depression, respiratory depression, constipation, vertigo, change in appetite, headache.

INTERACTIONS: CNS-depressant effects with barbiturates, alcohol. Diminished tolerance to alcohol and other CNS depressants. Increased plasma levels with valproate and probenecid, decrease dose by 50%.

PREGNANCY: Not for use in pregnancy or nursing.

MECHANISM OF ACTION: Benzodiazepine; antianxiety agent, interacts with GABA-benzodiazepine receptor complex.

PHARMACOKINETICS: Absorption: Absolute bioavailability (90%); C_{max}=20ng/mL (2mg PO); T_{max}=2 hrs. **Distribution:** Plasma protein binding (85%). **Metabolism:** Glucuronidation. **Elimination:** Urine; $T_{1/2}$=12 hrs.

ATRACURIUM BESYLATE RX
atracurium besylate (Various)

THERAPEUTIC CLASS: Skeletal muscle relaxant (nondepolarizing)

INDICATIONS: Adjunct to general anesthesia to facilitate endotracheal intubation and to provide skeletal muscle relaxation during surgery or mechanical ventilation.

DOSAGE: *Adults:* Initial: 0.4-0.5mg/kg IV bolus. Prolonged Procedure: Maint: 0.08-0.1mg/kg at regular intervals to meet needs; give after 1st dose. Operating Room Infusion: Initial: 0.3-0.5mg/kg IV bolus. Maint: 9-10mcg/kg/min initial infusion to counteract recovery from bolus followed by 5-9mcg/kg/min. ICU: 11-13mcg/kg/min IV. Isoflurane/Enflurane at Steady State: Reduce dose by 1/3. Significant Cardiovascular Disease/Histamine Release Sensitive Patients: Initial: 0.3-0.4mg/kg IV slowly or in divided doses. Following Succinylcholine: Initial: 0.3-0.4mg/kg IV.
Pediatrics: >2 yrs: Initial: 0.4-0.5mg/kg IV bolus. Prolonged Procedure: Maint: 0.08-0.1mg/kg at regular intervals to meet needs; give after 1st dose. Operating Room Infusion: Initial: 0.3-0.5mg/kg IV bolus. Maint: 9-10mcg/kg/min initial infusion to counteract recovery from bolus followed by 5-9mcg/kg/min. Isoflurane/Enflurane at Steady State: Reduce dose by 1/3. 1 month-2 yrs (under halothane): Initial: 0.3-0.4mg/kg IV bolus. Maint: Slightly greater frequency than adults. ≥1 month: Significant Cardiovascular Disease/Histamine Release Sensitive Patients: Initial: 0.3-0.4mg/kg IV slowly or in divided doses.

HOW SUPPLIED: Inj: 10mg/mL

WARNINGS/PRECAUTIONS: Avoid IM administration or administration before uncon-sciousness has been induced. Use with adequate anesthesia. The 10mL vial contains benzyl alcohol. May release histamines; caution in those where substantial histamine release would be hazardous (eg, severe cardiovascular disease) or if at a greater risk of histamine release (eg, anaphylactoid reactions, asthma). Use peripheral nerve stimu-lators to assess neuromuscular block in myasthenia gravis, Eaton-Lambert syndrome, other neuromuscular diseases, severe electrolyte disorders, elderly, carcinomatosis. Malignant hyperthermia (rare) reported. Resistance may develop in burn patients; increase dose. Monitor neuromuscular transmission of ICU patients continuously with a nerve stimulator.

ADVERSE REACTIONS: Allergic reactions, inadequate/prolonged block, hypotension, vasodilation (flushing), tachycardia, bradycardia, dyspnea, bronchospasm, laryngo-spasm, rash, urticaria, injection site pain.

INTERACTIONS: Enhanced neuromuscular blocking action with enflurane, isoflurane, hal-othane, certain antibiotics (eg, aminoglycosides, polymixins), lithium, magnesium salts, procainamide, quinidine. Possible synergistic or antagonistic effects with other muscle relaxants. Prior succinylcholine may quicken onset and increase depth of neuromuscu-lar block. Do not mix with alkaline solutions.

PREGNANCY: Category C, caution in nursing.

ATRALIN   RX
tretinoin (DPT Laboratories)

THERAPEUTIC CLASS: Retinoid

INDICATIONS: Topical treatment of acne vulgaris.

DOSAGE: *Adults:* Cleanse area(s) thoroughly, then apply thin layer qd before bedtime. *Pediatrics:* ≥10 yrs: Cleanse area(s) thoroughly, then apply thin layer qd before bed-time.

HOW SUPPLIED: Gel: 0.05% (45g)

WARNINGS/PRECAUTIONS: Avoid eyes, mouth, paranasal creases, and mucous mem-branes. Skin may become dry, red, or exfoliated. If degree of irritation warrants, tempo-rarily reduce amount/frequency, or d/c use temporarily or altogether. May cause mild to moderate dryness; use appropriate moisturizer. Caution with eczematous or sun-burned skin, with high levels of exposure to sun, wind, or cold, or with known sensitivity to fish allergy.

ADVERSE REACTIONS: Dry skin, peeling, scaling, flaking skin, burning sensation, ery-thema.

INTERACTIONS: Caution with topical medications, medicated or abrasive soaps and cleansers, products with strong drying effects, high concentrations of alcohol, astrin-gents, spices, or lime. Caution with benzoyl peroxide, sulfur, resorcinol, or salicylic acid; allow effects of these agents to subside before use.

PREGNANCY: Category C, caution in nursing.

MECHANISM OF ACTION: Retinoic acid derivative: Binds with high affinity to three spe-cific retinoic acid nuclear receptors (RARα, RARβ, and RARγ) which are located in both the cytosol and nucleus. Acts to modify gene expression, subsequent protein synthesis, and epithelial cell growth and differentiation. Decreases the cohesiveness of follicular epithelial cells with decreased microcomedo formation. Stimulates mitotic activity and increases turnover of follicular epithelial cells causing extrusion of the comedones.

PHARMACOKINETICS: Absorption: Tretinoin: Baseline plasma concentrations=0.68ng/mL, Day 14 plasma concentrations=0.69-2.88ng/mL. **Metabolism:** Major metabolites: 13-cis-retinoic acid and 4-oxo-13-cis-retinoic acid.

ATROPINE SULFATE   RX
atropine sulfate (Various)

THERAPEUTIC CLASS: Anticholinergic

INDICATIONS: Antisialagogue for preanesthetic medication to prevent or reduce secretions of the respiratory tract. To restore cardiac rate and arterial pressure during anesthesia when vagal stimulation produced by intra-abdominal surgical traction causes a sudden decrease in pulse rate and cardiac action. To lessen degree of AV heart block when increased vagal tone is a major factor in the conduction defect (possibly due to digitalis). To overcome severe bradycardia and syncope due to hyperactive carotid sinus reflex, as an antidote (with external cardiac massage) for cardiovascular collapse from the injudicious use of choline ester (cholinergic) drug. In the treatment of anticholinesterase poisoning from organophosphorus insecticides, and as an antidote for the "rapid" type of mushroom poisoning due to presence of the alkaloid muscarine, in certain species of fungus such as *Amanita muscaria*.

DOSAGE: *Adults:* Usual: 0.5mg IM/IV/SC. Range: 0.4-0.6mg. If used as an antisialagogue, inject IM prior to anesthesia induction. Bradyarrhythmias: 0.4-1mg every 1-2 hrs prn. Max: 2mg/dose. May be used as antidote for cardiovascular collapse resulting from injudicious administration of choline ester. When cardiac arrest has occurred, external cardiac massage or other method of resuscitation is required to distribute the drug after IV injection. Anticholinesterase Poisoning From Insecticide Poisoning: 2-3mg IV. Repeat until signs of atropine intoxication appear. Mushroom Poisoning: Administer sufficient doses to control parasympathomimetic signs before coma and cardiovascular collapse supervene.
Pediatrics: Range: 0.1mg (newborn) to 0.6mg (>12 yrs). Inject SC 30 min before surgery. Bradyarrhythmias: Range: 0.01-0.03mg/kg IV.

HOW SUPPLIED: Inj: 0.05mg/mL, 0.1mg/mL, 0.4mg/mL, 0.5mg/mL, 1mg/mL

CONTRAINDICATIONS: Glaucoma, pyloric stenosis, or prostatic hypertrophy except in doses used for preanesthetic medication.

WARNINGS/PRECAUTIONS: Avoid overdose in IV administration. Increased susceptibility to toxic effects in children. Caution in patients >40 yrs. Conventional doses may precipitate glaucoma in susceptible patients, convert partial organic pyloric stenosis into complete obstruction, lead to complete urinary retention in patients with prostatic hypertrophy or cause inspissation of bronchial secretions and formation of dangerous viscid plugs in patients with chronic lung disease.

ADVERSE REACTIONS: Dryness of the mouth, blurred vision, photophobia, tachycardia, anhidrosis.

PREGNANCY: Category C, safety in nursing not known.

MECHANISM OF ACTION: Anticholinergic; inhibits smooth muscle and glands innervated by postganglionic cholinergic nerves; stimulates/depresses CNS activity depending upon the dose.

PHARMACOKINETICS: Distribution: Plasma protein binding (44%), crosses placental barrier. **Metabolism:** Via enzymatic hydrolysis in liver. Noratropine, atropin-n-oxide, tropine, and tropic acid (major metabolites). **Elimination:** Urine (50% unchanged); $T_{1/2}$=2.5 hrs.

ATROVENT NASAL   RX
ipratropium bromide (Boehringer Ingelheim)

THERAPEUTIC CLASS: Anticholinergic

INDICATIONS: (0.03%) Relief of rhinorrhea associated with allergic and nonallergic perennial rhinitis in adults and children ≥6 yrs. (0.06%) Relief of rhinorrhea associated with the common cold or seasonal allergic rhinitis in adults and children ≥5 yrs.

DOSAGE: *Adults:* Rhinorrhea w/Allergic/Nonallergic Perennial Rhinitis: (0.03%) 2 sprays per nostril bid-tid. Rhinorrhea w/Common Cold: (0.06%) 2 sprays per nostril tid-qid. Rhinorrhea w/Seasonal Allergic Rhinitis: (0.06%) 2 sprays per nostril qid.
Pediatrics: Rhinorrhea w/Allergic/Nonallergic Perennial Rhinitis: ≥6 yrs: (0.03%) 2 sprays per nostril bid-tid. Rhinorrhea w/Common Cold: ≥12 yrs: (0.06%) 2 sprays per nostril tid-qid. 5-11 yrs: (0.06%) 2 sprays per nostril tid. Rhinorrhea w/Seasonal Allergic Rhinitis: ≥5 yrs: (0.06%) 2 sprays per nostril qid.

HOW SUPPLIED: Spray: (0.03%) 21mcg/spray (31g), (0.06%) 42mcg/spray (16.6g)

CONTRAINDICATIONS: Hypersensitivity to atropine or its derivatives.

WARNINGS/PRECAUTIONS: Immediate hypersensitivity reaction reported. Caution with narrow-angle glaucoma, prostatic hyperplasia or bladder-neck obstruction.

ADVERSE REACTIONS: Epistaxis, nasal dryness, dry mouth, dry throat, headache, upper respiratory infection, pharyngitis.

INTERACTIONS: May produce additive effects with other anticholinergic agents.

PREGNANCY: Category B, caution in nursing.

MECHANISM OF ACTION: Anticholinergic; inhibits secretions from serous and seromucous glands lining the nasal mucosa.

PHARMACOKINETICS: Absorption: 6-18 yrs old: C_{max}=undetectable up to 0.49 ng/mL. **Distribution:** Plasma protein binding (0-9%). **Elimination:** 6-18 yrs old: Urine (8.6-11.1% unchanged). *Adults:* Urine (3.7-5.6% unchanged).

ATTENUVAX   RX
measles vaccine live (Merck)

THERAPEUTIC CLASS: Vaccine

INDICATIONS: Vaccination against measles.

DOSAGE: *Pediatrics:* 0.5mL SQ in the upper arm at 12-15 months old. If vaccinated <12 months old, revaccinate at 12-15 months old. Revaccinate prior to school entry.

HOW SUPPLIED: Inj: 1000TCID$_{50}$/vial

CONTRAINDICATIONS: Pregnancy, anaphylactic reaction to neomycin, febrile respiratory illness or other active febrile infection, immunosuppressive therapy, blood dyscrasias, leukemia, lymphomas, malignant neoplasms affecting bone marrow or lymphatic systems, immunodeficiency states.

WARNINGS/PRECAUTIONS: Caution with egg hypersensitivity, history of cerebral injury, individual or family history of convulsions, and avoid conditions that cause stress due to fever. May potentiate thrombocytopenia. Defer for 3 months or longer after blood or plasma transfusions, or immune globulin administration. Have epinephrine injection (1:1000) available.

ADVERSE REACTIONS: Panniculitis, atypical measles, fever, syncope, headache, vasculitis, diarrhea, thrombocytopenia, lymphadenopathy, Guilliain-Barre syndrome, febrile convulsion, pneumonitis, cough, rhinitis, Stevens-Johnson syndrome, erythema multiforme, rash.

INTERACTIONS: Immune globulins may interfere with immune response. Temporary depression of tuberculin skin sensitivity.

PREGNANCY: Category C, caution in nursing.

MECHANISM OF ACTION: Stimulates immune response to produce antibodies that may protect against measles (rubeola).

AUGMENTIN   RX
amoxicillin - clavulanate potassium (GlaxoSmithKline)

THERAPEUTIC CLASS: Aminopenicillin/beta lactamase inhibitor

INDICATIONS: Treatment of lower respiratory tract (LRTI), skin and skin structure (SSSI), and urinary tract infections (UTI), otitis media (OM), sinusitis caused by susceptible strains of microorganisms.

DOSAGE: *Adults:* (Dose based on amoxicillin) 500mg q12h or 250mg q8h. Severe Infections/RTI: 875mg q12h or 500mg q8h. May use 125mg/5mL or 250mg/5mL sus in place of 500mg tab and 200mg/5mL sus or 400mg/5mL sus in place of 875mg tab. CrCl <30mL/min: Do not give 875mg tab. CrCl 10-30mL/min: 250-500mg q12h. CrCl <10mL/min: 250-500mg q24h. Hemodialysis: 250-500mg q24h, give additional dose during and at end of dialysis.
Pediatrics: (Dose based on amoxicillin) ≥40kg: Use adult dose. ≥12 weeks: Sinusitis/Otitis Media/LRTI/Severe Infections: (Sus/Tab, Chewable) 45mg/kg/day given q12h or 40mg/

kg/day given q8h. Treat otitis media for 10 days. Less Severe Infections: 25mg/kg/day given q12h or 20mg/kg/day given q8h. <12 weeks: 15mg/kg q12h (use 125mg/5mL sus).

HOW SUPPLIED: (Amoxicillin-Clavulanate) Sus: 125-31.25mg/5mL (75mL, 100mL, 150mL), 200-28.5mg/5mL (50mL, 75mL, 100mL), 250-62.5mg/5mL (75mL, 100mL, 150mL), 400-57mg/5mL (50mL, 75mL, 100mL); Tab: 250-125mg, 500-125mg, 875-125mg*; Tab, Chewable: 200-28.5mg, 250-62.5mg, 400-57mg *scored

CONTRAINDICATIONS: History of PCN allergy or amoxicillin-clavulanate associated cholestatic jaundice/hepatic dysfunction.

WARNINGS/PRECAUTIONS: Serious, sometimes fatal, hypersensitivity reactions reported with PCN therapy. *Clostridium difficile*-associated diarrhea reported. Possibility of superinfection. Caution with hepatic dysfunction. Monitor renal, hepatic, and hematopoietic functions with prolonged use. Avoid with mononucleosis. Take with food to reduce GI upset. The 200mg and 400mg chewable tabs and 200mg/5mL and 400mg/5mL sus contain phenylalanine. The 250mg tab and chewable tab are not interchangeable due to unequal clavulanic acid amounts. Only use 250mg tab in pediatrics ≥40kg. False (+) for urine glucose with Clinitest® and Benedict's or Fehling's solution.

ADVERSE REACTIONS: Diarrhea/loose stools, NV, skin rashes, urticaria, vaginitis.

INTERACTIONS: Increased and prolonged plasma levels with probenecid. May reduce effects of oral contraceptives. Allopurinol may increase incidence of rash. May increase PT with anticoagulant therapy.

PREGNANCY: Category B, caution in nursing.

MECHANISM OF ACTION: Amoxicillin: Semisynthetic antibiotic with broad-spectrum of bactericidal activity against gram-positive and gram-negative organisms. Clavulanate: β-lactamase inhibitor; possesses ability to inactivate a wide range of β-lactamase enzymes commonly found in microorganisms resistant to PCN and cephalosporins.

PHARMACOKINETICS: Absorption: Well absorbed from GI tract. C_{max} and AUC varied according to dose and regimen; see Full PI for more information. (Tab, Sol) T_{max}=1.5 hrs, 1 hr. **Distribution:** Found in breast milk. Amoxicillin: Diffuses readily in body tissues and fluids. Clavulanic: Well distributed in body tissues. Plasma protein binding: Amoxicillin (18%), clavulanic (25%). **Elimination:** Urine, (amoxicillin) (50-70% unchanged), (clavulanic) (25-40% unchanged); $T_{1/2}$=1.3 hrs (amoxicillin), 1 hr (clavulanic).

Augmentin ES-600   RX
amoxicillin - clavulanate potassium (GlaxoSmithKline)

THERAPEUTIC CLASS: Aminopenicillin/beta lactamase inhibitor

INDICATIONS: Treatment of pediatric patients with recurrent or persistent acute otitis media due to susceptible strains of microorganisms.

DOSAGE: *Pediatrics:* 3 months-12 yrs: <40kg: (Dose based on amoxicillin content) 45mg/kg q12h for 10 days.

HOW SUPPLIED: Sus: (Amoxicillin-Clavulanate) 600mg-42.9mg/5mL (75mL, 125mL, 200mL)

CONTRAINDICATIONS: History of PCN allergy or amoxicillin-clavulanate associated cholestatic jaundice/hepatic dysfunction.

WARNINGS/PRECAUTIONS: Serious, sometimes fatal, hypersensitivity reactions reported with PCN therapy. *Clostridium difficile*-associated diarrhea reported. Possibility of superinfection. Caution with hepatic dysfunction. Monitor renal, hepatic, and hematopoietic functions with prolonged use. Avoid with mononucleosis. Contains phenylalanine. False (+) for urine glucose with Clinitest® and Benedict's or Fehling's solution.

ADVERSE REACTIONS: Diaper rash, diarrhea, vomiting, moniliasis, rash.

INTERACTIONS: Increased and prolonged plasma levels with probenecid. May reduce effects of oral contraceptives. Allopurinol may increase incidence of rash. May increase PT with anticoagulant therapy.

PREGNANCY: Category B, caution in nursing.

MECHANISM OF ACTION: Amoxicillin: Semisynthetic antibiotic with broad spectrum of bactericidal activity against gram-positive and gram-negative organisms. Clavulanate: β-lactamase inhibitor. Possesses ability to inactivate a wide range of β-lactamase enzymes commonly found in microorganisms resistant to PCN and cephalosporins.

PHARMACOKINETICS: Absorption: Amoxicillin: C_{max}=15.7mcg/mL; T_{max}=2.0 hr; AUC=59.8mcg•hr/mL. Clavulanic acid: C_{max}=1.7mcg/mL; T_{max}=1.1 hr; AUC=4.0mcg•hr/mL. **Distribution:** Plasma protein binding 18% (amoxicillin), 25% (clavulanic acid). Well distributed in bodily tissues except brain and spinal fluid. **Elimination:** Urine (unchanged) amoxicillin (50-70%); clavulanic acid (25-40%).

AUGMENTIN XR   RX
amoxicillin - clavulanate potassium (GlaxoSmithKline)

THERAPEUTIC CLASS: Aminopenicillin/beta lactamase inhibitor

INDICATIONS: Treatment of community-acquired pneumonia (CAP) or acute bacterial sinusitis due to confirmed or suspected β-lactamase producing pathogens and S.pneumoniae with reduced susceptibility to PCN.

DOSAGE: *Adults:* Sinusitis: 2 tabs q12h for 10 days. CAP: 2 tabs q12h for 7-10 days. Take at start of a meal.
Pediatrics: ≥16 yrs: Sinusitis: 2 tabs q12h for 10 days. CAP: 2 tabs q12h for 7-10 days. Take at the start of a meal.

HOW SUPPLIED: Tab, Extended-Release: (Amoxicillin-Clavulanate) 1000mg-62.5mg

CONTRAINDICATIONS: History of PCN allergy or amoxicillin-clavulanate associated cholestatic jaundice/hepatic dysfunction, severe renal impairment (CrCl <30mL/min), hemodialysis.

WARNINGS/PRECAUTIONS: Serious, sometimes fatal, hypersensitivity reactions reported with PCN therapy. *Clostridium difficile*-associated diarrhea reported. Possibility of superinfection. Caution with hepatic dysfunction. Monitor renal, hepatic, and hematopoietic functions with prolonged use. Avoid with mononucleosis. Not interchangeable with other Augmentin products due to unequal clavulanic acid amounts. False (+) for urine glucose with Clinitest and Benedict's or Fehling's solution.

ADVERSE REACTIONS: Diarrhea, nausea, genital moniliasis, abdominal pain, vaginal mycosis.

INTERACTIONS: Increased and prolonged plasma levels with probenecid. May reduce effects of oral contraceptives. Allopurinol may increase incidence of rash. May increase PT with anticoagulant therapy.

PREGNANCY: Category B, caution in nursing.

MECHANISM OF ACTION: Amoxicillin: Semisynthetic antibiotic with broad spectrum of bactericidal activity against gram-positive and gram-negative organisms. Clavulanate: β-lactamase inhibitor; possesses ability to inactivate a wide range of β-lactamase enzymes commonly found in microorganisms resistant to PCN and cephalosporins.

PHARMACOKINETICS: Absorption: Well-absorbed. Amoxicillin: C_{max}=17 mcg/mL, T_{max}=1.5 hrs, AUC=71.6mcg•hr/mL. Clavulanate potassium: C_{max}=2.05mcg/mL, T_{max}=1.03 hrs, AUC=5.29mcg•hr/mL. **Distribution:** Plasma protein binding: Amoxicillin (18%); Clavulante potassium (25%). Found in breast milk. Well distributed to body tissues except brain and spinal fluid. **Elimination:** Urine: Amoxicillin (60-80% unchanged); $T_{1/2}$=1.27 hrs. Clavulanate potassium: (30-50% unchanged); $T_{1/2}$=1.03 hrs.

AVAPRO   RX
irbesartan (Bristol-Myers Squibb/Sanofi-Aventis)

> **Can cause death/injury to developing fetus during 2nd and 3rd trimesters. Stop therapy if pregnancy detected.**

THERAPEUTIC CLASS: Angiotensin II receptor antagonist

INDICATIONS: Hypertension, alone or with other antihypertensives. Diabetic nephropathy with an elevated serum creatinine and proteinuria (>300mg/day) in patients with type 2 diabetes and hypertension.

DOSAGE: *Adults:* HTN: Initial: 150mg qd. Titrate: May increase to 300mg qd. Intravascular Volume/Salt Depletion: Initial: 75mg qd. Nephropathy: Maint: 300mg qd.
Pediatrics: HTN: ≥17 yrs: Initial: 150mg qd. Titrate: May increase to 300mg qd. Intravascular Volume/Salt Depletion: Initial: 75mg qd.

HOW SUPPLIED: Tab: 75mg, 150mg, 300mg

WARNINGS/PRECAUTIONS: Can cause fetal injury/death. Correct volume or salt depletion before therapy. Changes in renal function may occur; caution with renal artery stenosis, severe CHF. Angioedema reported.

ADVERSE REACTIONS: Diarrhea, dyspepsia/heartburn, musculoskeletal trauma, fatigue, upper respiratory infection.

PREGNANCY: Category C (1st trimester) and D (2nd and 3rd trimesters), not for use in nursing.

AXID   RX
nizatidine (GlaxoSmithKline)

OTHER BRAND NAME: Axid Oral Solution (Reliant)

THERAPEUTIC CLASS: H_2-blocker

INDICATIONS: Short term treatment of active duodenal ulcer (DU) and benign gastric ulcer (GU). Maintenance therapy for duodenal ulcers. Treatment of endoscopically diagnosed esophagitis, including erosive and ulcerative esophagitis, and heartburn due to GERD.

DOSAGE: *Adults:* Active DU/Active Benign GU: Usual: 300mg qhs or 150mg bid up to 8 weeks. Healed DU: Maint: 150mg qhs, up to 1 year. GERD: 150mg bid up to 12 weeks. Renal Impairment: Treatment: CrCl 20-50mL/min: 150mg/day. CrCl <20mL/min: 150mg every other day. Maint: CrCl 20-50mL/min: 150mg every other day. CrCl <20mL/min: 150mg every 3 days.
Pediatrics; ≥12 yrs: (Sol) Erosive Esophagitis/GERD: 150mg bid up to 8 weeks. Max: 300mg/day. Renal Impairment: Treatment: CrCl 20-50mL/min: 150mg/day. CrCl <20mL/min: 150mg every other day. Maint: CrCl 20-50mL/min: 150mg every other day. CrCl <20mL/min: 150mg every 3 days.

HOW SUPPLIED: Cap: 150mg, 300mg; Sol: 15mg/mL

WARNINGS/PRECAUTIONS: Caution with renal dysfunction; reduce dose. Symptomatic response does not preclude the presence of gastric malignancy. False positive tests for urobilinogen with Multistix.

ADVERSE REACTIONS: Headache, abdominal pain, pain, asthenia, diarrhea, nausea, flatulence, vomiting, dyspepsia, rhinitis, pharyngitis, dizziness, headache.

INTERACTIONS: May elevate serum salicylate levels with high dose ASA.

PREGNANCY: Category B, not for use in nursing.

MECHANISM OF ACTION: H_2 receptor antagonist; competitive, reversible inhibitor of histamine at the histamine H_2 receptors, particularly those in gastroparietal cells.

PHARMACOKINETICS: Absorption: Absolute bioavailability (>70%); (150mg, 300mg) C_{max}=700-1800mcg/L, 1400-3600mcg/L; T_{max}=0.5-3 hrs. (12-18 yrs, 150mg) C_{max}=1422.9ng/mL; T_{max}=1.3 hrs; AUC=3764ng•hr/mL. **Distribution:** (Adult) V_d=0.8-1.5L/kg; (12-18 yrs) V_d=71.4L. Plasma protein binding (35%); found in breast milk. **Metabolism:** N_2-monodesmethylnizatidine (major). **Excretion:** Urine (90%, 60% unchanged); feces (6%). (Adult) $T_{1/2}$=1-2 hrs; (12-18 yrs) $T_{1/2}$=1.2 hrs.

AZACTAM   RX
aztreonam (Elan)

THERAPEUTIC CLASS: Monobactam

INDICATIONS: Treatment of septicemia and lower respiratory tract (eg, pneumonia, bronchitis), skin and skin-structure, urinary tract (UTI), gynecologic (eg, endometritis), and intra-abdominal (eg, peritonitis) infections caused by susceptible microorganisms. Adjunct therapy to surgery for management of infections caused by susceptible microorganisms.

DOSAGE: *Adults:* UTI: 500mg-1g IM/IV q8-12h. Moderately Severe Systemic Infections: 1-2g IM/IV q8-12h. Severe Systemic/Life-Threatening Infections/*Pseudomonas aeruginosa:* 2g IV q6-8h. Max: 8g/day. CrCl 10-30mL/min/1.73m²: Initial: LD: 1 or 2g. Maint: 50% of usual dose. CrCl <10mL/min/1.73m²: Initial: LD: 500mg, 1g or 2g. Maint: 25% of usual initial dose at usual intervals. Serious/Life-Threatening Infections: In addition to maint dose, give 1/8 initial dose after each hemodialysis session. IV route recommended for single doses >1g or for bacterial septicemia, localized parenchymal abscess (eg, intra-abdominal abscess), peritonitis, or other severe systemic or life-threatening infections. Continue for at least 48 hrs after patient is asymptomatic or evidence of bacterial eradication.

Pediatrics: 9 months-16 yrs: Mild-Moderate Infections: 30mg/kg IV q8h. Moderate-Severe Infections: 30mg/kg IV q6-8h. Max: 120mg/kg/day. IV route is recommended for single doses >1g or for bacterial septicemia, localized parenchymal abscess (eg, intra-abdominal abscess), peritonitis, or other severe systemic or life-threatening infections. Continue for at least 48 hrs after patient is asymptomatic or evidence of bacterial eradication.

HOW SUPPLIED: Inj: 1g, 2g, 1g/50mL, 2g/50mL

WARNINGS/PRECAUTIONS: Caution with hypersensitivity to other β-lactams or allergens. *Clostridium difficile*-associated diarrhea reported. May promote overgrowth of nonsusceptible organisms. Monitor with renal or hepatic impairment. Toxic epidermal necrolysis reported (rarely) in bone marrow transplant with multiple risk factors including sepsis.

ADVERSE REACTIONS: Diarrhea, NV, rash, abdominal cramps, vaginal candidiasis, discomfort/swelling at injection site, hypersensitivity reaction.

INTERACTIONS: Monitor renal function with aminoglycosides; increased risk of nephrotoxicity, ototoxicity. Toxic epidermal necrolysis reported (rarely) in bone marrow transplant with radiation therapy and other drugs associated with toxic epidermal necrolysis.

PREGNANCY: Category B, not for use in nursing.

MECHANISM OF ACTION: Monobactam; synthetic bactericidal antibiotic. Inhibits bacterial cell-wall synthesis due to high affinity of aztreonam for penicillin-binding protein 3 (PBP3).

PHARMACOKINETICS: Absorption: C_{max}=90μ/ml (1g dose), 204μ/ml (2g dose); T_{max}=1 hr. **Distribution:** V_d=12.6L; found in breast milk. **Elimination:** Urine; $T_{1/2}$=1.7 hr.

AZASITE
azithromycin (Inspire)

RX

THERAPEUTIC CLASS: Macrolide

INDICATIONS: Treatment of bacterial conjunctivitis caused by susceptible strains of microorganisms.

DOSAGE: *Adults:* Initial: 1 drop bid, 8 to 12 hrs apart, for first 2 days. Maint: 1 drop qd for next 5 days.

Pediatrics: ≥1 yr: Initial: 1 drop bid, 8 to 12 hrs apart, for first 2 days. Maint: 1 drop qd for next 5 days.

HOW SUPPLIED: Sol: 1% (2.5mL)

WARNINGS/PRECAUTIONS: Not for injection; do not give systemically, inject subconjunctivally or into chamber of eye. Caution may cause hypersensitivity reactions. Growth of resistant organisms including fungi may occur with prolonged use. Avoid contact lens use.

ADVERSE REACTIONS: Eye irritation, burning, stinging and irritation upon instillation, contact dermatitis, corneal erosion, dry eye, dysgeusia, nasal congestion, ocular discharge, punctate keratitis, sinusitis.

PREGNANCY: Category B, caution in nursing.

MECHANISM OF ACTION: Macrolide: binds to the 50S ribosomal subunit of susceptible microorganisms and interferes with microbial protein synthesis.

PHARMACOKINETICS: Absorption: C_{max}≤10ng/mL

AZELEX

azelaic acid (Allergan)

RX

THERAPEUTIC CLASS: Dicarboxylic acid antimicrobial

INDICATIONS: Mild to moderate inflammatory acne vulgaris.

DOSAGE: *Adults:* Wash and dry skin. Massage gently into affected area bid (am and pm).
Pediatrics: ≥12 yrs: Wash and dry skin. Massage gently into affected area bid (am and pm).

HOW SUPPLIED: Cre: 20% (30g, 50g)

WARNINGS/PRECAUTIONS: Avoid mouth, eyes, mucous membranes, and occlusive dressings.

ADVERSE REACTIONS: Pruritus, burning, stinging, tingling, hypopigmentation.

PREGNANCY: Category B, caution in nursing.

MECHANISM OF ACTION: Dicarboxylic acid antimicrobial; not established. Possesses antimicrobial activity that may be attributable to inhibition of microbial cellular protein synthesis. A normalization of keratinization leading to an anticomedonal effect of azelaic acid may also contribute to clinical activity.

PHARMACOKINETICS: Absorption: Penetrates stratum corneum (3-5%), up to 10% of dose found in dermis and epidermis; systemic absorption (4%); C_{max}=20-80ng/mL. **Metabolism:** Cutaneous (negligible), beta-oxidation. **Elimination:** Urine (mainly unchanged); $T_{1/2}$=12 hrs (after topical dosing).

AZMACORT
triamcinolone acetonide (Abbott)

RX

THERAPEUTIC CLASS: Corticosteroid

INDICATIONS: Maintenance treatment of asthma as prophylactic therapy in patients ≥6 yrs; to reduce or eliminate the need for oral corticosteroidal therapy.

DOSAGE: *Adults:* 2 inh (150mcg) tid-qid or 4 inh (300mcg) bid. Severe Asthma: Initial: 12-16 inh/day. Max: 16 inh/day (1200mcg). Rinse mouth after use.
Pediatrics: >12 yrs: 2 inh (150mcg) tid-qid or 4 inh (300mcg) bid. Severe Asthma: Initial: 12-16 inh/day. Max: 16 inh/day (1200mcg). 6-12 yrs: 1-2 inh (75-150mcg) tid-qid or 2-4 (150-300mcg) inh bid. Max: 12 inh/day (900mcg). Rinse mouth after use.

HOW SUPPLIED: MDI: 75mcg/inh (20g)

CONTRAINDICATIONS: Primary treatment of status asthmaticus or other acute asthma attacks.

WARNINGS/PRECAUTIONS: Deaths due to adrenal insufficiency have occurred with transfer from systemic corticosteroids to inhaled corticosteroids. Resume oral corticosteroids during stress or severe asthma attack. Observe for adrenal insufficiency, systemic corticosteroid withdrawal effects, hypercorticism and growth suppression (children). More susceptible to infections. Not for acute bronchospasm. D/C if bronchospasm occurs after dosing. Caution with TB of respiratory tract; untreated systemic fungal, bacterial, viral or parasitic infections; or ocular herpes simplex. *Candida* infection of mouth and pharynx reported.

ADVERSE REACTIONS: Pharyngitis, sinusitis, headache, flu syndrome.

INTERACTIONS: Caution with prednisone.

PREGNANCY: Category C, caution in nursing.

MECHANISM OF ACTION: Corticosteroid; not established. Inhaled route makes possible to provide local anti-inflammatory activity.

PHARMACOKINETICS: Absorption: T_{max}=1.5-2 hrs. **Distribution:** V_d=99.5L; plasma protein binding (68%). **Elimination:** Urine (40%), feces (60%); $T_{1/2}$=88 min.

AZULFIDINE
sulfasalazine (Pharmacia & Upjohn)

RX

THERAPEUTIC CLASS: 5-Aminosalicylic acid derivative/sulfapyridine

INDICATIONS: Treatment of mild to moderate ulcerative colitis. Adjunct therapy in severe ulcerative colitis. To prolong remission period between acute attacks of ulcerative colitis.

DOSAGE: *Adults:* Initial: 3-4g/day in divided doses. May initiate at 1-2g/day to reduce GI intolerance. Maint: 2g/day.
Pediatrics: ≥2 yrs: 40-60mg/kg/day divided into 3-6 doses. Maint: 7.5mg/kg qid.

HOW SUPPLIED: Tab: 500mg* *scored

CONTRAINDICATIONS: <2 yrs, intestinal or urinary obstruction, porphyria, hypersensitivity to sulfonamides, salicylates.

WARNINGS/PRECAUTIONS: Caution with hepatic/renal impairment, blood dyscrasias, severe allergy, bronchial asthma, G6PD deficiency. Monitor CBC, WBC, LFTs, at baseline, every 2nd week for 1st 3 months, monthly for next 3 months, and every 3 months thereafter. Monitor renal function periodically. Maintain adequate fluid intake to prevent crystalluria and stone formation. D/C if hypersensitivity or toxic reaction occurs.

ADVERSE REACTIONS: Anorexia, headache, nausea, vomiting, gastric distress, reversible oligospermia.

INTERACTIONS: Reduces absorption of folic acid, digoxin.

PREGNANCY: Category B, caution in nursing.

MECHANISM OF ACTION: 5-aminosalicylic acid (5-ASA) derivative/sulfapyridine (SP); not established, may be related to anti-inflammatory and/or immunodulatory properties of sulfasalazine (SSZ) or its metabolites (5-ASA and SP), its affinity for connective tissue, and/or to relatively high concentration reached in serous fluids, liver, and intestinal wall.

PHARMACOKINETICS: Absorption: SSZ: C_{max}=6mcg/mL, T_{max}=6 hrs; 5-ASA; SP: T_{max}=10 hrs. SSZ: Absolute bioavailability <15%; SP: Well absorbed from colon, estimated bioavailability 60%. 5-ASA: Much less well absorbed from GI tract, estimated bioavailability 10-30%. **Distribution:** SSZ: V_d=7.5L; plasma protein binding >99.3%. SP: Plasma protein binding 70%. **Metabolism:** Intestinal bacteria to 5-ASA and SP; liver (acetylation). **Elimination:** Urine (37%), feces. SSZ: $T_{1/2}$=7.6 hrs; SP: $T_{1/2}$=10.4 hrs (slow acetylators), 14.8 hrs (fast acetylators).

AZULFIDINE EN
sulfasalazine (Pharmacia & Upjohn)

RX

THERAPEUTIC CLASS: 5-Aminosalicylic acid derivative/sulfapyridine

INDICATIONS: Mild to moderate ulcerative colitis, as an adjunct treatment of severe ulcerative colitis, and for the prolongation of the remission period between acute attacks of ulcerative colitis. Rheumatoid arthritis and polyarticular-course juvenile rheumatoid arthritis that has responded inadequately to salicylates or other NSAIDs.

DOSAGE: *Adults:* Ulcerative Colitis: Initial: 1-4g/day in divided doses at intervals not exceeding 8 hrs. Maint: 2g/day. Rheumatoid Arthritis: Initial: 0.5-1g/day. Maint: 2g/day given bid. Swallow tabs whole after meals.
Pediatrics: ≥6 yrs: Ulcerative Colitis: Initial: 40-60mg/kg/24 hrs in 3-6 divided doses. Maint: 7.5mg/kg qid. Juvenile Rheumatoid Arthritis: 30-50mg/kg/day given bid. To reduce GI effects give 1/4 to 1/3 initial dose; increase weekly for 1 month. Max: 2g/day. Swallow tabs whole after meals.

HOW SUPPLIED: Tab, Delayed-Release: 500mg

CONTRAINDICATIONS: Intestinal or urinary obstruction, porphyria, hypersensitivity to sulfonamides or salicylates.

WARNINGS/PRECAUTIONS: Caution with hepatic or renal impairment, blood dyscrasias, severe allergy, bronchial asthma or G6PD deficiency. Monitor CBC, WBC, and LFTs prior to therapy and every other week for the 1st 3 months, once monthly for next 3 months, then every 3 months. Monitor renal function periodically. Maintain adequate fluid intake. Fatal hypersensitivity reactions reported. D/C if tabs pass undisintegrated or if hypersensitivity reactions occur.

ADVERSE REACTIONS: Anorexia, headache, nausea, vomiting, gastric distress, oligospermia, rash, pruritus, urticaria, fever, orange-yellow urine or skin.

INTERACTIONS: Reduces absorption of folic acid and digoxin. Increased incidence of GI adverse events with combination of sulfasalazine (2g/day) and MTX (7.5mg/week).

PREGNANCY: Category B, caution in nursing.

MECHANISM OF ACTION: 5-aminosalicylic acid (5-ASA) derivative/sulfapyridine (SP); not established, may be related to the anti-inflammatory and/or immunodulatory properties of sulfasalazine (SSZ) or its metabolites (5-ASA and SP), its affinity for connective tissue, and/or to relatively high concentration reached in serous fluids, liver and intestinal wall.

PHARMACOKINETICS: Absorption: SSZ: C_{max}=6mcg/mL, T_{max}=6 hrs; 5-ASA. SP: T_{max}=10 hrs. SSZ: Absolute bioavailability <15%; SP: Well absorbed from colon, estimated bioavailability 60%. 5-ASA: Much less well absorbed from GI tract, estimated bioavailability 10-30%. **Distribution:** SSZ: V_d=7.5L; plasma protein binding >99.3%. SP: Plasma protein binding 70%. **Metabolism:** Intestinal bacteria to 5-ASA and SP; liver (acetylation). **Elimination:** Urine (37%), feces. SSZ: $T_{1/2}$=7.6 hrs, SP: $T_{1/2}$=10.4 hrs (slow acetylators), 14.8 hrs (fast acetylators).

BACITRACIN INJECTION RX
bacitracin (Pharmacia & Upjohn)

> May cause renal failure due to tubular and glomerular necrosis. Monitor renal function prior to, and daily during therapy. Fluid intake and urinary output should be maintained at proper levels to avoid kidney toxicity. Discontinue if renal toxicity occurs. Avoid other nephrotoxic drugs.

THERAPEUTIC CLASS: Antibiotic

INDICATIONS: Treatment of pneumonia and empyema caused by staphylococci.

DOSAGE: *Pediatrics:* <2500g: 900U/kg/24h IM. >2500g: 1000U/kg/24h IM. Administer in 2-3 divided doses. Inject in upper outer quadrant of buttocks.

HOW SUPPLIED: Inj: 50,000U

WARNINGS/PRECAUTIONS: Use appropriate therapy if superinfection occurs.

ADVERSE REACTIONS: Albuminuria, cylindruria, azotemia, NV, pain at injection site, skin rashes, rising blood levels without increase in dosage.

INTERACTIONS: Avoid with other nephrotoxic drugs (eg, streptomycin, kanamycin, polymyxin B, polymyxin E, neomycin).

PREGNANCY: Safety in pregnancy or nursing not known.

MECHANISM OF ACTION: Exerts antibacterial action *in vitro* against variety of gram-positive and some gram-negative organisms.

PHARMACOKINETICS: Absorption: Rapid and complete. **Distribution:** Widely distributed in all body organs; found in ascitic and pleural fluid.

BACLOFEN RX
baclofen (Various)

OTHER BRAND NAME: Kemstro (Schwarz)

THERAPEUTIC CLASS: GABA analog

INDICATIONS: Treatment of spasticity associated with multiple sclerosis. May be effective in spinal cord injuries and other spinal cord diseases.

DOSAGE: *Adults:* Initial: 5mg tid for 3 days. Titrate: May increase dose by 5mg tid every 3 days. Usual: 40-80mg/day. Max: 80 mg/day (20mg qid). Renal Impairment: Reduce dose.
Pediatrics: ≥12 yrs: Initial: 5mg tid for 3 days. Titrate: May increase dose by 5mg tid every 3 days. Usual: 40-80mg/day. Max: 80 mg/day (20mg qid). Renal Impairment: Reduce dose.

HOW SUPPLIED: Tab: (Generic) 10mg, 20mg; Tab, Disintegrating (ODT): (Kemstro) 10mg, 20mg

WARNINGS/PRECAUTIONS: Caution with psychosis, schizophrenia, confusional states; may exacerbate conditions. Caution with bladder sphincter hypertonia, peptic ulceration, seizures, elderly, cerebrovascular disorder, respiratory failure, hepatic or renal failure. Abnormal AST, alkaline phosphatase and blood glucose reported. Caution when used to maintain locomotion or to obtain increased function. Decreased alertness with operating machinery. Has not significantly benefited stroke patients. Avoid abrupt discontinuation; reduce dose slowly over 1-2 weeks.

ADVERSE REACTIONS: Drowsiness, dizziness, weakness, fatigue, confusion, daytime sedation, headache, insomnia, hypotension, nausea, constipation, urinary frequency.

INTERACTIONS: May potentiate antihypertensives. May increase CNS depressant effects with MAO inhibitors. Potentiated by TCAs. Mental confusion, hallucinations and agitation with levodopa plus carbidopa therapy. May increase blood glucose and require dosage adjustment of antidiabetic agents. Synergistic effects with magnesium sulfate and other neuromuscular blockers. Additive CNS effects with alcohol and other CNS depressants.

PREGNANCY: Category C, caution in nursing.

MECHANISM OF ACTION: A GABA analog; muscle relaxant/antispastic agent; not fully known; capable of inhibiting both monosynaptic and polysynaptic reflexes at the spinal level, possibly by hyperpolarization of afferent terminals, although actions at supraspinal sites may also occur and contribute to its clinical effect.

Bactrim

RX

sulfamethoxazole - trimethoprim (AR Scientific)

OTHER BRAND NAME: Bactrim DS (AR Scientific)

THERAPEUTIC CLASS: Sulfonamide/tetrahydrofolic acid inhibitor

INDICATIONS: Treatment of urinary tract infection (UTI), acute otitis media, acute exacerbation of chronic bronchitis (AECB), traveler's diarrhea, shigellosis, and *Pneumocystis carinii* pneumonia (PCP).

DOSAGE: *Adults:* UTI: 800mg SMX-160mg TMP or 2 tabs of 400mg SMX-80mg TMP q12h for 10-14 days. Shigellosis: 800mg SMX-160mg TMP or 2 tabs of 400mg SMX-80mg TMP q12h for 5 days. AECB: 800mg SMX-160mg TMP or 2 tabs of 400mg SMX-80mg TMP q12h for 14 days. PCP Treatment: 15-20mg/kg TMP and 75-100mg/kg SMX per 24 hrs given q6h for 14-21 days. PCP Prophylaxis: 800mg SMX-160mg TMP qd. Traveler's Diarrhea: 800mg SMX-160mg TMP q12h for 5 days. CrCl: 15-30mL/min: 50% usual dose. CrCl: <15mL/min: Not recommended.
Pediatrics: ≥2 months: UTI/Otitis Media: 4mg/kg TMP and 20mg/kg SMX q12h for 10 days. Shigellosis: 8mg/kg TMP and 40mg/kg SMX per 24 hrs given q12h for 5 days. PCP Treatment: 15-20mg/kg TMP and 75-100mg/kg SMX per 24 hrs given q6h for 14-21 days. PCP Prophylaxis: 150mg/m^2/day TMP with 750mg/m^2/day SMX given bid, on 3 consecutive days/week. Max: 320mg TMP/1600mg SMX/day. CrCl: 15-30mL/min: 50% usual dose. CrCl: <15mL/min: Not recommended.

HOW SUPPLIED: (Sulfamethoxazole (SMX)-Trimethoprim (TMP)) Tab: 400mg-80mg*; Tab, DS: 800mg-160mg* *scored

CONTRAINDICATIONS: Megaloblastic anemia due to folate deficiency, pregnancy, nursing, infants <2 months, marked hepatic damage, severe renal insufficiency if cannot monitor renal status.

WARNINGS/PRECAUTIONS: Fatal hypersensitivity reactions (eg, Stevens-Johnson syndrome, toxic epidermal necrolysis, fulminant hepatic necrosis, agranulocytosis, aplastic anemia) may occur. Pseudomembranous colitis, cough, SOB, and pulmonary infiltrates reported. Avoid with group A β-hemolytic streptococcal infections. Caution with hepatic/renal impairment, elderly, folate deficiency (eg, chronic alcoholics, anticonvulsants, malabsorption, malnutrition), bronchial asthma, and other allergies. In G6PD deficiency, hemolysis may occur. Increased incidence of adverse events with AIDS. Ensure adequate fluid intake and urinary output. Caution with porphyria, thyroid dysfunction.

ADVERSE REACTIONS: NV, anorexia, rash, urticaria.

INTERACTIONS: Diuretics (especially thiazides) may increase risk of thrombocytopenia with purpura in elderly patients. Caution with warfarin, may prolong PT. Increased effects of phenytoin, oral hypoglycemics. Increased plasma levels of methotrexate, digoxin (especially in elderly). Marked but reversible nephrotoxicity reported with cyclosporine. May develop megaloblastic anemia with pyrimethamine >25mg/week. Increased levels with indomethacin. May decrease effects of TCAs. Single case of toxic delirium with amantadine.

PREGNANCY: Category C, contraindicated in nursing.

MECHANISM OF ACTION: Sulfamethoxazole: Inhibits bacterial synthesis of dyhydrofolic acid by competing with PABA. Trimethoprim: Blocks the production of tetrahydrofolic acid from dihydrofolic acid by binding to and reversibly inhibiting the required enzyme, dihydrofolate reductase.

PHARMACOKINETICS: Absorption: Rapid; T_{max}=1-4 hrs; Sulfamethoxazole: C_{max}=57.4mcg/mL (free), 68.0mcg/mL (total); Trimethoprim: C_{max}=1.72mcg/mL. **Distribution:** Sulfamethoxazole: Plasma protein binding (70%); Trimethoprim: Plasme protein binding (44%). Both pass placental barrier and excreted in breast milk. **Metabolism:** Sulfamethoxazole: N_4-acetylation; Trimethoprim: 1- and 3-oxides, 3′-4′-hydroxy derivatives (principal metabolites). **Elimination:** Sulfamethoxazole: $T_{1/2}$=0.72 hrs. Urine: Total sulfonamide (84.5%), 30% (free), and the remaining (N_4-acetylated metabolite); 66.8% (trimethoprim); $T_{1/2}$=10 hrs (sulfamethoxazole), 8-10 hrs (trimethoprim).

BACTROBAN   RX
mupirocin (GlaxoSmithKline)

THERAPEUTIC CLASS: Bacterial protein synthesis inhibitor

INDICATIONS: (Oint) Topical treatment of impetigo due to *S.aureus* and *S.pyogenes*. (Cre) Treatment of secondarily infected traumatic skin lesions (up to 10cm in length or $100cm^2$) due to *S.aureus* and *S.pyogenes*.

DOSAGE: *Adults:* (Oint) Apply tid. (Cre) Apply tid for 10 days. May cover with gauze. Re-evaluate if no response within 3-5 days.
Pediatrics: (Oint) 2 months -16 yrs: Apply tid. (Cre) 3 months-16 yrs: Apply tid for 10 days. May cover with gauze. Re-evaluate if no response within 3-5 days.

HOW SUPPLIED: Cre: 2% (15g, 30g); Oint: 2% (22g)

WARNINGS/PRECAUTIONS: Avoid eyes. D/C if sensitization or irritation occurs. May cause superinfection with prolonged use. Caution with oint in renal dysfunction. Avoid mucosal surfaces. Avoid open wounds or damaged skin with oint.

ADVERSE REACTIONS: Burning, pain, pruritus, headache, rash, nausea.

PREGNANCY: Category B, caution in nursing.

MECHANISM OF ACTION: Bacterial protein synthesis inhibitor; inhibits bacterial protein synthesis by reversibly and specifically binding to bacterial isoleucyl transfer-RNA synthetase. Active against a wide range of gram-positive bacteria including methicillin-resistant *Staphylococcus aureus* (MRSA). Also active against certain gram-negative bacteria.

PHARMACOKINETICS: Absorption: Minimal percutaneous absorption. **Metabolism:** Rapid. Monic acid (inactive metabolite). **Elimination:** Renal (metabolite).

BACTROBAN NASAL   RX
mupirocin calcium (GlaxoSmithKline)

THERAPEUTIC CLASS: Antibacterial agent

INDICATIONS: Eradication of nasal colonization of MRSA in adults and healthcare workers in certain institutional settings during outbreaks of MRSA.

DOSAGE: *Adults:* Apply 1/2 of the single-use tube into each nostril bid for 5 days. Spread oint by pressing together and releasing the sides of the nose repetitively for 1 min. Do not re-use tube.
Pediatrics: ≥12 yrs: Apply 1/2 of the single-use tube into each nostril bid for 5 days. Spread oint by pressing together and releasing the sides of the nose repetitively for 1 min. Do not re-use tube.

HOW SUPPLIED: Oint: 2% (1g pkt)

WARNINGS/PRECAUTIONS: Avoid eyes. D/C if sensitization or irritation occurs. May cause superinfection with prolonged use.

ADVERSE REACTIONS: Headache, rhinitis, respiratory disorder, pharyngitis, taste perversion.

INTERACTIONS: Avoid use with other intranasal products.

PREGNANCY: Category B, caution in nursing.

MECHANISM OF ACTION: Antibacterial agent; inhibits protein synthesis by reversibly and specifically binding to bacterial isoleucyl transfer-RNA synthetase.

PHARMACOKINETICS: Absorption: Significant in neonates and premature infants. **Elimination:** Urine.

BARACLUDE

RX

entecavir (Bristol-Myers Squibb)

> Lactic acidosis and severe, possibly fatal, hepatomegaly with steatosis reported. Reports of severe acute exacerbations of hepatitis B upon discontinuation of therapy. Follow-up liver function monitoring required. Limited clinical experience suggests there is a potential for the development of resistance to HIV nucleoside reverse transcriptase inhibitors if Baraclude is used to treat chronic hepatitis B virus infection in patients with HIV infection that is not being treated. Not recommended for HIV/HBV coinfected patients who are not receiving highly active antiretroviral therapy (HAART).

THERAPEUTIC CLASS: Guanosine nucleoside analogue

INDICATIONS: Treatment of chronic hepatitis B virus (HBV) infection with active viral replication and persistent elevations in serum aminotransferases (ALT or AST) or histologically active disease.

DOSAGE: *Adults:* Nucleoside-Treatment-Naive: 0.5mg qd. CrCl 30 to <50mL/min: 0.25mg qd or 0.5mg q48h. CrCl 10 to <30mL/min: 0.15mg qd or 0.5mg q72h. CrCl <10mL/min: 0.05mg qd or 0.5mg q7 days. Receiving Lamivudine or Known Lamivudine Resistance Mutation: 1mg qd. CrCl 30 to <50mL/min: 0.5mg qd or 1mg q48h. CrCl 10 to <30mL/min: 0.3mg qd or 1mg q72h. CrCl <10mL/min: 0.1mg qd or 1mg q7 days. Take on empty stomach.
Pediatrics: ≥16 yrs: Nucleoside-Treatment-Naive:0.5mg qd. CrCl 30 to <50mL/min: 0.25mg qd or 0.5mg q48h. CrCl 10 to <30mL/min: 0.15mg qd or 0.5mg q72h. CrCl <10mL/min: 0.05mg qd or 0.5mg q7 days. Receiving Lamivudine or Known Lamivudine Resistance Mutation: 1mg qd. CrCl 30 to <50mL/min: 0.5mg qd or 1mg q48h. CrCl 10 to <30mL/min: 0.3mg qd or 1mg q72h. CrCl <10mL/min: 0.1mg qd or 1mg q7 days. Take on empty stomach.

HOW SUPPLIED: Sol: 0.05mg/mL; Tab: 0.5mg, 1mg

WARNINGS/PRECAUTIONS: See BlackBox Warning. Reduce dose in renal dysfunction (CrCl <50mL/min) including patients on hemodialysis or CAPD (continuous ambulatory peritoneal dialysis). Exacerbations of hepatitis after discontinuation of treatment.

ADVERSE REACTIONS: Headache, fatigue, dizziness, nausea, hyperglycemia, lipase ≥2.1 X ULN, glycosuria, hematuria and increase in total bilirubin.

INTERACTIONS: May increase serum concentrations of entecavir or coadministered drug with drugs that reduce renal function or compete for active tubular secretion.

PREGNANCY: Category C, not for use in nursing.

MECHANISM OF ACTION: Guanosine nucleoside analogue; inhibits base priming, reverse transcription of negative strand from pregenomic mRNA, and synthesis of positive strand of HBV DNA.

PHARMACOKINETICS: Absorption: (0.5mg) C_{max}=4.2ng/mL; T_{max}=0.5-1.5 hrs. (1.0mg) C_{max}=8.2ng/mL. Bioavailability (100%). **Distribution:** Plasma protein binding (13%). **Metabolism:** Hepatic. **Elimination:** Kidneys; urine (62-73%); $T_{1/2}$=128-149 hrs.

BAYER ASPIRIN

OTC

aspirin (Bayer Healthcare)

OTHER BRAND NAMES: Bayer Aspirin Children's (Bayer Healthcare) - Bayer Aspirin Regimen (Bayer Healthcare) - Bayer Aspirin Regimen with Calcium (Bayer Healthcare) - Genuine Bayer Aspirin (Bayer Healthcare)

THERAPEUTIC CLASS: Salicylate

INDICATIONS: To reduce the risk of death and nonfatal stroke with previous ischemic stroke or transient ischemia of the brain. To reduce risk of vascular mortality with suspected acute MI. To reduce risk of death and nonfatal MI with previous MI or unstable angina. To reduce risk of MI and sudden death in chronic stable angina pectoris. For patients who have undergone revascularization procedures with a pre-existing condition for which ASA is indicated. Relief of signs of rheumatoid arthritis (RA), juvenile rheumatoid arthritis (JRA), osteoarthritis (OA), spondyloarthropathies, arthritis, and pleurisy associated with systemic lupus erythematosus (SLE). For minor aches and pains.

DOSAGE: *Adults:* Ischemic Stroke/TIA: 50-325mg qd. Suspected Acute MI: Initial: 160-162.5mg qd as soon as suspect MI. Maint: 160-162.5mg qd for 30 days post-infarction, consider further therapy for prevention/recurrent MI. Prevention or Recurrent MI/Unstable Angina/Chronic Stable Angina: 75-325mg qd. CABG: 325mg qd, start 6 hrs post-surgery. Continue for 1 yr. PTCA: Initial: 325mg, 2 hrs pre-surgery. Maint: 160-325mg qd. Carotid Endarterectomy: 80mg qd to 650mg bid, start pre-surgery. RA: Initial: 3g qd in divided doses. Increase for anti-inflammatory efficacy to 150-300mcg/mL plasma salicylate level. Spondyloarthropathies: Up to 4g/day in divided doses. OA: Up to 3g/day in divided doses. Arthritis/SLE Pleurisy: Initial: 3g/day in divided doses. Increase for anti-inflammatory efficacy to 150-300mcg/mL plasma salicylate level. Pain: 325-650mg q4-6h. Max: 4g/day.
Pediatrics: JRA: Initial: 90-130mg/kg/day in divided doses. Increase for anti-inflammatory efficacy to 150-300mcg/mL plasma salicylate level. Pain: ≥12 yrs: 325-650mg q4-6h. Max: 4g/day.

HOW SUPPLIED: Tab: (Genuine Bayer Aspirin) 325mg; Tab: (Bayer Aspirin Regimen with Calcium) 81mg; Tab, Chewable: (Bayer Aspirin Children's) 81mg; Tab, Delayed-Release: (Bayer Aspirin Regimen) 81mg, 325mg

CONTRAINDICATIONS: NSAID allergy, viral infections in children or teenagers, syndrome of asthma, rhinitis, and nasal polyps.

WARNINGS/PRECAUTIONS: Increased risk of bleeding with heavy alcohol use (≥3 drinks/day). May inhibit platelet function; can adversely affect inherited (hemophilia) or acquired (hepatic disease, vitamin K deficiency) bleeding disorders. Monitor for bleeding and ulceration. Avoid in history of active peptic ulcer, severe renal failure, severe hepatic insufficiency, and sodium restricted diets. Associated with elevated LFTs, BUN, and serum creatinine; hyperkalemia; proteinuria; and prolonged bleeding time. Avoid 1 week before and during labor.

ADVERSE REACTIONS: Fever, hypothermia, dysrhythmias, hypotension, agitation, cerebral edema, dehydration, hyperkalemia, dyspepsia, GI bleed, hearing loss, tinnitus, problems in pregnancy.

INTERACTIONS: Diminished hypotensive and hyponatremic effects of ACE inhibitors. May increase levels of acetazolamide, valproic acid. Increased bleeding risk with heparin, warfarin. Decreased levels of phenytoin. Decreased hypotensive effects of β-blockers. Decreased diuretic effects with renal or cardiovascular disease. Decreased methotrexate clearance; increased risk of bone marrow toxicity. Avoid NSAIDs. Increased effects of hypoglycemic agents. Antagonizes uricosuric agents.

PREGNANCY: Avoid in 3rd trimester of pregnancy and nursing.

MECHANISM OF ACTION: Provides temporary relief from arthritis pain and arthritis inflammation.

BAYER ASPIRIN EXTRA STRENGTH   OTC

aspirin (Bayer Healthcare)

THERAPEUTIC CLASS: Salicylate

INDICATIONS: Temporary relief of headache, pain and fever of colds, muscle aches and pains, menstrual pain, toothache pain, minor aches and arthritis pain.

DOSAGE: *Adults:* 500-1000mg q4-6h prn. Max: 4g/24hrs.
Pediatrics: ≥12 yrs: 500-1000mg q4-6h prn. Max: 4g/24hrs.

HOW SUPPLIED: Tab: 500mg

WARNINGS/PRECAUTIONS: Avoid in children or teenagers for chickenpox or flu symptoms; Reye's syndrome may occur. Do not take >10 days for pain or >3 days for fever. Avoid in asthma, stomach problems that persist or recur, gastric ulcers, or bleeding problems. Stop therapy if ringing in the ears or loss of hearing occurs.

INTERACTIONS: Avoid with drugs for anticoagulation, diabetes, gout, or arthritis. Increased risk of stomach bleeding with alcohol use (≥3 drinks/day).

PREGNANCY: Avoid in 3rd trimester of pregnancy; safety in nursing not known.

BECONASE AQ

RX

beclomethasone dipropionate (GlaxoSmithKline)

THERAPEUTIC CLASS: Corticosteroid

INDICATIONS: Relief of symptoms of seasonal or perennial allergic and nonallergic rhinitis. Prevention of nasal polyp recurrence following surgical removal.

DOSAGE: *Adults:* 1-2 sprays per nostril bid. Max: 2 sprays per nostril bid.
Pediatrics: ≥6 yrs: 1-2 sprays per nostril bid. Max: 2 sprays per nostril bid.

HOW SUPPLIED: Spray: 42mcg/spray (25g)

WARNINGS/PRECAUTIONS: Risk of adrenal insufficiency and withdrawal symptoms when replacing systemic corticosteroids with topical corticosteroids. Caution with active or quiescent TB, ocular herpes simplex, or untreated bacterial, fungal and systemic viral infections. Avoid with recent nasal trauma/surgery or septum ulcers. Risk for more severe/fatal course of infections (eg, chickenpox, measles) and for *Candida* infection of the nose and pharynx. Potential for growth velocity reduction in pediatrics.

ADVERSE REACTIONS: Nasopharyngeal irritation, sneezing, headache, nausea, lightheadedness, irritated/dry nose and throat, unpleasant taste/smell.

INTERACTIONS: Concomitant systemic corticosteroids increase risk of hypercorticism and/or HPA axis suppression.

PREGNANCY: Category C, caution in nursing.

MECHANISM OF ACTION: Corticosteroid; not established; anti-inflammatory and vaso-constrictor effects.

PHARMACOKINETICS: Absorption: Absolute bioavailability (44%) (for the active metabolite B-17-MP). $C_{max} \leq 50$pg/mL. **Distribution:** V_d=20L (parent drug); V_d=424L (B-17-MP). Plasma protein binding (87%). **Metabolism:** B-17-MP (active metabolite) via esterase enzymes.

BENADRYL ALLERGY

OTC

diphenhydramine HCl (McNeil)

THERAPEUTIC CLASS: Antihistamine

INDICATIONS: Relief of hay fever or upper respiratory allergies, and rhinorrhea/sneezing due to the common cold.

DOSAGE: *Adults:* 25-50mg q4-6h. Max: 300mg/24hrs.
Pediatrics: ≥12 yrs: 25-50mg q4-6h. Max: 300mg/24 hrs. 6-11 yrs: 12.5-25mg q4-6h. Max: 150mg/24hrs.

HOW SUPPLIED: Cap: 25mg; Sol: 12.5mg/5mL; Tab: 25mg; Tab, Chewable: 12.5mg

WARNINGS/PRECAUTIONS: Caution with emphysema, chronic bronchitis, glaucoma, or difficulty in urination due to prostate gland enlargement. May impair mental/physical abilities.

ADVERSE REACTIONS: Drowsiness, excitability (especially in children).

INTERACTIONS: Increased drowsiness with alcohol, sedatives, tranquilizers.

PREGNANCY: Safety in pregnancy and nursing not known.

BENZACLIN

RX

benzoyl peroxide - clindamycin (Dermik)

THERAPEUTIC CLASS: Antibacterial/keratolytic

INDICATIONS: Topical treatment of acne vulgaris.

DOSAGE: *Adults:* Wash face and pat dry. Apply bid (am and pm).
Pediatrics: ≥12 yrs: Wash face and pat dry. Apply bid (am and pm).

HOW SUPPLIED: Gel: (Clindamycin-Benzoyl Peroxide) 1%-5% (25g, 50g)

CONTRAINDICATIONS: Hypersensitivity to lincomycin. History of regional enteritis, ulcerative colitis, and antibiotic-associated colitis.

WARNINGS/PRECAUTIONS: Severe colitis reported with oral and parenteral clindamycin. D/C if severe diarrhea occurs. Avoid contact with eyes and mucous membranes.

ADVERSE REACTIONS: Dry skin, pruritus, peeling, erythema, sunburn.

INTERACTIONS: Cumulative irritancy possible with other topical acne agents. Avoid erythromycin agents.

PREGNANCY: Category C, not for use in nursing.

MECHANISM OF ACTION: Antibacterial/keratolytic; acts against *Propionibacterium acnes*.

PHARMACOKINETICS: Absorption: Benzoyl peroxide: Systemic bioavailability (<2%). Clindamycin: Systemic bioavailability (≤1%).

BENZAGEL
benzoyl peroxide (Dermik)

RX

THERAPEUTIC CLASS: Antibacterial/keratolytic

INDICATIONS: Treatment of mild to moderate acne, used alone or as an adjunct.

DOSAGE: *Adults:* Apply qd or more often to clean affected area. Very fair patients should start with single application qhs.
Pediatrics: ≥12 yrs: Apply qd or more often to clean affected area. Very fair patients should start with single application qhs.

HOW SUPPLIED: Gel: 5%, 10% (42.5g)

WARNINGS/PRECAUTIONS: D/C if itching, redness, burning, swelling, or undue dryness occurs. Avoid contact with eyes and mucous membranes. May bleach colored fabrics or hair.

ADVERSE REACTIONS: Irritation, contact dermatitis.

PREGNANCY: Category C, caution in nursing.

MECHANISM OF ACTION: Antibacterial/keratolytic agent. Effective against *Propionibacterium acnes*.

BENZAMYCIN
benzoyl peroxide - erythromycin (Dermik)

RX

THERAPEUTIC CLASS: Antibacterial/keratolytic

INDICATIONS: Topical treatment of acne vulgaris.

DOSAGE: *Adults:* Wash skin and dry. Apply bid (am and pm).
Pediatrics: ≥12 yrs: Wash skin and dry. Apply bid (am and pm).

HOW SUPPLIED: Gel: (Benzoyl Peroxide-Erythromycin) 5%-3% (0.8g/pkt, 60³)

WARNINGS/PRECAUTIONS: D/C if severe irritation occurs. Avoid eyes, mouth, and mucous membranes. Keep refrigerated after reconstitution and discard after 3 months.

ADVERSE REACTIONS: Dryness, urticaria, skin irritation, skin discoloration, oiliness, tenderness.

INTERACTIONS: Additive irritation with peeling, desquamating, or abrasive agents.

PREGNANCY: Category C, caution in nursing.

MECHANISM OF ACTION: Antibacterial/keratolytic agent; mechanism not fully known. Erythromycin: Antibacterial agent; inhibits protein synthesis by reversibly binding to 50S ribosomal subunits, thereby inhibiting translocation of aminoacyl transfer-RNA and inhibiting polypeptide synthesis. Benzoyl peroxide: Believed to act by releasing active oxygen.

PHARMACOKINETICS: Absorption: Benzoyl peroxide shown to be absorbed by skin, where it is converted to benzoic acid. **Distribution:** Orally and parenterally administered erythromycin found in breast milk.

BETAMETHASONE DIPROPIONATE RX

betamethasone dipropionate (Various)

THERAPEUTIC CLASS: Corticosteroid

INDICATIONS: Corticosteroid-responsive dermatoses.

DOSAGE: *Adults:* (Cre, Oint) Apply qd-bid. (Lot) Apply a few drops bid, am and pm. *Pediatrics:* (Cre, Oint) Apply qd-bid. (Lot) Apply a few drops bid, am and pm.

HOW SUPPLIED: Cre, Oint: 0.05% (15g, 45g); Lot: 0.05% (60mL)

WARNINGS/PRECAUTIONS: May produce reversible HPA axis suppression, manifestations of Cushing's syndrome, hyperglycemia, and glucosuria. Avoid occlusive dressings. Pediatrics are more prone to systemic toxicity. D/C if irritation occurs. Avoid eyes.

ADVERSE REACTIONS: Burning, itching, irritation, dryness, folliculitis, hypertrichosis, acneiform eruptions, hypopigmentation, perioral dermatitis, allergic contact dermatitis, skin maceration, secondary infection, skin atrophy, striae, miliaria.

PREGNANCY: Category C, caution in nursing.

MECHANISM OF ACTION: Corticosteroid: Not established. Possesses anti-inflammatory, anti-pruritic, and vasoconstrictive actions. Effective in treating corticosteroid-responsive dermatoses.

PHARMACOKINETICS: Absorption: Percutaneous; inflammation, other disease states, and occlusive dressings increase absorption. **Metabolism:** Liver. **Elimination:** Kidney, bile.

BETAPACE RX

sotalol HCl (Bayer Healthcare)

> To minimize risk of arrhythmia, place patients initiated or reinitiated on therapy for minimum of 3 days in a facility that can provide ECG monitoring and cardiac resuscitation. Perform CrCl before therapy. Do not substitute Betapace for Betapace AF.

THERAPEUTIC CLASS: Beta-blocker (group II/III antiarrhythmic)

INDICATIONS: Treatment of documented life-threatening ventricular arrhythmias.

DOSAGE: *Adults:* Initial: 80mg bid. Titrate: Increase to 120-160mg bid if needed. Allow 3 days between dose increments. Usual: 160-320mg/day given bid-tid. Refractory Patients: 480-640mg/day. CrCl 30-59mL/min: Dose q24h. CrCl 10-29mL/min: Dose q36-48h. CrCl <10mL/min: Individualize dose. May increase dose with renal impairment after at least 5-6 doses.
Pediatrics: ≥2 yrs: Initial: 30mg/m^2 tid. Titrate: Wait at least 36 hrs between dose increases. Guide dose by response, HR, and QTc. Max: 60mg/m^2. <2 yrs: See dosing chart in PI. Reduce dose or d/c if QTc >550msec. Renal Impairment: Reduce dose or increase interval. Preparation of 5mg/mL Oral Solution: Add five 120mg tabs to 120mL simple syrup in a 6oz plastic, amber bottle. Shake bottle to wet all tabs. Allow tabs to hydrate for 2 hrs then shake bottle intermittently over 2 hrs until tabs are completely disintegrated. Shake before administration. Store at room temp for 3 months.

HOW SUPPLIED: Tab: 80mg*, 120mg*, 160mg* *scored

CONTRAINDICATIONS: Bronchial asthma, sinus bradycardia, 2nd- and 3rd-degree AV block (unless a functioning pacemaker is present), long QT syndromes, cardiogenic shock, uncontrolled CHF.

WARNINGS/PRECAUTIONS: Caution with heart failure controlled by digitalis and/or diuretics, DM, left ventricular dysfunction, non-allergic bronchospasm, sick sinus syndrome, renal impairment, 2-weeks post-MI. Avoid with hypokalemia, hypomagnesemia, excessive QT interval prolongation (>550msec). Correct electrolyte imbalances before therapy. May provoke new or worsen ventricular arrhythmias. Avoid abrupt withdrawal. Use in surgery is controversial. May mask hypoglycemia, hyperthyroidism symptoms. Proarrhythmic events reported.

ADVERSE REACTIONS: Dyspnea, fatigue, dizziness, bradycardia, chest pain, palpitation, asthenia, abnormal ECG, hypotension, headache, lightheadedness, edema.

INTERACTIONS: May block epinephrine effects. Caution with drugs that prolong the QT interval (eg, Class I and III antiarrhythmics, phenothiazines, TCAs, bepridil, certain quinolones and oral macrolides, astemizole). Avoid within 2 hrs of aluminum- or magnesium-containing antacids. Potentiates rebound HTN with clonidine withdrawal. May potentiate bradycardia or hypotension with catecholamine-depleting drugs (eg, reserpine). Antidiabetic agents may need adjustment. Avoid Class 1A and Class III antiarrhythmics; potential to prolong refractoriness. β_2-agonists (eg, terbutaline) may need dose increase. Additive Class II effects with β-blockers. Additive conduction abnormalities with digoxin and CCBs. Caution with diuretics.

PREGNANCY: Category B, not for use in nursing.

MECHANISM OF ACTION: Has both β-adrenoceptor blocking and cardiac action potential duration prolongation antiarrhythmic property. It prolongs the plateau phase of the cardiac action potential.

PHARMACOKINETICS: Absorption: T_{max}=2.5-4 hrs. **Distribution:** Crosses blood-brain barrier (poor); found in breast milk. **Elimination:** Urine (unchanged); $T_{1/2}$=12 hrs.

BETAPACE AF   RX
sotalol HCl (Bayer Healthcare)

> To minimize risk of arrhythmia, place patients initiated or reinitiated on therapy for minimum of 3 days in a facility that can provide CrCl, ECG monitoring, and cardiac resuscitation. Do not substitute Betapace for Betapace AF.

THERAPEUTIC CLASS: Beta-blocker (group II/III antiarrhythmic)

INDICATIONS: Maintenance of normal sinus rhythm with symptomatic atrial fibrillation/atrial flutter (AFIB/AFL) in patients who are currently in sinus rhythm.

DOSAGE: *Adults:* Initiate with continuous ECG monitoring. Give dose qd for CrCl 40-60mL/min and bid for CrCl >60mL/min. Initial: 80mg. Monitor QT 2-4hrs after each dose. Reduce dose or d/c if QT ≥500msec. If QT <500msec after 3 days (after 5th or 6th dose if receiving qd dosing), discharge on current treatment. Alternately, may increase dose to 120mg during hospitalization, and follow for 3 days with bid dose and for 5 or 6 doses if receiving qd dose. Max: 160mg qd or bid depending on CrCl. *Pediatrics:* ≥2 yrs: Initial: 30mg/m² tid. Titrate: Wait at least 36 hrs between dose increases. Guide dose by response, heart rate and QTc. Max: 60mg/m². <2 yrs: See dosing chart in PI. Reduce dose or d/c if QTc >550msec. Renal Impairment: Reduce dose or increase interval. Preparation of 5mg/mL Oral Solution: Add five 120mg tabs to 120mL simple syrup in a 6oz plastic, amber bottle. Shake bottle to wet all tabs. Allow tabs to hydrate for 2 hrs then shake bottle intermittently over 2 hrs until tabs are completely disintegrated. Shake before administration. Store at room temp for 3 months.

HOW SUPPLIED: Tab: 80mg*, 120mg*, 160mg* *scored

CONTRAINDICATIONS: Sinus bradycardia (<50bpm during waking hrs), sick sinus syndrome or 2nd- or 3rd-degree AV block (unless a functioning pacemaker is present), long QT syndromes, baseline QT interval >450msec, cardiogenic shock, uncontrolled heart failure, hypokalemia (<4meq/L), CrCl <40mL/min, bronchial asthma.

WARNINGS/PRECAUTIONS: Can cause serious ventricular arrhythmias. Avoid with hypokalemia, hypomagnesemia. Correct electrolyte imbalances before therapy. Bradycardia reported. Caution with heart failure controlled by digitalis and/or diuretics, non-allergic bronchospasm, sick sinus syndrome, left ventricular dysfunction, DM, renal dysfunction, post-MI. Avoid abrupt withdrawal. Use in surgery is controversial. May mask hypoglycemia, hyperthyroidism symptoms.

ADVERSE REACTIONS: Bradycardia, dyspnea, fatigue, dose-related QT interval prolongation, abnormal ECG, chest pain, diarrhea, NV, hyperhidrosis, dizziness.

INTERACTIONS: May block epinephrine effects. Avoid drugs that prolong the QT interval (eg, antiarrhythmics, phenothiazines, TCAs, bepridil, certain oral macrolides). Avoid within 2 hrs of aluminum- or magnesium-containing antacids. Potentiates rebound HTN with clonidine withdrawal. May potentiate bradycardia or hypotension with catecholamine-depleting drugs (eg, reserpine). Antidiabetic agents may need adjustment. β_2-agonists (eg, terbutaline) may need dose increase. Additive conduction abnormalities with digoxin and CCBs. Caution with diuretics.

PREGNANCY: Category B, not for use in nursing.

MECHANISM OF ACTION: Antiarrhythmic drug (Class II and III properties); has both β-adrenoceptor blocking and cardiac action potential duration prolongation property.

PHARMACOKINETICS: Absorption: T_{max}=2.5-4 hrs. **Distribution:** Crosses blood brain barrier (poor); found in breast milk. **Elimination:** Urine (unchanged); $T_{1/2}$=12 hrs.

BIAXIN
RX
clarithromycin (Abbott)

THERAPEUTIC CLASS: Macrolide

INDICATIONS: Treatment of the following infections caused by susceptible strains of microorganisms: (Adults): Pharyngitis/tonsillitis, acute maxillary sinusitis, acute bacterial exacerbation of chronic bronchitis (ABECB), community-aquired pneumonia (CAP), uncomplicated skin and skin structure infections (SSSI), and disseminated mycobacterial infections. Combination therapy for *H.pylori* infection with duodenal ulcers. MAC prophylaxis in advanced HIV. (Pediatrics): Pharyngitis/tonsillitis, CAP, acute maxillary sinusitis, acute otitis media, uncomplicated SSSI, disseminated mycobacterial infections. MAC prophylaxis in advanced HIV.

DOSAGE: *Adults:* Pharyngitis/Tonsillitis: 250mg q12h for 10 days. Sinusitis: 500mg q12h for 14 days. ABECB: 250-500mg q12h for 7-14 days. SSSI/CAP: 250mg q12h for 7-14 days. MAC Prophylaxis/Treatment: 500mg bid. CrCl <30mL/min: Give 50% dose or double interval. *H.pylori:* Triple Therapy: 500mg + amoxicillin 1g + omeprazole 20mg, all q12h for 10 days; or 500mg + amoxicillin 1g + lansoprazole 30mg, all q12h for 10-14 days. Give additional omeprazole 20mg qd for 18 days with active ulcer. Dual Therapy: 500mg q8h + omeprazole 40mg qd for 14 days (give additional omeprazole 20mg qd for 14 days with active ulcer); or 500mg q8h or q12h + ranitidine bismuth citrate 400mg q12h for 14 days (give additional ranitidine bismuth citrate 400mg bid for 14 days with active ulcer). Avoid combination with ranitidine bismuth citrate if CrCl<25mL/min. *Pediatrics:* ≥6 months: Usual: 7.5mg/kg q12h for 10 days. MAC Prophylaxis/Treatment: ≥20 months: 7.5mg/kg bid, up to 500mg bid. CrCl <30mL/min: Give 50% dose or double interval.

HOW SUPPLIED: Sus: 125mg/5mL, 250mg/5mL (50mL, 100mL); Tab: 250mg, 500mg

CONTRAINDICATIONS: Concomitant cisapride, pimozide, astemizole, terfenadine, ergotamine or dihydroergotamine, or other macrolide antibiotics.

WARNINGS/PRECAUTIONS: Avoid in pregnancy. *Clostridium difficile*-associated diarrhea reported. Adjust dose with severe renal impairment. Colchicine toxicity reported; avoid concomitant use especially in elderly.

ADVERSE REACTIONS: Diarrhea, NV, abnormal taste, dyspepsia, abdominal pain, headache, rash.

INTERACTIONS: See Contraindications. Increases serum levels of theophylline, digoxin, HMG-CoA reductase inhibitors, omeprazole, carbamazepine, drugs metabolized by CYP450. Decreases zidovudine plasma levels. Potentiates oral anticoagulant effects. Decreased clearance of triazolam. Avoid ranitidine, bismuth citrate if CrCl <25mL/min or history of porphyria. Reduce dose with ritonavir if CrCl <60mL/min. Increased levels with fluconazole. Caution with concomitant colchicine use.

PREGNANCY: Category C, caution in nursing.

MECHANISM OF ACTION: Macrolide antibiotic; exerts antibacterial action by binding to the 50S ribosomal subunit of susceptible microorganisms, resulting in inhibition of protein synthesis. Active against aerobic and anaerobic gram-positive and gram-negative microorganisms.

PHARMACOKINETICS: Absorption: Rapid; absolute bioavailability (50%); C_{max}=1-2mcg/mL (250mg tab), 3-4mcg/mL (500mg tab), 2mcg/mL (sus); T_{max}=2-3 hrs. **Metabolism:** 14-OH clarithromycin (principal metabolite). **Elimination:** Urine: 20% (250mg tab), 40% (500mg tab), 10-15% (14-OH). Parent drug; $T_{1/2}$=3-4 hrs (250mg tab, sus), 5-7 hrs (500mg tab). 14-OH: $T_{1/2}$=5-6 hrs (250mg tab, sus), 7-9 hrs (500mg tab).

BICILLIN C-R

RX

penicillin G benzathine - penicillin G procaine (King)

> **Not for IV use nor for admix with other IV solutions. Cardiorespiratory arrest and death reported with inadvertent IV administration.**

THERAPEUTIC CLASS: Penicillin

INDICATIONS: Treatment of moderately severe to severe upper-respiratory tract (URTI) and skin and soft-tissue infections (SSTI), scarlet fever and erysipelas due to streptococci. Treatment of moderately severe pneumonia and otitis media due to pneumococci.

DOSAGE: *Adults:* Group A Strep: URTI/SSTI/Scarlet Fever/Erysipelas: 2.4MU IM. Treat at a single session using multiple IM sites, or use an alternative schedule and give 1/2 of the total dose on Day 1 and 1/2 on Day 3. Pneumococcal Infections (Except Meningitis): 1.2MU IM, repeat every 2-3 days until temperature is normal for 48 hrs. Administer IM into upper, outer quadrant of buttock.
Pediatrics: Group A Strep: URTI/SSTI/Scarlet Fever/Erysipelas: >60 lbs: 2.4MU IM. 30-60 lbs: 900,000U-1.2MU IM. <30 lbs: 600,000U IM. Treat at a single session using multiple IM sites, or use an alternative schedule and give 1/2 of the total dose on Day 1 and 1/2 on Day 3. Pneumococcal Infections (Except Meningitis): 600,000U IM, repeat every 2-3 days until temperature is normal for 48 hrs. Administer IM into upper, outer quadrant of buttock. Use the midlateral aspect of thigh in neonates, infants, and small children.

HOW SUPPLIED: Inj: (Penicillin G Benzathine-Penicillin G Procaine) 300,000-300,000U/mL (2mL)

CONTRAINDICATIONS: Do not inject into or near an artery or nerve.

WARNINGS/PRECAUTIONS: Serious, fatal anaphylactic reactions reported; increased risk with hypersensitivity to PCN, cephalosporins, and other allergens. *Clostridium difficile* associated with diarrhea reported. reported. Avoid IV, intra-arterial administration, or injection into/near major peripheral nerves or blood vessels may cause severe neurovascular and neurological damage. IM administration into anterolateral thigh may cause quadriceps femoris fibrosis and atrophy. Caution with asthma. Avoid with procaine sensitivity. May result in overgrowth of nonsusceptible organisms. Monitor culture after therapy completion to determine eradication. Monitor renal and hematopoietic systems periodically with prolonged and high-dose therapy.

ADVERSE REACTIONS: Maculopapular/exfoliative dermatitis, urticaria, laryngeal edema, fever, pseudomembranous colitis, hemolytic anemia, leukopenia, thrombocytopenia, neuropathy, nephropathy.

INTERACTIONS: Increased and prolonged levels with probenecid. Tetracycline may antagonize bacterial effect; avoid concomitant use.

PREGNANCY: Category B, caution in nursing.

MECHANISM OF ACTION: Penicillin; exerts bactericidal action against susceptible organisms during the active multiplication stage. Acts through inhibition of biosynthesis of cell-wall mucopepetide.

PHARMACOKINETICS: Absorption: Slow; C_{max}=1-3 U/mL (600,000 U), 2.1-2.6 units/mL (1,200,000 U); T_{max}=3 hrs. **Distribution:** Plasma protein binding (60%); found in breast milk, high cocentration in kidney, lesser extent in liver, skin, and intestines. **Metabolism:** Hydrolysis. **Elimination:** Urine.

BICILLIN C-R 900/300

RX

penicillin G benzathine - penicillin G procaine (King)

> **Not for IV use nor for admix with other IV solutions. Cardiorespiratory arrest and death reported with inadvertent IV administration.**

THERAPEUTIC CLASS: Penicillin

INDICATIONS: Treatment of moderately severe to severe upper-respiratory tract (URTI) and skin and soft-tissue infections (SSTI), scarlet fever and erysipelas due to streptococci. Treatment of moderately severe pneumonia and otitis media due to pneumococci. Not for treatment of venereal diseases.

DOSAGE: *Pediatrics:* Group A Strep: URTI/SSTI/Scarlet Fever/Erysipelas: 1.2MU IM single dose. Pneumococcal Infections (Except Meningitis): 1.2MU IM every 2-3 days until temperature is normal for 48 hrs. Administer IM into upper, outer quadrant of buttock. Use midlateral aspect of thigh in neonates, infants, and small children.

HOW SUPPLIED: Inj: (Penicillin G Benzathine-Penicillin G Procaine) 900,000-300,000U/2mL

CONTRAINDICATIONS: Do not inject into or near an artery or nerve.

WARNINGS/PRECAUTIONS: Serious, fatal anaphylactic reactions reported; increased risk with hypersensitivity to penicillin, cephalosporins, and other allergens. *Clostridium difficile* associated with diarrhea reported. Avoid IV, intra-arterial administration, or injection into/near major peripheral nerves or blood vessels may cause severe neurovascular and neurological damage. IM administration into anterolateral thigh may cause quadriceps femoris fibrosis and atrophy. Caution with asthma. Avoid with procaine sensitivity. May result in overgrowth of nonsusceptible organisms. Monitor culture after therapy completion to determine eradication. Monitor renal and hematopoietic systems periodically with prolonged and high-dose therapy.

ADVERSE REACTIONS: Maculopapular/exfoliative dermatitis, urticaria, laryngeal edema, fever, pseudomembranous colitis, hemolytic anemia, leukopenia, thrombocytopenia, neuropathy, nephropathy.

INTERACTIONS: Increased and prolonged levels with probenecid. Tetracycline may antagonize bactericidal effect; avoid concurrent use.

PREGNANCY: Category B, caution in nursing.

MECHANISM OF ACTION: Penicillin; exerts bactericidal action against susceptible organisms during the active multiplication stage. Acts through inhibition of biosynthesis of cell-wall mucopepetide.

PHARMACOKINETICS: Absorption: Slow. **Distribution:** Plasma protein binding (60%); found in breast milk, high concentration in kidney, lesser extent in liver, skin, and intestines. **Metabolism** : Hyrolysis. **Elimination**: Urine.

BICILLIN L-A
penicillin G benzathine (King)

RX

> Not for IV use nor for admix with other IV solutions. Cardiorespiratory arrest and death reported with inadvertent IV administration.

THERAPEUTIC CLASS: Penicillin

INDICATIONS: Treatment of mild to moderate upper respiratory tract infections (URTI) due to streptococci and venereal infections (eg, syphilis, yaws, bejel, pinta). Prophylaxis to prevent recurrence of rheumatic fever or chorea.

DOSAGE: *Adults:* Group A Strep: URTI: 1.2MU IM single dose. Primary/Secondary/Latent Syphilis: 2.4MU IM single dose. Late Syphilis (Tertiary/Neurosyphilis): 2.4MU IM every 7 days for 3 doses. Yaws/Bejel/Pinta: 1.2MU IM single dose. Rheumatic Fever/Glomerulonephritis Prophylaxis: 1.2MU IM once a month or 600,000U IM every 2 weeks. Administer IM into upper, outer quadrant of buttock.
Pediatrics: Group A Strep: URTI: Older *Pediatrics:* 900,000U IM single dose. <60 lbs: 300,000-600,000U IM single dose. Congenital Syphilis: 2-12 yrs: Adjust dose based on adult schedule. <2 yrs: 50,000U/kg IM single dose. Rheumatic Fever/Glomerulonephritis Prophylaxis: 1.2MU IM once a month or 600,000U every 2 weeks. Administer IM into upper, outer quadrant of buttock. Use the midlateral aspect of thigh in neonates, infants, and small children.

HOW SUPPLIED: Inj: 600,000U/mL

CONTRAINDICATIONS: Do not inject into or near an artery or nerve.

WARNINGS/PRECAUTIONS: Serious, fatal anaphylactic reactions reported; increased risk with hypersensitivity to PCNs, cephalosporins, and other allergens. Pseudomembranous colitis reported. Avoid IV, intra-arterial administration, or injection into/near major peripheral nerves or blood vessels may cause severe neurovascular and neurological damage. IM administration into anterolateral thigh may cause quadriceps femoris fibrosis and atrophy. Caution with asthma. May result in overgrowth of nonsusceptible organisms. Monitor culture after therapy completion to determine eradication.

ADVERSE REACTIONS: Maculopapular/exfoliative dermatitis, urticaria, laryngeal edema, fever, pseudomembranous colitis, hemolytic anemia, leukopenia, thrombocytopenia, neuropathy, nephropathy.

INTERACTIONS: Increased and prolonged levels with probenecid. Tetracycline may antagonize bactericidal effect.

PREGNANCY: Category B, caution in nursing.

MECHANISM OF ACTION: Pencillin; exerts bactericidal action against susceptible organisms during the active multiplication stage. Acts through inhibition of biosynthesis of cell-wall mucopepetide.

PHARMACOKINETICS: Absorption: Slow. **Distribution:** Plasma protein binding (60%). **Metabolism:** Hydrolysis. **Elimination:** Urine.

BILTRICIDE RX
praziquantel (Schering)

INDICATIONS: Treatment of infections due to all species of schistosoma and due to liver flukes.

DOSAGE: *Adults:* Schistosomiasis: 20mg/kg tid for 1 day. Clonorchiasis/Opisthorchiasis: 25mg/kg tid for 1 day. Take with fluids during meals; do not chew. Dosage interval should not be <4 hrs or >6 hrs.
Pediatrics: ≥4 yrs: Schistosomiasis: 20mg/kg tid for 1 day. Clonorchiasis/Opisthorchiasis: 25mg/kg tid for 1 day. Take with fluids during meals; do not chew. Dosage interval should not be <4 hrs or >6 hrs.

HOW SUPPLIED: Tab: 600mg (6s)

CONTRAINDICATIONS: Ocular cysticercosis.

WARNINGS/PRECAUTIONS: Avoid driving or operating machinery until one day after treatment. Minimal increases in liver enzymes reported. Hospitalize if schistosomiasis or fluke infection is associated with cerebral cysticercosis. Monitor during treatment with cardiac irregularities.

ADVERSE REACTIONS: Malaise, headache, dizziness, abdominal discomfort, nausea, rise in temperature.

INTERACTIONS: CYP450 inducers, eg antiepileptic drugs (phenytoin, phenobarbital, carbamazepine), dexamethasone, may reduce plasma levels. Avoid concomitant rifampin. CYP450 inhibitors, eg cimetidine, ketoconazole, itraconazole, erythromycin may increase plasma levels. Chloroquine, may lead to lower concentrations of praziquantel in blood. Grapefruit juice can increase Cmax and AUC.

PREGNANCY: Category B, not for use in nursing.

MECHANISM OF ACTION: Praziquantel; antihelminthic that induces rapid contraction of schistosomes by a specific effect on permeability of the cell membrane. Drug further causes vacuolisation and disintegration of the schistosome tegument.

PHARMACOKINETICS: Absorption: Rapid. PO administration in different groups of people with varying degrees of hepatic dysfunction resulted in different pharmacokinetic parameters. **Distribution:** Appears in breast milk. **Elimination:** Urine (approximately 80% drug), (>99% metabolites); $T_{1/2}$=0.8-1.5 hrs.

BLEPH-10 RX
sulfacetamide sodium (Allergan)

OTHER BRAND NAME: AK-Sulf (Akorn)

THERAPEUTIC CLASS: Sulfonamide

INDICATIONS: (Oint, Sol) Treatment of conjunctivitis and other superficial ocular infections. (Sol) Adjunct to systemic sulfonamide therapy of trachoma.

DOSAGE: *Adults:* Conjunctivitis/Superficial Infections: (Sol) 1-2 drops q2-3h initially. (Oint) Apply 1/2 inch q3-4h and hs. Taper dose by decreasing frequency with improvement. Treat for 7-10 days. Trachoma: (Sol) 2 drops q2h with systemic therapy.
Pediatrics: ≥2 months: Conjunctivitis/Superficial Infections: (Sol) 1-2 drops q2-3h initially. (Oint) Apply 1/2 inch q3-4h and hs. Taper dose by decreasing frequency with improvement. Treat for 7-10 days. Trachoma: (Sol) 2 drops q2h with systemic therapy.

HOW SUPPLIED: Oint: (AK-Sulf) 10% (3.5g); Sol: (Bleph-10) 10% (5mL, 15mL)

WARNINGS/PRECAUTIONS: Fatalities reported from severe reactions to sulfonamides. D/C if develop sign of hypersensitivity. Ointments may retard corneal wound healing.

ADVERSE REACTIONS: Local irritation, stinging, burning.

INTERACTIONS: Incompatible with silver preparations.

PREGNANCY: Category C, not for use in nursing.

MECHANISM OF ACTION: Sulfonamide: inhibits bacterial synthesis of dihydrofolic acid by preventing the condensation of pteridine with aminobenzoic acid through competitive inhibition of enzyme dihydropteroate synthetase.

BLEPHAMIDE

RX

prednisolone acetate - sulfacetamide sodium (Allergan)

OTHER BRAND NAME: Blephamide S.O.P. (Allergan)

THERAPEUTIC CLASS: Sulfonamide/corticosteroid

INDICATIONS: For steroid-responsive inflammatory ocular conditions associated with bacterial infection or risks of bacterial infection (eg, corneal injury).

DOSAGE: *Adults:* (Sus) 2 drops into conjunctival sac q4h and qhs. (Oint) Apply 1/2 inch into conjunctival sac tid-qid and qd-bid at night. Re-evaluate if no improvement after 2 days. Decrease dose as condition improves. Max: 20mL or 8g prescribed initially. *Pediatrics:* ≥6 yrs: (Sus) 2 drops into conjunctival sac q4h and qhs. (Oint) Apply 1/2 inch into conjunctival sac tid-qid and qd-bid at night. Re-evaluate if no improvement after 2 days. Decrease dose as condition improves. Max: 20mL or 8g prescribed initially.

HOW SUPPLIED: (Sulfacetamide-Prednisolone) Oint: 10%-0.2% (3.5g); Sus: 10%-0.2% (5mL, 10mL)

CONTRAINDICATIONS: Most viral diseases of the cornea and conjunctiva (eg, epithelial herpes simplex keratitis, vaccinia, and varicella), mycobacterial infection of the eye, fungal diseases of ocular structures.

WARNINGS/PRECAUTIONS: Not for injection. Ocular HTN, glaucoma, secondary infections may occur with prolonged use. Acute anterior uveitis may occur. May mask or enhance infection with acute purulent conditions. Caution with glaucoma, treatment of herpes simplex. Monitor IOP. Staphylococcal isolates may be resistant to sulfonamides. Not effective in mustard gas keratitis and Sjogren's keratoconjunctivitis. Sensitization may recur with sulfonamides. May delay healing after cataract surgery. Fatalities reported due to adverse effects.

ADVERSE REACTIONS: Local irritation, intraocular pressure elevation, acute anterior uveitis, mydriasis, allergic sensitization (Stevens-Johnson syndrome, toxic epidermal necrolysis, fulminant hepatic necrosis, etc.).

INTERACTIONS: Incompatible with silver preparations. Local anesthetics related to p-amino benzoic acid may antagonize sulfonamides.

PREGNANCY: Category C, not for use in nursing.

MECHANISM OF ACTION: Prednisolone: corticosteroid. Suppresses inflammatory response and probably delays or slows healing. Sulfacetamide: antibacterial. Exerts bacteriostatic effect by restricting synthesis of folic acid required for growth through competition with p-aminobenzoic acid.

BONTRIL SLOW-RELEASE

CIII

phendimetrazine tartrate (Valeant)

OTHER BRAND NAME: Bontril PDM (Valeant)

THERAPEUTIC CLASS: Anorectic sympathomimetic amine

INDICATIONS: Short-term adjunct treatment of exogenous obesity.

DOSAGE: *Adults:* (Slow-Release) 105mg qam, 30-60 min before breakfast. (PDM) 35mg bid-tid, 1 hr before meals; may reduce to 17.5mg/dose. Max: 70mg tid. *Pediatrics:* ≥12 yrs: (Slow-Release) 105mg qam, 30-60 min before breakfast. (PDM) 35mg bid-tid, 1 hr before meals; may reduce to 17.5mg/dose. Max: 70mg tabs tid.

HOW SUPPLIED: Cap, Extended-Release: (Slow-Release) 105mg; Tab: (PDM) 35mg*
*scored

CONTRAINDICATIONS: Advanced arteriosclerosis, symptomatic cardiovascular disease, moderate and severe HTN, hyperthyroidism, glaucoma, agitated states, history of drug abuse, concomitant CNS stimulants including MAOIs.

WARNINGS/PRECAUTIONS: Tolerance to anorectic effect develops within a few weeks, d/c if this occurs. Fatigue and depression with abrupt withdrawal after prolonged high dose therapy. Caution with mild HTN.

ADVERSE REACTIONS: Palpitation, tachycardia, BP elevation, overstimulation, restlessness, dizziness, dry mouth, diarrhea, constipation, nausea, libido changes, dysuria, insomnia.

INTERACTIONS: Hypertensive crisis if used within 14 days of MAOIs. May decrease hypotensive effects of guanethidine. May alter insulin requirements.

PREGNANCY: Not for use in pregnancy, safety in nursing not known.

MECHANISM OF ACTION: Anorectic sympathomimetic amine; CNS stimulant, elevates BP. As anorectic, appetite suppression as primary action not established.

PHARMACOKINETICS: Elimination: Urine; $T_{1/2}$=9.8 hrs (slow release), 3.7 hrs (PDM).

BOOSTRIX RX
diphtheria toxoid - pertussis vaccine, acellular - tetanus toxoid (GlaxoSmithKline)

THERAPEUTIC CLASS: Vaccine/toxoid combination

INDICATIONS: Active booster immunization against tetanus, diphtheria, and pertussis as a single dose in individuals 10-18 yrs of age.

DOSAGE: *Pediatrics:* 10-18 yrs: 0.5mL IM into the deltoid muscle.

HOW SUPPLIED: Inj: (Tetanus-Diphtheria-Pertussis) 5LF-2.5LF-8mcg/0.5mL.

CONTRAINDICATIONS: Hypersensitivity to any component; serious allergic reaction (eg, anaphylaxis) associated with previous dose. Encephalopathy not due to an identifiable cause within 7 days prior to pertussis immunization and progressive neurologic disorder, uncontrolled epilepsy, or progressive encephalopathy.

WARNINGS/PRECAUTIONS: May cause allergic reactions in latex sensitive patients. Caution if within 48 hrs of fever ≥105°F not due to another identifiable cause; collapse or shock-like state; persistent, inconsolable crying lasting ≥3 hrs. Caution if within 3 days of seizure with or without fever. Do not administer in patients with bleeding disorders such as hemophilia or thrombocytopenia, or patients on anticoagulant therapy unless potential benefit outweighs risk. Caution if Guillain-Barre syndrome within 6 weeks of tetanus toxoid vaccine. Do not give Td, Tdap, or emergency dose of Td more frequently then every 10 yrs if patient has experienced Arthus-type reaction. Hypersensitivity reaction possible: epinephrine injection (1:1000) should be readily available.

ADVERSE REACTIONS: Local: pain, redness, swelling. Systemic: headache, fatigue, fever, nausea, vomiting, diarrhea, abdominal pain.

INTERACTIONS: Immunosuppressive therapies, including irradiation; antimetabolites, alkylating agents, cytotoxic drugs, and corticosteroids may reduce the immune response to vaccines.

PREGNANCY: Category C, caution in nursing.

MECHANISM OF ACTION: Stimulates immune system to elicit immune response, which produces antibodies that may protect against tetanus, diphtheria, and pertussis.

BOTOX RX
botulinum toxin type A (Allergan)

THERAPEUTIC CLASS: Purified neurotoxin complex

INDICATIONS: Treatment of strabismus and blepharospasm associated with dystonia, including benign essential blepharospasm or VII nerve disorders. Treatment of cervical dystonia to decrease severity of abnormal head position and neck pain. Treatment of severe primary axillary hyperhidrosis that is inadequately managed with topical agents

DOSAGE: *Adults:* Cervical Dystonia: Average Dose: 236U divided among affected muscles. Adjust to individual response. Max: 100U total dose in sternocleidomastoid muscles. Strabismus: Initial: Vertical Muscle and Horizontal Strabismus <20 Prism Diopters: 1.25-2.5U in any muscle. Horizontal Strabismus of 20-50 Prism Diopters: 2.5-5U in any one muscle. Persistent VI Nerve Palsy ≥1 Month: 1.25-2.5U into medial rectus muscle. Increase dose by 2-fold if previous dose results in incomplete paralysis. Max: 25U/muscle. Reassess 7-14 after each injection. Blepharospasm: Initial: 1.25-2.5U into medial and lateral pre-tarsal orbicularis oculi of the upper lid and into lateral pre-tarsal orbicularis oculi of the lower lid. Max: 200U/30 day. Primary Axillary Hyperhidrosis: 50 units per axilla.

Pediatrics: ≥16 yrs: Cervical Dystonia: 236U divided among affected muscles. Adjust dose to individual response. Max: 100U in sternocleidomastoid muscles. ≥12 yrs: Strabismus: Initial: Vertical Muscle and Horizontal Strabismus <20 Prism Diopters: 1.25-2.5U in any muscle. Horizontal Strabismus of 20-50 Prism Diopters: 2.5-5U in any one muscle. Persistent VI Nerve Palsy ≥1 Month: 1.25-2.5U into medial rectus muscle. Increase dose by 2-fold if previous dose results in incomplete paralysis. Max: 25U/muscle. Reassess 7-14 after each injection. Blepharospasm: Initial: 1.25-2.5U into medial and lateral pre-tarsal orbicularis oculi of the upper lid and into lateral pre-tarsal orbicularis oculi of the lower lid. Max: 200U/30 day.

HOW SUPPLIED: Inj: 100U

WARNINGS/PRECAUTIONS: Do not exceed dosing recommendations. Caution with peripheral motor neuropathic diseases (eg, amyotrophic lateral sclerosis, motor neuropathy), neuromuscular junctional disorders (eg, myasthenia gravis, Lambert-Eaton syndrome); increased risk of dysphagia and respiratory compromise. Contains albumin. Have epinephrine available if anaphylactic reaction occurs. Caution with inflammation at injection sites, excessive weakness or atrophy in target muscles. Injection of orbicularis muscle may reduce blinking. Caution to resume activities gradually. Retrobulbar hemorrhages compromising retinal circulation reported; have instruments to decompress orbit accessible. Increased risk of dysphagia in patients with smaller neck muscle mass and those with bilateral injections into sternocleidomastoid muscle; limit dose. Caution in elderly.

ADVERSE REACTIONS: (Cervical Dystonia) dysphagia, upper respiratory infection, neck pain, headache, (Blepharospasm) ptosis, keratitis, eye dryness, (Strabismus) ptosis, vertical deviation.

INTERACTIONS: May be potentiated with aminoglycosides, agents interfering with neuromuscular transmission (eg, curare-like compounds). Excessive neuromuscular weakness may be exacerbated if administer another botulinum toxin before effects resolve from the previous botulinum toxin injection.

PREGNANCY: Category C, caution in nursing.

BREVITAL
methohexital sodium (King)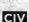

> Should be used only in hospital or ambulatory care settings that provide for continuous monitoring of respiratory and cardiac function. Immediate availability of resuscitative drugs and age- and size-appropriate equipment for bag/valve/mask ventilation and intubation and personnel trained in their use and skilled in airway management should be assured. For deeply sedated patients, a designated individual other than practitioner performing procedure should be present to continuously monitor patient.

THERAPEUTIC CLASS: Barbiturate

INDICATIONS: IV induction of anesthesia prior to the use of other general anesthetic agents. IV induction of anesthesia and as adjunct to subpotent inhalational anesthetic agents (such as nitrous oxide in oxygen) for short surgical procedures. For use along with other parenteral agents, usually narcotic analgesics, to supplement subpotent inhalational anesthetic agents (such as nitrous oxide in oxygen) for longer surgical procedures. IV anesthesia for short surgical, diagnostic, or therapeutic procedures associated with minimal painful stimuli. Agent for inducing a hypnotic state. Pediatrics (>1 month): Rectal or IM induction of anesthesia prior to the use of other general anesthetic agents; rectal or IM induction of anesthesia and as adjunct to subpotent inhalational anesthetic agents for surgical procedures; rectal or IM anesthesia for short surgical, diagnostic, or therapeutic procedures associated with minimal painful stimuli.

DOSAGE: *Adults;* Individualize dose. Induction: 1% sol administered at rate of 1mL/5 sec. Range: 50-120mg or more (average: 70mg). Usual dose: 1-1.5mg/kg. Maint: Intermittent: 20-40mg (2-4mL of 1% sol) q 4-7 min. Continuous drip: Average rate of administration is 3mL of a 0.2% sol/min (1 drop/sec).
Pediatrics: ≥1 month: Individualize dose: Induction: IM: 6.6 to 10mg/kg IM of 5% concentration. Rectal: 25mg/kg rectally of the 1% sol.

HOW SUPPLIED: Inj: 500mg, 2.5g

CONTRAINDICATIONS: Patients with latent or manifest porphyria.

WARNINGS/PRECAUTIONS: Seizures may be elicited in patients with previous history of convulsive activity. Caution in severe hepatic dysfunction, severe cardiovascular instability, shock-like condition, asthma, COPD, severe HTN or hypotension, MI, CHF, severe anemia, status asthmaticus, extreme obesity, debilitated patients or those with impaired function of respiratory, circulatory, renal, hepatic, or endocrine system. Unintended intra-arterial injection may produce platelet aggregates and thrombosis at site of injection.

ADVERSE REACTIONS: Circulatory depression, thrombophlebitis, hypotension, tachycardia, respiratory depression, skeletal muscle hypersensitivity (twitching), emergence delirium.

INTERACTIONS: May influence metabolism of other concomitantly used drugs, such as phenytoin, halothane, anticoagulants, corticosteroids, ethyl alcohol, and propylene glycol-containing solutions. Prior chronic administration of barbituates or phenytoin may reduce effectiveness of methohexital. Additive CNS effects with other CNS depressants, including ethyl alcohol and propylene alcohol.

PREGNANCY: Category B, caution in nursing.

MECHANISM OF ACTION: Ultra-short acting barbiturate anesthetic; rapid uptake by the brain and rapid induction of sleep.

PHARMACOKINETICS: Absorption: *Pediatrics:* (IM) C_{max}=3mcg/mL; T_{max}=15 min. (PR) C_{max}=6.9-7.9mcg/mL; T_{max}=15 min; absolute bioavailability (17%). **Metabolism:** Liver; (demethylation and oxidation). **Elimination:** Urine.

BREVOXYL   RX
benzoyl peroxide (Stiefel)

THERAPEUTIC CLASS: Antibacterial/keratolytic

INDICATIONS: Topical treatment of mild to moderate acne vulgaris.

DOSAGE: *Adults:* (Gel) Apply qd-bid to clean affected area. (Lot) Shake well. Wet affected area and wash qd for 1st week, then bid thereafter if tolerated.
Pediatrics: ≥12 yrs: (Gel) Apply qd-bid to clean affected area. (Lot) Shake well. Wet affected area and wash qd for 1st week, then bid thereafter if tolerated.

HOW SUPPLIED: Gel: 4%, 8% (42.5g, 90g); Lot: (Cleanser) 4%, 8% (297g); Lot: (Creamy Wash) 4%, 8% (170g)

WARNINGS/PRECAUTIONS: Avoid contact with hair, eyes, mucous membranes, carpeting, and fabrics.

ADVERSE REACTIONS: Erythema, peeling.

PREGNANCY: Category C, caution in nursing.

MECHANISM OF ACTION: Antibacterial/keratolytic agent; not established; demonstrated activity against *Propionibacterium acnes.* Has also shown to have a mild keratolytic effect.

PHARMACOKINETICS: Absorption: Absorbed by skin. **Metabolism:** Metabolized in skin to benzoic acid. **Elimination:** Urine (benzoate; metabolite).

BROMFED   RX
brompheniramine maleate - pseudoephedrine HCl (Muro)

OTHER BRAND NAMES: Bromfed-PD (Muro) - Bromfenex (Ethex) - Bromfenex-PD (Ethex)
THERAPEUTIC CLASS: Antihistamine/decongestant

INDICATIONS: Treatment of symptoms of seasonal and perennial allergic rhinitis, and vasomotor rhinitis, including nasal congestion.

DOSAGE: *Adults:* (12mg-120mg) 1 cap q12h. (6mg-60mg) 1-2 caps q12h. *Pediatrics:* ≥12 yrs: (12mg-120mg) 1 cap q12h. (6mg-60mg) 1-2 caps q12h. 6-11 yrs: (6mg-60mg) 1 cap q12h.

HOW SUPPLIED: (Brompheniramine-Pseudoephedrine) Cap, Extended-Release: (PD) 6mg- 60mg, (Bromfed, Bromfenex) 12mg-120mg

CONTRAINDICATIONS: Severe HTN, CAD, narrow-angle glaucoma, MAOI therapy, urinary retention, peptic ulcer, during an asthmatic attack.

WARNINGS/PRECAUTIONS: Caution with HTN, DM, ischemic heart disease, hyperthyroidism, increased IOP, prostatic hypertrophy, and elderly. Caution while operating machinery.

ADVERSE REACTIONS: Drowsiness, lassitude, nausea, giddiness, dryness of the mouth, blurred vision, palpitations, flushing, increased irritability or excitement.

INTERACTIONS: Potentiated by MAOIs and β-blockers. Reduced antihypertensive effects of methyldopa, mecamylamine, reserpine, and veratrum alkaloids. Additive effects with alcohol and other CNS depressants.

PREGNANCY: Safety in pregnancy and nursing not known.

MECHANISM OF ACTION: Brompheniramine: Histamine antagonist; specifically an H_1-receptor blocking agent, also has anticholinergic and sedative effects and antagonizes the allergic response of nasal tissues. Pseudoephedrine: Sympathomimetic; acts predominantly on α-receptor, has a little action on β-receptor. Functions as an oral nasal decongestant with minimal CNS stimulation.

BUPRENEX `CIII`
buprenorphine HCl (Reckitt Benckiser)

THERAPEUTIC CLASS: Opioid analgesic

INDICATIONS: Relief of moderate to severe pain.

DOSAGE: *Adults:* 0.3mg IM/IV q6h prn. Repeat if needed, 30-60 min after initial dose and then prn. High Risk Patients/Concomitant CNS depressants: Reduce dose by approximately 50%. May use single doses ≤0.6mg IM if not at high-risk. *Pediatrics:* ≥13 yrs: 0.3mg IM/IV q6h prn. Repeat if needed, 30-60 min after initial dose and then prn. High Risk Patients/Concomitant CNS depressants: Reduce dose by approximately 50%. May use single doses ≤0.6mg IM if not at high-risk. 2-12 yrs: 2-6mcg/kg IM/IV q4-6h.

HOW SUPPLIED: Inj: 0.3mg/mL

WARNINGS/PRECAUTIONS: Significant respiratory depression reported; caution with compromised respiratory function. May increase CSF pressure; caution with head injury, intracranial lesions. Caution with debilitated, BPH, biliary tract dysfunction, myxedema, hypothyroidism, urethral stricture, acute alcoholism, Addison's disease, CNS disease, coma, toxic psychoses, delirium tremens, elderly, pediatrics, kyphoscoliosis or hepatic/renal/pulmonary impairment. May impair mental or physical abilities. May precipitate withdrawal in narcotic-dependence. May lead to psychological dependence.

ADVERSE REACTIONS: Sedation, NV, dizziness, sweating, hypotension, headache, miosis, hypoventilation.

INTERACTIONS: Caution with MAOIs, CNS and respiratory depressants. Respiratory and cardiovascular collapse reported with diazepam. Increased CNS depression with other narcotic analgesics, general anesthetics, antihistamines, benzodiazepines, phenothiazines, other tranquilizers, sedative-hypnotics. Decreased clearance with CYP3A4 inhibitors (eg, macrolides, azole antifungals, protease inhibitors). Increased clearance with CYP3A4 inducers (eg, rifampin, carbamazepine, phenytoin).

PREGNANCY: Category C, not for use in nursing.

MECHANISM OF ACTION: Opioid analgesic; high affinity binding to µ opiate receptors in CNS. Possesses slow rate of dissociation from its receptor. Also possesses narcotic antagonist activity.

PHARMACOKINETICS: Absorption: $T_{max}=1$ hr. **Distribution:** Found in breast milk. **Metabolism:** Liver. **Elimination:** $T_{1/2}=1.2-7.2$ hrs.

CADUET

RX

amlodipine besylate - atorvastatin calcium (Pfizer)

THERAPEUTIC CLASS: Calcium channel blocker/HMG-CoA reductase inhibitor

INDICATIONS: When treatment with both amlodipine and atorvastatin is appropriate. (Amlodipine) Treatment of hypertension, chronic stable or vasospastic angina (Prinzmetal's or Variant Angina). (Atorvastatin) Adjunct to diet to reduce total cholesterol (total-C), LDL-C, TG, and Apo B levels, and to increase HDL-C in primary hypercholesterolemia (heterozygous familial and nonfamilial) and mixed dyslipidemia (Types IIa and IIb). Adjunct to diet for elevated serum TG levels (Type IV). Treatment of primary dysbetalipoproteinemia (Type III) inadequately responding to diet. Adjunct to other lipid-lowering treatments or if treatments are unavailable, to reduce total-C and LDL-C in homozygous familial hypercholesterolemia. Adjunct to diet to lower total-C, LDL-C and Apo B in boys and postmenarchal girls with heterozygous familial hypercholesterolemia.

DOSAGE: *Adults:* Dosing should be individualized and based on the appropriate combination of recommendations for the monotherapies. (Amlodipine): HTN: Initial: 5mg qd. Titrate over 7-14 days. Max: 10mg qd. Small, Fragile, or Elderly/Hepatic Dysfunction/ Concomitant Antihypertensive: Initial: 2.5mg qd. Angina: 5-10mg qd. Elderly/Hepatic Dysfunction: 5mg qd. (Atorvastatin): Hypercholesterolemia/Mixed Dyslipidemia: Initial: 10-20mg qd (or 40mg qd for LDL-C reduction >45%). Titrate: Adjust dose if needed at 2-4 week intervals. Usual: 10-80mg qd. Homozygous Familial Hypercholesterolemia: 10-80mg qd.
Pediatrics: ≥10 yrs (postmenarchal): (Amlodipine): HTN: 2.5-5mg qd. 10-17 yrs (postmenarchal): (Atorvastatin): Heterozygous Familial Hypercholesterolemia: Initial: 10mg/day. Titrate: Adjust dose if needed at intervals of ≥4 weeks. Max: 20mg/day.

HOW SUPPLIED: Tab: (Amlodipine-Atorvastatin) 2.5mg-10mg, 2.5mg-20mg, 2.5mg-40mg, 5mg-10mg, 5mg-20mg, 5mg-40mg, 5mg-80mg, 10mg-10mg, 10mg-20mg, 10mg-40mg, 10mg-80mg

CONTRAINDICATIONS: Active liver disease, unexplained persistent elevations of serum transaminases, pregnancy, nursing mothers.

WARNINGS/PRECAUTIONS: May rarely increase angina or MI with severe obstructive CAD. Monitor LFTs prior to therapy, at 12 weeks after initiation, with dose elevation, and periodically thereafter. Reduce dose or withdraw if AST or ALT >3x ULN persist. Caution with heavy alcohol use and/or history of hepatic disease, severe aortic stenosis, CHF. D/C if markedly elevated CPK levels occur, if myopathy is diagnosed or suspected, or if predisposition to renal failure secondary to rhabdomyolysis. Increased risk of hemorrhagic stroke in patients with recent stroke or TIA.

ADVERSE REACTIONS: Headache, edema, palpitation, dizziness, fatigue, constipation, flatulence, dyspepsia, abdominal pain.

INTERACTIONS: Increases levels with erythromycin. Increases levels of oral contraceptives (norethindrone, ethinyl estradiol), digoxin. Cyclosporine, fibric acid derivatives, niacin, erythromycin, azole antifungals may increase risk of myopathy. Caution with drugs that decrease levels or activity of endogenous steroid hormones (eg, ketoconazole, spironolactone, cimetidine). Decreased levels with Maalox TC, but LDL-C reduction not altered. Colestipol decreases levels when coadministered, but greater LDL-C reduction with coadministration than when each given alone. Avoid fibrates.

PREGNANCY: Category X, not for use in nursing

CAFCIT

RX

caffeine citrate (Mead Johnson)

THERAPEUTIC CLASS: Methylxanthine

INDICATIONS: Short-term treatment of apnea of prematurity in infants.

DOSAGE: *Pediatrics:* 28-<33 weeks: LD: 1mL/kg (20mg/kg) IV over 30 min. Maint: 0.25mL/kg (5mg/kg) IV over 30 min or PO q24h beginning 24 hrs after LD.

HOW SUPPLIED: Inj: 20mg/mL (3mL); Sol: 20mg/mL (3mL)

WARNINGS/PRECAUTIONS: Necrotizing enterocolitis, seizures reported. Rule out other possible causes of apnea before initiating therapy. Caution with CVD, seizure disorder, renal/hepatic impairment. Monitor baseline caffeine levels if previously exposed to theophylline.

ADVERSE REACTIONS: Feeding intolerance, sepsis, hemorrhage, necrotizing enterocolitis, gastritis, GI hemorrhage, DIC, acidosis, abnormal healing, dyspnea, cerebral hemorrhage, dyspnea, lung edema, dry skin, rash, skin breakdown, retinopathy of prematurity.

INTERACTIONS: Potential for interaction with CYP450 1A2 substrates, inducers, inhibitors. May need lower dose with cimetidine, ketoconazole. May need dose increase with phenobarbital, phenytoin.

PREGNANCY: Category C, safety in nursing not known.

MECHANISM OF ACTION: Bronchial smooth muscle relaxant, CNS stimulant, cardiac muscle stimulant, and diuretic. Preventing apnea in prematurity not established; believed it has been attributed to antagonism of adenosine receptors, both A_1 and A_2 subtypes.

PHARMACOKINETICS: Absorption: C_{max}=6-10mg/L, T_{max}=30 min-2 hrs. **Distribution:** V_d=0.8-0.9L/kg (infants), V_d=0.6L/kg (adults); plasma protein binding (approximately 36%); crosses placental barrier. **Metabolism:** Liver via CYP1A2. **Elimination:** Urine, (neonates) $T_{1/2}$=approximately 3-4 days, (86%) unchanged, (>9months, adults) $T_{1/2}$=5 hrs, (1%) unchanged.

CARBATROL   RX
carbamazepine (Shire)

> Serious and fatal dermatologic reactions, including toxic epidermal necrolysis (TEN), Stevens-Johnson syndrome (SJS) and presence of HLA-B*1502 allele reported. Aplastic anemia and agranulocytosis reported. Obtain complete pretreatment hematological testing as a baseline. D/C if evidence of bone marrow depression develops.

THERAPEUTIC CLASS: Carboxamide

INDICATIONS: Treatment of partial seizures with complex symptomatology, generalized tonic-clonic seizures, and mixed seizure patterns of these or other partial or generalized seizures. Treatment of trigeminal neuralgia pain.

DOSAGE: *Adults:* Epilepsy: Initial: 200mg bid. Titrate: May increase weekly by 200mg/day. Maint: 800-1200mg/day. Max: 1200mg/day. Trigeminal Neuralgia: Initial (Day 1): 200mg qd. Titrate: May increase by 200mg/day q12h. Maint: 400-800mg/day. Max: 1200mg/day. Re-evaluate every 3 months.
Pediatrics: Epilepsy: >12 yrs: Initial: 200mg bid. Titrate: May increase weekly by 200mg/day. Max: 12-15 yrs: 1000mg/day. >15 yrs: 1200mg/day. 6 months-12 yrs: May convert immediate-release dose ≥400mg/day to equal daily dose using bid regimen. Usual/Max: ≤35mg/kg/day.

HOW SUPPLIED: Cap, Extended-Release:100mg, 200mg, 300mg

CONTRAINDICATIONS: History of bone marrow depression, MAOI use within 14 days, sensitivity to TCAs.

WARNINGS/PRECAUTIONS: Toxic epidermal necrolysis (Lyell's syndrome), Stevens-Johnson syndrome (SJS), multi-organ hypersensitivity reactions, and presence of HLA-B*1502 reported. Caution with history of adverse hematologic reaction to any drug, increased IOP, the elderly, mixed seizure with atypical absence seizure. Fetal harm with pregnancy. May activate latent psychosis. Caution with cardiac, hepatic, or renal damage. Perform eye exam and monitor LFTs and renal function at baseline and periodically.

ADVERSE REACTIONS: Dizziness, drowsiness, unsteadiness, nausea, vomiting, bone marrow depression, rash, urticaria, hypersensitivity reactions, photosensitivity reactions, CHF, edema, HTN, hypotension.

INTERACTIONS: See Contraindications. Metabolism is inhibited by CYP3A4 inhibitors (eg, cimetidine, macrolides, etc.) and induced by CYP3A4 inducers (eg, rifampin, phenytoin, trazodone, etc.). Decreases oral contraceptive effectiveness. Increases plasma levels of clomipramine, phenytoin, and primidone. Decreases levels of APAP, alprazolam, clonazepam, clozapine, dicumarol, doxycycline, ethosuximide, haloperi-dol, methsuximide, phensuximide, phenytoin, theophylline, valproate, warfarin. Increased risk of neurotoxic side effects with lithium.

PREGNANCY: Category D, not for use in nursing.

MECHANISM OF ACTION: Carboxamide anticonvulsant; suspected to reduce polysyn-aptic responses and blocks post-tetanic potentiation.

PHARMACOKINETICS: Absorption: C_{max}=1.9mcg/mL (200mg); T_{max}=19 hrs (200mg). **Distribution:** Plasma protein binding (76%). **Metabolism:** Liver, via CYP3A4 to carbamazepine-10,11-epoxide (metabolite). **Elimination:** Urine (72%), feces (28%); $T_{1/2}$=35-40 hrs.

CARNITOR
levocarnitine (Sigma-Tau)

RX

OTHER BRAND NAME: Carnitor SF (Sigma-Tau)

THERAPEUTIC CLASS: Carnitine supplement

INDICATIONS: (Tab) Primary carnitine deficiency. (Inj/Tab) Acute and chronic treatment of inborn error of metabolism in secondary carnitine deficiency. (Inj) Prevention and treatment of carnitine deficiency in dialysis patients with end stage renal disease (ESRD).

DOSAGE: *Adults:* (Inj) Usual: 50mg/kg/day IV bolus or infusion. Max: 300mg/kg/day. Severe Metabolic Crisis: LD: 50mg/kg, then 50mg/kg over the next 24 hrs given q3-4h, and never less than q6h by infusion or IV injection. ESRD: Initial: 10-20mg/kg bolus into venous return line after dialysis. Adjust dose based on trough (pre-dialysis) levocarnitine levels. Can make downward dose adjustments the 3rd or 4th week of therapy. (Tab) 990mg PO bid-tid. (Sol) Initial: 1g/day. Usual: 1-3g/day per 50kg. Take after meals. May dissolve solution in fluids/liquid foods; drink slowly.
Pediatrics: (Inj) Usual: 50mg/kg/day IV bolus or infusion. Max: 300mg/kg/day. Severe Metabolic Crisis: LD: 50mg/kg, then 50mg/kg over the next 24 hrs given q3-4h, and never less than q6h by infusion or IV injection. ESRD: Initial: 10-20mg/kg bolus into venous return line after dialysis. Adjust dose based on trough (pre-dialysis) levocarnitine levels. Can make downward dose adjustments the 3rd or 4th week of therapy. (Sol/Tab) Infants/Children: Initial: 50mg/kg/day. Maint: 50-100mg/kg/day in divided doses. Max: 3g/day. Take after meals. May dissolve solution in fluids/liquid foods; drink slowly.

HOW SUPPLIED: Inj: 200mg/mL; Sol: 100mg/mL (118mL); Tab: 330mg; Sol: (Carnitor SF) 100mg/mL (118mL)

WARNINGS/PRECAUTIONS: Avoid long term, high oral dose therapy with severely compromised renal function or ESRD with dialysis. Monitor carnitine levels periodically.

ADVERSE REACTIONS: Nausea, vomiting, abdominal cramps, diarrhea, gastritis, seizures.

PREGNANCY: Category B, not for use in nursing.

MECHANISM OF ACTION: Carnitine supplement; facilitates long-chain fatty acid entry into cellular mitochondria, thereby delivering substrate for oxidation and subsequent energy production.

PHARMACOKINETICS: Absorption: Absolute bioavailability: 15.1% (Tab), 15.9% (Oral Sol); C_{max}=80µmol/L, T_{max}=3.3 hrs. **Distribution:** Not bound to plasma protein. **Metabolism:** Trimethylamine N-oxide and (hydrogen-3)-gamma-butyrobetaine (major metabolites). **Elimination:** Urine (approximately 4-8% of dose); feces (<1%, total drug); $T_{1/2}$=17.4 hrs.

CATHFLO ACTIVASE
alteplase (Genentech)

RX

THERAPEUTIC CLASS: Thrombolytic agent

INDICATIONS: To restore function to central venous access devices as assessed by ability to withdraw blood.

DOSAGE: *Adults:* ≥30kg: 2mg in 2mL. <30kg: 110% of catheter internal lumen volume, not to exceed 2mg in 2mL. If function not restored after 120 min, may instill 2nd dose. Max: 2mg/dose. Reconstitute to final concentration of 1mg/mL.

Pediatrics: ≥2 yrs: ≥30kg: 2mg in 2mL. 10 to <30kg: 110% of catheter internal lumen volume, not to exceed 2mg in 2mL. If function not restored after 120 min, may instill 2nd dose. Max: 2mg/dose. Reconstitute to final concentration of 1mg/mL.

HOW SUPPLIED: Inj: 2mg

WARNINGS/PRECAUTIONS: Before therapy, consider catheter dysfunction due to causes other than thrombus formation. Avoid excessive pressure when instilling alteplase into catheter. D/C and withdraw drug from catheter if serious bleeding in critical location occurs. Caution if active internal bleeding, infection in the catheter, any bleeding condition that is difficult to manage, thrombocytopenia, hemostatic defects, or if high risk for embolic complications. Caution if any of the following occurred within 48 hrs: surgery, OB delivery, percutaneous biopsy of viscera or deep tissues, or puncture of noncompressible vessels.

ADVERSE REACTIONS: Sepsis, GI bleeding, venous thrombosis.

PREGNANCY: Category C, caution in nursing.

MECHANISM OF ACTION: Thrombolytic agent; enzyme produces fibrin-enhanced conversion of plasminogen to plasmin. Produces limited conversion of plasminogen in the absence of fibrin. Binds to fibrin in thrombus and converts the entrapped plasminogen to plasmin, thereby initiating local fibrinolysis.

PHARMACOKINETICS: Metabolism: Liver. **Elimination:** $T_{1/2}$=5 min (initial); $T_{1/2}$=72 minutes (terminal).

Cᴇᴅᴀx
ceftibuten (Shionogi)

RX

THERAPEUTIC CLASS: Cephalosporin (3rd generation)

INDICATIONS: Acute bacterial exacerbations of chronic bronchitis (ABECB), acute bacterial otitis media, pharyngitis and tonsillitis.

DOSAGE: *Adults:* ABECB/Otitis Media/Pharyngitis/Tonsillitis: 400mg qd for 10 days. Max: 400mg/day. CrCl 30-49mL/min: 4.5mg/kg or 200mg qd. CrCl 5-29mL/min: 2.25mg/kg or 100mg qd. Take 2 hrs before or at least 1 hr after a meal.
Pediatrics: ≥6 months: Pharyngitis/Tonsillitis/Otitis Media: 9mg/kg qd for 10 days. Max: 400mg. ABECB/Otitis Media/Pharyngitis/Tonsillitis: ≥12 yrs: 400mg qd for 10 days. Max: 400mg/day. CrCl 30-49mL/min: 4.5mg/kg or 200mg qd. CrCl 5-29mL/min: 2.25mg/kg or 100mg qd. Take 2 hrs before or at least 1 hr after a meal.

HOW SUPPLIED: Cap: 400mg; Sus: 90mg/5mL (30mL, 60mL, 90mL, 120mL)

WARNINGS/PRECAUTIONS: Pseudomembranous colitis (toxin produced by *Clostridium difficile* is the primary cause) reported. Caution with history of GI disease. Cross-sensitivity with cephalosporins and penicillins.

ADVERSE REACTIONS: Diarrhea, NV, abdominal pain, anorexia, dizziness, dyspepsia, dry mouth, dyspnea, dysuria, fatigue, flatulence, loose stools, headache, pruritus, rash, rigors, urticaria, superinfection (prolonged use).

PREGNANCY: Category B, caution in nursing.

MECHANISM OF ACTION: 3rd generation cephalosporin; binds to essential target proteins of bacterial cell wall, leading to inhibition of cell-wall synthesis.

PHARMACOKINETICS: Absorption: Rapid. C_{max}=15.0(3.3)mcg/mL (Cap), 13.3mcg/mL (Sus). AUC=73.7mcg•hr/mL (Cap), 56.0mcg•hr/mL (Sus). T_{max}=2.6 hrs. (Cap), 2 hrs. (Sus). **Distribution:** Vd=0.21L/kg (Cap), 0.5L/kg (Sus); plasma protein binding (65%). **Metabolism:** Cis-ceftibuten (metabolite). **Elimination:** Urine (56%), feces (39%).

CᴇᴇNU
lomustine (Bristol-Myers Squibb)

RX

> **Bone-marrow suppression (eg, thrombocytopenia, leukopenia) may contribute to bleeding and infections in compromised patients. Monitor blood counts weekly for 6 weeks after each dose. Adjust dose based on nadir blood counts from prior dose.**

THERAPEUTIC CLASS: Nitrosourea alkylating agent

CEFACLOR

INDICATIONS: Single or adjunct treatment in primary/metastatic brain tumors in patients who already received surgical and/or radiation therapy. Secondary combination therapy of Hodgkin's disease in patients who relapse/fail primary therapy.

DOSAGE: *Adults:* Single Regimen/Previously Untreated: 130mg/m^2 PO single dose every 6 weeks. Compromised Bone Marrow: 100mg/m^2 PO single dose every 6 weeks. Subsequent Doses: Adjust according to hematologic response. Leukocytes 2000-2999, platelets 25,000-74,999: Give 70% of dose. Leukocytes <2000, platelets <25,000: Give 50% of dose.
Pediatrics: Single Regimen/Previously Untreated: 130mg/m^2 PO single dose every 6 weeks. Compromised Bone Marrow: 100mg/m^2 PO single dose every 6 weeks. Subsequent Doses: Adjust according to hematologic response. Leukocytes 2000-2999, platelets 25,000-74,999: Give 70% of dose. Leukocytes <2000, platelets <25,000: Give 50% of dose.

HOW SUPPLIED: Cap: 10mg, 40mg, 100mg

WARNINGS/PRECAUTIONS: Pulmonary toxicity is dose-related. May develop secondary malignancies with long-term use. Monitor hepatic and renal function. Caution in elderly.

ADVERSE REACTIONS: Delayed myleosuppression, pulmonary infiltrates/fibrosis, nausea, vomiting, hepatotoxicity, azotemia, renal failure, stomatitis, alopecia, optic atrophy, visual disturbances, lethargy, ataxia.

PREGNANCY: Category D, not for use in nursing.

MECHANISM OF ACTION: Nitrosourea alkylating agent; alkylates DNA and RNA. Inhibits several key enzymatic processes by carbamyolation of amino acids in proteins.

PHARMACOKINETICS: Elimination: Urine, T$_{1/2}$=16 hrs-2 days.

CEFACLOR
cefaclor (Various)

RX

THERAPEUTIC CLASS: Cephalosporin (2nd generation)

INDICATIONS: Treatment of otitis media, pharyngitis, tonsillitis, lower respiratory tract, urinary tract, and skin and skin structure infections caused by susceptible strains of microorganisms.

DOSAGE: *Adults:* Usual: 250mg q8h. Severe Infections/Pneumonia: 500mg q8h. Treat β-hemolytic strep for 10 days.
Pediatrics: ≥1 month: Usual: 20mg/kg/day given q8h. Otitis Media/Serious Infections/ Infections Caused by Less Susceptible Organisms: 40mg/kg/day. Max: 1g/day. May administer q12h for otitis media and pharyngitis. Treat β-hemolytic strep for 10 days.

HOW SUPPLIED: Cap: 250mg, 500mg; Sus: 125mg/5mL (75mL, 150mL), 187mg/5mL (50mL, 100mL), 250mg/5mL (75mL, 150mL), 375mg/5mL (50mL, 100mL)

WARNINGS/PRECAUTIONS: Cross-sensitivity to PCNs and other cephalosporins may occur. *Clostridium difficile*-associated diarrhea reported. Positive direct Coombs' test reported. Caution with markedly impaired renal function, history of GI disease. False (+) for urine glucose with Benedict's, Fehling's solution, and Clinitest tablets.

ADVERSE REACTIONS: Hypersensitivity reactions, diarrhea, eosinophilia, genital pruritus and vaginitis, serum-sickness-like reactions, superinfection.

INTERACTIONS: Renal excretion inhibited by probenecid. May potentiate warfarin and other anticoagulants; monitor PT/INR.

PREGNANCY: Category B, caution in nursing.

MECHANISM OF ACTION: Cephalosporin; bactericidal agent, inhibits cell-wall synthesis.

PHARMACOKINETICS: Absorption: Well-absorbed; (Fasting): C$_{max}$=7mcg/mL (250mg), 13mcg (500mg), 23mcg (1g); T$_{max}$=30-60 min. **Elimination:** Urine (60-85% unchanged); T$_{1/2}$= 0.6-0.9 hrs.

CEFACLOR ER

RX

cefaclor (Various)

THERAPEUTIC CLASS: Cephalosporin (2nd generation)

INDICATIONS: Treatment of acute bacterial exacerbation of chronic bronchitis (ABECB), secondary bacterial infections of acute bronchitis, pharyngitis, tonsillitis, and uncomplicated skin and skin structure infections (SSSI) caused by susceptible strains of microorganisms.

DOSAGE: *Adults:* ABECB/Acute Bronchitis: 500mg q12h for 7 days. Pharyngitis/Tonsillitis: 375mg q12h for 10 days. SSSI: 375mg q12h for 7-10 days. Take with meals. Do not crush, cut, or chew tab.
Pediatrics: ≥16 yrs: ABECB/Acute Bronchitis: 500mg q12h for 7 days. Pharyngitis/Tonsillitis: 375mg q12h for 10 days. SSSI: 375mg q12h for 7-10 days. Take with meals. Do not crush, cut, or chew tab.

HOW SUPPLIED: Tab, Extended-Release: 500mg

WARNINGS/PRECAUTIONS: Cross-sensitivity to PCNs and other cephalosporins may occur. *Clostridium difficile*-associated diarrhea reported. Positive direct Coombs' test reported. Caution with markedly impaired renal function, history of GI disease. False (+) for urine glucose with Benedict's, Fehling's solution, and Clinitest tablets.

ADVERSE REACTIONS: Headache, rhinitis, diarrhea, nausea, vaginitis, abdominal pain, pharyngitis, increased cough, pruritus, back pain, serum-sickness-like reactions, superinfection (prolonged use).

INTERACTIONS: Decreased absorption with aluminum or magnesium hydroxide-containing antacids; space dose by 1 hr. Potentiated by probenecid. May potentiate warfarin, and other anticoagulants; monitor PT/INR.

PREGNANCY: Category B, caution in nursing.

MECHANISM OF ACTION: Cephalosporin; bactericidal, inhibits cell-wall synthesis.

PHARMACOKINETICS: Absorption: Fed: (375mg) C_{max}=3.7mcg/ml, T_{max}=2.7 hr, AUC=9.9mcg•hr/mL. (500mg) C_{max}=4.2mcg/ml, T_{max}=2.5 hr, AUC=18.1mcg•hr/mL. Fasting: C_{max}=5.4, T_{max}=1.5 hrs, AUC=14.8mcg•hr/mL.

CEFADROXIL

RX

cefadroxil monohydrate (Various)

THERAPEUTIC CLASS: Cephalosporin (1st generation)

INDICATIONS: Treatment of skin and skin structure (SSSI) and urinary tract infections (UTI), pharyngitis, and tonsillitis caused by susceptible strains of microorganisms.

DOSAGE: *Adults:* Uncomplicated Lower UTI: 1-2g/day given qd or bid. Other UTI: 1g bid. SSSI: 1g qd or 500mg bid. Group A β-hemolytic Strep Pharyngitis/Tonsillitis: 1g qd or 500mg bid for 10 days. CrCl ≤50mL/min: Initial: 1g. Maint: CrCl 25-50mL/min: 500mg q12h; CrCl 10-25mL/min: 500mg q24h; CrCl 0-10mL/min: 500mg q36h.
Pediatrics: UTI/SSSI: 15mg/kg q12h. Pharyngitis/Tonsillitis/Impetigo: 30mg/kg qd or 15mg/kg q12h. Treat β-hemolytic strep infections for at least 10 days.

HOW SUPPLIED: Cap: 500mg; Sus: 250mg/5mL (100mL), 500mg/5mL (75mL, 100mL); Tab: 1g* *scored

WARNINGS/PRECAUTIONS: Caution with markedly impaired renal function, history of GI disease. Cross-sensitivity with cephalosporins and PCNs. False (+) direct Coombs' tests, colitis, and *Clostridium difficile*-associated diarrhea (CDAD) reported.

ADVERSE REACTIONS: Diarrhea, rash, hypersensitivity reactions, pruritus, hepatic dysfunction, genital moniliasis, vaginitis, fever, superinfection (prolonged use).

PREGNANCY: Category B, caution in nursing.

CEFAZOLIN RX
cefazolin (Various)

THERAPEUTIC CLASS: Cephalosporin (1st generation)

INDICATIONS: Treatment of respiratory tract, urinary tract (UTI), skin and skin structure, biliary tract, bone and joint, and genital infections, septicemia, and endocarditis caused by susceptible strains of microorganisms. Perioperative prophylaxis for surgical procedures classified as contaminated or potentially contaminated.

DOSAGE: *Adults:* Moderate-Severe Infections: 500mg-1g q6-8h. Mild Gram-Positive Cocci Infection: 250-500mg q8h. Acute, Uncomplicated UTI: 1g q12h. Pneumococcal Pneumonia: 500mg q12h. Severe Life-Threatening Infection (eg, Endocarditis, Septicemia): 1-1.5g q6h; Max: 12g/day (rare). Perioperative Prophylaxis: 1g IM/IV 0.5-1 hr before surgery. For Procedures ≥2 hrs: 500mg-1g IM/IV during surgery. Maint: 500mg-1g IM/IV q6-8h for 24 hrs post-op. Continue for 3-5 days post-op for devastating procedures (eg, open-heart surgery and prosthetic arthroplasty). Renal Impairment: CrCl 35-54mL/min: Full dose q8h. CrCl 11-34mL/min: 1/2 usual dose q12h. CrCl <10mL/min: 1/2 usual dose q18-24h. Apply reduced dosage recommendations after initial LD is given.
Pediatrics: Mild-Moderately Severe Infection: 25-50mg/kg/day in 3-4 equal doses. Severe Infection: 100mg/kg/day in divided doses. Renal Impairment: CrCl 40-70mL/min: 60% of normal daily dose in equally divided doses q12h. CrCl 20-40mL/min: 25% of normal daily dose in equally divided doses q12h. CrCl 5-20mL/min: 10% of normal daily dose q24h. Apply reduced dosage recommendations after initial LD is given.

HOW SUPPLIED: Inj: 500mg, 1g, 10g, 20g

WARNINGS/PRECAUTIONS: Prolonged use may result in overgrowth of nonsusceptible organisms. Possible cross-sensitivity between PCNs, cephalosporins, and other β-lactam antibiotics. Pseudomembranous colitis reported. Elevated levels with renal insufficiency can lead to seizures. Caution with colitis and other GI diseases. Safety in premature infants and neonates not established.

ADVERSE REACTIONS: Diarrhea, oral candidiasis, NV, stomach cramps, anorexia, allergic reactions, blood dyscrasias, renal failure, transient rise in SGOT/SGPT/BUN/SCr/alkaline phosphatase, local reactions.

INTERACTIONS: Decreased renal tubular secretion with probenecid.

PREGNANCY: Category B, caution in nursing.

MECHANISM OF ACTION: Cephalosporin; inhibits cell wall synthesis.

PHARMACOKINETICS: Absorption: C_{max}=185mcg/mL. **Distribution:** Crosses placenta; found in breast milk. **Elimination:** Urine (unchanged); $T_{1/2}$=1.8 hrs.

CEFIZOX RX
ceftizoxime (Astellas)

THERAPEUTIC CLASS: Cephalosporin (3rd generation)

INDICATIONS: Treatment of lower respiratory tract, skin and skin structure, intra-abdominal, bone and joint, and urinary tract infections (UTI), gonorrhea, pelvic inflammatory disease (PID), meningitis, and septicemia.

DOSAGE: *Adults:* Uncomplicated UTI: 500mg q12h IM/IV. Other Sites: 1g q8-12h IM/IV. Severe/Refractory Infections: 1-2g IM/IV q8-12h. PID: 2g IV q8h. Life Threatening Infections: 3-4g IV q8h. Uncomplicated Gonorrhea: 1g IM as single dose. Renal Impairment: LD: 500mg-1g IM/IV. Less Severe Infection: Maint: CrCl 50-79mL/min: 500mg q8h. CrCl 5-49mL/min: 250-500mg q12h. CrCl 0-4mL/min (Dialysis): 500mg q48h or 250mg q24h. Life-Threatening Infection: Maint: CrCl 50-79mL/min: 0.75-1.5g q8h. CrCl 5-49mL/min: 0.5-1g q12h. CrCl 0-4mL/min (Dialysis): 0.5-1g q48h or 0.5g q24h.
Pediatrics: ≥6 months: 50mg/kg IM/IV q6-8h, up to 200mg/kg/day. Max: 6g/day for serious infections.

HOW SUPPLIED: Inj: 500mg, 1g, 2g

WARNINGS/PRECAUTIONS: *Clostridium difficile*-associated diarrhea reported. Caution with history of GI disease. Cross-sensitivity with cephalosporins and PCNs may occur. Prolonged use may result in overgrowth of superinfection, (+) Coombs' test.

ADVERSE REACTIONS: Rash, pruritus, fever, BUN elevation, injection site reactions (eg, burning, cellulitis, phlebitis, pain, induration, tenderness), eosinophilia, thrombocytosis, elevated liver enzymes, GI effects.

INTERACTIONS: Risk of nephrotoxicity with aminoglycosides and other cephalosporins.

PREGNANCY: Category B, caution in nursing.

MECHANISM OF ACTION: 3rd-generation cephalosporin; inhibits cell wall systhesis.

PHARMACOKINETICS: Absorption: IV administration of variable doses resulted in different parameters. **Distribution:** Plasma protein binding (30%); found in various bodily fluids and tissues and breast milk; CSF only if meninges inflamed. **Elimination:** Urine (unchanged); $T_{1/2}$=1.7 hrs.

CEFOXITIN RX
cefoxitin sodium (Various)

OTHER BRAND NAME: Mefoxin (Merck)

THERAPEUTIC CLASS: Cephalosporin (2nd generation)

INDICATIONS: Treatment of lower respiratory tract, urinary tract, intra-abdominal, gyne-cological, skin and skin structure, and bone and joint infections, and septicemia caused by susceptible strains of microorganisms. Prophylaxis of infection in patients undergoing uncontaminated GI surgery, abdominal/vaginal hysterectomy, or cesarean section.

DOSAGE: *Adults:* Usual: 1-2g IV q6-8h. Uncomplicated Infections: 1g IV q6-8h. Moderate-Severe: 1g IV q4h or 2g IV q6-8h. Gas Gangrene/Other Infections Requiring Higher Dose: 2g IV q4h or 3g IV q6h. Renal Insufficiency: LD: 1-2g IV. Maint: CrCl 30-50mL/min: 1-2g IV q8-12h. CrCl 10-29mL/min: 1-2g IV q12-24h. CrCl 5-9mL/min: 0.5-1g IV q12-24h. CrCl <5mL/min: 0.5-1g IV q24-48h. Hemodialysis: LD: 1-2g IV after dialysis. Maint: See renal insufficiency doses above. Prophylaxis: Uncontaminated GI Surgery/Hysterectomy: 2g IV 0.5-1 hr prior to surgery (1/2-1 hr before initial incision), then 2g IV q6h after 1st dose up to 24 hrs. C-Section: 2g IV single dose as soon as umbilical cord is clamped, or 2g IV as soon as umbilical cord is clamped, followed by 2g IV at 4 and 8 hrs after initial dose.
Pediatrics: ≥3 months: 80-160mg/kg/day divided into 4-6 equal doses. Max: 12g/day. Prophylaxis: Uncontaminated GI Surgery/Hysterectomy: 30-40mg/kg IV 0.5-1 hr prior to surgery, then 30-40mg/kg IV q6h after first dose for up to 24 hrs.

HOW SUPPLIED: Inj: 1g, 1g/50mL, 2g, 2g/50mL, 10g

WARNINGS/PRECAUTIONS: Possible cross-sensitivity between PCNs and cephalosporins. *Clostridium difficile*-associated diarrhea reported. Caution with allergies, GI disease, particularly colitis. Prolonged use may result in overgrowth of nonsusceptible organisms. Monitor renal, hepatic, hematopoietic functions, especially with prolonged therapy. False (+) for urine glucose with Clinitest tabs.

ADVERSE REACTIONS: Thrombophlebitis, rash, pseudomembranous colitis, pruritus, fever, dyspnea, hypotension, diarrhea, blood dyscrasias, elevated LFTs, changes in renal function tests, exacerbation of myasthenia gravis.

INTERACTIONS: Increased nephrotoxicity with concomitant aminoglycosides.

PREGNANCY: Category B, caution use in nursing.

MECHANISM OF ACTION: 2nd generation cephalosporin; inhibits bacterial cell-wall syn-thesis.

PHARMACOKINETICS: Metabolism: Passes pleural and joint fluids; found in bile and breast milk. **Elimination:** Urine (85% unchanged); $T_{1/2}$=41-59 min.

CEFTAZIDIME RX
ceftazidime (Various)

THERAPEUTIC CLASS: Cephalosporin (3rd generation)

INDICATIONS: Treatment of lower respiratory tract (eg, pneumonia), skin and skin struc-ture (SSSI), bone and joint, gynecologic, CNS (eg, meningitis), intra-abdominal, and uri-nary tract infections (UTI), and septicemia caused by susceptible strains of microorganisms. For use in sepsis.

DOSAGE: *Adults:* Usual: 1g IM/IV q8-12h. Uncomplicated UTI: 250mg IM/IV q12h. Complicated UTI: 500mg IM/IV q8-12h. Bone and Joint Infection: 2g IV q12h. Uncomplicated Pneumonia/SSSI: 500mg-1g IM/IV q8h. Gynecological/Intra-Abdominal/Meningitis/ Severe Life-Threatening Infection: 2g IV q8h. Lung Infection caused by Pseudomonas spp. in Cystic Fibrosis (normal renal function): 30-50mg/kg IV q8h. Max: 6g/day. CrCl 31-50mL/min: 1g q12h. CrCl 16-30mL/min: 1g q24h. CrCl 6-15mL/min: 500mg q24h. CrCl <5mL/min: 500mg q48h. For severe infections (6g/day), increase renal impairment dose by 50% or increase dosing interval. Apply reduced dosage recommendations after initial 1g LD is given. Hemodialysis: Give 1g before then 1g after each hemodialysis. Intra-Peritoneal Dialysis/Continuous Ambulatory Peritoneal Dialysis: Give 1g followed by 500mg q24h.

Pediatrics: ≥12 yrs: Usual: 1g IM/IV q8-12h. Uncomplicated UTI: 250mg IM/IV q12h. Complicated UTI: 500mg IM/IV q8-12h. Bone and Joint Infection: 2g IV q12h. Uncomplicated Pneumonia/SSSI: 500mg-1g IM/IV q8h. Gynecological/Intra-Abdominal/Meningitis/ Severe Life-Threatening Infection: 2g IV q8h. Lung Infection caused by Pseudomonas spp. in Cystic Fibrosis (normal renal function): 30-50mg/kg IV q8h. Max: 6g/day. CrCl 31-50mL/min: 1g q12h. CrCl 16-30mL/min: 1g q24h. CrCl 6-15mL/min: 500mg q24h. CrCl <5mL/min: 500mg q48h. For severe infections (6g/day), increase renal impairment dose by 50% or increase dosing interval. Apply reduced dosage recommendations after initial 1g LD is given. Hemodialysis: Give 1g before then 1g after each hemodialysis. Intra-Peritoneal Dialysis/Continuous Ambulatory Peritoneal Dialysis: Give 1g followed by 500mg q24h.

HOW SUPPLIED: Inj: 1g, 2g, 6g

WARNINGS/PRECAUTIONS: Monitor renal function; potential for nephrotoxicity. Prolonged use may result in overgrowth of nonsusceptible organisms. Possible cross-sensitivity between PCNs, cephalosporins, and other β-lactam antibiotics. Pseudomembranous colitis reported. Elevated levels with renal insufficiency can lead to seizures, encephalopathy, asterixis, coma, and neuromuscular excitability. Possible decrease in PT; caution with renal or hepatic impairment, poor nutritional state; monitor PT and give vitamin K if needed. Caution with colitis and other GI diseases. Distal necrosis can occur after inadvertent intra-arterial administration. Continue therapy for 2 days after the signs and symptoms of infection have disappeared, but in complicated infections longer therapy may be required. False positive for urine glucose with Benedict's, Fehling's solution, and Clinitest® tablets.

ADVERSE REACTIONS: Phlebitis and inflammation at injection site, pruritus, rash, fever, diarrhea.

INTERACTIONS: Nephrotoxicity reported with aminoglycosides or potent diuretics (eg, furosemide). Avoid with chloramphenicol; may decrease effect of β-lactam antibiotics.

PREGNANCY: Category B, not for use in nursing.

MECHANISM OF ACTION: Broad spectrum, β-lactam antibiotic; exerts effects by inhibiting enzymes responsible for cell-wall synthesis.

PHARMACOKINETICS: Absorption: (IV) C_{max}=45mcg/mL (500mg), 90mcg/mL (1g). (IM) C_{max}=17mcg/mL (500mg), 39mcg/mL (1g), T_{max}=1 hr. **Distribution:** Plasma protein binding (<10%); found in breast milk. **Elimination:** Urine, (80-90% unchanged). $T_{1/2}$=1.9 hrs (IV), 2 hrs (IM).

CEFTIN   RX
cefuroxime axetil (GlaxoSmithKline)

THERAPEUTIC CLASS: Cephalosporin (2nd generation)

INDICATIONS: Treatment of the following infections caused by susceptible strains of microorganisms: (Sus/Tab) Pharyngitis/tonsillitis, acute otitis media, and impetigo. (Tab) Uncomplicated skin and skin structure (SSSI), and urinary tract infection (UTI), gonorrhea, early Lyme disease, acute bacterial maxillary sinusitis, acute bacterial exacerbations of chronic bronchitis (ABECB) and secondary bacterial infections of acute bronchitis.

DOSAGE: *Adults:* (Tab) Pharyngitis/Tonsillitis/Sinusitis: 250mg bid for 10 days. ABECB/SSSI: 250-500mg bid for 10 days. Acute Bronchitis: 250-500mg bid for 5-10 days. UTI: 250mg bid for 7-10 days. Gonorrhea: 1000mg single dose. Lyme Disease: 500mg bid for 20 days.

Pediatrics: ≥13 yrs: (Tab) Pharyngitis/Tonsillitis/Sinusitis: 250mg bid for 10 days. ABECB/ SSSI: 250-500mg bid for 10 days. Acute Bronchitis: 250-500mg bid for 5-10 days. UTI: 250mg bid for 7-10 days. Gonorrhea: 1000mg single dose. Lyme Disease: 500mg bid for 20 days. 3 months-12 yrs: (Sus) Pharyngitis/Tonsillitis: 10mg/kg bid for 10 days. Max: 500mg/day. Otitis Media/Sinusitis/Impetigo: 15mg/kg bid for 10 days. Max: 1000mg/ day. (Tab-if can swallow whole) Otitis Media/Sinusitis: 250mg bid for 10 days.

HOW SUPPLIED: Sus: 125mg/5mL (100mL), 250mg/5mL (50mL, 100mL); Tab: 250mg, 500mg

WARNINGS/PRECAUTIONS: Tabs are not bioequivalent to sus. Caution with colitis, renal impairment. Cross-sensitivity with cephalosporins and PCNs. False (+) for urine glucose with Benedict's, Fehling's solution, and Clinitest® tablets. May cause fall in PT; risk in patients stable on anticoagulants, if receiving protracted course of antibiotics, renal/ hepatic impairment, or a poor nutritional state; give vitamin K as needed. Watery, bloody stools (with or without stomach cramps and fever) may develop after starting treatment; notify physician. *Clostridium difficile*-associated diarrhea (CDAD) reported.

ADVERSE REACTIONS: Diarrhea, NV, vaginitis, (suspension in peds) taste aversion, super-infection (prolonged use).

INTERACTIONS: Probenecid increases plasma levels. Lower bioavailability with drugs that lower gastric acidity. Caution with agents causing adverse effects on renal function (diuretics). Reduced efficacy of combined oral estrogen/progesterone contraceptives.

PREGNANCY: Category B, not for use in nursing.

MECHANISM OF ACTION: 2nd-generation cephalosporin; binds to essential target proteins and inhibits cell-wall synthesis.

PHARMACOKINETICS: Absorption: Absolute bioavailability (52% with food). PO administration of variable doses resulted in different parameters. **Distribution:** Plasma protein binding (50%). **Metabolism:** Rapid hydrolysis, via nonspecific esterases in the intestinal mucosa and blood. **Elimination:** Urine (50% unchanged).

CEFZIL   RX
cefprozil (Bristol-Myers Squibb)

THERAPEUTIC CLASS: Cephalosporin (2nd generation)

INDICATIONS: Treatment of mild to moderate pharyngitis/tonsillitis, otitis media, acute sinusitis, secondary bacterial infection of acute bronchitis, acute bacterial exacerbation of chronic bronchitis (ABECB), and uncomplicated skin and skin structure infections (SSSI) caused by susceptible strains of microorganisms.

DOSAGE: *Adults:* Pharyngitis/Tonsillitis: 500mg q24h for 10 days. Acute Sinusitis: 250-500mg q12h for 10 days. ABECB/Acute Bronchitis: 500mg q12h for 10 days. SSSI: 250-500mg q12h or 500mg q24h for 10 days. CrCl <30mL/min: 50% of standard dose. *Pediatrics:* ≥13 yrs: Use adult dose. 2-12 yrs: Pharyngitis/Tonsillitis: 7.5mg/kg q12h for 10 days. SSSI: 20mg/kg q24h for 10 days. 6 months-12 yrs: Otitis Media: 15mg/kg q12h for 10 days. Acute Sinusitis: 7.5-15mg/kg q12h for 10 days. Do not exceed adult dose. CrCl <30mL/min: 50% of standard dose.

HOW SUPPLIED: Sus: 125mg/5mL (50mL, 75mL, 100mL), 250mg/5mL (50mL, 75mL, 100mL); Tab: 250mg, 500mg

WARNINGS/PRECAUTIONS: Cross-sensitivity with cephalosporins and PCNs. False (+) direct Coombs' tests reported. *Clostridium difficile*-associated diarrhea reported. Caution with GI disease, renal impairment, elderly. False (+) for urine glucose with Benedict's, Fehling's solution, and Clinitest tablets. Sus contains phenylalanine.

ADVERSE REACTIONS: Diarrhea, nausea, hepatic enzyme elevations, eosinophilia, genital pruritus, vaginitis, superinfection (prolonged use).

INTERACTIONS: Nephrotoxicity with aminoglycosides reported. Probenecid may increase plasma levels. Caution with agents causing adverse effects on renal function (diuretics).

PREGNANCY: Category B, caution in nursing.

MECHANISM OF ACTION: 2nd-generation cephalosporin; inhibits bacterial cell-wall synthesis.

PHARMACOKINETICS: Absorption: C_{max}=6.1mcg/mL (250mg), 10.5mcg/mL (500mg), 18.3mcg/mL(1g); T_{max}=1.5 hrs (adults), 1-2 hrs (peds). Plasma concentration (peds) at 7.5, 15, and 30mg/kg doses similar to those observed within same time frame in normal adults at 250, 500, and 1000mg doses, respectively. **Distribution:** V_d=0.23L/kg; plasma protein binding (36%); found in breast milk. **Elimination:** Urine (60%); $T_{1/2}$=1.3 hrs (adults), 1.5 hrs (peds).

CELEBREX RX

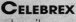
celecoxib (G.D. Searle)

> NSAIDs may cause an increased risk of serious cardiovascular thrombotic events, MI, stroke and serious GI adverse events including bleeding, ulceration, and perforation of the stomach or intestines. Contraindicated for the treatment of perioperative pain in the setting of coronary artery bypass graft (CABG) surgery.

THERAPEUTIC CLASS: COX-2 inhibitor

INDICATIONS: Relief of signs and symtoms of rheumatoid arthritis (RA) in adults, osteoarthritis (OA), and ankylosing spondylitis (AS). Management of acute pain in adults. Treatment of primary dysmenorrhea. To reduce the number of adematous colorectal polyps in familial adenomatous polyposis (FAP). Relief of signs and symptoms of juvenile rheumatoid arthritis (JRA) in patients ≥2 yrs.

DOSAGE: *Adults:* ≥18 yrs: OA: 200mg qd or 100mg bid. RA: 100-200mg bid. AS: 200mg qd or 100mg bid. Titrate: May increase to 400mg/day after 6 weeks. FAP: 400mg bid with food. Acute Pain/Primary Dysmenorrhea: Day 1: 400mg, then 200mg if needed. Maint: 200mg bid prn. Moderate Hepatic Insufficiency: Reduce daily dose by 50%. *Pediatrics:* JRA: ≥2 yrs: 10-25kg: 50mg bid. >25kg: 100mg bid.

HOW SUPPLIED: Cap: 50mg, 100mg, 200mg, 400mg

CONTRAINDICATIONS: Sulfonamide hypersensitivity. Asthma, urticaria, or allergic type reactions after ASA or NSAID use. Treatment of perioperative pain in the setting of CABG surgery.

WARNINGS/PRECAUTIONS: Increased risk of serious adverse cardiovascular thrombotic events, MI, and stroke. May lead to onset of new HTN or worsening of pre-existing HTN; monitor BP closely. Fluid retention and edema reported; caution with fluid retention or heart failure. Renal papillary necrosis and other renal injury reported after long-term use. Not recommended for use with advanced renal disease; if therapy must be initiated, monitor renal function. Greatest risk with those taking diuretics and ACE-inhibitors. Anaphylactoid reactions may occur. May cause serious skin adverse events (eg, exfoliative dermatitis, Stevens-Johnson syndrome, and toxic epidermal necrolysis). Avoid in late pregnancy; may cause premature closure of ductus arteriosus. May cause elevations of LFTs; d/c if liver disease develops or systemic manifestations occur. Caution in elderly. Anemia may occur; with long-term use, monitor Hgb/Hct if signs or symptoms of anemia or blood loss develop. May inhibit platelet aggregation and prolong bleeding time (prolonged APTT); monitor with coagulation disorders. Caution with asthma and avoid with ASA-sensitive asthma. Caution in pediatric patients with systemic onset JRA due to increased possibly of DIC.

ADVERSE REACTIONS: Dyspepsia, diarrhea, abdominal pain, nausea, dizziness, headache, sinusitis, upper respiratory infection, rash, fever, cough, arthralgia, HTN, insomnia, pharyngitis.

INTERACTIONS: Monitor oral anticoagulants; reports of serious bleeding, some fatal, with warfarin. Decrease effects of ACE-inhibitors, furosemide, and thiazides. Increased levels with fluconazole. Monitor lithium. Caution with CYP2C9 inhibitors and drugs metabolized by CYP2D6. Celecoxib is not a substitute for ASA for cardiovascular prophylaxis; may use with low-dose ASA but may increase GI complications.

PREGNANCY: Category C, not for use in nursing.

MECHANISM OF ACTION: NSAID; inhibits prostaglandin synthesis primarily via inhibition of COX-2.

PHARMACOKINETICS: Absorption: C_{max}=705ng/mL, T_{max}=2.8 hrs. **Distribution:** V_d=429L; plasma protein binding (97%). **Metabolism:** CYP2C9. Primary alcohol, carboxylic acid, glucuronide conjugate (metabolites). **Elimination:** Urine (27%), feces (57%); $T_{1/2}$=11.2 hrs.

CELESTONE
betamethasone (Schering)

RX

THERAPEUTIC CLASS: Glucocorticoid

INDICATIONS: Steroid responsive disorders.

DOSAGE: *Adults:* Initial: 0.6-7.2mg/day depending on disease. Maintain until sufficient response. Maint: Decrease dose by small amounts to lowest effective dose. D/C gradually.
Pediatrics: Initial: 0.6-7.2mg/day depending on disease. Maintain until sufficient response. Maint: Decrease dose by small amounts to lowest effective dose. D/C gradually.

HOW SUPPLIED: Syrup: 0.6mg/5mL (118mL)

CONTRAINDICATIONS: Systemic fungal infections.

WARNINGS/PRECAUTIONS: May need to increase dose before, during, and after stressful situations. May mask signs of infection or cause new infections. Prolonged use may produce posterior subcapsular cataracts, glaucoma, optic nerve damage, secondary ocular infections. Increases BP, salt/water retention, potassium and calcium excretion. More severe/fatal course of infections reported with chickenpox, measles. Caution with threadworm infestation, latent TB, hypothyroidism, cirrhosis, ocular herpes simplex, HTN, diverticulitis, fresh intestinal anastomosis, ulcerative colitis, osteoporosis, myasthenia gravis, renal insufficiency, peptic ulcer disease. Growth and development of children on prolonged therapy should be monitored. Monitor for psychic disturbances. Avoid abrupt withdrawal.

ADVERSE REACTIONS: Sodium retention, fluid retention, potassium loss, muscle weakness, myopathy, peptic ulcer, impaired wound healing, thin fragile skin, convulsions, menstrual irregularities, cataracts.

INTERACTIONS: Caution with ASA in hypoprothrombinemia. Increased susceptibility to infections with immunosuppressives. Avoid smallpox vaccines and other immunization procedures at high doses. Increased requirements of insulin or oral hypoglycemic agents.

PREGNANCY: Safety in pregnancy and nursing not known.

MECHANISM OF ACTION: Glucocorticoid; has16β-methyl group that enhaces anti-inflammatory action and reduces sodium- and water-retaining properties of fluorine atom bound at carbon 9.

PHARMACOKINETICS: Absorption: Readily absorbed. **Distribution:** Found in breast milk. **Metabolism:** Liver.

CELESTONE SOLUSPAN
betamethasone (augmented) sodium phosphate - betamethasone acetate
(Schering)

RX

THERAPEUTIC CLASS: Glucocorticoid

INDICATIONS: When oral therapy is not feasible, use IM route for steroid-responsive treatment of endocrine, rheumatic, collagen, dermatologic, respiratory, ophthalmic, neoplastic, hematologic, and GI disorders, allergic and edematous states and Tuberculous meningitis with subarachnoid block and trichinosis with neurologic/myocardial involvement. Intra-articular or soft tissue administration for short-term adjunct treatment of synovitis, osteoarthritis (OA), rheumatoid arthritis (RA), bursitis, acute gouty arthritis, epicondylitis, acute nonspecific tenosynovitis. Intralesional injection for keloids, discoid lupus erythematosus, necrobiosis lipoidica diabeticorum, alopecia areata, lesions of: lichen planus, psoriatic plaques, granuloma, annulare, lichen simplex chronicus.

DOSAGE: *Adults:* Initial: 0.5-9mg/day IM. Parenteral dose is usually 1/2-1/3 the oral dose given q12h. Maintain until sufficient response occurs. Maint: Decrease in small increments at appropriate time intervals until lowest effective dose. D/C gradually. Bursitis/Tenosynovitis/Peritendinitis: 1mL intrabursal injection. Tenosynovitis/Tendinitis: Give 3-4 injections every 1-2 weeks. Chronic Bursitis: Reduce initial dose. Ganglion Cysts: 0.5mL into cyst. RA/OA: 0.5-2mL intra-articularly. Dermatologic Conditions: 0.2mL/sq cm intradermally. Max: 1mL/week.

Pediatrics: Initial: 0.5-9mg/day IM. Parenteral dose is usually 1/2-1/3 the oral dose given q12h. Maintain until sufficient response. Maint: Decrease in small increments at appropriate time intervals until reach lowest dose that sustains response. D/C gradually.

HOW SUPPLIED: Inj: (Betamethasone Acetate-Betamethasone Sodium Phosphate) 3mg-3mg/mL

CONTRAINDICATIONS: Systemic fungal infections.

WARNINGS/PRECAUTIONS: May need to increase dose before, during, and after stressful situations. May mask signs of infection or cause new infections. Prolonged use may produce posterior subcapsular cataracts, glaucoma, optic nerve damage, secondary ocular infections. Increases BP, salt/water retention, potassium and calcium excretion. More severe/fatal course of infections reported with chickenpox, measles. Caution with threadworm infestation, latent TB, hypothyroidism, cirrhosis, ocular herpes simplex, HTN, diverticulitis, fresh intestinal anastomosis, ulcerative colitis, osteoporosis, myasthenia gravis, renal insufficiency, peptic ulcer disease. Growth and development of children on prolonged therapy should be monitored. Monitor for psychic disturbances. Avoid abrupt withdrawal. (Intra-articular) Examine joint fluid to rule out a septic process. Avoid injection into previously infected joint.

ADVERSE REACTIONS: Sodium retention, fluid retention, potassium loss, muscle weakness, myopathy, peptic ulcer, impaired wound healing, thin fragile skin, convulsions, menstrual irregularities, cataracts.

INTERACTIONS: Caution with ASA in hypoprothrombinemia. Increased susceptibility to infections with immunosuppressives. Avoid smallpox vaccines and other immunization procedures at high doses. Increased requirements of insulin or oral hypoglycemic agents. Avoid diluents containing methylparaben, phenol, propylparaben; may cause flocculation of steroid.

PREGNANCY: Safety in pregnancy and nursing not known.

MECHANISM OF ACTION: Glucocorticoid; has 16β-methyl group that enhances anti-inflammatory action and reduces sodium- and water-retaining properties of flourine atom bound at carbon 9.

PHARMACOKINETICS: Absorption: GI tract (Readily absorbed). **Distribution:** Found in breast milk. **Metabolism:** Liver.

CELLCEPT   RX
mycophenolate mofetil (Roche Labs)

> Immunosuppression may lead to increased susceptibility to infection and possible development of lymphoma. Female users of childbearing potential must use contraception. Use of CellCept during pregnancy is associated with increased risk of pregnancy loss and congenital malformations.

THERAPEUTIC CLASS: Inosine monophosphate dehydrogenase inhibitor

INDICATIONS: Prophylaxis of organ rejection in allogeneic renal, cardiac, or hepatic transplants. Use with cyclosporine and corticosteroids.

DOSAGE: *Adults:* Renal Transplant: 1g IV/PO bid. Cardiac Transplant: 1.5g IV/PO bid. Hepatic Transplant: 1g IV bid or 1.5g PO bid. Start PO as soon as possible after transplant. Start IV within 24 hrs after transplant; can continue for up to 14 days. Switch to oral when tolerated. Give on an empty stomach.
Pediatrics: Renal Transplant: (Sus) 600mg/m^2 PO bid. Max: 2g/day (10 mL/day). (Cap) BSA 1.25m^2 to 1.5m^2: 750mg PO bid. (Cap/Tab) BSA >1.5m^2: 1g bid.

HOW SUPPLIED: Cap: 250mg; Inj: 500mg; Sus: 200mg/mL (175mL); Tab: 500mg

CONTRAINDICATIONS: (Inj) Hypersensitivity to Polysorbate 80 (TWEEN).

WARNINGS/PRECAUTIONS: Risk of lymphomas and other malignancies, especially of the skin. Avoid sunlight to decrease risk of skin cancer. May cause fetal harm during pregnancy. Must have negative serum/urine pregnancy test within 1 week before therapy. Two reliable forms of contraception required before and during therapy, and 6 weeks following discontinuation. Monitor for bone marrow suppression. Risk of GI ulceration, hemorrhage, and perforation; caution with active digestive system disease. Caution with delayed renal graft function post-transplant. Oral suspension contains phenylalanine; caution with phenylketonurics. Monitor CBC weekly during the 1st month, twice monthly for the 2nd and 3rd months, and then monthly through 1st year. Avoid with rare hereditary deficiency of hypoxanthine-guanine phosphoribosyl-transferase (eg, Lesch-Nyhan and Kelley-Seegmiller syndrome). Increased susceptibility infections/ sepsis.

ADVERSE REACTIONS: Infections, diarrhea, leukopenia, sepsis, vomiting, GI bleeding, pain, abdominal pain, fever, headache, asthenia, chest pain, back pain, anemia, leukopenia, thrombocytopenia.

INTERACTIONS: Additive bone marrow suppression with azathioprine; avoid use. Reduced efficacy with drugs that interfere with enterohepatic recirculation (eg, cholestyramine). Efficacy/safety with other immunosuppressive agents not determined. Avoid live attenuated vaccines. Increased levels of both drugs with acyclovir, ganciclovir. Decreased levels with magnesium- and aluminum-containing antacids; space dosing. Decreased effects of oral contraceptives. Increased levels with probenecid. Other drugs that compete for renal tubular secretion may raise levels of both drugs.

PREGNANCY: Category D, not for use in nursing.

MECHANISM OF ACTION: Prolongs the survival of allogeneic transplants (kidney, heart, liver, intestine, limb, small bowel, pancreatic islets, and bone marrow). Inhibits proliferative arteriopathy in experimental models of aortic and cardiac allografts in rats as well as in primate cardiac xenografts. Inhibits immunologically mediated inflammatory responses and tumor development and prolongs survival in tumor transplant models.

PHARMACOKINETICS: Absorption: Oral; rapid and complete, absolute bioavailability (94%). MPA C_{max} decreased by 40% with food. **Distribution:** V_d=3.6L/kg (IV), 4L/kg (oral); plasma protein binding of MPA (97%), MPAG (82%). **Metabolism:** MPA (active metabolite) metabolized by glucuronyl transferase to MPAG, which is converted to MPA via entrohepatic recirculation. **Elimination:** Oral: Urine (93%), feces (6%). Urine: MPA (<1%) and MPAG (87%). MPA: (Oral) $T_{1/2}$=17.9 hrs. (Oral) and (IV) $T_{1/2}$=16.6 hrs. In pediatrics: Oral administarion in different age groups ranging between 1-18 years results in different pharmacokinetics.

CELONTIN   RX
methsuximide (Parke-Davis)

THERAPEUTIC CLASS: Succinimide

INDICATIONS: Management of absence (petit mal) seizures refractory to other drugs.

DOSAGE: *Adults:* Initial: 300mg qd for 7 days. Titrate: Increase weekly by 300mg/day for 3 weeks if needed. Max: 1.2g/day.
Pediatrics: Initial: 300mg qd for 7 days. Titrate: Increase weekly by 300mg/day 3 weeks if needed. Max: 1.2g/day. Use 150mg caps in small children.

HOW SUPPLIED: Cap: 150mg, 300mg

WARNINGS/PRECAUTIONS: Fatal blood dyscrasias reported; monitor blood counts periodically or if signs of infection. SLE reported. Withdraw slowly if altered behavior appears. May increase frequency of grand mal seizures if given alone in mixed type of seizures. Avoid abrupt withdrawal. Caution with renal/hepatic disease. May impair mental/physical abilities.

ADVERSE REACTIONS: GI effects, blood dyscrasias, dermatologic manifestations, drowsiness, ataxia, dizziness, hyperemia, proteinuria, periorbital edema.

INTERACTIONS: May interact with other anticonvulsants; monitor serum levels periodically.

PREGNANCY: Safety in pregnancy and nursing not known.

MECHANISM OF ACTION: Anticonvulsant succinamide; supresses the paroxysmal three cycle/second spike and wave activity associated with lapses of conciousness. Also depresses the motor cortex and elevation of the CNS threshold to convulsive stimuli.

CEREZYME   RX
imiglucerase (Genzyme)

THERAPEUTIC CLASS: Beta-glucocerebrosidase
INDICATIONS: Long-term enzyme replacement therapy in Type 1 Gaucher disease.

DOSAGE: *Adults:* Initial: 2.5U/kg TIW to 60U/kg once every 2 weeks IV infusion over 1-2 hours. Adjust dose based on therapeutic goals.
Pediatrics: ≥2 yrs: Initial: 2.5U/kg TIW to 60U/kg once every 2 weeks IV infusion over 1-2 hours. Adjust dose based on therapeutic goals.

HOW SUPPLIED: Inj: 200U, 400U

WARNINGS/PRECAUTIONS: Monitor for IgG antibody formation during the 1st year of therapy. Reduce rate of infusion and pretreat with antihistamines and/or corticosteroids if anaphylactoid reactions occur. Caution in patients who developed antibodies or hypersensitivity reactions to alglucerase.

ADVERSE REACTIONS: Injection site reactions, pruritus, flushing, urticaria, angioedema, chest discomfort, dyspnea, coughing, cyanosis, hypotension, nausea, vomiting, rash, headache, fever.

PREGNANCY: Category C, caution in nursing.

MECHANISM OF ACTION: β-glucocerebrosidase; catalyzes hydrolysis of the glycolipid glucocerebroside to glucose and ceramide.

PHARMACOKINETICS: Distribution: V_d=0.09-0.15L/kg. **Elimination:** $T_{1/2}$=3.6-10.4 min.

CERUBIDINE   RX
daunorubicin HCl (Bedford)

> Avoid IM/SQ route. Severe local tissue necrosis with extravasation. Myocardial toxicity may occur during or after terminate therapy; increased risk if cumulative dose >400-550mg/m² in adults, >300mg/m² in pediatrics >2 yrs, or >10mg/m² in pediatrics <2 yrs. Severe myelosuppression may occur. Reduce dose with impaired hepatic or renal function.

THERAPEUTIC CLASS: Anthracycline

INDICATIONS: In combination with other anticancer drugs, for remission induction in acute nonlymphocytic leukemia (ANLL) in adults, and for remission induction in acute lymphocytic leukemia (ALL) in children and adults.

DOSAGE: *Adults:* ANLL: Combination Therapy: <60 yrs: 45mg/m²/day IV on Days 1, 2, 3 of 1st course and on Days 1, 2 of subsequent courses. ≥60 yrs: 30mg/m²/day IV on Days 1, 2, 3 of 1st course and on Days 1, 2 of subsequent courses. ALL: Combination Therapy: 45mg/m²/day IV on Days 1, 2, 3. Renal Impairment: If SCr >3mg%, reduce dose by 50%. Hepatic Impairment: If serum bilirubin 1.2-3mg%, reduce dose by 25%. If >3mg%, reduce dose by 50%.
Pediatrics: ALL: Combination Therapy: 25mg/m² IV on Day 1 every week. If complete remission not obtained after 4 courses, may give additional 1-2 courses. If <2 yrs or <0.5m² BSA, calculate dose based on weight (1mg/kg) instead of BSA.

HOW SUPPLIED: Inj: 20mg

WARNINGS/PRECAUTIONS: Avoid if pre-existing drug-induced bone-marrow suppression occurs unless benefit warrants the risk. May cause fetal harm during pregnancy. May impart red color to urine. Monitor blood uric acid levels. Determine CBC frequently. Evaluate cardiac, renal, and hepatic function before each course.

ADVERSE REACTIONS: Cardiotoxicity, myelosuppression, alopecia, nausea, vomiting, diarrhea, abdominal pain, hyperuricemia, mucositis (3-7 days after therapy).

INTERACTIONS: Possible secondary leukemias with other antineoplastics or radiation therapy. Increased risk of cardiotoxicity with previous doxorubicin therapy or with concomitant cyclophosphamide. May need dose reduction with other myelosuppressants. Hepatotoxic agents (eg, high dose MTX) may increase risk of toxicity.

PREGNANCY: Category D, not for use in nursing.

MECHANISM OF ACTION: Anthracycline antineoplastic agent; inhibits topoisomerase II activity by stabilizing the DNA-topoisomerase II complex, preventing the religation portion of the ligation-religation reaction that topoisomerase II catalyzes, and resulting in single-strand and double-strand DNA breaks.

PHARMACOKINETICS: Distribution: Widely distributed in tissues. **Metabolism:** Liver (extensively), via cytoplasmic aldo-keto reductases, 4-O demethylation, conjugation. Daunorubicinol (major metabolite). **Elimination:** Urine and bile (40%). $T_{1/2}$(daunorubicinol)=26.7 hrs.

CHERACOL W/CODEINE

codeine phosphate - guaifenesin (Lee Pharmaceuticals)

OTHER BRAND NAMES: Cheratussin AC (Vintage) - Guaituss AC (Alpharma) - Halotussin AC (Watson) - Mytussin AC (Morton Grove)

THERAPEUTIC CLASS: Cough suppressant/expectorant

INDICATIONS: Relief of cough due to minor throat and bronchial irritation from a cold or inhaled irritants. Loosens phlegm and thins bronchial secretions to make coughs more productive.

DOSAGE: *Adults:* 10mL q4h. Max: 60mL/24 hrs.
Pediatrics: ≥12 yrs: 10mL q4h. Max: 60mL/24 hrs. 6 to <12 yrs: 5mL q4h. Max: 30mL/24 hrs.

HOW SUPPLIED: Syrup: (Codeine-Guaifenesin) 10-100mg/5mL (120mL)

WARNINGS/PRECAUTIONS: Use caution with persistant/chronic cough, cough with excessive phlegm, chronic pulmonary disease, or shortness of breath. May cause or aggravate constipation.

ADVERSE REACTIONS: Constipation, sedation.

INTERACTIONS: Increased sedation with sedatives, tranquilizers and antidepressants, especially MAOIs.

PREGNANCY: Safety in pregnancy and nursing not known.

CHILDREN'S MYLANTA

OTC

calcium carbonate (J&J -- Merck)

THERAPEUTIC CLASS: Antacid

INDICATIONS: For the relief of acid indigestion, sour stomach, and upset stomach due to these symptoms or overindulgence in food and drink.

DOSAGE: *Pediatrics:* 24-47 lbs or 2-5 yrs: 1 tab; 48-95 lbs or 6-11 yrs: 2 tabs. Max: 2-5 yrs: 3 tabs/24hrs; 6-11 yrs: 6 tabs/24hrs. Repeat as needed. Do not use for >2 weeks unless under supervision of a doctor.

HOW SUPPLIED: Tab, Chewable: 400mg

INTERACTIONS: Antacids may interact with other prescription drugs.

CHLORAL HYDRATE

chloral hydrate (Pharmaceutical Associates)

THERAPEUTIC CLASS: Trichloroacetaldehyde monohydrate

INDICATIONS: Short-term sedative/hypnotic (<2 weeks). To allay anxiety or induce sedation preoperatively or prior to EEG evaluations. Alone or with paraldehyde to prevent or suppress alcohol withdrawal syndrome. To reduce anxiety associated with withdrawal of other drugs such as narcotics or barbiturates.

DOSAGE: *Adults:* Dilute in half glass of water, fruit juice, or ginger ale. Hypnotic: Usual: 500mg-1g 15-30 min before bedtime. Sedative: Usual: 250mg tid pc. Alcohol Withdrawal: Usual: 500mg-1g q6h prn. Max: 2g/day.
Pediatrics: Hypnotic: 50mg/kg. Max: 1g/dose. Sedative: 8mg/kg tid. Max: 500mg tid. Prior to EEG: 20-25mg/kg.

HOW SUPPLIED: Syrup: 500mg/5mL

CONTRAINDICATIONS: Marked hepatic or renal impairment.

WARNINGS/PRECAUTIONS: May be habit forming. Caution with depression, suicidal tendencies, history of drug abuse. Avoid with esophagitis, gastritis or gastric or duodenal ulcers, large doses with severe cardiac disease. May impair mental/physical abilities. Risk of gastritis, skin eruptions, parenchymatous renal damage with prolonged use. Withdraw gradually with chronic use.

ADVERSE REACTIONS: Nausea, vomiting, diarrhea, ataxia, dizziness.

INTERACTIONS: Reduces effectiveness of coumarin anticoagulants. May result in transient potentiation of warfarin-induced hypoprothrombinemia. Additive CNS effects with other CNS depressants (eg, paraldehyde, barbiturates, alcohol). Use with IV furosemide may cause diaphoresis, flushes, variable BP; use alternative hypnotic.

PREGNANCY: Category C, caution in nursing.

MECHANISM OF ACTION: Sedative/hypnotic agent, confined to cerebral hemispheres.

PHARMACOKINETICS: Distribution: Found in breast milk. **Metabolism:** Liver. **Elimination:** Kidneys.

CHLORPROMAZINE   RX
chlorpromazine (Various)

THERAPEUTIC CLASS: Phenothiazine

INDICATIONS: Treatment of schizophrenia. Control of nausea and vomiting. Relief of restlessness and apprehension before surgery. Treatment of acute intermittent porphyria. Adjunct treatment of tetanus. To control the manic type of manic-depressive illness. Relief of intractable hiccups. Treatment of severe behavioral problems in children. Short-term treatment of hyperactivity in children.

DOSAGE: *Adults:* Severe Behavioral Problems: Inpatient: Acute Schizophrenic/Manic State: 25mg IM, then 25-50mg IM in 1 hr if needed. Titrate: Increase over several days up to 400mg q4-6h until controlled then switch to PO. Usual: 500mg/day PO. Max: 1000mg/day PO. Less Acutely Disturbed: 25mg PO tid. Titrate: Increase gradually to 400mg/day. Outpatient: 10mg PO tid-qid or 25mg PO bid-tid. More Severe: 25mg PO tid. Titrate: After 1-2 days, increase by 20-50mg twice weekly until calm. Prompt Control of Severe Symptoms: 25mg IM, may repeat in 1 hr then 25-50mg PO tid. Nausea/Vomiting: Usual: 10-25mg PO q4-6h prn; 25mg IM then, if no hypotension, 25-50mg q3-4h prn until vomiting stops then switch to PO; 100mg rectally q6-8h prn. Nausea/Vomiting in Surgery: 12.5mg IM, may repeat in 1/2 hr; 2mg IV per fractional injection at 2 min intervals. Max: 25mg. Presurgical Apprehension: 25-50mg PO 2-3 hrs pre-op; 12.5-25mg IM 1-2 hrs pre-op. Intractable Hiccups: 25-50mg PO tid-qid; if symptoms persist after 2-3 days, give 25-50mg IM; if symptoms still persist, give 25-50mg slow IV. Porphyria: 25-50mg PO tid-qid; 25mg IM tid-qid until PO therapy. Tetanus: 25-50mg IM tid-qid; 25-50mg IV. Elderly: Use lower doses, increase dose more gradually, monitor closely. *Pediatrics:* 6 months-12 yrs: Severe Behavioral Problems: Outpatient: 0.25mg/lb PO q4-6h prn; 0.5mg/lb sup rectally q6-8h prn; 0.25mg/lb IM q6-8h prn. Inpatient: Start low and increase gradually to 50-100mg/day; ≥200mg/day in older children. Max: 500mg/day. <5 yrs (<50lbs): Max: ≤40mg/day IM; 5-12 yrs (50-100lbs): Max: ≤75mg/day IM. Nausea/Vomiting: 0.25mg/lb PO q4-6h; 0.5mg/lb sup rectally q6-8 prn. 0.25mg/lb IM q6-8h prn. Max: 6 months-5 yrs (or 50 lbs): <40mg/day. 5-12 yrs (or 50-100lbs): <75mg/day except in severe cases. During Surgery: 0.125mg/lb IM repeat in 1/2 hr if needed; 1mg IV per fractional injection at 2 min intervals and not exceeding recommended IM dosage. Presurgical Apprehension: 0.25mg/lb PO 2-3 hrs (or IM 1-2 hrs) before operation. Tetanus: 0.25mg/lb IM/IV q6-8h. <50lbs: Max: ≤40mg/day; 50-100lbs: Max: ≤75mg/day.

HOW SUPPLIED: Cap, Extended-Release: 30mg, 75mg, 150mg; Inj: 25mg/mL; Sup: 25mg, 100mg; Syrup: 10mg/5mL (120mL); Tab: 10mg, 25mg, 50mg, 100mg, 200mg

CONTRAINDICATIONS: Comatose states, or with large amounts of CNS depressants. Hypersensitivity to phenothiazines.

WARNINGS/PRECAUTIONS: Tardive dyskinesia, NMS may occur. Caution with chronic respiratory disorders, acute respiratory infections (especially in children), glaucoma, cardiovascular, hepatic, or renal disease, history of hepatic encephalopathy due to cirrhosis. Suppresses cough reflex; aspiration of vomitus possible. Caution if exposed to extreme heat or organophosphates. Avoid in children/adolescents with signs of Reye's syndrome. Lowers seizure threshold. Reduce dose gradually to prevent side effects. May mask signs of overdoses to other drugs and obscure diagnosis of other conditions (eg, intestinal obstruction, brain tumor, Reye's syndrome). May produce false-positive PKU test. May elevate prolactin levels. Injection contains sulfites.

ADVERSE REACTIONS: Drowsiness, jaundice, agranulocytosis, hypotensive effects, EKG changes, dystonias, motor restlessness, pseudo-parkinsonism, tardive dyskinesia, anticholinergic effects, NMS, ocular changes.

INTERACTIONS: See Contraindications. May decrease effects of oral anticoagulants, guanethidine. Propranolol increases plasma levels of both agents. Thiazide diuretics may potentiate orthostatic hypotension. Potentiates effects of CNS depressants (eg, anesthetic, barbiturates, narcotics); reduce doses of these drugs by 1/4 to 1/2. Anticonvulsants may need adjustment; phenytoin toxicity reported. Do not use with Amipaque®; discontinue at least 48 hrs before myelography and resume at least 24 hrs after. Can cause α-adrenergic blockade. Caution with atropine or related drugs. Encephalopathic syndrome reported with lithium.

PREGNANCY: Safety in pregnancy not known. Not for use in nursing.

MECHANISM OF ACTION: Phenothiazine; not established. Suspected to act at all levels of CNS, primarily at subcortical levels as well as on multiple organ systems. Exerts psychotropic, sedative, and antiemetic activity. Has strong antiadrenergic and weaker peripheral anticholinergic activity and ganglionic blocking action.

CHLOR-TRIMETON OTC
chlorpheniramine maleate (Schering)

THERAPEUTIC CLASS: Antihistamine

INDICATIONS: Allergic rhinitis and conjunctivitis.

DOSAGE: *Adults:* (Tab/Syrup) 4mg q4-6h. (Tab, ER) 8mg q8-12h or 12mg q12h. Max: 24mg/day.
Pediatrics: ≥12 yrs: (Tab/Syrup) 4mg q4-6h. Tab, ER: 8mg q8-12h or 12mg q12h. Max: 24mg/day. 6-12 yrs: (Tab/Syrup) 2mg q4-6h. Max: 12mg/24hrs.

HOW SUPPLIED: Syrup: 2mg/5mL; Tab: 4mg; Tab, Extended-Release: 8mg, 12mg

WARNINGS/PRECAUTIONS: Avoid with emphysema, chronic bronchitis, glaucoma, and difficulty in urination due to prostate gland enlargement.

ADVERSE REACTIONS: Drowsiness, excitability.

INTERACTIONS: Alcohol, sedatives, hypnotics potentiate CNS depression.

PREGNANCY: Safety in pregnancy or nursing not known.

CILOXAN RX
ciprofloxacin HCl (Alcon)

THERAPEUTIC CLASS: Fluoroquinolone

INDICATIONS: Bacterial conjunctivitis and corneal ulcers.

DOSAGE: *Adults:* Bacterial Conjunctivitis: Sol: 1-2 drops q2h while awake for 2 days, then 1-2 drops q4h while awake for 5 days. Oint: 1/2 inch tid for 2 days, then bid for 5 days. Corneal Ulcer: Sol: 2 drops every 15 min for 1st 6 hrs, then 2 drops every 30 min for rest of Day 1, then 2 drops every hr on Day 2, then 2 drops q4h on Days 3-14. May continue if re-epithelialization has not occurred.
Pediatrics: Bacterial Conjunctivitis: ≥1 yr: Sol: 1-2 drops q2h while awake for 2 days, then 1-2 drops q4h while awake for 5 days. ≥2 yrs: Oint: 1/2 inch tid for 2 days, then bid for 5 days. Corneal Ulcer: Sol: ≥1 yr: 2 drops every 15 min for 1st 6 hrs, then 2 drops every 30 min for rest of Day 1, then 2 drops every hr on Day 2, then 2 drops q4h on Days 3-14. May continue if re-epithelialization has not occurred.

HOW SUPPLIED: Oint: 0.3% (3.5g); Sol: 0.3% (2.5mL, 5mL, 10mL)

WARNINGS/PRECAUTIONS: Not for injection into eye. Superinfection may result with prolonged use. Fatal hypersensitivity reactions reported after 1st dose of systemic quinolone therapy. Avoid allowing tip of container to contact eye or surrounding structures. Avoid contact lenses with conjunctivitis. Risk of crystalline precipitate in cornea. Ointment may slow corneal healing and cause visual blurring.

ADVERSE REACTIONS: Local burning, white crystalline precipitants, lid margin crusting, crystals/scales, foreign body sensation, itching, conjunctival hyperemia, bad taste.

INTERACTIONS: Systemic quinolone therapy may increase theophylline levels, interfere with caffeine metabolism, enhance warfarin effects, and elevate serum creatinine with cyclosporine.

PREGNANCY: Category C, caution in nursing.

MECHANISM OF ACTION: Fluoroquinolone antibacterial agent. Bactericidal; interferes with the enzyme DNA gyrase which is needed for synthesis of bacterial DNA.

PHARMACOKINETICS: Absorption: $C_{max} \leq 5ng/mL$.

CIMETIDINE   RX
cimetidine (Various)

OTHER BRAND NAME: Tagamet (GlaxoSmithKline)

THERAPEUTIC CLASS: H_2-blocker

INDICATIONS: Short-term treatment of active duodenal ulcer (DU), active benign gastric ulcer (GU). Maintenance of healed duodenal ulcer. Treatment of GERD and/or pathological hypersecretory conditions (eg, Zollinger-Ellison syndrome). Prevention of upper GI bleeding in critically ill patients.

DOSAGE: *Adults:* (PO) Active DU: 800mg qhs or 300mg qid or 400mg bid for 4-8 weeks. Maint: 400mg qhs. Active Benign GU: 800mg qhs or 300mg qid for 6 weeks. GERD: 800mg bid or 400mg qid for 12 weeks. Hypersecretory Conditions: 300mg qid. Max: 2400mg/day. (Inj) 300mg IM/IV q6-8h. Max: 2400mg/day. Rapid Gastric pH Elevation: LD: 150mg IV, then 37.5mg/hr IV. Upper GI Bleed Prevention: Continuous IV infusion of 50mg/hr for 7 days. CrCl <30mL/min: Give half the recommended dose.
Pediatrics: ≥16 yrs: (PO) Active DU: 800mg qhs or 300mg qid or 400mg bid for 4-8 weeks. Maint: 400mg qhs. Active Benign GU: 800mg qhs or 300mg qid for 6 weeks. GERD: 800mg bid or 400mg qid for 12 weeks. Hypersecretory Conditions: 300mg qid. Max: 2400mg/day. (Inj) 300mg IM/IV q6-8h. Max: 2400mg/day. Rapid Gastric pH Elevation: LD: 150mg IV, then 37.5mg/hr IV. Upper GI Bleed Prevention: Continuous IV infusion of 50mg/hr for 7 days. CrCl <30mL/min: Give half the recommended dose.

HOW SUPPLIED: Inj: (HCl) 150mg/mL, 300mg/5mL; Sol: (HCl) 300mg/5mL; Tab: 200mg, 300mg, 400mg*, 800mg* *scored

WARNINGS/PRECAUTIONS: Cardiac arrhythmias and hypotension reported following rapid IV administration (rare). Symptomatic response does not preclude the presence of gastric malignancy. Reversible confusional states reported, especially in severely ill patients. Elderly, renal and/or hepatic impairment are risk factors for confusional states. Risk of hyperinfection of strongyloidiasis in immunocompromised patients.

ADVERSE REACTIONS: Diarrhea, headache, dizziness, somnolence, reversible confusional states, impotence, increased serum transaminases, rash, gynecomastia, blood dyscrasias.

INTERACTIONS: Reduces metabolism of warfarin-type anticoagulants, phenytoin, propranolol, nifedipine, chlordiazepoxide, diazepam, certain TCAs, lidocaine, theophylline and metronidazole. Monitor PT/INR. Adverse effects reported with phenytoin, lidocaine and theophylline; monitor levels. May affect absorption of drugs (eg, ketoconazole) affected by gastric pH; give 2 hrs before cimetidine. Antacids may interfer with absorption of cimetidine; space the dosing.

PREGNANCY: Category B, not for use in nursing.

MECHANISM OF ACTION: H_2-receptor antagonist; competitively inhibits the action of histamine at the histamine H_2 receptors of the parietal cells.

PHARMACOKINETICS: Absorption: (PO) Rapid. T_{max}=45-90 mins. (IV) C_{max}=0.9mcg/mL. **Metabolism:** Sulfoxide (major metabolite). **Elimination:** Urine, (PO 48%); (IV/IM 75%); $T_{1/2}$=2 hrs.

CIPRO HC   RX
ciprofloxacin HCl - hydrocortisone (Alcon)

THERAPEUTIC CLASS: Antibacterial/corticosteroid combination

INDICATIONS: Acute otitis externa in adults and pediatric patients ≥1 year.

DOSAGE: *Adults:* 3 drops into affected ear bid for 7 days. Warm bottle in hand for 1-2 min to avoid dizziness. Shake well before use.
Pediatrics: ≥1 yr: 3 drops into affected ear bid for 7 days. Warm bottle in hand for 1-2 min to avoid dizziness. Shake well before use.

HOW SUPPLIED: Sus: (Ciprofloxacin-Hydrocortisone) 0.2%-1% (10mL)

CONTRAINDICATIONS: Perforated tympanic membrane, viral infections of external ear canal (eg, varicella and herpes simplex infections).

WARNINGS/PRECAUTIONS: D/C if hypersensitivity reaction occurs. Re-evaluate if no improvement after one week.

ADVERSE REACTIONS: Headache, pruritus.

PREGNANCY: Category C, not for use in nursing.

MECHANISM OF ACTION: Broad-spectrum anti-inflammatory antibiotic; exerts antimicrobial activity against gram-positive and gram-negative bacteria.

CIPRO IV   RX
ciprofloxacin (Bayer/Schering)

THERAPEUTIC CLASS: Fluoroquinolone

INDICATIONS: Treatment of skin and skin structure (SSSI), bone and joint, complicated intra-abdominal infections, lower respiratory tract infections (LRTI), urinary tract infections (UTI), nosocomial pneumonia, acute sinusitis, chronic bacterial prostatitis, postexposure inhalational anthrax, empirical therapy for febrile neutropenia, complicated UTI and pyelonephritis in pediatrics.

DOSAGE: *Adults:* ≥18 yrs: IV: UTI: Mild-Moderate: 200mg q12h for 7-14 days. Complicated/Severe: 400mg q12h for 7-14 days. LRTI/SSSI: Mild-Moderate: 400mg q12h for 7-14 days. Complicated/Severe: 400mg q8h for 7-14 days. Bone and Joint: Mild-Moderate: 400mg q12h for ≥4-6 weeks. Complicated/Severe: 400mg q8h for ≥4-6 weeks. Nosocomial Pneumonia: 400mg q8h for 10-14 days. Complicated Intra-Abdominal: 400mg q12h (w/metronidazole) for 7-14 days. Acute Sinusitis: 400mg q12h for 10 days. Chronic Bacterial Prostatitis: 400mg q12h for 28 days. Febrile Neutropenia: 400mg q8h (w/piperacillin 50mg/kg q4h) for 7-14 days. Max: 24g/day. Inhalational Anthrax: 400mg q12h for 60 days. Administer over 60 min. CrCl 5-29mL/min: 200-400mg q18-24h.
Pediatrics: <18 yrs: Inhalational Anthrax: 10mg/kg q12h for 60 days. Max: 400mg/dose; 800mg/day. 1-17 yrs: Complicated UTI/Pyelonephritis: 6-10mg/kg q8h for 10-21 days. Max: 400mg/dose.

HOW SUPPLIED: Inj: 10mg/mL, 200mg/100mL, 400mg/200mL

CONTRAINDICATIONS: Concomitant administration with tizanidine.

WARNINGS/PRECAUTIONS: Convulsions, increased ICP, and toxic psychosis reported. Caution with CNS disorders or if predisposed to seizures. Severe, fatal hypersensitivity reactions may occur. *Clostridium difficile*-associated diarrhea, achilles and other tendon ruptures reported. D/C at first sign of rash/hypersensitivity or if pain, inflammation, or ruptured tendon occur. May permit overgrowth of clostridia. Maintain hydration; avoid alkaline urine. Avoid excessive sunlight and UV light. Do not give via feeding tube. Monitor renal, hepatic and hematopoietic function with prolonged use. Adust dose with renal dysfunction. Caution with concomitant drugs that may result in prolongation of QT interval or in patients with risk factors for torsade de pointes.

ADVERSE REACTIONS: Nausea, diarrhea, CNS disturbances, local IV site reactions, hepatic enzyme abnormalities, eosinophilia, headache, restlessness, rash.

INTERACTIONS: See Contraindications. Increases theophylline and caffeine levels and prolongs effects. Altered serum levels of phenytoin. Severe hypoglycemia with glyburide (rare). Potentiated by probenecid. Transient serum creatinine elevations with cyclosporine. Enhances oral anticoagulant effects. Caution with drugs that lower seizure threshold. Severe tendon disorder risks are increased with concomitant corticosteroid therapy. Caution with concomitant drugs that may result in prolongation of QT interval.

PREGNANCY: Category C, not for use in nursing.

MECHANISM OF ACTION: Synthetic broad-spectrum antimicrobial agent. Inhibits the enzymes topoisomerase II (DNA gyrase) and topoisomerase IV, which are required for bacterial DNA replication, transcription, repair, and recombination.

PHARMACOKINETICS: Absorption: Absolute bioavailability (70-80%); C_{max}=0.1, 002µg/mL (200mg, 400mg, after 12 hrs). **Distribution:** Plasma protein binding (20-40%). **Metabolism:** CYP1A2. **Elimination:** Urine (unchanged), feces (15%). $T_{1/2}$=5-6 hrs.

CIPRO ORAL

RX

ciprofloxacin HCl (Bayer/Schering)

THERAPEUTIC CLASS: Fluoroquinolone

INDICATIONS: Treatment of lower respiratory tract (LRTI), complicated intra-abdominal, skin and skin structure (SSSI), bone and joint, and urinary tract infections (UTI), acute exacerbations of chronic bronchitis, acute sinusitis, acute uncomplicated cystitis in females, chronic bacterial prostatitis, infectious diarrhea, typhoid fever, postexposure inhalational anthrax, uncomplicated cervical and urethral gonorrhea, complicated UTI and pyelonephritis in pediatrics.

DOSAGE: *Adults:* ≥18 yrs: Acute Sinusitis/Typhoid Fever: 500mg q12h for 10 days. LRTI/SSSI: Mild-Moderate: 500mg q12h for 7-14 days. Severe/Complicated: 750mg q12h for 7-14 days. Cystitis/Acute Uncomplicated UTI: 250mg q12h for 3 days. Mild-Moderate UTI: 250mg q12h for 7-14 days. Severe/Complicated UTI: 500mg q12h for 7-14 days. Chronic Bacterial Prostatitis: 500mg q12h for 28 days. Intra-Abdominal: 500mg q12h (w/ metronidazole) for 7-14 days. Bone and Joint: Mild-Moderate: 500mg q12h for ≥4-6 weeks. Severe/Complicated: 750mg q12h for ≥4-6 weeks. Infectious Diarrhea: 500mg q12h for 5-7 days. Uncomplicated Urethral/Cervical Gonococcal Infections: 250mg single dose. Inhalational Anthrax: 500mg q12h for 60 days. CrCl 30-50mL/min: 250-500mg q12h. CrCl 5-29mL/min: 250-500mg q18h. Hemodialysis/Peritoneal Dialysis: 250-500mg q24h (after dialysis). Administer at least 2 hrs before or 6 hrs after magnesium- or aluminum-containing antacids, sucralfate, Videx (didanosine) chewable/buffered tablets or pediatric powder, or other products containing calcium, iron, or zinc.
Pediatrics: <18 yrs: Inhalational Anthrax: 15mg/kg q12h for 60 days. Max: 500mg/dose. 1-17 yrs: Complicated UTI/Pyelonephritis: 10-20mg/kg q12h for 10-21 days. Max: 750mg/dose.

HOW SUPPLIED: Sus: 250mg/5mL, 500mg/5mL (100mL); Tab: 250mg, 500mg, 750mg

CONTRAINDICATIONS: Concomitant administration with tizanidine.

WARNINGS/PRECAUTIONS: Convulsions, increased ICP, and toxic psychosis reported. Caution with CNS disorders or if predisposed to seizures. Severe, fatal hypersensitivity reactions may occur. *Clostridium difficile*-associated diarrhea, colitis, achilles and other tendon ruptures reported. D/C at first sign of rash or if pain, inflammation, or ruptured tendon occurs. Maintain hydration; avoid alkaline urine. Avoid excessive sunlight and UV light. Do not give via feeding tube. Monitor renal, hepatic, and hematopoietic function with prolonged use. Adjust dose with renal dysfunction. Caution with concomitant drugs that may result in prolongation of the QT interval or in patients with risk factors for torsade de pointes.

ADVERSE REACTIONS: Nausea, dizziness, headache, CNS disturbances, vomiting, diarrhea, rash, abdominal pain/discomfort, pain, swelling, tendon tears.

INTERACTIONS: See Contraindications. Increases theophylline and caffeine levels and prolongs effects. Fatal reactions have occurred with theophylline. Magnesium- or aluminum-containing antacids, sucralfate, Videx (didanosine) chewable/buffered tablets or pediatric powder, and products containing calcium, iron, or zinc decrease serum and urine levels; space doses at least 2 hrs before or 6 hrs after administration. Altered serum levels of phenytoin. Severe hypoglycemia with glyburide (rare). Potentiated by probenecid. Transient serum creatinine elevations with cyclosporine. Enhances oral anticoagulant effects. Monitor PT. Caution with drugs that lower seizure threshold. Severe tendon disorder risks increased with concomitant corticosteroid therapy. Caution with concomitant drugs that may result in prolongation of the QT interval.

PREGNANCY: Category C, not for use in nursing.

MECHANISM OF ACTION: Synthetic broad-spectrum antimicrobial agent; inhibits enzymes topoisomerase II (DNA gyrase) and topoisomerase IV, which are required for bacterial DNA replication.

PHARMACOKINETICS: Absorption: Absolute bioavailability (70%); C_{max}=0.1, 0.2, 0.4mcg/mL (250mg, 500mg, 750mg, after 12 hrs); T_{max}=1-2 hrs. **Distribution:** Plasma protein binding (20-40%). **Metabolism:** CYP1A2. **Elimination:** Urine (40-50%); $T_{1/2}$=4 hrs.

CIPRODEX RX
ciprofloxacin - dexamethasone (Alcon)

THERAPEUTIC CLASS: Antibacterial/corticosteroid combination

INDICATIONS: Acute otitis media in pediatric patients with tympanostomy tubes. Acute otitis externa.

DOSAGE: *Adults:* Acute Otitis Externa: 4 drops in affected ear(s) bid for 7 days. Warm bottle in hand for 1-2 min to avoid dizziness. Shake well before use.
Pediatrics: ≥6 months: 4 drops in affected ear(s) bid for 7 days. Warm bottle in hand for 1-2 min to avoid dizziness. Shake well before use.

HOW SUPPLIED: Sus: (Ciprofloxacin-Dexamethasone) 0.3%-0.1% (5mL, 7.5mL)

CONTRAINDICATIONS: Viral infections of external ear canal including herpes simplex infections.

WARNINGS/PRECAUTIONS: D/C if hypersensitivity reaction occurs. Re-evaluate if no improvement after one week.

ADVERSE REACTIONS: Ear pain/discomfort/pruritus.

PREGNANCY: Category C, not for use in nursing.

MECHANISM OF ACTION: Fluoroquinolone, corticosteroid; antibacterial/anti-inflammatory; bactericidal action results from interference with the enzyme (DNA gyrase), which is needed for the synthesis of bacterial DNA.

PHARMACOKINETICS: Absorption: Ciprofloxacin: C_{max}=1.39ng/mL, T_{max}=15 min-2 hrs. Dexamethasone: C_{max}=1.14ng/mL, T_{max}=15 min-2 hrs.

CLAFORAN RX
cefotaxime sodium (Sanofi-Aventis)

THERAPEUTIC CLASS: Cephalosporin (3rd generation)

INDICATIONS: Treatment of lower respiratory tract, genitourinary, gynecologic, intra-abdominal, skin and skin structure, bone and joint, and CNS infections (eg, meningitis), bacteremia, and septicemia caused by susceptible strains of microorganisms. For surgical prophylaxis of certain infections.

DOSAGE: *Adults:* Gonococcal Urethritis/Cervicitis (Males/Females): 500mg single dose IM. Rectal Gonorrhea: 0.5g (females) or 1g (males) single dose IM. Uncomplicated Infections: 1g IM/IV q12h. Moderate-Severe Infections: 1-2g IM/IV q8h. Septicemia: 2g IV q6-8h. Life-Threatening Infections: 2g IV q4h. Max: 12g/day. Surgical Prophylaxis: 1g IM/IV 30-90 min before surgery. Cesarean Section: 1g IV when umbilical cord is clamped, then 1g IV at 6 and 12 hrs after 1st dose. CrCl <20mL/min/1.73m^2: Give 1/2 of usual dose.
Pediatrics: ≥50kg: Use adult dose. Max: 12g/day. 1 month-12 yrs and ≤50kg: 50-180mg/kg/day IM/IV divided in 4-6 doses. 1-4 weeks: 50mg/kg IV q8h. 0-1 week: 50mg/kg IV q12h. CrCl <20mL/min/1.73m^2: Give 1/2 of usual dose.

HOW SUPPLIED: Inj: 500mg, 1g, 2g, 10g

WARNINGS/PRECAUTIONS: Cross sensitivity to PCNs and other cephalosporins may occur. *Clostridium difficile*-associated diarrhea reported. May result in overgrowth of nonsusceptible organisms. Caution with history of GI disease. Reduce dose with renal dysfunction. Granulocytopenia may occur with long-term use. Monitor blood counts if therapy >10 days. Monitor injection site for tissue inflammation. False (+) direct Coombs' tests reported.

ADVERSE REACTIONS: Injection site reactions, rash, pruritus, fever, eosinophilia, colitis, diarrhea.

INTERACTIONS: Increased nephrotoxicity with aminoglycosides.

PREGNANCY: Category B, caution in nursing.

MECHANISM OF ACTION: 3rd-generation cephalosporin; inhibits cell-wall synthesis.

PHARMACOKINETICS: Absorption: IM: C_{max} (500mg, 1g)=11.7, 20.5mcg/mL; T_{max}=30min. **Elimination:** Unchanged, cefotaxime and desacetyl derivative (major metabolite) are excreted by kidneys; $T_{1/2}$=1 hr.

CLARINEX
desloratadine (Schering)

RX

OTHER BRAND NAMES: Clarinex RediTabs (Schering) - Clarinex Syrup (Schering)

THERAPEUTIC CLASS: H_1-antagonist

INDICATIONS: Relief of perennial allergic rhinitis and chronic idiopathic urticaria in patients ≥ 6 months. Relief of seasonal allergic rhinitis in patients ≥ 2 yrs.

DOSAGE: *Adults:* 5mg qd. Hepatic/Renal Impairment: 5mg every other day. Dissolve RediTabs on tongue with or without water.
Pediatrics: Tabs: ≥ 12 yrs: 5mg qd. 6-11 yrs: 2.5mg qd. Syrup: ≥ 12 yrs: 10mL (5mg) qd. 6-11 yrs: 5mL (2.5mg) qd. 12 months-5 yrs: 2.5mL (1.25mg) qd. 6-11 months: 2mL (1mg) qd. Dissolve RediTabs on tongue with or without water.

HOW SUPPLIED: Tab: 5mg; Tab, Disintegrating: (RediTabs) 2.5mg, 5mg; Syrup: 0.5mg/mL

WARNINGS/PRECAUTIONS: Adjust dose with renal or hepatic impairment. Caution in elderly.

ADVERSE REACTIONS: Pharyngitis, dry mouth, headache, fever, diarrhea, cough, upper respiratory tract infection, cough, irritability, somnolence, bronchitis, otitis media, vomiting, nausea, fatigue.

INTERACTIONS: Erythromycin, ketoconazole increase plasma levels.

PREGNANCY: Category C, not for use in nursing.

MECHANISM OF ACTION: Long-acting tricyclic histamine antagonist with selective H_1-receptor histamine antagonist activity; inhibits histamine release from human mast cells.

PHARMACOKINETICS: Absorption: T_{max}=3 hrs., C_{max}=4ng/mL, AUC=56.9ng•hr/mL. **Distribution:** Found in breast milk; plasma protein binding (82-87% of desloratadine), (85-89% of 3-hydroxydesloratadine). **Metabolism:** Extensive. Desloratadine (major metabolite), 3-hydroxydesloratadine (active metabolite). **Elimination:** Urine and feces (metabolites); $T_{1/2}$=27 hrs.

CLARINEX-D
desloratadine - pseudoephedrine sulfate (Schering)

RX

THERAPEUTIC CLASS: H_1-antagonist/sympathomimetic amine

INDICATIONS: Relief of nasal and non-nasal symptoms of seasonal allergic rhinitis including nasal congestion.

DOSAGE: *Adults:* 2.5mg-120mg tab bid or 5mg-240mg tab qd w/ or w/o food. Hepatic Impairment: 12-Hour/24-Hour: Avoid use. Renal Impairment: 12-Hour: Avoid use. 24-Hour: 1 tab qod.
Pediatrics: ≥ 12 yrs: 2.5mg-120mg tab bid or 5mg-240mg tab qd w/ or w/o food. Hepatic Impairment: 12-Hour/24-Hour: Avoid use. Renal Impairment: 12-Hour: Avoid use. 24-Hour: 1 tab qod.

HOW SUPPLIED: Tab, Extended-Release: (Desloratadine-Pseudoephedrine) (12-Hour) 2.5mg-120mg, (24-Hour) 5mg-240mg

CONTRAINDICATIONS: Narrow-angle glaucoma, urinary retention, MAOI therapy or within 14 days of discontinuation, severe HTN, severe CAD, hypersensitivity or idiosyncrasy to adrenergic agents, or to other drugs of similar chemical structures.

WARNINGS/PRECAUTIONS: Caution with HTN, DM, ischemic heart disease, increased intraocular pressure, hyperthyroidism, renal impairment, or prostatic hypertrophy. CNS stimulation with convulsions or cardiovascular collapse with accompanying hypotension may be produced by sympathomimetic amines. Avoid with hepatic insufficiency.

ADVERSE REACTIONS: Dry mouth, headache, insomnia, fatigue, pharyngitis, somnolence

INTERACTIONS: Do not use with MAOIs or within 14 days of discontinuation. Antihypertensive effects of β-adrenergic blocking agents, methyldopa, mecamylamine, reserpine, and veratrum alkaloids may be reduced by sympathomimetics (eg, pseudoephedrine). Increased ectopic pacemaker activity with digitalis.

PREGNANCY: Category C, not for use in nursing.

MECHANISM OF ACTION: Desloratadine: Long acting tricyclic histamine antagonist with selective H_1-receptor antagonist activity. Inhibits histamine release from human mast cells *in vitro*. Pseudoephedrine: Orally active sympathomimetic amine, which exerts a decongestant action on nasal mucosa.

PHARMACOKINETICS: Absorption: Desloratadine: (24 hr) C_{max}=approximately 1.79ng/mL; T_{max}=approximately 6-7 hrs, AUC=approximately 61.1ng•hr/mL. (12 hr) C_{max}=approximately 1.09ng/ml; T_{max}=approximately 4-5 hrs, AUC=31.6ng•hr/ml. Pseudoephedrine: (24 hr) C_{max}=approximately 328ng/mL, T_{max}=8-9 hrs, AUC=6438ng•hr/mL. (12 hr) C_{max}=263ng/ml, T_{max}=approximately 6-7 hr, AUC=approximately 4588ng•hr/ml. **Distribution:** Desloratadine: Found in breast milk, plasma protein binding (approximately 82-87%), 3-hydroxydesloratadine (85%-89%). **Metabolism:** Desloratadine (major metabolite): Extensive, 3-hydroxydesloratadine (active metabolite) and glucuronidation pathway. Pseudoephedrine: Liver (incomplete), through N-demethylation. **Elimination:** Desloratadine: (24 hr) $T_{1/2}$=approximately 24 hrs, (12 hr) $T_{1/2}$=27 hrs. Pseudoephedrine: Urine (55-96%, unchanged). If urinary pH=5, ($T_{1/2}$=3-6 hrs); if urinary pH=8, ($T_{1/2}$=9-16 hrs).

CLARIPEL
hydroquinone (Stiefel)

RX

THERAPEUTIC CLASS: Depigmenting agent

INDICATIONS: Gradual treatment of ultraviolet induced dyschromia and discoloration resulting from use of oral contraceptives, pregnancy, hormone replacement therapy, or skin trauma.

DOSAGE: *Adults:* Apply bid.
Pediatrics: ≥12 yrs: Apply bid.

HOW SUPPLIED: Cre: 4% (28g, 45g)

WARNINGS/PRECAUTIONS: Avoid sun exposure on bleached skin. Claripel contains sunscreen. May produce unwanted cosmetic effects if not used as directed. Test for skin sensitivity. D/C if no lightening effect after 2 months of therapy, if blue-black skin discoloration occurs, or if itching, vesicle formation, or excessive inflammatory reactions occur. Contains sodium metabisulfite; may cause serious allergic type reactions. Avoid contact with eyes.

ADVERSE REACTIONS: Cutaneous hypersensitivity (contact dermatitis).

PREGNANCY: Category C, caution in nursing.

MECHANISM OF ACTION: Produces a reversible depigmentation of the skin by inhibition of the enzymatic oxidation of tyrosine to 3-(3,4-dihydroxyphenyl) alanine (dopa)[1] and suppression of other melanocyte metabolic processes.

CLARITIN OTC
loratadine (Schering)

OTC

OTHER BRAND NAME: Claritin Reditab OTC (Schering)

THERAPEUTIC CLASS: H_1-antagonist

INDICATIONS: Relief of symptoms due to hay fever or other upper respiratory allergies.

DOSAGE: *Adults:* (Reditab, Syrup, Tab) 10mg qd. Max: 10mg/d. Dissolve Reditab on tongue. Hepatic/Renal Impairment: May need to adjust dose.
Pediatrics: ≥6 yrs: (Reditab, Syr, Tab) 10mg qd. Max: 10mg/d. 2-5 yrs: (Syr) 5mg qd. Max: 5mg/d. Dissolve Reditab on tongue. Hepatic/Renal Impairment: May need to adjust dose.

HOW SUPPLIED: Syrup: 1mg/mL; Tab, Extended-Release: (24 hr) 10mg; Tab, Disintegrating: (Reditab) 10mg

WARNINGS/PRECAUTIONS: Caution with hepatic or renal impairment.

PREGNANCY: Safety in pregnancy and nursing is not known.

CLARITIN-D OTC

OTC

loratadine - pseudoephedrine sulfate (Schering)

THERAPEUTIC CLASS: H_1-antagonist/sympathomimetic amine

INDICATIONS: Relief of symptoms due to hay fever or other upper respiratory allergies. Reduces swelling of nasal passages. Relief of sinus congestion and pressure.

DOSAGE: *Adults:* 5-120mg tab q12h or 10-240mg tab qd (with full glass of water). Max: 10-240mg/24 hrs. Hepatic/Renal Impairment: May need to adjust dose. Do not divide, crush, chew or dissolve tabs.
Pediatrics: ≥12 yrs: 5-120mg tab q12h, or 10-240mg tab qd (with full glass of water). Max: 10-240mg/24 hrs. Hepatic/Renal Impairment: May need to adjust dose. Do not divide, crush, chew or dissolve tabs.

HOW SUPPLIED: Tab, Extended-Release: (Loratadine-Pseudoephedrine) (12-Hour) 5-120mg, (24-Hour) 10-240mg

WARNINGS/PRECAUTIONS: Caution with hepatic or renal impairment, heart disease, thyroid disease, high BP, diabetes, enlarged prostate.

ADVERSE REACTIONS: Dizziness, insomnia, nervousness.

INTERACTIONS: Avoid during or within 14 days MAOIs.

PREGNANCY: Safety in pregnancy and nursing is not known.

CLENIA

RX

sulfacetamide sodium - sulfur (Upsher-Smith)

THERAPEUTIC CLASS: Sulfonamide/sulfur combination

INDICATIONS: Topical treatment of acne vulgaris, acne rosacea, and seborrheic dermatitis.

DOSAGE: *Adults:* (Cleanser) Wash qd-bid. Massage into skin for 10-20 seconds, then rinse and dry. (Cre) Initial: Apply qd. Titrate: Increase up to bid-tid prn.
Pediatrics: ≥12 yrs: (Cleanser) Wash qd-bid. Massage into skin for 10-20 seconds, then rinse and dry. (Cre) Initial: Apply qd. Titrate: Increase up to bid-tid prn.

HOW SUPPLIED: Cleanser: (Sulfacetamide-Sulfur) 10%-5% (170g, 340g); Cre: 10%-5% (28g)

CONTRAINDICATIONS: Kidney disease.

WARNINGS/PRECAUTIONS: D/C if excessive irritation occurs. Avoid contact with eyes, eyelid, lips, or mucous membranes. Caution with denuded or abraded skin. Can cause reddening and scaling of epidermis.

ADVERSE REACTIONS: Dryness, erythema, itching, edema.

PREGNANCY: Category C, caution in nursing.

MECHANISM OF ACTION: Sulfacetamide: Believed to block bacterial growth by acting as a competitive antagonist of para-aminobenzoic acid (PABA). Sulfur: Not established. Keratolytic activity reported to result from the interaction with the cysteine content of keratinocytes. In combination with sulfacetamide, it inhibits *Propionibacterium acnes*, thereby reducing associated inflammation.

PHARMACOKINETICS: Absorption: 1% of topically applied sulfur is absorbed through intact skin. **Distribution:** Small amounts of orally administered sulfonamides have been found in breast milk.

CLEOCIN

RX

clindamycin HCl (Pharmacia & Upjohn)

> *Clostridium difficile*-associated diarrhea (CDAD) reported with use of nearly all antibacterial agents, including clindamycin, and may range in severity from mild diarrhea to fatal colitis. If CDAD is suspected or confirmed, ongoing antibiotic use not directed against *C.difficile* may need to be discontinued.

THERAPEUTIC CLASS: Lincomycin derivative

INDICATIONS: Serious infections caused by anaerobes, streptococci, pneumococci, and staphylococci.

DOSAGE: *Adults:* Serious Infection: 150-300mg PO q6h or 600-1200mg/day IM/IV given bid-qid. More Severe Infection: 300-450mg PO q6h or 1200-2700mg/day IM/IV given bid-qid. Life-Threatening Infections: Up to 4800mg/day IV. Max: 600mg per IM injection. Take caps with full glass of water. Treat β-hemolytic strep for at least 10 days. *Pediatrics:* Give tid or qid. Cap: Serious Infections: 8-16mg/kg/day. More Severe Infections: 16-20mg/kg/day. Sol: Serious Infections: 8-12mg/kg/day. Severe Infections: 13-16mg/kg/day. More Severe Infections: 17-25mg/kg/day. IM/IV: 1 month-16 yrs: 20-40mg/kg/day; use the higher dose for more severe infections. <1 month: 15-20mg/ kg/day. Take caps with full glass of water. Treat β-hemolytic strep for at least 10 days.

HOW SUPPLIED: Cap: (HCl) 75mg, 150mg, 300mg; Inj: (Phosphate) 150mg/mL, 300mg/ 50mL, 600mg/50mL, 900mg/50mL; Sol: (Palmitate HCl) 75mg/5mL (100mL)

WARNINGS/PRECAUTIONS: May permit overgrowth of clostridia. Not for treatment of meningitis. Caution with atopic patients, GI disease (eg, colitis), hepatic disease, and the elderly. Monitor blood, hepatic and renal function with long-term use. Do not give injection undiluted as bolus. The 75mg and 100mg caps contain tartrazine.

ADVERSE REACTIONS: Abdominal pain, colitis, esophagitis, NV, diarrhea, hypersensitivity reactions, jaundice, blood dyscrasias, pruritus, vaginitis, superinfection (prolonged use).

INTERACTIONS: Antagonism may occur with erythromycin. May potentiate neuromuscular blockers.

PREGNANCY: Category B, not for use in nursing.

MECHANISM OF ACTION: Inhibits bacterial protein synthesis at the level of the bacterial ribosome and binds preferentially to the 50S ribosomal subunit affecting process of peptide chain initiation.

PHARMACOKINETICS: Absorption: Cap: Rapid, complete; C_{max}=2.5mcg/mL, T_{max}=45 min. Inj: C_{max}=10.8mcg/mL (adults, IV 600mg q8h), 9mcg/mL (adults, IM q12h), 10mcg/ml (peds, IV), 8mcg/mL (peds, IM); T_{max}=3 hrs (adults), 1 hr (peds). Oral Sol: C_{max}=1.24mcg/mL (peds, 8mg/kg/day), 2.25mcg/mL (12mg/kg/day). **Distribution:** Wide; body fluids, tissues, and bones; found in breast milk. **Elimination:** Cap: Urine (10% unchanged), feces (3.6% unchanged); $T_{1/2}$=3.2 hr. Inj: $T_{1/2}$=3 hrs (adults), 2.5 hrs (peds). Oral Sol: $T_{1/2}$=2 hrs (peds).

Cleocin T   RX
clindamycin phosphate (Pharmacia & Upjohn)

THERAPEUTIC CLASS: Lincomycin derivative

INDICATIONS: Acne vulgaris.

DOSAGE: *Adults:* Apply thin film bid.
Pediatrics: ≥12 yrs: Apply thin film bid. May use more than 1 pledget.

HOW SUPPLIED: Gel: 1% (30g, 60g); Lot: 1% (60mL); Sol: 1% (30mL, 60mL); Swab (Pledgets): 1% (60ˢ)

CONTRAINDICATIONS: Hypersensitivity to lincomycin. History of regional enteritis, ulcerative colitis, or antibiotic-associated colitis.

WARNINGS/PRECAUTIONS: Avoid eyes, abraded skin, mucous membranes, and mouth. Caution in atopic patients. D/C if significant diarrhea occurs.

ADVERSE REACTIONS: Dryness, oily skin, erythema, peeling, burning, itching, pseudomembranous colitis (rare).

INTERACTIONS: May potentiate neuromuscular blockers.

PREGNANCY: Category B, not for use in nursing.

MECHANISM OF ACTION: Inhibits growth of *Propionibacterium acnes* and decreases free fatty acids on the skin surface.

PHARMACOKINETICS: Absorption: Following topical administration of multiple doses, serum levels of clindamycin were measured at 0-3ng/mL. **Distribution:** Orally and parenterally administered clindamycin has been found in breast milk. **Metabolism:** Hydrolysis. **Elimination:** Urine (≤0.2% found as clindamycin).

CLEOCIN VAGINAL RX
clindamycin phosphate (Pharmacia & Upjohn)

OTHER BRAND NAMES: Cleocin Vaginal Ovules (Pharmacia & Upjohn) - Clindamax Vaginal (PharmaDerm)

THERAPEUTIC CLASS: Lincomycin derivative

INDICATIONS: (Cream) Treatment of bacterial vaginosis in non-pregnant women and pregnant women during the 2nd and 3rd trimester. (Sup) Treatment of bacterial vaginosis in non-pregnant women.

DOSAGE: *Adults:* (Cream) 1 applicatorful intravaginally qhs. Treat non-pregnant females for 3 or 7 days. Treat pregnant females (2nd and 3rd trimester) for 7 days. (Sup) 1 suppository intravaginally qhs for 3 days.
Pediatrics: Post-Menarchal: (Sup) 1 suppository intravaginally qhs for 3 days.

HOW SUPPLIED: Cre: 2% (40g); Sup, Vaginal: (Ovules) 100mg (3's)

CONTRAINDICATIONS: Hypersensitivity to lincomycin. History of regional enteritis, ulcerative colitis, or antibiotic-associated colitis.

WARNINGS/PRECAUTIONS: Do not use condoms or contraceptive diaphragms within 72 hrs following treatment. Monitor for pseudomembranous colitis. Avoid eye contact. Do not engage in vaginal intercourse or use other vaginal products (such as tampons or douches) during treatment. Monitor for pseudomembranous colitis. May result in overgrowth of nonsusceptible organisms in vagina.

ADVERSE REACTIONS: Vaginitis, vulvovaginal disorder, candidiasis, moniliasis, pruritus, abnormal labor.

INTERACTIONS: May potentiate neuromuscular blockers.

PREGNANCY: Category B, not for use in nursing.

MECHANISM OF ACTION: Antibiotic; inhibits bacterial protein synthesis at the level of the bacterial ribosome and binds preferentially to the 50S ribosomal subunit affecting peptide chain initiation.

PHARMACOKINETICS: Absorption: (Day 1) C_{max} =13ng/ml; (Day 7) C_{max}=16ng/mL, T_{max}=14 hrs. **Elimination:** $T_{1/2}$=1.5-2.6 hrs.

CLINDAGEL RX
clindamycin phosphate (Galderma)

THERAPEUTIC CLASS: Lincomycin derivative

INDICATIONS: Acne vulgaris.

DOSAGE: *Adults:* Apply thin film once daily.
Pediatrics: ≥12 yrs: Apply thin film once daily.

HOW SUPPLIED: Gel: 1% (40mL, 75mL)

CONTRAINDICATIONS: Hypersensitivity to lincomycin. History of regional enteritis, ulcerative colitis, or antibiotic-associated colitis.

WARNINGS/PRECAUTIONS: D/C if significant diarrhea occurs. Caution in atopic individuals.

ADVERSE REACTIONS: Peeling, pruritus, pseudomembranous colitis (rare).

INTERACTIONS: May potentiate neuromuscular blockers.

PREGNANCY: Category B, not for use in nursing.

MECHANISM OF ACTION: Lincomycin derivative; inhibits bacteria protein synthesis at ribosomal level by binding to the 50S ribosomal subunit and affecting the process of peptide chain initiation.

PHARMACOKINETICS: Absorption: C_{max}≤5.5ng/mL. **Distribution:** Orally and parenterally administered clindamycin appears in breast milk. **Excretion:** Urine (<0.4% of total dose).

CLINDAMYCIN PHOSPHATE
clindamycin phosphate (Various)

THERAPEUTIC CLASS: Lincomycin derivative

INDICATIONS: Treatment of acne vulgaris.

DOSAGE: *Adults:* Apply thin film bid.
Pediatrics: ≥12 yrs: Apply thin film bid.

HOW SUPPLIED: Swab: 1% (69 pads)

CONTRAINDICATIONS: History of regional enteritis, ulcerative colitis, or antibiotic-associated colitis.

WARNINGS/PRECAUTIONS: Avoid eyes, abraded skin, mucous membranes and mouth. Caution in atopic patients. Diarrhea, bloody diarrhea and colitis reported with systemic and topical use. D/C if significant diarrhea occurs.

ADVERSE REACTIONS: Burning, itching, dryness, erythema, oily skin, peeling.

INTERACTIONS: May potentiate neuromuscular blockers.

PREGNANCY: Category B, not for use in nursing.

CLOBEVATE
clobetasol propionate (Stiefel)

THERAPEUTIC CLASS: Corticosteroid

INDICATIONS: Inflammatory and pruritic manifestations of corticosteroid-responsive dermatoses.

DOSAGE: *Adults:* Apply thin layer bid. Limit treatment to 2 consecutive weeks. Max: 50g/week. Avoid with occlusive dressings.
Pediatrics: ≥12 yrs: Apply thin layer bid. Limit treatment to 2 consecutive weeks. Max: 50g/week. Avoid with occlusive dressings.

HOW SUPPLIED: Gel: 0.05% (45g)

WARNINGS/PRECAUTIONS: May produce reversible HPA axis suppression, manifestations of Cushing's syndrome, hyperglycemia, and glucosuria. Pediatrics may be more susceptible to systemic toxicity. D/C if irritation occurs. Use appropriate antifungal or anti-bacterial with concomitant skin infections; d/c if infection does not clear. Should not be used to treat rosacea or perioral dermatitis. Avoid use on face, groin, or axillae.

ADVERSE REACTIONS: Burning, stinging, irritation, pruritus, erythema, folliculitis, cracking and fissuring of the skin, numbness of fingers, skin atrophy, telangiectasia.

PREGNANCY: Category C, caution in nursing.

MECHANISM OF ACTION: Corticosteroid; not established. Has anti-inflammatory, antipruritic, and vasoconstrictive properties. Anti-inflammatory not established; thought to induct phospholipase A_2 inhibitory proteins called lipocortins. Lipocortins control the biosynthesis of potent mediators of inflammation (eg, prostaglandins, leukotrienes) through inhibition of their common precursor, arachidonic acid. Arachidonic acid is released from membrane phospholipids by phospholipase A_2.

PHARMACOKINETICS: Absorption: Absorbed through skin. Occlusive dressings ≤24 hrs, no effect. Occlusive dressings at 96 hrs, markedly enhances penetration. **Distribution:** Systemically administered corticosteroids appear in human breast milk.

CLODERM
clocortolone pivalate (Healthpoint)

THERAPEUTIC CLASS: Topical corticosteroid

INDICATIONS: Corticosteroid-responsive dermatoses.

DOSAGE: *Adults:* Apply tid. Use with occlusive dressing for management of psoriasis or recalcitrant conditions.
Pediatrics: Apply TID. Use with occlusive dressing for management of psoriasis or recalcitrant conditions.

HOW SUPPLIED: Cre: 0.1% (15g, 45g, 90g)

WARNINGS/PRECAUTIONS: May produce reversible HPA axis suppression, manifestations of Cushing's syndrome, hyperglycemia, glucosuria. Caution when applied to large surface areas or under occlusive dressings. Use appropriate antifungal or antibacterial agent with dermatological infections. D/C if infection is not adequately controlled or if irritation develops.

ADVERSE REACTIONS: Burning, itching, irritation, dryness, folliculitis, hypertrichosis, acneform eruptions, hypopigmentation, perioral/allergic contact dermatitis, secondary infection, skin atrophy.

PREGNANCY: Category C, caution in nursing.

MECHANISM OF ACTION: Topical corticosteroid; not established. Possesses anti-inflammatory, anti-pruritic, and vasoconstrictive actions.

PHARMACOKINETICS: Absorption: Percutaneous; occlusion, inflammation, and other skin diseases, increase absorption. **Distribution:** Bound to plasma protein to varying degrees. Systemically administered corticosteroids found in breast milk. **Metabolism:** Liver. **Elimination:** Kidney and bile.

CLOLAR   RX
clofarabine (Genzyme)

THERAPEUTIC CLASS: Antimetabolite

INDICATIONS: Treatment of pediatric patients 1-21 years old with relapsed or refractory acute lymphoblastic leukemia after at least two prior regimens.

DOSAGE: *Pediatrics:* 1-21 yrs: 52mg/m^2 IV over 2 hours daily for 5 consecutive days. Treatment cycles are repeated following recovery or return to baseline organ function, approximately 2-6 weeks. Continuous IV fluids throughout 5 days of clofarabine therapy is recommended. The use of prophylactic steroids (eg, 100mg/m^2 hydrocortisone on Days 1-3) may be of benefit in preventing signs and symptoms of systemic inflammatory response syndrome (SIRS) or capillary leak. If patient develops signs and symptoms of SIRS or capillary leak, clofarabine therapy should be discontinued and appropriate supportive measures should be provided. Close monitoring of renal and hepatic function is required. If substantial increases in creatine or bilirubin occur, clofarabine therapy should be discontinued.

HOW SUPPLIED: Inj: 1mg/mL

WARNINGS/PRECAUTIONS: Suppression of bone marrow function should be anticipated. Increased risk of infection, including severe sepsis is possible. Monitor for signs and symptoms of tumor lysis syndrome, as well as cytokine release that could develop into SIRS/capillary leak syndrome and organ dysfunction. D/C immediately if SIRS or capillary leak syndrome develop. Severe bone marrow suppression, including neutropenia, anemia and thrombocytopenia have been observed. Dehydration may occur due to vomiting and diarrhea. Clofarabine should be discontinued if patient develops hypotension for any reason during the 5 days of administration. Since clofarabine is excreted primarily by the kidneys, drugs with known renal toxicity should be avoided during the 5 days of administration. Since the liver is a known target of clofarabine, concomitant use of medications known to induce hepatic toxicity should also be avoided. Patients taking medications known to affect BP or cardiac function should be closely monitored during administration.

ADVERSE REACTIONS: Vomiting, nausea, diarrhea, anemia, leukopenia, thrombocytopenia, neutropenia, febrile neutropenia, and infection.

PREGNANCY: Category D, not for use in nursing.

MECHANISM OF ACTION: Antimetabolite; inhibits DNA synthesis by decreasing cellular deoxynucleotide triphosphate pools through an inhibitory action on ribonucleotide reductase, and by terminating DNA chain elongation and inhibiting repair through incorporation into DNA chain by competitive inhibition of DNA polymerases.

PHARMACOKINETICS: Distribution: V_d=172L/m^2; plasma protein binding (47%). **Elimination:** Urine (unchanged); $T_{1/2}$=5.2 hrs.

CLOTRIMAZOLE TOPICAL

clotrimazole (Various)

THERAPEUTIC CLASS: Azole antifungal

INDICATIONS: Topical treatment of candidiasis caused by *Candida albicans* and tinea versicolor caused by *Malassezia furfur*.

DOSAGE: *Adults:* Apply bid (am and pm). Re-evaluate if no improvement after 4 weeks.
Pediatrics: Apply bid (am and pm). Re-evaluate if no improvement after 4 weeks.

HOW SUPPLIED: Cre: 1% (15g, 30g); Sol: 1% (10mL)

WARNINGS/PRECAUTIONS: D/C if irritation or sensitivity occurs. Not for ophthalmic use.

ADVERSE REACTIONS: Erythema, stinging, blistering, peeling, edema, pruritus, urticaria, burning, irritation.

PREGNANCY: Category B, caution in nursing.

MECHANISM OF ACTION: Broad spectrum antifungal agent; primary action is against dividing and growing organisms. Causes leakage of intracellular phosphorus compounds into the ambient medium with concomitant breakdown of cellular nucleic acids and accelerated potassium efflux.

PHARMACOKINETICS: **Absorption:** Minimally absorbed. **Elimination:** Urine (≤0.5%).

CODICLEAR DH

guaifenesin - hydrocodone bitartrate (Victory)

THERAPEUTIC CLASS: Opioid antitussive

INDICATIONS: Temporary relief of non-productive cough associated with upper and lower respiratory tract congestion.

DOSAGE: *Adults:* 1 teaspoonful q4-6h. Max: 6 teaspoonsful/24hrs.
Pediatrics: >12 yrs: 1 teaspoonful q4-6h. Max: 6 teaspoonfuls/24hrs. 6-12 yrs: 1/2 teaspoonful q4-6h. Max: 3 teaspoonsful/24 hrs.

HOW SUPPLIED: Syrup: (Hydrocodone-Guaifenesin) 3.5mg-300mg/5mL

CONTRAINDICATIONS: (Hydrocodone) Increased ICP and whenever ventilatory function is depressed

WARNINGS/PRECAUTIONS: Hydrocodone is potentially habit-forming. Extreme caution with severe respiratory impairment or impaired respiratory drive. May cause respiratory depression; caution with COPD. Caution with renal, hepatic, or gall bladder disease, asthma, glaucoma, urinary retention, prostatic hypertrophy, hypothyroidism, seizures or epilepsy, head injury, or Addison's disease. May cause drowsiness or dizziness; caution when operating heavy machinery or other hazardous activities.

ADVERSE REACTIONS: Drowsiness, nausea, giddiness, constipation, respiratory depression, dizziness, restlessness, irritability, blurred vision, dry mouth, vomiting, decreased appetite, sweating, itching, decreased urination.

INTERACTIONS: Additive CNS depression with other narcotic analgesics, general anesthetics, phenothiazines, tranquilizers, sedative hypnotics, alcohol, other CNS depressants (including alcohol).

PREGNANCY: Category C, not for use in nursing.

MECHANISM OF ACTION: Hydrocodone: Unknown. Suppresess the cough reflex by depressing the medullary cough center. Guaifenesin: Increases the output of phlegm and bronchial secretions by reducing adhesiveness and surface tension.

COLACE

docusate sodium (Purdue Products)

THERAPEUTIC CLASS: Stool softener

INDICATIONS: (PO) Stool softener for constipation, painful anorectal conditions and in cardiac conditions.

DOSAGE: *Adults:* 50-200mg/day. (Retention or Flushing Enema) Add 5-10mL of liquid to enema fluid. Mix Liq/Syr into 6-8 oz of milk or juice.
Pediatrics: ≥12 yrs: 50-200mg/day. 6-12 yrs: 40-120mg/day Liq. 3-6 yrs: 2mL Liq tid. Mix Liq/Syr into 6-8 oz of milk, juice or formula. (Retention/Flushing Enema) Add 5-10mL of liquid to enema fluid.

HOW SUPPLIED: Cap: 50mg, 100mg; Liq: 10mg/mL; Syrup: 20mg/5mL

WARNINGS/PRECAUTIONS: Avoid with abdominal pain, nausea, or vomiting. D/C enema if rectal bleeding occurs or fail to have a bowel movement.

ADVERSE REACTIONS: Bitter taste, throat irritation, nausea, rash.

PREGNANCY: Safety in pregnancy and nursing not known.

COLAZAL
balsalazide disodium (Salix)

RX

THERAPEUTIC CLASS: Anti-inflammatory Agent

INDICATIONS: Treatment of mild-to-moderate active ulcerative colitis in patients ≥5 yrs.

DOSAGE: *Adults:* 3 caps tid for up to 8 weeks (or 12 weeks if needed). May open cap and sprinkle on applesauce.
Pediatrics: 5-17 yrs: 1 or 3 caps tid for 8 weeks. May open cap and sprinkle on applesauce.

HOW SUPPLIED: Cap: 750mg

CONTRAINDICATIONS: Hypersensitivity to salicylates.

WARNINGS/PRECAUTIONS: May exacerbate symptoms of colitis. Prolonged gastric retention with pyloric stenosis. Caution with renal dysfunction or history of renal disease.

ADVERSE REACTIONS: Headache, abdominal pain, diarrhea, nausea, vomiting, respiratory problems, arthralgia, rhinitis, insomnia, fatigue, rectal bleeding, flatulence, fever, dyspepsia.

INTERACTIONS: Oral antibiotics may interfere with the release of mesalamine in the colon.

PREGNANCY: Category B, caution in nursing.

MECHANISM OF ACTION: Not established; a prodrug enzymatically cleaved in colon to produce mesalamine (5-ASA), an anti-inflammatory drug that acts locally to block production of arachidonic acid metabolites in the colon.

PHARMACOKINETICS: Absorption: Different dosing conditions (fasted, fed, sprinkled) resulted in variable parameters. **Distribution:** Plasma protein binding (≥99%). **Metabolism:** Key metabolites: 5-ASA and N-acetyl-5-ASA. **Elimination:** Urine, feces.

COLY-MYCIN M
colistimethate sodium (King)

RX

THERAPEUTIC CLASS: Antibacterial agent

INDICATIONS: Treatment of acute or chronic infections due to certain gram-negative bacilli (eg, *Pseudomonas aeruginosa, Enterobacter aerogenes, E. coli, Klebsiella pneumoniae*).

DOSAGE: *Adults:* Usual: 2.5-5mg/kg/day IV/IM in 2-4 divided doses. Max: 5mg/kg/day. SCr 1.3-1.5mg/dL: 2.5-3.8mg/kg/day IV/IM in 2 divided doses. SCr 1.6-2.5mg/dL: 2.5mg/kg/day IV/IM in 1-2 divided doses. SCr 2.6-4mg/dL: 1.5mg/kg/day IV/IM q36h. Obesity: Base dose on IBW.
Pediatrics: Usual: 2.5-5mg/kg/day IV/IM in 2-4 divided doses. Max: 5mg/kg/day. SCr 1.3-1.5mg/dL: 2.5-3.8mg/kg/day IV/IM in 2 divided doses. SCr 1.6-2.5mg/dL: 2.5mg/kg/day IV/IM in 1-2 divided doses. SCr 2.6-4mg/dL: 1.5mg/kg/day IV/IM q36h. Obesity: Base dose on IBW.

HOW SUPPLIED: Inj: 150mg

WARNINGS/PRECAUTIONS: Transient neurological disturbances may occur; dose reduction may alleviate symptoms. Respiratory arrest reported after IM administration. Increased risk of apnea and neuromuscular blockade with renal impairment. Reversible dose-dependent nephrotoxicity reported. Pseudomembranous colitis reported. May permit overgrowth of clostridia. Use extreme caution with renal impairment; d/c with further impairment.

ADVERSE REACTIONS: GI upset, tingling of extremities and tongue, slurred speech, dizziness, vertigo, paresthesia, itching, urticaria, rash, fever, increased BUN and creatinine, decreased creatinine clearance, respiratory distress, apnea, nephrotoxicity, decreased urine output.

INTERACTIONS: Avoid certain antibiotics (eg, aminoglycosides, polymyxin); may interfere with nerve transmission at neuromuscular junction. Extreme caution with curariform muscle relaxants (eg, tubocurarine), succinylcholine, gallamine, decamethonium and sodium citrate; may potentiate neuromuscular blocking effect. Avoid sodium cephalothin; may enhance nephrotoxicity.

PREGNANCY: Category C, caution in nursing.

MECHANISM OF ACTION: Antibacterial agent; penetrates into and disrupts the bacterial cell membrane.

PHARMACOKINETICS: Elimination: $T_{1/2}$=2-3 hrs.

COMBIGAN
brimonidine tartrate - timolol maleate (Allergan)

RX

THERAPEUTIC CLASS: Alpha$_{2\text{-agonist/beta-blocker}}$

INDICATIONS: Reduction of elevated intraocular pressure (IOP) in patients with glaucoma or ocular hypertension who require adjunctive or replacement therapy due to inadequately controlled IOP.

DOSAGE: *Adults:* 1 drop in affected eye(s) bid approximately 12 hrs apart. Instill other topical ophthalmic products at least 5 min apart.
Pediatrics: ≥2 yrs: 1 drop in affected eye(s) bid approximately 12 hrs apart. Instill other topical ophthalmic products at least 5 min apart.

HOW SUPPLIED: Sol: (Brimonidine-Timolol) 2mg-5mg/mL

CONTRAINDICATIONS: Bronchial asthma, history of bronchial asthma, severe COPD, sinus bradycardia, second or third degree AV block, overt cardiac failure, cardiogenic shock.

WARNINGS/PRECAUTIONS: Systemic absorption, leading to adverse reactions (including severe respiratory reactions) may occur. Caution with cardiac failure; d/c if cardiac failure develops. Avoid with bronchospastic disease and/or mild-to-moderate COPD. May potentiate syndromes associated with vascular insufficiency; caution with depression, cerebral or coronary insufficiency, Raynaud's phenomenon, orthostatic hypotension, or thromboangiitis obliterans. May increase reactivity to allergens. May potentiate muscle weakness consistent with certain myasthenic symptoms. May mask signs/symptoms of acute hypoglycemia; caution in patients subject to spontaneous hypoglycemia or diabetic patients receiving insulin or hypoglycemic agents. May mask signs of hyperthyroidism. Bacterial keratitis reported with use of multiple dose containers of topical ophthalmic products. May need to gradually withdraw β-blocking agents in patients undergoing elective surgery.

ADVERSE REACTIONS: Allergic conjunctivitis, conjunctival folliculosis, conjunctival hyperemia, eye pruritus, ocular burning/stinging.

INTERACTIONS: May reduce BP; caution with antihypertensives and/or cardiac glycosides. Monitor with concomitant oral β-blockers; avoid concomitant use of 2 topical β-blocking agents. Caution with concomitant oral or IV calcium antagonists; avoid concomitant use with impaired cardiac function. Monitor closely with concomitant catecholamine-depleting drugs (eg, reserpine). Possibility of additive or potentiating effect with CNS depressants (eg, alcohol, barbiturates, opiates, sedatives, anesthetics). Concomitant use of β-blockers with digitalis and/or calcium antagonists may have additive effects in prolonging AV-conduction time. Potentiated systemic β-blockade reported with CYP2D6 inhibitors and timolol. Caution with TCAs and/or MAOIs.

PREGNANCY: Category C, not for use in nursing.

MECHANISM OF ACTION: Decreases elevated IOP. Brimonidine: Selective α-2 adrenergic receptor. Timolol: Non selective β-blocker.

PHARMACOKINETICS: Absorption: Brimonidine: C_{max}=30pg/mL; T_{max}= 1-4 hrs. Timolol: C_{max}=400pg/mL; T_{max}=1-3 hrs. **Distribution:** Timolol: Plasma protein binding (60%). **Metabolism:** Brimonidine: Liver (extensive). Timolol: Liver (partial). **Elimination:** Brimonidine: Urine (74%); $T_{1/2}$=3 hrs. Timolol: Excreted mainly by kidney; $T_{1/2}$=7 hrs.

COMBIVIR RX
lamivudine - zidovudine (GlaxoSmithKline)

> Zidovudine has been associated with hematologic toxicity (eg, granulocytopenia, severe ane-mia), especially with advanced HIV disease, and symptomatic myopathy reported with pro-longed use. Lactic acidosis and severe, fatal hepatomegaly with steatosis reported with nucleoside analogues. Severe acute exacerbations of hepatitis B reported in patients coinfected with hepatitis B virus and HIV who discontinued lamivudine (a component of Combivir); monitor hepatic function closely after discontinuation.

THERAPEUTIC CLASS: Nucleoside analog combination

INDICATIONS: Treatment of HIV infection in combination with other antiretrovirals.

DOSAGE: *Adults:* 1 tab bid. Do not give if CrCl ≤50mL/min or with dose-limiting adverse events.
Pediatrics: ≥12 yrs: 1 tab bid. Do not give if CrCl ≤50mL/min or with dose-limiting adverse events.

HOW SUPPLIED: Tab: (Lamivudine-Zidovudine) 150mg-300mg

WARNINGS/PRECAUTIONS: Caution with granulocyte count <1000cells/mm³ or Hgb <9.5g/dL; monitor blood counts frequently with advanced HIV and periodically with asymptomatic or early HIV. Hepatic decompensation occured when used with inter-feron alfa w/ or w/o ribavirin. Avoid with CrCl ≤50mL/min, and hepatic impairment. Myopathy, myositis may occur. Posttreatment exacerbation of hepatitis reported. Lamivudine-resistant hepatitis B virus reported. Caution in elderly. Possible redistribution or accumulation of body fat. Immune reconstitution syndrome reported.

ADVERSE REACTIONS: Headache, malaise, fatigue, fever, chills, nausea, diarrhea, anorexia, abdominal pain/cramps, neuropathy, insomnia, dizziness, neutropenia, mus-culoskeletal pain, myalgia, rash, cough, aplastic anemia, gynecomastia, oral mucosal pigmentation.

INTERACTIONS: Ganciclovir, interferon-α, other bone marrow suppressives and cytotoxic agents may increase the hematologic toxicity of zidovudine. Increased lamivudine exposure with trimethoprim 160mg/sulfamethoxazole 800mg. Avoid with zalcitabine, stavudine, doxorubicin, ribavirin, zidovudine, lamivudine, and fixed-dose combinations of abacavir, lamivudine, and zidovudine.

PREGNANCY: Category C, not for use in nursing.

MECHANISM OF ACTION: Nucleoside analogue; inhibits reverse transcriptase via DNA chain termination.

PHARMACOKINETICS: Absorption: Lamivudine: Rapid. Absolute bioavailabilty (86%). Zidovudine: Rapid. Absolute bioavialiabilty (64%). **Distribution:** Lamivudine: V_d=1.3L/kg; plasma protein binding (<36%). Zidovudine: V_d=1.6L/kg; plasma protein binding (<38%). **Metabolism:** Lamivudine: Trans-sulfoxide (metabolite). Zidovudine: Hepatic. 3'azido-3'-deoxy-5'-O-β-D-glucopyranurosylthymidine (metabolite). **Elimination:** Lamivudine: Urine (70%, unchanged), $T_{1/2}$=5-7 hrs. Zidovudine: Urine (14-74%); $T_{1/2}$=0.5-3 hrs.

COMVAX RX
haemophilus B conjugate - hepatitis B (recombinant) (Merck)

THERAPEUTIC CLASS: Vaccine

INDICATIONS: Vaccination against diseases caused by *Haemophilus influenza* type b and hepatitis B virus in infants born to HBsAg negative mothers.

DOSAGE: *Pediatrics:* ≥6 weeks: 0.5mL IM at 2, 4, and 12-15 months of age. If schedule cannot be followed, wait at least 6 weeks between 1st 2 doses. 2nd and 3rd dose should be close to 8-11 months apart.

HOW SUPPLIED: Inj: (Haemophilus B Conjugate Vaccine-Hepatitis B Recombinant Vaccine) 7.5mcg-5mcg-125mcg/0.5mL

WARNINGS/PRECAUTIONS: Possible suboptimal response with malignancy, immunosuppression, or immunocompromised patients. Delay vaccine in acute febrile illness. Have epinephrine injection (1:1000) available.

ADVERSE REACTIONS: Injection site pain, irritability, somnolence, anorexia, fever, seizures, febrile seizures.

INTERACTIONS: Immunosuppressive therapies may reduce effectiveness.

PREGNANCY: Category C, safety in nursing not known.

MECHANISM OF ACTION: Vaccine; elicits the formation of antibodies that may protect against *H.influenzae* type b and hepatitis B infections.

CONCERTA
methylphenidate HCl (McNeil Pediatrics)   `CII`

THERAPEUTIC CLASS: Sympathomimetic amine

INDICATIONS: Treatment of attention deficit hyperactivity disorder (ADHD) in patients ≥6 yrs.

DOSAGE: *Adults:* Methylphenidate-Naive or Receiving Other Stimulant: Initial: 18mg qam. Titrate: Adjust dose at weekly intervals. Previous Methylphenidate Use: Initial: 18mg qam if previous dose 10-15mg/day; 36mg qam if previous dose 20-30mg/day; 54mg qam if previous dose 30-45mg/day. Initial conversion should not exceed 54mg/day. Titrate: Adjust dose at weekly intervals. Max: 72mg/day. Reduce dose or discontinue if paradoxical aggravation of symptoms occurs. Discontinue if no improvement after appropriate dosage adjustments over 1 month. Swallow whole with liquids. Do not crush, chew, or divide.
Pediatrics: ≥6 yrs: Methylphenidate-Naive or Receiving Other Stimulant: Initial: 18mg qam. Titrate: Adjust dose at weekly intervals. Max: 6-12 yrs: 54mg/day; 13-17 yrs: 72mg/day not to exceed 2mg/kg/day. Previous Methylphenidate Use: Initial: 18mg qam if previous dose 10-15mg/day; 36mg qam if previous dose 20-30mg/day; 54mg qam if previous dose 30-45mg/day. Initial conversion should not exceed 54mg/day. Titrate: Adjust dose at weekly intervals. Max: 72mg/day. Reduce dose or discontinue if paradoxical aggravation of symptoms occurs. Discontinue if no improvement after appropriate dosage adjustments over 1 month. Swallow whole with liquids. Do not crush, chew, or divide.

HOW SUPPLIED: Tab, Extended-Release: 18mg, 27mg, 36mg, 54mg

CONTRAINDICATIONS: Marked anxiety, tension, and agitation; glaucoma; motor tics or family history or diagnosis of Tourette's syndrome, during or within 14 days of MAOI use.

WARNINGS/PRECAUTIONS: Monitor growth during treatment in children. Not for severe depression or fatigue. May exacerbate symptoms of behavior disturbance and thought disorder in psychotic patients. Avoid with severe GI narrowing (eg, esophageal motility disorders, small bowel inflammatory disease, short-gut syndrome). May lower seizure threshold, especially in known EEG abnormalities. Caution with HTN, conditions affected by BP or HR elevation, history of drug abuse or alcoholism. Monitor during withdrawal from abusive use. Visual disturbances may occur (rare). Monitor CBC, differential, and platelets with prolonged use. Caution when using stimulants to treat patients with comorbid bipolar disorder because of concern for possible induction of mixed/manic episode in such patients. Stimulants at usual dose can cause treatment emergent psychotic or manic symptoms (eg, hallucinations, delusional thinking, mania) in children and adolescents without prior history of psychotic illness. Aggressive behavior or hostility reported in clinical trials and postmarketing experience of some medications indicated for the treatment of ADHD. Avoid with known structural cardiac abnormalities or other serious cardiac problems.

ADVERSE REACTIONS: Headache, abdominal pain, anorexia, insomnia, upper respiratory tract infection, vomiting, rhinitis, fever, cough, pharyngitis, sinusitis.

INTERACTIONS: Avoid MAOIs. Potentiates anticoagulants, anticonvulsants (eg, phenobarbital, phenytoin, primidone), TCAs, and SSRIs. Caution with α_2-agonists (eg, clonidine) and pressor agents.

PREGNANCY: Category C, caution in nursing.

MECHANISM OF ACTION: Sympathomimetic amine; blocks reuptake of norepinephrine and dopamine into presynaptic neuron and increases release of these monoamines into extraneuronal space.

PHARMACOKINETICS: Absorption: (PO) Readily absorbed; T_{max}=6-10 hrs. **Metabolism:** De-esterification; α-phenyl-piperidine acetic acid (metabolite). **Elimination:** Urine (90%); $T_{1/2}$=3.5 hrs.

CORDRAN
flurandrenolide (Watson)

RX

OTHER BRAND NAME: Cordran SP (Watson)

THERAPEUTIC CLASS: Corticosteroid

INDICATIONS: Treatment of corticosteroid responsive dermatoses.

DOSAGE: *Adults:* (Cre, Lot) Apply qd-qid depending on severity. For moist lesions, apply cream bid-tid. Apply lotion bid-tid. (Tape) Clean and dry skin. Shave or clip hair. Apply tape q12-24h.
Pediatrics: (Cre, Lot) Apply qd-qid depending on severity. For moist lesions, apply cream bid-tid. Apply lotion bid-tid. (Tape) Clean and dry skin. Shave or clip hair. Apply tape q12-24h.

HOW SUPPLIED: Cre (SP): 0.05% (15g, 30g, 60g); Lot: 0.05% (15mL, 60mL); Tape: 4mcg/cm^2

CONTRAINDICATIONS: (Tape) Not for lesions exuding serum or in intertriginous areas.

WARNINGS/PRECAUTIONS: Systemic absorption may produce reversible HPA axis suppression, manifestations of Cushing's syndrome, hyperglycemia, and glucosuria. Application of more potent steroids, use on large surfaces, prolonged use, or occlusive dressings may augment systemic absorption. Evaluate periodically for HPA suppression if large dose applied to large area or with occlusive dressings. Pediatrics are more susceptible to toxicity. D/C if irritation develops. May use occlusive dressing for psoriasis or recalcitrant conditions.

ADVERSE REACTIONS: Burning, itching, irritation, dryness, folliculitis, hypertrichosis, acneform eruptions, hypopigmentation, dermatitis. Occlusive dressing may cause skin maceration, secondary infection, skin atrophy, miliaria.

PREGNANCY: Category C, caution in nursing.

MECHANISM OF ACTION: Corticosteroid; possesses anti-inflammatory, antipruritic, and vasoconstrictive properties. Suspected to stabilize cellular and lysosomal membranes, thereby preventing release of proteolytic enzymes, and consequently reducing inflammation.

PHARMACOKINETICS: Absorption: Extent of percutaneous absorption depends on integrity of skin, vehicle, and use of occlusive dressings. **Distribution:** Plasma protein binding (variable). **Metabolism:** Liver. **Elimination:** Kidney (major), bile.

CORLOPAM
fenoldopam mesylate (Hospira)

RX

THERAPEUTIC CLASS: Dopamine D_1-like receptor agonist

INDICATIONS: (Adults) For short-term (up to 48 hrs), in-hospital management of severe hypertension when rapid, but quickly reversible, emergency reduction of BP is clinically indicated, including malignant hypertension with deteriorating end-organ function. (Pediatrics) For in-hospital, short-term (up to 4 hours) reduction in BP.

DOSAGE: *Adults:* Range: Initial: 0.01-0.8 mcg/kg/min IV. Titrate: Increase/decrease by 0.05-0.1mcg/kg/min no more frequently than every 15 min. May use for up to 48 hrs. Refer to PI for detailed dosing info.
Pediatrics: <1 month-12 years: Initial: 0.2mcg/kg/min. May increase dose every 20-30 min up to 0.3-0.5 mcg/kg/min. Refer to PI for detailed dosing info.

HOW SUPPLIED: Inj: 10mg/mL

WARNINGS/PRECAUTIONS: Contains sodium metabisulfite; may cause allergic-type reactions especially in asthmatics. Caution in glaucoma or intraocular HTN. Dose-related tachycardia reported. Symptomatic hypotension may occur; monitor BP. Avoid hypotension with acute cerebral infarction or hemorrhage. Hypokalemia reported; monitor serum electrolytes.

ADVERSE REACTIONS: Headache, nausea, flushing, extrasystoles, palpitations, bradycardia, heart failure, elevated BUN/glucose/transaminase, chest pain, leukocytosis, bleeding, dyspnea.

INTERACTIONS: Avoid β-blockers; unexpected hypotension may occur.

PREGNANCY: Category B, caution in nursing.

MECHANISM OF ACTION: Dopamine D_1-like receptor agonist; rapid-acting vasodilator.

PHARMACOKINETICS: Metabolism: Conjugation. **Elimination:** (Adults) Urine (4%), feces; $T_{1/2}$=5 min. (Pediatrics) $T_{1/2}$=3-5 min.

CORMAX   RX
clobetasol propionate (Watson)

OTHER BRAND NAME: Cormax Scalp (Watson)

THERAPEUTIC CLASS: Corticosteroid

INDICATIONS: Corticosteroid-responsive dermatoses.

DOSAGE: *Adults:* Apply bid. Limit treatment to 2 consecutive weeks. Max: 50g/week or 50mL/week.
Pediatrics: ≥12 yrs: (Cre, Sol) Apply bid. Limit treatment to 2 consecutive weeks. Max: 50g/week or 50mL/week.

HOW SUPPLIED: Cre: 0.05% (15g, 30g, 45g); Sol (Scalp): 0.05% (25mL, 50mL)

CONTRAINDICATIONS: Primary infections of the scalp with solution.

WARNINGS/PRECAUTIONS: Not for treatment of rosacea or perioral dermatitis. May produce reversible HPA axis suppression, manifestations of Cushing's syndrome, hyperglycemia, and glucosuria. Reassess diagnosis if no improvement after 2 weeks. D/C if irritation occurs. Pediatrics may be more susceptible to systemic toxicity. Use appropriate antifungal or antibacterial agent with dermatological infections. Avoid occlusive dressings.

ADVERSE REACTIONS: Burning, stinging, pruritus, skin atrophy, cracking/fissuring of skin, irritation, (sol) tingling, (sol) folliculitis.

PREGNANCY: Category C, caution in nursing.

MECHANISM OF ACTION: Corticosteroid; possesses anti-inflammatory, antipruritic, and vasoconstrictive properties. Suspected to stabilize cellular and lysosomal membranes, thereby preventing release of proteolytic enzymes, and consequently reducing inflammation.

PHARMACOKINETICS: Absorption: Extent of percutaneous absorption depends on integrity of skin, vehicle, and use of occlusive dressings. **Distribution:** Plasma protein binding (variable). **Metabolism:** Liver. **Elimination:** Kidney (major), bile.

CORTANE-B   RX
chloroxylenol - hydrocortisone - pramoxine HCl (Blansett)

OTHER BRAND NAME: Zoto HC (Sciele)

THERAPEUTIC CLASS: Antimicrobial/Corticosteroid/Topical anesthetic

INDICATIONS: Treatment of superficial infections of the external ear and to control inflammation and itching.

DOSAGE: *Adults:* Instill 4-5 drops tid-qid. Gauze or wick may be inserted into ear canal after 1st administration. Add additional drops to saturate wick q4h. Remove wick after 24 hrs and continue to instill. Do not treat for >10 days.
Pediatrics: Instill 3 drops tid-qid. Gauze or wick may be inserted into ear canal after 1st administration. Add additional drops to saturate wick q4h. Remove wick after 24 hrs and continue to instill. Do not treat for >10 days.

HOW SUPPLIED: Sol: (Chloroxylenol-Hydrocortisone-Pramoxine) 1mg-10mg-10mg/mL (10mL)

CONTRAINDICATIONS: Varicella, vaccinia, perforated ear drum or when medication can reach the middle ear.

WARNINGS/PRECAUTIONS: Caution in long-standing otitis media. D/C if local irritation or sensitization occur. Systemic absorption has produced HPA axis, manifestations of Cushing's syndrome, hyperglycemia, and glucosuria.

ADVERSE REACTIONS: Itching, burning, irritation, dryness, folliculitis, hypertrichosis, acneform eruptions, hypopigmentations.

PREGNANCY: Category C, caution in nursing.

MECHANISM OF ACTION: Chloroxylenol: Bactericidal agent. Hydrocortisone: Glucocorticoid, anti-inflammatory, and antipruritic agent. Pramoxine: Topical anesthetic.

PHARMACOKINETICS: Distribution: Secreted in breast milk.

CORTEF

RX

hydrocortisone (Pharmacia & Upjohn)

THERAPEUTIC CLASS: Corticosteroid

INDICATIONS: Steroid-responsive disorders.

DOSAGE: *Adults:* Initial: 20-240mg/day depending on disease. Adjust until a satisfactory response. Maint: Decrease in small amounts to lowest effective dose. Acute Exacerbations of Multiple Sclerosis: Initial: (Tab) 200mg/day of prednisolone for 1 week, then 80mg every other day for 1 month (20mg hydrocortisone=5mg prednisolone). *Pediatrics:* Initial: 20-240mg/day depending on disease. Adjust until a satisfactory response. Maint: After favorable response, decrease in small amounts to lowest effective dose. Acute Exacerbations of Multiple Sclerosis: Initial: (Tab) 200mg/day of prednisolone for 1 week, then 80mg every other day for 1 month (20mg hydrocortisone=5mg prednisolone).

HOW SUPPLIED: Sus: (Hydrocortisone Cypionate) 10mg/5mL (120mL); Tab: (Hydrocortisone) 5mg, 10mg, 20mg

CONTRAINDICATIONS: Systemic fungal infections.

WARNINGS/PRECAUTIONS: May need to increase dose before, during, and after stressful situations. May mask signs of infections. Avoid abrupt withdrawal. Prolonged use may produce glaucoma, optic nerve damage, secondary ocular infections. Increases BP, salt/water retention, potassium excretion. More severe/fatal course of infections reported with chickenpox, measles. Caution with TB, hypothyroidism, cirrhosis, ocular herpes simplex, HTN, diverticulitis, fresh intestinal anastomosis, ulcerative colitis, osteoporosis, myasthenia gravis, renal insufficiency, peptic ulcer disease. Growth and development of children on prolonged therapy should be monitored. Monitor for psychic disturbances. Kaposi's sarcoma reported.

ADVERSE REACTIONS: Fluid and electrolyte disturbances, HTN, osteoporosis, muscle weakness, cushingoid state, menstrual irregularities, nervousness, insomnia, impaired wound healing, DM, ulcerative esophagitis, excessive sweating, increases intracranial pressure, carbohydrate intolerance, glaucoma, cataracts.

INTERACTIONS: Reduced efficacy and increased clearance with hepatic enzyme inducers (eg, phenobarbital, phenytoin, and rifampin). Decreased clearance with ketoconazole and troleandomycin. Increases clearance of chronic high dose ASA; caution with hypoprothrombinemia. Effects on oral anticoagulants are variable; monitor PT. Increased insulin and oral hypoglycemic requirements in DM. Avoid live vaccines with immunosuppressive doses. Possible decreased vaccine response with killed or inactivated vaccines with immunosuppressive doses.

PREGNANCY: Safety in pregnancy and nursing not known.

MECHANISM OF ACTION: Anti-inflammatory glucocorticoid; causes profound and varied metabolic effects and modifies the body's immune responses to diverse stimuli.

CORTISPORIN-TC OTIC RX
colistin sulfate - hydrocortisone acetate - neomycin sulfate - thonzonium bromide (King)

THERAPEUTIC CLASS: Antibacterial/corticosteroid combination

INDICATIONS: Treatment of infections of the external auditory canal, mastoidectomy and fenestration cavities.

DOSAGE: *Adults:* Clean and dry ear canal. Dropper: 5 drops (calibrated dropper) or 4 drops (dropper bottle) tid-qid. Alternate Regimen: Insert cotton wick into ear canal, then saturate cotton. Repeat q4h to keep cotton moist. Replace wick q24h.
Pediatrics: Clean and dry ear canal. Dropper: 4 drops (calibrated dropper) or 3 drops (dropper bottle) tid-qid. Alternate Regimen: Insert cotton wick into ear canal, then saturate cotton. Repeat q4h to keep cotton moist. Replace wick q24h.

HOW SUPPLIED: (Colistin-Hydrocortisone-Neomycin-Thonzonium) Sus: 3mg-10mg-3.3mg-0.5mg/mL (10mL)

CONTRAINDICATIONS: Herpes simplex, vaccinia, and varicella infections.

WARNINGS/PRECAUTIONS: Caution with perforated eardrum, chronic otitis media. Prolonged use may result in secondary infection. Re-evaluate if no improvement after 1 week. D/C after 10 days.

ADVERSE REACTIONS: Cutaneous sensitization.

PREGNANCY: Safety in pregnancy and nursing not known.

MECHANISM OF ACTION: Colistin: Polypeptide antibiotic; penetrates into and disrupts bacterial cell membrane. Neomycin: Aminoglycoside antibiotic; inhibits protein synthesis, disrupting normal cycle of ribosomal function. Hydrocortisone: Corticosteroid hormone; thought to act by regulating rate of protein synthesis and controls inflammation. Thonzonium: Surfactant; promotes tissue contact by dispersion and penetration of the cellular debris and exudate.

CORTROSYN RX
cosyntropin (Amphastar)

THERAPEUTIC CLASS: Synthetic ACTH

INDICATIONS: Diagnostic agent used to screen for adrenocortical insufficiency.

DOSAGE: *Adults:* 0.25-0.75mg IM/IV injection or 0.25-0.75mg IV over 4-8 hrs. (See PI for method details).
Pediatrics: >2 yrs: 0.25-0.75mg IM/IV injection or 0.25-0.75mg IV over 4-8 hrs. ≤2 yrs: 0.125mg IM/IV injection or IV over 4-8 hrs. (See PI for method details).

HOW SUPPLIED: Inj: 0.25mg

WARNINGS/PRECAUTIONS: Exhibits slight immunologic activity. Patients known to be sensitized to natural ACTH with markedly positive skin tests will, with few exceptions, react negatively when tested intradermally. Falsely high fluorescence measurements with high plasma bilirubin or if plasma contains free Hgb.

ADVERSE REACTIONS: Hypersensitivity/anaphylactic reactions (rare), bradycardia, tachycardia, HTN, peripheral edema, rash.

INTERACTIONS: May potentiate electrolyte loss associated with diuretics.

PREGNANCY: Category C, caution in nursing.

MECHANISM OF ACTION: Synthetic ACTH; a diagnostic agent used to screen for adrenocortical insufficiency.

COSMEGEN
dactinomycin (Ovation)

RX

> Administer only under supervision of physician experienced in the use of cancer chemothera-peutic agents. Drug is highly toxic; handle and administer with care. Avoid inhalation of dust or vapors and contact with skin or mucous membranes. Avoid exposure during pregnancy. Extremely corrosive to soft tissue. Severe damage to soft tissue will occur with extravasation during IV use.

THERAPEUTIC CLASS: Actinomycin antibiotic

INDICATIONS: Concomitant treatment of Wilms' tumor, childhood rhabdomyosarcoma, Ewing's sarcoma, and metastatic nonseminomatous testicular carcinoma. Monotherapy for gestational trophoblastic neoplasia, and as palliative and/or adjunctive treatment of solid malignancies.

DOSAGE: *Adults:* Wilms' Tumor/Childhood Rhabdomyosarcoma/Ewing's Sarcoma: 15mcg/kg IV daily for 5 days. Testicular Cancer: 1000mcg/m^2 IV on Day 1 of combination therapy. Gestational Trophoblastic Neoplasia: Monotherapy: 12mcg/kg IV daily for 5 days. Combination Therapy: 500mcg/m^2 IV on Days 1 and 2. Solid Malignancies: 50mcg/kg IV for lower extremity or pelvis. 35mcg/kg IV for upper extremity. May need lower dose with obese patients, or with previous chemotherapy or radiation use. Dose intensity per 2-week cycle should not exceed 15mcg/kg/day or 400-600mcg/m^2 daily for 5 days. Calculate dose for obese or edematous patients based on BSA. Elderly: Start at low end of dosing range.
Pediatrics: >6-12 months: Wilms' Tumor, Childhood Rhabdomyosarcoma/Ewing's Sarcoma: 15mcg/kg IV daily for 5 days. Testicular Carcinoma: 1000mcg/m^2 IV on Day 1 of combination therapy. Gestational Trophoblastic Neoplasia: Monotherapy: 12mcg/kg IV daily for 5 days. Combination Therapy: 500mcg/m^2 IV on Days 1 and 2. Solid Malignancies: 50mcg/kg IV for lower extremity or pelvis. 35mcg/kg IV for upper extremity. May need lower dose with obese patients, or with previous chemotherapy or radiation use. Dose intensity per 2-week cycle should not exceed 15mcg/kg/day or 400-600mcg/m^2 daily for 5 days. Calculate dose for obese or edematous patients based on BSA.

HOW SUPPLIED: Inj: 0.5mg

CONTRAINDICATIONS: At or about the time of infection with chickenpox or herpes zoster.

WARNINGS/PRECAUTIONS: Monitor renal, hepatic, and bone marrow functions frequently. Can cause fetal harm during pregnancy. Possible anaphylactoid reactions. If stomatitis, diarrhea, or severe hematopoietic depression occurs; d/c until recovery. Caution in elderly; increased risk of myelosuppression. Veno-occlusive disease (primarily hepatic) reported. Not for oral administration.

ADVERSE REACTIONS: Nausea, vomiting, fatigue, lethargy, fever, cheilitis, esophagitis, abdominal pain, liver toxicity, anemia, blood dyscrasias, skin eruptions, acne, alopecia.

INTERACTIONS: Increased GI toxicity, marrow suppression, and incidence of secondary tumors with radiation. May reactivate erythema from previous radiation therapy. Caution if used within 2 months of irradiation for treatment of right-sided Wilms' tumor; hepatomegaly and elevated AST levels reported. Only use with radiotherapy for Wilms' tumor if benefit outweighs risks.

PREGNANCY: Category D, not for use in nursing.

MECHANISM OF ACTION: Actinomycin antibiotic; bindd to DNA and inhibits RNA synthesis.

PHARMACOKINETICS: Metabolism: Minimally metabolized. **Elimination:** Feces (30%), urine; T$_{1/2}$=36 hrs.

COSOPT
dorzolamide HCl - timolol maleate (Merck)

RX

THERAPEUTIC CLASS: Carbonic anhydrase inhibitor/nonselective beta-blocker

INDICATIONS: Treatment of ocular hypertension and open-angle glaucoma insufficiently responsive to β-blockers.

DOSAGE: *Adults:* 1 drop bid. Space dosing of other ophthalmic drugs by 10 min. *Pediatrics:* ≥2 yrs: 1 drop bid. Space dosing of other ophthalmic drugs by 10 min.

HOW SUPPLIED: Sol: (Dorzolamide-Timolol) 2%-0.5% (5mL, 10mL)

CONTRAINDICATIONS: Bronchial asthma, history of bronchial asthma, severe COPD, sinus bradycardia, 2nd- or 3rd-degree AV block, overt cardiac failure, cardiogenic shock.

WARNINGS/PRECAUTIONS: Caution with sulfonamide allergy, cardiac failure, DM, COPD, bronchospastic disease, surgery and hepatic impairment. May mask symptoms of hypoglycemia and thyrotoxicosis. Bacterial keratitis reported with contaminated containers. Avoid in severe renal impairment. D/C if hypersensitivity or ocular reaction occur. Reinsert contact lenses 15 minutes after applying drops.

ADVERSE REACTIONS: Taste perversion, ocular burning, conjunctival hyperemia, blurred vision, superficial punctate keratitis, eye itching.

INTERACTIONS: Avoid oral carbonic anhydrase inhibitors, oral β-blockers, or topical β-blockers due to potential additive effects. Oral/IV calcium antagonists can cause AV-conduction disturbances, left ventricular failure or hypotension. Potentiated systemic β-blockade with concomitant CYP2D6 inhibitors. Reserpine can cause additive effects, hypotension and/or bradycardia. AV conduction time prolonged with digitalis. Quinidine may potentiate β-blockade. Increased risk of hypoglycemia with insulin or oral hypoglycemic agents. Wait 10 minutes before using another ophthalmic drug.

PREGNANCY: Category C, not for use in nursing.

MECHANISM OF ACTION: Dorzolamide: Inhibitor of human carbonic anhydrase II; decreases aqueous humor secretion, presumably by slowing formation of bicarbonate ions with subsequent reduction in Na^+ and fluid transport. Timolol: β_1 and β_2 (nonselective) adrenergic receptor blocking agent; decrease elevated IOP by reducing aqueous humor secretion.

PHARMACOKINETICS: Absorption: Timolol: C_{max}=0.46ng/mL. **Distribution:** Dorzolamide: Plasma protein binding (33%). **Elimination:** Dorzolamide: Urine (unchanged).

COZAAR
losartan potassium (Merck)
RX

> Can cause death/injury to developing fetus during 2nd and 3rd trimesters. Stop therapy if pregnancy detected.

THERAPEUTIC CLASS: Angiotensin II receptor antagonist

INDICATIONS: Treatment of hypertension (HTN), alone or with other antihypertensives. To reduce the risk of stroke in patients with HTN and left ventricular hypertrophy (LVH), but evidence shows this does not apply to black patients. Diabetic nephropathy with an elevated serum creatinine and proteinuria (urinary albumin to creatinine ratio ≥300mg/g) in patients with type 2 diabetes and HTN.

DOSAGE: *Adults:* HTN: Initial: 50mg qd. Usual: 25-100mg/day given qd-bid. Intravascular Volume Depletion/Hepatic Impairment: Initial: 25mg qd. HTN with LVH: Initial: 50mg qd. Add hydrochlorothiazide (HCTZ) 12.5mg qd and/or increase losartan to 100mg qd, followed by an increase in HCTZ to 25mg qd based on BP response. Nephropathy: Initial: 50 mg qd. Titrate: Increase to 100mg qd based on BP response.
Pediatrics: ≥6 yrs: HTN: Initial: 0.7mg/kg qd (up to 50mg/day). Max: 1.4mg/kg/day (100mg/day).

HOW SUPPLIED: Tab: 25mg, 50mg, 100mg

WARNINGS/PRECAUTIONS: Can cause fetal injury/death. Correct volume or salt depletion before therapy. Changes in renal function may occur; caution with renal artery stenosis, severe CHF. Angioedema reported. Consider dose adjustment with hepatic dysfunction.

ADVERSE REACTIONS: Dizziness, cough, upper respiratory infection, diarrhea.

INTERACTIONS: K^+-sparing diuretics (eg, spironolactone, triamterene, amiloride), K^+ supplements, or K^+-containing salt substitutes may increase serum K^+. May reduce excreation of lithium; monitor lithium levels. Combination with NSAIDs, including COX-2 inhibitors, may lead to further deterioration of renal function and diminish antihypertensive effect.

PREGNANCY: Category C (1st trimester) and D (2nd and 3rd trimesters), not for use in nursing.

MECHANISM OF ACTION: Angiotensin II receptor antagonist; blocks vasoconstrictor and aldosterone-secreting effects of angiotensin II by selectively blocking binding of angiotensin II to AT_1 receptor.

PHARMACOKINETICS: Absorption: Bioavailability (33%). *Adults:* C_{max}=224ng/mL, T_{max}=0.9 hrs, AUC=442ng•h/mL. (Metabolite) C_{max}=212ng/mL, T_{max}=3.5 hrs, AUC= 1685 ng•h/mL. *Pediatrics:* C_{max}=141ng/mL, T_{max}=2 hrs, AUC=368ng•h/mL. (Metabolite) C_{max}=222ng/ mL, T_{max}=4.1 hrs, AUC=1866ng•h/mL. **Distribution:** V_d=34L, 12L (metabolite). **Metabolism:** Liver via CYP2C9, 3A4; carboxylic acid (active metabolite). **Elimination:** Urine (4% unchanged; 6% metabolite). *Adults:* $T_{1/2}$=2.1 hrs, 7.4 hrs (metabolite). *Pediatrics:* $T_{1/2}$=2.3 hrs, 5.6 hrs (metabolite).

CREON
amylase - lipase - protease (Solvay)

RX

THERAPEUTIC CLASS: Pancreatic enzyme supplement

INDICATIONS: Treatment of pancreatic exocrine insufficiency, often associated with cystic fibrosis (CF), chronic pancreatitis, post-pancreatectomy, post-GI bypass surgery, and ductal obstruction from neoplasm.

DOSAGE: *Adults:* Initial: (Creon 5) 2-4 caps per meal/snack. (Creon 10) 1-2 caps per meal/snack. (Creon 20) 1 cap per meal/snack. CF: Usual: 1500-3000 U lipase/kg/meal. Adjust dose to disease severity, control of steatorrhea, and maintenance of good nutritional status. Do not chew/crush caps. May add capsule contents to soft food (pH <5.5) and swallow immediately without chewing; take with water.
Pediatrics: <6yrs: Initial: (Creon 5) 1-2 caps per meal/snack. (Creon 10) 1 cap per meal/snack. (Creon 20) Dose based on clinical experience for age group. >6 yrs: Initial: (Creon 5) 2-4 caps per meal/snack. (Creon 10) 1-2 caps per meal/snack. (Creon 20) 1 cap per meal/snack. CF: Usual: 1500-3000 U lipase/kg/meal. Adjust dose to disease severity, control of steatorrhea, and maintenance of good nutritional status. Max: 6000 U lipase/kg/meal. Do not chew/crush caps. May add capsule contents to soft food (pH <5.5) and swallow immediately without chewing; take with water.

HOW SUPPLIED: Cap, Delayed-Release: (Amylase-Lipase-Protease) (Creon 5) 16,600 U-5000 U-18,750 U, (Creon 10) 33,200 U-10,000 U-37,500 U, (Creon 20) 66,400 U-20,000 U-75,000 U

CONTRAINDICATIONS: Pork protein hypersensitivity and early stages of acute pancreatitis.

WARNINGS/PRECAUTIONS: Strictures in the ileo-cecal region and/or ascending colon reported with ≥20,000 U lipase/cap in CF patients. Caution if >6000 U lipase/kg/meal fails to resolve symptoms especially with history of intestinal complications. Maintain adequate fluid intake. D/C if hypersensitivity occurs.

ADVERSE REACTIONS: Nausea, vomiting, bloating, cramping, constipation, diarrhea.

INTERACTIONS: Do not add capsule contents to food with pH >5.5.

PREGNANCY: Category C, caution in nursing.

MECHANISM OF ACTION: Pancreatic enzyme; catalyzes the hydrolysis of fats to glycerol and fatty acids, proteins into proteoses, and derived substances and starch into dextrins and short chain sugars.

CROFAB
crotalidae polyvalent immune fab (Ovine) (Savage)

RX

THERAPEUTIC CLASS: Venom specific immunoglobulin Fab fragment

INDICATIONS: Management of minimal to moderate North American crotalid envenomation. Use within 6 hrs to prevent clinical deterioration and systemic coagulation abnormalities.

DOSAGE: *Adults:* Initial: 4-6 vials IV over 60 min. Observe patient for 1 hr following dose to determine if envenomation is controlled. If needed, administer additional 4-6 vials until envenomation controlled. Once control is achieved, give 2 vials q6h for up to 18

hrs (3 doses). Additional 2-vial doses may be given based on clinical course.
Pediatrics: Initial: 4-6 vials IV over 60 min. Observe patient for 1 hr following dose to determine if envenomation is controlled. If needed, administer additional 4-6 vials until envenomation controlled. Once control is achieved, give 2 vials q6h for up to 18 hrs (3 doses). Additional 2-vial doses may be given based on clinical course.

HOW SUPPLIED: Inj: 1g/vial

CONTRAINDICATIONS: Hypersensitivity to papaya or papain.

WARNINGS/PRECAUTIONS: Recurrent coagulopathy may persist for 1-2 weeks; monitor for symptoms. Risk of anaphylactic reaction. Sensitization may occur; caution with a repeat course of treatment for subsequent envenomation episode. Contains ethyl mercury; use with caution in children. Use caution with conditions that cause coagulation defects (eg, cancer, collagen disease, CHF, diarrhea, elevated temperature, hepatic disorders, hyperthyroidism, poor nutritional state, steatorrhea, vitamin K deficiency).

ADVERSE REACTIONS: Urticaria, rash.

PREGNANCY: Category C, caution in nursing.

MECHANISM OF ACTION: Venom-specific immunoglobulin Fab fragment; acts by binding and neutralizing venom toxins, facilitating their redistribution away from target tissues and their elimination from the body.

PHARMACOKINETICS: Distribution: V_d=0.3L/kg. **Elimination:** $T_{1/2}$=approximately 12-23 hrs.

CROLOM
cromolyn sodium (Bausch & Lomb)

RX

THERAPEUTIC CLASS: Mast cell stabilizer

INDICATIONS: Treatment of vernal keratoconjunctivitis, vernal conjunctivitis, and vernal keratitis.

DOSAGE: *Adults:* 1-2 drops 4-6x/day at regular intervals.
Pediatrics: ≥4 yrs: 1-2 drops 4-6x/day at regular intervals.

HOW SUPPLIED: Sol: 4% (10mL)

WARNINGS/PRECAUTIONS: Do not wear contacts during therapy. Do not exceed recommended frequency.

ADVERSE REACTIONS: Transient burning or stinging.

PREGNANCY: Category B, caution in nursing.

MECHANISM OF ACTION: Mast cell stabilizer: inhibits degranulation of sensitized mast cells which occur after exposure to specific antigens. Inhibits release of histamine and SRS-A mast cells.

CROMOLYN
cromolyn sodium (Various)

RX

THERAPEUTIC CLASS: Mast cell stabilizer

INDICATIONS: Treatment of vernal keratoconjunctivitis, vernal conjunctivitis, and vernal keratitis.

DOSAGE: *Adults:* 1-2 drops 4-6x/day at regular intervals.
Pediatrics: ≥4 yrs: 1-2 drops 4-6x/day at regular intervals.

HOW SUPPLIED: Sol: 4% (10mL)

WARNINGS/PRECAUTIONS: Do not wear contacts during therapy. Do not exceed recommended frequency.

ADVERSE REACTIONS: Transient burning or stinging.

PREGNANCY: Category B, caution in nursing.

CROMOLYN SODIUM INHALATION
cromolyn sodium (Various)

RX

OTHER BRAND NAME: Intal (King)

THERAPEUTIC CLASS: Mast cell stabilizer

INDICATIONS: Prophylactic treatment of bronchial asthma and of acute bronchocon-striction due to exercise, environmental agents, and known antigens.

DOSAGE: *Adults:* Asthma: (Inhaler) Usual/Max: 2 inh qid. (Sol) 20mg nebulized qid. Acute Bonchospasm Prevention: (Inhaler) Usual: 2 inh 10-60 min before exposure to precipitant. (Sol) 20mg nebulized shortly before exposure to precipitant. Renal/Hepatic Dysfunction: Decrease inhaler dose.
Pediatrics: Asthma: (Inhaler) ≥5 yrs: Usual/Max: 2 inh qid. (Sol) ≥2 yrs: 20mg nebulized qid. Acute Bronchospasm Prevention: (Inhaler) ≥5 yrs: Usual: 2 inh 10-60 min before exposure to precipitant. (Sol) ≥2 yrs: 20mg nebulized shortly before exposure to precipitant. Renal/Hepatic Dysfunction: Decrease inhaler dose.

HOW SUPPLIED: MDI: (Intal) 0.8mg/inh (8.1g, 14.2g); Sol: (Cromolyn, neb) 10mg/mL (2mL, 10^s 60^s)

WARNINGS/PRECAUTIONS: Not for treatment of acute attack. Severe anaphylaxis may occur. D/C if eosinophilic pneumonia or pulmonary infiltrates with eosinophilia develop. May experience cough and/or bronchospasm. Caution with inhaler in CAD or history of cardiac arrhythmias. Decrease dose or d/c with renal/hepatic dysfunction.

ADVERSE REACTIONS: Throat irritation/dryness, bad taste, cough, nausea, broncho-spasm, sneezing, wheezing.

INTERACTIONS: Avoid with isoproterenol during pregnancy.

PREGNANCY: Category B, caution in nursing.

MECHANISM OF ACTION: Mast cell stabilizer; inhibits sensitized mast cell degranulation, release of mediators from mast cells, and both immediate and non-immediate bronchoconstrictive reactions to inhaled antigen.

PHARMACOKINETICS: Absorption: 8% absorbed. **Elimination:** Urine, bile.

CUPRIMINE RX
penicillamine (Aton)

Supervise closely due to toxicity, special dosage considerations, and therapeutic benefits.

OTHER BRAND NAME: Depen (Wallace)

THERAPEUTIC CLASS: Copper chelating agent

INDICATIONS: Treatment of Wilson's disease, cystinuria, and severe, active rheumatoid arthritis (RA) when conventional therapy has failed.

DOSAGE: *Adults:* Wilson's Disease: Determine dosage by 24-hr urinary copper excretion. Maint: 0.75-1.5g/day for 3 months. Max: Up to 2g/day, based on serum free copper. Cystinuria: Initial: 250mg qd. Usual: 250mg-1g qid. RA: Initial: 125-250mg/day. Titrate: May increase by 125-250mg/day every 1-3 months. If needed after 2-3 months, increase by 250mg/day every 2-3 months. D/C if no improvement after 3-4 months at dose of 1-1.5g/day. Maint: 500-750mg/day. Max: 1.5g/day. Give on empty stomach, 1 hr before or 2 hrs after meals, and 1 hr apart from any other drug, food or milk. Supple-mental pyridoxine 25mg/day recommended.
Pediatrics: Cystinuria: 30mg/kg/day given qid.

HOW SUPPLIED: Cap: (Cuprimine): 250mg; Tab: (Depen) 250mg* *scored

CONTRAINDICATIONS: Pregnancy (except for treatment of Wilson's disease or certain cases of cystinuria), nursing, RA patients with renal insufficiency, history of penicillamine-related aplastic anemia or agranulocytosis.

WARNINGS/PRECAUTIONS: Aplastic anemia, agranulocytosis, drug fever, thrombocyto-penia, Goodpasture's syndrome, myasthenia gravis, pemphigus foliaceus/vulgaris, oblit-erative bronchiolitis, proteinuria and hematuria reported. Routine urinalysis, CBC with differentials, Hgb and platelet count every 2 weeks for 6 months, then monthly.

ADVERSE REACTIONS: Rash, urticaria, anorexia, epigastric pain, NV, diarrhea, leukope-nia, thrombocytopenia, proteinuria.

INTERACTIONS: Hematologic and renal adverse reactions increase with gold therapy, antimalarial or cytotoxic drugs, oxyphenbutazone and phenylbutazone. Systemic levels lowered by iron; separate doses by 2 hrs. Mineral supplements may block response to therapy.

PREGNANCY: Category D, not for use in nursing.

MECHANISM OF ACTION: Chelator: (Wilson's disease) removes excess copper; (cystinuria) reduces excess cystine excretion by disulfide interchange; interferes with formation of cross-links between tropocollagen molecules; (RA) not established, appears to suppress disease activity.

PHARMACOKINETICS: Absorption: Rapid, incomplete; C_{max}=1-2mg/mL (250mg); T_{max}=1-3 hrs. **Distribution:** Plasma protein binding (80%). **Metabolism:** Liver, **Elimination:** Renal; elimination phase=4-6 days.

CUTIVATE
fluticasone propionate (PharmaDerm)

RX

THERAPEUTIC CLASS: Corticosteroid

INDICATIONS: (Cre, Oint) Relief of the inflammatory and pruritic manifestations of corticosteroid-responsive dermatoses. Cre may be used with caution in pediatric patients ≥3 months of age. (Lot) Relief of the inflammatory and pruritic manifestations of atopic dermatitis in patients ≥1 yr of age.

DOSAGE: *Adults:* Atopic Dermatitis: (Cre) Apply qd-bid. (Lot) Apply qd. Other Dermatoses: (Cre) Apply bid. (Oint) Apply bid. (Cre, Lot, Oint) Avoid occlusive dressings and re-evaluate if no improvement after 2 weeks.
Pediatrics: ≥3 months: Atopic Dermatitis: (Cre) Apply qd-bid. Other Dermatoses: (Cre) Apply bid. Avoid in diaper area. ≥1 yr: Atopic Dermatitis: (Lot) Apply qd. (Cre, Lot): Avoid occlusive dressings and re-evaluate if no improvement after 2 weeks. Oint not approved in peds.

HOW SUPPLIED: Cre: 0.05% (30g, 60g); Lot: 0.05% (120mL); Oint: 0.005% (30g, 60g)

WARNINGS/PRECAUTIONS: Caution with cre in peds. May produce reversible HPA axis suppression, manifestations of Cushing's syndrome, hyperglycemia, and glucosuria. D/C if irritation occurs. Use appropriate antifungal or antibacterial agent with dermatological infections. Peds may be more susceptible to systemic toxicity. Caution when applied to large surface areas. Avoid with pre-existing skin atrophy. Not for use in rosacea or perioral dermatitis.

ADVERSE REACTIONS: (Cre) Pruritus, dryness, numbness of fingers, burning. (Oint) Pruritus, burning, hypertrichosis, increased erythema, hives, irritation, light-headedness. (Lot) Burning, stinging, dryness, common cold, upper respiratory tract infection, cough, fever.

PREGNANCY: Category C, caution in nursing.

MECHANISM OF ACTION: Corticosteroid; not fully established. Possesses anti-inflammatory, antipruritic, and vasoconstrictive properties. Suspected to act by the induction of phospholipase A_2 inhibitory proteins, called lipocortins. Lipocortins control biosynthesis of potent mediators of inflammation (eg, prostaglandins, leukotrienes) by inhibiting release of common precursor, arachidonic acid. Arachidonic acid is released from membrane phospholipids by phospholipase A_2.

PHARMACOKINETICS: Absorption: Extent of percutaneous absorption depends on skin integrity, vehicle, and use of occlusive dressings. **Distribution:** (IV) V_d=4.2L/kg; plasma protein binding (91%). **Metabolism:** Liver via CYP3A4 (hydrolysis). **Elimination:** (IV) $T_{1/2}$=7.2 hrs.

CYANIDE ANTIDOTE PACKAGE
amyl nitrite - sodium nitrite - sodium thiosulfate (Akorn)

RX

THERAPEUTIC CLASS: Antidote

INDICATIONS: Treatment of cyanide poisoning.

DOSAGE: *Adults:* Apply 1 amp of Amyl Nitrite to handkerchief and hold in front of patient's mouth for 15 sec followed by rest for 15 sec. Then reapply until Sodium Nitrite can be administered. D/C Amyl Nitrite and give Sodium Nitrite IV 300mg at rate of 2.5-5mL/min. Immediately after, inject 12.5g of Sodium Thiosulfate. If poison taken by mouth, gastric lavage should be performed as soon as possible. If signs of poisoning reappear, repeat Sodium Nitrite and Sodium Thiosulfate at one-half original dose.
Pediatrics: Apply 1 amp of Amyl Nitrite to handkerchief and hold in front of patient's mouth for 15 sec followed by rest for 15 sec. Then reapply until Sodium Nitrite can be administered. D/C Amyl Nitrite and give 6-8mL/m² of Sodium Nitrite IV; Max: 10mL.

Immediately after, inject 7g/m^2 of Sodium Thiosulfate; max: 12.5g. If poison taken by mouth, gastric lavage should be performed as soon as possible. If signs of poisoning reappear, repeat Sodium Nitrite and Sodium Thiosulfate at one-half original dose.

HOW SUPPLIED: Sodium Nitrite: 300mg/10mL (2 amps); Sodium Thiosulfate: 12.5mg/50mL (2 vials); Amyl Nitrite Inhalant: 0.3mL (12 amps)

WARNINGS/PRECAUTIONS: Sodium Nitrite and Amyl Nitrite in high doses induce methemoglobinemia and can cause death.

PREGNANCY: Safety in pregnancy and nursing is not known.

MECHANISM OF ACTION: Sodium nitrate: Reacts with Hgb to form methemoglobin. Sodium thiosulfate: Converts cyanide to thiocyanate, probably by rhodanese.

CYPROHEPTADINE   RX
cyproheptadine HCl (Various)

THERAPEUTIC CLASS: Serotonin/histamine antagonist

INDICATIONS: Perennial and seasonal rhinitis, vasomotor rhinitis, allergic conjunctivitis, uncomplicated allergic skin manifestations, blood or plasma allergic reactions, cold urticaria, and dermatographism. Adjunct to anaphylaxis.

DOSAGE: *Adults:* Initial: 4mg tid. Usual: 4-20mg/day. Max: 0.5mg/kg/day.
Pediatrics: 7-14 yrs: Usual: 4mg bid-tid. Max: 16mg/day. 2-6 yrs: Usual: 2mg bid-tid or 0.25mg/kg/day. Max: 12mg/day.

HOW SUPPLIED: Syrup: 2mg/5mL; Tab: 4mg* *scored

CONTRAINDICATIONS: Newborn or premature infants, nursing mothers, concomitant MAOIs, angle-closure glaucoma, stenosing peptic ulcer, symptomatic prostatic hypertrophy, bladder neck obstruction, pyloroduodenal obstruction, elderly, debilitated.

WARNINGS/PRECAUTIONS: Caution with bronchial asthma, increased IOP, hyperthyroidism, CVD, HTN, and elderly. May impair mental/physical abilities.

ADVERSE REACTIONS: Drowsiness, somnolence, sedation, dizziness, confusion, restlessness, excitation, nervousness, insomnia, blurred vision, hypotension, palpitation, dry mouth, urinary frequency and retention.

INTERACTIONS: Avoid MAOIs. Additive effects with alcohol and other CNS depressants.

PREGNANCY: Category B, not for use in nursing.

MECHANISM OF ACTION: Serotonin and histamine antagonist.

PHARMACOKINETICS: Metabolism: Quaternary ammonium glucuronide conjugate (principal metabolite). **Elimination:** Feces, urine.

CYTARABINE   RX
cytarabine (Various)

> Associated with bone marrow suppression, nausea, vomiting, oral ulceration, hepatic dysfunction, diarrhea, and abdominal pain. For induction therapy, treat in a facility able to monitor drug tolerance and toxicity.

THERAPEUTIC CLASS: Antimetabolite

INDICATIONS: Adjunct therapy for remission induction in acute non-lymphocytic leukemia (ANLL). Found useful in the treatment of acute lymphocytic leukemia (ALL) and blast phase of chronic myelocytic leukemia (CML). Prophylaxis and treatment of meningeal lymphoma.

DOSAGE: *Adults:* ANLL: Induction: 100mg/m^2/day continuous infusion or 100mg/m^2 IV q12h for Days 1-7. Meningeal Leukemia: Give intrathecally. Range: 5-75mg/m^2 given qd to every 4 days. Usual: 30mg/m^2 every 4 days until CSF normal, followed by 1 additional treatment.
Pediatrics: ANLL: Induction: 100mg/m^2/day continuous infusion or 100mg/m^2 IV q12h for Days 1-7. Meningeal Leukemia: Give intrathecally. Range: 5-75mg/m^2 given qd to every 4 days. Usual: 30mg/m^2 every 4 days until CSF normal, followed by 1 additional treatment.

HOW SUPPLIED: Inj: 100mg, 500mg, 1g, 2g

WARNINGS/PRECAUTIONS: Caution with pre-existing drug-induced bone marrow suppression, hepatic or renal dysfunction. Perform leukocyte and platelet counts daily during induction therapy. Monitor bone marrow, hepatic and renal functions, platelets, and leukocytes frequently. Sudden respiratory distress, cardiomyopathy, alopecia reported with high dose therapy. Severe and fatal CNS, GI, and pulmonary toxicity reported. Contains benzyl alcohol; fatal "Gasping Syndrome" in premature infants reported. Acute pancreatitis, hyperuricemia reported.

ADVERSE REACTIONS: Anorexia, nausea, vomiting, diarrhea, oral/anal inflammation or ulceration, hepatic dysfunction, fever, rash, thrombophlebitis, bleeding (all sites).

INTERACTIONS: Antagonizes susceptibility of gentamicin for *K.pneumoniae*. May inhibit efficacy of flucytosine. Monitor digoxin. Acute pancreatitis reported in patients receiving prior L-asparaginase treatment. Cardiomyopathy and death reported during high dose therapy with cyclophosphamide.

PREGNANCY: Category D, not for use in nursing.

MECHANISM OF ACTION: Antineoplastic; not established. Appears to act through inhibition of DNA polymerase. Also incorporates into both RNA and DNA.

PHARMACOKINETICS: Absorption: (SQ/IM) T_{max}=20-60 min. **Metabolism:** Rapid metabolism; 1-β-D-arabinofuranosyluracil (inactive metabolite). **Excretion:** Urine (80%); $T_{1/2}$=1-3 hrs.

CYTOMEL   RX
liothyronine sodium (King)

THERAPEUTIC CLASS: Thyroid replacement hormone

INDICATIONS: Hypothyroidism. As a pituitary TSH suppressant in the treatment and prevention of euthyroid goiters, including thyroid nodules, and Hashimoto's and multinodular goiter. Diagnostic agent in suppression tests to differentiate mild hyperthyroidism or thyroid gland autonomy.

DOSAGE: *Adults:* Mild Hypothyroidism: Initial: 25mcg qd. Titrate: May increase by up to 25mcg qd every 1-2 weeks. Maint: 25-75mcg qd. Myxedema: Initial: 5mcg qd. Titrate: May increase by 5-10mcg qd every 1-2 weeks up to 25mcg qd, then increase by 5-25mcg qd every 1-2 weeks. Maint: 50-100mcg/day. Goiter: Initial: 5mcg qd. Titrate: May increase by 5-10mcg qd every 1-2 weeks up to 25mcg qd, then by 12.5-25mcg qd every 1-2 weeks. Maint: 75mcg qd. Elderly/Coronary Artery Disease: Initial: 5mcg qd. Titrate: Increase by no more than 5mcg qd every 2 weeks. Thyroid Suppression Therapy: 75-100mcg qd for 7 days. Radioactive iodine uptake is determined before and after administration of hormone.
Pediatrics: Congenital Hypothyroidism: Initial: 5mcg qd. Titrate: Increase by 5mcg qd every 3-4 days until desired response. Maint: <1 yr: 20mcg qd. 1-3 yrs: 50mcg qd. >3 yrs: 25-75mcg/day.

HOW SUPPLIED: Tab: 5mcg, 25mcg*, 50mcg* *scored

CONTRAINDICATIONS: Uncorrected adrenal cortical insufficiency and untreated thyrotoxicosis.

WARNINGS/PRECAUTIONS: Do not use in the treatment of obesity; larger doses in euthyroid patients can cause serious or even life threatening toxicity. Caution with angina pectoris and elderly; use lower doses. Rule out hypogonadism and nephrosis prior to therapy. With prolonged and severe hypothyroidism supplement with adrenocortical steroids. May aggravate diabetes mellitus or insipidus and adrenal cortical insufficiency. Add glucocorticoid with myxedema coma. Excessive doses may cause craniosynostosis in infants.

ADVERSE REACTIONS: Allergic skin reactions (rare).

INTERACTIONS: Hypothyroidism decreases and hyperthyroidism increases sensitivity to oral anticoagulants; monitor PT/INR. Monitor insulin and oral hypoglycemic requirements. Decreased absorption with cholestyramine; space dosing by 4-5 hrs. Large dose may cause life-threatening toxicities with sympathomimetic amines. Estrogens increase thyroxine-binding globulin; increase in thyroid dose may be needed. Additive effects of both agents with TCAs. HTN and tachycardia with ketamine. May potentiate digitalis toxicity. Increased adrenergic effects of catecholamines; caution with CAD.

PREGNANCY: Category A, caution in nursing.

MECHANISM OF ACTION: Synthetic thyroid hormone; not established, suspected to enhance oxygen consumption by tissues, increases the basal metabolic rate and metabolism of carbohydrates, lipids, and proteins.

PHARMACOKINETICS: Elimination: $T_{1/2}$=2.5 days.

CYTOXAN

RX

cyclophosphamide (Bristol-Myers Squibb)

THERAPEUTIC CLASS: Nitrogen mustard alkylating agent

INDICATIONS: Treatment of malignant lymphomas, Hodgkin's disease, lymphocytic lymphoma, mixed-cell type or histiocytic lymphoma, Burkitt's lymphoma, multiple myeloma, chronic lymphocytic leukemia, chronic granulocytic leukemia, acute myelogenous and monocytic leukemia, acute lymphoblastic leukemia in children, mycosis fungoides, neuroblastoma, ovary adenocarcinoma, retinoblastoma, breast carcinoma. Treatment of biopsy proven "minimal change" nephrotic syndrome in children, but not as primary therapy.

DOSAGE: *Adults:* Malignant Diseases (Without Hematologic Deficiency): Monotherapy: Initial: 40-50mg/kg IV in divided doses over 2-5 days, or 10-15mg/kg IV given every 7-10 days, or 3-5mg/kg twice weekly. Oral Dosing: Initial/Maint: 1-5mg/kg/day PO. Adjust dose according to antitumor activity and/or leukopenia. May need to reduce dose when combined with other cytotoxic drugs.
Pediatrics: Malignant Diseases (Without Hematologic Deficiency): Monotherapy: Initial: 40-50mg/kg IV in divided doses over 2-5 days, or 10-15mg/kg IV given every 7-10 days, or 3-5mg/kg twice weekly. Oral Dosing: Initial/Maint: 1-5mg/kg/day PO. Adjust dose according to antitumor activity and/or leukopenia. May need to reduce dose when combined with other cytotoxic drugs. Nephrotic Syndrome: 2.5-3mg/kg/day PO for 60-90 days.

HOW SUPPLIED: Inj (Lyophilized): 500mg, 1g, 2g; Tab: 25mg, 50mg

CONTRAINDICATIONS: Severely depressed bone marrow function.

WARNINGS/PRECAUTIONS: Second malignancies, cardiac dysfunction, and hemorrhagic cystitis reported. May cause fetal harm in pregnancy. Serious, fatal infections may develop if severely immunosuppressed. Monitor for toxicity with leukopenia, thrombocytopenia, tumor cell infiltration of bone marrow, previous x-ray therapy or cytotoxic therapy, and impaired hepatic and/or renal function. Monitor hematologic profile for hematopoietic suppression. Examine urine for red blood cells. Anaphylactic reactions reported. Possible cross-sensitivity with other alkylating agents. May cause sterility. May interfere with normal wound healing. Consider dose adjustment with adrenalectomy.

ADVERSE REACTIONS: Impairment of fertility, amenorrhea, nausea, vomiting, anorexia, abdominal discomfort, diarrhea, alopecia, leukopenia, thrombocytopenia, hemorrhagic ureteritis, interstitial pneumonitis, malaise, asthenia, renal tubular necrosis.

INTERACTIONS: Chronic, high doses of phenobarbital increase metabolism and leukopenic activity. Potentiates succinylcholine chloride effects and doxorubicin-induced cardiotoxicity. Alert anesthesiologist if treated within 10 days of general anesthesia.

PREGNANCY: Category D, not for use in nursing.

MECHANISM OF ACTION: Nitrogen mustard alkylating agent; exerts action by cross linking of tumor cell DNA.

PHARMACOKINETICS: Absorption: Well absorbed; bioavailability ($\geq$75%). **Distribution:** Plasma protein binding ($\geq$60% as metabolites). **Metabolism:** Liver; active metabolites. **Elimination:** Urine (5-25% unchanged); $T_{1/2}$=3-12 hrs.

DALLERGY

RX

chlorpheniramine maleate - methscopolamine nitrate - phenylephrine HCl
(Laser)

THERAPEUTIC CLASS: Antihistamine/anticholinergic/sympathomimetic

INDICATIONS: Relief of upper respiratory symptoms associated with allergies and the common cold.

DOSAGE: *Adults:* 1 tab or 10mL q4-6h. Max: 4 doses/24hrs.
Pediatrics: ≥12 yrs: 1 tab or 10mL q4-6h. 6-12 yrs: 1/2 tab or 5mL q4-6h. Max: 4 doses/24hrs.

HOW SUPPLIED: (Chlorpheniramine-Methscopolamine-Phenylephrine) Syrup: 2mg-0.625mg-10mg/5mL; Tab: 4mg-1.25mg-10mg*; Tab, Extended-Release: 12mg-2.5mg-20mg *scored

CONTRAINDICATIONS: Severe HTN, severe CAD, MAOI therapy, narrow angle glaucoma, urinary retention, PUD, during asthma attack.

WARNINGS/PRECAUTIONS: Caution in HTN, DM, ischemic heart disease, hyperthyroidism, increased IOP, prostatic hypertrophy. Adverse events are more common in elderly. May cause excitability in children.

ADVERSE REACTIONS: Drowsiness, lassitude, nausea, giddiness, dry mouth, blurred vision, cardiac palpitations, flushing, increased irritability or excitement.

INTERACTIONS: Increased effect of sympathomimetic amines with MAOIs and β-blockers. May reduce antihypertensive effect of methyldopa, mecamylamine, reserpine, and veratrum alkaloids. Additive effect with alcohol, other CNS depressants.

PREGNANCY: Category C, caution in nursing.

DALLERGY JR   RX
chlorpheniramine maleate - phenylephrine HCl (Laser)

THERAPEUTIC CLASS: Antihistamine/sympathomimetic amine

INDICATIONS: Relief of upper respiratory symptoms associated with allergies and the common cold.

DOSAGE: *Adults:* 2 caps q12h. Max: 2 doses/24h.
Pediatrics: >12 yrs: 2 caps q12h. 6-12 yrs: 1 cap q12h. Max: 2 doses/24h.

HOW SUPPLIED: Cap: (Chlorpheniramine-Phenylephrine) 4mg-20mg

CONTRAINDICATIONS: Severe HTN, severe CAD, MAOI therapy, narrow angle glaucoma, urinary retention, PUD, during asthma attack.

WARNINGS/PRECAUTIONS: Caution with HTN, DM, ischemic heart disease, hyperthyroidism, increased IOP, prostatic hypertrophy, the elderly. May cause excitability especially in children.

ADVERSE REACTIONS: Drowsiness, lassitude, nausea, giddiness, dry mouth, blurred vision, cardiac palpitations, flushing, increased irritability or excitement.

INTERACTIONS: Increased sympathomimetic effect with MAOIs and β-blockers. May reduce antihypertensive effect of methyldopa, mecamylamine, reserpine, and veratum alkaloids. Additive effect with alcohol and other CNS depressants.

PREGNANCY: Category C, caution in nursing.

DALMANE   CIV
flurazepam HCl (Valeant)

THERAPEUTIC CLASS: Benzodiazepine

INDICATIONS: Treatment of insomnia.

DOSAGE: *Adults:* Usual: 15-30mg at bedtime. Elderly/Debilitated: Initial: 15mg at bedtime.
Pediatrics: ≥15 yrs: Usual: 15-30mg at bedtime.

HOW SUPPLIED: Cap: 15mg, 30mg

CONTRAINDICATIONS: Pregnancy.

WARNINGS/PRECAUTIONS: Caution in elderly, debilitated, severely depressed, those with suicidal tendencies, hepatic/renal impairment, respiratory disease. Ataxia and falls reported in elderly and debilitated.Withdrawal symptoms after discontinuation; avoid abrupt discontinuation. Rare cases of angioedema involving the tongue, glottis, or larynx reported. Complex behaviors such as sleep driving, and other complex behaviors (eg, preparing and eating food, making phone calls, and having sex) reported.

ADVERSE REACTIONS: Confusion, dizziness, drowsiness, lightheadedness, ataxia.

INTERACTIONS: Additive effects with alcohol and other CNS depressants.

PREGNANCY: Not for use in pregnancy or nursing.

MECHANISM OF ACTION: Benzodiazepine; hypnotic.

PHARMACOKINETICS: Absorption: Rapid; C_{max}=4.0ng/mL; T_{max}=1 hr. **Metabolism:** N_1-desalkyl-flurazepam (active metabolite); conjugation. **Elimination:** Urine; $T_{1/2}$=2.3 hrs, 47-100 hrs (active metabolite).

DANTRIUM

RX

dantrolene sodium (Procter & Gamble Pharmaceuticals)

> Associated with hepatotoxicity; monitor hepatic function. Discontinue if no benefit after 45 days.

THERAPEUTIC CLASS: Direct acting skeletal muscle relaxant

INDICATIONS: To control manifestations of clinical spasticity from upper motor neuron disorders (eg, spinal cord injury, stroke, cerebral palsy, multiple sclerosis). Preoperatively to prevent or attenuate development of malignant hyperthermia, and after a malignant hyperthermia crisis.

DOSAGE: *Adults:* Chronic Spasticity: Initial: 25mg qd for 7 days. Titrate: Increase to 25mg tid for 7 days, then 50mg tid for 7 days, then 100mg tid. Max: 100mg qid. If no further benefit at next higher dose, decrease to previous lower dose. Malignant Hyperthermia: Pre-Op: 4-8mg/kg/day given tid-qid for 1-2 days before surgery, with last dose given 3-4 hrs before surgery. Post-Op Following Malignant Hyperthermia Crisis: 4-8mg/kg/day given qid for 1-3 days.
Pediatrics: ≥5 yrs: Chronic Spasticity: Initial: 0.5mg/kg qd for 7 days. Titrate: Increase to 0.5mg/kg tid for 7 days, then 1mg/kg tid for 7 days, then 2mg/kg tid. Max: 100mg qid. If no further benefit at next higher dose, decrease to previous lower dose.

HOW SUPPLIED: Cap: 25mg, 50mg, 100mg

CONTRAINDICATIONS: Active hepatic disease, where spasticity is utilized to sustain upright posture and balance in locomotion, when spasticity is utilized to obtain or maintain increased function.

WARNINGS/PRECAUTIONS: Monitor LFTs at baseline, then periodically. Increased risk of hepatocellular disease in females and patients >35 yrs. Caution with pulmonary, cardiac, and liver dysfunction. Photosensitivity reaction may occur; limit sunlight exposure.

ADVERSE REACTIONS: Drowsiness, dizziness, weakness, malaise, fatigue, diarrhea, hepatitis, tachycardia, aplastic anemia, thrombocytopenia, depression, seizure.

INTERACTIONS: Increased drowsiness with CNS depressants. Caution with estrogens; risk of hepatotoxicity. Avoid with CCBs; risk of cardiovascular collapse. May potentiate vecuronium-induced neuromuscular block.

PREGNANCY: Safety in nursing not known. Not for use in nursing.

MECHANISM OF ACTION: Direct acting skeletal muscle relaxant; interferes with the release of calcium ions from the sarcoplasmic reticulum.

PHARMACOKINETICS: Absorption: Incomplete/slow but consistent. **Metabolism:** Hepatic microsomal enzymes; 5-hydroxy and acetamido analog (major metabolites). **Elimination:** Urine; $T_{1/2}$=8.7 hrs.

DANTRIUM **IV**

RX

dantrolene sodium (Procter & Gamble Pharmaceuticals)

THERAPEUTIC CLASS: Direct acting skeletal muscle relaxant

INDICATIONS: Adjunct management of fulminant hypermetabolism of skeletal muscle characteristic of malignant hyperthermia crises. For pre- and post-operative use to prevent or attenuate development of malignant hyperthermia.

DOSAGE: *Adults:* Malignant Hyperthermia: Initial: Minimum 1mg/kg IV push. Continue until symptoms subside or max cumulative dose 10mg/kg. Pre-Op Malignant Hyperthermia Prophylaxis: 2.5mg/kg 1.25 hrs before anesthesia and infuse over 1 hr. May need additional therapy during anesthesia/surgery if symptoms arise. Post-Op Prophylaxis: Initial: 1mg/kg or more as clinical situation dictates.
Pediatrics: Malignant Hyperthermia: Initial: Minimum 1mg/kg IV push. Continue until symptoms subside or max cumulative dose 10mg/kg.

HOW SUPPLIED: Inj: 20mg

WARNINGS/PRECAUTIONS: Use with supportive therapies to treat malignant hyperthermia. Take steps to prevent extravasation. Fatal and non-fatal hepatic disorders reported. Do not operate automobile or engage hazardous activity for 48 hrs after therapy. Caution at meals on day of administration because difficulty in swallowing/choking reported. Monitor vital signs if receive pre-operatively.

ADVERSE REACTIONS: Loss of grip strength, weakness in legs, drowsiness, dizziness, pulmonary edema, thrombophlebitis, urticaria, erythema.

INTERACTIONS: Plasma protein-binding reduced by warfarin and clofibrate, and increased by tolbutamide. Avoid with CCBs; possible risk of cardiovascular collapse. Caution with tranquilizers. Possible increased metabolism by drugs known to induce hepatic microsomal enzymes. May potentiate vecuronium-induced neuromuscular block.

PREGNANCY: Category C, safety in nursing not known.

MECHANISM OF ACTION: Direct acting skeletal muscle relaxant; interferes with release of calcium ions from sarcoplasmic reticulum.

PHARMACOKINETICS: Distribution: Found in breast milk. **Metabolism:** Hydrolysis and oxidation; 5-hydroxy dantrolene and acetylamino analog (major metabolites). **Elimination:** Urine; $T_{1/2}$=4-8 hrs.

DAPSONE   RX
dapsone (Jacobus)

THERAPEUTIC CLASS: Leprostatic agent

INDICATIONS: Treatment of dermatitis herpetiformis and leprosy.

DOSAGE: *Adults:* Dermatitis Herpetiformis: Initial: 50mg/day. Usual: 50-300mg/day, may increase dose if needed. Reduce to minimum maintenance dose. Leprosy: Give with 1 or more antileprosy drugs. Maint: 100mg/day.
Pediatrics: Same schedule as adults but with correspondingly smaller doses.

HOW SUPPLIED: Tab: 25mg* 100mg* *scored

WARNINGS/PRECAUTIONS: Agranulocytosis, aplastic anemia and other blood dyscrasias reported. CBC weekly for the 1st month, monthly for 6 months and semi-annually thereafter. D/C if significant reduction in leukocytes, platelets or hemopoiesis occurs. Treat severe anemia prior to therapy. D/C if sensitivity occurs. Caution in those with G6PD deficiency, methemoglobin reductase deficiency, or hemoglobin M. Toxic hepatitis and cholestatic jaundice reported. Monitor LFT's.

ADVERSE REACTIONS: Hemolysis, peripheral neuropathy, NV, abdominal pain, pancreatitis, vertigo, blurred vision, tinnitus, insomnia, fever, headache, psychosis, phototoxicity, pulmonary eosinophilia, tachycardia, albuminuria, renal papillary necrosis, male infertility.

INTERACTIONS: Rifampin lowers plasma levels. Folic acid antagonists (eg, pyrimethamine) may increase hematologic reactions. Dapsone and trimethoprim each raise the level of the other.

PREGNANCY: Category C, not for use in nursing.

MECHANISM OF ACTION: Antibacterial agent; not established.

PHARMACOKINETICS: Absorption: Rapid, almost complete; T_{max}=4-8 hrs. **Elimination:** $T_{1/2}$=28 hrs.

DAPTACEL   RX
diphtheria toxoid - pertussis vaccine acellular, adsorbed - tetanus toxoid
(Sanofi Pasteur)

THERAPEUTIC CLASS: Vaccine

INDICATIONS: Active immunization against diphtheria, tetanus, and pertussis as a five-dose series in infants and children 6 weeks through 6 years of age (prior to seventh birthday).

DOSAGE: *Pediatrics:* 6 weeks-up to 7 yrs: 0.5mL IM at 2, 4, 6 months (at intervals of 6-8 weeks), at 15-20 months, and at 4-6 years of age. The interval between 3rd and 4th dose should be at least 6 months. May use to complete series in infants who received ≥1 dose of whole-cell pertussis (DTP). First dose given early as 6 weeks of age.

HOW SUPPLIED: Inj: 0.5mL

CONTRAINDICATIONS: Adults and pediatrics ≥7yrs. Administration after immediate anaphylactic reaction, or encephalopathy not attributable to another identifiable cause within 7 days from initial vaccination. Progressive neurological disorder, including infantile spasms, uncontrolled epilepsy, or progressive encephalopathy.

WARNINGS/PRECAUTIONS: Stopper contains dry natural latex rubber. Evaluate risks/ benefits of subsequent doses if temperature ≥105°F, or if collapse/shock occurs, or persistent crying for ≥3 hrs within 48 hrs, and convulsions with or without fever within 3 days of vaccine. Epinephrine and other appropriate agents and equipments should be available. Continue with DT vaccine if pertussis must be withheld. Caution if Guillain-Barre syndrome occurred within 6 weeks of receipt of prior vaccine containing tetanus toxoid. Increased risk of neurological events with family history of convulsions; administer antipyretic at time of and for 24 hrs after immunization. May not achieve expected immune response in immunosuppressed patients. May not protect all individuals. Avoid injection into blood vessel.

ADVERSE REACTIONS: Local tenderness, fever, fretfulness, anorexia, drowsiness, vomiting.

INTERACTIONS: Immunosuppressives (eg, irradiation, antimetabolites, alkylating agents, cytotoxic drugs, corticosteroids) may reduce immune response to vaccine. Adequate immune response may not occur after recent immune globulin injection.

PREGNANCY: Category C, safety in nursing not known.

MECHANISM OF ACTION: Vaccine: develops neutralizing antibodies against diphtheria, tetanus, and pertussis.

DARAPRIM RX
pyrimethamine (GlaxoSmithKline)

THERAPEUTIC CLASS: Folic acid antagonist

INDICATIONS: Adjunct treatment of toxoplasmosis and acute malaria. Chemoprophylaxis of malaria.

DOSAGE: *Adults:* Toxoplasmosis: Initial: 50-75mg qd with 1-4g/day of sulfonamide. After 1-3 weeks, reduce dose of each drug to 1/2 of previous dose for additional 4-5 weeks. Acute Malaria: 25mg qd for 2 days with sulfonamide. As monotherapy in semi-immune persons, 50mg for 2 days. Follow with prophylaxis dose through periods of early recrudescence and late relapse. Malaria Prophylaxis: 25mg once weekly.
Pediatrics: Toxoplasmosis: 0.5mg/kg bid. After 2-4 days, reduce to 0.25mg/kg bid for 1 month. Use with usual pediatric sulfonamide dose. Acute Malaria: 4-10 yrs: As monotherapy in semi-immune persons, 25mg for 2 days. Follow with prophylaxis dose through periods of early recrudescence and late relapse. Malaria Prophylaxis: >10 yrs: 25mg once weekly. 4-10 yrs: 12.5 once weekly. <4 yrs: 6.25mg once weekly.

HOW SUPPLIED: Tab: 25mg* *scored

CONTRAINDICATIONS: Megaloblastic anemia due to folate deficiency.

WARNINGS/PRECAUTIONS: Dose for toxoplasmosis approaches toxic levels; reduce dose or d/c if develop folate deficiency. Administer leucovorin 5-15mg qd (po, IV, or IM) until normal hematopoiesis. May be carcinogenic. Pediatric deaths reported with accidental ingestion. Use small initial dose with convulsive disorders to avoid nervous system toxicity. Caution with renal or hepatic dysfunction or if possible folate deficiency (eg, pregnancy, malabsorption syndrome, alcoholism). Perform semiweekly blood counts, including platelets with high doses.

ADVERSE REACTIONS: Hypersensitivity reactions (eg, Stevens-Johnson syndrome, toxic epidermal necrolysis) hyperphenylalinemia (with sulfonamides), anorexia, vomiting, blood dyscrasias, cardiac rhythm disorders.

INTERACTIONS: Concurrent phenytoin may affect folate levels. Increased risk of bone marrow suppression with antifolic drugs (eg, sulfonamides or trimethoprim-sulfamethoxazole). Mild hepatotoxicity reported with lorazepam.

PREGNANCY: Category C, not for use in nursing.

MECHANISM OF ACTION: Folic acid antagonist highly selective against Toxoplasma gondii and plasmodia.

PHARMACOKINETICS: Absorption: Well absorbed; T_{max}=2-6hrs. **Distribution:** Plasma protein binding (87%). **Elimination:** $T_{1/2}$=96 hrs.

DAYPRO

RX

oxaprozin (Pharmacia & Upjohn)

> **NSAIDs may cause an increased risk of serious cardiovascular thrombotic events, MI, stroke and serious GI adverse events including bleeding, ulceration, and perforation of the stomach or intestines. Contraindicated for the treatment of perioperative pain in the setting of coronary artery bypass graft (CABG) surgery.**

THERAPEUTIC CLASS: NSAID

INDICATIONS: Relief of signs and symptoms of osteoarthritis (OA), rheumatoid arthritis (RA), and juvenile rheumatoid arthritis (JRA).

DOSAGE: *Adults:* RA: 1200mg qd. Max: 1800mg/day in divided doses (not to exceed 26mg/kg/day). OA: 1200mg qd, give 600mg qd for low weight or milder disease. Max: 1800mg/day in divided doses (not to exceed 26mg/kg/day). Renal Dysfunction/ Hemodialysis: Initial: 600mg qd.
Pediatrics: 6-16yrs: JRA: ≥55kg: 1200mg qd. 32-54kg: 900mg qd. 22-31kg: 600mg qd.

HOW SUPPLIED: Tab: 600mg* *scored

CONTRAINDICATIONS: Complete or partial syndrome of nasal polyps, angioedema and bronchospastic reactivity to ASA or other NSAIDs. Treatment of perioperative pain in the setting of CABG surgery.

WARNINGS/PRECAUTIONS: May lead to onset of new HTN or worsening of pre-existing HTN; monitor BP closely. Fluid retention and edema reported; caution with fluid retention or heart failure. Renal papillary necrosis and other renal injury reported after long-term use. Not recommended for use with advanced renal disease; if therapy must be initiated, monitor renal function. Anaphylactoid reactions may occur. May cause serious skin adverse events (eg, exfoliative dermatitis, Stevens-Johnson syndrome, and toxic epidermal necrolysis). Avoid in late pregnancy; may cause premature closure of ductus arteriosis. May cause elevations of LFTs; d/c if liver disease develops or systemic manifestations occur. Caution in elderly. Anemia may occur; with long-term use, monitor Hgb/Hct if signs or symptoms of anemia develop. May inhibit platelet aggregation and prolong bleeding time; monitor with coagulation disorders. Caution with asthma and avoid with ASA-sensitive asthma. Rash and/or mild photosensitivity reactions reported.

ADVERSE REACTIONS: Constipation, diarrhea, dyspepsia, flatulence, nausea, rash.

INTERACTIONS: Avoid with ASA. Caution with oral anticoagulants. Reduces effects of ACE-inhibitors, furosemide, and thiazides. Increases lithium levels and toxicity of methotrexate. Monitor BP with β-blockers.

PREGNANCY: Category C, not for use in nursing.

MECHANISM OF ACTION: NSAIDs; unknown, suspected to inhibit prostaglandin synthetase.

PHARMACOKINETICS: Absorption: 95% absorbed. **Distribution:** V_d/F=11-17L/70kg; plasma protein binding (99%); exreted in human milk. **Metabolism:** Liver via oxidation (65%) and glucuronic acid conjugation (35%). **Elimination:** Feces (35%), urine (5% unchanged, 65% as metabolite); $T_{1/2}$=22 hrs.

DAYTRANA

methylphenidate (Shire)

THERAPEUTIC CLASS: Sympathomimetic amine

INDICATIONS: Treatment of attention deficit hyperactivity disorder (ADHD).

DOSAGE: *Adults:* Individualize dose. Apply to hip area 2 hrs before effect is needed and remove 9 hrs after application. Recommended Titration Schedule: Week 1: 10mg/9 hrs. Week 2: 15mg/9 hrs. Week 3: 20mg/9 hrs. Week 4: 30mg/9 hrs.

DDAVP

Pediatrics: ≥6 yrs: Individualize dose. Apply to hip area 2 hrs before effect is needed and remove 9 hrs after application. Recommended Titration Schedule: Week 1: 10mg/9 hrs. Week 2: 15mg/9 hrs. Week 3: 20mg/9 hrs. Week 4: 30mg/9 hrs.

HOW SUPPLIED: Patch: 10mg/9 hrs, 15mg/9 hrs, 20mg/9 hrs, 30mg/9 hrs (10^s, 30^s)

CONTRAINDICATIONS: Marked anxiety, tension, and agitation; glaucoma; motor tics or family history or diagnosis of Tourette's syndrome; treatment with MAOIs and within minimum of 14 days following discontinuation.

WARNINGS/PRECAUTIONS: Avoid use with known structural cardiac abnormalities; sudden death reported. D/C if contact sensitization is suspected. Monitor growth during treatment. May exacerbate symptoms of behavior disturbance and thought disorder in psychotic patients. Caution when using stimulants to treat patients with comorbid bipolar disorder because of concern for possible induction of mixed/manic episode in such patients. Stimulants at usual doses can cause treatment emergent psychotic or manic symptoms (eg, hallucinations, delusional thinking, mania) in children and adolescents without prior history of psychotic illness. Aggressive behavior or hostility reported in clinical trials and postmarketing experience of some medications indicated for the treatment of ADHD. May lower convulsive threshold; d/c in the presence of seizures. Caution with HTN; monitor BP. Caution when underlying medical conditions might be compromised by increases in BP or HR (eg, pre-existing HTN, heart failure, recent MI, or hyperthyroidism). Visual disturbances reported. Caution with history of drug dependence or alcoholism. Avoid exposing application site to external heat sources (eg, heating pads, electric blankets, heated water beds, etc). Monitor CBC, differential, and platelet counts during prolonged therapy.

ADVERSE REACTIONS: Nausea, vomiting, nasopharyngitis, weight decrease, anorexia, decreased appetite, affect lability, insomnia, tic, nasal congestion.

INTERACTIONS: See Contraindications. Caution with pressor agents. May decrease effectiveness of antihypertensive agents. May inhibit metabolism of coumarin anticoagulants, anticonvulsants (eg, phenobarbital, phenytoin, primidone), some tricyclic drugs (eg, imipramine, clomipramine, desipramine), and SSRIs. Monitor drug levels (or coagulation times with coumarin) and consider dose adjustments with concomitant use. Serious adverse events reported with concomitant clonidine use.

PREGNANCY: Category C, caution in nursing.

MECHANISM OF ACTION: Sympathomimetic amine; CNS stimulant. Suspected to block reuptake of norepinephrine and dopamine into presynaptic neuron; increases release of monoamines into neuronal spaces.

PHARMACOKINETICS: Absorption: C_{max}=39ng/mL; T_{max}=7.5-10.5 hrs. **Distribution:** Plasma concentrations decline in biexponential manner due to continued distribution from skin after patch removal. **Metabolism:** De-esterification; ritalinic acid (metabolite). **Elimination:** $T_{1/2}$=3-4 hrs (*d*-methylphenidate); $T_{1/2}$=1.4-2.9 hrs (*l*-methylphenidate).

DDAVP   RX
desmopressin acetate (Sanofi-Aventis)

OTHER BRAND NAMES: DDAVP Nasal Spray (Sanofi-Aventis) - DDAVP Rhinal Tube (Sanofi-Aventis)

THERAPEUTIC CLASS: Synthetic vasopressin analog

INDICATIONS: (Tab) Management of primary nocturnal enuresis. (Inj/Nasal Spray/Rhinal Tube/Tab) As antidiuretic replacement therapy in management of central (cranial) diabetes insipidus. Management of temporary polyuria and polydipsia following head trauma or surgery in pituitary region. (Inj) Hemophilia A with factor VIII coagulant activity levels >5% and mild to moderate classic von Willebrand's disease (Type I) with factor VIII levels >5%.

DOSAGE: *Adults:* Diabetes Insipidus: (Tab) Initial: 0.05mg bid. Titrate: May increase/decrease by 0.1-1.2mg/day given bid-tid. Maint: 0.1-0.8mg/day in divided doses. (Spray/Tube) Usual: 0.1-4mL/day given qd-tid. (Inj) 0.5-1mL/day IV/SQ given bid. Hemophilia A/von Willebrand's Disease: (Inj) 0.3mcg/kg IV over 15-30 min. Add 50mL diluent. If used pre-op, give 30 min before procedure.
Pediatrics: Diabetes Insipidus: (Tab) ≥4 yrs: Initial: 0.05mg bid. Titrate: May increase/decrease by 0.1-1.2mg/day given bid-tid. Maint: 0.1-0.8mg/day in divided doses. (Spray/Tube) 3 months-12 yrs: Usual: 0.05-0.3mL/day given qd-bid. (Inj) ≥12 yrs: 0.5-1mL/

day IV/SQ given bid. Hemophilia A/von Willebrand's Disease: (Inj) ≥3 months: 0.3mcg/kg IV over 15-30 min. Add 50mL diluent (>10kg) or 10mL diluent (≤10kg). If used pre-op, give 30 min before procedure.

HOW SUPPLIED: Inj: 4mcg/mL; Nasal Spray: 10mcg/inh (5mL); Tab: 0.1mg*, 0.2mg*; Rhinal Tube: 0.01% (2.5mL) *scored

CONTRAINDICATIONS: Moderate to severe renal impairment (CrCL<50mL/min), hyponatremia, or history of hyponatremia.

WARNINGS/PRECAUTIONS: Mucosal changes with nasal forms may occur; d/c until resolved. Decrease fluid intake in pediatrics and elderly to decrease risk of water intoxication and hyponatremia; monitor osmolality. Caution with coronary artery insufficiency, hypertensive cardiovascular disease, fluid and electrolyte imbalance (eg, cystic fibrosis). Anaphylaxis reported with IV use. Caution with IV use if history of thrombus formation. For diabetes insipidus, dosage must be adjusted according to diurnal pattern of response; estimate response by adequate duration of sleep and adequate, not excessive, water turnover.

ADVERSE REACTIONS: Inj: Headache, nausea, abdominal cramps, vulval pain, injection site reactions, facial flushing, BP changes. Spray: Headache, dizziness, rhinitis, nausea, nasal congestion, sore throat, cough, respiratory infection, epistaxis. Tab: Nausea, flushing, abdominal cramps, headache, increased SGOT, water intoxication, hyponatremia.

INTERACTIONS: Caution with other pressor agents.

PREGNANCY: Category B, caution in nursing.

MECHANISM OF ACTION: Synthetic vasopressin analog; antidiuretic affecting renal water conservation.

PHARMACOKINETICS: Absorption: (Inj) Rapid, T_{max}=90 min-2 hrs; (Tab, Nasal) Rapid, T_{max}=0.9-1.5 hrs. **Elimination:** Urine; (Inj, Nasal) $T_{1/2}$=3 hrs; (Tab) 1.5-2.5 hrs.

DECLOMYCIN RX
demeclocycline HCl (Wyeth)

THERAPEUTIC CLASS: Tetracycline derivative

INDICATIONS: Treatment of infections due to rickettsiae, *Mycoplasma pneumoniae*, *B.recurrentis*, agents of psittacosis, ornithosis, lymphomagranuloma venereum or granuloma inguinale. Treatment of gram-negative infections (eg, respiratory, urinary tract), gram-positive infections (eg, respiratory tract, skin and soft tissue), trachoma, inclusion conjunctivitis. When PCN is contraindicated, treatment of gonorrhea, syphilis, listeriosis, anthrax, *Clostridium* species, and others. Adjunct therapy for amebicides.

DOSAGE: *Adults:* Usual: 150mg qid or 300mg bid. Gonorrhea: 600mg followed by 300mg q12h for 4 days to a total of 3g. Renal/Hepatic Impairment: Reduce dose and/or extend dose intervals. Continue therapy for at least 24-48 hrs after symptoms subside. Treat strep infections for at least 10 days. Take at least 1 hr before or 2 hrs after meals with plenty of fluids.
Pediatrics: >8 yrs: Usual: 7-13mg/kg/day divided bid-qid. Max: 600mg/day. Renal/Hepatic Impairment: Reduce dose and/or extend dose intervals. Continue therapy for at least 24-48 hrs after symptoms subside. Treat strep infections for at least 10 days. Take at least 1 hr before or 2 hrs after meals with plenty of fluids.

HOW SUPPLIED: Tab: 150mg, 300mg

CONTRAINDICATIONS: Hypersensitivity to any of the tetracyclines.

WARNINGS/PRECAUTIONS: May cause fetal harm during pregnancy. Use during tooth development (last half of pregnancy, infancy, <8 yrs), or long-term use, or repeated short-term use may cause permanent discoloration of the teeth. Pseudotumor cerebri (adults), bulging fontanels (infants) reported. Caution with renal or hepatic impairment. Long-term use may cause reversible, nephrogenic diabetes insipidus syndrome. May result in overgrowth of nonsusceptible organisms; d/c if superinfection develops. CNS symptoms may occur; caution when operating machinery. May decrease bone growth in premature infants. Monitor hematopoietic, renal, and hepatic function with long-term use. D/C at first evidence of skin erythema after sun/UV light exposure.

ADVERSE REACTIONS: GI problems, rash, esophageal ulceration, hypersensitivity reactions, dizziness, headache, tinnitus, blood dyscrasias, photosensitivity reactions, enamel hypoplasia, elevated BUN, acute renal failure.

INTERACTIONS: Decreases PT; may need to decrease dose of anticoagulants. May interfere with bactericidal action of PCN; avoid concomitant use. May decrease efficacy of oral contraceptives; use alternate method. Decreased absorption with antacids and iron-containing products. Fatal renal toxicity with methoxyflurane reported. Foods/dairy products interfere with absorption.

PREGNANCY: Category D, not for use in nursing.

MECHANISM OF ACTION: Tetracycline; thought to inhibit protein synthesis.

PHARMACOKINETICS: Absorption: T_{max}=4 hrs. **Distribution:** Plasma protein binding (40%), found in breast milk. **Elimination:** Feces (13 and 46%); active drug and urine (44%); $T_{1/2}$=10-16 hrs.

DECONAMINE   RX
chlorpheniramine maleate - pseudoephedrine HCl (Kenwood Therapeutics)

OTHER BRAND NAMES: Deconamine SR (Kenwood Therapeutics) - De-Congestine TR (Qualitest) - Kronofed-A (Ferndale)

THERAPEUTIC CLASS: Antihistamine/decongestant

INDICATIONS: Temporary relief of symptoms associated with rhinorrhea, sneezing, and nasal congestion.

DOSAGE: *Adults:* (Cap, SR) 1 cap q12h. (Tab) 1 tab tid-qid. (Syrup) 5-10mL tid-qid. *Pediatrics:* ≥12 yrs: (Cap, SR) 1 cap q12h. (Tab) 1 tab tid-qid. (Syrup) 5-10mL tid-qid. 2-6 yrs: (Syrup) 2.5mL tid-qid. Max: 10mL/24hrs. 6-12 yrs: 2.5-5mL tid-qid. Max: 20mL/24hrs.

HOW SUPPLIED: (Chlorpheniramine-Pseudoephedrine) Cap, Sustained Release: 8mg-120mg; Syrup: 2mg-30mg/5mL; Tab: 4mg-60mg

CONTRAINDICATIONS: Severe HTN, severe CAD, concomitant MAOIs.

WARNINGS/PRECAUTIONS: Extreme caution in narrow-angle glaucoma, stenosing peptic ulcer, pyloroduodenal obstruction, symptomatic prostatic hypertrophy, bladder neck obstruction. Caution in bronchial asthma, emphysema, chronic pulmonary disease, HTN, ischemic heart disease, DM, increased IOP, hyperthyroidism. May cause excitability in children. May produce CNS stimulation with convulsions or cardiovascular collapse with hypotension.

ADVERSE REACTIONS: Drowsiness, urticaria, drug rash, hypotension, hemolytic anemia, sedation, epigastric distress, urinary frequency, nervousness, dizziness.

INTERACTIONS: Hypertensive crisis may occur with MAOIs. May reduce antihypertensive effect of methyldopa, reserpine, veratrum alkaloids, mecamylamine. Sedative effects potentiated by alcohol, other CNS depressants.

PREGNANCY: Category C, not for use in nursing.

MECHANISM OF ACTION: Chlorpheniramine: Antihistaminic; antagonizes the physiological action of histamine by acting as an H_1 receptor blocking agent. Pseudoephedrine: Sympathomimetic; exerts a decongestant action on nasal mucosa by vasoconstriction.

DELATESTRYL   CIII
testosterone enanthate (Indevus)

THERAPEUTIC CLASS: Androgen

INDICATIONS: Testosterone replacement in males with primary hypogonadism and hypogonadotropic hypogonadism. To stimulate puberty in males with delayed puberty. May also be used secondarily in females with advancing inoperable metastatic (skeletal) mammary cancer who are 1-5 years postmenopausal.

DOSAGE: *Adults:* Dose based on age, sex, and diagnosis. Adjust dose according to response and adverse reactions. Male Hypogonadism: 50-400mg IM every 2-4 weeks. Delayed Puberty: 50-200mg every 2-4 weeks for a limited duration (eg, 4-6 months). Breast Cancer: 200-400mg every 2-4 weeks.
Pediatrics: Dose based on age, sex, and diagnosis. Adjust dose according to response and adverse reactions. Male Hypogonadism: 50-400mg IM every 2-4 weeks. Delayed Puberty: 50-200mg every 2-4 weeks for a limited duration (eg, 4-6 months). Caution in children.

HOW SUPPLIED: Inj: 200mg/mL

CONTRAINDICATIONS: Breast or prostate carcinoma in men. Pregnancy.

WARNINGS/PRECAUTIONS: D/C if hypercalcemia occurs in breast cancer or immobilized patients; monitor calcium levels. Risk of hepatic adenomas, hepatocellular carcinoma, and peliosis hepatitis with prolonged high doses. D/C if jaundice, cholestatic hepatitis, or abnormal LFTs occur. Avoid use in elderly who has age related hypogonadism. D/C if edema occurs in patients with pre-existing cardiac, renal, or hepatic disease; restart at lower dose. Risk of compromised stature in children; monitor bone growth every 6 months. Monitor for virilization in females. Caution with a history of MI or CAD due to altered serum cholesterol levels. Monitor cholesterol, LFTs, Hct, Hgb periodically.

ADVERSE REACTIONS: Amenorrhea, virilization, menstrual irregularities, gynecomastia, excessive frequency/duration of penile erections, male pattern baldness, increased/decreased libido, oligospermia, hirsutism, acne, fluid and electrolyte disturbances, nausea, hypercholesterolemia, clotting factor suppression, polycythemia, altered LFTs, oligospermia, anxiety, depression.

INTERACTIONS: Potentiates oral anticoagulants and oxyphenbutazone. May decrease blood glucose and insulin requirements. ACTH and corticosteroids may enhance edema.

PREGNANCY: Category X, not for use in nursing.

MECHANISM OF ACTION: Endogenous androgen; responsible for normal growth and development of male sex organs and for maintenance of secondary sex characteristics.

PHARMACOKINETICS: Absorption: Slow. **Distribution:** Plasma protein binding (98%). **Metabolism:** Liver. **Elimination:** Urine (90%), feces (6%); $T_{1/2}$=10-100 minutes.

DEMEROL INJECTION `CII`
meperidine HCl (Hospira)

THERAPEUTIC CLASS: Opioid analgesic

INDICATIONS: For relief of moderate to severe pain. For preoperative medication, anesthesia support, and obstetrical analgesia.

DOSAGE: *Adults:* Pain: Usual: 50-150mg IM/SQ q3-4h prn. Preoperative: Usual: 50-100mg IM/SQ 30-90 min before anesthesia. Anesthesia Support: Use repeated slow IV inj of fractional doses (eg, 10mg/mL) or continuous IV infusion of a more dilute solution (eg, 1mg/mL). Titrate as needed. Obstetrical Analgesia: Usual: 50-100mg IM/SQ when pain is regular, may repeat at 1- to 3-hr intervals. Elderly: Start at lower end of dosage range and observe. With Phenothiazines/Other Tranquilizers: Reduce dose by 25 to 50%). IM method preferred with repeated use. For IV injection: Reduce dose and administer slowly, preferably using diluted solution.
Pediatrics: Pain: Usual: 0.5-0.8mg/lb IM/SQ, up to 50-150mg, q3-4h prn. Preoperative: Usual: 0.5-1mg/lb IM/SQ, up to 50-100mg, 30-90 min before anesthesia. With Phenothiazines/Other Tranquilizers: Reduce dose by 25 to 50%). IM method preferred with repeated use. For IV injection: Reduce dose and administer slowly, preferably using diluted solution.

HOW SUPPLIED: Inj: 25mg/mL, 50mg/mL, 75mg/mL, 100mg/mL

CONTRAINDICATIONS: MAOIs during or within 14 days of use.

WARNINGS/PRECAUTIONS: May develop tolerance and dependence; abuse potential. Extreme caution with head injury, increased ICP, intracranial lesions, acute asthmatic attack, chronic COPD or cor pulmonale, decreased respiratory reserve, respiratory depression, hypoxia, and hypercapnia. Rapid IV infusion may result in increased adverse reactions. Caution with acute abdominal conditions, atrial flutter, supraventricular tachycardias. May aggravate convulsive disorders. Caution and reduce initial dose with elderly or debilitated, renal/hepatic impairment, hypothyroidism, Addison's disease, prostatic hypertrophy or urethral stricture. Severe hypotension may occur post-op or if depleted blood volume. Orthostatic hypotension may occur. May impair mental/physical abilities. Not for use in pregnancy prior to labor. May produce depression of respiration and psychophysiologic functions in newborn when used as an obstetrical analgesic.

ADVERSE REACTIONS: Lightheadedness, dizziness, sedation, NV, sweating, respiratory/circulatory depression.

INTERACTIONS: See Contraindications. Caution and reduce dose with other CNS depressants (eg, narcotics, anesthetics, phenothiazines, tranquilizers, sedative-hypnotics, TCAs, alcohol).

PREGNANCY: Safety in pregnancy and nursing not known.

MECHANISM OF ACTION: Narcotic analgesic; produces actions similiar to morphine. Principle actions involve the CNS and organs composed of smooth muscle. Produces analgesic and sedative effects.

PHARMACOKINETICS: Distribution: Crosses placental barrier; found in breast milk.

DEMEROL ORAL · CII
meperidine HCl (Sanofi-Aventis)

THERAPEUTIC CLASS: Opioid analgesic

INDICATIONS: Moderate to severe pain.

DOSAGE: *Adults:* Usual: 50-150mg q3-4h prn. Concomitant Phenothiazines/Other Tranquilizers: Reduce dose by 25-50%. Dilute syrup in 1/2 glass of water.
Pediatrics: Usual: 1.1-1.8mg/kg up to 50-150mg q3-4h prn. Concomitant Phenothiazines/Other Tranquilizers: Reduce dose by 25-50%. Dilute syrup in 1/2 glass of water.

HOW SUPPLIED: Syrup: 50mg/5mL; Tab: 50mg*, 100mg *scored

CONTRAINDICATIONS: MAOI during or within 14 days of use.

WARNINGS/PRECAUTIONS: May develop tolerance and dependence; abuse potential. Extreme caution with head injury, increased ICP, intracranial lesions, acute asthma attack, chronic COPD, cor pulmonale, decreased respiratory reserve, respiratory depression, hypoxia, and hypercapnia. Caution with sickle cell anemia, pheochromocytoma, acute alcoholism, Addison's disease, CNS depression or coma, delirium tremens, elderly or debilitated, kyphoscoliosis associated with respiratory depression, myxedema, hypothyroidism, acute abdominal conditions, epilepsy, atrial flutter, other supraventricular tachycardias, renal/hepatic impairment, prostatic hypertrophy, urethral stricture, drug dependencies, neonates, and young infants. Severe hypotension may occur post-op or if depleted blood volume. Orthostatic hypotension may occur. Not for use in pregnancy prior to labor.

ADVERSE REACTIONS: Lightheadedness, dizziness, sedation, NV, sweating, respiratory depression.

INTERACTIONS: See Contraindications. Reduce dose with other CNS depressants (eg, narcotics, anesthetics, phenothiazines, tranquilizers, sedative-hypnotics, TCAs, alcohol). Mixed agonist/antagonist analgesics (eg, pentazocine, nalbuphine, butorphanol, buprenorphine) may reduce analgesic effects and/or precipitate withdrawal symptoms. Caution with acyclovir, cimetidine. Phenytoin may enhance hepatic metabolism. May enhance neuroblocking action of skeletal muscle relaxants. Increased levels with ritonavir; avoid concurrent administration.

PREGNANCY: Category C, not for use in nursing.

MECHANISM OF ACTION: Narcotic analgesic; produces actions similiar to morphine. Principle actions involve the CNS and organs composed of smooth muscle. Produces analgesic and sedative effects.

PHARMACOKINETICS: Distribution: Crosses placental barrier; found in breast milk.

DEMSER · RX
metyrosine (Aton)

THERAPEUTIC CLASS: Tyrosine hydroxylase inhibitor

INDICATIONS: Treatment of pheochromocytoma for preoperative preparation and when surgery is contraindicated. Chronic treatment with malignant pheochromocytoma.

DOSAGE: *Adults:* Initial: 250mg qid. Titrate: May increase by 250-500mg/day. Max: 4g/day. Titrate based on clinical symptoms and catecholamine excretion. Usual: 2-3g/day. Preoperative Preparation: Take 5-7 days before surgery.

Pediatrics: ≥12 yrs: Initial: 250mg qid. Titrate: May increase by 250-500mg/day. Max: 4g/day. Titrate based on clinical symptoms and catecholamine excretion. Usual: 2-3g/day. Preoperative Preparation: Take 5-7 days before surgery.

HOW SUPPLIED: Cap: 250mg

WARNINGS/PRECAUTIONS: When used preoperatively or with α-adrenergic blockers, maintain intravascular volume intra- and post-operatively to avoid hypotension and decreased perfusion. Maintain adequate water intake to achieve urine volume of ≥2000mL to prevent crystalluria. Risk of hypertensive crisis or arrhythmias during tumor manipulation. Monitor BP and ECG continuously during surgery.

ADVERSE REACTIONS: Sedation, EPS, anxiety, depression, hallucinations, disorientation, confusion, diarrhea.

INTERACTIONS: Additive sedative effects with alcohol and other CNS depressants (eg, hypnotics, sedatives, tranquilizers). May potentiate EPS with phenothiazines and haloperidol.

PREGNANCY: Category C, caution in nursing.

MECHANISM OF ACTION: Tyrosine hydroxylase inhibitor; inhibits conversion of tyrosine to dihydroxyphenylalanine (DOPA), resulting in decreased catecholamines.

PHARMACOKINETICS: Elimination: Urine (69%); $T_{1/2}$=3-3.7 hrs.

Denavir
penciclovir (Novartis)

RX

THERAPEUTIC CLASS: Nucleoside analogue

INDICATIONS: Treatment of recurrent herpes labialis (cold sores) in adults and children ≥12 yrs.

DOSAGE: *Adults:* Apply q2h while awake for 4 days. Start with earliest sign or symptom. *Pediatrics:* ≥12 yrs: Apply q2h while awake for 4 days. Start with earliest sign or symptom.

HOW SUPPLIED: Cre: 1% (1.5g)

WARNINGS/PRECAUTIONS: Only use on herpes labialis on the lips and face. Avoid mucous membranes or near the eyes. Effectiveness not established in immunocompromised patients.

ADVERSE REACTIONS: Headache, application site reaction, local anesthesia, taste perversion, rash.

PREGNANCY: Category B, not for use in nursing.

MECHANISM OF ACTION: Antiviral agent. Active against herpes simplex virus types 1 (HSV-1) and 2 (HSV-2). Inhibits HSV polymerase competitively with deoxyguanosine triphosphate. Consequently, herpes viral DNA synthesis and replication are selectively inhibited.

Depacon
valproate sodium (Abbott)

RX

> Fatal hepatic failure (<2 yrs at considerable risk), teratogenic effects (eg, neural tube defects), and life-threatening pancreatitis reported.

THERAPEUTIC CLASS: Carboxylic acid derivative

INDICATIONS: Monotherapy and adjunctive therapy for treatment of simple and complex absence seizures, and complex partial seizures. Adjunct therapy for multiple seizure types.

DOSAGE: *Adults:* Simplex/Complex Absence Seizure: Initial: 15mg/kg/day. Titrate: Increase weekly by 5-10mg/kg/day until optimal response. Max: 60mg/kg/day. Complex Partial Seizure: Initial: 10-15mg/kg/day. Titrate: Increase weekly by 5-10mg/kg/day until optimal response. Max: 60mg/kg/day. Elderly: Reduce initial dose and titrate slowly. If dose >250mg/day, give in divided doses. Administer as 60 min IV infusion, not >20mg/min. Not for use >14 days; switch to oral route as soon as clinically feasible. Decrease dose or d/c if decreased food or fluid intake or if excessive somnolence occurs.

Pediatrics: ≥2 yrs: Simplex/Complex Absence Seizure: Initial: 15mg/kg/day. Titrate: Increase weekly by 5-10mg/kg/day until optimal response. Max: 60mg/kg/day. ≥10 yrs: Complex Partial Seizure: Initial: 10-15mg/kg/day. Titrate: Increase weekly by 5-10mg/kg/day until optimal response. Max: 60mg/kg/day. If dose >250mg/day, give in divided doses. Administer as 60 min IV infusion, not >20mg/min. Not for use >14 days; switch to oral route as soon as clinically feasible. Decrease dose or d/c with decreased food or fluid intake and if excessive somnolence.

HOW SUPPLIED: Inj: 100mg/mL

CONTRAINDICATIONS: Hepatic disease, significant hepatic dysfunction, known urea cycle disorders (UCD).

WARNINGS/PRECAUTIONS: Hyperammonemic encephalopathy in UCD patients; d/c if this occurs. Prior to therapy, evaluate for UCD in high risk patients (eg, history of unexplained encephalopathy, coma, etc). Measure ammonia levels if develop unexplained lethargy, vomiting, or mental status changes. Caution in elderly; monitor for fluid/nutritional intake, dehydration, somnolence. Monitor LFTs before therapy and during 1st 6 months. D/C if develop hepatic dysfunction, pancreatitis. Increased risk of hepatotoxicity with multiple anticonvulsants, congenital metabolic disorders, severe seizure disorder with mental retardation, organic brain disease, children <2 yrs. Avoid abrupt withdrawal. Monitor platelets and coagulation tests before therapy and periodically thereafter. Elevated liver enzymes and thrombocytopenia may be dose-related. Not for prophylaxis of post-traumatic seizures in acute head trauma. May interfere with urine ketone and thyroid function tests.

ADVERSE REACTIONS: Dizziness, headache, nausea, local reactions.

INTERACTIONS: Clonazepam may induce absence status in patients with absence seizures. Potentiates amitriptyline, nortriptyline, carbamazepine, diazepam, ethosuximide, lamotrigine, phenobarbital, primidone, phenytoin, tolbutamide, warfarin, zidovudine. Potentiated by ASA and felbamate. Antagonized by rifampin, carbamazepine, phenobarbital, phenytoin. Additive CNS depression with other CNS depressants (eg, alcohol).

PREGNANCY: Category D, not for use in nursing.

MECHANISM OF ACTION: Anticonvulsant; increases GABA concentrations in the brain.

PHARMACOKINETICS: Absorption: T_{max}=1 hr. **Distribution:** Plasma protein binding (10%-18.5%). **Metabolism:** Liver; glucuronidation, mitochondrial β-oxidation. **Elimination:** Urine (<3% unchanged); $T_{1/2}$=16 hrs.

DEPAKENE RX
valproic acid (Abbott)

> **Fatal hepatic failure (<2 yrs at considerable risk), teratogenic effects (eg, neural tube defects), and life-threatening pancreatitis reported.**

THERAPEUTIC CLASS: Carboxylic acid derivative

INDICATIONS: Monotherapy and adjunctive therapy for treatment of simple and complex absence seizures, and complex partial seizures. Adjunct therapy for multiple seizure types.

DOSAGE: *Adults:* Simplex/Complex Absence Seizure: Initial: 15mg/kg/day. Titrate: Increase weekly by 5-10mg/kg/day until optimal response. Max: 60mg/kg/day. Complex Partial Seizure: Initial: 10-15mg/kg/day. Titrate: Increase weekly by 5-10mg/kg/day until optimal response. Max: 60mg/kg/day. If dose >250mg/day, give in divided doses. Elderly: Reduce initial dose. Swallow caps whole, do not chew.
Pediatrics: ≥10 yrs: Complex Partial Seizure: Initial: 10-15mg/kg/day. Titrate: Increase weekly by 5-10mg/kg/day until optimal response. Max: 60mg/kg/day. If dose >250mg/day, give in divided doses. Swallow caps whole, do not chew.

HOW SUPPLIED: Cap: 250mg; Syrup: 250mg/5mL

CONTRAINDICATIONS: Hepatic disease, significant hepatic dysfunction, known urea cycle disorders (UCD).

WARNINGS/PRECAUTIONS: Hyperammonemic encephalopathy in UCD patients; d/c if this occurs. Prior to therapy, evaluate for UCD in high risk patients (eg, history of unexplained encephalopathy, coma, etc). Measure ammonia levels if develop unexplained lethargy, vomiting, or mental status changes. Caution in elderly; monitor for fluid/nutritional intake, dehydration, somnolence. Monitor LFTs before therapy and during 1st

6 months. D/C if develop hepatic dysfunction, pancreatitis. Increased risk of hepatotoxicity with multiple anticonvulsants, congenital metabolic disorders, severe seizure disorder with mental retardation, organic brain disease, children <2 yrs. Avoid abrupt withdrawal. Hyperammonemia reported. Monitor platelets and coagulation tests before therapy and periodically thereafter. Elevated liver enzymes and thrombocytopenia may be dose-related. May interfere with urine ketone and thyroid function tests.

ADVERSE REACTIONS: Headache, asthenia, nausea, vomiting, diarrhea, abdominal pain, somnolence, tremor, dizziness, thrombocytopenia, ecchymosis, nystagmus, alopecia.

INTERACTIONS: Clonazepam may induce absence status in patients with absence seizures. Potentiates amitriptyline, nortriptyline, carbamazepine, diazepam, ethosuximide, lamotrigine, phenobarbital, primidone, phenytoin, tolbutamide, warfarin, zidovudine. Potentiated by ASA and felbamate. Antagonized by rifampin, carbamazepine, phenobarbital, phenytoin. Additive CNS depression with other CNS depressants (eg, alcohol).

PREGNANCY: Category D, not for use in nursing.

MECHANISM OF ACTION: Anticonvulsant; increases GABA concentration in the brain.

PHARMACOKINETICS: Absorption: T_{max}=4-8 hrs (tab), T_{max}=3.3-4.8 hrs (caps). **Distribution:** V_d=11L/1.73m^2; plasma protein binding (10%-18.5%). **Metabolism:** Liver; glucuronidation, mitochondrial β-oxidation. **Elimination:** Urine (<3% unchanged); $T_{1/2}$=9-16 hrs.

DEPAKOTE
divalproex sodium (Abbott)

RX

> Fatal hepatic failure (<2 yrs at considerable risk), teratogenic effects (eg, neural tube defects), and life-threatening pancreatitis reported.

THERAPEUTIC CLASS: Valproate compound

INDICATIONS: (Tab, Cap) Management of simple and complex absence seizures; complex partial seizures; and adjunctively with multiple seizure types including absence seizures. (Tab) Treatment of mania associated with bipolar disorder and migraine prophylaxis.

DOSAGE: *Adults:* (Cap/Tab) Complex Partial Seizures: Initial: 10-15mg/kg/day. Titrate: Increase by 5-10mg/kg/week. Max: 60mg/kg/day. Absence Seizures: Initial: 15mg/kg/day. Titrate: Increase weekly by 5-10mg/kg/day. Max: 60mg/kg/day. Give in divided doses if >250mg/day. (Tab) Migraine: Initial: ≥16 yrs: 250mg bid. Max: 1000mg/day. Mania: 750mg daily in divided doses. Titrate: Increase dose rapidly to clinical effect. Max: 60mg/kg/day. Elderly: Reduce initial dose and titrate slowly. Decrease dose or d/c if decreased food or fluid intake or if excessive somnolence occurs.
Pediatrics: ≥10 yrs: (Cap/Tab) Complex Partial Seizures: Initial: 10-15mg/kg/day. Titrate: Increase by 5-10mg/kg/week. Max: 60mg/kg/day. Absence Seizures: Initial: 15mg/kg/day. Titrate: Increase weekly by 5-10mg/kg/day. Max: 60mg/kg/day. Give in divided doses if >250mg/day.

HOW SUPPLIED: Cap, Delayed-Release: (Sprinkle) 125mg; Tab, Delayed-Release: 125mg, 250mg, 500mg

CONTRAINDICATIONS: Hepatic disease, significant hepatic dysfunction, known urea cycle disorders (UCD).

WARNINGS/PRECAUTIONS: Hyperammonemic encephalopathy in UCD patients; d/c if this occurs. Prior to therapy, evaluate for UCD in high risk patients (eg, history of unexplained encephalopathy, coma, etc). Measure ammonia levels if develop unexplained lethargy, vomiting, or mental status changes. Caution with hepatic disease. Check LFTs prior to therapy, then frequently during 1st six months. Dose-related thrombocytopenia and elevated liver enzymes reported. Monitor platelet and coagulation tests prior to therapy, then periodically. Altered thyroid function tests and urine ketone test. May stimulate replication of HIV and CMV viruses. Avoid abrupt discontinuation.

ADVERSE REACTIONS: Nausea, vomiting, diarrhea, somnolence, dyspepsia, thrombocytopenia, asthenia, abdominal pain, tremor, headache, anorexia, diplopia, blurred vision, weight gain, ataxia, nystagmus.

INTERACTIONS: Potentiates carbamazepine, amitriptyline, nortriptyline, diazepam, ethosuximide, primidone, lamotrigine, phenobarbital, phenytoin, tolbutamide, zidovudine, lorazepam. Efficacy potentiated by ASA, felbamate. Efficacy reduced by rifampin, carbamazepine, phenobarbital, phenytoin, primidone. Clonazepam may induce absence status in patients with absence type seizures. CNS depression with alcohol and other CNS depressants. Monitor PT/INR with warfarin.

PREGNANCY: Category D, not for use in nursing.

MECHANISM OF ACTION: Anticonvulsant; increases GABA concentrations in the brain.

PHARMACOKINETICS: Absorption: T_{max}=4-8 hrs (tab), T_{max}=3.3-4.8 hrs (cap). **Distribution:** Plasma protein binding (10%-18.5%). **Metabolism:** Liver; glucuronidation, mitochondrial β-oxidation. **Elimination:** Urine (<3% unchanged); $T_{1/2}$=9-16 hrs.

Depakote ER   RX
divalproex sodium (Abbott)

> Fatal hepatic failure (<2 yrs at considerable risk), teratogenic effects (eg, neural tube defects), and life-threatening pancreatitis reported.

THERAPEUTIC CLASS: Valproate compound

INDICATIONS: Migraine prophylaxis. Monotherapy and adjunct therapy for treatment of complex partial seizures, and simple and complex absence seizures. Adjunct for multiple seizure types that include absence seizures. Acute manic or mixed episodes associated with bipolar disorder.

DOSAGE: *Adults:* For qd dosing. Migraine: Initial: 500mg qd for 1 week. Titrate: Increase to 1000mg qd. Max: 1000mg/day. Complex Partial Seizures: Monotherapy/Adjunct Therapy: Initial: 10-15mg/kg/day. Titrate: Increase by 5-10mg/kg/week to optimal response. Usual: Less than 60mg/kg/day (accepted therapeutic range 50-100mcg/mL). When converting to monotherapy, reduce concomitant antiepilepsy drug by 25% every 2 weeks starting at initiation or delay 1-2 weeks after start of therapy. Simple and Complex Absence Seizures: Initial: 15mg/kg/day. Titrate: Increase weekly by 5-10mg/kg/day to optimal response. Max: 60mg/kg/day. Bipolar Disorder: Initial: 25mg/kg/day given once daily. Titrate: Increase dose rapidly to clinical effect. Max: 60mg/kg/day. Conversion from Depakote: Administer Depakote ER qd using a dose 8-20% higher than the total daily dose of Depakote. If cannot directly convert to Depakote ER, consider increasing to next higher Depakote total daily dose before converting to appropriate total daily Depakote ER dose. Elderly: Give lower initial dose and titrate slowly. Decrease dose or d/c if decreased food or fluid intake or if excessive somnolence occurs. Swallow whole; do not crush or chew.

Pediatrics: ≥10yrs: For qd dosing. Complex Partial Seizures: Monotherapy/Adjunct Therapy: Initial: 10-15mg/kg/day. Titrate: Increase by 5-10mg/kg/week to optimal response. Usual: Less than 60mg/kg/day (accepted therapeutic range 50-100mcg/mL). When converting to monotherapy, reduce concomitant antiepilepsy drug by 25% every 2 weeks starting at initiation or delay 1-2 weeks after start of therapy. Simple and Complex Absence Seizures: Initial: 15mg/kg/day. Titrate: Increase weekly by 5-10mg/kg/day to optimal response. Max: 60mg/kg/day. Conversion from Depakote: Administer Depakote ER qd using a dose 8-20% higher than the total daily dose of Depakote. If cannot directly convert to Depakote ER, consider increasing to next higher Depakote total daily dose before converting to appropriate total daily Depakote ER dose. Swallow whole; do not crush or chew.

HOW SUPPLIED: Tab, Extended-Release: 250mg, 500mg

CONTRAINDICATIONS: Hepatic disease, significant hepatic dysfunction, known urea cycle disorders (UCD).

WARNINGS/PRECAUTIONS: Hyperammonemic encephalopathy in UCD patients; d/c if this occurs. Prior to therapy, evaluate for UCD in high risk patients (eg, history of unexplained encephalopathy, coma, etc). If unexplained lethargy, vomiting, or mental status changes occur measure ammonia levels. Caution with hepatic disease and elderly. Check LFTs prior to therapy, then frequently during 1st 6 months. Dose-related thrombocytopenia and elevated liver enzymes reported. Thrombocytopenia significantly increases with plasma trough levels >110mcg/mL in females and >135mcg/mL in males. Monitor platelet and coagulation tests prior to therapy, then periodically. Altered thyroid function tests and urine ketone test. May stimulate replication of HIV and CMV viruses. Avoid abrupt discontinuation.

ADVERSE REACTIONS: Nausea, dyspepsia, diarrhea, vomiting, abdominal pain, increased appetite, asthenia, somnolence, infection, dizziness, tremor, weight gain, back pain, alopecia.

INTERACTIONS: Potentiates carbamazepine, amitriptyline, nortriptyline, diazepam, ethosuximide, primidone, lamotrigine, phenobarbital, phenytoin, tolbutamide, zidovudine, lorazepam. Efficacy potentiated by ASA, felbamate. Efficacy reduced by rifampin, carbamazepine, phenobarbital, phenytoin, primidone. Clonazepam may induce absence status in patients with history of absence type seizures. CNS depression with alcohol and other CNS depressants. Monitor PT/INR with warfarin.

PREGNANCY: Category D, not for use in nursing.

MECHANISM OF ACTION: Anti-convulsant; increases GABA concentrations in the brain.

PHARMACOKINETICS: Absorption: Bioavailability (90%); T_{max}=4-17 hrs. **Distribution:** Plasma protein binding (10-18.5%). **Metabolism:** Liver; glucuronidation, mitochondrial β-oxidation. **Elimination:** Urine (<3% unchanged); $T_{1/2}$=9-16 hrs.

DEPO-MEDROL   RX
methylprednisolone acetate (Pharmacia & Upjohn)

THERAPEUTIC CLASS: Glucocorticoid

INDICATIONS: Steroid-responsive disorders.

DOSAGE: *Adults:* Local Effect: Rheumatoid/Osteoarthritis: Large Joint: 20-80mg. Medium Joint: 10-40mg. Small Joint: 4-10mg. Administer intra-articularly into synovial space every 1-5 weeks or more depending on relief. Ganglion/Tendinitis/Epicondylitis: 4-30mg into cyst/area of greatest tenderness. May repeat if necessary. Dermatologic Conditions: Inject 20-60mg into lesion. Distribute 20-40mg doses by repeated injections into large lesions. Usual: 1-4 injections. Systemic Effect: Substitute for Oral Therapy: IM dose should equal total daily PO methylprednisolone dose q24h. Prolonged Therapy: Administer weekly PO dose as single IM injection. Androgenital Syndrome: 40mg IM every 2 weeks. Rheumatoid Arthritis: 40-120mg IM weekly. Dermatologic Lesions: 40-120mg IM weekly for 1-4 weeks. Acute Severe Dermatitis (Poison Ivy): 80-120mg IM single dose. Chronic Contact Dermatitis: May repeat injections every 5-10 days. Seborrheic Dermatitis: 80mg IM weekly. Multiple Sclerosis: 200mg/day prednisolone for 1 week, then 80mg every other day for 1 month (4mg methylprednisolone=5mg prednisolone). Asthma/Allergic Rhinitis: 80-120mg IM.
Pediatrics: Use lower adult doses. Determine dose by severity of condition and response.

HOW SUPPLIED: Inj: 20mg/mL, 40mg/mL, 80mg/mL

CONTRAINDICATIONS: Intrathecal administration, systemic fungal infections.

WARNINGS/PRECAUTIONS: Dermal and subdermal atrophy reported; do not exceed recommended doses. May need to increase dose before, during, and after stressful situations. May mask signs of infection or cause new infections. Prolonged use may produce cataracts, glaucoma, secondary ocular infections. Increases BP, salt/water retention, potassium and calcium excretion. More severe/fatal course of infections reported with chickenpox, measles. Caution with Strongyloides, latent TB, hypothyroidism, cirrhosis, ocular herpes simplex, HTN, diverticulitis, fresh intestinal anastomoses, ulcerative colitis, osteoporosis, myasthenia gravis, renal insufficiency, peptic ulcer disease. Kaposi's sarcoma reported. Growth and development of children on prolonged therapy should be monitored. Monitor for psychic disturbances. Avoid abrupt withdrawal. Do not use intra-articularly, intrabursally, or for intratendinous administration in acute infection. Avoid injection into unstable and previously infected joints. Monitor urinalysis, blood sugar, BP, weight, chest X-ray, and upper GI x-ray (if ulcer history) regularly during prolonged therapy.

ADVERSE REACTIONS: Fluid and electrolyte disturbances, HTN, osteoporosis, muscle weakness, cushingoid state, menstrual irregularities, impaired wound healing, DM, ulcerative esophagitis, excessive sweating, increases intracranial pressure, carbohydrate intolerance, glaucoma, cataracts, urticaria, subcutaneous/cutaneous atrophy.

INTERACTIONS: Reduced efficacy with hepatic enzyme inducers (eg, phenobarbital, phenytoin, and rifampin). Increases clearance of chronic high dose ASA. Caution with ASA in hypoprothrombinemia. Effects on oral anticoagulants are variable; monitor PT. Increased insulin and oral hypoglycemic requirements in DM. Avoid live vaccines with immunosuppressive doses. Possible decreased vaccine response with killed or inactivated vaccines with immunosuppressive doses. Mutual inhibition of metabolism with cyclosporine; convulsions reported. Potentiated by ketoconazole and troleandomycin. Do not dilute or mix with other solutions.

PREGNANCY: Safety in pregnancy and nursing not known.

MECHANISM OF ACTION: Anti-inflammatory glucocorticoid; causes profound and varied metabolic effects and modifies the body's immune responses to diverse stimuli.

PHARMACOKINETICS: Absorption: C_{max}=11.8ng/mL; AUC=1286ng•hr/mL. **Elimination:** 139 hrs.

DEPO-TESTOSTERONE CIII
testosterone cypionate (Pharmacia & Upjohn)

THERAPEUTIC CLASS: Androgen

INDICATIONS: Testosterone replacement in males with primary hypogonadism and hypogonadotropic hypogonadism.

DOSAGE: *Adults:* Male Hypogonadism: 50-400mg IM every 2-4 weeks. Dose based on age, sex, and diagnosis. Adjust dose according to response and adverse reactions. *Pediatrics:* ≥12 yrs: Male Hypogonadism: 50-400mg IM every 2-4 weeks. Dose based on age, sex, and diagnosis. Adjust dose according to response and adverse reactions.

HOW SUPPLIED: Inj: 100mg/mL, 200mg/mL

CONTRAINDICATIONS: Severe renal, hepatic and cardiac disease. Males with carcinoma of the breast or prostate gland. Pregnancy.

WARNINGS/PRECAUTIONS: May accelerate bone maturation without linear growth; monitor bone growth every 6 months. Risk of hepatic damage with long-term use. D/C if hypercalcemia occurs in immobilized patients. D/C with acute urethral obstruction, priapism, excessive sexual stimulation, or oligospermia; restart at lower doses. Risk of edema; caution with pre-existing cardiac, renal or hepatic disease. Caution in the elderly; increased risk of prostatic hypertrophy and prostatic carcinoma. Caution with BPH. Should not be used for enhancement of athletic performance. Do not administer IV. Monitor Hct, Hgb, cholesterol periodically.

ADVERSE REACTIONS: Gynecomastia, excessive frequency/duration of penile erections, male pattern baldness, increased/decreased libido, oligospermia, hirsutism, acne, fluid and electrolyte disturbances, nausea, hypercholesterolemia, clotting factor suppression, polycythemia, altered LFTs, priapism, anxiety, depression.

INTERACTIONS: May potentiate oral anticoagulants (eg, warfarin) and oxyphenbutazone. May decrease blood glucose and insulin requirements in diabetics.

PREGNANCY: Category X, not for use in nursing.

MECHANISM OF ACTION: Endogenous androgen; responsible for normal growth and development of male sex organs and for maintenance of secondary sex characteristics.

PHARMACOKINETICS: Distribution: Plasma protein binding (98%). **Elimination:** Urine (90%), feces (6%). $T_{1/2}$=8 days.

DERMA-SMOOTHE/FS RX
fluocinolone acetonide (Hill Dermaceuticals)

THERAPEUTIC CLASS: Topical corticosteroid

INDICATIONS: Treatment of atopic dermatitis in adults and pediatrics ≥3 months.

DOSAGE: *Adults:* Atopic Dermatitis: Apply to affected area(s) tid.
Pediatrics: 3 months-17 yrs: Atopic Dermatitis: Moisten skin and apply bid for up to 4 weeks.

HOW SUPPLIED: Oil: 0.01% (120mL)

WARNINGS/PRECAUTIONS: May produce reversible hypothalamic-pituitary-adrenal (HPA) axis suppression, manifestations of Cushing's syndrome, hyperglycemia, and glucosuria. Children may be more susceptible to systemic toxicity. Use appropriate antifungal or antibacterial agent with dermatological infections. Contains refined peanut oil. D/C if hypersensitivity develops and treat accordingly. Avoid face, diaper area, and intertriginous areas with pediatrics.

ADVERSE REACTIONS: Atrophy, striae, telangiectasias, burning, itching, irritation, dryness, folliculitis, acneiform eruptions, hypopigmentation, perioral dermatitis, allergic contact dermatitis, secondary infections, miliaria.

PREGNANCY: Category C, caution in nursing.

MECHANISM OF ACTION: Corticosteroid; possesses anti-inflammatory, antipruritic, and vasoconstrictive properties. Anti-inflammatory action not established. Suspected to act by induction of phospholipase A_2 inhibitory proteins, lipocortins. Lipocortins control biosynthesis of prostaglandins and leukotrienes by inhibiting release of arachidonic acid. Arachidonic acid is released from membrane phospholipids by phospholipase A_2.

PHARMACOKINETICS: Absorption: Percutaneous; occlusion, inflammation, and other disease states may increase absorption. **Distribution:** Systemically administered corticosteroids found in breast milk.

DERMATOP
prednicarbate (Dermik)

RX

THERAPEUTIC CLASS: Corticosteroid

INDICATIONS: Corticosteroid responsive dermatoses.

DOSAGE: *Adults:* (Cre, Oint) Apply bid.
Pediatrics: ≥1 yr: (Cre) Apply bid. Max: 3 weeks of therapy. ≥10 yrs: (Oint) Apply bid.

HOW SUPPLIED: Cre, Oint: 0.1% (15g, 60g)

WARNINGS/PRECAUTIONS: May produce reversible HPA axis suppression, manifestations of Cushing's syndrome, hyperglycemia, and glucosuria. D/C if irritation occurs. Use appropriate antifungal or antibacterial agent with dermatological infections. Pediatrics may be more susceptible to systemic toxicity. Re-evaluate if no improvement after 2 weeks. Avoid eyes, occlusive dressings. Not for treatment of diaper dermatitis.

ADVERSE REACTIONS: Stinging, burning, dry skin, pruritus, urticaria, allergic contact dermatitis, edema, paresthesia, rash, skin atrophy.

PREGNANCY: Category C, caution in nursing.

MECHANISM OF ACTION: Corticosteroid; not established. Possesses anti-inflammatory, anti-pruritic, and vasoconstrictive properties. Suspected to act by induction of phospholipase A_2 inhibitory proteins, called lipocortins. Lipocortins control synthesis of potent inflammation mediators (eg, prostaglandins, leukotrienes) through inhibiting release of their common precursor, arachidonic acid. Arachidonic acid is released from membrane phospholipids by phospholipase A_2.

PHARMACOKINETICS: Absorption: Percutaneous; inflammation and/or other disease states increase absorption. Occlusive dressings for <24 hrs not shown to increase drug penetration; for 96 hrs markedly enhances penetration. **Distribution:** Systemically administered corticosteroids found in breast milk.

DESFERAL
deferoxamine mesylate (Novartis)

RX

THERAPEUTIC CLASS: Iron-chelating agent

INDICATIONS: Treatment of acute iron intoxication and of chronic iron overload due to transfusion-dependent anemias.

DOSAGE: *Adults:* See PI for solution preparation. Iron Intoxication: IM preferred for all patients not in shock. Only use IV slow infusion with cardiovascular collapse, and do not exceed 15mg/kg/hr for 1st 1g. Subsequent IV dosing should not exceed 125mg/hr. IM: Initial: 1g, then 500mg q4h for 2 doses. Give subsequent 500mg doses q4-12h depending upon clinical response. Max: 6g/24 hrs. IV: 1g, then 500mg over 4 hrs for 2 doses. Give subsequent 500mg doses over 4-12 hrs depending upon clinical response. Max: 6g/24 hrs. Iron Overload: IM: 500mg-1g/day IM. In addition, 2g IV per unit of blood transfused; not to exceed 15mg/kg/hr. Max: 1g without transfusion or 6g even with ≥3 units of blood or PRBC. SQ: 1-2g (20-40mg/kg/day) SQ over 8-24 hrs using small pump for continuous infusion. Individualize duration.

Pediatrics: ≥3 yrs: See PI for solution preparation. Iron Intoxication: IM preferred for all patients not in shock. Only use IV slow infusion with cardiovascular collapse, and do not exceed 15mg/kg/hr for 1st 1g. Subsequent IV dosing should not exceed 125mg/hr. IM: Initial: 1g, then 500mg q4h for 2 doses. Give subsequent 500mg doses q4-12h depending upon clinical response. Max: 6g/24 hrs. IV: 1g, then 500mg over 4 hrs for 2 doses. Give subsequent 500mg doses over 4-12 hrs depending upon clinical response. Max: 6g/24 hrs. Iron Overload: IM: 500mg-1g/day IM. In addition, 2g IV per unit of blood transfused; not to exceed 15mg/kg/hr. Max: 1g without transfusion or 6g even with ≥3 units of blood or PRBC. SQ: 1-2g (20-40mg/kg/day) SQ over 8-24 hrs using small pump for continuous infusion. Individualize duration.

HOW SUPPLIED: Inj: 500mg, 2g

CONTRAINDICATIONS: Severe renal disease, anuria.

WARNINGS/PRECAUTIONS: Ocular and auditory disturbances reported with prolonged use, high doses, or low ferritin levels. Periodic visual acuity tests, slit-lamp exams, funduscopy, and audiometry with prolonged treatment. High doses with low ferritin levels associated with growth retardation. Adult respiratory distress syndrome, also in children, reported after high IV doses in acute iron intoxication or thalassemia. Give IM, slow SQ, or IV infusion; skin flushing, urticaria, hypotension, and shock reported with rapid IV injection. High dose may exacerbate neurological dysfunction in aluminum-related encephalopathy. May precipitate onset of dialysis dementia. Aluminum overload with deferoxamine may decrease serum calcium and aggravate hyperparathyroidism. D/C with mucormycosis, *Yersinia enterocolitica* or *Yersinia pseudotuberculosis* infections. Monitor pediatrics body weight and growth every 3 months. Caution in elderly patients.

ADVERSE REACTIONS: Injection-site reactions, hypersensitivity reactions, tachycardia, hypotension, shock, abdominal discomfort, diarrhea, NV, blood dyscrasia, leg cramps, growth retardation, bone changes, reddish urine.

INTERACTIONS: Cardiac dysfunction reported with high dose vitamin C (>500mg/day in adults) in patients with severe chronic iron overload; avoid vitamin C supplements in cardiac failure patients. Only give vitamin C after 1 month of deferoxamine therapy and monitor cardiac function. Do not exceed vitamin C 200mg/day in adults; 50mg/day for pediatrics <10 yrs and 100mg/day for older children usually suffices. Concurrent prochlorperazine may lead to temporary impairment of consciousness. May distort imaging results with gallium-67; discontinue deferoxamine 48 hrs before scintigraphy.

PREGNANCY: Category C, caution in nursing.

MECHANISM OF ACTION: Iron chelating agent; chelates iron by forming a stable complex that prevents iron from entering into further chemical reactions.

PHARMACOKINETICS: Metabolism: Metabolized primarily by plasma enzymes. **Elimination:** Urine, feces, bile.

DESMOPRESSIN ACETATE RX
desmopressin acetate (Ferring)

THERAPEUTIC CLASS: Synthetic vasopressin analog

INDICATIONS: Management of primary nocturnal enuresis, central cranial diabetes insipidus and temporary polyuria and polydipsia following head trauma or surgery.

DOSAGE: *Adults:* Central Cranial Diabetes Insipidus: 0.1-0.4mL/day intranasally as single dose or divided into 2-3 doses. *Pediatrics:* Primary Nocturnal Enuresis: ≥6 yrs: 20mcg (0.2mL) intranasally hs. Administer 1/2 the dose into each nostril. Max: 40mcg/day. Central Cranial Diabetes Insipidus: >12 yrs: 0.1-0.4mL/day as single dose or divided into 2-3 doses. 3 months-12 yrs: 0.05-0.3mL/day as single dose or divided into 2-3 doses.

HOW SUPPLIED: Sol, Intranasal: 0.1mg/mL (2.5mL).

WARNINGS/PRECAUTIONS: For intranasal use only. Adjust fluid intake downward in order to decrease the potential for water intoxication and hyponatremia. May increase BP, caution in coronary insufficiency and cardiovascular disease. Caution in fluid and electrolyte imbalance. Anaphylaxis reported. Changes in the nasal mucosa may cause erratic absorption; use IV administration in these cases.

ADVERSE REACTIONS: Transient headache, nausea, nasal congestion, rhinitis, flushing, abdominal cramps, nosebleed, sore throat, cough, upper respiratory tract infection, water intoxication, hyponatremia, asthenia, dizziness, epistaxis, GI disorder, conjunctivitis, edema lachrymation disorder.

INTERACTIONS: Caution with pressor agents.

PREGNANCY: Category B, caution in nursing.

MECHANISM OF ACTION: Synthetic vasopressin analog; antidiuretic affecting renal water conservation.

DESONATE
RX

desonide (SkinMedica)

THERAPEUTIC CLASS: Corticosteroid

INDICATIONS: Mild to moderate atopic dermatitis.

DOSAGE: *Adults:* Apply thin layer bid to affected area(s) and rub in gently. Not recommended beyond 4 consecutive weeks.
Pediatrics: ≥3 months: Apply a thin layer bid to the affected area(s) and rub in gently. Not recommended beyond 4 consecutive weeks.

HOW SUPPLIED: Gel: 0.05% (15g, 30g, 60g)

WARNINGS/PRECAUTIONS: May produce reversible HPA axis suppression, manifestations of Cushing's syndrome, hyperglycemia, and glucosuria. D/C if irritation occurs. Pediatrics may be more susceptible to systemic toxicity. Caution when applied to large surface areas. Avoid occlusive dressings. Avoid use beyond 4 wks.

ADVERSE REACTIONS: Burning, rash, application site pruritus.

PREGNANCY: Category C, caution in nursing.

MECHANISM OF ACTION: Corticosteroid; not established. Possesses anti-inflammatory, antipruritic, and vasoconstrictive properties. Suspected to act by the induction of phospholipase A_2 inhibitory proteins called lipocortins. Lipocortins control the biosynthesis of potent mediators of inflammation (eg, prostaglandins, leukotrienes) by inhibiting the release of their common precursor, arachidonic acid. Arachidonic acid is released from membrane phospholipids by phospholipase A_2.

PHARMACOKINETICS: Absorption: Percutaneous. Occlusion, inflammation and/or other disease processes may increase absorption. **Distribution:** Systemically administered corticosteroids appear in breast milk. **Metabolism:** Liver. **Elimination:** Kidneys and bile.

DESOXYN
CII

methamphetamine HCl (Ovation)

High potential for abuse. Avoid prolonged therapy in obesity.

THERAPEUTIC CLASS: Sympathomimetic amine

INDICATIONS: Attention deficit disorder with hyperactivity. Short-term adjunct to treat exogenous obesity.

DOSAGE: *Adults:* Obesity: 5mg, 1/2 hr before each meal. Do not exceed a few weeks of treatment.
Pediatrics: ADHD: ≥6 yrs: Initial: 5mg qd-bid. Titrate: Increase weekly by 5mg/day until optimum response. Usual: 20-25mg/day given bid. Obesity: ≥12 yrs: 5mg, 1/2 hr before each meal. Do not exceed a few weeks of treatment.

HOW SUPPLIED: Tab: 5mg

CONTRAINDICATIONS: Advanced arteriosclerosis, symptomatic cardiovascular disease, moderate to severe HTN, hyperthyroidism, glaucoma, agitated states, history of drug abuse, during or within 14 days of MAOI use.

WARNINGS/PRECAUTIONS: Tolerance to anorectic effect develops within a few weeks, do not exceed recommended dose to increase effect. Monitor growth in children. Caution with HTN. Do not use to combat fatigue or replace rest. Exacerbation of motor and phonic tics and Tourette's syndrome. May exacerbate behavior disturbance and thought disorder in psychotic pediatrics. Emergence of new psychotic symptoms may warrant discontinuation of therapy. Monitor for the appearance or worsening of aggressive behavior in children. Therapy may lower the convulsive threshold and cause blurred vision and difficulty with accommodation. Interrupt occasionally to determine if patient requires continued therapy. Misuse may cause sudden death and serious cardiovascular adverse events. Caution in patients with underlying cardiovascular conditions and comorbid bipolar disorder.

ADVERSE REACTIONS: BP elevation, tachycardia, palpitation, dizziness, insomnia, tremor, diarrhea, constipation, dry mouth, urticaria, impotence, changes in libido.

INTERACTIONS: May alter insulin requirements. May decrease hypotensive effect of guanethidine. Avoid MAOIs. Caution with TCAs and indirect acting sympathomimetic amines. Antagonized by phenothiazines.

PREGNANCY: Category C, not for use in nursing.

MECHANISM OF ACTION: Sympathomimetic amine; CNS stimulant. Peripheral actions involve elevation of BP, weak bronchodilation, and respiratory stimulant actions.

PHARMACOKINETICS: Absorption: Rapid. **Metabolism:** Liver; aromatic hydroxylation, N-dealkylation and deamination. **Elimination:** Urine (62%); $T_{1/2}$=4-5 hrs.

DEXAMETHASONE   RX
dexamethasone (Various)

OTHER BRAND NAME: Decadron (Merck)

THERAPEUTIC CLASS: Glucocorticoid

INDICATIONS: (PO) Treatment of steroid-responsive disorders. (Inj) Treatment of steroid responsive disorders when oral therapy not feasible.

DOSAGE: *Adults:* Individualize for disease and patient response. Withdraw gradually. (Tab) Initial: 0.75-9mg/day PO. Maint: Decrease in small amounts to lowest effective dose. Cushing's Syndrome Test: 1mg PO at 11pm; draw blood at 8am next morning. Or, 0.5mg PO q6h for 48 hrs; or 2mg (to distinguish if excess pituitary ACTH or other causes) PO q6h for 48 hrs; obtain 24-hr urine collections. (Inj) Initial: 0.5-9mg/day IV/IM. Cerebral Edema: Initial: 10mg IV, then 4mg IM q6h until edema subsides. Reduce dose after 2-4 days and gradually d/c over 5-7 days. Palliative Management of Recurrent/Inoperable Brain Tumors: Maint: 2mg IV/PO bid-tid. Acute Allergic Disorders: 4-8mg IM on 1st day, then 1.5mg PO bid for 2 days, then 0.75mg PO bid for 1 day, then 0.75mg PO qd for 2 days. (Inj) Usual: 0.2-9mg. Maint: Decrease in small amounts to lowest effective dose. Intra-Articular/Intralesional/Soft Tissue Injection: Usual: 0.2-6mg once every 3-5 days to once every 2-3 weeks. See PI for Shock Treatment. Take with meals and antacids to prevent peptic ulcer.
Pediatrics: Individualize for disease and patient response. Withdraw gradually. (Tab) Initial: 0.75-9mg/day PO. Maint: Decrease in small amounts to lowest effective dose. Cushing's Syndrome Test: 1mg PO at 11pm; draw blood at 8am next morning. Or, 0.5mg PO q6h for 48 hrs; or 2mg (to distinguish if excess pituitary ATCH or other causes) PO q6h for 48 hrs; obtain 24-hr urine collections. (Inj) Initial: 0.5-9mg/day IV/IM. Cerebral Edema: Initial: 10mg IV, then 4mg IM q6h until edema subsides. Reduce dose after 2-4 days and gradually d/c over 5-7 days. Palliative Management of Recurrent/Inoperable Brain Tumors: Maint: 2mg IV/PO bid-tid. Acute Allergic Disorders: 4-8mg IM on 1st day, then 1.5mg PO bid for 2 days, then 0.75mg PO bid for 1 day, then 0.75mg PO qd for 2 days. (Inj) Usual: 0.2-9mg. Maint: Decrease in small amounts to lowest effective dose. Intra-Articular/Intralesional/Soft Tissue Injection: Usual: 0.2-6mg once every 3-5 days to once every 2-3 weeks. See PI for shock treatment. Take with meals and antacids to prevent peptic ulcer.

HOW SUPPLIED: Inj: (Dexamethasone Sodium Phosphate) 4mg/mL, 10mg/mL; Sol: (Dexamethasone) 0.5mg/5mL, 1mg/mL; Tab: (Dexamethasone) 0.5mg*, 0.75mg*, 1mg*, 1.5mg*, 2mg*, 4mg*, 6mg* *scored

CONTRAINDICATIONS: Systemic fungal infections.

WARNINGS/PRECAUTIONS: Increase dose before, during, and after stressful situations. Avoid abrupt withdrawal. May mask signs of infection, activate latent amebiasis, elevate BP, cause salt/water retention, increase excretion of potassium and calcium. Prolonged use may produce cataracts, glaucoma, secondary ocular infections. Caution with recent MI, ocular herpes simplex, emotional instability, nonspecific ulcerative colitis, diverticulitis, peptic ulcer, renal insufficiency, HTN, osteoporosis, myasthenia gravis, threadworm infection, active tuberculosis. Enhanced effect with hypothyroidism, cirrhosis. Consider prophylactic therapy if exposed to measles or chickenpox. Risk of glaucoma, cataracts, and eye infections. False negative dexamethasone suppression test with indomethacin.

ADVERSE REACTIONS: Fluid/electrolyte disturbances, muscle weakness, osteoporosis, peptic ulcer, pancreatitis, ulcerative esophagitis, impaired wound healing, headache, psychic disturbances, growth suppression (pediatrics), glaucoma, hyperglycemia, weight gain, nausea, malaise.

INTERACTIONS: Caution with ASA. Inducers of CYP3A4 (eg, phenytoin, phenobarbital, carbamazepine, rifampin) and ephedrine enhance clearance; increase steroid dose. Inhibitors of CYP3A4 (ketoconazole, macrolides) may increase plasma levels. Drugs that affect metabolism may interfere with dexamethasone suppression tests. Increased clearance of drugs metabolized by CYP3A4 (eg, indinavir, erythromycin). May increase or decrease phenytoin levels. Ketoconazole may inhibit adrenal corticosteroid synthesis and cause adrenal insufficiency during corticosteroid withdrawal. Antagonizes or potentiates coumarins. Hypokalemia with potassium-depleting diuretics. Live virus vaccines are contraindicated with immunosuppressive doses.

PREGNANCY: Category C, not for use in nursing.

MECHANISM OF ACTION: Adrenocortical steroid; produces anti-inflammatory effects.

PHARMACOKINETICS: Distribution: Found in breast milk. **Metabolism**: Liver; CYP3A4.

DEXEDRINE `CII`
dextroamphetamine sulfate (GlaxoSmithKline)

> High potential for abuse. Avoid prolonged use. Misuse may cause sudden death and serious CV adverse events.

OTHER BRAND NAME: Dexedrine Spansules (GlaxoSmithKline)

THERAPEUTIC CLASS: Sympathomimetic amine

INDICATIONS: Treatment of attention deficit disorder with hyperactivity (ADHD) and narcolepsy.

DOSAGE: *Adults:* Narcolepsy: Initial: 10mg/day. Titrate: May increase by 10mg/day every week. Usual: 5-60mg/day. For tabs, give 1st dose upon awakening and additional every 4-6 hrs. May give caps once daily.
Pediatrics: Narcolepsy: 6-12 yrs: Initial: 5mg qd. Titrate: Increase weekly by 5mg/day. ≥12 yrs: Initial: 10mg qd. Titrate: Increase weekly by 10mg/day. Usual: 5-60mg/day in divided doses. ADHD: Initial: 3-5 yrs: 2.5mg qd. Titrate: Increase weekly by 2.5mg/day. ≥6 yrs: 5mg qd-bid. Titrate: Increase weekly by 5mg/day. Max: 40mg/day. For tabs, give 1st dose upon awakening and additional every 4-6 hrs. May give caps once daily.

HOW SUPPLIED: Cap, Extended-Release: (Spansules) 5mg, 10mg, 15mg; Tab: 5mg*
*scored

CONTRAINDICATIONS: Advanced arteriosclerosis, symptomatic cardiovascular disease, moderate to severe HTN, hyperthyroidism, glaucoma, agitated states, history of drug abuse, during or within 14 days of MAOI use.

WARNINGS/PRECAUTIONS: May exacerbate symptoms of behavior disturbance and thought disorder in psychotic patients. Caution when using stimulants to treat patients with comorbid bipolar disorder because of concern for possible induction of mixed/manic episode in such patients. Stimulants at usual doses can cause treatment emergent psychotic or manic symptoms (eg, hallucinations, delusional thinking, mania) in children and adolescents without prior history of psychotic illness. Aggressive behavior or hostility reported in clinical trials and the postmarketing experience of some medications indicated for the treatment of ADHD. Caution with HTN. Tablets contain tartrazine; may cause allergy reactions. Exacerbation of motor and phonic tics and Tourette's syndrome. Monitor growth in children. Avoid with serious structural cardiac abnormalities, cardiomyopathy, serious heart rhythm abnormalities, CAD, or other serious cardiac problems. Avoid use in the presence of seizure. Visual disturbances reported with stimulant treatment.

ADVERSE REACTIONS: Palpitations, tachycardia, BP elevation, CNS overstimulation, restlessness, insomnia, dry mouth, GI disturbances, anorexia, urticaria, impotence.

INTERACTIONS: GI acidifying agents (guanethidine, reserpine, glutamic acid, etc.) and urinary acidifying agents (ammonium chloride, etc) decrease efficacy. MAOIs may cause hypertensive crisis. Potentiated by GI and urinary alkalinizers, propoxyphene overdose. Potentiated effects of both agents with TCAs. May delay absorption of phenytoin, ethosuximide, phenobarbital. Potentiates meperidine, norepinephrine, phenobarbital, phenytoin. Antagonized by haloperidol, chlorpromazine, lithium. Antagonizes adrenergic blockers, antihistamines, antihypertensives, veratrum alkaloids (antihypertensive).

PREGNANCY: Category C, not for use in nursing.

MECHANISM OF ACTION: Amphetamine; noncatecholamine sympathomimetic amine with CNS stimulant activity. Peripheral actions involve elevation of BP, weak bronchodilation, and respiratory stimulant actions.

PHARMACOKINETICS: Absorption: (15mg Tab) C_{max}=36.6ng/mL, T_{max}=3 hrs. (15mg Cap-ER) C_{max}=23.5ng/mL, T_{max}=8 hrs. **Elimination:** $T_{1/2}$=12 hrs.

DextroStat `CII`
dextroamphetamine sulfate (Shire)

> **High potential for abuse. Avoid prolonged use.**

THERAPEUTIC CLASS: Sympathomimetic amine

INDICATIONS: Treatment of narcolepsy and attention deficit disorder with hyperactivity (ADHD).

DOSAGE: *Adults:* Narcolepsy: Initial: 10mg/day. Titrate: May increase by 10mg/day every week. Usual: 5-60mg/day. Give 1st dose upon awakening, and additional doses every 4-6 hrs.
Pediatrics: Narcolepsy: 6-12 yrs: Initial: 5mg/day. Titrate: Increase weekly by 5mg/day. ≥12 yrs: Initial: 10mg/day. Titrate: Increase weekly by 10mg/day. Usual: 5-60mg/day in divided doses. ADHD: 3-5 yrs: Initial: 2.5mg/day. Titrate: Increase weekly by 2.5mg/day until optimum response. 6-16 yrs: Initial 5mg qd-bid. Titrate: Increase weekly by 5mg/day until optimum response. Give 1st dose upon awakening, and additional doses q4-6h.

HOW SUPPLIED: Tab: 5mg*, 10mg* *scored

CONTRAINDICATIONS: Advanced arteriosclerosis, symptomatic cardiovascular disease, moderate to severe HTN, hyperthyroidism, glaucoma, agitated states, history of drug abuse, during or within 14 days of MAOI use.

WARNINGS/PRECAUTIONS: Caution in HTN. Contains tartrazine, may cause allergic reactions. Exacerbation of motor and phonic tics and Tourette's syndrome. May exacerbate behavior disturbance and thought disorder in psychotic pediatrics. Interrupt occasionally to determine if patient requires continued therapy. Monitor growth in children.

ADVERSE REACTIONS: BP elevation, tachycardia, palpitation, dizziness, insomnia, tremor, diarrhea, constipation, dry mouth, urticaria, impotence, changes in libido.

INTERACTIONS: GI acidifying agents (guanethidine, reserpine, glutamic acid, etc.) and urinary acidifying agents (ammonium chloride, etc.) decrease efficacy. MAOIs may cause hypertensive crisis. Potentiated by GI and urinary alkalinizers, propoxyphene overdose. Potentiated effects of both agents with TCAs. May delay absorption of phenytoin, ethosuximide, phenobarbital. Potentiates meperidine, norepinephrine, phenobarbital, phenytoin. Antagonized by haloperidol, chlorpromazine, lithium. Antagonizes adrenergic blockers, antihistamines, antihypertensives, veratrum alkaloids (antihypertensive).

PREGNANCY: Category C, not for use in nursing.

MECHANISM OF ACTION: Sympathomimetic amine; CNS stimulant activity. Peripheral actions involve elevation of BP, weak bronchodilation, and respiratory stimulant actions.

PHARMACOKINETICS: Absorption: C_{max}=29.2ng/mL, T_{max}=2 hrs. **Elimination:** Urine (45%); $T_{1/2}$=10.25 hrs.

DIASTAT
diazepam (Valeant) `CIV`

THERAPEUTIC CLASS: Benzodiazepine

INDICATIONS: Management of refractory patients with epilepsy, on stable regimens of anti-epileptic drugs, who require intermittent use to control bouts of increased seizure activity.

DOSAGE: *Adults:* 0.2mg/kg rectally. Calculate amount and round upwards to next available dose. May give 2nd dose 4-12 hrs later. Max: 5 episodes/month or 1 episode every 5 days.
Pediatrics: ≥12 yrs: 0.2mg/kg. 6-11yrs: 0.3mg/kg. 2-5 yrs: 0.5mg/kg. Calculate amount and round upwards to next available dose. May give 2nd dose 4-12 hrs later. For rectal administration. Max: 5 episodes/month and 1 episode every 5 days.

HOW SUPPLIED: Kit: 2.5mg, 5mg, 10mg, 15mg, 20mg

CONTRAINDICATIONS: Acute narrow angle glaucoma, untreated open angle glaucoma.

WARNINGS/PRECAUTIONS: Produces CNS depression. Avoid abrupt withdrawal. Caution with elderly, hepatic/renal dysfunction, compromised respiratory function, neurologic damage. Not for daily chronic use. Withdrawal symptoms reported with discontinuation.

ADVERSE REACTIONS: Somnolence, dizziness, headache, pain, abdominal pain, nervousness, vasodilation, diarrhea, ataxia, euphoria, incoordination, asthma, rhinitis, rash.

INTERACTIONS: Potentiated by phenothiazines, narcotics, barbiturates, valproate, MAOIs, and other antidepressants. Potential inhibitors of CYP450 2C19 (eg, cimetidine, quinidine, tranylcypromine) and CYP450 3A4 (eg, ketoconazole, troleandomycin, clotrimazole) may decrease elimination. CYP450 2C19 (eg, rifampin) and CYP450 3A4 (eg, carbamazepine, phenytoin, dexamethasone, phenobarbital) inducers could increase elimination. May interfere with metabolism of substrates for CYP450 2C19 (eg, omeprazole, propranolol, imipramine) and CYP450 3A4 (eg, cyclosporine, paclitaxel, terfenadine, theophylline, warfarin).

PREGNANCY: Category D, not for use in nursing.

MECHANISM OF ACTION: Benzodiazepine; unknown, suspected to suppress seizures through an interaction with GABA receptors (A-type). GABA acts at this receptor to allow entry of chloride ions, which causes an inhibitory potential that reduces the ability of neurons to depolarize to the threshold potential necessary to produce action potentials.

PHARMACOKINETICS: Absorption: Absolute bioavailability (90%); T_{max}=1.5 hrs. **Distribution:** V_d=1L/kg; plasma protein binding (95-98%). **Metabolism:** Hepatic (CYP3A4, CYP2C19) to form desmethyldiazepam (major active metabolite), temazepam and oxazepam (minor active metabolites). **Elimination:** $T_{1/2}$=46 hrs (15mg rectal).

DIAZEPAM INJECTION
diazepam (Various) `CIV`

THERAPEUTIC CLASS: Benzodiazepine

INDICATIONS: Management of anxiety disorders and short-term relief of anxiety symptoms. Symptomatic relief of acute alcohol withdrawal. Adjunct prior to endoscopic procedures, surgical procedures and cardioversion. Adjunct therapy in skeletal muscle spasm (eg, tetanus, etc), status epilepticus and severe recurrent convulsive disorders.

DOSAGE: *Adults:* Anxiety (moderate): 2-5mg IM/IV, may repeat in 3-4 hrs. Anxiety (severe): 5-10mg IM/IV, may repeat in 3-4 hrs. Alcohol Withdrawal (acute): 10mg IM/IV, then 5-10mg in 3-4 hrs if needed. Endoscopic Procedures: Usual: ≤10mg IV (up to 20mg) or 5-10mg IM 30 min prior to procedure. Muscle Spasm: 5-10mg IM/IV, then 5-10mg in 3-4 hrs if needed. Status Epilepticus/Severe Seizures: Initial: 5-10mg IM. Maint: May repeat at 10-15 min intervals. Max: 30mg. Preoperative: 10mg IM. Cardioversion: 5-15mg IV, 5-10 min prior to procedure. Elderly/Debilitated: Usual: 2-5mg.
Pediatrics: Tetanus: 30 days-5 yrs: 1-2mg IM/IV (slowly), may repeat every 3-4 hrs prn. ≥5

yrs: 5-10mg IM/IV, may repeat every 3-4 hrs. Status Epilepticus/Severe Seizures: 30 days-5 yrs: 0.2-0.5mg IV (slowly) every 2-5 min up to 5mg. ≥5 yrs: 1mg IV (slowly) every 2-5 min up to 10mg, may repeat in 2-4 hrs.

HOW SUPPLIED: Inj: 5mg/mL

CONTRAINDICATIONS: Acute narrow angle glaucoma, untreated open angle glaucoma.

WARNINGS/PRECAUTIONS: Inject slowly and avoid small veins with IV. Do not mix or dilute with other products in syringe or infusion flask. Extreme caution in elderly, severely ill and those with limited pulmonary reserve. Avoid if in shock, coma or acute alcohol intoxication with depressed vital signs. May impair mental/physical abilities. Increase in grand mal seizures reported. Caution with kidney or hepatic dysfunction. Not for obstetrical use. Withdrawal symptoms may occur. Hypotension and muscular weakness reported. Monitor blood counts and LFTs. Not for maintenance of seizures once controlled.

ADVERSE REACTIONS: Drowsiness, fatigue, ataxia, venous thrombosis and phlebitis (injection site).

INTERACTIONS: Phenothiazines, narcotics, barbiturates, MAOIs, and other antidepressants may potentiate effects. Delayed clearance with cimetidine. Reduce narcotic dose by at least one-third. Risk of apnea with concomitant barbiturates, alcohol, or other CNS depressants.

PREGNANCY: Not for use during pregnancy, safety in nursing unknown.

MECHANISM OF ACTION: Antianxiety/hypnotic agent; induces calming effect on parts of the limbic system, the thalamus and the hypothalamus (animal study).

DICLOXACILLIN   RX
dicloxacillin sodium (Various)

THERAPEUTIC CLASS: Penicillin (penicillinase-resistant)

INDICATIONS: Infections caused by penicillinase-producing staphylococci.

DOSAGE: *Adults:* Mild-Moderate Infection: 125mg q6h. Severe Infection: 250mg q6h for at least 14 days.
Pediatrics: <40kg: Mild-Moderate Infection: 12.5mg/kg/day in divided doses q6h. Severe Infection: 25mg/kg/day in divided doses q6h for at least 14 days.

HOW SUPPLIED: Cap: 250mg, 500mg

WARNINGS/PRECAUTIONS: Serious, fatal hypersensitivity reactions reported. Pseudomembranous colitis has been reported; toxin produced by *Clostridium difficile* is the primary cause. Caution with history of allergy and/or asthma. Monitor renal, hepatic, and hematopoietic function with prolonged use. Not for use as initial therapy with serious, life-threatening infections, or with nausea, vomiting, gastric dilation, cardiospasm, or intestinal hypermotility.

ADVERSE REACTIONS: Allergic reactions, NV, diarrhea, stomatitis, black or hairy tongue, superinfection (prolonged use), hepatotoxicity.

INTERACTIONS: Tetracycline may antagonize the bactericidal effects. Potentiated by probenecid.

PREGNANCY: Category B, caution in nursing.

MECHANISM OF ACTION: Penicillin (penicillinase-resistant); bactericidal against penicillin-susceptible microorganisms during state of active multiplication. Inhibits biosynthesis of bacterial cell-wall.

PHARMACOKINETICS: Absorption: Rapid, incomplete; C_{max}=1-1.5 hrs; T_{max}=10-17mcg/mL. **Distribution:** Serum protein binding (95%-99%); found in breast milk. **Elimination:** Urine (unchanged); $T_{1/2}$=0.7 hrs.

DIDREX   
benzphetamine HCl (Pharmacia & Upjohn)

THERAPEUTIC CLASS: Anorectic sympathomimetic amine

INDICATIONS: Short-term adjunct treatment of exogenous obesity.

DOSAGE: *Adults:* Initial: 25-50mg qd. Usual: 25-50mg qd-tid.
Pediatrics: ≥12 yrs: Initial: 25-50mg qd. Usual: 25-50mg qd-tid.

HOW SUPPLIED: Tab: 50mg* *scored

CONTRAINDICATIONS: Advanced arteriosclerosis, symptomatic cardiovascular disease, moderate to severe HTN, agitated states, hyperthyroidism, glaucoma, history of drug abuse, concomitant CNS stimulants, MAOI use within 14 days, pregnancy.

WARNINGS/PRECAUTIONS: Caution with mild HTN. D/C if tolerance develops. Psychological disturbances reported with restrictive dietary regimen.

ADVERSE REACTIONS: Palpitations, tachycardia, BP elevation, restlessness, dizziness, insomnia, headache, tremor, sweating, dry mouth, nausea, diarrhea, unpleasant tastes, urticaria, altered libido.

INTERACTIONS: Hypertensive crisis risk if used within 14 days of MAOIs. Potentiates TCAs. Avoid with other CNS stimulants. Decreases effects of antihypertensives. Potentiated by urinary alkalinizing agents and reduced effect with urinary acidifying agents. May alter insulin requirements.

PREGNANCY: Category X, not for use in nursing.

MECHANISM OF ACTION: Anorectic sympathomimetic amine; CNS stimulant, elevates BP. As anorectic, appetite suppression as primary action not established.

DIETHYLPROPION   CIV
diethylpropion HCl (Various)

THERAPEUTIC CLASS: Sympathomimetic amine

INDICATIONS: Short-term adjunct for exogenous obesity in patients with initial BMI ≥30kg/m^2.

DOSAGE: *Adults:* (Tab) 25mg tid 1 hour before meals, and mid-evening if needed for night hunger. (Tab, ER): 75mg at qd in mid-morning, swallowed whole.
Pediatrics: ≥16 yrs: (Tab) 25mg tid 1 hour before meals, and mid-evening if needed for night hunger. (Tab, ER): 75mg at qd in mid-morning, swallowed whole.

HOW SUPPLIED: Tab: 25mg; Tab, Extended-Release: 75mg

CONTRAINDICATIONS: Advanced arteriosclerosis, hyperthyroidism, glaucoma, pulmonary HTN, severe HTN, within 14 days of MAOI use, agitated states, history of drug abuse, other concomitant anorectics.

WARNINGS/PRECAUTIONS: Possible risk of pulmonary HTN and valvular heart disease. Caution with HTN, symptomatic cardiovascular disease. Avoid with heart murmur, valvular heart disease, severe HTN. May increase convulsions with epilepsy. Prolonged use may induce dependence with withdrawal symptoms. D/C if tolerance develops or insignificant weight loss after 4 weeks of therapy.

ADVERSE REACTIONS: Palpitations, tachycardia, arrhythmias, blurred vision, dizziness, anxiety, insomnia, depression, urticaria, gynecomastia, nausea, vomiting, GI disturbances, bone marrow depression, impotence.

INTERACTIONS: See Contraindications. MAOIs may cause hypertensive crisis. Avoid with other anorectic agents (prescription, OTC, herbal products) or if used within prior year. Phenothiazines may antagonize anorectic effects. Potential for arrhythmias with general anesthetics. May interfere with antihypertensives (eg, guanethidine, methyldopa). Adverse reactions with alcohol. Antidiabetic drug requirements may be altered. Valvular heart disease reported with fenfluramine or dexfenfluramine.

PREGNANCY: Category B, caution in nursing.

MECHANISM OF ACTION: Anorectic sympathomimetic amine; not established as appetite suppressor; causes CNS stimulation and elevation of BP.

PHARMACOKINETICS: Absorption: Rapid. **Distribution:** Crosses placenta; found in breast milk. **Metabolism:** N-dealkylation, reduction; aminoketone (metabolites). **Elimination:** Urine; $T_{1/2}$=4-6 hrs (aminoketone).

DIFFERIN
adapalene (Galderma)

RX

THERAPEUTIC CLASS: Naphthoic acid derivative (retinoid-like)

INDICATIONS: Topical treatment of acne vulgaris.

DOSAGE: *Adults:* Apply qhs after washing.
Pediatrics: ≥12 yrs: Apply qhs after washing.

HOW SUPPLIED: Cre: 0.1% (45g); Gel: 0.1%, 0.3% (45g, 75g)

WARNINGS/PRECAUTIONS: Avoid contact with eyes, lips, paranasal creases, mucous membranes, cuts, abrasions, eczematous or sunburned skin. Minimize sun exposure. Extreme weather may increase skin irritation.

ADVERSE REACTIONS: Erythema, scaling, dryness, pruritus, burning, sunburn; acne flares.

INTERACTIONS: Caution with other topicals with strong drying effects, high concentration of alcohol, astringents, spices, or lime. Allow effects of sulfur, resorcinol, or salicylic acid to subside before use.

PREGNANCY: Category C, caution in nursing.

MECHANISM OF ACTION: Naphthoic acid derivative; not established. Suspected to normalize differentiation of follicular epithelial cells resulting in decreased microcomedone formation.

PHARMACOKINETICS: Absorption: Low. **Elimination:** Bile.

DIFLUCAN
fluconazole (Pfizer)

RX

THERAPEUTIC CLASS: Azole antifungal

INDICATIONS: Treatment of vaginal, oropharyngeal, and esophageal candidiasis. Treatment of systemic *Candida* infections. Treatment of peritonitis and UTI caused by *Candida.* Treatment of cryptococcal meningitis. Prophylaxis in patients undergoing BMT.

DOSAGE: *Adults:* Vaginal Candidiasis: 150mg PO single dose. IV/PO: Oropharyngeal Candidiasis: 200mg on 1st day, then 100mg qd for at least 2 weeks. Esophageal Candidiasis: 200mg on 1st day, then 100mg qd for at least 3 weeks and for at least 2 weeks following resolution of symptoms. Max: 400mg/day. Systemic *Candida* Infections: Up to 400mg/day. UTI/Peritonitis: 50-200mg/day. Cryptococcal Meningitis: 400mg on 1st day, then 200mg qd for 10-12 weeks after negative CSF culture. Suppression of Cryptococcal Meningitis Relapse in AIDS: 200mg qd. Prophylaxis in BMT: 400mg qd. Renal Impairment: CrCl ≤50mL/min (no dialysis): Initial: LD 50-400mg. Maint: Give 50% of recommended dose. Dialysis: Give 100% of dose after each dialysis.
Pediatrics: IV/PO: Oropharyngeal Candidiasis: 6mg/kg on 1st day, then 3mg/kg/day for at least 2 weeks. Esophageal Candidiasis: 6mg/kg on 1st day, then 3mg/kg/day for at least 3 weeks and for at least 2 weeks following resolution of symptoms. Max: 12mg/kg/day. Systemic *Candida* Infections: 6-12mg/kg/day. Cryptococcal Meningitis: 12mg/kg 1st day, then 6mg/kg/day for 10-12 weeks after negative CSF culture. Suppression of Cryptococcal Meningitis Relapse in AIDS: 6mg/kg qd. Renal Impairment: CrCl <50mL/min (no dialysis): Initial: LD: 50-400mg. Maint: Give 50% of recommended dose. Dialysis: Give 100% of dose after each dialysis.

HOW SUPPLIED: Inj: 200mg/100mL, 400mg/200mL; Sus: 50mg/5mL, 200mg/5mL (35mL); Tab: 50mg, 100mg, 150mg, 200mg

CONTRAINDICATIONS: Coadministration with cisapride or terfenadine (with multiple Diflucan doses of ≥400mg). Caution if hypersensitive to other azoles.

WARNINGS/PRECAUTIONS: Monitor LFTs. D/C if hepatic dysfunction develops or exfoliative skin disorder progresses. Anaphylaxis reported. Rare cases of QT prolongation and torsades de pointes reported.

ADVERSE REACTIONS: Headache, NV, abdominal pain, diarrhea, skin rash.

INTERACTIONS: See Contraindications. Severe hypoglycemia with oral hypoglycemics. May increase PT with coumarin-type drugs. Increases levels of phenytoin, cyclosporine, cisapride, astemizole, zidovudine and theophylline. Rifampin enhances metabolism of fluconazole. Cimetidine may decrease levels. HCTZ may increase levels. Contraindicated with terfenadine and cisapride due to prolongation of QTc interval. Cardiac events (torsade de pointes) reported with cisapride. Uveitis reported with rifabutin. Nephrotoxicity reported with tacrolimus. May increase or decrease levels of ethinyl estradiol- and levonorgestrel-containing oral contraceptives.

PREGNANCY: Category C, not for use in nursing.

MECHANISM OF ACTION: Antifungal; inhibits fungal CYP450 sterol C-14 α-demethylation. Subsequent loss of normal sterol correlates with accumulation of 14 α-methyl sterols in fungi and may be responsible for its fungistatic activity.

PHARMACOKINETICS: Absorption: Oral: Absolute bioavailability (90%); C_{max}=6.72mcg/mL (50-400mg), T_{max}=1-2 hrs (fasted). **Distribution:** Plasma protein binding (11-12%). **Elimination:** Urine (80% unchanged and 11% metabolites); $T_{1/2}$=30 hrs. Refer to PI for pediatric pharmacokinetic parameters.

Digibind
digoxin immune fab (ovine) (GlaxoSmithKline)

RX

THERAPEUTIC CLASS: Antidote, digoxin toxicity

INDICATIONS: Treatment of life-threatening digoxin intoxication. Also has been successfully used to treat digitoxin overdose.

DOSAGE: *Adults:* Acute Ingestion of Unknown Amount: Usual: Administer 10 vials, observe response, then additional 10 vials if clinically indicated. Calculation: # vials = total digitalis body load (mg)/0.5mg of digitalis bound per vial. 1 vial will bind approximately 0.5mg of digoxin (or digitoxin). Steady-State Serum Digoxin Concentrations: # of vials = (serum dig conc in ng/mL) x (wt in kg)/100. Steady-State Digitoxin Concentrations: # of vials = (serum digitoxin conc in ng/mL) x (wt in kg)/1000. If toxicity not adequately reversed after several hrs or appears to recur, may need readministration. See PI for details.

Pediatrics: Acute Ingestion of Unknown Amount: Usual: Administer 10 vials, observe response, then additional 10 vials if clinically indicated. Calculation: # vials = total digitalis body load (mg)/0.5mg of digitalis bound per vial. 1 vial will bind approximately 0.5mg of digoxin (or digitoxin). Steady-State Serum Digoxin Concentrations: Dose (mg) = (# vials) (38mg/vial). Steady-State Digitoxin Concentrations: # of vials = (serum digitoxin conc in ng/mL) x (wt in kg)/1000. If toxicity not adequately reversed after several hrs or appears to recur, may need readministration. See PI for details.

HOW SUPPLIED: Inj: 38mg

WARNINGS/PRECAUTIONS: Obtain digoxin level before initiation. Do not overlook possibility of multiple drug overdose. Risk of hypersensitivity is greater with allergies to papain, chymopapain, or other papaya extracts; skin testing may be appropriate for high-risk individuals. K^+ levels may drop rapidly after administration; monitor closely. Digitalis toxicity may recur with renal dysfunction; caution and monitor closely. Caution with cardiac dysfunction, further deterioration may occur from digoxin withdrawal. Consider additional support with inotropes or vasodilators. Monitor for volume overload in children. D/C if anaphylactoid reaction occurs and treat appropriately.

ADVERSE REACTIONS: Allergic reactions, exacerbation of low cardiac output, CHF, hypokalemia.

PREGNANCY: Category C, caution in nursing.

MECHANISM OF ACTION: Antidote; digoxin toxicity. Binds to molecules of digoxin, making them unavailable for binding at their site of action on cells.

PHARMACOKINETICS: Elimination: Urine; $T_{1/2}$=15-20 hrs.

Dilantin
phenytoin (Parke-Davis)

RX

THERAPEUTIC CLASS: Hydantoin

INDICATIONS: (CER, CTB) Control of generalized tonic-clonic (grand mal) and complex partial (psychomotor, temporal lobe) seizures. Prevention and treatment of neurosurgically induced seizures. (Sus) Control of tonic-clonic (grand mal) and psychomotor (temporal lobe) seizures.

DIOVAN

DOSAGE: *Adults:* (CER) Initial: 100mg tid. Titrate: May increase at 7-10 day intervals. Max: 200mg tid. May give once daily with extended-release if controlled on 300mg daily. LD (clinic/hospital): 1g in 3 divided doses (400mg, 300mg, 300mg) given 2 hrs apart. Start maintenance 24 hrs later. (CTB) Initial: 100mg tid. Titrate: May increase at 7-10 day intervals. Usual: 300-400mg/day. Max: 600mg/day. May chew or swallow tab whole. Not for once daily dosing. (Sus) Initial: 125mg tid. Titrate: May increase at 7-10 day intervals. Max: 625mg/day.
Pediatrics: (CER, CTB, Sus) Initial: 5mg/kg/day given bid-tid. Titrate: May increase at 7-10 day intervals. Maint: 4-8mg/kg/day. Max: 300mg/day. >6 yrs: May require the minimum adult dose (300mg/day).

HOW SUPPLIED: Cap, Extended-Release (CER): 30mg, 100mg; Sus: 125mg/5mL (237mL); Tab, Chewable (CTB): 50mg* *scored

WARNINGS/PRECAUTIONS: Avoid abrupt discontinuation. Caution with porphyria, hepatic dysfunction, elderly, diabetes, debilitated. D/C if rash occurs. Lymphadenopathy reported. Serum sickness may occur with lymph node involvement. Gingival hyperplasia reported; maintain proper dental hygiene. Hyperglycemia, birth defects and osteomalacia reported. Monitor levels. Confusional states reported with increased levels. Increased seizure frequency during pregnancy. Neonatal coagulation defects reported within first 24 hrs of birth. Give vitamin K to mother before delivery and to neonate after birth. Avoid use with seizures due to hypoglycemia or other metabolic causes.

ADVERSE REACTIONS: Nystagmus, ataxia, slurred speech, decreased coordination, confusion, dizziness, insomnia, transient nervousness, motor twitchings, headaches, nausea, vomiting, constipation, rash, hypersensitivity reactions.

INTERACTIONS: Increased levels with acute alcohol intake, amiodarone, chloramphenicol, chlordiazepoxide, diazepam, dicumarol, disulfiram, estrogens, H_2-antagonists, halothane, isoniazid, methylphenidate, phenothiazines, phenylbutazone, salicylates, succinamides, sulfonamides, tolbutamide, trazodone. Decreased levels with chronic alcohol abuse, carbamazepine, reserpine, sucralfate. Decreases effects of corticosteroids, coumarin anticoagulants, digitoxin, doxycycline, estrogens, furosemide, oral contraceptives, quinidine, rifampin, theophylline, vitamin D. Phenobarbital, sodium valproate, valproic acid may increase or decrease levels. May increase or decrease levels of phenobarbital, sodium valproate, valproic acid. Calcium antacids decrease absorption; space dosing. Moban® contains calcium ions that interfere with absorption. TCAs may precipitate seizures. Increased risk of phenytoin hypersensitivity with barbiturates, succinamides, oxazolidinediones.

PREGNANCY: Possibly teratogenic, weigh benefits versus risk; not for use in nursing.

MECHANISM OF ACTION: Anticonvulsant; inhibits seizure activity by promoting sodium efflux from neurons, stabilizing threshold against hyperexcitability caused by excessive stimulation of environmental changes capable of reducing membrane sodium gradient.

PHARMACOKINETICS: Absorption: T_{max}=1.5-3 hrs. **Distribution:** Highly protein bound. **Metabolism:** Liver (hydroxylation). **Elimination:** Bile, urine; $T_{1/2}$=22 hrs.

DIOVAN   RX
valsartan (Novartis)

> When used in pregnancy, drugs that act directly on the renin-angiotensin system can cause injury and even death to the developing fetus. D/C therapy when pregnancy is detected.

THERAPEUTIC CLASS: Angiotensin II receptor antagonist

INDICATIONS: Treatment of hypertension, alone or with other antihypertensives. Treatment of heart failure (NYHA Class II-IV). Reduction of cardiovascular mortality in clinically stable patients with left ventricular failure or dysfunction following MI.

DOSAGE: *Adults:* HTN: Monotherapy Without Volume Depletion: Initial: 80mg or 160mg qd. Titrate: May increase to 320mg qd or add diuretic (greater effect than increasing dose >80mg). Hepatic/Severe Renal Dysfunction: Use with caution. Heart Failure: Initial: 40mg bid. Titrate: May increase to 80mg or 160mg bid (use highest dose tolerated). Max: 320mg/day in divided doses. Post-MI: Initial: 20mg bid. Titrate: May increase to 40mg bid within 7 days, with subsequent titrations up to 160mg bid.
Pediatrics: 6-16 yrs: HTN: Initial: 1.3mg/kg qd (up to 40mg total). Adjust dose according

to BP response. Max: 2.7mg/kg (up to 160mg) qd. Use of a sus recommended for children who cannot swallow tabs, or children for whom calculated dosage (mg/kg) does not correspond to available tab strengths. Adjust dose accordingly when switching dosage forms. Hepatic/Severe Renal Impairment: Use with caution. Avoid use in pediatrics with GFR <30mL/min/1.73m^2.

HOW SUPPLIED: Tab: 40mg*, 80mg, 160mg, 320mg *scored

WARNINGS/PRECAUTIONS: Changes in renal function may occur; caution with renal artery stenosis, severe CHF. Caution with hepatic dysfunction, renal dysfunction, and obstructive biliary disorder. Risk of hypotension; caution when initiating therapy in heart failure or post-MI. Correct volume or salt depletion before therapy. Avoid use in pediatric patients with GFR <30mL/min/1.73m^2. May cause fetal harm when administered to pregnant women.

ADVERSE REACTIONS: (HTN) Headache, dizziness, viral infection, fatigue, abdominal pain. (Heart Failure) dizziness, hypotension, diarrhea, arthralgia, fatigue, back pain, hyperkalemia. (Post-MI) hypotension, cough, increased blood creatinine.

INTERACTIONS: Concomitant use of K$^+$-sparing diuretics, K$^+$ supplements, or salt substitutes containing K$^+$ may increase serum K$^+$ levels, and in heart failure patients increase SrCr.

PREGNANCY: Category D, not for use in nursing.

MECHANISM OF ACTION: Angiotensin II receptor antagonist; blocks vasoconstrictor and aldosterone-secreting effects of angiotensin II by selectively blocking binding of angiotensin II to AT$_1$ receptor.

PHARMACOKINETICS: Absorption: Absolute bioavailability (25%); T$_{max}$=2-4 hrs. **Distribution:** (IV) V$_d$=17L; plasma protein binding (95%). **Metabolism:** Valeryl 4-hydroxy valsartan (metabolite). **Elimination:** Feces, urine; T$_{1/2}$=6 hrs.

DIPHENHYDRAMINE HCL INJECTION RX
diphenhydramine HCl (Various)

THERAPEUTIC CLASS: Antihistamine

INDICATIONS: Amelioration of allergic reactions to blood or plasma. Adjunct to epinephrine in anaphylaxis. For other uncomplicated immediate type allergic conditions when oral therapy is contraindicated. Treatment of motion sickness. For parkinsonism when oral therapy is not possible or contraindicated.

DOSAGE: *Adults:* Usual: 10-50mg IV or up to 100mg IM if needed. Max: 400mg/day. *Pediatrics:* Usual: 5mg/kg/24hrs or 150mg/m^2/24hrs IV/IM in 4 divided doses. Max: 300mg/day.

HOW SUPPLIED: Inj: 50mg/mL

CONTRAINDICATIONS: Neonates, premature infants, nursing, as a local anesthetic.

WARNINGS/PRECAUTIONS: Caution with narrow-angle glaucoma, stenosing peptic ulcer, pyloroduodenal obstruction, symptomatic prostatic hypertrophy, or bladder-neck obstruction. May cause excitation in pediatrics. Increased risk of dizziness, sedation, and hypotension in elderly. Caution with lower respiratory diseases, bronchial asthma, increased IOP, hyperthyroidism, cardiovascular disease, or HTN. Local necrosis with SQ or intradermal use.

ADVERSE REACTIONS: Sedation, drowsiness, dizziness, disturbed coordination, epigastric distress, thickening of bronchial secretions.

INTERACTIONS: Additive effects with alcohol, CNS depressants. MAOIs prolong and intensify anticholinergic effects.

PREGNANCY: Category B, contraindicated in nursing.

MECHANISM OF ACTION: Antihistamine; competes with histamine for cell receptor sites on effector cells.

PHARMACOKINETICS: Metabolism: Liver. **Elimination:** Urine.

DIPRIVAN
propofol (Abraxis)

RX

THERAPEUTIC CLASS: General anesthetic

INDICATIONS: Sedative-hypnotic agent used for both induction and maintenance of anesthesia. For initiation and maintenance of monitored anesthesia care (MAC) sedation during diagnostic procedures and in conjunction with local/regional anesthesia in patients undergoing surgical procedures. To provide continuous sedation and control of stress responses in intubated, mechanically ventilated adult patients in ICU.

DOSAGE: *Adults:* General Anesthesia: <55 yrs: 40mg IV every 10 seconds until induction onset. Maint: 100-200mcg/kg/min IV or 20-50mg intermittently byIV bolus prn. Elderly/Debilitated/ASA III & IV: 20mg IV every 10 seconds until induction onset. Maint: 50-100mcg/kg/min IV. Cardiac Anesthesia: 20mg IV every 10 seconds until induction onset. Maint: 100-150mcg/kg/min IV with secondary opioid or 50-100mcg/kg/min IV with primary opioid. Neurosurgical Patients: 20mg IV every 10 seconds until induction onset. Maint: 100-200mcg/kg/min IV. MAC Sedation: 100-150mcg/kg/min IV infusion or 0.5mg/kg slow IV injection over 3-5 min followed immediately by maintenance infusion. Maint: 25-75mcg/kg/min IV infusion or 10-20mg incremental IV boluses. Elderly/Debilitated/ASA III & IV: Use doses similar to healthy adults. Avoid rapid boluses. Maint: 80% of the usual adult dose. ICU Sedation: Initial: 5mcg/kg/min IV infusion for 5 min. Increase 5-10mcg/kg/min IV over 5-10 min. Maint: 5-50mcg/kg/min IV or higher may be required.
Pediatrics: 3-16 yrs: General Anesthesia: 2.5-3.5mg/kg IV over 20-30 seconds. Maint: 2 months-16 yrs: 125-300mcg/kg/min IV.

HOW SUPPLIED: Inj: 10mg/mL

WARNINGS/PRECAUTIONS: Avoid rapid bolus administration in elderly, debilitated or ASA III/IV patients. Monitor oxygen saturation and for signs of significant hypotension, bradycardia, cardiovascular depression, apnea or airway obstruction. Caution with hyperlipoproteinemia, diabetic hyperlipemia, pancreatitis, epilepsy. Rare reports of anaphylaxis reactions, pulmonary edema, perioperative myoclonia, postoperative pancreatitis, bradycardia, asystole, cardiac arrest, rhabdomyolysis. Minimize transient local pain by using larger veins of forearm or antecubital fossa and/or prior lidocaine injection. May elevate serum TG. Do not infuse for >5 days without drug holiday to replace zinc losses; consider supplemental zinc with chronic use in those predisposed to zinc deficiency. In renal impairment, perform baseline urinalysis/urinary sediment then monitor on alternate days during sedation. (Neurosurgical Anesthesia) Use infusion or slow bolus to avoid significant hypotension and decreases in cerebral perfusion pressure. (Cardiac Anesthesia) Use slower rates of administration in premedicated and geriatric patients, patients with recent fluid shifts or those hemodynamically unstable. Correct fluid deficits prior to use.

ADVERSE REACTIONS: Bradycardia, arrhythmia, hypotension, HTN, tachycardia nodal, decreased cardiac output, CNS movement, injection site burning/stinging/pain, hyperlipemia, apnea, rash, pruritus, respiratory acidosis during weaning.

INTERACTIONS: Increased effects with narcotics (eg, morphine, meperidine, fentanyl), combinations of opioids and sedatives (eg, benzodiazepines, barbiturates, chloral hydrate, droperidol) and potent inhalational agents (eg, isoflurane, enflurane, halothane). Concomitant fentanyl may cause bradycardia in pediatrics.

PREGNANCY: Category B, not for use in nursing.

MECHANISM OF ACTION: Sedative-hypnotic agent; uses in induction and maintenance of anesthesia or sedation.

PHARMACOKINETICS: Distribution: Crosses placenta; found in breast milk.

DIPROLENE
betamethasone (augmented) dipropionate (Schering)

RX

OTHER BRAND NAME: Diprolene AF (Schering)

THERAPEUTIC CLASS: Corticosteroid

INDICATIONS: Relief of inflammatory and pruritic manifestations of corticosteroid-responsive dermatoses.

DOSAGE: *Adults:* (Lot) Apply qd-bid for no more than 2 weeks. Max: 50mL/week. (Cre, Oint) Apply qd-bid, up to 45g/week.
Pediatrics: ≥13 yrs: (Cre) Apply qd-bid for no more than 2 weeks. Limit to 45g/week. ≥12 yrs: (Lot) Apply qd-bid for no more than 2 weeks. Limit to 50mL/week. (Oint) Apply qd-bid, up to 45g/week.

HOW SUPPLIED: Cre (AF), Oint: 0.05% (15g, 50g); Lot: 0.05% (30mL, 60mL)

WARNINGS/PRECAUTIONS: May produce reversible HPA axis suppression, manifestations of Cushing's syndrome, hyperglycemia and glucosuria. D/C if irritation occurs. Use appropriate antifungal or antibacterial agent with dermatological infections. Pediatrics may be more susceptible to systemic toxicity. Caution when applied to large surface areas. Not for use with occlusive dressings. Gel is not for use in rosacea or perioral dermatitis or on the face, groin, or in the axillae.

ADVERSE REACTIONS: Stinging, burning, dry skin, pruritus, folliculitis, acneiform papules, irritation, hypopigmentation, skin maceration, secondary infection, skin atrophy, striae, miliaria.

PREGNANCY: Category C, (Cre, Lot) not for use in nursing; (Oint) caution in nursing.

MECHANISM OF ACTION: Corticosteroid; not established. Possesses anti-inflammatory, antipruritic, and vasoconstrictive actions.

PHARMACOKINETICS: Absorption: Percutaneous. Inflammation, use of occlusive dressings, and/or other disease states may increase absorption. **Distribution:** Systemically administered corticosteroids appear in breast milk. **Metabolism:** Liver. **Elimination:** Kidneys, bile.

DISPERMOX   RX
amoxicillin (Ranbaxy)

THERAPEUTIC CLASS: Semisynthetic ampicillin derivative

INDICATIONS: Treatment of the following infections due to susceptible microorganisms: ear, nose, throat; genitourinary tract; skin and skin structure; lower respiratory tract due to susceptible (β-lactamase negative) organisms; gonorrhea (acute uncomplicated). *H. pylori* eradication to reduce the risk of duodenal ulcer recurrence.

DOSAGE: *Adults:* ENT/SSSI/GU: (Mild/Moderate): 500mg q12h or 250mg q8h. (Severe): 875mg q12h or 500mg q8h. LRTI: 875mg q12h or 500mg q8h. Gonorrhea: 3g as single oral dose. Do not chew or swallow dispersible tabs. *H. pylori* Eradication: (Dual Therapy) 1g + 30mg lansoprazole, both tid for 14 days. (Triple Therapy): 1g + 30mg lansoprazole + 500mg clarithromycin, all q12h for 14 days.
Pediatrics: Neonates: ≤12 weeks: Max: 30mg/kg/day divided q12h. >3 months: ENT/ SSSI/GU: (Mild/Moderate): 25mg/kg/day given q12h or 20mg/kg/day given q8h. (Severe): 45mg/kg/day given q12h or 40 mg/kg/day given q8h. LRTI: 45mg/kg/day given q12h or 40mg/kg/day given q8h. Gonorrhea: (Prepubertal) 50mg/kg with 25mg/kg probenecid as single dose (regimen not for use if <2 yrs). >40kg: Dose as adult. Do not chew or swallow dispersible tabs.

HOW SUPPLIED: Tab, Dispersible: 200mg, 400mg, 600mg

WARNINGS/PRECAUTIONS: Serious and fatal hypersensitivity reactions have been reported. Pseudomembranous colitis has been reported; toxin produced by *Clostridium difficile* is the primary cause. Monitor renal, hepatic, and blood with prolonged use. Dispersible tabs contain phenylalanine.

ADVERSE REACTIONS: NV, diarrhea, pseudomembranous colitis, hypersensitivity reactions, blood dyscrasias, superinfection (prolonged use).

INTERACTIONS: Increased levels with probenecid. Chloramphenicol, macrolides, sulfonamides, tetracyclines may interfere with bactericidal effects. False (+) for urine glucose with Clinitest, Benedict's or Fehling's solution. Decreased plasma concentration of total conjugated estriol, estril-glucuronide, conjugated estrone, and estradiol.

PREGNANCY: Category B, caution in nursing.

MECHANISM OF ACTION: Semi-synthetic antibiotic; has a broad spectrum bactericidal activity against susceptible organisms during active multiplication; inhibits biosynthesis of cell-wall mucopeptide.

PHARMACOKINETICS: Absorption: Rapid; administration of different doses resulted in different parameters. **Distribution:** Plasma protein binding (20%). **Elimination:** Urine (unchanged); $T_{1/2}$=61.3 min.

DITROPAN XL   RX
oxybutynin chloride (Ortho-McNeil)

OTHER BRAND NAME: Ditropan (Ortho-McNeil)

THERAPEUTIC CLASS: Anticholinergic

INDICATIONS: (All) Overactive bladder/bladder instability with symptoms of urge urinary incontinence, urgency, and frequency. (Tab, Extended-Release) Detrusor overactivity associated with a neurological condition in pediatrics ≥6 yrs.

DOSAGE: *Adults:* (Tab, Syrup) Usual: 5mg bid-tid. Max: 5mg qid. Frail Elderly: 2.5mg bid-tid.(Tab, Extended-Release) Initial: 5 or 10mg qd. Titrate: May increase by 5mg weekly. Max: 30mg/day. Swallow XL whole with liquid; do not chew, divide or crush tab. *Pediatrics:* >5 yrs: (Tab, Syrup) Usual: 5mg bid. Max: 5mg tid. ≥6 yrs: (Tab, Extended-Release) Initial: 5mg qd. Titrate: May increase by 5mg weekly. Max: 20mg/day. Swallow XL whole with liquid; do not chew, divide, or crush tab.

HOW SUPPLIED: Syrup: 5mg/5mL; Tab: 5mg*; Tab, Extended-Release: 5mg, 10mg, 15mg
*scored

CONTRAINDICATIONS: Urinary retention, gastric retention and other severe decreased GI motility conditions, uncontrolled narrow-angle glaucoma, and in patients at risk for these conditions.

WARNINGS/PRECAUTIONS: Caution with hepatic or renal impairment, bladder outflow obstruction, GI obstruction/narrowing, ulcerative colitis, intestinal atony, myasthenia gravis, hyperthyroidism, CHD, CHF, arrhythmias, HTN, tachycardia, prostatic hypertrophy, and GERD. Heat prostration can occur with high environmental temperatures. Tab, Extended-Release shell may be excreted in the stool. Reduce dose or d/c if anticholinergic CNS effects occur. Caution in preexisting dementia.

ADVERSE REACTIONS: Dry mouth, constipation, somnolence, headache, diarrhea, nausea, blurred vision, dyspepsia, asthenia, pain, dizziness, dry eyes, UTI, insomnia, nervousness.

INTERACTIONS: Increased adverse effects with other anticholinergics. Increased drowsiness with alcohol or other sedatives. May alter GI absorption of other drugs due to GI motility effects. Increased levels with ketoconazole; caution with CYP3A4 inhibitors (eg, antimycotics, macrolides). Caution with bisphosphonates or other drugs that may exacerbate esophagitis.

PREGNANCY: Category B, caution in nursing.

MECHANISM OF ACTION: Antispasmodic/anticholinergic agent; inhibits muscarinic action of acetylcholine on smooth muscle exerting direct antispasmodic effect; relaxes smooth muscle of bladder.

PHARMACOKINETICS: Absorption: (Tab, Syrup) Rapid; absolute bioavailability (6%). Refer to PI for pediatric, isomer, and metabolite parameters. **Distribution:** V_d=193L. **Metabolism:** Liver via CYP3A4; desethyloxybutynin (active metabolite). **Elimination:** Urine (<0.1% unchanged); $T_{1/2}$=13.2 hrs.

DIURIL   RX
chlorothiazide (Salix)

THERAPEUTIC CLASS: Thiazide diuretic

INDICATIONS: (PO/IV) Adjunct therapy in edema associated with CHF, hepatic cirrhosis, corticosteroid and estrogen therapy, renal dysfunction. (PO) Management of hypertension.

DOSAGE: *Adults:* (PO/IV) Edema: 0.5-1g qd-bid. May give every other day or 3-5 days/week. Substitute IV for oral using same dosage. (PO) HTN: 0.5-1g qd or in divided doses. Max: 2g/day.
Pediatrics: (PO) Diuresis/HTN: Usual: 10-20mg/kg/day given qd-bid. Max: Infants up to 2 yrs: 375mg/day. 2-12 yrs: 1g/day. <6 months: Up to 15mg/kg bid may be required.

HOW SUPPLIED: Inj: 0.5g; Sus: 250mg/5mL (237mL)

CONTRAINDICATIONS: Anuria, sulfonamide hypersensitivity.

WARNINGS/PRECAUTIONS: Caution in severe renal disease, liver dysfunction, electrolyte/fluid imbalance. Monitor electrolytes. Hyperuricemia, hyperglycemia, hypokalemia, hyponatremia, hypomagnesemia, hypercalcemia may occur. Increases in cholesterol and triglyceride levels reported. May exacerbate SLE. Sensitivity reactions reported. D/C prior to parathyroid test. Enhanced effects in post-sympathectomy patient. IV use not recommended in infants or children.

ADVERSE REACTIONS: Weakness, hypotension, pancreatitis, jaundice, diarrhea, vomiting, blood dyscrasias, rash, photosensitivity, electrolyte imbalance, impotence.

INTERACTIONS: May potentiate orthostatic hypotension with alcohol, barbiturates, narcotics. Adjust antidiabetic drugs. Possible decreased response to pressor amines. Corticosteroids, ACTH increase electrolyte depletion. May potentiate nondepolarizing skeletal muscle relaxants, antihypertensives. Lithium toxicity. NSAIDs including selective cyclooxygenase-2 (COX-2) inhibitors decrease effects. Decreased PO absorption with cholestyramine, colestipol.

PREGNANCY: Category C, not for use in nursing.

MECHANISM OF ACTION: Thiazide diuretic; not established. Affects distal renal tubular mechanism of electrolyte reabsorption.

PHARMACOKINETICS: Elimination: Kidney; $T_{1/2}$=45-120 min. PO: Urine (10-15%); IV: Urine (96%).

DOLOBID

RX

diflunisal (Merck)

NSAIDs may cause an increased risk of serious cardiovascular thrombotic events, MI, stroke and serious GI adverse events including bleeding, ulceration, and perforation of the stomach or intestines. Contraindicated for the treatment of perioperative pain in the setting of coronary artery bypass graft (CABG) surgery.

THERAPEUTIC CLASS: NSAID

INDICATIONS: Acute or long-term symptomatic treatment of mild to moderate pain, osteoarthritis (OA), rheumatoid arthritis (RA).

DOSAGE: *Adults:* Pain: Initial: 1g, then 500mg q8-12h. OA/RA: 250-500mg bid. Max: 1500mg/day.
Pediatrics: ≥12 yrs: Pain: Initial: 1g, then 500mg q12h or 500mg q8h. OA/RA: 250-500mg bid. Max: 1500mg/day.

HOW SUPPLIED: Tab: 250mg, 500mg

CONTRAINDICATIONS: ASA or other NSAID allergy that precipitates acute asthmatic attack, urticaria, or rhinitis. Treatment of perioperative pain in the setting of CABG surgery.

WARNINGS/PRECAUTIONS: May lead to onset of new HTN or worsening of pre-existing HTN; monitor BP closely. Fluid retention and edema reported; caution with fluid retention or heart failure. Renal papillary necrosis and other renal injury reported after long-term use. Not recommended for use with advanced renal disease; if therapy must be initiated, monitor renal function. Anaphylactoid reactions may occur. May cause serious skin adverse events (eg, exfoliative dermatitis, Stevens-Johnson syndrome, and toxic epidermal necrolysis). Avoid in late pregnancy; may cause premature closure of ductus arteriosis. May cause elevations of LFTs; d/c if liver disease develops or systemic manifestations occur. Caution in elderly. Anemia may occur; with long-term use, monitor Hgb/Hct if signs or symptoms of anemia develop. May inhibit platelet aggregation and prolong bleeding time; monitor with coagulation disorders. Caution with asthma and avoid with ASA-sensitive asthma. Adverse eye findings reported. Hypersensitivity syndrome reported; d/c if hypersensitivity occurs. Reye's syndrome may develop.

ADVERSE REACTIONS: Nausea, dyspepsia, GI pain, diarrhea, rash, headache, insomnia, dizziness, tinnitus, fatigue.

INTERACTIONS: May prolong PT with oral anticoagulants. Decreases hyperuricemic effect of HCTZ, furosemide. Antacids may reduce plasma levels. Avoid other NSAIDs. May potentiate methotrexate, cyclosporine toxicities. Increased plasma levels of APAP. Decreased plasma levels with ASA. Caution with nephrotoxic or hepatotoxic drugs.

PREGNANCY: Category C, not for use in nursing.

MECHANISM OF ACTION: NSAID; suspected to inhibit prostaglandin synthetase; exerts anti-inflammatory, analgesic, and antipyretic actions.

PHARMACOKINETICS: Absorption: Rapid and complete; C_{max}=41mcg/mL (250mg), 87mcg/mL (500mg), 124mcg/mL (1000mg); T_{max}=2-3 hrs. **Distribution:** Plasma protein binding (99%); found in breast milk. **Elimination:** Urine (90% glucuronide conjugates); $T_{1/2}$=8-12 hrs.

DONNATAL   RX
atropine sulfate - hyoscyamine sulfate - phenobarbital - scopolamine hydrobromide (PBM Pharmaceuticals)

OTHER BRAND NAME: Donnatal Extentabs (PBM Pharmaceuticals)

THERAPEUTIC CLASS: Anticholinergic/barbiturate

INDICATIONS: Adjunct therapy for irritable bowel syndrome, acute enterocolitis, duodenal ulcers.

DOSAGE: *Adults:* (Elixir/Tab) 1-2 tabs or 5-10mL tid-qid. (Extentabs) 1 tab q8-12h. Hepatic Disease: Use lower doses.
Pediatrics: (Elixir) 4.5kg: 0.5mL q4h or 0.75mL q6h. 9.1kg: 1mL q4h or 1.5mL q6h. 13.6kg: 1.5mL q4h or 2mL q6h. 22.7kg: 2.5mL q4h or 3.75mL q6h. 34kg: 3.75mL q4h or 5mL q6h. 45.4kg: 5mL q4h or 7.5mL q6h. Hepatic Disease: Use lower doses.

HOW SUPPLIED: (Atropine-Hyoscyamine-Phenobarbital-Scopolamine) Elixir: 0.0194mg-0.1037mg-16.2mg-0.0065mg/5mL; Tab: 0.0194mg-0.1037mg-16.2mg-0.0065mg; Tab, Extended-Release: (Extentabs) 0.0582mg-0.3111mg-48.6mg-0.0195mg

CONTRAINDICATIONS: Glaucoma, obstructive uropathy, obstructive GI disease, paralytic ileus, intestinal atony in elderly or debilitated, unstable cardiovascular status in acute hemorrhage, severe ulcerative colitis, myasthenia gravis, hiatal hernia with reflux esophagitis, intermittent porphyria, and for patients in whom phenobarbital produces restlessness and/or excitement.

WARNINGS/PRECAUTIONS: Inconclusive whether anticholinergic/antispasmodic drugs aid in duodenal ulcer healing, decrease recurrence rate, or prevent complications. Heat prostration can occur with high environmental temperatures. Avoid with intestinal obstruction. May be habit forming; caution with history of physical and/or psychological drug dependence. Caution with hepatic disease, renal disease, autonomic neuropathy, hyperthyroidism, coronary heart disease, CHF, arrhythmias, tachycardia, HTN. May delay gastric emptying. Diarrhea may be an early symptom of incomplete intestinal obstruction, especially with ileostomy or colostomy; treatment would be inappropriate.

ADVERSE REACTIONS: Xerostomia, urinary hesitancy/retention, blurred vision, tachycardia/palpitation, mydriasis, cycloplegia, increased ocular tension, loss of taste, headache, nervousness, drowsiness, weakness, dizziness, insomnia, nausea, vomiting, impotence, suppression of lactation, constipation, bloated feeling, musculoskeletal pain, allergic reaction/drug idiosyncrasies, decreased sweating.

INTERACTIONS: Phenobarbital may decrease anticoagulant effects; adjust dose.

PREGNANCY: Category C, caution in nursing.

MECHANISM OF ACTION: Anticholinergic/Barbiturate; drug combination that provides peripheral anticholinergic, antispasmodic action and mild sedation.

DORYX   RX
doxycycline hyclate (Warner Chilcott)

THERAPEUTIC CLASS: Tetracycline derivative

INDICATIONS: Treatment of the following infections: respiratory, urinary, lymphogranuloma, psittacosis, trachoma, uncomplicated urethral/endocervical/rectal, nongonococcal urethritis, Rocky Mountain spotted fever, typhus fever and the typhus group, Q fever, rickettsialpox, tick fevers, inclusion conjunctivitis, tularemia, campylobacter fetus infections, bartonellosis, granuloma chancroid, plague, cholera, brucellosis, anthrax (including inhalational anthrax, post-exposure). When penicillin is contraindicated, treatment of uncomplicated gonorrhea, syphilis, yaws, listeriosis, Vincent's infection, actinomycosis, and infections caused by *Clostridium* species. Adjunct therapy for intestinal amebiasis and severe acne. Prophylaxis of malaria in short-term travelers (<4 months) to areas with chloroquine and/or pyrimethamine-sulfadoxine resistant strains.

DOSAGE: *Adults:* Usual: 100mg q12h on 1st day, followed by 100mg/day (single dose or as 50mg q12h). Severe Infections/Chronic UTI: 100mg q12h. Uncomplicated Gonococcal Infections (Men, except anorectal infections): 100mg bid for 7 days, or 300mg followed 300mg 1 hr later. Acute Epididymo-Orchitis: 100mg bid for at least 10 days. Early Syphilis: 100mg bid for 14 days. Syphilis >1 yr: 100mg bid for 28 days. Nongonococcal Urethritis, Uncomplicated Urethral/Endocervical/Rectal Infection: 100mg bid for at least 7 days. Inhalational Anthrax (post-exposure): 100mg bid for 60 days. Treat Strep infections for 10 days. Malaria Prophylaxis: 100mg qd, begin 1-2 days before travel and continue daily during travel and for 28 days after travel to malarious area.
Pediatrics: >8 yrs: >100 lbs: 100mg q12h on 1st day, followed by 100mg/day (single dose or as 50mg q12h). Severe Infections/Chronic UTI: 100mg q12h. ≤100lbs: 2mg/lb in divided doses bid on Day 1, followed by 1mg/lb/day (single dose or divided bid) thereafter. Severe Infections: Up to 2mg/lb. Inhalational Anthrax (post-exposure): <100 lbs: 1mg/lb bid for 60 days. ≥100 lbs: 100mg bid for 60 days. Malaria Prophylaxis: 2mg/kg (up to adult dose) qd, begin 1-2 days before travel and continue daily during travel and for 28 days after travel to malarious area.

HOW SUPPLIED: Tab, Delayed-Release: 75mg, 100mg

WARNINGS/PRECAUTIONS: *Clostrium difficile*-associated diarrhea has been reported. May decrease bone growth in premature infants, and cause fetal harm during pregnancy. May cause permanent discoloration of the teeth or enamel hypoplasia if used in last half of pregnancy, infancy, or <8 yrs. Photosensitivity, increased BUN, superinfection may occur. Monitor hematopoietic, renal and hepatic values periodically with long term therapy. Bulging fontanels in infants and benign intracranial HTN in adults reported. May increase incidence of vaginal candidiasis.

ADVERSE REACTIONS: Anorexia, NV, diarrhea, dysphagia, enterocolitis, rash, inflammatory lesions, exfoliative dermatitis, renal toxicity, hypersensitivity reactions, blood dyscrasias, tooth discloration (<8 Yrs).

INTERACTIONS: Depress plasma PT, adjust anticoagulant dosage. May interfere with bactericidal action of penicillin; avoid concurrent use when possible. Avoid antacids containing aluminum, calcium, or magnesium, sodium bicarbonate, and iron-containing preparations. Reduced absorption with bismuth subsalicylate. Barbiturates, carbamazepine, and phenytoin decrease half-life. Fatal renal toxicity with Penthrane® (methoxyflurane). May render oral contraceptives less effective.

PREGNANCY: Category D, not for use in nursing.

MECHANISM OF ACTION: Tetracycline derivative; thought to inhibit protein synthesis.

PHARMACOKINETICS: Absorption: Complete; C_{max}=2.6 mcg/mL; T_{max}=2 hrs. **Distribution:** Crosses placenta. **Metabolism:** Liver. **Elimination:** Urine, feces.

DOXORUBICIN HCL
RX
doxorubicin HCl (Various)

Severe local tissue necrosis will occur if extravasation occurs. Do not give IM/SC route. Myocardial toxicity may occur during or after therapy. Increased risk of CHF with high cumulative doses, previous anthracycline/anthracenedione therapy, pre-existing heart disease, radiotherapy to mediastinal/pericardial area, concomitant cardiotoxic drugs. Increased risk of delayed cardiotoxicity in pediatrics. Secondary acute myelogenous leukemia reported. Reduce dose in hepatic impairment. Severe myelosuppression may occur.

THERAPEUTIC CLASS: Anthracycline

INDICATIONS: To produce regression in disseminated neoplastic conditions such as acute lymphoblastic and myeloblastic leukemias, Wilms' tumor, neuroblastoma, soft tissue/bone sarcomas, breast carcinoma, ovary, bladder and thyroid, gastric and bronchogenic carcinomas, Hodgkin's disease, malignant lymphoma in which the small-cell histologic type is the most responsive compared with other cell types. Adjuvant therapy in women with evidence of axillary lymph node involvement following resection of primary breast cancer.

DOSAGE: *Adults:* Monotherapy: 60-75mg/m² IV every 21 days. Use the lower dose with inadequate bone marrow reserves due to old age, prior therapy, or neoplastic marrow infiltration. Concomitant Chemotherapy: 40-60mg/m² IV every 21-28 days. Hyperbilirubinemia: Reduce dose by 50% if 1.2-3mg/dL; reduce dose by 75% if 3.1-5mg/dL.
Pediatrics: Monotherapy: 60-75mg/m² IV every 21 days. Use the lower dose with inadequate bone marrow reserves due to old age, prior therapy, or neoplastic marrow infiltration. Concomitant Chemotherapy: 40-60mg/m² IV every 21-28 days.
Hyperbilirubinemia: Reduce dose by 50% if 1.2-3mg/dL; reduce dose by 75% if 3.1-5mg/dL.

HOW SUPPLIED: Inj: (2mg/mL) 10mg, 20mg, 50mg

CONTRAINDICATIONS: Marked myelosuppression induced by previous treatment with other antitumor agents or radiotherapy. Previous therapy with complete cumulative doses of doxorubicin, daunorubicin, idarubicin, or other anthracyclines and anthracenes.

WARNINGS/PRECAUTIONS: Irreversible myocardial toxicity may occur. Bone marrow depression and arrhythmias reported. Enhanced toxicity with hepatic impairment; evaluate hepatic function before dosing. Imparts a red coloration to urine for 1-2 days after administration. May induce tumor lysis syndrome and hyperuricemia with rapidly growing tumors. Periodically monitor CBC, hepatic function, and radionuclide left ventricular ejection fraction. May cause prepubertal growth failure and gonadal impairment.

ADVERSE REACTIONS: Myelosuppression, cardiotoxicity, alopecia, nausea, vomiting, mucositis, ulceration and necrosis of colon, fever, chills, urticaria, phlebosclerosis, facial flushing.

INTERACTIONS: May potentiate toxicity of other anticancer therapies. May exacerbate cyclophosphamide-induced hemorrhagic cystitis. May enhance hepatotoxicity of 6-mercaptopurine. May increase radiation induced toxicity of the myocardium, mucosae, skin, and liver. Acute "recall" pneumonitis in pediatrics with actinomycin-D. Paclitaxel infused before doxorubicin may decrease clearance of doxorubicin and increase neutropenia and stomatitis episodes, than the reverse sequence of administration. Enhanced neutropenia and thrombocytopenia reported with IV progesterone. Cyclosporine may prolong and exacerbate hematologic toxicity. Phenobarbital increases elimination. May decrease phenytoin levels. Streptozocin may inhibit hepatic metabolism. Live vaccines may be hazardous in those undergoing cytotoxic chemotherapy. Necrotizing colitis reported with cytarabine. Seizures and coma reported with cyclosporine, cisplatin or vincristine. Possible increased risk of cardiotoxicity with CCBs. Increased risk of CHF with radiotherapy to mediastinal/pericardial area or cardiotoxic drugs.

PREGNANCY: Category D, not for use in nursing.

MECHANISM OF ACTION: Anthracycline antineoplastic agent; inhibits nucleotide replication and action of DNA and RNA polymerases.

PHARMACOKINETICS: Distribution: V_d=809-1214L/m². Plasma protein binding (74-76%), excreted in breast milk. **Metabolism:** Enzymatic reduction; doxorubicinol (major metabolite). **Elimination:** Bile (40%), urine (5-12%); $T_{1/2}$=20-48 hrs.

Doxycycline IV   RX
doxycycline hyclate (Bedford)

THERAPEUTIC CLASS: Tetracycline derivative

INDICATIONS: Treatment of rickettsiae, *Mycoplasma pneumoniae*, psittacosis, ornithosis, lymphogranuloma venereum, granuloma inguinale, relapsing fever, chancroid, *Pasteurella pestis*, *Pasturella tularensis*, *Bartonella bacilliformis*, *Bacteroides* species, *Vibrio comma*, *Vibrio fetus*, *Brucella* species, *E.coli*, *Enterobacter aerogenes*, *Shigella* species, *Mima* species, *Herellea* species, *Haemophilus influenzae*, *Klebsiella* species, *Streptococcus* species, *Diplococcus pneumoniae*, *Staphylococcus aureus*, anthrax, and trachoma. When PCN is contraindicated; treatment of *Neisseria gonorrhoeae*, *N.meningitis*, syphilis, yaws, *Listeria monocytogenes*, *Clostridium* species, *Fusobacterium fusiforme*, and *Actinomyces* species. Adjunct therapy for amebiasis.

DOSAGE: *Adults:* Usual: 200mg IV divided qd-bid on Day 1 then 100-200mg/day IV depending on severity, with 200mg administered in 1 or 2 infusions. Primary/Secondary Syphilis: 300mg/day IV for at least 10 days. Inhalational Anthrax (post-exposure): 100mg

IV bid. Institute oral therapy as soon as possible and continue therapy for a total of 60 days.

Pediatrics: >8 yrs: >100 lbs: Usual: 200mg IV divided qd-bid on Day 1 then 100-200mg/day IV depending on severity, with 200mg administered in 1 or 2 infusions. ≤100 lbs: 2mg/lb IV divided qd-bid on Day 1 then 1-2mg/lb/day IV divided qd-bid depending on severity. Inhalational Anthrax (post-exposure): <100 lbs: 1 mg/lb IV bid. Institute oral therapy as soon as possible and continue therapy for total of 60 days.

HOW SUPPLIED: Inj: 100mg

WARNINGS/PRECAUTIONS: May cause fetal harm during pregnancy. Permanent tooth discoloration during tooth development (last half of pregnancy and children <8 yrs) reported; avoid use in this age group except for anthrax treatment. Decreased bone growth in premature infants reported. May increase BUN. Photosensitivity, enamel hypoplasia reported. Superinfection with prolonged use. Monitor hematopoietic, renal and hepatic values periodically with long term therapy. Bulging fontanels in infants and benign intracranial HTN in adults reported.

ADVERSE REACTIONS: GI effects, increased BUN, rash, hypersensitivity reactions, hemolytic anemia, thrombocytopenia.

INTERACTIONS: May decrease PT; adjust anticoagulants. Avoid use with bactericidal agents (eg, penicillin).

PREGNANCY: Safety in pregnancy not known; not for use in nursing.

MECHANISM OF ACTION: Tetracycline derivative; thought to inhibit protein synthesis.

PHARMACOKINETICS: Absorption: Readily absorbed; C_{max}=2.5 mcg/mL. **Elimination:** $T_{1/2}$=18-22 hrs.

DRYVAX

RX

smallpox vaccine, dried (Wyeth)

> **Acute myopericarditis has been observed after administration. Encephalitis and progressive vaccinia have occured following smallpox immunization, almost always in immunocompromised patients. Severe vaccinal skin infections have occured among persons with eczema. Do not administer in persons with eczema, cardiac disease and immunocompromised.**

THERAPEUTIC CLASS: Vaccine

INDICATIONS: For active immunization against smallpox disease.

DOSAGE: *Adults:* Give IM into deltoid muscle or posterior aspect of arm over triceps muscle. Use 2 or 3 needle punctures for primary vaccination and 15 punctures for revaccination. May cover vaccination site with a porous bandage, until scab separates and underlying skin has healed. Inspect vaccination site 6-8 days later to interpret response.

Pediatrics: ≥12 months: Give IM into deltoid muscle or posterior aspect of arm over triceps muscle. Use 2 or 3 needle punctures for primary vaccination and 15 punctures for revaccination. May cover vaccination site with a porous bandage, until scab separates and underlying skin has healed. Inspect vaccination site 6-8 days later to interpret response.

HOW SUPPLIED: Inj: 100 million PFU

CONTRAINDICATIONS: (Routine non-emergency use) Hypersensitivity to polymyxin B sulfate, dihydrostreptomycin sulfate, chlortetracycline HCl, and neomycin sulfate; infants <12 months of age; eczema, history of eczema, or other acute, chronic, or exfoliative skin conditions (including household contacts of such persons); systemic corticosteroid use at doses ≥2mg/kg or ≥20mg/day of prednisone for ≥2 weeks, or immunosuppressive use (eg, alkylating agents, antimetabolites), or radiation (including household contacts of such persons); congenital or acquired immune deficiencies (including household contacts of such persons); immunosuppressed individuals (including household contacts of such persons); pregnancy (including household contacts of such persons).

WARNINGS/PRECAUTIONS: Vial stopper contains dry natural rubber; caution with latex sensitivity. Patients susceptible to adverse effects of caccinia virus should avoid contact with persons with active vaccination lesions. Vaccinia virus may be cultured from site of primary vaccine from time of papule development until scab separates from skin lesion. Not recommended for elderly in non-emergency conditions.

ADVERSE REACTIONS: Fever, rash, secondary pyogenic infections at vaccination site, inadvertent inoculation at other sites, regional lymphadenopathy, malaise.

INTERACTIONS: Avoid salves or ointments on vaccination site.

PREGNANCY: Category C, not for use in nursing in non-emergency conditions.

MECHANISM OF ACTION: Stimulates the immune system to produce antibodies that may prevent against smallpox disease.

DUAC   RX
benzoyl peroxide - clindamycin (Stiefel)

THERAPEUTIC CLASS: Antibacterial/keratolytic

INDICATIONS: Topical treatment of inflammatory acne vulgaris.

DOSAGE: *Adults:* Wash face and pat dry. Apply qd in evening.
Pediatrics: ≥12 yrs: Wash face and pat dry. Apply qd in evening.

HOW SUPPLIED: Gel: (Clindamycin-Benzoyl Peroxide) 1%-5% (45g)

CONTRAINDICATIONS: Hypersensitivity to lincomycin. History of regional enteritis, ulcerative colitis, pseudomembranous colitis, or antibiotic-associated colitis.

WARNINGS/PRECAUTIONS: Severe colitis reported with oral and parenteral clindamycin. D/C if severe diarrhea occurs. Avoid contact with eyes and mucous membranes. May bleach hair or colored fabric. Limit sunlight exposure.

ADVERSE REACTIONS: Dry skin, erythema, peeling, burning.

INTERACTIONS: Cumulative irritancy possible with other topical acne agents. Avoid erythromycin agents.

PREGNANCY: Category C, not for use in nursing.

MECHANISM OF ACTION: Clindamycin: Antibacterial; binds to 50S ribosomal subunits of susceptible bacteria and prevents elongation of peptide chains by interfering with peptidyl transfer, thereby suppressing protein synthesis. Benzoyl peroxide: Keratolytic; potent oxidizing agent.

PHARMACOKINETICS: Distribution: Orally and parenterally administered clindamycin found in breast milk.

DULCOLAX   OTC
bisacodyl (Boehringer Ingelheim)

THERAPEUTIC CLASS: Stimulant laxative

INDICATIONS: Relief of occasional constipation and irregularity. For bowel cleansing regimen for surgery or endoscopic exam.

DOSAGE: *Adults:* (Tab) Take 2-3 tabs qd. Do not crush/chew. (Sup) Insert 1 sup rectally; retain for 15-20 min. May coat tip with petroleum jelly with anal fissures or hemorrhoids. X-Ray Endoscopy For Barium Enema: Avoid food after tab administration. Insert 1 sup rectally 1-2 hrs before exam.
Pediatrics ≥12 yrs: (Tab) 2-3 tabs qd. 6-12 yrs: 1 tab qd. Do not crush/chew. (Sup) ≥12 yrs: Insert 1 sup rectally; retain for 15-20 min. 6-12 yrs: Insert 1/2 sup rectally qd. May coat tip with petroleum jelly with anal fissures or hemorrhoids. X-Ray Endoscopy for Barium Enema: ≥6 yrs: Avoid food after tab administration. Insert 1 sup 1-2 hrs before exam. <6 yrs: Avoid tab. Insert 1/2 sup rectally 1-2 hrs before exam.

HOW SUPPLIED: Sup: 10mg; Tab, Delayed-Release: 5mg

CONTRAINDICATIONS: Acute abdominal surgery, appendicitis, rectal bleeding, gastroenteritis, intestinal obstruction.

WARNINGS/PRECAUTIONS: Avoid with abdominal pain, nausea, or vomiting. Not for long-term use (>7 days). D/C with rectal bleeding or fail to have bowel movement.

ADVERSE REACTIONS: Abdominal discomfort.

INTERACTIONS: Avoid tabs within 1 hr after antacids or milk.

PREGNANCY: Safety in pregnancy and nursing not known.

DURAGESIC
fentanyl (Janssen)   CII

> Life-threatening hypoventilation can occur. Contraindicated for acute or post-op pain and mild/intermittent pain. Avoid in patients <2 yrs. Only for use in opioid tolerant patients. Concomitant use with potent CYP450 3A4 inhibitors may result in an increase in fentanyl plasma concentrations which may cause potentially fatal respiratory depression. Monitor patients receiving potent CYP450 3A4 inhibitors.

THERAPEUTIC CLASS: Opioid analgesic

INDICATIONS: Management of persistent, moderate to severe chronic pain when continuous, around-the-clock opioid administration for an extended period of time is required and cannot be managed by other means such as nonsteroidal analgesics, opioid combination products, or immediate-release opioids.

DOSAGE: *Adults:* Individualize dose. Determine dose based on opioid tolerance. Initial: 25mcg/hr for 72 hr.
Pediatrics: ≥2 yrs: Individualize dose. Determine dose based on opioid tolerance. Initial: 25mcg/hr for 72 hr.

HOW SUPPLIED: Patch: 12.5mcg/hr, 25mcg/hr, 50mcg/hr, 75mcg/hr, 100mcg/hr (5^s)

CONTRAINDICATIONS: Non opioid-tolerant patients, management of acute/post-op pain, mild/intermittent pain. Diagnosis or suspicion of paralytic ileus. Patients who have acute or severe broncial asthma, significant respiratory depression especially in settings where there is lack of resuscitative equipment.

WARNINGS/PRECAUTIONS: Monitor patients with serious adverse events for at least 24 hrs after removal. Avoid exposing application site to direct external heat. Hypoventilation may occur; caution with chronic pulmonary diseases. Caution with brain tumors, bradyarrhythmias, renal/hepatic impairment, pancreatic/biliary tract disease. Avoid with increased ICP, impaired consciousness, or coma. May obscure clinical course of head injury. Tolerance and physical dependence can occur. May impair mental/physical abilities.

ADVERSE REACTIONS: Hypoventilation, HTN, fever, NV, constipation, dry mouth, somnolence, confusion, asthenia, sweating, nervousness, application site reaction, apnea, dyspnea.

INTERACTIONS: See Black Box Warning. Concomitant use with CNS depressants (opioids, sedatives, hypnotics, tranquilizers, general anesthetics, phenothiazines, skeletal muscle relaxants, alcohol) may cause respiratory depression, hypotension, profound sedation, or potentially coma or death. May increase clearance with CYP3A4 inducers (eg, rifampin, carbamazepine, phenytoin). Avoid use within 14 days of MAOI.

PREGNANCY: Category C, not for use in nursing.

MECHANISM OF ACTION: Opioid analgesic; interacts predominantly with the opioid μ-receptor. Exerts principle pharmacological actions on CNS.

PHARMACOKINETICS: Absorption: T_{max}=24-72 hrs. Transdermal administration of variable doses resulted in different parameters. **Distribution:** V_d=6 L/kg; found in breast milk. Accumulates in skeletal muscle and fat; released slowly into the blood; readily crosses placenta. **Metabolism:** Liver via CYP3A4; oxidative N-dealkylation to norfentanyl and other metabolites. **Elimination:** Urine (75%), feces (9%); $T_{1/2}$=3-12 hrs.

DURATUSS
guaifenesin - pseudoephedrine HCl (Victory)   RX

THERAPEUTIC CLASS: Expectorant/decongestant

INDICATIONS: Relief of nasal congestion due to the common cold, hay fever, sinusitis, or other upper respiratory allergies. Relief of eustachian tube congestion and cough. Adjunct therapy in serious otitis media.

DOSAGE: *Adults:* 1 tab q12h.
Pediatrics: ≥12 yrs: 1 tab q12h. 6-12 yrs: 1/2 tab q12h.

HOW SUPPLIED: Tab, Extended-Release: (Guaifenesin-Pseudoephedrine) 600mg-120mg*
*scored

CONTRAINDICATIONS: Hypersensitivity to sympathomimetics, severe HTN, with MAOIs.

WARNINGS/PRECAUTIONS: Do not crush or chew tabs. Caution with HTN, hyperthyroidism, DM, heart disease, peripheral vascular disease, glaucoma, prostatic hypertrophy.

ADVERSE REACTIONS: Nervousness, insomnia, restlessness, headache.

INTERACTIONS: Avoid MAOIs. May reduce effects of antihypertensive drugs which interfere with sympathetic activity (eg, methyldopa, mecamylamine, reserpine). Increased ectopic pacemaker activity with digitalis. Caution with concomitant sympathomimetic amines.

PREGNANCY: Category C, not for use in nursing.

DYNACIN   RX
minocycline HCl (Medicis)

THERAPEUTIC CLASS: Tetracycline derivative

INDICATIONS: Treatment of inclusion conjunctivitis, nongonococcal urethritis, and other infections (eg, respiratory tract, endocervical, rectal, urinary tract, skin and skin structure) caused by susceptible strains of microorganisms. Alternative treatment in certain other infections (eg, urethritis, gonococcal, syphilis, anthrax). Adjunctive therapy in acute intestinal amebiasis and severe acne. Treatment of *Mycobacterium marinum* and asymptomatic carriers of *Neisseria meningitidis*.

DOSAGE: *Adults:* Usual: 200mg initially, then 100mg q12h; alternative is 100-200mg initially, then 50mg qid. Uncomplicated Gonococcal Infection (Men, other than urethritis and anorectal infections): 200mg initially, then 100mg q12h for minimum 4 days. Uncomplicated Gonococcal Urethritis (Men): 100mg q12h for 5 days. Syphilis: Administer usual dose for 10-15 days. Meningococcal Carrier State: 100mg q12h for 5 days. *Mycobacterium marinum:* 100mg q12h for 6-8 weeks. Uncomplicated urethral, endocervical, or rectal infection: 100mg q12h for at least 7 days. Renal Dysfunction: Reduce dose and/or extend dose intervals.
Pediatrics: >8 yrs: 4mg/kg initially followed by 2mg/kg q12h. Take with plenty of fluids.

HOW SUPPLIED: Tab: 50mg, 75mg, 100mg

WARNINGS/PRECAUTIONS: May cause fetal harm during pregnancy. Use during tooth development (last half of pregnancy, infancy, <8 yrs) may cause permanent discoloration of the teeth or enamel hypoplasia; avoid use during this period. Renal toxicity, hepatotoxicity, photosensitivity, increased BUN, superinfection, pseudotumor cerebri may occur; perform hematopoietic, renal, and hepatic monitoring. May impair mental/physical abilities. Use alternate form of contraception other than oral contraceptives. May decrease bone growth in premature infants.

ADVERSE REACTIONS: Anorexia, NV, diarrhea, dysphagia, enterocolitis, pancreatitis, increased LFTs, hepatitis, liver failure, renal toxicity, rash, exfoliative dermatitis, Stevens-Johnson syndrome, skin and mucous membrane pigmentation, blood dyscrasias, headache, tooth discoloration.

INTERACTIONS: May require downward adjustments of anticoagulant dosage. May interfere with bactericidal action of penicillin; avoid concurrent use when possible. May decrease efficacy of oral contraceptives. Impaired absorption with antacids containing aluminum, calcium, or magnesium and iron-containing products. Fatal renal toxicity with methoxyflurane has been reported.

PREGNANCY: Category D, not for use in nursing.

MECHANISM OF ACTION: Tetracycline derivative; thought to inhibit protein synthesis.

PHARMACOKINETICS: Absorption: Rapid. **Distribution:** Crosses placenta, excreted in breast milk. **Elimination:** Urine, feces.

E.E.S.

RX

erythromycin ethylsuccinate (Abbott)

THERAPEUTIC CLASS: Macrolide

INDICATIONS: Treatment of mild to moderate upper/lower respiratory tract and skin and skin structure infections, listeriosis, pertussis, diphtheria, erythrasma, intestinal amebiasis, acute pelvic inflammatory disease (PID) (*N.gonorrhoeae*), primary syphilis (if PCN allergy), Legionnaires' disease, chlamydial infections (eg, newborn conjunctivitis, pneumonia of infancy, urogenital infections during pregnancy, or urethral, endocervical, or rectal infections when tetracyclines are contraindicated or not tolerated), and nongonococcal urethritis caused by susceptible strains of microorganisms. Prophylaxis of initial and recurrent attacks of rheumatic fever if PCN allergy.

DOSAGE: *Adults:* Usual: 1600mg/day in divided doses given q6h, q8h, or q12h. Max: 4g/day. Treat strep infections for at least 10 days. Streptococcal Infection Prophylaxis with Rheumatic Heart Disease: 400mg bid. Urethritis (*C.trachomatis* or *U.urealyticum*): 800mg tid for 7 days. Primary Syphilis: 48-64g in divided doses over 10-15 days. Intestinal Amebiasis: 400mg qid for 10-14 days. Pertussis: 40-50mg/kg/day in divided doses for 5-14 days. Legionnaires' Disease: 1.6-4g/day in divided doses.
Pediatrics: Usual: 30-50mg/kg/day in divided doses q6h, q8h, or q12h. Severe Infections: May double dose. Treat strep infections for at least 10 days. Streptococcal Infection Prophylaxis with Rheumatic Heart Disease: 400mg bid. Intestinal Amebiasis: 30-50mg/kg/day in divided doses for 10-14 days.

HOW SUPPLIED: Sus: 200mg/5mL, 400mg/5mL; Tab: 400mg

CONTRAINDICATIONS: Concomitant terfenadine, astemizole, cisapride, or pimozide.

WARNINGS/PRECAUTIONS: *Clostridium difficile*-associated diarrhea, hepatic dysfunction reported. Caution with impaired hepatic function. May aggravate weakness of patients with myasthenia gravis.

ADVERSE REACTIONS: N/V, abdominal pain, diarrhea, anorexia, hepatic dysfunction, abnormal LFTs, allergic reactions, superinfection (prolonged use).

INTERACTIONS: See Contraindications. Rhabdomyolysis reported with lovastatin. May increase levels of theophylline, digoxin, drugs metabolized by CYP450 (eg, carbamazepine, cyclosporine, tacrolimus, phenytoin, alfentanil, disopyramide, lovastatin, bromocriptine, valproate, etc). Increases effects of oral anticoagulants, triazolam, midazolam. Risk of acute ergot toxicity with ergotamine or dihydroergotamine. May increase AUC of sildenafil; consider dose reduction of sildenafil.

PREGNANCY: Category B, caution in nursing.

MECHANISM OF ACTION: Macrolide antibiotic; inhibits protein synthesis by binding 50S ribosomal subunits of susceptible organisms.

PHARMACOKINETICS: Absorption: Readily absorbed. **Distribution:** Diffuses into most body fluids, crosses placental barrier. **Metabolism:** Liver. **Elimination:** Biliary excretion, urine (≤5%).

ECOTRIN

OTC

aspirin (GlaxoSmithKline Consumer)

THERAPEUTIC CLASS: Salicylate

INDICATIONS: To reduce the risk of death and nonfatal stroke with previous ischemic stroke or transient ischemia of the brain. To reduce risk of vascular mortality with suspected acute MI. To reduce risk of death and nonfatal MI with previous MI or unstable angina. To reduce risk of MI and sudden death in chronic stable angina. Indicated for patients who have undergone revascularization procedures with a pre-existing condition for which ASA is indicated. Relief of signs of rheumatoid arthritis (RA), juvenile rheumatoid arthritis (JRA), osteoarthritis (OA), spondyloarthropathies, arthritis, and pleurisy associated with systemic lupus erythematosus (SLE).

DOSAGE: *Adults:* Ischemic Stroke/TIA: 50-325mg qd. Suspected Acute MI: Initial: 160-162.5mg qd as soon as suspect MI. Maint: 160-162.5mg for 30 days post-infarction, consider further therapy for prevention/recurrent MI. Prevention or Recurrent MI/Unstable Angina/Chronic Stable Angina: 75-325mg qd. CABG: 325mg qd, start 6 hrs post-surgery. Continue for 1 yr. PTCA: Initial: 325mg, 2 hrs pre-surgery. Maint: 160-325mg qd. Carotid

155

Endarterectomy: 80mg qd to 650mg bid, start pre-surgery. RA/Arthritis/SLE Pleurisy: Initial: 3g qd in divided doses. Increase for anti-inflammatory efficacy to 150-300mcg/mL plasma salicylate level. Spondyloarthropathies: Up to 4g/day in divided doses. OA: Up to 3g/day in divided doses.

Pediatrics: JRA: Initial: 90-130mg/kg/day in divided doses. Increase for anti-inflammatory efficacy to 150-300mcg/mL plasma salicylate level.

HOW SUPPLIED: Tab, Delayed-Release: 81mg, 325mg, 500mg

CONTRAINDICATIONS: NSAID allergy, children or teenagers for viral infections with or without fever, syndrome of asthma, rhinitis, and nasal polyps.

WARNINGS/PRECAUTIONS: Increased risk of bleeding with heavy alcohol use (≥3 drinks/day). May inhibit platelet function; can adversely affect inherited (hemophilia) or acquired (hepatic disease, vitamin K deficiency) bleeding disorders. Monitor for bleeding and ulceration. Avoid in history of active peptic ulcer, severe renal failure, severe hepatic insufficiency, and sodium restricted diets. Associated with elevated LFTs, BUN, and serum creatinine; hyperkalemia; proteinuria; and prolonged bleeding time. Avoid 1 week before and during labor.

ADVERSE REACTIONS: Fever, hypothermia, dysrhythmias, hypotension, agitation, cerebral edema, dehydration, hyperkalemia, dyspepsia, GI bleed, hearing loss, tinnitus, problems in pregnancy.

INTERACTIONS: Diminished hypotensive and hyponatremic effects of ACE inhibitors. May increase levels of acetazolamide, valproic acid. Increased risk of bleeds with heparin, warfarin. Decreased levels of phenytoin. Decreased hypotensive effects of β-blockers. Decreased diuretic effects with renal or cardiovascular disease. Decreased methotrexate clearance; increased risk of bone marrow toxicity. Avoid NSAIDs. Increased effects of hypoglycemic agents. Antagonizes uricosuric agents.

PREGNANCY: Avoid in 3rd trimester of pregnancy and nursing.

EDECRIN
ethacrynic acid (Aton)

RX

THERAPEUTIC CLASS: Aryloxyacetic acid derivative

INDICATIONS: Treatment of edema when agent of greater diuretic potential is required. Treatment of edema in CHF, hepatic cirrhosis, and renal disease. Short-term management of ascites due to malignancy, idiopathic edema, lymphedema; congenital heart disease and nephrotic syndrome in hospitalized pediatrics.

DOSAGE: *Adults:* Initial: 50-100mg qd. Titrate: 25-50mg increments. Usual: 50-200mg/day. After diuresis achieved, give smallest effective dose continuously or intermittently. *Pediatrics:* Initial: 25mg. Titrate: Increase by 25mg increments. Maint: Reduce dose and frequency once dry weight achieved; may give intermittently.

HOW SUPPLIED: Tab: 25mg* *scored

CONTRAINDICATIONS: Anuria, infants. D/C if increasing electrolyte imbalance, azotemia, or oliguria develops during treatment of severe, progressive renal disease. D/C if severe, watery diarrhea occurs.

WARNINGS/PRECAUTIONS: Caution in advanced liver cirrhosis. Monitor serum electrolytes, CO2, BUN early in therapy and periodically during active diuresis. Vigorous diuresis may induce acute hypotensive episode and in elderly cardiac patients, hemoconcentration resulting in thromboembolic disorders. Ototoxicity reported with severe renal dysfunction. Hypomagnesemia and transient increase in serum urea nitrogen may occur. Reduce dose or withdraw if excessive electrolyte loss occurs. Initiate therapy in the hospital for cirrhotic patients with ascites. Liberalize salt intake and supplement with K+ if needed. Reduced responsiveness in renal edema with hypoproteinemia; use salt poor albumin.

ADVERSE REACTIONS: Anorexia, malaise, abdominal discomfort, gout, deafness, tinnitus, vertigo, headache, fatigue, rash, chills.

INTERACTIONS: Risk of lithium toxicity. May increase ototoxic potential of aminoglycosides and some cephalosporins. Displaces warfarin from plasma protein; may need dose reduction. NSAIDs may decrease effects. Orthostatic hypotension may occur with antihypertensives. Increased risk of gastric hemorrhage with corticosteroids. Excessive K+ loss may precipitate digitalis toxicity. Caution with K+-depleting steroids.

PREGNANCY: Category B, not for use in nursing.

MECHANISM OF ACTION: Aryloxyacetic acid derivative; inhibits reabsorption of filtered sodium.

ELDOPAQUE FORTE

RX

hydroquinone (Valeant)

OTHER BRAND NAME: Eldoquin Forte (Valeant)

THERAPEUTIC CLASS: Depigmenting agent

INDICATIONS: For the gradual bleaching of hyperpigmented skin conditions (eg, chloasma, melasma, freckles, senile lentigines).

DOSAGE: *Adults:* Apply bid. Do not rub in Eldopaque Forte. Use sunscreen with Eldoquin Forte.
Pediatrics: ≥12 yrs: Apply bid. Do not rub in Eldopaque Forte. Use sunscreen with Eldoquin Forte.

HOW SUPPLIED: Cre: 4% (28.4g)

WARNINGS/PRECAUTIONS: Avoid sun exposure on bleached skin. Eldopaque Forte contains sunblock; use sunscreen. May produce unwanted cosmetic effects if not used as directed. Test for skin sensitivity. D/C if no lightening effect after 2 months. Contains sodium metabisulfite; may cause serious allergic type reactions. Limit treatment to small areas of body at one time. Avoid contact with eyes.

ADVERSE REACTIONS: Cutaneous hypersensitivity (contact dermatitis).

PREGNANCY: Category C, caution in nursing.

MECHANISM OF ACTION: Produces a reversible depigmentation of the skin by inhibiting the enzymatic oxidation of tyrosine to 3,4-dihydroxyphenylalanine and suppressing the melanocyte metabolic processes.

ELESTAT

RX

epinastine HCI (Allergan)

THERAPEUTIC CLASS: H_1-antagonist

INDICATIONS: For the prevention of itching associated with allergic conjunctivitis.

DOSAGE: *Adults:* 1 drop in each eye bid.
Pediatrics: ≥3 yrs: 1 drop in each eye bid.

HOW SUPPLIED: Sol: 0.05% (5mL)

WARNINGS/PRECAUTIONS: Not for contact lens related irritation. May reinsert contact lens 10 minutes after dosing if eye is not red.

ADVERSE REACTIONS: Burning sensation in the eye, folliculosis, hyperemia, pruritus.

PREGNANCY: Category C, caution in nursing.

MECHANISM OF ACTION: Antihistaminic; topically active; direct H_1-receptor antagonist and an inhibitor of histamine release from the mast cell; selective for the histamine H_1-receptor and has affinity for the histamine H_2-receptor and possesses affinity for the α_1-α_2-and 5-HT_2-receptors.

PHARMACOKINETICS: Absorption: C_{max}=0.04ng/ml. T_{max}=2 hrs. **Distribution:** Plasma protein binding (64%). **Elimination:** Urine, feces; $T_{1/2}$=12 hrs.

ELIDEL

RX

pimecrolimus (Novartis)

THERAPEUTIC CLASS: Macrolactam ascomycin derivative

INDICATIONS: Short-term and intermittent long-term therapy of moderate to severe atopic dermatitis in nonimmunocompromised patients intolerant to or unresponsive to conventional therapy.

DOSAGE: *Adults:* Apply bid. Re-evaluate if symptoms persist after 6 weeks.
Pediatrics: ≥2 yrs: Apply bid. Re-evaluate if symptoms persist after 6 weeks.

HOW SUPPLIED: Cre: 1% (30g, 60g, 100g)

WARNINGS/PRECAUTIONS: Increased risk of varicella zoster infection, herpes simplex virus infection or eczema herpeticum. Lymphadenopathy reported; d/c if unknown etiology of lymphadenopathy or acute mononucleosis presents. Skin papilloma or warts reported; consider discontinuation if worsening or unresponsive skin papilloma. Minimize or avoid natural or artificial sunlight exposure. Avoid with Netherton's syndrome, areas of active cutaneous viral infections, or occlusive dressings. Long-term safety has not been established. Rare cases of malignancy (eg, skin and lymphoma) reported with topical calcineurin inhibitors; therefore, continuous long-term use should be avoided and application limited to areas of involvement. Not indicated for use in children <2 yrs.

ADVERSE REACTIONS: Application site burning, headache, nasopharyngitis, influenza, pharyngitis, viral infection, pyrexia, cough, skin discoloration.

INTERACTIONS: Caution with CYP3A4 inhibitors (eg, erythromycin, itraconazole, ketoconazole, fluconazole, CCBs, cimetidine) in widespread and/or erythrodermic disease.

PREGNANCY: Category C, not for use in nursing.

MECHANISM OF ACTION: Macrolactam ascomycin derivative; not fully established. Suspected to bind with high affinity to macrophilin-12 (FKBP-12) and inhibit the calcium-dependent phosphatase, calcineurin. Consequently, this inhibits T cell activation by blocking the transcription of early cytokines.

PHARMACOKINETICS: Absorption: C_{max}=1.4ng/mL. **Distribution:** Plasma protein binding (99.5%). **Metabolism:** Liver by CYP3A. **Elimination:** Feces (78.4% metabolites) and (≤1% unchanged).

ELIMITE   RX
permethrin (Allergan)

THERAPEUTIC CLASS: Pyrethroid scabicidal agent

INDICATIONS: Treatment of scabies.

DOSAGE: *Adults:* Massage into skin from head to soles of feet. Wash off after 8-14 hrs. One treatment should be adequate. Retreat if living mites present after 14 days. *Pediatrics:* ≥2 months: Massage into skin from head (scalp, temples and forehead) to soles of feet. Wash off after 8-14 hrs. One treatment should be adequate. Retreat if living mites present after 14 days.

HOW SUPPLIED: Cre: 5% (60g)

CONTRAINDICATIONS: Allergy to synthetic pyrethroid or pyrethrin.

WARNINGS/PRECAUTIONS: May temporarily exacerbate infection (eg, pruritus, edema, erythema). Avoid eyes. D/C if hypersensitivity occurs.

ADVERSE REACTIONS: Burning, stinging, pruritus, erythema, numbness, tingling, rash.

PREGNANCY: Category B, not for use in nursing.

ELITEK   RX
rasburicase (Sanofi-Aventis)

> May cause serious hypersensitivity reactions including anaphylaxis; discontinue if this occurs. Hemolysis may occur in G6PD deficiency; discontinue with hemolysis. Before initiate, screen patients at high risk for G6PD deficiency. Discontinue if develop methemoglobinemia. Causes enzymatic degradation of uric acid within blood samples left at room temperature. Collect blood in pre-chilled tubes containing heparin; immediately immerse and maintain in ice water bath and assay sample within 4 hrs of collection.

THERAPEUTIC CLASS: Recombinant urate-oxidase enzyme

INDICATIONS: Initial management of plasma uric acid levels in pediatrics with leukemia, lymphoma, and solid tumor malignancies who are receiving anti-cancer therapy expected to result in tumor lysis and subsequent elevation of plasma uric acid.

DOSAGE: *Pediatrics:* 1 month-17 yrs: 0.15 or 0.2mg/kg IV as single daily dose for 5 days. Administer over 30 min, not as bolus. Dosing >5 days or >1 course not recommended. Initiate chemotherapy 4-24 hrs after 1st dose.

HOW SUPPLIED: Inj: 1.5mg, 7.5mg

CONTRAINDICATIONS: G6PD deficiency, history of anaphylaxis or hypersensitivity reactions, hemolytic or methemoglobinemia reactions to rasburicase or any of the excipients.

WARNINGS/PRECAUTIONS: Screen patients at high risk for G6PD deficiency (eg, African or Mediterranean ancestry) prior to initiation. Administer IV hydration.

ADVERSE REACTIONS: Vomiting, fever, nausea, headache, abdominal pain, constipation, diarrhea, mucositis, rash, respiratory distress, sepsis, neutropenia with or without fever.

PREGNANCY: Category C, not for use in nursing.

MECHANISM OF ACTION: A recombinant urate-oxidase enzyme; catalyses enzymatic oxidation of uric acid into an inactive and soluble metabolite.

PHARMACOKINETICS: Distribution: V_d=110-127mL/kg. **Elimination:** $T_{1/2}$=18 hrs.

ELMIRON
pentosan sodium (Ortho-McNeil)

RX

THERAPEUTIC CLASS: Analgesic, urinary

INDICATIONS: Relief of bladder pain/discomfort associated with interstitial cystitis.

DOSAGE: *Adults:* Take 1 hr before or 2 hrs after meals with water. 100mg tid for 3 months. Re-evaluate after 3 months; may continue for another 3 months. *Pediatrics:* ≥16 yrs: Take 1 hr before or 2 hrs after meals with water. 100mg tid for 3 months. Re-evaluate after 3 months; may continue for another 3 months.

HOW SUPPLIED: Cap: 100mg

WARNINGS/PRECAUTIONS: Bleeding complications (eg, ecchymosis, epistaxis, gum hemorrhage), alopecia, increased PT/PTT reported. Caution with invasive procedures, coagulopathy, aneurysms, thrombocytopenia, hemophilia, GI ulcers, polyps, diverticula, history of heparin-induced thrombocytopenia, and hepatic impairment. Transient liver enzyme elevation reported.

ADVERSE REACTIONS: Nausea, diarrhea, alopecia, headache, rash, dyspepsia, abdominal pain.

INTERACTIONS: Increased risk of bleeding with anticoagulants, heparin, t-PA, streptokinase, high-dose ASA, and NSAIDs.

PREGNANCY: Category B, caution in nursing.

MECHANISM OF ACTION: Low molecular weight heparin-type compound; not fully established. Possesses anticoagulant and fibrinolytic effects.

PHARMACOKINETICS: Absorption: 3% of administered dose. **Distribution:** Mainly into uroepithelium. **Metabolism:** Liver and spleen, partial desulfation; depolymerization in kidney. **Elimination:** Urine (3% unchanged); $T_{1/2}$=4.8 hrs.

ELOCON
mometasone furoate (Schering)

RX

THERAPEUTIC CLASS: Corticosteroid

INDICATIONS: Corticosteroid-responsive dermatoses.

DOSAGE: *Adults:* (Cre, Oint) Apply qd. (Lot) Apply a few drops qd. Re-assess if no improvement within 2 weeks. *Pediatrics:* (Cre, Oint) ≥2 yrs: Apply qd for up to 3 weeks if needed. Avoid in diaper area. Re-assess if no improvement within 2 weeks.

HOW SUPPLIED: Cre, Oint: 0.1% (15g, 45g); Lot: 0.1% (30mL, 60mL)

WARNINGS/PRECAUTIONS: May produce reversible HPA axis suppression, manifestations of Cushing's syndrome, hyperglycemia and glucosuria. D/C if irritation occurs. Use appropriate antifungal or antibacterial agent with dermatological infections. Pediatrics may be more susceptible to systemic toxicity. Caution when applied to large surface areas or with occlusive dressings.

ADVERSE REACTIONS: Burning, pruritus, skin atrophy, rosacea, acneiform reaction, tingling, stinging, furunculosis, folliculitis.

PREGNANCY: Category C, caution in nursing.

MECHANISM OF ACTION: Corticosteroid; possesses anti-inflammatory, antipruritic, and vasoconstrictive properties. Mechanism of anti-inflammatory effects not established. Suspected to induce phospholipase A_2 inhibitory proteins, lipocortins. Lipocortins control biosynthesis of potent mediators of inflammation (eg, prostaglandins and leukotrienes) by inhibiting release of their precursor, arachidonic acid.

PHARMACOKINETICS: Absorption: Extent of absorption depends on skin integrity, vehicle, and use of occlusive dressing.

EMADINE
emedastine difumarate (Alcon)

RX

THERAPEUTIC CLASS: H_1-receptor antagonist

INDICATIONS: Temporary relief of signs and symptoms of allergic conjunctivitis.

DOSAGE: *Adults:* 1 drop in affected eye up to qid.
Pediatrics: ≥3 yrs: 1 drop in affected eye up to qid.

HOW SUPPLIED: Sol: 0.05% (5mL)

WARNINGS/PRECAUTIONS: Wait at least 10 min after application to insert contact lens (if eye is not red). Not for irritation due to contact lens.

ADVERSE REACTIONS: Headache, abnormal dreams, asthenia, bad taste, blurred vision, burning, stinging, corneal infiltrates, corneal staining, dermatitis, discomfort, dry eye, foreign body sensation, hyperemia, keratitis, pruritus, rhinitis, sinusitis, tearing.

PREGNANCY: Category B, caution in nursing.

MECHANISM OF ACTION: Antihistaminic; relatively selective histamine H_1 antagonist; inhibits histamine-stimulated vascular permeability in the conjuctiva.

PHARMACOKINETICS: Metabolism: 5- and 6-hydroxymedastine (primary metabolites).

EMBELINE E
clobetasol propionate (Healthpoint)

RX

THERAPEUTIC CLASS: Corticosteroid

INDICATIONS: Corticosteroid-responsive dermatoses.

DOSAGE: *Adults:* Apply bid. Limit to 2 consecutive weeks. Max: 50g/week. Moderate-Severe Psoriasis: Apply to 5%-10% BSA up to 4 weeks. Max: 50g/week.
Pediatrics: ≥12 yrs: Apply bid. Limit to 2 consecutive weeks. Max: 50g/week. Moderate-Severe Psoriasis: ≥16 yrs: Apply to 5%-10% BSA up to 4 weeks. Max: 50g/week.

HOW SUPPLIED: Cre: 0.05% (15g, 30g, 60g)

WARNINGS/PRECAUTIONS: Not for use on the face, groin, or axillae, or for treatment of rosacea or perioral dermatitis. May produce reversible HPA axis suppression, manifestations of Cushing's syndrome, hyperglycemia, and glucosuria. Reassess if no improvement after 2 weeks. D/C if irritation occurs. Peds may be more susceptible to systemic toxicity. Avoid occlusive dressings.

ADVERSE REACTIONS: Burning/stinging, pruritus, irritation, erythema, folliculitis, cracking/fissuring of skin, numbness of fingers, tenderness in elbows, telangiectasia, skin atrophy.

PREGNANCY: Category C, caution in nursing.

MECHANISM OF ACTION: Corticosteroid; posssess anti-inflammatory, antipruritic, and vasoconstrictive properties. Mechanism not established; suspected to inhibit phospholipase A_2 inhibitory proteins, lipocortins. Lipocortins control biosynthesis of potent mediators of inflammation (eg, prostaglandins, leukotrienes) by inhibiting release of their precursor, arachidonic acid.

PHARMACOKINETICS: Absorption: Percutaneous; inflammation and other disease states may increase absorption. Use of occlusive dressings <24 hrs not shown to increase penetration. Use of occlusive dressings for up to 96 hrs significantly increases penetration. **Distribution:** Systemically administered corticosteroids found in breast milk.

EMLA
lidocaine - prilocaine (AstraZeneca)

RX

THERAPEUTIC CLASS: Acetamide local anesthetic

INDICATIONS: Topical anesthetic for use on normal intact skin or on genital mucous membranes for minor surgery. Pretreatment for infiltration anesthesia.

DOSAGE: *Adults:* Apply thick layer of cream to intact skin and cover with occlusive dressing. Minor Dermal Procedure: Apply 2.5g (1/2 tube) over 20-25cm^2 of skin surface. Major Dermal Procedure: Apply 2g/10cm^2 of skin for 2 hrs. Adult Male Genital Skin: Apply 1g/10cm^2 of skin surface for 15 min. Female External Genitalia: Apply 5-10g for 5-10 min.
Pediatrics: 7-12 yrs and >20kg: Max: 20g/200cm^2 for up to 4 hrs.1-6 yrs and >10 kg: Max:10g/100cm^2 for up to 4 hrs. 3-12 months and ≥5 kg: Max: 2g/20cm^2 for up to 4 hrs. 3-12 months and ≥5 kg: Max: 2g/20cm^2 for up to 4 hrs. 0-3 months or <5kg: Max: 1g/10cm^2 for up to 1 hr.

HOW SUPPLIED: Cre: (Lidocaine-Prilocaine) 2.5%-2.5%

WARNINGS/PRECAUTIONS: Avoid application for longer than recommended times or on large areas. Avoid with methemoglobinemia. Risk of methemoglobinemia in very young or with G6P deficiency. Avoid eye contact, use in ear. Caution with severe hepatic disease, acutely ill, debilitated, elderly, history of drug sensitivities. Avoid in neonates with a gestational age <37 weeks and infants <12 months receiving treatment with methemoglobin-inducing agents.

ADVERSE REACTIONS: Local reactions such as: erythema, edema, abnormal sensations, paleness (pallor or blanching), altered temperature sensations, itching, rash.

INTERACTIONS: Caution with Class I (eg, tocainide, mexiletine) and Class III (eg, amiodarone, bretylium, sotalol) antiarrhythmic drugs. Avoid drugs associated with drug-induced methemoglobinemia (eg, sulfonamides, APAP, nitrates/nitrites, nitrofurantoin, phenobarbital, phenytoin, quinine). Caution with other products containing local anesthetics; consider the amount absorbed from all formulations.

PREGNANCY: Category B, caution in nursing.

MECHANISM OF ACTION: Amide-type local anesthetic; provides dermal analgesia by releasing lidocaine and prilocaine into epidermal and dermal layers of skin and by accumulation in vicinity of dermal pain receptors and nerve endings. Also stabilizes neuronal membranes by inhibiting ionic fluxes required for initiation and conduction impulses, thereby effecting local anesthetic action.

PHARMACOKINETICS: Absorption: Lidocaine: (3 hrs 400cm^2) C_{max}=0.12mcg/mL, T_{max}=4 hrs; (24 hrs 400cm^2) C_{max}=0.28mcg/mL, T_{max}=10 hrs. Prilocaine: (3 hrs 400cm^2) C_{max}=0.07mcg/mL, T_{max}=4 hrs; (24 hrs 400 cm^2) C_{max}=0.14mcg/mL, T_{max}=10 hrs. **Distribution:** V_d=1.5L/kg (lidocaine), 2.6L/kg (prilocaine); plasma protein binding 70% (lidocaine), 55% (prilocaine). Crosses placental and blood-brain barrier; found in breast milk. **Metabolism:** Lidocaine: Liver (rapid); monoethylglycinexylidide and glycinexylidide (active metabolites). Prilocaine: Liver and kidneys by amidases; *ortho*-toluidine and propylalanine (metabolites). **Elimination:** Lidocaine: Urine (>98%); $T_{1/2}$=110 min. Prilocaine: $T_{1/2}$=70 min.

EMTRIVA
emtricitabine (Gilead)

RX

> Lactic acidosis and severe hepatomegaly with steatosis, including fatal cases, reported with nucleoside analogs alone or with concomitant antiretrovirals. Not indicated for the treatment of chronic HBV infection; severe acute exacerbations of hepatitis B reported in patients co-infected with HBV and HIV upon discontinuation of emtricitabine.

THERAPEUTIC CLASS: Nucleoside analogue

INDICATIONS: Treatment of HIV-1 infection in combination with other antivirals.

DOSAGE: *Adults:* ≥18 yrs: Cap: 200mg qd. CrCl 30-49mL/min: 200mg q48h. CrCl 15-29mL/min: 200mg q72h. CrCl <15mL/min (including hemodialysis): 200mg q96h. Sol: 240mg (24mL) qd. CrCl 30-49mL/min: 120mg (12mL) qd. CrCl 15-29mL/min: 80mg (8mL)

qd. CrCl <15mL/min (including hemodialysis): 60mg (6mL) qd.
Pediatrics: 0-3 months: Sol: 3mg/kg qd. 3 months-17 yrs: Cap: >33kg: 200mg qd. Sol: 6mg/kg qd. Max: 240mg (24mL).

HOW SUPPLIED: Cap: 200mg; Sol: 10mg/mL (170mL)

WARNINGS/PRECAUTIONS: Test for chronic hepatitis B prior to initiation; post-treatment exacerbations reported. Monitor hepatic function for several months in patients who d/c the drug and are co-infected with HIV and HBV. Reduce dose with renal dysfunction. Monitor changes in fasting cholesterol, serum amylase, creatinine kinase, and neutrophil count. Redistribution/accumulation of body fat reported. Immune reconstitution syndrome reported.

ADVERSE REACTIONS: Headache, diarrhea, NV, rash, dyspepsia, asthenia, abdominal pain, dizziness, insomnia, neuropathy, paresthesia, increased cough, rhinitis.

INTERACTIONS: Avoid co-administration with Atripla, Truvada, or lamivudine-containing products.

PREGNANCY: Category B, not for use in nursing.

MECHANISM OF ACTION: Nucleoside analog of cytidine; inhibits the activity of HIV-1 reverse transcriptase by competing with the natural substrate deoxycytidine 5'-triphosphate and incorporating into nascent viral DNA, resulting in chain termination.

PHARMACOKINETICS: Absorption: Rapid and extensive. C_{max}=1.8mcg/mL, T_{max}=1-2 hrs, AUC=10.0mcg•hr/mL. (Cap) Absolute bioavailability (93%). (Sol) Absolute bioavailability (75%). **Distribution:** Plasma protein binding (<4%). **Metabolism:** Hepatic (conjugation and oxidation). Metabolites: 3'sulfoxide diastereomers and 2'O-glucuronide. **Elimination:** Urine (86%), feces (14%); $T_{1/2}$=10 hrs.

ENBREL   RX
etanercept (Amgen)

> **Serious infections, including bacterial sepsis and TB, reported; d/c if severe infection develops. Evaluate for TB risk factors and test for latent TB infection prior to initiation.**

THERAPEUTIC CLASS: TNF-receptor blocker

INDICATIONS: To reduce signs/symptoms, induce major clinical response, improve physical function, and inhibit progression of structural damage in moderate to severe rheumatoid arthritis (RA) (may be initiated in combination with methotrexate (MTX) or alone). To reduce signs/symptoms, inhibit progression of structural damage of active arthritis, and improve physical function in psoriatic arthritis (may be used with MTX in patients not responding to MTX alone). To reduce signs/symptoms of moderate to severe polyarticular-course juvenile rheumatoid arthritis (JRA) unresponsive to one or more DMARDs. To reduce signs/symptoms of active ankylosing spondylitis (AS). Chronic moderate to severe plaque psoriasis for candidates of systemic therapy or phototherapy.

DOSAGE: *Adults:* ≥18 yrs: RA/Psoriatic Arthritis/AS: 50mg SQ per week, given as one SQ injection. May continue MTX, glucocorticoids, salicylates, NSAIDs, or analgesics. Psoriasis: Initial: 50mg SQ twice weekly given 3 or 4 days apart for 3 months. May begin with 25-50mg/week. Maint: 50mg/week.
Pediatrics: 2-17 yrs: JRA: 0.8mg/kg SQ per week. Max: 50mg/week. May continue glucocorticoids, NSAIDs, or analgesics.

HOW SUPPLIED: Inj: (MDV) 25mg, (Syringe) 50mg/mL

CONTRAINDICATIONS: Sepsis.

WARNINGS/PRECAUTIONS: May cause autoimmune antibodies. Avoid with active infections. Monitor closely if new infection develops. Caution with pre-existing or recent onset CNS demyelinating disorders. Rare cases of pancytopenia including aplastic anemia reported; d/c if significant hematologic abnormalities occur. May cause reactivation of hepatitis B virus; evaluate prior to therapy initiation. Caution in patients with heart failure; monitor closely. JRA patients should be brought up to date with current immunization guidelines prior to initiating therapy. D/C temporarily with significant varicella virus exposure and consider prophylaxis. Avoid with Wegener's granulomatosis. Needle cap on prefilled syringe and autoinjector contains dry natural rubber; caution with latex allergy.

ADVERSE REACTIONS: (*Adults/Pediatrics*) Injection site reactions, infections, headache. (Pediatrics) Varicella, gastroenteritis, depression, cutaneous ulcer, esophagitis.

INTERACTIONS: Do not give live vaccines. Avoid with cyclophosphamide. May cause neutropenia with anakinra.

PREGNANCY: Category B, not for use in nursing.

MECHANISM OF ACTION: TNF-receptor blocker; binds specifically to tumor necrosis factor (TNF) and blocks its interaction with cell surface TNF-receptors.

PHARMACOKINETICS: Absorption: SQ administration of different doses resulted in different parameters.

ENGERIX-B
hepatitis B (recombinant) (GlaxoSmithKline)

RX

OTHER BRAND NAME: Engerix-B Pediatric/Adolescent (GlaxoSmithKline)

THERAPEUTIC CLASS: Vaccine

INDICATIONS: Immunization against all known hepatitis B virus subtypes.

DOSAGE: *Adults:* >19 yrs: 20mcg IM in deltoid or thigh at 0, 1, 6 months. Hemodialysis: 40mcg IM at 0, 1, 2, 6 months. Booster: 20mcg IM. Hemodialysis Booster: 40mcg IM. May give SQ with risk of hemorrhage.
Pediatrics: ≤19 yrs: 10mcg/0.5mL IM at 0, 1, 6 months. Booster: ≤10 yrs: 10mcg IM. 11-19 yrs: 20mcg IM. See PI for special populations. May give SQ with risk of hemorrhage.

HOW SUPPLIED: Inj: 10mcg/0.5mL, 20mcg/mL

CONTRAINDICATIONS: Yeast hypersensitivity.

WARNINGS/PRECAUTIONS: Will not prevent hepatitis A, C, and E viruses infection. Vaccine may be ineffective with unrecognized hepatitis. Delay vaccine with moderate or severe febrile illnesses. May exacerbate MS (rare). Suboptimal immune response may occur with immunosuppressed persons. Have epinephrine injection (1:1000) available.

ADVERSE REACTIONS: Injection site induration, erythema, swelling, fever, headache, dizziness.

INTERACTIONS: Suboptimal immune response may occur with immunosuppressants; defer vaccine ≥3 months after immunosuppressive therapy.

PREGNANCY: Category C, caution in nursing.

MECHANISM OF ACTION: Stimulates the immune system to induce antibodies that may protect against infection caused by all known subtypes of Hepatitis B virus.

ENTEX HC
guaifenesin - hydrocodone bitartrate - phenylephrine HCl (Andrx)

CIII

THERAPEUTIC CLASS: Opioid antitussive

INDICATIONS: Temporary relief of nonproductive cough.

DOSAGE: *Adults:* 5-10mL q4-6h. Max 40mL/24 hrs.
Pediatrics: ≥12 yrs: 5-10mL q4-6h. Max 40mL/24 hrs. 6-12 yrs: 5mL q4-6h. Max 20mL/24 hrs. 2-6 yrs: 2.5mL q4-6h. Max 10mL/24 hrs.

HOW SUPPLIED: Liq: (Guaifenesin-Hydrocodone-Phenylephrine) 100mg-5mg-7.5mg/5mL (473mL)

CONTRAINDICATIONS: Infants, newborns, severe HTN or CAD, hyperthyroidism, or MAOI therapy.

WARNINGS/PRECAUTIONS: May be habit-forming. May cause respiratory depression or increase CSF pressure in the presence of other intracranial pathology. May obscure head injuries or acute abdominal conditions. Caution in elderly, debilitated, hepatic/renal dysfunction, Addison's disease, hypothyroidism, postoperative use, prostatic hypertrophy, pulmonary disease, and urethral stricture. Suppresses cough reflex.

ADVERSE REACTIONS: CNS stimulation, constipation, drowsiness, dizziness, excitability, headache, insomnia, lightheadedness, nausea, vomiting, nervousness, respiratory depression, restlessness, tachycardia, tremors, urinary retention, weakness, arrhythmias, and cardiovascular.

INTERACTIONS: Additive CNS effects with alcohol, antianxiety agents, antihistamines, antipsychotics, narcotics, tranquilizers, or other CNS depressants. Increased sympathomimetic effects with MAOIs or β-blockers. Sympathomimetics may reduce antihypertensive effects of methyldopa, mecamylamine, reserpine, veratrum alkaloids. May enhance the effects of TCAs, barbiturates, alcohol, other CNS depressants.

PREGNANCY: Category C, not for use in nursing.

ENTEX LA   RX
guaifenesin - phenylephrine HCl (Andrx)

THERAPEUTIC CLASS: Expectorant/decongestant

INDICATIONS: Temporary relief of symptoms associated with upper respiratory tract disorders and cough associated with respiratory tract infections and related disorders when complicated by tenacious mucous or mucous plugs and congestion.

DOSAGE: *Adults:* 1 tab q12h. Max: 2 tabs/24hrs.
Pediatrics: ≥12 yrs: 1 tab q12h. Max: 2 tabs/24hrs. 6-12 yrs: 1/2 tab q12h. Max: 1 tab/24hrs.

HOW SUPPLIED: Tab, Extended-Release: (Guaifenesin-Phenylephrine) 400mg-30mg*
*scored

CONTRAINDICATIONS: HTN, ventricular tachycardia, MAOI use within 14 days. Extreme caution in elderly, hyperthyroidism, bradycardia, partial heart block, myocardial disease, severe arteriosclerosis.

WARNINGS/PRECAUTIONS: Caution in HTN, DM, ischemic heart disease, increase IOP, hyperthyroidism, or prostatic hypertrophy. May produce CNS stimulation with convulsions or cadiovascular collapse with hypotension. Adverse effects occur more often in elderly.

ADVERSE REACTIONS: Palpitations, headache, dizziness, nausea, anxiety, restlessness, tremor, weakness, pallor, dysuria, respiratory difficulty.

INTERACTIONS: β-blockers and MAOIs may potentiate pressor response. Increased risk of arrhythmias with digitalis glycosides and halothane anesthesia. May reduce hypotensive effects of guanethidine, mecamylamine, methyldopa, reserpine, and veratrum alkaloids. TCAs may antagonize effects.

PREGNANCY: Category C, not for use in nursing.

ENTEX PSE   RX
guaifenesin - pseudoephedrine HCl (Andrx)

OTHER BRAND NAMES: Ami-Tex PSE (Amide) - Guaifenex PSE 120 (Ethex)

THERAPEUTIC CLASS: Expectorant/decongestant

INDICATIONS: Relief of nasal congestion due to common cold, hay fever, upper respiratory allergies, and nasal congestion associated with sinusitis. To promote nasal or sinus drainage. For symptomatic relief of respiratory conditions characterized by dry nonproductive cough and in the presence of tenacious mucous plugs in the respiratory tract.

DOSAGE: *Adults:* 1 tab q12h.
Pediatrics: ≥12 yrs: 1 tab q12h. 6 to <12 yrs: 1/2 tab q12h.

HOW SUPPLIED: Tab, Extended-Release: (Guaifenesin-Pseudoephedrine) 400mg-120mg*
*scored

CONTRAINDICATIONS: Nursing, severe HTN, severe CAD, prostatic hypertrophy, concomitant MAOIs.

WARNINGS/PRECAUTIONS: Caution in HTN, DM, heart disease, peripheral vascular disease, increased IOP, hyperthyroidism, or prostatic hypertrophy.

ADVERSE REACTIONS: Nausea, vomiting, nervousness, dizziness, sleeplessness, lightheadedness, tremor, palpitations, tachycardia, weakness, respiratory difficulties.

INTERACTIONS: MAOI and β-blockers increase sympathomimetic effects. May reduce antihypertensive effects of methyldopa, guanethidine, mecamylamine, reserpine, and veratrum alkaloids.

PREGNANCY: Category C, contraindicated in nursing.

MECHANISM OF ACTION: Pseudoephedrine: Sympathomimetic, decongestant; produces vasoconstriction by stimulating α-receptors within the mucosa of the respiratory tract. Guaifenesin: Expectorant; promotes lower respiratory tract drainage.

EPIFOAM
hydrocortisone acetate - pramoxine HCl (Schwarz)

RX

THERAPEUTIC CLASS: Corticosteroid

INDICATIONS: Corticosteroid responsive dermatoses.

DOSAGE: *Adults:* Apply tid-qid. Use occlusive dressings for management of psoriasis or recalcitrant conditions.
Pediatrics: Use least amount necessary for effective regimen. Use occlusive dressings for management of psoriasis or recalcitrant conditions.

HOW SUPPLIED: Foam: (Hydrocortisone-Pramoxine) 1%-1% (10g)

WARNINGS/PRECAUTIONS: Avoid prolonged use. D/C use if irritation persists. May produce reversible HPA axis suppression, manifestations of Cushing's syndrome, hyperglycemia, glucosuria. Pediatrics more susceptible to systemic toxicity.

ADVERSE REACTIONS: Burning, itching, irritation, dryness, folliculitis, hypertrichosis, acneiform eruptions, hypopigmentation, perioral dermatitis, maceration, secondary infection, skin atrophy, striae, miliaria.

PREGNANCY: Category C, caution in nursing.

MECHANISM OF ACTION: Hydrocortisone: Corticosteroid; possesses anti-inflammatory, antipruritic, and vasoconstrictive properties. Anti-inflammatory activity not established. Pramoxine: Local anesthetic.

PHARMACOKINETICS: Absorption: Percutaneous; inflammation, other disease states, and use of occlusive dressings may increase absorption. **Distribution:** Systemically administered corticosteroids are found in breast milk. **Metabolism:** Liver. **Elimination:** Kidneys, bile.

EPIPEN
epinephrine (Dey)

RX

OTHER BRAND NAME: EpiPen Jr. (Dey)

THERAPEUTIC CLASS: Sympathomimetic catecholamine

INDICATIONS: Emergency treatment of allergic reactions (anaphylaxis) to insect stings or bites, foods, drugs, other allergens, and idiopathic or exercise-induced anaphylaxis.

DOSAGE: *Adults:* 0.3mg IM in thigh. May repeat with severe anaphylaxis.
Pediatrics: 0.15mg or 0.3mg (0.01mg/kg) IM in thigh. May repeat with severe anaphylaxis.

HOW SUPPLIED: Inj: (Epipen Jr) 0.5mg/mL, (Epipen) 1mg/mL

WARNINGS/PRECAUTIONS: Not for IV use. Contains sulfites. Extreme caution with heart disease. Anginal pain may be induced with coronary insufficiency. Increased risk of adverse reactions with hyperthyroidism, CVD, HTN, DM, elderly, pregnancy, pediatrics <30kg with Epipen and <15kg with Epipen, Jr.

ADVERSE REACTIONS: Palpitations, tachycardia, sweating, nausea, vomiting, respiratory difficulty, pallor, dizziness, weakness, tremor, headache, apprehension, anxiety.

INTERACTIONS: Potentiated by TCAs and MAOIs. Increased risk of arrhythmias with digitalis, mercurial diuretics, or quinidine. Pressor effects may be counteracted by rapidly acting vasodilators.

PREGNANCY: Category C, safety in nursing not known.

MECHANISM OF ACTION: Sympathomimetic drug; acts on both α and β receptors.

EPIQUIN MICRO

RX

hydroquinone (SkinMedica)

THERAPEUTIC CLASS: Depigmenting agent

INDICATIONS: Gradual treatment of UV-induced dyschromia and discoloration resulting from the use of oral contraceptives, pregnancy, hormone replacement therapy, or skin trauma.

DOSAGE: *Adults:* Apply bid (am and hs). Use sunscreen.
Pediatrics: ≥12yrs: Apply bid (am and hs). Use sunscreen.

HOW SUPPLIED: Cre: 4% (30g)

WARNINGS/PRECAUTIONS: Avoid sun exposure on bleached skin. Use sunscreen. May produce unwanted cosmetic effects if not used as directed. Test for skin sensitivity. D/C if no lightening effect after 2 months of therapy, if blue-black darkening of the skin occurs, or if itching, vesicle formation, or excessive inflammatory reactions occur. Contains sodium metabisulfite; may cause serious allergic type reactions. Avoid contact with eyes.

ADVERSE REACTIONS: Cutaneous hypersensitivity (contact dermitits).

PREGNANCY: Category C, caution in nursing.

MECHANISM OF ACTION: Produces a reversible depigmentation of the skin by inhibition of the enzymatic oxidation of tyrosine to 3-(3,4-dihydroxyphenyl) alanine (dopa)[2] and suppresses the melanocyte metabolic processes.

EPIVIR

RX

lamivudine (GlaxoSmithKline)

> Lactic acidosis and severe hepatomegaly with steatosis, including fatal cases, reported. Epivir tablets and solution, used to treat HIV, contain higher dose of lamivudine than Epivir-HBV, used to treat hepatitis B; only use appropriate dosing forms for HIV treatment. Severe acute exacerbations of hepatitis B reported in patients coinfected with hepatitis B virus and HIV who discontinued therapy; monitor hepatic function closely.

THERAPEUTIC CLASS: Nucleoside analogue

INDICATIONS: Treatment of HIV infection in combination with other antiretrovirals.

DOSAGE: *Adults:* >16 yrs: 150mg bid or 300mg qd, concomitantly with other antiretrovirals. CrCl 30-49mL/min: 150mg qd. CrCl 15-29mL/min: 150mg first dose, then 100mg qd. CrCl 5-14mL/min: 150mg first dose, then 50mg qd. CrCl <5mL/min: 50mg first dose, then 25mg qd.
Pediatrics: Sol: 3 months-16 yrs: 4mg/kg bid, concomitantly with other antiretrovirals. Max: 150mg bid. Scored Tab: 14-21kg: 1/2 tab (75mg) in am and 1/2 tab (75mg) in pm. 21-30kg: 1/2 tab (75mg) in am and 1 tab (150mg) in pm. ≥30kg: 1 tab (150mg) in am and 1 tab (150mg) in pm. Adolescents: CrCl 30-49mL/min: 150mg qd. CrCl 15-29mL/min: 150mg first dose, then 100mg qd. CrCl 5-14mL/min: 150mg 1st dose, then 50mg qd. CrCl <5mL/min: 50mg 1st dose, then 25mg qd.

HOW SUPPLIED: Sol: 10mg/mL (240mL); Tab: 150mg, 300mg

WARNINGS/PRECAUTIONS: Caution in pediatrics with history of prior antiretroviral nucleoside exposure, history of pancreatitis, or other significant risk factors for developing pancreatitis. D/C if pancreatitis develops. Post-treatment exacerbations of hepatitis reported. Hepatic decompensation occured when used with interferon-α w/ or w/o ribavirin. Suspend therapy if lactic acidosis or pronounced hepatotoxicity occurs. Reduce dose in renal dysfunction. Possible redistribution or accumulation of body fat. Immune reconstitution syndrome reported.

ADVERSE REACTIONS: Headache, malaise, fatigue, fever, chills, NV, diarrhea, anorexia, abdominal pain, neuropathy, dizziness, skin rash, musculoskeletal pain, cough.

INTERACTIONS: TMP/SMX increases levels of lamivudine. Avoid with zalcitabine, zidovudine, and fixed-dose combinations of abacavir, lamivudine, and zidovudine. Also avoid emtricitabine and fixed-dose combinations of emtricitabine, efavirenz, and tenofovir.

PREGNANCY: Category C, not for use in nursing.

MECHANISM OF ACTION: Nucleoside analogue; inhibits HIV-1 reverse transcriptase via DNA chain termination after incorporation into viral DNA.

PHARMACOKINETICS: Absorption: Rapid; (Tab) Absolute bioavailability (86%). (Sol) Absolute bioavailability (87%); C_{max}=1.5mcg/mL (HIV); T_{max}=0.9 hrs. **Distribution:** V_d=1.3L/kg; plasma protein binding (<36%). **Metabolism:** Hepatic (minor); trans-sulfoxide (metabolite). **Elimination:** Urine (unchanged); $T_{1/2}$=5-7 hrs.

EPIVIR-HBV
lamivudine (GlaxoSmithKline)

RX

> Lactic acidosis and severe, possibly fatal, hepatomegaly reported. If prescribed for patients with unrecognized or untreated HIV infection, rapid emergence of HIV resistance is likely; Epivir-HBV contains a lower dose of lamivudine than Epivir which is used to treat HIV. Severe acute exacerbations of hepatitis B reported upon discontinuation of therapy; follow-up liver function monitoring required.

THERAPEUTIC CLASS: Nucleoside analogue

INDICATIONS: Treatment of chronic hepatitis B associated with viral replication and active liver inflammation.

DOSAGE: *Adults:* 100mg qd. CrCl 30-49mL/min: 100mg Day 1, then 50mg qd. CrCl: 15-29mL/min: 100mg Day 1, then 25mg qd. CrCl 5-14mL/min: 35mg Day 1, then 15mg qd. CrCl <5mL/min: 35mg Day 1, then 10mg qd.
Pediatrics: 2-17 yrs: 3mg/kg qd. Max: 100mg/day.

HOW SUPPLIED: Sol: 5mg/mL (240mL); Tab: 100mg

WARNINGS/PRECAUTIONS: Reduce dose in renal dysfunction. Caution in elderly. This formulation is not appropriate in both HBV and HIV infections. Post-treatment exacerbations of hepatitis reported. Pancreatitis reported, especially in HIV-infected pediatrics with prior nucleoside exposure. Monitor patient regularly during treatment. Safety and efficacy of treatment after 1 yr is not known. Suspend therapy if lactic acidosis or pronounced hepatotoxicity develops. Emergence of resistance-associated HBV mutations.

ADVERSE REACTIONS: Pancreatitis, lactic acidosis, severe hepatomegaly, GI complaints, sore throat, infections, elevated LFTs, arthralgia.

INTERACTIONS: TMP/SMX may increase lamivudine levels. Avoid with zalcitabine.

PREGNANCY: Category C, not for use in nursing.

MECHANISM OF ACTION: Nucleoside analogue; phosphorylated to active 5'-triphosphate metabolite intracellularly; incorporation of monophosphate form into viral DNA by HBV reverse transcriptase results in DNA termination.

PHARMACOKINETICS: Absorption: Rapid; C_{max}=1.28mcg/mL (HBV), C_{max}=1.05mcg/mL (healthy); T_{max}=0.5-2.0 hrs; AUC=4.3mcg•h/mL (HBV), AUC=4.7mcg•h/mL (healthy). Tab: Absolute bioavailability (86%). Sol: Absolute bioavailability (87%). **Distribution:** Plasma protein binding (<36%); V_d=1.3L/kg. **Metabolism:** Hepatic (minor); trans-sulfoxide (metabolite). **Elimination:** Urine (unchanged); $T_{1/2}$=5-7 hrs.

EPOGEN
epoetin alfa (Amgen)

RX

> Increased mortality, serious cardiovascular/thromboembolic events, and tumor progression. (Renal Failure) Patients experienced greater risks for death and serious cardiovascular events when administered erythropoiesis-stimulating agents (ESAs) to target higher vs lower Hgb levels (13.5 vs 11.3 g/dL; 14 vs 10 g/dL) in 2 clinical studies. Individualize dosing to achieve and maintain Hgb levels within range of 10-12g/dL. (Cancer) ESAs shortened overall survival and/or time-to-tumor progression in clinical studies in patients with breast, head and neck, lymphoid, and non-small cell lung, and cervical cancers when dosed to target Hgb ≥12g/dL. The risks of shortened survival and tumor progression have not been excluded when ESAs are dosed to target Hgb <12g/dL. To minimize these risks, as well as the risk of serious cario- and thrombovascular events, use lowest dose needed to avoid RBC transfusions. Use only for treatment of anemia due to concomitant myelosuppressive chemotherapy. D/C following completion of a chemotherapy course. (Perisurgery) Epoetin alfa increased the rate of DVT in patients not receiving prophylactic anticoagulation. Consider DVT prophylaxis.

THERAPEUTIC CLASS: Erythropoiesis stimulator

Ertaczo

INDICATIONS: Treatment of anemia of chronic renal failure (CRF), anemia related to zidovudine in HIV (serum erythropoietin ≤500 mU/mL and zidovudine ≤4200mg/week), chemotherapy-induced anemia in patients with non-myeloid malignancies, and reduction of allogeneic blood transfusions in anemic (≤13 to >10 g/dL) patients scheduled for elective, noncardiac, nonvascular surgery.

DOSAGE: *Adults:* CRF: Initial: 50-100 U/kg IV/SQ 3x/week. IV is preferred route in dialysis patients. Maint: Individually titrate. Reduce dose by 25% when Hgb approaches 12g/dL or increases >1g/dL in any 2 week period. Increase dose by 25% if Hgb is <10g/dL and has not increased by 1g/dL after 4 weeks of therapy. Zidovudine-Treated HIV Patients: If serum erythropoietin ≤500 mU/mL and zidovudine ≤4200mg/week give100 U/kg IV/SQ 3x/week for 8 weeks. Titrate: Increase by 50-100 U/kg 3x/week after 8 weeks if necessary. Max: 300 U/kg 3x/week Maint: if Hgb >13g/dL, d/c until Hgb <12g/dL, then reduce dose by 25% when resume therapy. Chemotherapy-Induced Anemia: Initial: 150 U/kg SQ 3x/week. Titrate: Reduce by 25% when Hgb approaches 12g/dL or Hgb increases >1g/dL in any 2-week period. If Hgb >13g/dL, withhold until Hgb <12g/dL then restart at 25% below previous dose. May increase to 300 U/kg 3x/week if no response after 8 weeks of therapy. Max: 300 U/kg 3x/week. Weekly Dosing: 40,000 U SQ weekly. Titrate: If Hgb not increased by ≥1g/dL after 4 weeks, increase to 60,000 U weekly. If Hgb >13g/dL, withhold until Hgb <12g/dL then restart with 25% dose reduction. Reduce dose by 25% if very rapid Hgb response (eg, increase >1g/dL in any 2-week period. Max: 60,000 U weekly. Surgery: 300 U/kg/day SQ for 10 days before, on day of, and 4 days after surgery; or 600 U/kg SQ once weekly on 21, 14, and 7 days before surgery, and a 4th dose on day of surgery.
Pediatrics: CRF: Initial: 50 U/kg 3x/week IV/SQ. Maint: Individually titrate. Reduce dose by 25% when Hgb approaches 12g/dL or increases >1g/dL in any 2 week period. Increase dose by 25% if Hgb is <10g/dL and has not increased by 1g/dL after 4 weeks of therapy. Chemotherapy Induced Anemia: Initial: 600 U/kg IV weekly. Titrate: If Hgb not increased by ≥1g/dL after 4 weeks, increase to 900 U/kg IV weekly. If Hgb >13g/dL, withhold until Hgb <12g/dL then restart with 25% dose reduction. Reduce dose by 25% if very rapid Hgb response (eg, increase >1g/dL in any 2-week period. Max: 60,000 U weekly.

HOW SUPPLIED: Inj: 2000 U/mL, 3000 U/mL, 4000 U/mL, 10,000 U/mL, 20,000 U/mL, 40,000 U/mL

CONTRAINDICATIONS: Uncontrolled HTN. Hypersensitivity to mammalian cell-derived products and Albumin (human).

WARNINGS/PRECAUTIONS: Pure red cell aplasia and severe anemia (with or without other cytopenias) may occur. Caution with porphyria, HTN or a history of seizures. Evaluate iron stores prior to and during therapy. Most patients need iron supplementation. Monitor Hct, BP, iron levels, serum chemistry, and CBC. Menses may resume. Multidose formulation contains benzyl alcohol. Increased mortality, cardiovascular, and thrombo-embolic events in patients with CRF reported. ESAs shortened the time to tumor progression in patients with advanced head and neck cancer receiving radiation therapy. Dose should be carefully adjusted in patients with CRF and CHF.

ADVERSE REACTIONS: HTN, headache, fatigue, arthralgias, nausea, vomiting, diarrhea, edema, rash, pyrexia, clotted vascular access, respiratory congestion, dyspnea, asthenia, dizziness, seizures, thrombotic events.

INTERACTIONS: Adjust anticoagulant dose in dialysis patients.

PREGNANCY: Category C, caution in nursing.

MECHANISM OF ACTION: Erythropoiesis stimulator.

PHARMACOKINETICS: Absorption: (SC) T_{max}=5-24 hrs. **Elimination:** (IV) $T_{1/2}$=4-13 hrs.

Ertaczo   RX
sertaconazole nitrate (Ortho Neutrogena)

THERAPEUTIC CLASS: Azole antifungal
INDICATIONS: Treatment of interdigital tinea pedis in immunocompetent patients caused by *Trichophyton rubrum*, *Trichophyton mentagrophytes*, and *Epidermophyton floccosum*.

DOSAGE: *Adults:* Apply bid to affected areas between toes and adjacent areas for 4 weeks. Re-evaluate if no clinical improvement after 2 weeks.
Pediatrics: ≥12 yrs: Apply bid to affected areas between toes and adjacent areas for 4 weeks. Re-evaluate if no clinical improvement after 2 weeks.

HOW SUPPLIED: Cre: 2% (30g, 60g)

WARNINGS/PRECAUTIONS: Not for ophthalmic, oral, or intravaginal use. D/C if irritation or sensitivity occurs.

ADVERSE REACTIONS: Contact dermatitis, dry skin, burning skin, application site reaction, skin tenderness, hyperpigmentation.

PREGNANCY: Category C, caution in nursing.

MECHANISM OF ACTION: Azole antifungal agent; not established. Believed to act primarily by inhibiting CYP450-dependent synthesis of ergosterol, a key component of fungi cell membranes. Lack of egosterol leads to fungal cell injury through leakage of key constituents in cytoplasm from cell.

ERYC

RX

erythromycin (Warner Chilcott)

THERAPEUTIC CLASS: Macrolide

INDICATIONS: Treatment of mild to moderate upper/lower respiratory tract and skin and soft tissue infections, pertussis, diphtheria, erythrasma, intestinal amebiasis, acute pelvic inflammatory disease (PID) (*N. gonorrhea*), listeriosis, primary syphilis (if PCN allergy), Legionnaires' disease, chlamydial infections (eg, newborn conjunctivitis, pneumonia of infancy, urogenital infections during pregnancy, or urethral, endocervical, or rectal, infections in adults when tetracyclines are contraindicated or not tolerated), and nongonococcal urethritis caused by susceptible strains of microorganisms. Prophylaxis of initial or recurrent attacks of rheumatic fever if PCN allergy.

DOSAGE: *Adults:* Usual: 250mg q6h or 500mg q12h. Max: 4g/day. Do not take bid when dose is >1g/day. Treat strep infections for at least 10 days. Streptococcal Infection Prophylaxis with Rheumatic Heart Disease: 250mg bid. Chlamydial Urogenital Infection During Pregnancy: 500mg qid for at least 7 days or 250mg qid for 14 days. Urethral/Endocervical/Rectal Chlamydial Infections: 500mg qid for at least 7 days. Primary Syphilis: 30-40g in divided doses for 10-15 days. Acute PID: 500mg (erythromycin lactobionate) IV q6h for 3 days, then 250mg PO q6h for 7 days. Intestinal Amebiasis: 250mg qid for 10-14 days. Pertussis: 40-50mg/kg/day in divided doses for 5-14 days. Legionnaires' Disease: 1-4g/day in divided doses. Nongonococcal Urethritis: 500mg PO qid for at least 7 days.
Pediatrics: Usual: 30-50mg/kg/day in divided doses. Severe Infections: 60-100mg/kg/day in divided doses. Treat strep infections for at least 10 days. Streptococcal Infection Prophylaxis with Rheumatic Heart Disease: 250mg bid. Intestinal Amebiasis: 30-50mg/kg/day in divided doses for 10-14 days.

HOW SUPPLIED: Cap, Delayed-Release: 250mg

CONTRAINDICATIONS: Concomitant terfenadine or astemizole.

WARNINGS/PRECAUTIONS: *Clostridium difficile*-associated diarrhea, hepatic dysfunction, and prolonged QT syndrome reported. Caution with impaired hepatic function. May aggravate weakness of patients with myasthenia gravis.

ADVERSE REACTIONS: NV, abdominal pain, diarrhea, anorexia, abnormal LFTs, allergic reaction, superinfection (prolonged use).

INTERACTIONS: See Contraindications. May increase levels of theophylline, digoxin, drugs metabolized by CYP450 (eg, carbamazepine, cyclosporine, phenytoin, tacrolimus, hexobarbital). May increase effects of oral anticoagulants and triazolam. Risk of acute ergot toxicity with ergotamine or dihydroergotamine.

PREGNANCY: Category B, caution in nursing.

MECHANISM OF ACTION: Macrolide; inhibits protein synthesis by binding 50S ribosomal subunits of susceptible organisms.

PHARMACOKINETICS: Absorption: Readily absorbed; C_{max}=1.13-1.68mcg/mL; T_{max}=3 hrs. **Distribution:** Largely bound to plasma proteins. Crosses blood-brain barrier, placenta, breast milk. Diffuses into most body fluids. **Elimination:** Bile, urine (≤5%).

EryPed
RX

erythromycin ethylsuccinate (Abbott)

THERAPEUTIC CLASS: Macrolide

INDICATIONS: Treatment of mild to moderate upper and lower respiratory tract and skin and skin structure infections, listeriosis, pertussis, diphtheria, erythrasma, intestinal amebiasis, acute pelvic inflammatory disease (PID) (*N.gonorrhea*), primary syphilis in PCN allergy, Legionnaires' disease, chlamydial infections (eg, newborn conjunctivitis, urethral, endocervical, or rectal, etc.), and nongonococcal urethritis. Prophylaxis of endocarditis or rheumatic fever.

DOSAGE: *Adults:* Usual: 1600mg/day given q6h, q8h or q12h. Max: 4g/day. Treat strep infections for 10 days. Streptococcal Infection Prophylaxis with Rheumatic Heart Disease: 400mg bid. Urethritis (*C.trachomatis* or *U.urealyticum*): 800mg tid for 7 days. Primary Syphilis: 48-64g in divided doses over 10-15 days. Intestinal Amebiasis: 400mg qid for 10-14 days. Pertussis: 40-50mg/kg/day in divided doses for 5-14 days. Legionnaires' Disease: 1.6-4g/day in divided doses.
Pediatrics: Usual: 30-50mg/kg/day in divided doses q6h, q8h or q12h. Double dose for more severe infections. Treat strep infections for 10 days. Intestinal Amebiasis: 30-50mg/kg/day in divided doses for 10-14 days. Pertussis: 40-50mg/kg/day in divided doses for 5-14 days.

HOW SUPPLIED: Sus: 100mg/2.5mL (50mL), 200mg/5mL, 400mg/5mL (5mL, 100mL, 200mL); Tab, Chewable: 200mg* *scored

CONTRAINDICATIONS: Concomitant terfenadine, astemizole, cisapride, pimozide.

WARNINGS/PRECAUTIONS: *Clostridium difficile*-associated diarrhea, hepatic dysfunction, infantile hypertrophic pyloric stenosis reported. May aggravate myasthenia gravis.

ADVERSE REACTIONS: NV, abdominal pain, diarrhea, anorexia, hepatic dysfunction, abnormal LFTs, allergic reactions, superinfection (prolonged use).

INTERACTIONS: Rhabdomyolysis reported with lovastatin. May increase levels of theophylline, digoxin, drugs metabolized by CYP450 (eg, carbamazepine, cyclosporine, tacrolimus, phenytoin, alfentanil, disopyramide, lovastatin, bromocriptine, valproate, etc). Increases effects of oral anticoagulants, triazolam, midazolam. Risk of acute ergot toxicity with ergotamine or dihydroergotamine. May potentiate sildenafil. Avoid terfenadine, astemizole, cisapride, pimozide.

PREGNANCY: Category B, caution in nursing.

MECHANISM OF ACTION: Macrolide; inhibits protein synthesis by binding 50S ribosomal subunits of susceptible organisms.

PHARMACOKINETICS: Absorption: Readily and reliably absorbed (both fasting and nonfasting conditions). **Distribution:** Diffuses into most body fluids, crosses placenta, excreted in breast milk. **Elimination:** Bile, feces, urine (<5%, active form).

Ery-Tab
RX

erythromycin (Abbott)

THERAPEUTIC CLASS: Macrolide

INDICATIONS: Treatment of mild to moderate upper/lower respiratory tract and skin and skin structure infections, listeriosis, pertussis, diphtheria, erythrasma, intestinal amebiasis, acute pelvic inflammatory disease (PID) (*N.gonorrhea*), primary syphilis (if PCN allergy), Legionnaires' disease, chlamydial infections (eg, newborn conjunctivitis, pneumonia of infancy, urogenital infections during pregnancy, or urethral, endocervical, or rectal infections when tetracyclines are contraindicated or not tolerated), and nongonococcal urethritis caused by susceptible strains of microorganisms. Prophylaxis of initial and recurrent attacks of rheumatic fever if PCN allergy.

DOSAGE: *Adults:* Usual: 250mg qid, 333mg q8h or 500mg q12h. Max: 4g/day. Do not take bid when dose is >1g/day. Treat strep infections for at least 10 days. Streptococcal Infection Long-Term Prophylaxis with Rheumatic Fever: 250mg bid. Chlamydial Urogenital Infection During Pregnancy: 500mg qid or 666mg q8h for at least 7 days, or 500mg q12h, 333mg q8h or 250mg qid for at least 14 days. Urethral/Endocervical/Rectal Chlamydial Infections and Nongonococcal Urethritis: 500mg qid or 666mg q8h for at least 7 days. Primary Syphilis: 30-40g in divided doses for 10-15 days. Acute PID:

500mg (erythromycin lactobionate) IV q6h for 3 days, then 500mg PO q12h or 333mg q8h for 7 days. Intestinal Amebiasis: 500mg q12h, 333mg q8h or 250mg q6h for 10-14 days. Pertussis: 40-50mg/kg/day in divided doses for 5-14 days. Legionnaires' Disease: 1-4g/day in divided doses.

Pediatrics: Usual: 30-50mg/kg/day in divided doses. Severe Infections: May double dose. Max: 4g/day. Treat strep infections for at least 10 days. Streptococcal Infection Long-Term Prophylaxis with Rheumatic Fever: 250mg bid. Chlamydial Conjunctivitis of Newborns/Chlamydial Pneumonia in Infancy: 12.5mg/kg qid for 2 weeks and 3 weeks, respectively. Intestinal Amebiasis: 30-50mg/kg/day in divided doses for 10-14 days.

HOW SUPPLIED: Tab, Delayed-Release: 250mg, 333mg, 500mg

CONTRAINDICATIONS: Concomitant terfenadine, astemizole, pimozide, or cisapride.

WARNINGS/PRECAUTIONS: Pseudomembranous colitis, hepatic dysfunction reported. Caution with impaired hepatic function. May aggravate weakness of patients with myasthenia gravis. Erythromycin does not reach adequate concentrations in fetus to prevent congenital syphilis.

ADVERSE REACTIONS: NV, abdominal pain, diarrhea, anorexia, abnormal LFTs, allergic reactions, superinfection (prolonged use).

INTERACTIONS: See Contraindications. Rhabdomyolysis reported with lovastatin. May increase levels of theophylline, digoxin, drugs metabolized by CYP450 (eg, carbamazepine, cyclosporine, phenytoin, alfentanil, disopyramide, lovastatin, bromocriptine, valproate, etc). Increases effects of oral anticoagulants, triazolam, midazolam. Risk of acute ergot toxicity with ergotamine or dihydroergotamine. May increase AUC of sildenafil; consider dose reduction of sildenafil.

PREGNANCY: Category B, caution in nursing.

MECHANISM OF ACTION: Macrolide antibiotic; inhibits protein synthesis by binding 50S ribosomal subunits of susceptible organisms.

PHARMACOKINETICS: Absorption: (PO) readily absorbed. **Distribution:** Largely bound to plasma proteins. Crosses blood-brain barrier, placenta, and breast milk. Diffuses into most bodily fluids. **Elimination:** Biliary and urinary excretion ($<5\%$).

ERYTHROCIN RX
erythromycin stearate (Abbott)

THERAPEUTIC CLASS: Macrolide

INDICATIONS: Treatment of mild to moderate upper/lower respiratory tract, and skin and skin structure infections, listeriosis, pertussis, diphtheria, erythrasma, intestinal amebiasis, acute pelvic inflammatory disease (PID) (*N.gonorrhea*), primary syphilis (if PCN allergy), Legionnaires' disease, chlamydial infections (eg, newborn conjunctivitis, pneumonia of infancy, urogenital infections during pregnancy or urethral, endocervical, or rectal infections when tetracyclines are contraindicated or not tolerated), and nongonococcal urethritis caused by susceptible strains of microorganisms. Prophylaxis of initial and recurrent attacks of rheumatic fever if PCN allergy.

DOSAGE: *Adults:* Usual: 250mg q6h or 500mg q12h without food. Max: 4g/day. Treat strep infections for at least 10 days. Streptococcal Infection Long-Term Prophylaxis in Rheumatic Fever: 250mg bid. Chlamydial Urogenital Infection During Pregnancy: 500mg qid or 666mg q8h for at least 7 days or 500mg q12h, 333mg q8h, or 250mg qid for at least 14 days. Urethral/Endocervical/Rectal Chlamydial Infections and Nongonococcal Urethritis: 500mg qid or 666mg q8h for at least 7 days. Primary Syphilis: 30-40g in divided doses over 10-15 days. Acute PID: 500mg (erythromycin lactobionate) IV q6h for 3 days, then 500mg PO q12h or 333mg PO q8h for 7 days. Intestinal Amebiasis: 500mg q12h, 333mg q8h, or 250mg q6h for 10-14 days. Pertussis: 40-50mg/kg/day in divided doses for 5-14 days. Legionnaires' Disease: 1-4g/day in divided doses.

Pediatrics: Usual: 30-50mg/kg/day in divided doses without food. Severe Infections: May double dose. Max: 4g/day. Treat strep infections for at least 10 days. Chlamydial Conjunctivitis of Newborns/Chlamydia Pneumonia in Infancy: (Sus) 12.5mg/kg qid for 2 weeks and 3 weeks, respectively. Intestinal Amebiasis: 30-50mg/kg/day in divided doses for 10-14 days.

HOW SUPPLIED: Tab: 250mg, 500mg

CONTRAINDICATIONS: Concomitant terfenadine, astenizole, pimozide, or cisapride.

WARNINGS/PRECAUTIONS: Hepatic dysfunction, pseudomembranous colitis reported. Caution with impaired hepatic function.

ADVERSE REACTIONS: NV, abdominal pain, diarrhea, anorexia, abnormal LFTs, superinfection (prolonged use).

INTERACTIONS: See Contraindications. Rhabdomyolysis reported with lovastatin. May increase levels of theophylline, digoxin, drugs metabolized by CYP450 (eg, carbamazepine, cyclosporine, phenytoin, etc). Increases effects of oral anticoagulants, triazolam. Risk of acute ergot toxicity with ergotamine or dihydroergotamine. May increase AUC of sildenafil; consider dose reduction of sildenafil.

PREGNANCY: Category B, caution in nursing.

MECHANISM OF ACTION: Macrolide; inhibits protein synthesis by binding 50S ribosomal subunits of susceptible organisms.

PHARMACOKINETICS: Absorption: (PO) Readily absorbed. **Distribution:** Largely bound to plasma proteins; crosses placenta, blood-brain barrier, and is excreted in breast milk. **Metabolism:** Liver via CYP3A. **Elimination:** Bile and urine (<5% unchanged).

ERYTHROMYCIN BASE

RX

erythromycin (Various)

THERAPEUTIC CLASS: Macrolide

INDICATIONS: Treatment of mild to moderate upper/lower respiratory tract and skin and skin structure infections, listeriosis, pertussis, diphtheria, erythrasma, intestinal amebiasis, acute pelvic inflammatory disease (PID) (*N.gonorrhea*), primary syphilis (if PCN allergy), Legionnaires' disease, chlamydial infections (eg, newborn conjunctivitis, pneumonia of infancy, urogenital infections during pregnancy or urethral, endocervical, or rectal infections when tetracyclines are contraindicated or not tolerated), and nongonococcal urethritis caused by susceptible strains of microorganisms. Prophylaxis of initial and recurrent attacks of rheumatic fever if PCN allergy.

DOSAGE: *Adults:* Usual: 250mg qid or 500mg q12h without food. Max: 4g/day. Treat strep infections for at least 10 days. Streptococcal Infection Long-Term Prophylaxis of Rheumatic Fever: 250mg bid. Chlamydial Urogenital Infection During Pregnancy: 500mg qid for at least 7 days or 500mg q12h or 250mg qid for at least 14 days. Urethral/Endocervical/Rectal Chlamydial Infections and Nongonococcal Urethritis: 500mg qid for at least 7 days. Primary Syphilis: 30-40g in divided doses over 10-15 days. Acute PID: 500mg (erythromycin lactobionate) IV q6h for 3 days, then 500mg PO q12h for 7 days. Intestinal Amebiasis: 500mg q12h or 250mg q6h for 10-14 days. Pertussis: 40-50mg/kg/day in divided doses for 5-14 days. Legionnaires' Disease: 1-4g/day in divided doses.
Pediatrics: Usual: 30-50mg/kg/day in divided doses without food. Severe Infections: May double dose. Max: 4g/day. Treat strep infections for at least 10 days. Streptococcal Infection Long-Term Prophylaxis of Rheumatic Fever: 250mg bid. Chlamydial Conjunctivitis of Newborns/Chlamydial Pneumonia in Infancy: (Sus) 12.5mg/kg qid for 2 weeks and 3 weeks, respectively. Intestinal Amebiasis: 30-50mg/kg/day in divided doses for 10-14 days.

HOW SUPPLIED: Tab: 250mg, 500mg

CONTRAINDICATIONS: Concomitant terfenadine, astemizole, pimozide, or cisapride.

WARNINGS/PRECAUTIONS: Pseudomembranous colitis, hepatic dysfunction reported. Caution with impaired hepatic function. May aggravate weakness of patients with myasthenia gravis.

ADVERSE REACTIONS: NV, abdominal pain, diarrhea, anorexia, abnormal LFTs, allergic reactions, superinfection (prolonged use).

INTERACTIONS: See Contraindications. Rhabdomyolysis reported with lovastatin. May increase levels of theophylline, digoxin, drugs metabolized by CYP450 (eg, carbamazepine, cyclosporine, phenytoin, etc). Increases effects of oral anticoagulants, triazolam. Risk of acute ergot toxicity with ergotamine or dihydroergotamine. May increase AUC of sildenafil; consider dose reduction of sildenafil.

PREGNANCY: Category B, caution in nursing.

MECHANISM OF ACTION: Macrolide; inhibits protein synthesis by binding 50S ribosomal subunits of susceptible organisms.

PHARMACOKINETICS: Absorption: (PO) readily absorbed. **Distribution:** Largely bound to plasma proteins. Crosses blood-brain barrier, placenta, breast milk. Diffuses into most body fluids. **Elimination:** Bile, urine (<5% unchanged).

ERYTHROMYCIN DELAYED-RELEASE
erythromycin (Various)

RX

THERAPEUTIC CLASS: Macrolide

INDICATIONS: Treatment of mild to moderate upper/lower respiratory tract and skin and skin structure infections, listeriosis, pertussis, diphtheria, erythrasma, intestinal amebiasis, acute pelvic inflammatory disease (PID) (*N.gonorrhea*), primary syphilis (if PCN allergy), Legionnaires' disease, chlamydial infections (eg, newborn conjunctivitis, pneumonia of infancy, urogenital infections during pregnancy, or urethral, endocervical, or rectal infections when tetracyclines are contraindicated or not tolerated), and nongonococcal urethritis caused by susceptible strains of microorganisms. Prophylaxis of initial and recurrent attacks of rheumatic fever if PCN allergy.

DOSAGE: *Adults:* Usual: 250mg q6h or 500mg q12h without food. Max: 4g/day. Treat strep infections for 10 days. Streptococcal Infection Prophylaxis with Rheumatic Heart Disease: 250mg bid. Primary Syphilis: 30-40g in divided doses over 10-15 days. Intestinal Amebiasis: 250mg q6h for 10-14 days. Legionnaires' Disease: 1-4g/day in divided doses. Chlamydial Urogenital Infection During Pregnancy: 500mg qid for 7 days or 250mg qid for 14 days. Urethral/Endocervical/Rectal Chlamydial Infections and Nongonococcal Urethritis: 500mg qid for at least 7 days. Pertussis: 40-50mg/kg/day in divided doses for 5-14 days. Acute PID: 500mg (erythromycin lactobionate) IV q6h for 3 days, then 250mg PO q6h for 7 days.
Pediatrics: Usual: 30-50mg/kg/day in divided doses without food. Severe Infections: May double dose. Max: 4g/day. Treat strep infections for 10 days. Streptococcal Infection Prophylaxis with Rheumatic Heart Disease: 250mg bid. Intestinal Amebiasis: 30-50mg/kg/day in divided doses for 10-14 days.

HOW SUPPLIED: Cap, Delayed-Release: 250mg

CONTRAINDICATIONS: Concomitant terfenadine, astenizole, pimozide, or cisapride.

WARNINGS/PRECAUTIONS: Hepatic dysfunction and pseudomembranous colitis reported. May aggravate weakness of patients with myasthenia gravis.

ADVERSE REACTIONS: NV, abdominal pain, diarrhea, anorexia, hepatic dysfunction, abnormal LFTs, superinfection (prolonged use).

INTERACTIONS: See Contraindications. Rhabdomyolysis reported with lovastatin. May increase levels of theophylline, digoxin, drugs metabolized by CYP450 (eg, carbamazepine, cyclosporine, phenytoin, etc). Increases effects of oral anticoagulants, triazolam. Risk of acute ergot toxicity with ergotamine or dihydroergotamine. Extreme caution with terfenadine.

PREGNANCY: Category B, caution in nursing.

MECHANISM OF ACTION: Macrolide; inhibits protein synthesis by binding 50S ribosomal subunits of susceptible organisms.

PHARMACOKINETICS: Absorption: (PO) readily absorbed; C_{max}=1.13-1.68mcg/mL; T_{max}=3 hrs. **Distribution:** Largely bound to plasma proteins; diffuses into most bodily fluids; crosses blood-brain barrier, placenta, and breast milk. **Elimination:** Bile, urine (<5% unchanged).

ERYTHROMYCIN OPHTHALMIC
erythromycin (Various)

RX

THERAPEUTIC CLASS: Macrolide

INDICATIONS: Superficial ocular infections of the conjunctiva and/or cornea. Prophylaxis of ophthalmia neonatorum due to *N.gonorrhoeae* or *C.trachomatis*.

DOSAGE: *Adults:* Superficial Ocular Infections: Apply 1cm to eye up to 6x/day, depending on severity. Do not flush ointment from eye.
Pediatrics: Superficial Ocular Infections: Apply 1 cm to eye up to 6 times/day, depending on severity. Neonatal Gonococcal or Chlamydial Ophthalmia Prophylaxis: Apply 1 cm into lower conjunctival sac. Do not flush oint from eye.

HOW SUPPLIED: Oint: 5mg/g (1g, 3.5g)

ADVERSE REACTIONS: Minor ocular irritations, redness, hypersensitivity reactions, superinfection (prolonged use).

PREGNANCY: Category B, caution in nursing.

MECHANISM OF ACTION: Macrolide; binds to 50S ribosomal subunits of susceptible organisms and inhibits protein synthesis

ESGIC
acetaminophen - butalbital - caffeine (Forest)

RX

THERAPEUTIC CLASS: Barbiturate/analgesic

INDICATIONS: Tension or muscle contraction headaches.

DOSAGE: *Adults:* 1-2 caps/tabs q4h prn. Max: 6 caps/tabs/day.
Pediatrics: ≥12 yrs: 1-2 caps/tabs q4h prn. Max: 6 caps/tabs/day.

HOW SUPPLIED: Cap/Tab: (Butalbital-APAP-Caffeine) 50mg-325mg-40mg* *scored

CONTRAINDICATIONS: Porphyria.

WARNINGS/PRECAUTIONS: May be habit-forming; potential for abuse. Not for long-term use. Caution in elderly, debilitated, severe renal or hepatic impairment, acute abdominal conditions, suicidal tendencies, history of drug abuse.

ADVERSE REACTIONS: Drowsiness, lightheadedness, dizziness, sedation, SOB, NV, abdominal pain, intoxicated feeling.

INTERACTIONS: Enhanced CNS effects with MAOIs. May enhance CNS depressant effects of other narcotic analgesics, alcohol, general anesthetics, tranquilizers, sedative hypnotics, or other CNS depressants.

PREGNANCY: Category C, not for use in nursing.

MECHANISM OF ACTION: Butalbital: Short to intermediate acting barbiturate. Acetaminophen: Nonopiate, nonsalicylate analgesic, antipyretic. Caffeine: CNS stimulant.

PHARMACOKINETICS: Absorption: APAP, caffeine: Rapid. **Distribution:** Butalbital: Plasma protein binding (45%); crosses placenta, found in breast milk. Caffeine: Found in breast milk. **Metabolism:** APAP: Conjugation. Caffeine: Biotransformation. **Elimination:** Butalbital: Urine (3.6%); $T_{1/2}$=35 hrs. APAP: Urine; $T_{1/2}$=1.25-3 hrs. Caffeine: Urine (3%); $T_{1/2}$=3 hrs.

ESGIC-PLUS
acetaminophen - butalbital - caffeine (Forest)

RX

THERAPEUTIC CLASS: Barbiturate/analgesic

INDICATIONS: Tension or muscle contraction headaches.

DOSAGE: *Adults:* 1 cap/tab q4h prn. Max: 6 caps/tabs/day.
Pediatrics: ≥12 yrs: 1 cap/tab q4h prn. Max: 6 caps/tabs/day.

HOW SUPPLIED: Cap/Tab: (Butalbital-APAP-Caffeine) 50mg-500mg-40mg* *scored

CONTRAINDICATIONS: Porphyria.

WARNINGS/PRECAUTIONS: May be habit-forming; potential for abuse. Not for long-term use. Caution in elderly, debilitated, severe renal or hepatic impairment, acute abdominal conditions, suicidal tendencies, history of drug abuse.

ADVERSE REACTIONS: Drowsiness, lightheadedness, dizziness, sedation, SOB, NV, abdominal pain, intoxicated feeling.

INTERACTIONS: Enhanced CNS effects with MAOIs. May enhance CNS depressant effects of other narcotic analgesics, alcohol, general anesthetics, tranquilizers, sedative hypnotics, or other CNS depressants.

PREGNANCY: Category C, not for use in nursing.

MECHANISM OF ACTION: Butalbital: Short to intermediate acting barbiturate. Acetaminophen: Nonopiate, nonsalicylate analgesic, antipyretic. Caffeine: CNS stimulant.

PHARMACOKINETICS: Absorption: APAP, caffeine: Rapid. **Distribution:** Butalbital: Plasma protein binding (45%); crosses placenta; found in breast milk. Caffeine: Found in breast milk. **Metabolism:** APAP: Conjugation. Caffeine: Biotransformation. **Elimination:** Butalbital: Urine (3.6%); $T_{1/2}$=35 hrs. APAP: Urine; $T_{1/2}$=1.25-3 hrs. Caffeine: Urine (3%); $T_{1/2}$=3 hrs.

ESKALITH   RX
lithium carbonate (GlaxoSmithKline)

| Lithium toxicity is related to serum levels, and can occur at doses close to therapeutic levels. |

OTHER BRAND NAME: Eskalith CR (GlaxoSmithKline)

THERAPEUTIC CLASS: Antimanic agent

INDICATIONS: Treatment of manic episodes of manic-depressive illness.

DOSAGE: *Adults:* (Cap) 300mg tid-qid. (Tab, Extended-Release) 450mg q12h. Monitor every 1-2 weeks and adjust dose if needed. When stable, monitor every 2 months to achieve levels of 0.6-1.2mEq/L. Maint: 900-1200mg/day. Acute Mania: 1800mg/day in divided doses. Monitor levels twice weekly to achieve 1-1.5mEq/L. When switching to extended-release tabs, give same total daily dose when possible.
Pediatrics: ≥12 yrs: (Cap) 300mg tid-qid. (Tab, Extended-Release) 450mg q12h. Monitor every 1-2 weeks and adjust dose if needed. When stable, monitor every 2 months to achieve levels of 0.6-1.2 mEq/L. Maint: 900-1200mg/day. Acute Mania: 1800mg/day in divided doses. Monitor levels twice weekly to achieve 1-1.5mEq/L. When switching to extended-release tabs, give same total daily dose when possible.

HOW SUPPLIED: Cap: (Eskalith) 300mg; Tab, Extended-Release: (Eskalith CR) 450mg*
*scored

WARNINGS/PRECAUTIONS: Avoid with significant renal or cardiovascular disease, severe debilitation, dehydration, or sodium depletion. Risk of encephalopathic syndrome (eg, weakness, lethargy, fever, tremulousness, confusion, EPS); d/c therapy. Maintain normal diet, adequate salt/fluid intake. Reduce dose or d/c with sweating, diarrhea, infection with elevated temperatures. Caution with hypothyroidism; may need supplemental therapy. Chronic therapy associated with diminution of renal concentrating ability, glomerular and interstitial fibrosis, and nephron atrophy.

ADVERSE REACTIONS: Fine hand tremor, polyuria, mild thirst, nausea, general discomfort, diarrhea, vomiting, drowsiness, muscular weakness.

INTERACTIONS: Increased risk of neurotoxicity with CCBs. Increased risk of toxicity with diuretics, metronidazole. Increased plasma levels with indomethacin, piroxicam, other NSAIDs, COX-2 inhibitors, ACE inhibitors, angiotensin II receptor antagonists. Caution with SSRIs. Decreased levels with acetazolamide, urea, xanthine agents, alkalinizing agents. Interacts with methyldopa, phenytoin, carbamazepine. May prolong effects of neuromuscular blockers.

PREGNANCY: Safety in pregnancy not known, not for use in nursing.

MECHANISM OF ACTION: Not established; suspected to alter sodium transport in nerve and muscle cells and effect a shift toward intraneuronal metabolism of catecholamines.

PHARMACOKINETICS: Distribution: Found in breast milk. **Elimination:** Urine (primary), feces (insignificant); $T_{1/2}$=24 hrs.

ESTROSTEP FE   RX
ethinyl estradiol - norethindrone acetate (Warner Chilcott)

THERAPEUTIC CLASS: Estrogen/progestogen combination

INDICATIONS: Prevention of pregnancy. Treatment of acne vulgaris in females ≥15 yrs who want contraception (for at least 6 months), have achieved menarche, and are unresponsive to topical acne agents.

DOSAGE: *Adults:* Contraception/Acne: 1 tab qd for 28 days, then repeat. Start 1st Sunday after menses begin or the 1st day of menses.
Pediatrics: ≥15 yrs: Contraception (Postpubertal Adolescents)/Acne: 1 tab qd for 28 days, then repeat. Start 1st Sunday after menses begins or the 1st day of menses.

HOW SUPPLIED: Tab: (Ethinyl Estradiol-Norethindrone) 0.035mg-1mg, 0.030mg-1mg, 0.020mg-1mg and 75mg ferrous fumarate

CONTRAINDICATIONS: Thrombophlebitis, history of DVT, active or history of thromboembolic disorders, pregnancy, cerebrovascular disease, CAD, undiagnosed abnormal genital bleeding, cholestatic jaundice of pregnancy, jaundice with prior pill use, hepatic adenoma or carcinoma, breast carcinoma, endometrium or other estrogen-dependent neoplasia.

WARNINGS/PRECAUTIONS: Cigarette smoking increases risk of serious cardiovascular side effects. This risk increases with age (especially >35 yrs) and heavy smoking. Increased risk of MI, vascular disease, thromboembolism, stroke, and gallbladder disease. Retinal thrombosis, hepatic neoplasia reported. May cause glucose intolerance. May increase BP, elevate LDL levels or cause other lipid changes, fluid retention, breakthrough bleeding, and spotting. May cause or exacerbate migraine. May develop visual changes with contact lenses. Increased risk of MI with HTN, hyperlipidemia, obesity, and diabetes. D/C if jaundice, significant depression, or ophthalmic irregularities develop. Perform annual physical exam. Use before menarche is not indicated. May affect certain endocrine, LFTs, and blood components.

ADVERSE REACTIONS: Nausea, vomiting, breakthrough bleeding, spotting, amenorrhea, migraine, depression, vaginal candidiasis, edema, weight changes.

INTERACTIONS: Reduced effects, increased breakthrough bleeding, and menstrual irregularities with rifampin, barbiturates, phenylbutazone, phenytoin, carbamazepine, St. John's wort, and possibly with griseofulvin, ampicillin, and tetracyclines. Increased plasma levels with atorvastatin. Ascorbic acid and APAP may increase plasma levels. Decreased plasma levels of APAP. Increased clearance of temazepam, salicylic acid, morphine, and clofibric acid. Increased plasma levels of cyclosporine, prednisolone, and theophylline.

PREGNANCY: Category X; not for use in nursing.

MECHANISM OF ACTION: Estrogen/progestogen oral contraceptive; acts by suppressing gonadotropins, inhibiting ovulation, and causing other alterations, including changes in the cervical mucus (increasing difficulty of sperm entry into the uterus) and the endometrium (reducing likelihood of implantation).

PHARMACOKINETICS: Absorption: Rapid and complete. Absolute bioavailability: Norethindrone (64%), ethinyl estradiol (43%); T_{max}=1-2 hrs. **Distribution:** V_d=2-4L/kg; plasma protein binding (>95%). **Metabolism:** Norethindrone: Extensive; reduction, sulfate/glucuronide conjugation. Ethinyl estradiol: CYP3A4; oxidation, conjugation. **Elimination:** Norethindrone: $T_{1/2}$=13 hrs. Ethinyl estradiol: Urine, feces; $T_{1/2}$=19 hrs.

ETODOLAC EXTENDED-RELEASE   RX
etodolac (Various)

> NSAIDs may cause an increased risk of serious cardiovascular thrombotic events, MI, stroke and serious GI adverse events including bleeding, ulceration, and perforation of the stomach or intestines. Contraindicated for the treatment of perioperative pain in the setting of coronary artery bypass graft (CABG) surgery.

THERAPEUTIC CLASS: NSAID

INDICATIONS: Relief of signs and symptoms of osteoarthritis (OA), rheumatoid arthritis (RA), and juvenile rheumatoid arthritis (JRA).

DOSAGE: *Adults:* Usual: 400-1000mg qd. Max: 1200mg/day.
Pediatrics: 6-16 yrs: JRA: >60kg: 1000mg/day. 46-60kg: 800mg/day. 31-45kg: 600mg/day. 20-30kg: 400mg/day.

HOW SUPPLIED: Tab, Extended-Release: 400mg, 500mg, 600mg

CONTRAINDICATIONS: ASA or other NSAID allergy that precipitates asthma, urticaria, or allergic reaction. Treatment of perioperative pain in the setting of CABG surgery.

WARNINGS/PRECAUTIONS: May lead to onset of new HTN or worsening of pre-existing HTN; monitor BP closely. Fluid retention and edema reported; caution with fluid retention or heart failure. Renal papillary necrosis and other renal injury reported after long-term use. Not recommended for use with advanced renal disease; if therapy must be initiated, monitor renal function. Anaphylactoid reactions may occur. May cause serious skin adverse events (eg, exfoliative dermatitis, Stevens-Johnson syndrome, and toxic epidermal necrolysis). Avoid in late pregnancy; may cause premature closure of ductus arteriosis. May cause elevations of LFTs; d/c if liver disease develops or systemic manifestations occur. Caution in elderly. Anemia may occur; with long-term use, monitor Hgb/Hct if signs or symptoms of anemia develop. May inhibit platelet aggregation and prolong bleeding time; monitor with coagulation disorders. Caution with asthma and avoid with ASA-sensitive asthma.

ADVERSE REACTIONS: Dyspepsia, abdominal pain, diarrhea, flatulence, NV, constipation, GI ulcers, gross bleeding/perforation.

INTERACTIONS: May elevate digoxin, lithium, and methotrexate serum levels. May enhance nephrotoxicity associated with cyclosporine. Avoid with phenylbutazone. Increased adverse effect potential with ASA. Caution with warfarin. May decrease antihypertensive effects with ACE inhibitors. May reduce natriuretic effect of furosemide and thiazides.

PREGNANCY: Category C, not for use in nursing.

MECHANISM OF ACTION: NSAID; inhibits prostaglandin synthetase; exhibits anti-inflammatory, analgesic, and antipyretic activities.

PHARMACOKINETICS: Absorption: T_{max}=6 hrs. **Distribution:** V_d=566mL/kg; plasma protein binding (99%). **Metabolism:** Hydroxylation, glucuronidation. **Elimination:** Urine, feces; $T_{1/2}$=8.4 hrs.

EVOCLIN   RX
clindamycin phosphate (Stiefel)

THERAPEUTIC CLASS: Lincomycin derivative

INDICATIONS: Treatment of acne vulgaris.

DOSAGE: *Adults*: Apply to affected area once daily.
Pediatrics: ≥12 yrs: Apply to affected area once daily.

HOW SUPPLIED: Foam: 1% (50g, 100g)

CONTRAINDICATIONS: History of regional enteritis, ulcerative colitis, or antibiotic-associated colitis.

WARNINGS/PRECAUTIONS: Diarrhea, bloody diarrhea, and colitis (including pseudomembranous colitis) reported with use of topical and systemic clindamycin. D/C if significant diarrhea occurs. Caution in atopic individuals. Avoid eye contact.

ADVERSE REACTIONS: Headache, application site burning/pruritus/dryness, pseudomembranous colitis (rare).

INTERACTIONS: May potentiate neuromuscular blockers; caution with concomitant use.

PREGNANCY: Category B, caution in nursing.

MECHANISM OF ACTION: Lincomycin derivative; shown to have activity against *Propionibacterium acnes*, which is associated with acne vulgaris.

PHARMACOKINETICS: Distribution: Orally and parenterally administered clindamycin has been found in breast milk. **Metabolism:** Liver. **Elimination:** Urine (0.024% total dose). $T_{1/2}$=2.4-3 hr.

EXJADE   RX
deferasirox (Novartis)

THERAPEUTIC CLASS: Iron-chelating agent

INDICATIONS: Treatment of chronic iron overload due to blood transfusions (transfusional hemosiderosis).

DOSAGE: *Adults*: Initial: 20mg/kg/day. Titrate: May increase 5-10mg/kg q 3-6 months. Max: 30mg/kg/day. Take on empty stomach at least 30 min before food at same time each day. Tabs should be completely dispersed in 3.5oz of liquid if dose <1g or in 7oz if dose >1g. If serum ferritin falls below 500µg/L, consider interrupting therapy.
Pediatrics: ≥2 yrs: Initial: 20mg/kg/day. Titrate: May increase 5-10mg/kg q 3-6 months. Max: 30mg/kg/day. Take on empty stomach at least 30 min before food at same time each day. Tabs should be completely dispersed in 3.5oz of liquid if dose <1g or in 7oz if dose >1g. If serum ferritin falls below 500µg/L, consider interrupting therapy.

HOW SUPPLIED: Tab: 125mg, 250mg, 500mg

WARNINGS/PRECAUTIONS: Assess SCr before therapy and monitor monthly therafter; reduce dose, interrupt or d/c therapy if necessary. Intermittent proteinuria reported; monitor closely. Acute renal failure and cytopenias reported. Use caution and monitor SCr in those at risk of complications, having preexisting renal or comorbid conditions, receiving medicinal products that depress renal function, or elderly. Caution with pre-existing hematologic disorders; monitor CBC regularly. Hepatic abnormalities, increased transaminases reported; monitor LFTs monthly; modify dose for severe or persistent elevations. Reports of auditory (high frequency hearing loss, decreased hearing) and ocular distrubances (lens opacities, cataracts, elevated IOP, retinal disorders); initial and yearly auditory and ophthalmic testing recommended. Reports of skin rashes; d/c if severe, may reinitiate with short period of oral steriod.

ADVERSE REACTIONS: Diarrhea, NV, headache, abdominal pain, pyrexia, cough, increased SCr, rash, b-thalassemia, rare anemias, sicke cell disease.

INTERACTIONS: Avoid with aluminum-containing antacids or other iron chelator therapies.

PREGNANCY: Category B, caution in nursing.

MECHANISM OF ACTION: Iron chelating agent.

PHARMACOKINETICS: Absorption: T_{max}=1.5-4 hrs. **Distribution:**V_d=14.37; plasma protein binding (99%). **Metabolism:** Glucoronidation, deconjugation. **Elimination:** Feces (84%), urine (8%); $T_{1/2}$=8-16 hrs.

EXTINA   RX
ketoconazole (Stiefel)

THERAPEUTIC CLASS: Azole antifungal

INDICATIONS: Topical treatment of seborrheic dermatitis in immunocompetent patients ≥12 yrs of age.

DOSAGE: *Adults:* Apply to affected area(s) bid for 4 weeks.
Pediatrics: ≥12 yrs: Apply to affected area(s) bid for 4 weeks.

HOW SUPPLIED: Foam: 2% (50g, 100g)

WARNINGS/PRECAUTIONS: Contact sensitization, including photoallergenicity. Contents are flammable.

ADVERSE REACTIONS: Application site burning, dryness, erythema, irritation, paresthesia, pruritis, rash, warmth, contact sensitization.

PREGNANCY: Category C, caution in nursing.

MECHANISM OF ACTION: Antifungal agent; MOA not established. Inhibits the synthesis of ergosterol, a key sterol in the cell membrane of *Malassezia furfur.*

FELBATOL   RX
felbamate (MedPointe)

> Associated with aplastic anemia and fatal hepatic failure. Monitor blood, LFTs. Avoid in history of hepatic dysfunction.

THERAPEUTIC CLASS: Dicarbamate anticonvulsant

INDICATIONS: Not for first line therapy. Monotherapy or adjunct therapy in partial seizures with and without generalization in adults. Adjunct therapy for partial and generalized seizures with Lennox-Gastaut syndrome in children.

DOSAGE: *Adults:* Initial Monotherapy: 300mg qid or 400mg tid. Titrate: Increase by 600mg every 2 weeks to 2.4g/day. Max: 3.6g/day. Initial Monotherapy Conversion/Adjunct Therapy: 300mg qid or 400mg tid while reducing present AED (see literature). Titrate: For conversion, increase at week 2 to 2.4g/day, at week 3 up to 3.6g/day. Adjunct Therapy: Increase by 1.2g/day every week up to 3.6mg/day. Renal Dysfunction: May need to reduce dose with concomitant AEDs.
Pediatrics: ≥14 yrs: Initial Monotherapy: 300mg qid or 400mg tid. Titrate: Increase by 600mg every 2 weeks to 2.4g/day. Max: 3.6g/day. Initial Monotherapy Conversion/Adjunct Therapy: 300mg qid or 400mg tid while reducing present AED (see literature).

Titrate: For conversion, increase at week 2 to 2.4g/day, at week 3 up to 3.6g/day. Adjunct Therapy: Increase by 1.2g/day every week up to 3.6g/day. 2-14 yrs: Lennox-Gastaut Adjunct Therapy: Initial: 15mg/kg/day in 3-4 divided doses. Titrate: Increase by 15mg/kg/day every week to 45mg/kg/day. Renal Dysfunction: May need to reduce dose with concomitant AEDs.

HOW SUPPLIED: Sus: 600mg/5mL (240mL, 960mL); Tab: 400mg*, 600mg* *scored

CONTRAINDICATIONS: History of blood dyscrasias, hepatic dysfunction.

WARNINGS/PRECAUTIONS: Avoid abrupt discontinuation. Caution with renal dysfunction. Obtain written, informed consent. Obtain full hematologic evaluations and LFTs before, during, and after discontinuation. D/C if bone marrow depression or liver abnormalities occur.

ADVERSE REACTIONS: Anorexia, vomiting, insomnia, nausea, headache, anemias, hepatic failure.

INTERACTIONS: Increases plasma levels of phenytoin, valproate, active carbamazepine metabolite and phenobarbital. Decreases carbamazepine levels. Decreased felbamate levels with phenytoin, carbamazepine, and phenobarbital. Caution with OCs.

PREGNANCY: Category C, safety in nursing not known.

MECHANISM OF ACTION: Anticonvulsant; weak inhibitory effects on GABA-receptor binding and benzodiazepine receptor binding. Acts as an antagonist at the strychnine-insensitive glycine recognition site of the NMDA receptor-ionophore complex.

PHARMACOKINETICS: Absorption: Well-absorbed. **Distribution:** V_d=756mL/kg; plasma protein binding (22-25%). **Metabolism:** Parahydroxyfelbamate, 2-hydroxyfelbamate, felbamatemonocarbamate (metabolites, little activity). **Elimination:** Urine (40-50% unchanged); $T_{1/2}$=20-23 hrs.

FEOSOL
ferrous sulfate - iron carbonyl (GlaxoSmithKline Consumer)
OTC

THERAPEUTIC CLASS: Iron supplement

INDICATIONS: Treatment of iron deficiency and iron deficiency anemia.

DOSAGE: *Adults:* 1 tab qd with food.
Pediatrics: ≥12 yrs: 1 tab qd with food.

HOW SUPPLIED: Tab: Feosol Caplet (Iron Carbonyl) 50mg (45mg elemental iron), Feosol Tablet (Ferrous Sulfate) 200mg (65mg elemental iron)

WARNINGS/PRECAUTIONS: Keep product out of reach of children. Accidental overdose of iron-containing products is a leading cause of fatal poisoning in children <6 yrs.

ADVERSE REACTIONS: Nausea, GI disturbance, constipation, diarrhea.

INTERACTIONS: Decreases absorption of tetracycline; space dose by 2 hrs.

PREGNANCY: Safety in pregnancy and nursing not known.

FERO-GRAD-500
ferrous sulfate - vitamin C (Abbott)
OTC

THERAPEUTIC CLASS: Iron/vitamin

INDICATIONS: Iron supplementation.

DOSAGE: *Adults:* 1 tab qd.
Pediatrics: ≥4 yrs: 1 tab qd.

HOW SUPPLIED: Tab, Extended-Release: Ferrous Sulfate 105mg-Vitamin C 500mg

FERRLECIT
sodium ferric gluconate complex (Watson)
RX

THERAPEUTIC CLASS: Hematinic

INDICATIONS: Treatment of iron deficiency anemia in patients ≥6 yrs old undergoing chronic hemodialysis and receiving supplemental epoetin therapy.

DOSAGE: *Adults:* 10mL (125mg) as IV infusion (diluted) over 1 hr or as slow IV injection (undiluted) at a rate of up to 12.5mg/min. Minimum Cumulative Dose: 1g elemental iron over 8 sequential dialysis sessions.
Pediatrics: ≥6 yrs: 0.12mL/kg (1.5mg/kg) as IV infusion over 1 hr at 8 sequential dialysis sessions. Max: 125mg/dose.

HOW SUPPLIED: Inj: 62.5mg elemental iron/5mL

CONTRAINDICATIONS: Anemia not associated with iron deficiency. Iron overload.

WARNINGS/PRECAUTIONS: Hypersensitivity reactions and hypotension reported. Iron overload is more common in patients with hemoglobinopathies and other refractory anemia. Should not be administered to patients with iron overload. Contains benzyl alcohol; avoid in neonates.

ADVERSE REACTIONS: Injection site reactions, nausea, vomiting, diarrhea, hypotension, cramps, HTN, dizziness, dyspnea, abnormal erythrocytes, leg cramps, pain, chest pain.

PREGNANCY: Category B, caution in nursing.

MECHANISM OF ACTION: Hematinic; used to replete the total body content of iron, which is critical for normal Hgb synthesis to maintain oxygen transport.

PHARMACOKINETICS: Absorption: *Adults:* Parameters varied by different dosage. (62.5mg) AUC=17.5mg-h/L; (125mg) C_{max}=19mg/L; T_{max}=7 min; AUC=35.6mg-h/L. *Pediatrics:* (1.5mg/kg) C_{max}=12.9mg/L; T_{max}=2 hrs; AUC=95mg•h/L. (3mg/kg) C_{max}=22.8mg/L; T_{max}=2.5 hrs; AUC=170.9mg•h/L. **Distribution:** V_d=6L. **Elimination:** $T_{1/2}$=1 hr.

FEVERALL
acetaminophen (Alpharma)

OTC

THERAPEUTIC CLASS: Analgesic

INDICATIONS: Treatment of pain and fever in patients who cannot tolerate oral meds due to nausea and vomiting.

DOSAGE: *Pediatrics:* Insert sup rectally. 3-11 months: 80mg q6h. Max: 480mg/24 hrs. 12-36 months: 80mg q4h. Max: 480mg/24 hrs. 3-6 yrs: 120mg q4-6h. Max: 720mg/24 hrs. 6-12 yrs: 325mg q4-6h. Max: 2600mg/24 hrs.

HOW SUPPLIED: Sup: 80mg, 120mg, 325mg, 650mg

PREGNANCY: Safety in pregnancy or nursing not known.

FINEVIN
azelaic acid (Bayer Healthcare)

RX

THERAPEUTIC CLASS: Dicarboxylic acid antimicrobial

INDICATIONS: Mild-to-moderate inflammatory acne vulgaris.

DOSAGE: *Adults:* Wash and dry skin. Massage gently into affected area bid (am and pm).
Pediatrics: ≥12 yrs: Wash and dry skin. Massage gently into affected area bid (am and pm).

HOW SUPPLIED: Cre: 20% (30g, 50g)

WARNINGS/PRECAUTIONS: Hypopigmentation reported after use. Avoid the mouth, eyes, mucous membranes, occlusive dressings, or wrappings.

ADVERSE REACTIONS: Pruritus, burning, stinging, tingling.

PREGNANCY: Category B, caution in nursing.

FIORICET
acetaminophen - butalbital - caffeine (Watson)

RX

THERAPEUTIC CLASS: Barbiturate/analgesic

INDICATIONS: Tension or muscle contraction headaches.

DOSAGE: *Adults:* 1-2 tabs q4h prn. Max: 6 tabs/day. Not for extended use. *Pediatrics:* ≥12 yrs: 1-2 tabs q4h prn. Max: 6 tabs/day. Not for extended use.

HOW SUPPLIED: Tab: (Butalbital-APAP-Caffeine) 50mg-325mg-40mg

CONTRAINDICATIONS: Porphyria.

WARNINGS/PRECAUTIONS: May be habit forming. Not for extended use. Caution in elderly, debilitated, severe renal or hepatic impairment, acute abdominal conditions. Caution in mentally depressed and suicidal tendencies, history of drug abuse.

ADVERSE REACTIONS: Drowsiness, lightheadedness, dizziness, sedation, SOB, NV, abdominal pain, intoxicated feeling.

INTERACTIONS: Enhanced CNS effects with MAOIs. May enhance CNS depressant effects of other narcotic analgesics, alcohol, general anesthetics, tranquilizers, sedative hypnotics, or other CNS depressants.

PREGNANCY: Category C, not for use in nursing.

MECHANISM OF ACTION: Butalbital: Short to intermediate acting barbiturate. APAP: Nonopiate, nonsalicylate analgesic, antipyretic. Caffeine: CNS stimulant.

PHARMACOKINETICS: Absorption: Well absorbed (butalbital), rapid (APAP, caffeine). **Distribution:** Butalbital: Plasma protein binding (45%); found in breast milk; crosses placenta. Caffeine: Found in CNS, placenta, and breast milk. **Metabolism:** APAP: Liver (conjugation). Caffeine: Hepatic; 1-methylxanthine, 1-methyluric acid. **Elimination:** Butalbital: Urine (59-88% unchanged or metabolite); $T_{1/2}$=35 hrs. APAP: Urine (85% metabolite, unchanged); $T_{1/2}$=1.25-3 hrs. Caffeine: Urine 70% (3% unchanged); $T_{1/2}$=3 hrs.

FLAGYL

RX

metronidazole (G.D. Searle)

> **Metronidazole has been shown to be carcinogenic in mice and rats. Unnecessary use of the drug should be avoided.**

THERAPEUTIC CLASS: Nitroimidazole

INDICATIONS: Treatment of symptomatic/asymptomatic trichomoniasis, asymptomatic consorts, acute intestinal amebiasis, amebic liver abscess, and anaerobic bacterial infections (following IV metronidazole therapy for serious infections) caused by susceptible strains of microorganisms. Treatment of intra-abdominal, skin and skin structure, bone/joint, CNS, lower respiratory tract, and gynecologic infections, septicemia, and endocarditis caused by susceptible strains of microorganisms.

DOSAGE: *Adults:* Trichomoniasis (Female/Male Sex Partner): Seven-Day Treatment: (Cap/Tab) 375mg bid or 250mg tid for 7 days. One-Day Therapy: (Tab) 2g as single dose or in two divided doses of 1g each given in the same day. If repeat course needed, reconfirm diagnosis and allow 4-6 weeks between courses. Acute Intestinal Amebiasis: 750mg PO tid for 5-10 days. Amebic Liver Abscess: 500mg or 750mg PO tid for 5-10 days. Anaerobic Bacterial Infection: Usually IV therapy initially if serious. 7.5mg/kg PO q6h for 7-10 days or longer. Max: 4g/24 hrs. Elderly: Adjust dose based on serum levels. Hepatic Disease: Give lower dose cautiously; monitor levels. *Pediatrics:* Amebiasis: 35-50mg/kg/24 hrs given tid for 10 days.

HOW SUPPLIED: Cap: 375mg; Tab: 250mg, 500mg

CONTRAINDICATIONS: Treatment during 1st trimester of pregnancy.

WARNINGS/PRECAUTIONS: Seizures and peripheral neuropathy reported. D/C if abnormal neurological signs occur. Caution with severe hepatic impairment, blood dyscrasias, or CNS diseases. Monitor leukocytes before and after therapy.

ADVERSE REACTIONS: Seizures, peripheral neuropathy, NV, headache, anorexia, urticaria, rash, metallic taste, dysuria, vaginal candidiasis, dizziness, leukopenia.

INTERACTIONS: Avoid alcohol during and for 3 days after use. Avoid within 2 weeks of disulfiram use; increased possibility of psychotic reactions. May potentiate anticoagulant effects of warfarin; monitor PT. Increased elimination with phenytoin, phenobarbital and other hepatic enzyme inducers. May impair phenytoin clearance. Potentiated by cimetidine and other hepatic enzyme inhibitors. May increase lithium levels.

PREGNANCY: Category B, not for use in nursing.

MECHANISM OF ACTION: Nitroimidazole antibacterial; exerts effect in anaerobic environment. Possesses bactericidal, amebicidal, and trichomonacidal activity.

PHARMACOKINETICS: Absorption: (PO) Well absorbed. PO administration of variable doses resulted in different parameters. **Distribution:** Plasma protein binding (<20%); excreted in breast milk. **Metabolism:** Side-chain oxidation and glucuronide conjugation. **Elimination:** Urine (60-80%), feces (6-15%); $T_{1/2}$=8 hrs.

FLEET BISACODYL   OTC
bisacodyl (Fleet)

THERAPEUTIC CLASS: Stimulant laxative

INDICATIONS: Relief of occasional constipation. For bowel cleansing for X-ray and endoscopic exam. Laxative in postoperative, antepartum, or postpartum care.

DOSAGE: *Adults:* (Enema) Use 1 rectally single dose qd. (Sup) Insert 1 rectally qd. Retain for 15-20 min. (Tab) 2-3 tabs single dose qd. Swallow tabs whole; do not chew or crush. *Pediatrics:* ≥12 yrs: (Enema) Use 1 rectally single dose qd. (Sup) Insert 1 rectally qd. Retain for 15-20 min. (Tab) 2-3 tabs single dose qd. 6-11 yrs: (Sup) Insert 1/2 sup rectally qd. Retain for 15-20 min. (Tab) 1 tab qd. Swallow tabs whole; do not chew or crush.

HOW SUPPLIED: Enema: 10mg; Sup: 10mg; Tab, Delayed-Release: 5mg

WARNINGS/PRECAUTIONS: Do not use with nausea, vomiting, or abdominal pain. Rectal bleeding or failure to have a bowel movement after use may indicate a serious condition. Should not be used longer than 1 week.

ADVERSE REACTIONS: Abdominal discomfort, faintness, cramps.

INTERACTIONS: Do not administer tabs within 1 hr after taking an antacid, milk, or milk products.

PREGNANCY: Safety in pregnancy and nursing is not known.

FLEET GLYCERIN LAXATIVES   OTC
glycerin (Fleet)

THERAPEUTIC CLASS: Laxative

INDICATIONS: Relief of constipation.

DOSAGE: *Adults:* 1 enema (5.6g) or 1 suppository (2g or 3g) rectally. *Pediatrics:* 2-5 yrs: 1 enema (2.3g) or 1 suppository (1g) rectally. ≥ 6 yrs: 1 enema (5.6g) or 1 suppository (2g or 3g) rectally.

HOW SUPPLIED: Enema: (Babylax) 2.3g, (Liquid Glycerin) 5.6g; Sup: 1g, 2g, 3g

WARNINGS/PRECAUTIONS: Rectal irritation may occur. Do not use with nausea, vomiting, or abdominal pain. Rectal bleeding or failure to have a bowel movement after use may indicate a serious condition. Do not use longer than 1 week.

ADVERSE REACTIONS: Rectal discomfort, burning sensation.

PREGNANCY: Safety in pregnancy and nursing in not known.

FLEXERIL   RX
cyclobenzaprine HCl (McNeil Consumer)

THERAPEUTIC CLASS: Skeletal muscle relaxant (central-acting)

INDICATIONS: Relief of muscle spasm associated with acute, painful musculoskeletal conditions.

DOSAGE: *Adults:* Usual: 5mg tid. Titrate: May increase to 10mg tid. Mild Hepatic Dysfunction/Elderly: Initial: 5mg qd, then slowly increase. Moderate/Severe Hepatic Dysfunction: Avoid use. Treatment should not exceed 2-3 weeks. *Pediatrics:* ≥15 yrs: Usual: 5mg tid. Titrate: May increase to 10mg tid. Mild Hepatic Dysfunction/Elderly: Initial: 5mg qd, then slowly increase. Moderate/Severe Hepatic Dysfunction: Avoid use. Treatment should not exceed 2-3 weeks.

HOW SUPPLIED: Tab: 5mg, 10mg

CONTRAINDICATIONS: Acute recovery phase of MI, arrhythmias, heart block or conduction disturbances, CHF, hyperthyroidism, MAOI use during or within 14 days.

WARNINGS/PRECAUTIONS: Caution with history of urinary retention, angle-closure glaucoma, increased IOP, hepatic dysfunction. Caution in elderly due to increased risk of CNS effects. May produce arrhythmias, sinus tachycardia and conduction time prolongation. May impair mental/physical abilities.

ADVERSE REACTIONS: Drowsiness, dry mouth, headache, fatigue.

INTERACTIONS: Enhances effects of alcohol, barbiturates, and other CNS depressants. May block antihypertensive action of guanethidine and similar compounds. May enhance seizure risk with tramadol. Contraindicated with MAOIs. Caution with anticholinergic medication.

PREGNANCY: Category B, caution in nursing.

MECHANISM OF ACTION: Centrally acting skeletal muscle relaxant; relieves skeletal muscle spasm of local origin without interfering with muscle function; reduces tonic somatic motor activity by influencing both gamma and α motor systems.

PHARMACOKINETICS: Absorption: Oral bioavailability (33-55%). C_{max}=25.9ng/mL, AUC=177ng•hr/mL. **Metabolism:** Extensive; through N-demethylation pathway. Via CYP3A4, 1A2, and 2D6. **Elimination:** Urine (glucuronides); $T_{1/2}$=18 hrs.

FLONASE
fluticasone propionate (GlaxoSmithKline)

RX

THERAPEUTIC CLASS: Corticosteroid

INDICATIONS: Management of the nasal symptoms of seasonal and perennial allergic rhinitis, and nonallergic rhinitis.

DOSAGE: *Adults:* Initial: 2 sprays per nostril qd or 1 spray per nostril bid. Maint: 1 spray per nostril qd. May dose as 2 sprays per nostril qd as needed for seasonal allergic rhinitis.
Pediatrics: ≥4 yrs: Initial: 1 sprays per nostril qd. If inadequate response, may increase to 2 sprays per nostril. Maint: 1 spray per nostril qd. Max: 2 sprays per nostril/day. ≥12 yrs: May dose as 2 sprays per nostril qd as needed for seasonal allergic rhinitis.

HOW SUPPLIED: Spray: 50mcg/spray (16g)

WARNINGS/PRECAUTIONS: Risk of adrenal insufficiency and withdrawal symptoms when replacing systemic corticosteroids with a topical corticosteroids. Caution with active or quiescent TB, ocular herpes simplex, or untreated bacterial, fungal and systemic viral infections. Avoid with recent nasal trauma, surgery or septum ulcers. Risk for more severe/fatal course of infections (eg, chickenpox, measles); avoid exposure in patients who have not had disease or been properly immunized. Candida infection of nose and pharynx reported (rare). Potential for growth velocity reduction in pediatrics. Excessive use may cause signs of hypercorticism or HPA suppression.

ADVERSE REACTIONS: Headache, pharyngitis, epistaxis, nasal burning/irritation, asthma symptoms, nausea/vomiting, cough.

INTERACTIONS: Caution with ketoconazole or other potent CYP3A4 inhibitors, may increase serum fluticasone levels. Concomitant inhaled corticosteroids increases risk of hypercorticism and/or HPA axis suppression. Increased levels with ritonavir; avoid use.

PREGNANCY: Category C, caution in nursing.

MECHANISM OF ACTION: Glucocorticosteroid; not established. Acts as anti-inflammatory agent with wide range of effects on multiple cell types (eg, mast cells, eosinophils, macrophages, and lymphocytes) and mediators (eg, histamine, eicosanoids, leukotrienes, and cytokines) involved in inflammation.

PHARMACOKINETICS: Absorption: Absolute bioavailability (<2%), C_{max}=50pg/mL.

FLOVENT HFA
fluticasone propionate (GlaxoSmithKline)

RX

THERAPEUTIC CLASS: Corticosteroid

INDICATIONS: Maintenance treatment of asthma as prophylactic therapy in patients ≥4 years; to reduce or eliminate the need for oral corticosteroidal therapy.

DOSAGE: *Adults:* Previous Bronchodilator Only: Initial: 88mcg bid. Max: 440mcg bid. Previous Inhaled Corticosteroids: Initial: 88-220mcg bid. Max: 440mcg bid. Previous Oral Corticosteroids: Initial: 440mcg bid. Max: 880mcg bid. Reduce PO prednisone no faster than 2.5 to 5mg/day weekly, beginning at least 1 week after starting fluticasone. Rinse mouth after use.

Pediatrics: ≥12 yrs: Previous Bronchodilator Only: Initial: 88mcg bid. Max: 440mcg bid. Previous Inhaled Corticosteroids: Initial: 88-220mcg bid. Max: 440mcg bid. Previous Oral Corticosteroids: Initial: 440mcg bid. Max: 880mcg bid. 4-11 yrs: Initial/Max: 88mcg bid. Reduce PO prednisone no faster than 2.5 to 5mg/day weekly, beginning at least 1 week after starting fluticasone. Rinse mouth after use.

HOW SUPPLIED: MDI: 44mcg/inh (10.6g), 110mcg/inh (12g), 220mcg/inh (12g)

CONTRAINDICATIONS: Primary treatment of status asthmaticus or other acute asthma attacks.

WARNINGS/PRECAUTIONS: Deaths due to adrenal insufficiency have occurred with transfer from systemic corticosteroids to inhaled corticosteroids. Resume oral corticosteroids during stress or severe asthma attack. Wean slowly from systemic corticosteroid therapy. Observe for adrenal insufficiency, systemic corticosteroid withdrawal effects, hypercorticism, adrenal suppression (including adrenal crisis), reduction in growth velocity (children and adolescents). May increase susceptibility to infections. Not for acute bronchospasm. D/C if bronchospasm occurs after dosing. Caution with TB of respiratory tract; untreated systemic fungal, bacterial, viral or parasitic infections; or ocular herpes simplex. *Candida* infection of mouth and pharynx reported. Glaucoma, increased IOP and cataracts reported. Rare cases of eosinophilic conditions.

ADVERSE REACTIONS: Pharyngitis, cough, bronchitis, nasal congestion, sinusitis, dysphonia, oral candidiasis, upper respiratory infection, influenza, headache, nasal discharge, allergic rhinitis, fever, paradoxical bronchospasm.

INTERACTIONS: Increased levels with ritonavir; avoid use. Caution with ketoconazole and other potent CYP3A4 inhibitors; may increase serum fluticasone levels.

PREGNANCY: Category C, caution in nursing.

MECHANISM OF ACTION: Synthetic trifluorinated corticosteroid; possesses potent anti-inflammatory activity and inhibits multiple cell types involved in asthmatic response.

PHARMACOKINETICS: Absorption: Acts locally in lung. **Distribution:** V_d=4.2 L/kg; plasma protein binding (99%). **Metabolism:** Liver via CYP3A4. **Elimination:** Feces (primary), urine (<5%); $T_{1/2}$=7.8 hrs.

FLOXIN OTIC   RX

ofloxacin (Daiichi Sankyo)

OTHER BRAND NAME: Floxin Otic Singles (Daiichi Sankyo)

THERAPEUTIC CLASS: Fluoroquinolone

INDICATIONS: Otitis externa in patients ≥6 mos. Chronic suppurative otitis media in patients ≥12 yrs with perforated tympanic membranes. Acute otitis media in patients ≥1 yr with tympanostomy tubes.

DOSAGE: *Adults:* Otitis Externa: 10 drops or 2 single-dispensing containers (SDCs) once daily for 7 days. Chronic Suppurative Otitis Media with Perforated Tympanic Membrane: 10 drops or 2 SDCs bid for 14 days.

Pediatrics: Otitis Externa: 6 mos-13 yrs: 5 drops or 1 single-dispensing container (SDC) once daily for 7 days. ≥13 yrs: 10 drops or 2 SDCs once daily for 7 days. Chronic Suppurative Otitis Media with Perforated Tympanic Membrane: ≥12 yrs: 10 drops or 2 SDCs bid for 14 days. Acute Otitis Media with Tympanostomy Tubes: 1-12 yrs: 5 drops or 1 SDC bid for 10 days.

HOW SUPPLIED: Sol: 0.3% (5mL, 10mL), (Singles) 0.3% (20^s)

WARNINGS/PRECAUTIONS: D/C if hypersensitivity reaction occurs. Re-evaluate if no improvement after one week.

ADVERSE REACTIONS: Pruritus, application site reaction, taste perversion.

PREGNANCY: Category C, not for use in nursing.

MECHANISM OF ACTION: Fluoroquinilone; exerts antibacterial activity; inhibits DNA gyrase (a bacterial topoisomerase), an essential enzyme which controls DNA topology and assists in DNA replication, repair, deactivation, and transcription.

PHARMACOKINETICS: Absorption: Perforated tympanic membrane; C_{max}=10ng/ml.

FLUMADINE
rimantadine HCl (Forest)

RX

THERAPEUTIC CLASS: Adamantane class antiviral

INDICATIONS: Prophylaxis and treatment of influenza A virus.

DOSAGE: *Adults:* Prophylaxis/Treatment: 100mg bid. Elderly/Severe Hepatic Dysfunction/CrCl ≤10mL/min: 100mg qd. Initiate treatment within 48 hrs of onset of symptoms. Treat for 7 days from initial onset of symptoms.
Pediatrics: Prophylaxis: 1-9 yrs: 5mg/kg qd. Max: 150mg qd. ≥10 yrs: 100mg bid.

HOW SUPPLIED: Syrup: 50mg/5mL (240mL); Tab: 100mg

WARNINGS/PRECAUTIONS: Caution with a history of epilepsy. D/C if seizures develop. Caution with renal or hepatic dysfunction.

ADVERSE REACTIONS: Insomnia, dizziness, nervousness, NV, anorexia, dry mouth, abdominal pain, asthenia.

INTERACTIONS: May be potentiated by cimetidine. APAP and ASA may decrease levels of rimantadine. Avoid use of Live Influenza Virus Vaccine within 2 weeks before or 48 hrs after use.

PREGNANCY: Category C, not for use in nursing.

MECHANISM OF ACTION: Antiviral; unknown, suspected to exert its inhibitory effect early in the viral replicative cycle, possibly inhibiting the uncoating of virus.

PHARMACOKINETICS: Absorption: C_{max}=74ng/mL; T_{max}=6 hrs. **Distribution:** Plasma protein binding (40%). **Metabolism:** Hepatic (extensive). **Elimination:** Urine (<25%); $T_{1/2}$=25.4 hrs.

FLUMIST
influenza virus vaccine live (MedImmune)

RX

THERAPEUTIC CLASS: Vaccine

INDICATIONS: Active immunization of individuals 2-49 years of age against influenza disease caused by influenza virus subtypes A and type B contained in the vaccine.

DOSAGE: *Adults:* ≤49 yrs: One 0.2mL (0.1mL per nostril) dose.
Pediatrics: ≥9 yrs: One 0.2mL (0.1mL per nostril) dose. 2-8 yrs: Not Previously Vaccinated With Influenza Vaccine: 0.2mL (0.1mL per nostril) for 2 doses at least 1 month apart. Previously Vaccinated With Influenza Vacine: One 0.2mL (0.1mL per nostril) dose.

HOW SUPPLIED: Nasal Spray: 0.2mL (10s)

CONTRAINDICATIONS: Parenteral use. Hypersensitivity to eggs or egg products. Children and adolescents 5-17 years of age receiving ASA or ASA-containing therapy. History of Guillain-Barre syndrome. Immune deficiency diseases such as combined immuno immunodeficiency, agammaglobulinemia, and thymic abnormalities, and conditions such as HIV infection, malignancy, leukemia, or lymphoma. Immunosuppressed or altered/compromised immune status due to treatment with systemic corticosteroids, alkylating drugs, antimetabolites, radiation, or other immunosuppressive therapies.

WARNINGS/PRECAUTIONS: Avoid with history of asthma or reactive airways disease, chronic disorders of the cardiovascular and pulmonary systems, second or third trimester of pregnancy, chronic metabolic diseases (including diabetes), renal dysfunction, hemoglobinopathies, congenital or acquired immunosuppression. Avoid close contact with immunocompromised individuals for at least 21 days. Have epinephrine available. Delay administration until after the acute phase (at least 72 hrs) of febrile and/or respiratory illnesses.

ADVERSE REACTIONS: Runny nose, congestion, cough, irritability, headache, sore throat, fever, chills, muscle aches, vomiting, tiredness/weakness.

INTERACTIONS: See Contraindications. Avoid concurrent use with other vaccines and within 48 hrs after cessation of antiviral therapy; antiviral agents until 2 weeks after vaccination unless medically indicated; ASA or ASA-containing products in children and adolescents 5-17 yrs.

PREGNANCY: Category C, caution in nursing.

MECHANISM OF ACTION: Stimulates the immune system to produce antibodies (influenza-specific T cells) that may protect against influenza virus infection.

FLUNISOLIDE NASAL SPRAY   RX
flunisolide (Various)

THERAPEUTIC CLASS: Corticosteroid

INDICATIONS: Relief of seasonal or perennial rhinitis.

DOSAGE: *Adults:* Initial: 2 sprays per nostril bid. Titrate: May increase to 2 sprays per nostril tid. Max: 8 sprays per nostril/day.
Pediatrics: 6-14 yrs: Initial: 1 spray per nostril tid or 2 sprays per nostril bid. Max: 4 sprays per nostril/day.

HOW SUPPLIED: Spray: 25mcg/spray (25mL)

CONTRAINDICATIONS: Untreated localized infection of the nasal mucosa.

WARNINGS/PRECAUTIONS: Risk of adrenal insufficiency and withdrawal symptoms when replacing systemic corticosteroids with a topical corticosteroids. Caution with active or quiescent TB, ocular herpes simplex, or untreated bacterial, fungal and systemic viral infections. Avoid with recent nasal trauma, surgery or septum ulcers. Risk for more severe/fatal course of infections (eg, chickenpox, measles) and for *Candida* infections of the nose and pharynx.

ADVERSE REACTIONS: Nasal congestion, sneezing, epistaxis, bloody mucous, nasal irritation, watery eyes, sore throat, nausea, vomiting, headache.

INTERACTIONS: Concomitant systemic corticosteroids increases risk of hypercorticism and/or HPA axis suppression.

PREGNANCY: Category C, caution in nursing.

MECHANISM OF ACTION: Glucocorticosteroid; not established, acts as anti-inflammatory agent with potent glucocorticoid and weak mineralocorticoid activity.

PHARMACOKINETICS: Absorption: Well absorbed. **Metabolism:** Liver. **Elimination:** Urine (65-70%, metabolites), feces, $T_{1/2}$=1-2 hrs.

FLUOCINONIDE   RX
fluocinonide (Various)

OTHER BRAND NAMES: Fluocinonide-E (Various) - Lidex (Medicis) - Lidex-E (Medicis)

THERAPEUTIC CLASS: Corticosteroid

INDICATIONS: Corticosteroid-responsive dermatoses.

DOSAGE: *Adults:* Apply bid-qid. May use occlusive dressing for psoriasis or recalcitrant conditions; d/c dressings if infection develops.
Pediatrics: Apply bid-qid. May use occlusive dressing for psoriasis or recalcitrant conditions; d/c dressings if infection develops.

HOW SUPPLIED: (Fluocinonide) Cre, Gel, Oint: 0.05% (15g, 30g, 60g); Sol: 0.05% (60mL); (Fluocinonide-E) Cre: 0.05% (15g, 30g, 60g)

WARNINGS/PRECAUTIONS: May produce reversible HPA axis suppression, manifestations of Cushing's syndrome, hyperglycemia, and glucosuria. Caution when applied to large surface areas or under occlusive dressings. Use appropriate antifungal or antibacterial agent with dermatological infections; d/c if infection does not clear. Pediatrics may be more susceptible to systemic toxicity. Avoid eyes. D/C if irritation occurs.

ADVERSE REACTIONS: Burning, itching, irritation, dryness, folliculitis, hypertrichosis, acneiform eruptions, hypopigmentation, perioral dermatitis, allergic contact dermatitis, skin maceration, secondary infection, skin atrophy, striae, miliaria.

PREGNANCY: Category C, caution in nursing.

MECHANISM OF ACTION: Corticosteroid; possesses anti-inflammatory, antipruritic, and vasoconstrictive actions.

PHARMACOKINETICS: Absorption: Extent of percutaneous absorption is determined by vehicle, integrity of skin, and use of occlusive dressings. **Metabolism:** Liver. **Elimination:** Urine, bile.

FLUORESCITE
fluorescein sodium (Alcon)

RX

THERAPEUTIC CLASS: Diagnostic dye

INDICATIONS: Indicated in diagnostic fluorescein angiography or angioscopy of the fundus and iris vasculature.

DOSAGE: *Adults:* Perform intradermal skin test before IV use if suspect potential allergy. Inject contents of ampule rapidly into antecubital vein. A syringe with fluorescein is attached to transparent tubing and a 25 gauge scalp vein needle for injection. Insert needle and draw patient's blood to hub of syringe so small air bubble separates patient's blood in tubing from fluorescein. With room lights on, inject blood back into vein while watching skin over needle tip. If needle extravasated, patient's blood will bulge skin; stop injection before injecting fluorescein. When certain there is no extravasation, turn room light off and complete fluorescein injection. Luminescence appears in retina and choroidal vessels in 9-14 seconds.
Pediatrics: Perform intradermal skin test before IV use if suspect potential allergy. Dose is 35mg/10lbs. Inject contents of ampule/vial rapidly into antecubital vein. A syringe with fluorescein is attached to transparent tubing and a 25 gauge scalp vein needle for injection. Insert needle and draw patient's blood to hub of syringe so small air bubble separates patient's blood in tubing from fluorescein. With room lights on, inject blood back into vein while watching skin over needle tip. If needle extravasated, patient's blood will bulge skin; stop injection before injecting fluorescein. When certain there is no extravasation, turn room light off and complete fluorescein injection. Luminescence appears in retina and choroidal vessels in 9-14 seconds.

HOW SUPPLIED: Inj: 10% (5mL), 25% (2mL)

WARNINGS/PRECAUTIONS: Not for intrathecal use. Avoid extravasation; severe local tissue damage can occur. Caution with history of allergy or bronchial asthma. Have emergency tray (eg, 0.1% epinephrine IV/IM, antihistamine, soluble steroid, IV aminophylline) and oxygen available. Avoid angiography in pregnancy, especially 1st trimester. Skin attains temporary yellowish discoloration and urine attains bright yellow color.

ADVERSE REACTIONS: Nausea, vomiting, headache, GI distress, syncope, hypotension, cardiac arrest, basilar artery ischemia, severe shock, convulsions, thrombophlebitis.

PREGNANCY: Safety in pregnancy not known, caution in nursing.

MECHANISM OF ACTION: Diagnostic dye; responds to electromagnetic radiation and light between wavelengths 465-490nm and fluoresces at wavelengths of 520-530nm.

PHARMACOKINETICS: Distribution: V_d=0.5L/kg. **Metabolism:** Rapid via conjugation. **Elimination:** Renal.

FLUVIRIN
influenza virus vaccine (Chiron)

RX

THERAPEUTIC CLASS: Vaccine

INDICATIONS: Immunization against influenza viruses containing antigens related to those in the vaccine.

DOSAGE: *Adults:* 0.5mL IM in deltoid or thigh single dose. Shake well.
Pediatrics: ≥4 yrs: 0.5mL IM. <9 yrs (Not Previously Vaccinated): Repeat dose minimum 1 month apart. Administer in deltoid muscle to older children and thigh muscle in infants and young children.

HOW SUPPLIED: Inj: 45mcg/0.5mL

CONTRAINDICATIONS: Allergy to chicken eggs, chicken, chicken feathers, chicken dander, or thimerosal (a mercury derivative). Delay administration to patients with an active neurological disorder or an acute febrile illness until disease stabilizes or symptoms subside. History of any neurological signs or symptoms following administration of any vaccine is contraindicated to further use.

WARNINGS/PRECAUTIONS: Do not administer in children younger than 6 months. Caution in children between the ages of 6 months through 4 years. Caution with thrombocytopenia, coagulation disorders, and impaired immune responses.

ADVERSE REACTIONS: Soreness at the injection site, fever, malaise, myalgia.

INTERACTIONS: Immunosuppressive therapies (eg, irradiation, corticosteroids, antimetabolites, alkylating and cytotoxic agents) may reduce effectiveness. May inhibit clearance of warfarin and theophylline.

PREGNANCY: Category C, safe for use in nursing.

MECHANISM OF ACTION: Stimulates the immune response to produce antibodies that may protect against influenza.

FLUVOXAMINE
fluvoxamine maleate (Various)

RX

Antidepressants increased the risk of suicidal thinking and behavior (suicidality) in short-term studies in children, adolescents, and young adults with major depressive disorder (MDD) and other psychiatric disorders. Fluvoxamine is not approved for use in pediatric patients except for pateints with obsessive compulsive disorder (OCD).

THERAPEUTIC CLASS: Selective serotonin reuptake inhibitor

INDICATIONS: Treatment of OCD.

DOSAGE: *Adults:* Initial: 50mg qhs. Titrate: Increase by 50mg every 4-7 days. Maint: 100-300mg/day. Give bid if total dose >100mg daily. Max: 300mg/day. Elderly/Hepatic Impairment: Modify initial dose and titration.
Pediatrics: 8-17 yrs: Initial: 25mg qhs. Titrate: Increase by 25mg every 4-7 days. Maint: 50-200mg/day. Max: 8-11 yrs: 200mg/day. Adolescents: 300mg/day. Give bid if total dose >50mg daily.

HOW SUPPLIED: Tab: 25mg, 50mg*, 100mg* *scored

CONTRAINDICATIONS: Co-administration of thioridazine, terfenadine, astemizole, cisapride, pimozide, alosetron, tizanidine.

WARNINGS/PRECAUTIONS: Activation of mania/hypomania, SIADH, and hyponatremia reported. Close supervision with high risk suicide patients. Caution with history of seizures, hepatic dysfunction, with conditions altering metabolism or hemodynamic responses. Smoking increases metabolism.

ADVERSE REACTIONS: Headache, asthenia, nausea, diarrhea, vomiting, anorexia, dyspepsia, insomnia, somnolence, nervousness, agitation, dizziness, anxiety, dry mouth, sweating, tremor, abnormal ejaculation.

INTERACTIONS: See Contraindications. May potentiate metoprolol, propranolol. Avoid alcohol, diazepam, terfenadine, astemizole, cisapride, pimozide. Increases serum levels of theophylline, warfarin, clozapine, carbamazepine, methadone. Bradycardia with diltiazem. Potential for serious, fatal interactions with MAOIs. Lithium may increase serotonergic effects. Reduces clearance of mexiletine and benzodiazepines metabolized by hepatic oxidation (eg, alprazolam, midazolam, triazolam). Caution with sumatriptan, TCAs, tryptophan. Avoid thioridazine; produces dose-related QTc interval prolongation. Increases tacrine serum levels.

PREGNANCY: Category C, not for use in nursing.

MECHANISM OF ACTION: SSRI; inhibits neuronal uptake of serotonin.

PHARMACOKINETICS: Absorption: Absolute bioavailability (53%). Administration of variable doses resulted in different parameters; T_{max}=3-8 hrs. **Distribution:** V_d=25L/kg; plasma protein binding (80%). **Metabolism:** Hepatic (oxidative demethylation and deamination). **Elimination:** Urine; $T_{1/2}$=15.6 hrs.

FLUZONE

RX

influenza virus vaccine (Sanofi Pasteur)

THERAPEUTIC CLASS: Vaccine

INDICATIONS: Active immunization against influenza disease caused by influenza virus types A and B contained in vaccine in subjects from 6 months of age and older.

DOSAGE: *Adults:* 0.5mL IM in the deltoid muscle.
Pediatrics: ≥9 yrs: 0.5mL IM. 3-8 yrs: 0.5mL IM. 6-35 months: 0.25mL IM. Children <9 yrs who have not previously been vaccinated should receive two doses of vaccine ≥1 month apart. Older children should be given the IM injection in deltoid muscle, infants and young children should receive the IM injection in the anterolateral aspect of the thigh.

HOW SUPPLIED: Inj: 0.25mL, 0.5mL

CONTRAINDICATIONS: Hypersensitivity reactions to egg proteins or to chicken proteins. Vaccination may be postponed in case of febrile or acute disease. Immunization should be delayed in patients with an active neurologic disorder.

WARNINGS/PRECAUTIONS: Avoid in individuals who have a prior history of Guillain-Barre syndrome and in patients with bleeding disorders, such as hemophilia or thrombocytopenia or if patients is on anticoagulant therapy. Immunosuppressed patients may not obtain expected antibody response. Have epinephrine injection (1:1000) available.

ADVERSE REACTIONS: Local: soreness, pain, swelling. Systemic: fever, malaise, myalgia.

PREGNANCY: Category C, safety in nursing not known.

MECHANISM OF ACTION: Stimulates the immune system to produce antibodies that may protect against influenza virus.

FML

RX

fluorometholone (Allergan)

OTHER BRAND NAME: FML Forte (Allergan)

THERAPEUTIC CLASS: Corticosteroid

INDICATIONS: Treatment of inflammation of the palpebral and bulbar conjunctiva, cornea, and anterior segment of the globe.

DOSAGE: *Adults:* (Sus) 1 drop bid-qid or (Oint) apply 1/2 inch qd-tid. May give 0.1% q4h during initial 24-48 hrs. Re-evaluate after 2 days if no improvement.
Pediatrics: ≥2 yrs: (Sus) 1 drop bid-qid or (Oint) apply 1/2 inch qd-tid. May give 0.1% q4h during initial 24-48 hrs. Re-evaluate after 2 days if no improvement.

HOW SUPPLIED: Oint: (S.O.P.) 0.1% (3.5g); Sus: 0.1% (5mL, 10mL, 15mL); (Forte) 0.25% (2mL, 5mL, 10mL, 15mL)

CONTRAINDICATIONS: Viral diseases of the cornea and conjunctiva including epithelial herpes simplex keratitis, vaccinia, and varicella. Mycobacterial infection and fungal diseases of the eye.

WARNINGS/PRECAUTIONS: Caution with glaucoma, herpes simplex, diseases causing thinning of cornea/sclera and other ocular viral infections. Prolonged use can cause glaucoma or secondary ocular infections (eg, fungal). Monitor IOP after 10 days of therapy. Re-evaluate if no response after 2 days. Ointment may retard corneal healing. May delay healing and increase incidence of bleb formation after cataract surgery. Avoid abrupt withdrawal with chronic use.

ADVERSE REACTIONS: Elevation of IOP, glaucoma, infrequent optic nerve damage, posterior subcapsular cataract formation, delayed wound healing, burning/stinging upon instillation, ocular irritation, taste perversion, visual disturbance.

PREGNANCY: Category C, not for use in nursing.

MECHANISM OF ACTION: Corticosteroid; suspected to act by induction of phospholipase A_2 inhibitory proteins called lipocortins which control the biosynthesis of potent inflammation mediators (eg, prostaglandins, leukotrienes) by inhibiting release of their precursor, arachidonic acid.

FOCALIN `CII`
dexmethylphenidate HCl (Novartis)

THERAPEUTIC CLASS: Sympathomimetic amine

INDICATIONS: Treatment of attention deficit hyperactivity disorder (ADHD).

DOSAGE: *Adults:* Take bid at least 4 hrs apart. Methylphenidate Naive: Initial: 2.5mg bid. Titrate: Increase weekly by 2.5-5mg/day. Max: 20mg/day. Currently on Methylphenidate: Initial: Take 1/2 of methylphenidate dose. Max: 20mg/day. Reduce or d/c if paradoxical aggravation of symptoms. D/C if no improvement after appropriate dosage adjustments over 1 month.
Pediatrics: ≥6 yrs: Take bid at least 4 hrs apart. Methylphenidate Naive: Initial: 2.5mg bid. Titrate: Increase weekly by 2.5-5mg/day. Max: 20mg/day. Currently on Methylphenidate: Initial: Take 1/2 of methylphenidate dose. Max: 20mg/day. Reduce or d/c if paradoxical aggravation of symptoms. D/C if no improvement after appropriate dosage adjustments over 1 month.

HOW SUPPLIED: Tab: 2.5mg, 5mg, 10mg

CONTRAINDICATIONS: Marked anxiety, tension, and agitation; glaucoma; motor tics or family history or diagnosis of Tourette's syndrome; during or within 14 days of MAOI use.

WARNINGS/PRECAUTIONS: Caution in drug dependence or alcoholism. Avoid with known serious structural cardiac abnormalities, cardiomyopathy, serious heart rhythm abnormalities, CAD, or other serious cardiac problems. May cause modest increase in BP; caution with HTN, heart failure, recent MI, or ventricular arrhythmia. May exacerbate symptoms of behavior disturbance and thought disorder with pre-existing psychotic disorder. Caution when using stimulants to treat patients with comorbid bipolar disorder because of concern for possible induction of mixed/manic episodes in such patients. Stimulants at usual doses may cause treatment-emergent psychotic or manic symptoms (eg, hallucinations, delusional thinking, mania) in children and adolescents without prior history of psychotic illness or mania. Aggressive behavior or hostility reported in clinical trials and the postmarketing experience of some medications indicated for the treatment of ADHD. Suppression of growth reported with long-term use; monitor growth. May lower convulsive threshold; d/c in the presence of seizures. Visual disturbances reported. Monitor CBC, differential, and platelets with prolonged therapy.

ADVERSE REACTIONS: Abdominal pain, fever, anorexia, nausea, nervousness, insomnia. (Pediatrics) Loss of appetite, weight loss, tachycardia.

INTERACTIONS: See Contraindications. May decrease the effectiveness of antihypertensives. Caution with pressor agents. May inhibit metabolism of coumarin anticoagulants, anticonvulsants, and some antidepressants; adjust dose. Adverse events reported with clonidine.

PREGNANCY: Category C, caution in nursing.

MECHANISM OF ACTION: Sympathomimetic amine; blocks the reuptake of norepinephrine and dopamine into the presynaptic neuron and increases the release of these monoamines into the extraneuronal space.

PHARMACOKINETICS: Absorption: Readily absorbed; T_{max}=2.9 hrs (fed), 1.5 hrs (fasting). **Metabolism:** Via de-esterification (d-ritalinic acid; primary metabolite). **Elimination:** Urine (approximately 90%); $T_{1/2}$=2.2 hrs.

FOCALIN XR `CII`
dexmethylphenidate HCl (Novartis)

THERAPEUTIC CLASS: Sympathomimetic amine

INDICATIONS: Treatment of attention deficit hyperactivity disorder (ADHD) in patients aged ≥6 yrs.

DOSAGE: *Adults:* Methylphenidate Naive: Initial: 10mg/day. Titrate: May adjust weekly by 10mg/day. Max: 20mg/day. Currently on Methylphenidate: Initial: Take 1/2 of methylphenidate dose. Max: 20mg/day. Reduce or d/c if paradoxical aggravation of symptoms. Swallow capsule whole or sprinkle contents on applesauce. Contents should not be crushed, chewed or divided. D/C if no improvement after appropriate dosage adjustments over 1 month.
Pediatrics: ≥6 yrs: Methylphenidate Naive: Initial: 5mg/day. Titrate: May adjust weekly

by 5mg/day. Max: 20mg/day. Currently on Methylphenidate: Initial: Take 1/2 of methylphenidate dose. Max: 20mg/day. Reduce or d/c if paradoxical aggravation of symptoms. Swallow capsule whole or sprinkle contents on applesauce: contents should not be crushed, chewed or divided. D/C if no improvement after appropriate dosage adjustments over 1 month.

HOW SUPPLIED: Cap, Extended-Release: 5mg, 10mg, 15mg, 20mg

CONTRAINDICATIONS: Marked anxiety, tension, and agitation; glaucoma; motor tics or family history or diagnosis of Tourette's syndrome; during or within 14 days of MAOI use.

WARNINGS/PRECAUTIONS: Caution in drug dependence or alcoholism. Avoid with known serious structural cardiac abnormalities, cardiomyopathy, serious heart rhythm abnormalities, CAD, or other serious cardiac problems. May cause modest increase in BP; caution with HTN, heart failure, recent MI, or ventricular arrhythmia. May exacerbate symptoms of behavior disturbance and thought disorder with pre-existing psychotic disorder. Caution when using stimulants to treat patients with comorbid bipolar disorder because of concern for possible induction of mixed/manic episodes in such patients. Stimulants at usual doses may cause treatment-emergent psychotic or manic symptoms (eg, hallucinations, delusional thinking, mania) in children and adolescents without prior history of psychotic illness or mania. Aggressive behavior or hostility reported in clinical trials and the postmarketing experience of some medications indicated for the treatment of ADHD. Suppression of growth reported with long-term use; monitor growth. May lower convulsive threshold; d/c in the presence of seizures. Visual disturbances reported. Monitor CBC, differential, and platelets with prolonged therapy.

ADVERSE REACTIONS: Dyspepsia, headache, anxiety. (Adults) dry mouth, pharyngolaryngeal pain, feeling jittery, dizziness. (Pediatrics) decreased appetite, nausea.

INTERACTIONS: See Contraindications. May decrease the effectiveness of antihypertensives. Caution with pressor agents. May inhibit metabolism of coumarin anticoagulants, anticonvulsants, and tricyclic drugs; adjust dose. Adverse events reported with clonidine. Antacids or acid supressants could alter the release of dexmethylphenidate.

PREGNANCY: Category C, caution in nursing.

MECHANISM OF ACTION: Sympathomimetic amine; CNS stimulant. Blocks reuptake of norepinephrine and dopamine into presynaptic neuron and increases release of these monoamines into extraneuronal space.

PHARMACOKINETICS: Absorption: Bimodal plasma concentration. T_{max}=1-4 hrs (first peak), 4-5.7 hrs (second peak). **Distribution:** V_d=2.65L/kg. **Metabolism:** Metabolized via de-esterification; d-ritalinic acid (metabolite). **Elimination:** Urine (90%); $T_{1/2}$=2-4.5 hrs.

FOLIC ACID
folic acid (Various)   RX

THERAPEUTIC CLASS: Erythropoiesis agent

INDICATIONS: Treatment of megaloblastic anemia due to folic acid deficiency and in anemias of nutritional origin, pregnancy, infancy or childhood.

DOSAGE: *Adults:* Usual: Up to 1mg/day. Maint: 0.4mg qd. Pregnancy/Nursing: Maint: 0.8mg qd. Max: 1mg/day. Increase maintenance dose with alcoholism, hemolytic anemia, anticonvulsant therapy, chronic infection.
Pediatrics: Usual: Up to 1mg/day. Maint: Infants: 0.1mg qd. <4 yrs: 0.3mg qd. ≥4 yrs: 0.4mg qd.

HOW SUPPLIED: Inj: 5mg/mL; Tab: (OTC) 0.4mg, 0.8mg, (RX) 1mg

WARNINGS/PRECAUTIONS: Not for monotherapy in pernicious anemia and other megaloblastic anemias with B_{12} deficiency. May obscure pernicious anemia in dosage >0.1 mg/day. Decreased B_{12} serum levels with prolonged therapy.

ADVERSE REACTIONS: Allergic sensitization.

INTERACTIONS: Antagonizes phenytoin effects. Methotrexate, phenytoin, primidone, barbiturates, alcohol, alcoholic cirrhosis, nitrofurantoin, and pyrimethamine increase loss of folate. Increased seizures with phenytoin, primidone and phenobarbital reported. Tetracycline may cause false low serum and red cell folate due to suppression of *Lactobacillus casei*.

PREGNANCY: Category A, requirement increases during nursing.

MECHANISM OF ACTION: Acts as cofactor for transformylation reactions in biosynthesis of purines and thymidylates of nucleic acids; acts on megaloblastic bone marrow to produce normo-blastic marrow; required for nucleo-protein synthesis and maintenance of normal erythropoiesis.

PHARMACOKINETICS: Absorption: Rapid (small intestine); T_{max}=1 hr. **Distribution:** Excreted in breast milk. **Metabolism:** Liver via reduced diphospho-pyridine nucleotide and folate reductase. **Elimination:** Urine, feces.

FORADIL

RX

formoterol fumarate (Schering)

Long-acting β_2-agonists may increase the risk of asthma-related death.

THERAPEUTIC CLASS: Beta$_2$-agonist

INDICATIONS: Long-term maintenance treatment of asthma and prevention of bronchospasm with reversible obstructive airway disease (including nocturnal asthma) in patients who require regular treatment with inhaled short acting β_2-agonists. Maintenance treatment of bronchoconstriction in chronic obstructive pulmonary disease (COPD). Acute prevention of exercise-induced bronchospasm (EIB).

DOSAGE: *Adults:* Do not swallow cap; give only by inhalation with Aerolizer Inhaler. Asthma/COPD: 12mcg q12h. Max: 24mcg/day. EIB: 12mcg 15 min before exercise (do not give added dose if already on q12h dose).
Pediatrics: ≥5 yrs: Do not swallow cap; give only by inhalation with Aerolizer™ Inhaler. Asthma/COPD: 12mcg q12h. Max: 24mcg/day. ≥12 yrs: EIB: 12mcg 15 min before exercise (do not give added dose if already on q12h dose).

HOW SUPPLIED: Cap (Inhalation): 12mcg (12^s, 60^s)

WARNINGS/PRECAUTIONS: Do not d/c inhaled corticosteroids. Only use short-acting β_2-agonist inhaler for acute symptoms. D/C if paradoxical bronchospasm occurs. D/C if ECG changes, QT interval increases, or ST depression occurs. Caution with cardiovascular disorders (eg, HTN, arrhythmias), thyrotoxicosis and convulsive disorders. Anaphylactic and other allergic reactions reported. Not for use in acute asthmatic conditions. Should not be used with other long-acting β_2-agonist medications. May cause hypokalemia.

ADVERSE REACTIONS: Viral infection, dyspnea, chest pain, tremor, HTN, hypotension, tachycardia, arrhythmias, headache, nausea, vomiting, fatigue, hypokalemia, hyperglycemia, exacerbation of asthma.

INTERACTIONS: Potentiates other sympathomimetics. Hypokalemia potentiated by xanthine derivatives (eg, theophylline), steroids and non-potassium sparing diuretics. Extreme caution with MAOIs, TCAs, and drugs known to prolong QT interval. Antagonized effect with β-blockers.

PREGNANCY: Category C, caution in nursing.

MECHANISM OF ACTION: Long-acting selective β_2-adrenergic receptor agonist; acts as a bronchodilator, activates adenyl cyclase on airway smooth muscles and increases the intracellular concentration of cyclic AMP. Increased cAMP levels are associated with relaxation of bronchial smooth muscle and inhibition of release of mediators of immediate hypersensitivity.

PHARMACOKINETICS: Absorption: Healthy: C_{max}=92pg/mL, T_{max}=5 min. COPD patient: (12mcg) C_{max}=4.0-8.8, 8, 17.3pg/mL at 10 min, 2 hrs, 6 hrs, respectively. **Distribution:** Plasma protein binding (61-64%), serum albumin binding (31-38%). **Metabolism:** Glucuronidation, O-methylation via CYP450 enzymes 2D6, 2C19, 2CP, 2A6. **Elimination:** Healthy: Urine (59-62%), feces (32-34%). With asthma: Urine (10% unchanged). COPD: Urine (7%). $T_{1/2}$=10 hrs.

FORTAZ

ceftazidime (GlaxoSmithKline)

RX

THERAPEUTIC CLASS: Cephalosporin (3rd generation)

INDICATIONS: Treatment of lower respiratory tract (eg, pneumonia), skin and skin structure (SSSI), bone/joint, gynecologic, CNS (eg, meningitis), intra-abdominal, and urinary tract infections (UTI); and septicemia caused by susceptible strains of microorganisms. Treatment of sepsis.

DOSAGE: *Adults:* Usual: 1g IM/IV q8-12h. Uncomplicated UTI: 250mg IM/IV q12h. Complicated UTI: 500mg IM/IV q8-12h. Bone and Joint Infection: 2g IV q12h. Uncomplicated Pneumonia/SSSI: 500mg-1g IM/IV q8h. Gynecological/Intra-Abdominal/Meningitis/Severe Life-Threatening Infection: 2g IV q8h. Lung Infection Caused by *Pseudomonas* spp. in Cystic Fibrosis (Normal Renal Function): 30-50mg/kg IV q8h. Max: 6g/day. CrCl 31-50mL/min: 1g q12h. CrCl 16-30mL/min: 1g q24h. CrCl 6-15mL/min: 500mg q24h. CrCl <5mL/min: 500mg q48h. For severe infections (6g/day), increase renal impairment dose by 50% or increase dosing interval. Apply reduced dosage recommendations after initial 1g LD is given. Hemodialysis: Give 1g before, then 1g after each hemodialysis. Intra-Peritoneal Dialysis/Continuous Ambulatory Peritoneal Dialysis: Give 1g followed by 500mg q24h, or add to fluid at 250mg/2L.
Pediatrics: 1 month-12 yrs: 30-50mg/kg IV q8h. Max: 6g/day. Neonates (0-4 weeks): 30mg/kg IV q12h. Higher doses for cystic fibrosis or meningitis. CrCl 31-50mL/min: 1g q12h. CrCl 16-30mL/min: 1g q24h. CrCl 6-15mL/min: 500mg q24h. CrCl <5mL/min: 500mg q48h. For severe infections (6g/day), increase renal impairment dose by 50% or increase dosing interval. Apply reduced dosage recommendations after initial 1g LD is given. Hemodialysis: Give 1g before, then 1g after each hemodialysis. Intra-Peritoneal Dialysis/Continuous Ambulatory Peritoneal Dialysis: Give 1g followed by 500mg q24h, or add to fluid at 250mg/2L.

HOW SUPPLIED: Inj: 500mg, 1g, 1g/50mL, 2g, 2g/50mL, 6g

WARNINGS/PRECAUTIONS: Monitor renal function; potential for nephrotoxicity. Prolonged use may result in overgrowth of nonsusceptible organisms. Possible cross-sensitivity between PCNs, cephalosporins, and other β-lactam antibiotics. *Clostridium difficile*-associated diarrhea reported and may range in severity from mild diarrhea to fatal colitis. Elevated levels with renal insufficiency can lead to seizures, encephalopathy, coma, asterixis and neuromuscular excitability. Possible decrease in PT; caution with renal/hepatic impairment, poor nutritional state; monitor PT and give vitamin K if needed. Caution with colitis, other GI diseases, and elderly. Distal necrosis may occur after inadvertent intra-arterial administration. Continue therapy for 2 days after the signs and symptoms of infection have disappeared, but in complicated infections longer therapy may be required. False (+) for urine glucose with Benedict's solution, Fehling's solution, and Clinitest® tablets.

ADVERSE REACTIONS: Phlebitis and inflammation at injection site, pruritus, rash, fever, diarrhea.

INTERACTIONS: Nephrotoxicity reported with aminoglycosides or potent diuretics (eg, furosemide). Avoid with chloramphenicol; may decrease effect of β-lactam antibiotics. Possible decrease in PT; caution with a protracted course of antimicrobial therapy; monitor PT and give vitamin K if needed. May reduce efficacy of oral contraceptives.

PREGNANCY: Category B, caution in nursing.

MECHANISM OF ACTION: 3rd-generation cephalosporin; bactericidal, inhibits cell-wall synthesis.

PHARMACOKINETICS: Absorption: (IV) Administration of variable doses resulted in different parameters. **Distribution:** Plasma protein binding (≤10%). **Elimination:** Urine (unchanged, 80-90%).

FURADANTIN

nitrofurantoin (Sciele)

RX

THERAPEUTIC CLASS: Imidazolidinedione antibacterial

INDICATIONS: Treatment of urinary tract infection (UTI).

DOSAGE: *Adults:* Usual: 50-100mg qid with food for 1 week or at least 3 days after sterility of urine. Use lower doses for uncomplicated UTI. Long-Term Suppressive Therapy: 50-100mg qhs.
Pediatrics: >1 month: Usual: 5-7mg/kg/day given qid with food for 1 week or at least 3 days after sterility of urine. Long-Term Suppressive Therapy: 1mg/kg/day qd or bid.

HOW SUPPLIED: Sus: 25mg/5mL

CONTRAINDICATIONS: Anuria, oliguria, CrCl <60 mL/min, pregnancy at term (38-42 weeks gestation), during labor and delivery, neonates <1 month of age.

WARNINGS/PRECAUTIONS: Acute, subacute or chronic pulmonary reactions have occurred. Enhanced occurrence of peripheral neuropathy with anemia, DM, renal dysfunction, electrolyte imbalance, vitamin B deficiency, and debilitating disease. D/C therapy with acute and chronic pulmonary reactions, hepatic disorders, hemolysis, or peripheral neuropathy. Monitor renal function, LFTs and pulmonary function periodically during long-term therapy. Pseudomembranous colitis reported.

ADVERSE REACTIONS: Pulmonary disorders, hepatic damage, peripheral neuropathy, nausea, emesis, anorexia, dizziness, exfoliative dermatitis, Stevens-Johnson syndrome, anaphylaxis, blood dyscrasias.

INTERACTIONS: Antacids, especially magnesium trisilicate, decrease rate and extent of absorption. Probenecid and sulfinpyrazone increase nitrofurantoin levels.

PREGNANCY: Category B, not for use in nursing.

MECHANISM OF ACTION: Imidazolidinedione antibacterial; inhibits protein synthesis, aerobic energy metabolism, DNA, RNA, and cell-wall synthesis.

PHARMACOKINETICS: Absorption: Readily absorbed (with food). **Elimination:** Urine.

FUROSEMIDE   RX
furosemide (Various)

Can lead to profound water and electrolyte depletion with excessive use.

OTHER BRAND NAME: Lasix (Sanofi-Aventis)

THERAPEUTIC CLASS: Loop diuretic

INDICATIONS: (Inj, PO) Treatment of edema associated with CHF, liver cirrhosis, and renal disease including nephrotic syndrome. (PO) Treatment of hypertension. (Inj) Adjunct therapy for acute pulmonary edema.

DOSAGE: *Adults:* (PO) HTN: Initial: 40mg bid. Edema: Initial: 20-80mg PO. May repeat or increase by 20-40mg after 6-8 hrs. Max: 600mg/day. Alternative Regimen: Dose on 2-4 consecutive days each week. Closely monitor if on >80mg/day. (Inj) Edema: Initial: 20-40mg IV/IM. May repeat or increase by 20mg after 2 hrs. Acute Pulmonary Edema: Initial: 40mg IV. May increase to 80mg IV after 1 hr.
Pediatrics: Edema: (PO) Initial: 2mg/kg single dose. May increase by 1-2mg/kg after 6-8 hrs. Max: 6mg/kg. (Inj) Initial: 1mg/kg IV/IM single dose. May increase by 1mg/kg IV/IM after 2 hrs. Max: 6mg/kg.

HOW SUPPLIED: Inj: 10mg/mL; Sol: 10mg/mL, 40mg/5mL; Tab: 20mg, 40mg*, 80mg
*scored

CONTRAINDICATIONS: Anuria.

WARNINGS/PRECAUTIONS: Monitor for fluid/electrolyte imbalance (eg, hypokalemia), renal or hepatic dysfunction. Initiate in hospital with hepatic cirrhosis and ascites. Tinnitus, hearing impairment, hyperglycemia, hyperuricemia reported. May activate SLE. Cross-sensitivity with sulfonamide allergy. Avoid excessive diuresis, especially in elderly.

ADVERSE REACTIONS: Pancreatitis, jaundice, anorexia, paresthesias, ototoxicity, blood dyscrasias, dizziness, rash, urticaria, photosensitivity, fever, thrombophlebitis, restlessness.

INTERACTIONS: Ototoxicity with aminoglycosides, ethacrynic acid. Caution with high dose salicylates. Lithium toxicity. Antagonizes tubocurarine. Potentiates antihypertensives, succinylcholine, ganglionic or peripheral adrenergic blockers. Decreases arterial response to norepinephrine. Separate sucralfate dose by 2 hrs. Indomethacin may decrease effects. Hypokalemia with ACTH, corticosteroids. Renal changes with NSAIDs. Orthostatic hypotension may be aggravated by alcohol, barbiturates, or narcotics.

PREGNANCY: Category C, caution in nursing.

MECHANISM OF ACTION: Anthranilic acid derivative (diuretic); primarly inhibits reabsorption of Na^+ and Cl^- in proximal and distal tubules and in loop of Henle.

PHARMACOKINETICS: Distribution: Plasma protein binding (91-99%). **Metabolism:** Biotransformation. Furosemide glucuronide (major metabolite). **Elimination:** Urine; $T_{1/2}=2$ hrs.

FUZEON   RX
enfuvirtide (Roche Labs)

THERAPEUTIC CLASS: Fusion inhibitor

INDICATIONS: Treatment of HIV-1 infection in combination with other antiretroviral agents in treatment-experienced patients with evidence of HIV-1 replication despite ongoing antiretroviral therapy.

DOSAGE: *Adults:* 90mg SQ bid. Inject SQ into upper arm, anterior thigh, or abdomen. Do not inject into moles, scar tissue, bruises, the navel, or near any blood vessels. Rotate sites; do not give if injection site reaction occurred from an earlier dose.
Pediatrics: 6-16 yrs: 2mg/kg SQ bid. Max: 90mg bid. 11-15.5kg: 27mg bid. 15.6-20.0kg: 36mg bid. 20.1-24.5kg: 45mg bid. 24.6-29.0kg: 54mg bid. 29.1-33.5kg: 63mg bid. 33.6-38.0kg: 72mg bid. 38.1-42.5kg: 81mg bid. ≥ 42.6kg: 90mg bid. Inject SQ into upper arm, anterior thigh, or abdomen. Do not inject into moles, scar tissue, bruises, or the navel. Rotate sites; do not give if injection site reaction occurred from an earlier dose.

HOW SUPPLIED: Inj: 90mg (60ˢ)

WARNINGS/PRECAUTIONS: Monitor for signs and symptoms of pneumonia, cellulitis, or local infection. D/C if hypersensitivity reactions occur. Theoretically may lead to production of anti-enfuvirtide antibodies; may result in false positive HIV test with an ELISA assay. Immune reconstitution syndrome reported. Increased risk of bleeding or bruising in patients with coagulation disorders.

ADVERSE REACTIONS: Diarrhea, nausea, fatigue, local injection site reactions, peripheral neuropathy, insomnia, depression, anxiety, cough, sinusitis, herpes simplex, decreased weight/appetite, pancreatitis, asthenia, pruritus, myalgia, nerve pain, bruising, hematomas.

PREGNANCY: Category B, not for use in nursing.

MECHANISM OF ACTION: Fusion inhibitor; inhibits the fusion of HIV-1 with $CD4^+$ cells by interfering with entry of HIV-1 into cells.

PHARMACOKINETICS: Absorption: (SQ) $C_{max}=4.59\mu g/mL$; $T_{max}=8$ hrs; $AUC=55.8\mu g \cdot hr/mL$. (IV) Absolute bioavailabilty (84.3%). Values obtained from different parameters are different when combined with other antiretroviral agents. **Distribution:** $V_d=5.5L$; plasma protein binding (92%). **Metabolism:** Hepatic (hydrolysis); metabolite (M_3). **Elimination:** (SQ) $T_{1/2}=3.8$ hrs.

GABITRIL   RX
tiagabine HCl (Cephalon)

THERAPEUTIC CLASS: Nipecotic acid derivative

INDICATIONS: Adjunctive therapy in the treatment of partial seizures.

DOSAGE: *Adults:* Initial: 4mg qd. Titrate: May increase weekly by 4-8mg until clinical response. Max: 56mg/day given bid-qid. Take with food.
Pediatrics: ≥12 yo: Initial: 4mg qd. Titrate: May increase to 8mg qd at beginning of Week 2, then increase weekly by 4-8mg until clinical response. Max: 32mg/day. Take with food.

HOW SUPPLIED: Tab: 2mg, 4mg, 12mg, 16mg

WARNINGS/PRECAUTIONS: Reports of new-onset seizure or status epilepticus in patients without epilepsy. D/C and evaluate for underlying seizure disorder. Avoid abrupt withdrawal. Monitor during initial titration for impaired concentration, speech problem, somnolence, fatigue; may require hospitalization if reaction is severe. May exacerbate EEG abnormalities; adjust dose. Status epilepticus and sudden death reported. Reduce dose or d/c if generalized weakness occurs. Reduce dose with hepatic impairment. Serious skin rash reported.

ADVERSE REACTIONS: Dizziness, asthenia, somnolence, nausea, vomiting, nervousness, tremor, abdominal pain, abnormal thinking, depression, confusion, pharyngitis, rash.

INTERACTIONS: May reduce valproate levels. Diminished effects with carbamazepine, phenytoin. Additive CNS depression with alcohol, triazolam, CNS depressants.

PREGNANCY: Category C, caution in nursing.

MECHANISM OF ACTION: Antiepileptic; not fully established. May enhance the activity of gamma aminobutytic acid (GABA), the major inhibitory neurotransmitter in the CNS. Binds to recognition sites associated with the GABA uptake carrier, thereby blocking GABA uptake into presynaptic neurons, permitting more GABA to be available for receptor binding on the surface of post-synaptic cells.

PHARMACOKINETICS: Absorption: Absolute bioavailability (90%). T_{max}=2.5 hrs. (with meals), T_{max}=45 min (fasting). **Distribution:** Plasma protein binding (96%). **Metabolism:** Hepatic via oxidation and glucoronidation, CYP3A. **Elimination:** Urine (25%), feces (63%); $T_{1/2}$=7-9 hrs. For pediatric parameters refer to full PI.

GAMMAR-P RX

immune globulin (CSL Behring)

THERAPEUTIC CLASS: Immunoglobulin

INDICATIONS: Patients with primary defective antibody synthesis (eg, agammaglobulinemia or hypogammaglobulinemia), who are at increased risk of infection.

DOSAGE: *Adults:* 200-400mg/kg IV every 3-4 weeks. Adjust dose to maintain desired IgG levels and clinical response.
Pediatrics/Adolescents: 200mg/kg IV every 3-4 weeks. Adjust dose to maintain desired IgG levels and clinical response.

HOW SUPPLIED: Inj: 5g, 10g

CONTRAINDICATIONS: History of allergic reactions to human albumin, anaphylactic or severe systemic response to IM/IV immune globulin, isolated IgA deficiency.

WARNINGS/PRECAUTIONS: Assure patient is not volume depleted before administration. Caution if predisposed to acute renal failure (eg, any degree of pre-existing renal insufficiency, DM, >65 yrs, volume depletion, sepsis, paraproteinemia, with nephrotoxic drugs). Monitor renal function and infusion rate. Aseptic meningitis syndrome reported. Made from human blood; risk of transmitting infection.

ADVERSE REACTIONS: Acute renal failure, acute tubular necrosis, proximal tubular nephropathy, osmotic nephrosis, chills, headache, backache, neck pain.

INTERACTIONS: May interfere with response to live viral vaccines (eg, measles, mumps, rubella).

PREGNANCY: Category C, safety in nursing not known.

MECHANISM OF ACTION: Immunoglobulin (IgG); provides broad range of antibodies capable of opsonization and neutralization of microbes and toxins against bacterial and viral antigens for prevention or attenuation of infectious disease.

PHARMACOKINETICS: Elimination: $T_{1/2}$=40 days.

GANTRISIN PEDIATRIC RX

sulfisoxazole (Roche Labs)

THERAPEUTIC CLASS: Sulfonamide

INDICATIONS: Treatment of acute, recurrent or chronic urinary tract infection. Treatment and prophylaxis in meningococcal meningitis. Adjunct treatment of Haemophilus influenzae meningitis, acute otitis media, malaria, and toxoplasmosis. Treatment of trachoma, inclusion conjunctivitis, nocardiosis, chancroid.

DOSAGE: *Pediatrics:* >2 months: Initial: 1/2 of 24hr dose. Maint: 150mg/kg/24hr or 4g/m^2/24hr given q4-6h. Max: 6g/24hr.

HOW SUPPLIED: Sus: 500mg/5mL

CONTRAINDICATIONS: Infants <2 months (except in congenital toxoplasmosis treatment), pregnancy at term, mothers nursing infants <2 months old.

WARNINGS/PRECAUTIONS: Fatalities reported due to Stevens-Johnson syndrome, toxic epidermal necrolysis, fulminant hepatic necrosis, agranulocytosis, aplastic anemia and other blood dyscrasias. D/C if skin rash or sign of an adverse reaction develops. Hypersensitivity reactions of the respiratory tract reported. Do not use in group A β-hemolytic streptococcal infections. Pseudomembranous colitis reported. Caution with renal/hepatic impairment, severe allergy or bronchial asthma. Hemolysis may occur in G6PD-deficient patients.

ADVERSE REACTIONS: Anaphylaxis, erythema multiforme, toxic epidermal necrolysis, tachycardia, hepatitis, nausea, anorexia, hematuria, crystalluria, BUN and creatinine elevations, blood dyscrasias, dizziness, psychosis, cough.

INTERACTIONS: May prolong PT with anticoagulants. May require less thiopental for anesthesia. May potentiate hypoglycemia effects of sulfonylureas. May displace methotrexate from plasma proteins.

PREGNANCY: Category C, not for use in nursing.

MECHANISM OF ACTION: Sulfonamide; bacteriostatic agent. Inhibits bacterial synthesis of dihydrofolic acid by preventing condensation of pteridine with aminobenzoic acid through competitive inhibition of enzyme dihydropteroate synthetase.

PHARMACOKINETICS: Absorption: Rapid, complete; $C_{max}(N^1$ acetyl sulfisoxazole, sulfisoxazole)=181, 169mcg/mL; $T_{max}(N^1$ acetyl sulfisoxazole, sulfisoxazole)=2-6 hrs, 2.5 hrs. **Distribution:** Plasma protein binding (85%); crosses placenta, blood brain barrier; excreted in breast milk. **Metabolism:** Metabolized to sulfisoxazole by digestive enzymes. **Elimination:** Urine; $T_{1/2}(N^1$ acetyl sulfisoxazole, sulfisoxazole)= 5.4-7.4, 4.6-7.8 hrs.

GARDASIL RX
human papillomavirus recombinant vaccine, quadrivalent (Merck)

THERAPEUTIC CLASS: Vaccine

INDICATIONS: Vaccination of girls and women ages 9-26 yrs for the prevention of cervical cancer, genital warts, cervical adenocarcinoma *in situ*, cervical intraepithelial neoplasia Grades 2 and 3, vulvar intraepithelial neoplasia Grades 2 and 3, vaginal intraepithelial neoplasia Grades 2 and 3, and cervical intraepithelial neoplasia Grade 1 caused by Human Papillomavirus types 6, 11, 16, and 18.

DOSAGE: *Adults:* Give 3 separate 0.5mL IM doses in the deltoid region of upper arm or higher anterolateral area of the thigh. First dose: At elected date; Second dose: 2 months after first dose; Third dose: 6 months after first dose.
Pediatrics: ≥9 yrs: Give 3 separate 0.5mL IM doses in the deltoid region of upper arm or higher anterolateral area of the thigh. First dose: At elected date; Second dose: 2 months after first dose; Third dose: 6 months after first dose.

HOW SUPPLIED: Inj: Vial/Syringe: 0.5mL

WARNINGS/PRECAUTIONS: Should not be administered with bleeding disorders or anticoagulant therapy unless the potential benefits outweight the risk. Patients with impaired immune responsiveness may have reduced antibody response to active immunization. Medical treatment should be readily available in case of rare anaphylactic reactions.

ADVERSE REACTIONS: Local site reactions, fever, pyrexia, nausea, nasopharyngitis, dizziness, diarrhea.

INTERACTIONS: Immunosuppressive therapies, including irradiation, antimetabolites, alkylating agents, cytotoxic drugs, and corticosteroids (used in greater than physiologic doses) may reduce the immune responses to vaccines.

PREGNANCY: Category B, caution in nursing.

MECHANISM OF ACTION: Develops humoral immune response that may protect against human papilloma virus types 6,11,16, and 18 (animal study).

GENOTROPIN RX
somatropin (Pharmacia & Upjohn)

OTHER BRAND NAME: Genotropin MiniQuick (Pharmacia & Upjohn)
THERAPEUTIC CLASS: Human growth hormone

INDICATIONS: Long-term treatment of pediatrics with growth failure due to growth hormone deficiency (GHD) or Prader-Willi syndrome (PWS) or who are born small for gestational age (SGA) and fail to catch-up by age 2. Long-term replacement therapy in adults with GHD of either childhood- or adult-onset etiology. Long-term treatment of growth failure associated with Turner Syndrome (TS) in patients who have open epiphyses.

DOSAGE: *Adults:* Individualize dose: GHD: Initial: Up to 0.04mg/kg/week. May increase at 4-8 week intervals. Max: 0.08mg/kg/week. Divide dose into 6-7 SQ injections. Elderly patients should receive a lower starting dose.
Pediatrics: Individualize dose. GHD: 0.16-0.24mg/kg/week. PWS: 0.24mg/kg/week. SGA: 0.48mg/kg/week. TS: 0.33mg/kg/week. Divide doses into 6-7 SQ injections.

HOW SUPPLIED: Inj: 1.5mg, 5.8mg, 13.8mg; Inj, MiniQuick: 0.2mg, 0.4mg, 0.6mg, 0.8mg, 1mg, 1.2mg, 1.4mg, 1.6mg, 1.8mg, 2mg

CONTRAINDICATIONS: Evidence of neoplastic activity. Pediatrics with closed epiphyses. Patients with diabetic retinopathy or active malignancy. Acute critical illness due to complications after open heart or abdominal surgery, multiple accidental trauma, or with acute respiratory failure. Patients with PWS who are severely obese or have severe respiratory impairment.

WARNINGS/PRECAUTIONS: In PWS, evaluate for upper airway obstruction prior to initiation; monitor weight, for sleep apnea, signs of upper airway obstruction (eg, suspend therapy with onset of or increased snoring), respiratory infections (treat early and aggressively if occur). Monitor GHD secondary to intracranial lesion for progression/recurrence. Monitor gait, glucose intolerance because insulin sensitivity is decreased, for malignant transformation of skin lesions, scoliosis progression, intracranial HTN (perform fundoscopic exam at start and periodically). Caution with DM, endocrine disorders, hypopituitarism, and Turner syndrome. Tissue atrophy may occur (rotate injection site).

ADVERSE REACTIONS: Peripheral swelling/edema, arthralgia, pain/stiffness in extremities, myalgia, upper respiratory infection, paresthesia.

INTERACTIONS: Antagonized by glucocorticoids. May alter clearance of CYP450 substrates (eg, corticosteroids, sex steroids, anticonvulsants, cyclosporine). May need dose adjustment if taking oral estrogen replacement. May need insulin dose adjustment.

PREGNANCY: Category B, caution in nursing.

MECHANISM OF ACTION: Human growth hormone; stimulates linear growth synthesis, metabolizes lipids, reduces body fat stores by increasing cellular protein, and increases plasma fatty acids.

PHARMACOKINETICS: Absorption: SQ administration of variable doses resulted in different parameters. **Distribution:** V_d=1.3L/kg. **Metabolism:** Liver and kidneys (protein catabolism). **Elimination:** (IV): $T_{1/2}$=0.4 hrs. (SC): $T_{1/2}$=3 hrs.

GENTAMICIN OPHTHALMIC   RX
gentamicin sulfate (Various)

THERAPEUTIC CLASS: Aminoglycoside

INDICATIONS: Treatment of ocular bacterial infections including conjunctivitis, keratitis, keratoconjunctivitis, corneal ulcers, blepharitis, blepharoconjunctivitis, acute meibomianitis and dacryocystitis.

DOSAGE: *Adults:* Usual: 1-2 drops q4h or apply 1/2 inch of oint bid-tid. Severe Infection: 2 drops every hour.
Pediatrics: Usual: 1-2 drops q4h or apply half-inch of oint bid-tid. Severe Infection: 2 drops every hour.

HOW SUPPLIED: Oint: 0.3% (3.5g); Sol: 0.3% (5mL)

WARNINGS/PRECAUTIONS: D/C if develop irritation, hypersensitivity, purulent discharge, inflammation or pain. Prolonged use may result in superinfection. Oint may retard corneal healing.

ADVERSE REACTIONS: Bacterial and fungal corneal ulcers, burning, irritation, conjunctivitis, conjunctival epithelial defects, conjunctival hyperemia.

PREGNANCY: Category C. Safety in nursing is not known.

MECHANISM OF ACTION: Aminoglycoside antibiotic: inhibits normal protein synthesis in susceptible microorganisms.

GENTAMICIN SULFATE INJECTION RX
gentamicin sulfate (Various)

Potential nephrotoxicity, neurotoxicity, ototoxicity. Risk of toxicity is greater with impaired renal function, high dosage, or prolonged therapy. Monitor serum concentrations closely. Avoid prolonged peak levels >12mcg/mL and trough levels >2mcg/mL. Monitor renal and eight cranial nerve function, urine, BUN, serum creatinine, and CrCl. Obtain serial audiograms. Advanced age and dehydration increase risk of toxicity. Adjust dose or D/C use with evidence of ototoxicity or nephrotoxicity. May cause fetal harm during pregnancy. Avoid concurrent and/or sequential systemic or topical use of other potentially neurotoxic and/or nephrotoxic drugs, such as cisplatin, cephaloridine, kanamycin, amikacin, neomycin, polymyxin B, colistin, paromomycin, streptomycin, tobramycin, vancomycin, and viomycin. Avoid concurrent use with potent diuretics, such as ethacrynic acid or furosemide.

THERAPEUTIC CLASS: Aminoglycoside

INDICATIONS: Treatment of bacterial neonatal sepsis, bacterial septicemia, and serious bacterial infections of the CNS (meningitis), urinary tract, respiratory tract, gastrointestinal tract (including peritonitis), skin, bone and soft tissue (including burns) caused by susceptible strains of microorganisms.

DOSAGE: *Adults:* IM/IV: Serious Infections: 3mg/kg/day given q8h. Life-Threatening Infections: 5mg/kg/day tid-qid; reduce to 3mg/kg/day as soon as clinically indicated. Treat for 7-10 days; may need longer course in difficult and complicated infections. Renal Impairment: Reduced dose given q8h or usual dose given at prolonged intervals based on either CrCl or serum creatinine. Dialysis: 1-1.7mg/kg, depending on severity of infection, at end of each dialysis period. Obese Patients: Calculate dose based on estimated lean body mass.
Pediatrics: 6-7.5mg/kg/day (2-2.5mg/kg given q8h). Infants and Neonates: 7.5mg/kg/day (2.5mg/kg given q8h). Premature and Full-Term Neonates ≤1 Week: 5mg/kg/day (2.5mg/kg given q12h). Treat for 7-10 days; may need longer course in difficult and complicated infections. Renal Impairment: Reduced dose given q8h or usual dose given at prolonged intervals based on either CrCl or serum creatinine. Dialysis: 2mg/kg at end of each dialysis period. Obese Patients: Calculate dose based on estimated lean body mass.

HOW SUPPLIED: Inj: 10mg/mL, 40mg/mL

WARNINGS/PRECAUTIONS: Contains metabisulfite. Neuromuscular blockade, respiratory paralysis, ototoxicity, and nephrotoxicity may occur after local irrigation or topical application during surgical procedures. Caution with neuromuscular disorders (eg, myasthenia gravis, parkinsonism). Caution in elderly; monitor renal function. Keep patients well-hydrated during treatment. May cause fetal harm when administered to pregnant women.

ADVERSE REACTIONS: Nephrotoxicity, neurotoxicity, rash, fever, urticaria, NV, headache, lethargy, confusion, depression, decreased appetite, weight loss, BP changes, blood dyscrasias, elevated LFTs.

INTERACTIONS: Increased nephrotoxicity with cephalosporins. Do not premix with other drugs; administer separately. Neuromuscular blockade and respiratory paralysis may occur in anesthetized patients or those receiving neuromuscular blockers (eg, succinylcholine, tubocurarine, decamethonium). See Black Box Warning.

PREGNANCY: Category D, safety not known in nursing.

MECHANISM OF ACTION: Aminoglycoside antibiotic; inhibits synthesis of proteins in bacterial cell.

PHARMACOKINETICS: Absorption: T_{max}=30-90 min. Administration of different doses resulted in different parameters. Distribution: Crosses placenta, distributed in body fluids. Elimination: Urine, bile.

GENTAMICIN TOPICAL

RX

gentamicin sulfate (Various)

THERAPEUTIC CLASS: Aminoglycoside

INDICATIONS: Treatment of primary skin infections such as impetigo contagiosa, folliculitis, ecthyma, furunculosis, sycosis barbae, and pyoderma gangrenosum; and secondary skin infections such as infectious eczematoid dermatitis, pustular acne, pustular psoriasis, infected seborrheic dermatitis, infected contact dermatitis, infected excoriations, and bacterial superinfections.

DOSAGE: *Adults:* Apply gently tid-qid. May apply gauze dressing.
Pediatrics: >1 yr: Apply gently tid-qid. May apply gauze dressing.

HOW SUPPLIED: Cre, Oint: 0.1% (15g, 30g)

WARNINGS/PRECAUTIONS: D/C if irritation, sensitization, or superinfection develops.

ADVERSE REACTIONS: Irritation (erythema and pruritus).

PREGNANCY: Unknown use in pregnancy and nursing.

MECHANISM OF ACTION: Aminoglycoside; wide-spectrum antibiotic that acts against primary and secondary bacterial infections of the skin.

GLEEVEC

RX

imatinib mesylate (Novartis)

THERAPEUTIC CLASS: Protein-tyrosine kinase inhibitor

INDICATIONS: (Adults) Treatment of newly diagnosed adult patients with Philadelphia chromosome positive (Ph+) chronic myeloid leukemia (CML) in chronic phase. Treatment of Ph+ CML in blast crisis, accelerated phase, or in chronic phase after failure of interferon-alpha therapy. Treatment of relapsed or refractory Ph+ acute lymphoblastic leukemia (ALL). Treatment of myelodysplastic/myeloproliferative diseases (MDS/MPD) associated with platelet-derived growth factor-receptor (PDGFR) gene re-arrangements. Treatment of aggressive systemic mastocytosis (ASM) patients without the D816V c-Kit mutation or with unknown cKit mutational status. Treatment of hypereosinophilic syndrome (HES) and/or chronic eosinophilic leukemia (CEL) patients who have the FIP1L1-PDGFRα fusion kinase (mutational analysis or FISH demonstration of CHIC2 allele deletion) and for patients with HES and/or CEL who are FIP1L1-PDGFRα fusion kinase negative or unknown. Treatment of patients with unresectable, recurrent, and/or metastatic dermatofibrosarcoma protuberans (DFSP). Treatment of patients with Kit (CD117) positive unresectable and/or metastatic malignant gastrointestinal stromal tumors (GIST). (Pediatrics) Treatment of patients with Ph+ chronic phase CML in chronic phase who are newly diagnosed or whose disease has recurred after stem cell transplant or who are resistant to interferon-alpha therapy.

DOSAGE: *Adults:* ≥18 yrs: CML: Chronic Phase: 400mg/d, may increase to 600mg qd. Accelerated Phase/Blast Crisis: 600mg/d, may increase to 400mg bid. Relapsed/Refractory Ph+ ALL: 600mg/d. MDS or MPD/ASM/HES and/or CEL: 400mg/d. DFSP: 800mg/d. GIST: 400mg/d or 600mg/d. Severe Hepatic Impairment: Reduce dose by 25%. Co-administration with Strong CYP3A4 Inducers: Increase dose by at least 50% and monitor carefully. Hepatotoxicity/Non-Hematologic Adverse Reaction: If bilirubin >3x ULN or transaminases >5x ULN, hold drug until bilirubin <1.5x ULN and transaminases <2.5x ULN. Continue at reduced dose. Neutropenia/Thrombocytopenia: See PI for dose adjustment. Take with food and plenty of water.
Pediatrics: ≥3 yrs: CML: Newly Diagnosed: 340mg/m2/d. Chronic Phase: 260mg/m2/day given qd or split into 2 doses (morning and evening). Severe Hepatic Impairment: Reduce dose by 25%. Co-administration with Strong CYP3A4 Inducers: Increase dose by at least 50% and monitor carefully. Hepatotoxicity/Non-Hematologic Adverse Reaction: If bilirubin >3x ULN or transaminases >5x ULN, hold drug until bilirubin <1.5x ULN and transaminases <2.5x ULN. Continue at reduced dose. Neutropenia/Thrombocytopenia: See PI for dose adjustments. Take with food and plenty of water.

HOW SUPPLIED: Tab: 100mg, 400mg

WARNINGS/PRECAUTIONS: Fluid retention/edema (pleural effusion, pericardial effusion, pulmonary edema and ascites) reported; monitor weight. Anemia/neutropenia/thrombocytopenia reported; monitor CBC weekly during 1st month, biweekly during

2nd month, and periodically thereafter. In pediatric patients, the most frequent toxicities observed were grade 3 and 4 cytopenias. May be hepatotoxic; monitor LFTs at baseline, then monthly or as needed. Avoid becoming pregnant. Interrupt treatment if severe non-hematologic adverse reaction develops (eg, severe hepatotoxicity, severe fluid retention); resume if appropriate. GI bleeds reported. Severe CHF and left ventricular dysfunction. Hypereosinophilic cardiac toxicity. Stevens-Johnson syndrome reported.

ADVERSE REACTIONS: Nausea, vomiting, fluid retention, neutropenia, thrombocytopenia, diarrhea, hemorrhage, pyrexia, rash, headache, fatigue, abdominal pain, elevated transaminases or bilirubin, edema, muscle cramps, musculoskeletal pain, flatulence, nasopharyngitis, insomnia, anemia, anorexia, rhinitis.

INTERACTIONS: Increased levels with CYP3A4 inhibitors (eg, ketoconazole, atazanavir, indinavir, nefazodone, nelfinavir, ritonavir, saquinavir, telithromycin, voriconazole, clarithromycin, itraconazole). Grapefruit juice may increase levels. Decreased levels with CYP3A4 inducers (eg, dexamethasone, phenytoin, carbamazepine, rifampin, phenobarbital, St. John's Wort). Caution with CYP3A4 substrates with narrow therapeutic windows (eg, alfentanil, cyclosporine, diergotamine, ergotamine, fentanyl, quinidine, sirolimus, tacrolimus, cyclosporine, pimozide). Increases levels of drugs metabolized by CYP3A4 (eg, dihydropyridines, triazolo-benzodiazepines, HMG-CoA reductase inhibitors). Switch patients on warfarin to low molecular weight or standard heparin.

PREGNANCY: Category D, not for nursing.

MECHANISM OF ACTION: Protein-tyrosine kinase inhibitor; inhibits the bcr-abl tyrosine kinase.

PHARMACOKINETICS: Absorption: Absolute bioavailability (98%). T_{max}=2-4 hrs. **Distribution:** Plasma protein binding (95%). **Metabolism:** Liver. N-demethyl derivative (major active metabolite). CYP3A4. **Elimination:** Urine and feces (predominant).

GLUCAGON
glucagon (Lilly)

RX

THERAPEUTIC CLASS: Glucagon

INDICATIONS: Treatment for severe hypoglycemia. Diagnostic aid for radiologic examination of the stomach, duodenum, small bowel, and colon.

DOSAGE: *Adults:* Severe Hypoglycemia: 1mg (1 U) SQ/IM/IV. May give another dose after 15 min if patient does not respond, but IV glucose would be a better alternative. Use immediately after reconstitution; discard unused portion. After patient responds give supplemental carbohydrate. Diagnostic Aid: Duodenum/Small Bowel: 0.25-0.5mg (0.25-0.5 U) IV, or 1mg (1 U) IM, or 2mg (2 U) IV/IM before procedure. Stomach: 0.5mg (0.5 U) IV or 2mg (2 U) IM before procedure. Colon: 2mg (2 U) IM 10 min before procedure.
Pediatrics: Severe Hypoglycemia: ≥20kg: 1mg (1 U) SQ/IM/IV. <20kg: 0.5mg (0.5 U) or 20-30mcg/kg. May give another dose after 15 min if patient does not respond, but IV glucose would be a better alternative. Use immediately after reconstitution; discard unused portion. After patient responds give supplemental carbohydrate.

HOW SUPPLIED: Inj: 1mg

CONTRAINDICATIONS: Pheochromocytoma.

WARNINGS/PRECAUTIONS: Caution with history suggestive of insulinoma and/or pheochromocytoma. Glucagon can cause pheochromocytoma tumor to release catecholamines, which may result in a sudden and marked increase in BP. Effective in treating hypoglycemia only if sufficient liver glycogen is present. Glucagon is not effective in states of starvation, adrenal insufficiency, or chronic hypoglycemia; use glucose to treat instead.

ADVERSE REACTIONS: Nausea, vomiting, allergic reactions, urticaria, respiratory distress, hypotension.

PREGNANCY: Category B, caution in nursing.

MECHANISM OF ACTION: Anti-hypoglycemic agent; polypeptide hormone that increases blood glucose levels. Acts on liver glycogen, converting it to glucose. Relaxes smooth muscle of GI tract.

PHARMACOKINETICS: Absorption: C_{max}=7.9ng/mL (SC), 6.9ng/mL (IM); T_{max}=20 min (SC), 13 min (IM). **Distribution:** V_d=0.25L/kg; found in breast milk. **Metabolism:** Extensively degraded in liver, kidneys, plasma. **Elimination:** Urine; $T_{1/2}$=8-18 min.

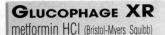

GLUCOPHAGE XR
metformin HCl (Bristol-Myers Squibb)

RX

OTHER BRAND NAMES: Glucophage (Bristol-Myers Squibb) - Riomet (Ranbaxy)

THERAPEUTIC CLASS: Biguanide

INDICATIONS: Adjunct to diet or with a sulfonylurea or insulin, to improve glycemic control in type 2 diabetes mellitus.

DOSAGE: *Adults:* (Sol, Tab) Initial: 500mg bid or 850mg qd with meals. Titrate: Increase by 500mg/week, or 850mg every 2 weeks, or may increase from 500mg bid to 850mg bid after 2 weeks. Max: 2550mg/day. Give in 3 divided doses with meals if dose is >2g/day. (Tab, Extended-Release) Initial: ≥17 yrs: 500mg qd with evening meal. Titrate: Increase by 500mg/week. Max: 2000mg/day. With Insulin: Initial: 500mg qd. Titrate: Increase by 500mg/week. Max: 2500mg/day and 2000mg/day (XR). Decrease insulin dose by 10-25% when FPG <120mg/dL. Swallow whole; do not crush or chew. Elderly/Debilitated/Malnourished: Conservative dosing; do not titrate to Max.
Pediatrics: 10-16 yrs: (Sol, Tab) Initial: 500mg bid with meals. Titrate: Increase by 500mg/week. Max: 2000mg/day.

HOW SUPPLIED: Sol: (Riomet) 500mg/5mL; Tab: 500mg, 850mg, 1000mg*; Tab, Extended-Release: 500mg, 750mg *scored

CONTRAINDICATIONS: Renal disease/dysfunction (SrCr ≥1.5mg/dL (males), ≥1.4mg/dL (females), or abnormal CrCl), CHF, metabolic acidosis, diabetic ketoacidosis. D/C temporarily (48 hrs) for radiologic studies with intravascular iodinated contrast materials.

WARNINGS/PRECAUTIONS: Lactic acidosis reported (rare); increased risk with renal dysfunction, increased age, DM, CHF, and other conditions with risk of hypoperfusion and hypoxemia. Avoid use in patients ≥80 yrs unless renal function is normal. Monitor renal function and for ketoacidosis and metabolic acidosis. Avoid in renal/hepatic impairment. D/C in hypoxic states (eg, CHF, shock, acute MI), loss of blood glucose control due to stress (give insulin), acidosis, dehydration, sepsis. Temporarily d/c prior to surgery (due to restricted food intake) and procedures requiring intravascular iodinated contrast materials. May decrease serum vitamin B_{12} levels. Increased risk of hypoglycemia in elderly, debilitated/malnourished, adrenal or pituitary insufficiency, or alcohol intoxication. Monitor renal function.

ADVERSE REACTIONS: Lactic acidosis, diarrhea, nausea, vomiting, flatulence, abdominal discomfort, abnormal stools, hypoglycemia, myalgia, dizziness, dyspnea, nail disorder, rash, sweating, taste disorder, chest discomfort, chills, flu syndrome, palpitations, asthenia, indigestion, headache.

INTERACTIONS: Furosemide, nifedipine, cimetidine, cationic drugs (eg, digoxin, amiloride, procainamide, quinidine, quinine, ranitidine, trimethoprim, vancomycin, triamterene, morphine) may increase metformin levels. Thiazides, other diuretics, corticosteroids, phenothiazines, thyroid products, estrogens, oral contraceptives, phenytoin, nicotinic acid, sympathomimetics, CCBs, isoniazid may cause hyperglycemia. Risk of hypoglycemia with alcohol. Excess alcohol may increase potential for lactic acidosis. May decrease furosemide levels.

PREGNANCY: Category B, not for use in nursing.

MECHANISM OF ACTION: Biguanide; decreases hepatic glucose production, decreases intestinal absorption of glucose, and improves insulin selectivity by increasing peripheral glucose uptake and utilization.

PHARMACOKINETICS: Absorption: Absolute bioavailability (50-60%). T_{max}=7 hrs. **Distribution:** V_d=654L. **Elimination:** Urine (90%); $T_{1/2}$=6.2 hrs (plasma). $T_{1/2}$=17.6 hrs (blood).

GRANULEX

RX

castor oil - peruvian balsam - trypsin (Mylan Bertek)

THERAPEUTIC CLASS: Debriding agent

INDICATIONS: Treatment of decubitus ulcers, varicose ulcers, debridement of eschar, dehiscent wounds and sunburn.

DOSAGE: *Adults:* Spray wound at least bid or more often prn.
Pediatrics: Spray wound at least bid or more often prn.

HOW SUPPLIED: Spray: (Castor Oil-Peruvian Balsam-Trypsin) 650mg-72.5mg-0.1mg/0.82mL (60mL, 120mL)

WARNINGS/PRECAUTIONS: Do not spray on fresh arterial clots. Avoid spraying in eyes. Wound may be left open or a wet bandage may be applied.

PREGNANCY: Safety in pregnancy and nursing is not known.

MECHANISM OF ACTION: Assists healing of external wounds by facilitating the removal of necrotic tissue, exudate, and organic debris.

GRIFULVIN V

RX

griseofulvin (Ortho Neutrogena)

THERAPEUTIC CLASS: *Penicillium*-derived antifungal

INDICATIONS: Management of tinea capitis, tinea corporis, tinea pedis, tinea unguium, tinea barbae, and tinea cruris. Inhibits the growth of fungi that commonly cause ringworm infections of hair, skin, and nails.

DOSAGE: *Adults:* Tinea Capitis: 500mg qd for 4-6 weeks. Tinea Corporis: 500mg qd for 2-4 weeks. Tinea Pedis: 1g qd for 4-8 weeks. Tinea Cruris: 500mg qd. Tinea Unguium: 1g qd for at least 4 months (fingernail) or at least 6 months (toenails).
Pediatrics: Usual: 5mg/lb/day. 30-50lb: 125-250mg qd. >50lb: 250-500mg qd. Tinea Capitis: Treat for 4-6 weeks. Tinea Corporis: Treat for 2-4 weeks. Tinea Pedis: Treat for 4-8 weeks. Tinea Unguium: Treat for at least 4 months (fingernail) or at least 6 months (toenails).

HOW SUPPLIED: Sus: 125mg/5mL (120mL); Tab: 250mg, 500mg

CONTRAINDICATIONS: Porphyria, hepatocellular failure, pregnancy.

WARNINGS/PRECAUTIONS: Confirm diagnosis. Not for prophylactic use. Monitor renal, hepatic, and hematopoietic functions periodically with prolonged therapy. Cross-sensitivity with PCN may exist. Photosensitivity reported. D/C if granulocytopenia occurs.

ADVERSE REACTIONS: Rash, urticaria, oral thrush, NV, epigastric distress, diarrhea, headache, dizziness, insomnia, mental confusion.

INTERACTIONS: Oral anticoagulants may need adjustment. Barbiturates decrease effects. Decreases effects of oral contraceptives; may increase incidence of breakthrough bleeding.

PREGNANCY: Not for use in pregnancy and in nursing.

GRIS-PEG

RX

griseofulvin (Pedinol)

THERAPEUTIC CLASS: *Penicillium*-derived antifungal

INDICATIONS: Treatment of t.capitis, t.corporis, t.pedis, t.unguium, t.barbae, and t.cruris.

DOSAGE: *Adults:* T.capitis: 375mg qd in single or divided doses for 4-6 weeks. T.corporis: 375mg qd in single or divided doses for 2-4 weeks. T.pedis: 375mg bid for 4-8 weeks. T.cruris: 375mg qd in single or divided doses. T.unguium: 375mg bid for at least 4 months (fingernail) or at least 6 months (toenails).
Pediatrics: Usual: 3.3mg/lb/day. 35-60lb: 125-187.5mg qd. >60lb: 187.5-375mg qd. T.capitis: Treat for 4-6 weeks. T.corporis: Treat for 2-4 weeks. T.pedis: Treat for 4-8 weeks. T.unguium: Treat for at least 4 months (fingernail) or at least 6 months (toenails).

HOW SUPPLIED: Tab: 125mg*, 250mg* *scored

CONTRAINDICATIONS: Porphyria, hepatocellular failure, pregnancy.

WARNINGS/PRECAUTIONS: Not for prophylactic use. Periodically monitor renal, hepatic, and hematopoietic functions in prolonged therapy. Cross-sensitivity with PCN may exist. Photosensitivity reported. D/C if granulocytopenia occurs.

ADVERSE REACTIONS: Rash, urticaria, oral thrush, NV, epigastric distress, diarrhea, headache, dizziness, insomnia, mental confusion.

INTERACTIONS: Oral anticoagulants may need dose adjustments. Decreased effects with barbiturates. Decreased effects of oral contraceptives. Increased alcohol effects.

PREGNANCY: Not for use in pregnancy and in nursing.

MECHANISM OF ACTION: Fungistatic agent. Active against various species of *Microsporum*, *Epidermophyton* and *Trichophyton*. Has greater affinity for depositing in keratin precursor cells of diseased tissue. Tightly binds to new keratin, which then becomes highly resistant to fungal invasions.

PHARMACOKINETICS: Absorption: C_{max}=600ng/mL; T_{max}=4 hrs; AUC=8618ng•hr/mL.

GUAIFED-PD   RX
guaifenesin - phenylephrine HCl (Victory)

THERAPEUTIC CLASS: Expectorant/decongestant

INDICATIONS: Temporary relief of nasal congestion and dry nonproductive cough associated with the common cold and other respiratory allergies.

DOSAGE: *Adults:* 1-2 caps q12h.
Pediatrics: ≥12 yrs: 1-2 caps q12h. 6 to <12yrs: 1 cap q12h.

HOW SUPPLIED: Cap: (Guaifenesin-Phenylephrine) 200mg-7.5mg

CONTRAINDICATIONS: Severe HTN, severe CAD, concomitant MAOIs, pregnancy, nursing mothers.

WARNINGS/PRECAUTIONS: Caution with HTN, DM, ischemic heart disease, hyperthyroidism, increased IOP, prostatic hypertrophy, and the elderly. Not for persistent or chronic cough such as occurs with smoking, asthma, emphysema, or where cough is accompanied by excessive secretions.

ADVERSE REACTIONS: Nausea, cardiac palpitations, increased irritability, headache, dizziness, tachycardia, diarrhea, drowsiness, stomach pain, seizures, slowed heart rate, shortness of breath.

INTERACTIONS: MAOIs and β-adrenergic blockers may increase the effect of sympathomimetics. Sympathomimetics may reduce the antihypertensive effects of methyldopa, mecamylamine, reserpine and veratrum alkaloids. Pseudoephedrine may increase the possibility of cardiac arrhythmias with digitalis glycosides.

PREGNANCY: Category B, not for use in nursing.

GUIATUSS DAC   CV
codeine phosphate - guaifenesin - pseudoephedrine HCl (Scientific Labs)

THERAPEUTIC CLASS: Cough suppressant/expectorant/ decongestant

INDICATIONS: Relief of nasal congestion and cough due to throat and bronchial irritation from a cold or inhaled irritants. Loosens phlegm and thins bronchial secretions to make coughs more productive.

DOSAGE: *Adults:* 10mL q4h. Max: 40mL/24 hrs.
Pediatrics: ≥12 yrs: 10mL q4h. Max: 40mL/24 hrs. 6 to <12 yrs: 5mL q4h. Max: 20mL/24 hrs.

HOW SUPPLIED: Syrup: (Codeine-Guaifenesin-Pseudoephedrine) 10mg-100mg-30mg/5mL

WARNINGS/PRECAUTIONS: Use caution with persistent/chronic cough, cough with excessive phlegm, chronic pulmonary disease, high BP, heart disease, DM, thyroid disease, or shortness of breath. May cause or aggravate constipation.

ADVERSE REACTIONS: Constipation, sedation.

INTERACTIONS: Caution with antidepressants, especially MAOIs.

PREGNANCY: Safety in pregnancy and nursing not known.

GYNE-LOTRIMIN
clotrimazole (Schering)

OTC

OTHER BRAND NAMES: Gyne-Lotrimin 3 (Schering) - Gyne-Lotrimin 3 Combination Pack (Schering) - Gyne-Lotrimin Combination Pack (Schering)

THERAPEUTIC CLASS: Azole antifungal

INDICATIONS: Treatment of vaginal candidiasis.

DOSAGE: *Adults:* 200mg sup or 2% cream intravaginally qhs for 3 days, or 100mg sup or 1% cream intravaginally qhs for 7 days. Apply 1% cream externally qd-bid prn.
Pediatrics: ≥12 yrs: 200mg sup or 2% cream intravaginally qhs for 3 days, or 100mg sup or 1% cream intravaginally qhs for 7 days. Apply 1% cream externally qd-bid prn.

HOW SUPPLIED: (Gyne-Lotrimin) Cre: 1% (5g, 45g); Sup: 100mg (7ˢ); (Combination Pack) Cre: 1% (7g); Sup: 100mg (7ˢ); (Gyne-Lotrimin 3) Sup: 200mg (3ˢ); (3 Combination Pack) Cre: 1% (7g); Sup: 200mg (3ˢ)

WARNINGS/PRECAUTIONS: Do not use if fever (>100°F), foul smelling vaginal discharge or abdominal, back or shoulder pain. Do not use with douches, spermicide or tampons. Do not rely on condoms or diaphragm to prevent STDs or pregnancy while using these products.

HALOG
halcinonide (Ranbaxy)

RX

THERAPEUTIC CLASS: Corticosteroid

INDICATIONS: Corticosteroid-responsive dermatoses.

DOSAGE: *Adults:* (Cre, Oint, Sol) Apply bid-tid. May use occlusive dressings for psoriasis and recalcitrant conditions.
Pediatrics: Limit to least amount compatible with an effective therapeutic regimen.

HOW SUPPLIED: Cre, Oint: 0.1% (15g, 30g, 60g); Sol: 0.1% (20mL, 60mL)

WARNINGS/PRECAUTIONS: May produce reversible HPA axis suppression, manifestations of Cushing's syndrome, hyperglycemia and glucosuria. Occlusive dressings and application to large surface areas may augment systemic absorption. Pediatrics may be more susceptible to systemic toxicity. D/C if irritation occurs.

ADVERSE REACTIONS: Burning, itching, irritation, dryness, folliculitis, hypertrichosis, acneiform eruptions, hypopigmentation, perioral dermatitis, contact dermatitis, skin maceration, secondary infection.

PREGNANCY: Category C, caution in nursing.

MECHANISM OF ACTION: Corticosteroid; possesses anti-inflammatory, antipruritic, and vasoconstrictive actions. Anti-inflammatory effects not established.

PHARMACOKINETICS: Absorption: Percutaneous; inflammation, other disease states, and occlusive dressings may increase percutaneous absorption. **Distribution:** Bound to plasma proteins to varying degrees. Systemically administered corticosteroids are found in breast milk. **Metabolism:** Liver. **Elimination:** Kidneys (major), bile.

HALOPERIDOL
haloperidol (Various)

RX

OTHER BRAND NAMES: Haldol (Ortho-McNeil) - Haldol Decanoate (Ortho-McNeil)

THERAPEUTIC CLASS: Butyrophenone

INDICATIONS: (Immediate-Release) Treatment of psychosis, Tourette's disorder, severe childhood behavioral problems. Short-term treatment of hyperactivity in children. (Decanoate) Prolonged management of psychosis.

DOSAGE: *Adults:* (Immediate-Release) PO: Moderate Symptoms/Elderly/Debilitated: 0.5-2mg bid-tid. Severe Symptoms/Resistant Patients: 3-5mg bid-tid. Max: 100mg/day. IM: Acute Agitation: 2-5mg every 4-8 hrs or hourly as needed for moderately severe or very severe symptoms. Max: 100mg/day. (Decanoate) For IM inj only. Give every 4 weeks or monthly. Initial:10-20 times daily oral dose up to 100mg. Give remainder of dose 3-7 days later if initial dose >100mg. Usual: 10-15 times daily oral dose. Max: 450mg/month.

Elderly/Debilitated: Initial: 10-15 times daily oral dose.
Pediatrics: 3-12 yrs: (15-40kg): PO: Psychosis: Initial: 0.05-0.15mg/kg/day given bid-tid.
Nonpsychotic Disorder/Tourette's: 0.05-0.075mg/kg/day given bid-tid. Max: 6mg/day.

HOW SUPPLIED: Inj: 5mg/mL; Inj: (Decanoate) 50mg/mL, 100mg/mL; Sol: 2mg/mL; Tab: 0.5mg*, 1mg*, 2mg*, 5mg*, 10mg*, 20mg** scored

CONTRAINDICATIONS: Comatose states, severe toxic CNS depression, Parkinson's disease.

WARNINGS/PRECAUTIONS: Risk of tardive dyskinesia, especially in elderly. NMS, hyperpyrexia, heat stroke, bronchopneumonia reported. Decreased cholesterol, cutaneous and/or ocular changes may occur. Neurotoxicity may occur with thyrotoxicosis. Caution with CV disease, seizures, EEG abnormalities, QT-prolonging conditions, elderly. Do not administer IV. Cases of sudden death and Torsades de Pointes reported.

ADVERSE REACTIONS: Extrapyramidal symptoms, tardive dyskinesia, tardive dystonia, ECG changes, QT prolongation, ventricular arrhythmias, tachycardia, hypotension, HTN, nausea, vomiting, constipation, diarrhea, dry mouth, blurred vision, urinary retention.

INTERACTIONS: Caution with rifampin, anticonvulsants, anticoagulants, anticholinergics, antiparkinson agents. May potentiate CNS depression with alcohol, opiates, anesthetics, and other CNS depressants. Antagonizes epinephrine. Monitor for neurological toxicity with lithium. Avoid concomitant alcohol use.

PREGNANCY: Category C, not for use in nursing.

MECHANISM OF ACTION: Butyrophenone; not established, suspected to block effects of dopamine and increase turnover rate.

PHARMACOKINETICS: Absorption: T_{max}=6 days (IM). **Elimination:** $T_{1/2}$=3 weeks (IM).

HALOTESTIN   CIII
fluoxymesterone (Pharmacia & Upjohn)

THERAPEUTIC CLASS: Androgen

INDICATIONS: Testosterone replacement therapy in males with primary hypogonadism or hypogonadotrophic hypogonadism. To stimulate puberty in males with delayed puberty. Palliation of androgen-responsive recurrent mammary cancer in females who are >1 to <5 yrs postmenopausal or who have a hormone-dependent tumor as shown by previous beneficial response to castration.

DOSAGE: *Adults:* Male Replacement Therapy: 5-20mg/day, qd or in divided doses tid-qid. Breast Cancer: 10-40mg/day in divided doses tid-qid. Continue therapy for at least 1 month for satisfactory subjective response, and for 2-3 months for objective response. *Pediatrics:* Male Replacement Therapy: 5-20mg/day, qd or in divided doses tid-qid. Delayed Puberty: Initial: Use low dose, titrate carefully; use for 4-6 months. Caution in children.

HOW SUPPLIED: Tab: 2mg*, 5mg*, 10mg* *scored

CONTRAINDICATIONS: Males with breast or prostate cancer, pregnancy, serious cardiac, hepatic or renal disease.

WARNINGS/PRECAUTIONS: D/C if hypercalcemia occurs in breast cancer or immobilized patients; monitor calcium levels. Risk of hepatic adenomas, hepatocellular carcinoma, and peliosis hepatitis with prolonged high doses. D/C if jaundice, cholestatic hepatitis occurs. Caution in the elderly; increased risk of prostatic hypertrophy and prostatic carcinoma. Risk of edema; caution with pre-existing cardiac, renal, or hepatic disease. Risk of compromised stature in children; monitor bone growth every 6 months. Should not be used for enhancement of athletic performance. Monitor for virilization in females. Patients with BPH may develop acute urethral obstruction. If priapism occurs, d/c and if restarted use lower dose. Contains tartrazine; may cause allergic type reactions especially in those with ASA hypersensitivity. Monitor LFTs, Hct, Hgb periodically.

ADVERSE REACTIONS: Amenorrhea, virilization, menstrual irregularities, gynecomastia, excessive frequency/duration of penile erections, male pattern baldness, increased/decreased libido, oligospermia, hirsutism, acne, fluid and electrolyte disturbances, nausea, hypercholesterolemia, clotting factor suppression, polycythemia, altered LFTs, oligospermia, priapism, anxiety, depression.

INTERACTIONS: May potentiate oral anticoagulants and oxyphenbutazone. May decrease blood glucose and insulin requirements.

PREGNANCY: Category X, not for use in nursing.

MECHANISM OF ACTION: Endogenous androgen; responsible for normal growth and development of male sex organs and for maintenance of secondary sex characteristics.

PHARMACOKINETICS: Elimination: $T_{1/2}$=9.2 hrs.

HAVRIX
hepatitis A Vaccine (Inactivated) (GlaxoSmithKline)

RX

THERAPEUTIC CLASS: Vaccine

INDICATIONS: Active immunization in persons ≥12 months against hepatitis A virus.

DOSAGE: *Adults:* ≥18 yrs: 1440 EL U IM (deltoid), then booster after 6-12 months. *Pediatrics:* 1-18 yrs: 720 EL U IM (deltoid), then booster after 6-12 months.

HOW SUPPLIED: Inj: 720 EL U/0.5mL, 1440 EL U/mL

CONTRAINDICATIONS: Hypersensitivity to any component, including neomycin.

WARNINGS/PRECAUTIONS: Epinephrine should be available for anaphylaxis. Delay with febrile illness. Caution with thrombocytopenia or bleeding disorders. Immunosuppressed may show suboptimal response. May not prevent hepatitis A in patients already infected.

ADVERSE REACTIONS: Injection site soreness, induration, redness, swelling, fever, fatigue, malaise, anorexia, nausea, headache.

INTERACTIONS: Caution with anticoagulant therapy and IM injection. Give immunoglobulins and other vaccines in different syringe and injection site.

PREGNANCY: Category C, caution in nursing.

MECHANISM OF ACTION: May produce immune response for protection against hepatitis A virus infection.

HEPARIN SODIUM
heparin sodium (Various)

RX

THERAPEUTIC CLASS: Glycosaminoglycan

INDICATIONS: Prophylaxis and treatment of venous thrombosis and its extension, PE in atrial fibrillation, and peripheral arterial embolism. Prevention of postoperative DVT and PE. Diagnosis and treatment of acute and chronic consumptive coagulopathies, for prevention of clotting in arterial and cardiac surgery.

DOSAGE: *Adults:* Based on 68kg: Initial: 5000 U IV, then 10,000-20,000 U SQ. Maint: 8000-10,000 U q8h or 15,000-20,000 U q12h. Intermittent IV Injection: Initial: 10,000 U. Maint: 5000-10,000 U q4-6h. Continuous IV Infusion: Initial: 5000U. Maint: 20,000-40,000 U/24 hrs. Adjust to coagulation test results. See PI for details in specific disease states. *Pediatrics:* Initial: 50 U/kg IV drip. Maint: 100 U/kg IV drip q4h or 20,000 U/m^2/24 hrs continuously.

HOW SUPPLIED: Inj: 1000 U/mL, 2500 U/mL, 5000 U/mL, 7500 U/mL, 10,000 U/mL

CONTRAINDICATIONS: Severe thrombocytopenia, if cannot perform appropriate blood-coagulation tests (with full-dose heparin), uncontrollable active bleeding state (except in DIC).

WARNINGS/PRECAUTIONS: Not for IM use. Hemorrhage can occur at any site; caution with increased danger of hemorrhage (severe HTN, bacterial endocarditis, surgery, etc.). Monitor blood coagulation tests frequently. Thrombocytopenia reported; d/c if platelets <100,000mm^3 or if recurrent thrombosis develops. Contains benzyl alcohol. "White-clot syndrome" reported. Monitor platelets, Hct, and occult blood in the stool. Increased heparin resistance with fever, thrombosis, thrombophlebitis, infections with thrombosing tendencies, MI, cancer, and post-op. Higher bleeding incidence in women >60 yrs.

ADVERSE REACTIONS: Hemorrhage, local irritation, erythema, mild pain, hematoma, chills, fever, urticaria.

INTERACTIONS: Wait ≥5 hrs after last IV dose or 24 hrs after last SQ dose before measure PT for dicumarol or warfarin. Platelet inhibitors (eg, acetylsalicylic acid, dextran, phenylbutazone, ibuprofen, indomethacin, dipyridamole, hydroxychloroquine) may induce bleeding. Digitalis, tetracyclines, nicotine, or antihistamines may counteract anticoagulant action.

PREGNANCY: Category C, safe in nursing.

MECHANISM OF ACTION: Glycosaminoglycan; inhibits reactions that lead to blood clotting and the formation of fibrin clots. Acts at multiple sites in the normal coagulation system.

PHARMACOKINETICS: Absorption: (SC) T_{max}=2-4 hrs. **Metabolism:** Liver and reticuloendothelial system. **Elimination:** $T_{1/2}$=10 min.

HEPSERA
RX
adefovir dipivoxil (Gilead Sciences)

> Discontinuation may result in severe acute exacerbations of hepatitis. Chronic use may result in nephrotoxicity in patients at risk of or having underlying renal dysfunction. HIV resistance may occur with unrecognized or untreated HIV infection. May cause lactic acidosis and severe hepatomegaly with steatosis.

THERAPEUTIC CLASS: Acyclic nucleotide analog

INDICATIONS: Treatment of chronic hepatitis B in patients ≥12 yrs of age with evidence of active viral replication and either evidence of persistent elevations in serum aminotransferases (ALT or AST) or histologically active disease.

DOSAGE: *Adults:* 10mg qd. Renal Impairment: CrCl 20-49mL/min: 10mg q48h. CrCl 10-19mL/min: 10mg q72h. Hemodialysis Patients: 10mg every 7 days following dialysis. *Pediatrics:* ≥12 yrs: 10mg qd.

HOW SUPPLIED: Tab: 10mg

WARNINGS/PRECAUTIONS: Monitor hepatic function at repeated intervals upon discontinuation. Monitor renal function in patients with pre-existing or risk factors for renal dysfunction; adjust dosage appropriately. May require HIV antibody testing prior to treatment. Suspend treatment if lactic acidosis and severe hepatomegaly are suspected.

ADVERSE REACTIONS: Asthenia, headache, abdominal pain, nausea, flatulence, diarrhea, dyspepsia, increased creatinine, hypophosphatemia.

INTERACTIONS: Coadministration with drugs that reduce renal function or compete for active tubular secretion may increase concentrations of adefovir or the coadministered drugs.

PREGNANCY: Category C, caution in nursing.

MECHANISM OF ACTION: Acyclic nucleotide analog; inhibits HBV DNA polymerase by competing with natural substrate deoxyadenosine triphosphate and by causing DNA chain termination after incorporation into viral DNA.

PHARMACOKINETICS: Absorption: Absolute bioavailability (59%); C_{max}=18.4ng/mL; T_{max}=1.75 hrs; AUC=220ng•h/mL. *Pediatrics:* C_{max}=23.3ng/mL; AUC=248.8ng•h/mL. **Distribution:** V_d=392mL/kg (1mg/kg/day), 352mL/kg (3mg/kg/day); plasma protein binding (≤4%). **Elimination:** Urine (45%); $T_{1/2}$=7.48 hrs.

HIPREX
RX
methenamine hippurate (Sanofi-Aventis)

THERAPEUTIC CLASS: Hippuric acid salt

INDICATIONS: Prophylaxis or suppression of recurrent urinary tract infections when long-term therapy is necessary. For use only after infection is eradicated by other appropriate antimicrobials.

DOSAGE: *Adults:* 1g bid.
Pediatrics: >12 yrs: 1g bid. 6 to 12 yrs: 0.5g-1g bid.

HOW SUPPLIED: Tab: 1g* *scored

CONTRAINDICATIONS: Renal insufficiency, severe hepatic insufficiency, severe dehydration, concomitant sulfonamides.

WARNINGS/PRECAUTIONS: Maintain acid urine. Doses of 8g/day may cause bladder irritation, painful and frequent micturition, albuminuria, gross hematuria. Monitor LFTs and repeated urine cultures. Contains tartrazine (FD&C Yellow No. 5), which may cause allergic-type reactions; caution with ASA hypersensitivity.

ADVERSE REACTIONS: Nausea, upset stomach, dysuria, rash.

INTERACTIONS: Avoid alkalinizing agents or foods. Sulfonamides may precipitate in the urine; avoid concomitant use.

PREGNANCY: Safety in pregnancy and nursing unknown.

MECHANISM OF ACTION: Hippuric acid salt; produces anti-bacterial effect through conversion of its methenamine component to formaldehyde in acid urine.

PHARMACOKINETICS: Absorption: Rapid. **Elimination:** Urine.

HISTA-VENT DA

RX

chlorpheniramine maleate - methscopolamine nitrate - phenylephrine HCl

(Ethex)

THERAPEUTIC CLASS: Antihistamine/anticholinergic/sympathomimetic

INDICATIONS: Temporary relief of symptoms of allergic rhinitis, vasomotor rhinitis, sinusitis, and the common cold.

DOSAGE: *Adults:* 1 tab q12h. Do not crush or chew.
Pediatrics: ≥12 yrs: 1 tab q12h. 6 to <12 yrs: 1/2 tab q12h. May cut in 1/2; do not crush or chew.

HOW SUPPLIED: Tab, Extended-Release: (Chlorpheniramine-Methscopolamine-Phenylephrine) 8mg-2.5mg-20mg* *scored

CONTRAINDICATIONS: Severe HTN, severe CAD, MAOI therapy, narrow angle glaucoma, urinary retention, PUD, during asthma attack.

WARNINGS/PRECAUTIONS: Caution in HTN, DM, ischemic heart disease, hyperthyroidism, increased IOP, prostatic hypertrophy. May produce CNS stimulation, convulsions, or cardiovascular collapse with accompanying hypotension; more common in the elderly. May cause excitability in children. May impair ability to operate machinery.

ADVERSE REACTIONS: Tachycardia, palpitations, nervousness, insomnia, restlessness, headache, gastric irritation, irritability, fear, anxiety, tenseness, restlessness, tremor.

INTERACTIONS: Increased effect of sympathomimetic amines with MAOI and β-blockers. May reduce antihypertensive effect of methyldopa, mecamylamine, and reserpine. Additive effect with alcohol, TCAs, barbiturates, other CNS depressants.

PREGNANCY: Category C, not for use in nursing.

MECHANISM OF ACTION: Clorpheniramine: Antihistaminic agent that possesses anticholinergic and sedative effects; antagonizes histamine at the H_1 receptor site, resulting in increased vascular permeability. Phenylephrine: Causes vasoconstriction by releasing norepinephrine from sympathetic nerve endings and by direct action on alpha adrenergic receptors. Methscopolamine: Anticholinergic; possesses peripheral actions of belladonna alkaloids.

HIVID

RX

zalcitabine (Roche Labs)

> Severe peripheral neuropathy, pancreatitis (rare), hepatic failure (rare), lactic acidosis, and severe hepatomegaly with steatosis, reported. Extreme caution with pre-existing neuropathy.

THERAPEUTIC CLASS: Nucleoside analogue

INDICATIONS: Treatment of HIV infection in combination with other antiretrovirals.

DOSAGE: *Adults:* 0.75mg q8h. CrCl 10-40mL/min: 0.75mg q12h. CrCl <10mL/min: 0.75mg q24h.
Pediatrics: ≥13 yrs: 0.75mg q8h.

HOW SUPPLIED: Tab: 0.375mg, 0.75mg

WARNINGS/PRECAUTIONS: Decreased CD4 counts increase risk of adverse effects including peripheral neuropathy, pancreatitis, lactic acidosis, severe hepatomegaly with steatosis, hepatic toxicity, oral/esophageal ulcers, cardiomyopathy and CHF. Caution in elderly. Reduce dose in renal impairment. Increased risk of lymphoma with high doses. D/C if moderate peripheral neuropathy develops; may reintroduce at 50% of dose if improve to mild symptoms. Interrupt or reduce dose if serious toxicities occur (eg, peripheral neuropathy, severe oral ulcers, pancreatitis, elevated LFTs). Monitor CBC and clinical chemistry tests before therapy and at appropriate intervals thereafter. Monitor hematologic indices frequently with poor bone marrow reserve. Interrupt therapy if severe anemia or granulocytopenia occurs; reduce dose if less severe. Possible redistribution or accumulation of body fat.

ADVERSE REACTIONS: Peripheral neuropathy, oral lesions/stomatitis, headache, elevated amylase, fatigue, abdominal pain, NV, hepatic dysfunction, blood dyscrasias, rash, urticaria, redistribution/accumulation of body fat.

INTERACTIONS: Avoid drugs associated with peripheral neuropathy. Monitor renal function and neuropathy development with amphotericin, foscarnet, aminoglycosides. Cimetidine and probenecid decrease clearance. Metoclopramide, aluminum- and magnesium-containing antacids reduce absorption. Interrupt therapy with pancreatitis causing agents (eg, intravenous pentamidine).

PREGNANCY: Category C, not for use in nursing.

MECHANISM OF ACTION: Pyrimidine nucleoside analog; inhibits activity of HIV-reverse transcriptase by competing for utilization of deoxycytidine 5'-triphosphate (dCTP) and by its incorporation into viral DNA.

PHARMACOKINETICS: Absorption: *Pediatrics:* Absolute bioavailability (54%). *Adults:* Absolute bioavailability (>80%); C_{max}=25.2ng/mL, T_{max}=0.8 hrs, AUC=72ng•h/mL (fasting); C_{max}=15.5ng/mL, T_{max}=1.6 hrs, AUC=62ng•h/mL (fed). **Distribution:** V_d=0.534L/kg. **Metabolism:** Phosphorylation (zalcitabine triphospate). Dideoxyuridine (metabolite). **Elimination:** Renal excretion: IV (80%), oral (60%); $T_{1/2}$=2 hrs.

HUMALOG RX
insulin lispro (Lilly)

THERAPEUTIC CLASS: Insulin

INDICATIONS: To control hyperglycemia in diabetes.

DOSAGE: *Adults:* Individualize dose. Inject SQ within 15 min before or immediately after a meal. May use with external insulin pump; do not dilute or mix with other insulin when used with pump.

Pediatrics: ≥3 yrs: Individualize dose. Inject SQ within 15 min before or immediately after a meal. May use with external insulin pump; do not dilute or mix with other insulin when used with pump.

HOW SUPPLIED: Cartridge: 100 U/mL; Inj: 100 U/mL; Pen: 100 U/mL

CONTRAINDICATIONS: Hypoglycemia.

WARNINGS/PRECAUTIONS: Any change of insulin should be made cautiously. Changes in strength, manufacturer, type or method of manufacture may result in the need for a change in dosage. Hypoglycemia may occur with taking too much insulin, missing or delaying meals, exercising or working more than usual. An infection or illness (especially with diarrhea or vomiting) may change insulin requirements. With type 1 DM a longer-acting insulin is usually required to maintain glucose control; not required with type 2 DM if regimen includes sulfonylureas. May be diluted with sterile diluent. Caution with potassium-lowering drugs or drugs sensitive to serum potassium levels.

ADVERSE REACTIONS: Hypoglycemia, hypokalemia, allergic reaction, injection site reaction, lipodystrophy, pruritus, rash.

INTERACTIONS: Increased insulin requirements with corticosteroids, isoniazid, niacin, estrogens, oral contraceptives, phenothiazines, thyroid replacement therapy. Decreased insulin requirements with oral hypoglycemics, salicylates, sulfa antibiotics, MAOIs, ACEIs, ARBs, β-blockers, octreotide and alcohol. β-blockers may mask symptoms of hypoglycemia.

PREGNANCY: Category B, caution in nursing.

MECHANISM OF ACTION: Insulin lispro (rDNA origin); regulates glucose metabolism.

PHARMACOKINETICS: Absorption: Absolute bioavailability (55-77%); T_{max}=30-90 min. **Distribution:** V_d=0.26-0.36L/kg. **Elimination:** $T_{1/2}$=1 hr.

HUMATROPE

RX

somatropin (Lilly)

THERAPEUTIC CLASS: Human growth hormone

INDICATIONS: Long-term treatment of pediatrics with growth failure due to growth hormone deficiency (GHD). For short stature associated with Turner syndrome if epiphyses are not closed. Long-term treatment of idiopathic short stature in pediatrics. Treatment of short stature or growth failure in children with SHOX (short stature homeobox-containing gene) deficiency whose epiphyses are not closed. Replacement therapy in adults.

DOSAGE: *Adults:* GHD: Up to 0.006mg/kg SQ qd. Titrate: Increase by individual requirements. Max: 0.0125mg/kg/day. Alternative Dose: Initial: 0.2mg/day (range, 0.15-0.30mg/day). Titrate: Increase gradually every 1-2 months to individual requirement. Max: 0.1-0.2mg/day
Pediatrics: GHD: 0.18mg/kg weekly SQ/IM. Max: 0.3mg/kg weekly in equally divided doses given either on 3 alternate days, 6 times per week, or daily. Turner Syndrome: Up to 0.375mg/kg SQ weekly equally divided, given either daily or on 3 alternate days. Idiopathic Short Stature: Up to 0.37mg/kg SQ weekly given 6 to 7 times per week equally divided. SHOX Deficiency: 0.35mg/kg SQ weekly given daily in equally divided doses.

HOW SUPPLIED: Inj: 5mg, 6mg, 12mg, 24mg

CONTRAINDICATIONS: Pediatrics with closed epiphyses. Proliferative or preproliferative diabetic retinopathy. Active malignancy. Hypersensitivity to Metacresol or glycerin. Acute critical illness due to complications after open heart or abdominal surgery, multiple accidental trauma or acute respiratory failure. Prader-Willi syndrome who are severely obese or have severe respiratory impairment.

WARNINGS/PRECAUTIONS: If sensitivity to diluent occurs reconstitute with bacteriostatic (contains benzyl alcohol; avoid in newborns) or sterile water for injection. Monitor GHD secondary to intracranial lesion for progression/recurrence. Monitor gait, glucose intolerance, for malignant transformation of skin lesions, scoliosis progression, intracranial HTN (perform fundoscopic exam at start and periodically). Caution with DM, endocrine disorders, hypopituitarism. With Turner syndrome monitor for otic or cardiovascular disorders, autoimmune thyroid disease. Caution with endocrine disorders, monitor for otic and cardiovascular disorder.

ADVERSE REACTIONS: Injection site pain, headache, edema, myalgia, pain, rhinitis. (Adults) Arthralgia, paresthesia, HTN, back pain. (Pediatrics) Flu-syndrome, AST/ALT increases, pharyngitis, gastritis, respiratory disorder.

INTERACTIONS: Antagonized by glucocorticoids. May alter clearance of CYP450 substrates (eg, corticosteroids, sex steroids, anticonvulsants, antipyrine, cyclosporine). May require larger dose with oral estrogen replacement. Adjust dose of insulin and/or oral agent in diabetic patients.

PREGNANCY: Category C, caution in nursing.

MECHANISM OF ACTION: Human growth hormone; stimulates linear growth synthesis, metabolizes lipids, reduces body fat stores by increasing cellular protein, and increases plasma fatty acids.

PHARMACOKINETICS: Absorption: (SQ) Absolute bioavailabilty (75%). (IM) Absolute bioavailabilty (63%). **Distribution:** (IV) V_d=0.07L/kg. **Metabolism:** Liver and kidney (protein catabolism). **Elimination:** Urine: (IV) $T_{1/2}$=0.36 hrs. (SQ) $T_{1/2}$=3.8 hrs. (IM) $T_{1/2}$=4.9 hrs.

HUMIRA

RX

adalimumab (Abbott)

> Reports of TB, invasive fungal infections, and other opportunistic infections. Evaluate for latent TB and treat if necessary prior to initiation of therapy.

THERAPEUTIC CLASS: Monoclonal antibody/TNF-blocker

INDICATIONS: For reducing signs and symptoms, inducing major clinical response, inhibiting structural damage progression, and improving physical function in moderately to severely active rheumatoid arthritis (RA). For reducing signs and symptoms of moderately to severely active polyarticular juvenile idiopathic arthritis in patients ≥4 yrs. For reducing signs and symptoms of active arthritis, inhibiting the progression of structural damage, and improving physical function in patients with psoriatic arthritis (PA). For reducing signs and symptoms of active ankylosing spondylitis (AS). For reducing signs and symptoms and inducing and maintaining clinical remission of moderately to severely active Crohn's disease in patients who have had an inadequate response to conventional therapy. For reducing signs and symptoms and inducing clinical remission in patients who have lost response to or are intolerant to infliximab. For treating moderate to severe chronic plaque psoriasis in patients who are candidates for systemic therapy or phototherapy.

DOSAGE: *Adults:* (RA/PA/AS): 40mg SQ every other week. Some patients with RA not taking concomitant MTX may derive additional benefit from increasing the dosing frequency to 40mg every week. Crohn's Disease: Initial: 160mg (may be given as 4 injections on Day 1, or 2 injections/day for 2 consecutive days); then 80mg after 2 weeks (Day 15). Maint: 40mg every other week beginning at Week 4 (Day 29). Plaque Psoriasis: Initial: 80mg. Maint: 40mg every other week starting 1 week after initial dose. *Pediatrics:* (4-17 yrs) 15kg-<30kg: 20mg every other week; ≥30kg: 40mg every other week.

HOW SUPPLIED: Inj: 20mg/0.4mL, 40mg/0.8mL

WARNINGS/PRECAUTIONS: Serious infections including sepsis and TB reported. Monitor for signs of infection during and after therapy; d/c if serious infection develops. Avoid with active infection. Monitor HBV carriers as reactivation may occur; if reactivation occurs, stop adalimumab and start antiviral therapy. Caution with history of recurrent infections or underlying conditions predisposing to infections or in areas where TB and histoplasmosis are endemic. Caution with pre-existing or recent-onset CNS demyelinating disorders. Lymphomas, allergic reactions observed. May affect host defenses against infections and malignancies. May result in autoantibody formation; d/c if lupuslike syndrome develops. Rare possibility of anaphylaxis and pancytopenia including aplastic anemia. May cause CHF or worsen pre-existing disease.

ADVERSE REACTIONS: URI, injection site pain/reactions, headache, rash, sinusitis, nausea, UTI, flu syndrome, abdominal pain, hyperlipidemia, hypercholesterolemia, back pain, hematuria, HTN, immunogenicity.

INTERACTIONS: Do not give concurrently with live vaccines. Reduced clearance with MTX. Do not use concurrently with anakinra due to increased risk of serious infections.

PREGNANCY: Category B, not for use in nursing.

MECHANISM OF ACTION: Monoclonal antibody/TNF-blocker; binds specifically to TNF-α and blocks its interaction with p55 and p75 cell surface TNF receptors. Lyses surface TNF-expressing cells in the presence of complement. Modulates biological responses that are induced or regulated by TNF. In plaque psoriasis, reduces the epidermal thickness and infiltration of inflammatory cells.

PHARMACOKINETICS: Absorption: Absolute bioavailability (64%); C_{max}=4.7mcg/mL; T_{max}=131 hrs. **Distribution:** V_d=4.7-6.0L. **Elimination:** $T_{1/2}$=2 weeks.

HUMULIN

OTC

insulin human, rDNA origin - insulin, human isophane - insulin, human regular (Lilly)

OTHER BRAND NAMES: Humulin N (Lilly) - Humulin R (Lilly)

THERAPEUTIC CLASS: Insulin

INDICATIONS: To control hyperglycemia in diabetes.

DOSAGE: *Adults:* Individualize dose.
Pediatrics: Individualize dose.

HOW SUPPLIED: Inj: 100 U/mL (Humulin N, Humulin R), 500 U/mL (Humulin R U-500); Pen: 100 U/mL (Humulin N).

CONTRAINDICATIONS: Hypoglycemia.

WARNINGS/PRECAUTIONS: Human insulin differs from animal source insulin. Any change of insulin should be made cautiously. Changes in strength, manufacturer, type or method of manufacture may result in the need for a change in dosage. Hypoglycemia may occur with taking too much insulin, missing or delaying meals, exercising or working more than usual. An infection or illness (especially with diarrhea or vomiting) may change insulin requirements. Administration of insulin SQ can result in lipoatrophy.

ADVERSE REACTIONS: Hypoglycemia, sweating, dizziness, palpitation, tremor, hunger, restlessness, lightheadedness, inability to concentrate, headache, injection site reaction, allergic reaction.

INTERACTIONS: Increased insulin requirements with oral contraceptives, corticosteroids, or thyroid replacement therapy. Reduced insulin requirements with oral hypoglycemics, salicylates, sulfa antibiotics, and certain antidepressants. Alcoholic beverages may change insulin requirements. β-blockers may mask symptoms of hypoglycemia.

PREGNANCY: Pregnancy category is not known.

MECHANISM OF ACTION: Insulin; regular insulin human injection of rDNA origin that helps in maintenance of blood glucose at near normal level.

HUMULIN 70/30 OTC
insulin human, rDNA origin - insulin, human (Isophane/Regular) (Lilly)

OTHER BRAND NAME: Humulin 50/50 (Lilly)

THERAPEUTIC CLASS: Insulin

INDICATIONS: To control hyperglycemia in diabetes.

DOSAGE: *Adults:* Individualize dose. Administer SQ.
Pediatrics: Individualize dose. Administer SQ.

HOW SUPPLIED: (Isophane-Regular) Inj: (Humulin 70/30) 70 U-30 U/mL, (Humulin 50/50) 50 U-50 U/mL

WARNINGS/PRECAUTIONS: Human insulin differs from animal source insulin. Make any change of insulin cautiously. Changes in strength, manufacturer, type, or method of manufacture may result in the need for a change in dosage. Hypoglycemia may occur with too much insulin, missing or delaying meals, exercising, or working more than usual. Infection or illness (especially with diarrhea or vomiting) may change insulin requirements. Administration of insulin SQ can result in lipoatrophy.

ADVERSE REACTIONS: Hypoglycemia, sweating, dizziness, palpitation, tremor, hunger, restlessness, lightheadedness, inability to concentrate, headache, injection site reaction, allergic reaction.

INTERACTIONS: Increased insulin requirements with oral contraceptives, corticosteroids, or thyroid replacement therapy. Reduced insulin requirements with oral hypoglycemics, salicylates, sulfa antibiotics, and certain antidepressants. Alcoholic beverages may change insulin requirements. β-blockers may mask symptoms of hypoglycemia.

PREGNANCY: Pregnancy category is not known.

MECHANISM OF ACTION: Insulin; lowers blood glucose levels by stimulating peripheral glucose uptake, especially by skeletal muscle and fat, and by inhibiting hepatic glucose production. Inhibits lipolysis and proteolysis, and enhances protein synthesis.

HYCODAN CIII
homatropine methylbromide - hydrocodone bitartrate (Endo)

OTHER BRAND NAME: Hydromet (Alpharma)

THERAPEUTIC CLASS: Opioid antitussive

INDICATIONS: Symptomatic relief of cough.

DOSAGE: *Adults:* 1 tab or 5mL q4-6h prn. Max: 6 tabs/24hrs or 30mL/24hrs.
Pediatrics: >12 yrs: 1 tab or 5mL q4-6h prn. Max: 6 tabs/24hrs or 30mL/24hrs. 6-12 yrs: 1/2 tab or 2.5mL q4-6h prn. Max: 3 tabs/24hrs or 15mL/24 hrs.

HOW SUPPLIED: (Hydrocodone-Homatropine) Syrup: 5mg-1.5mg/5mL; Tab: 5mg-1.5mg* *scored

WARNINGS/PRECAUTIONS: May be habit-forming. May cause respiratory depression. May obscure diagnosis or clinical course of acute abdominal conditions. Caution in elderly, debilitated, severe hepatic or renal impairment, hypothyroidism, Addison's disease, prostatic hypertrophy, urethral stricture, asthma, head injury, increased ICP, and narrow-angle glaucoma.

ADVERSE REACTIONS: Sedation, drowsiness, lethargy, mental/physical impairment, dizziness, psychic dependence, constipation, ureteral spasm, respiratory depression, rash.

INTERACTIONS: Narcotics, antihistamines, antipsychotics, antianxiety agents, MAOI's, TCAs, alcohol or other CNS depressants may potentiate CNS depression. Increased effect of antidepressant or hydrocodone with MAOIs or TCAs.

PREGNANCY: Category C, not for use in nursing.

MECHANISM OF ACTION: Hydrocodone: Semisynthetic opioid antitussive and analgesic; not established, believed to act directly on the cough center.

PHARMACOKINETICS: Absorption: Hydrocodone; C_{max}=23.6ng/mL, T_{max}=1.3 hrs. **Metabolism:** Hydrocodone: O-demethylation, N-demethylation and 6-keto reduction. **Elimination:** $T_{1/2}$=3.8 hrs.

Hycotuss   `CIII`
guaifenesin - hydrocodone bitartrate (Endo)

OTHER BRAND NAME: Vi-Q-Tuss (Vintage)

THERAPEUTIC CLASS: Cough suppressant/expectorant

INDICATIONS: Symptomatic relief of irritating nonproductive cough associated with upper and lower respiratory tract congestion.

DOSAGE: *Adults:* Initial: 5mL after meals and hs, not less than 4 hrs apart. Titrate: May increase up to 15mL after meals and hs. Max: 30mL/24 hrs.
Pediatrics: >12 yrs: Initial: 5mL after meals and hs, not less than 4 hrs apart. Max Single Dose: 10mL. 6-12 yrs: Initial: 2.5mL after meals and hs, not less than 4 hrs apart. Max Single Dose: 5mL.

HOW SUPPLIED: Syrup: (Hydrocodone-Guaifenesin) 5mg-100mg/5mL

CONTRAINDICATIONS: Cross sensitivity to other opioids. Intracranial lesion associated with increased ICP and whenever ventilatory function is depressed.

WARNINGS/PRECAUTIONS: May be habit forming. Risk of psychic dependence, physical dependence, tolerance, and potential for abuse. Dose-related respiratory depression. Caution with head injury, other intracranial lesions or a pre-existing increase in ICP. May obscure the clinical course head injuries, acute abdominal conditions.

ADVERSE REACTIONS: Respiratory depression, HTN, postural hypotension, palpitations, urinary retention, sedation, drowsiness, mental clouding, lethargy.

INTERACTIONS: Additive CNS depression with other narcotics, analgesics, general anesthetics, phenothiazines, other tranquilizers, sedative hypnotics or other CNS depressants (including alcohol).

PREGNANCY: Category C, not for use in nursing.

MECHANISM OF ACTION: Hydrocodone: Not established; believed to act directly by depressing the cough center. Guaifenesin: Not established; believed to act by stimulating receptors in gastric mucosa that initiate a reflex secretion of respiratory tract fluid, thereby increasing the volume and decreasing the viscosity of bronchial secretions.

PHARMACOKINETICS: Absorption: Hydrocodone: C_{max}=23.6ng/mL, T_{max}=1.3 hrs. Guaifenesin: GI tract (rapid). **Metabolism:** Hydrocodone: O-demethylation, N-demethylation and 6-keto reduction. **Elimination:** Hydrocodone: $T_{1/2}$=3.8 hrs. Guaifenesin: $T_{1/2}$=1 hr.

Hydralazine   RX
hydralazine HCl (Various)

THERAPEUTIC CLASS: Vasodilator

INDICATIONS: Management of hypertension.

DOSAGE: *Adults:* Initial: 10mg qid for 2-4 days. Titrate: Increase to 25mg qid for the rest of the week, then increase to 50mg qid. Maint: Use lowest effective dose. Resistant Patients: 300mg/day or titrate to lower dose combined with thiazide diuretic and/or reserpine, or β-blocker.

Pediatrics: Initial: 0.75mg/kg/day given qid. Titrate: Increase gradually over 3-4 weeks to a max of 7.5mg/kg/day or 200mg/day.

HOW SUPPLIED: Inj: 20mg/mL; Tab: 10mg, 25mg, 50mg, 100mg

CONTRAINDICATIONS: CAD and mitral valvular rheumatic heart disease.

WARNINGS/PRECAUTIONS: D/C if SLE symptoms occur. May cause angina and ECG changes of MI. Caution with suspected CAD, CVA, advanced renal impairment. May increase pulmonary artery pressure in mitral valvular disease. Postural hypotension reported. Add pyridoxine if peripheral neuritis develops. Monitor CBC and ANA titer before and periodically during therapy.

ADVERSE REACTIONS: Headache, anorexia, nausea, vomiting, diarrhea, tachycardia, angina.

INTERACTIONS: Caution with MAOIs. Profound hypotension with potent parenteral antihypertensives (eg, diazoxide). May reduce pressor response to epinephrine.

PREGNANCY: Category C, safety in nursing not known.

MECHANISM OF ACTION: Vasodilator; not established. Apparently lowers BP by direct relaxation of vascular smooth muscle; interferes with calcium movement within vascular smooth muscle responsible for initiating or maintaining contraction.

PHARMACOKINETICS: Absorption: Rapid; T_{max}=1-2 hrs. **Distribution:** Plasma protein binding (87%). **Metabolism:** Acetylation. **Elimination:** Urine; $T_{1/2}$=3-7 hrs.

HYDROCHLOROTHIAZIDE   RX
hydrochlorothiazide (Various)

THERAPEUTIC CLASS: Thiazide diuretic

INDICATIONS: Adjunct therapy in edema associated with CHF, hepatic cirrhosis, corticosteroid and estrogen therapy, renal dysfunction. Management of hypertension.

DOSAGE: *Adults:* Edema: 25-100mg qd or in divided doses. May give every other day or 3-5 days/week. HTN: Initial: 25mg qd. Titrate: May increase to 50mg/day.
Pediatrics: Diuresis/HTN: 1-2mg/kg/day given qd-bid. Max: Infants up to 2 yrs: 37.5mg/day. 2-12 yrs: 100mg/day. <6 months: Up to 1.5mg/kg bid may be required.

HOW SUPPLIED: Tab: 12.5mg, 25mg*, 50mg* *scored

CONTRAINDICATIONS: Anuria, sulfonamide hypersensitivity.

WARNINGS/PRECAUTIONS: Caution in severe renal disease, liver dysfunction, electrolyte/fluid imbalance. Monitor electrolytes. Hyperuricemia, hyperglycemia, hypokalemia, hyponatremia, hypomagnesemia, hypercalcemia may occur. Increases in cholesterol and triglyceride levels reported. May exacerbate SLE. Sensitivity reactions reported. D/C prior to parathyroid test. Enhanced effects in post-sympathectomy patients.

ADVERSE REACTIONS: Weakness, hypotension, pancreatitis, jaundice, diarrhea, vomiting, blood dyscrasias, rash, photosensitivity, electrolyte imbalance, impotence.

INTERACTIONS: May potentiate orthostatic hypotension with alcohol, barbiturates, narcotics. Adjust antidiabetic drugs. Possible decreased response to pressor amines. Corticosteroids, ACTH increase electrolyte depletion. May potentiate nondepolarizing skeletal muscle relaxants, antihypertensives. Lithium toxicity. NSAIDs decrease effects. Decreased PO absorption with cholestyramine, colestipol.

PREGNANCY: Category B, not for use in nursing.

MECHANISM OF ACTION: Thiazide diuretic; affects renal tubular mechanism of electrolyte reabsorption, increasing excretion of Na^+ and Cl^-.

PHARMACOKINETICS: Distribution: Crosses placenta and found in breast milk. **Elimination:** Kidneys (61%); $T_{1/2}$=5.6-14.8 hrs.

HYDROCORTISONE ACETATE   RX
hydrocortisone acetate (Truxton)

THERAPEUTIC CLASS: Corticosteroid

INDICATIONS: By intra-articular or soft tissue injection as adjunctive therapy for short-term administration in: synovitis of osteoarthritis, rheumatoid arthritis, bursitis, gouty arthritis, epicondylitis, nonspecific tenosynovitis, and post-traumatic osteoarthritis. By intralesional injection in: keloids, localized inflammatory lesions, discoid lupus erythematosus, necrobiosis lipoidica diabeticorum, alopecia areata, and cystic tumors of an aponeurosis or tendon.

DOSAGE: *Adults:* Usual: Large joints: 25-37.5mg. Max: 50mg. Small joints: 10-25mg. Bursae: 25-37.5mg. Tendon Sheaths: 5-12.5mg. Soft Tissue Infiltration: 25-50mg, occasionally 75mg. Ganglia: 12.5-25mg. For intra-articular, intralesional, and soft tissue injection only. Injection given once every 2-3 weeks; once a week for more severe conditions. *Pediatrics:* Usual: Large joints: 25-37.5mg. Max: 50mg. Small joints: 10-25mg. Bursae: 25-37.5mg. Tendon Sheaths: 5-12.5mg. Soft Tissue Infiltration: 25-50mg, occasionally 75mg. Ganglia: 12.5-25mg. For intra-articular, intralesional, and soft tissue injection only. Injection given once every 2-3 weeks; once a week for more severe conditions.

HOW SUPPLIED: Inj: 25mg/mL.

CONTRAINDICATIONS: Systemic fungal infections.

WARNINGS/PRECAUTIONS: May need to increase dose before, during, and after stressful situations. May mask signs of infection or cause new infections. Avoid with cerebral malaria. May activate latent amebiasis. Prolonged use may produce glaucoma, optic nerve damage, secondary ocular infections. Increases BP, salt/water retention, potassium excretion. More severe/fatal course of infections reported with chickenpox, measles. Caution with Strongyloides, latent TB, recent MI, hypothyroidism, cirrhosis, ocular herpes simplex, HTN, diverticulitis, fresh intestinal anastomosis, ulcerative colitis, osteoporosis, myasthenia gravis, renal insufficiency, peptic ulcer disease. May increase or decrease sperm count. Growth and development of children on prolonged therapy should be monitored. Monitor for psychic disturbances. Avoid abrupt withdrawal. Avoid injection into an infected site or unstable joint. Frequent intra-articular injections may cause joint tissue damage.

ADVERSE REACTIONS: Fluid and electrolyte disturbances, HTN, osteoporosis, muscle weakness, cushingoid state, menstrual irregularities, nervousness, insomnia, impaired wound healing, DM, ulcerative esophagitis, excessive sweating, increases intracranial pressure, carbohydrate intolerance, glaucoma, cataracts, weight gain, nausea, malaise.

INTERACTIONS: Reduced efficacy and increased clearance with hepatic enzyme inducers (eg, phenobarbital, phenytoin, ephedrine, and rifampin). Caution with ASA in hypoprothrombinemia. Effects on oral anticoagulants are variable; monitor PT. Increased insulin and oral hypoglycemic requirements in DM. Avoid live vaccines with immunosuppressive doses. Possible decreased vaccine response with killed or inactivated vaccines with immunosuppressive doses. Monitor for hypokalemia with potassium-depleting diuretics.

PREGNANCY: Safety in pregnancy not known, not for use in nursing.

HYDROXYZINE HCL   RX
hydroxyzine HCl (Various)

THERAPEUTIC CLASS: Piperazine antihistamine

INDICATIONS: (PO) Relief of anxiety associated with psychoneurosis and as adjunct in organic disease states with anxiety. As a sedative when used as premedication and following general anesthesia. Management of allergic pruritus. (Inj) Management of anxiety, tension, and psychomotor agitation in conditions of emotional stress. As pre-/postoperative and pre-/postpartum adjunctive medication to permit reduction in narcotic dosage, allay anxiety, and control emesis. To control nausea and vomiting, excluding pregnancy.

DOSAGE: *Adults:* PO: Anxiety: 50-100mg qid. Pruritus: 25mg tid-qid. Sedation: 50-100mg. IM: Nausea/Vomiting: 25-100mg. Pre-/Postoperative and Pre-/Postpartum Adjunct:

25-100mg. Psychiatric/Emotional Emergencies: 50-100mg q4-6h prn.
Pediatrics: PO: Anxiety/Pruritus: <6 yrs: 50mg/day in divided doses. ≥6 yrs: 50-100mg in divided doses. Sedation: 0.6mg/kg. IM: Nausea/Vomiting: 0.5mg/lb. Pre-/Postoperative Adjunct: 0.5mg/lb.

HOW SUPPLIED: Inj: 25mg/mL, 50mg/mL; Syrup: 10mg/5mL; Tab: 10mg, 25mg, 50mg, 100mg

CONTRAINDICATIONS: Early pregnancy. Injection is intended only for IM administration and should not, under any circumstances, be injected subcutaneously, intra-arterially, or IV.

WARNINGS/PRECAUTIONS: Caution in elderly. May impair mental/physical abilities. Effectiveness as an antianxiety agent for long term use (>4 months) has not been established.

ADVERSE REACTIONS: Dry mouth, drowsiness, involuntary motor activity.

INTERACTIONS: Potentiates CNS depression with other CNS depressants (eg, narcotics, non-narcotic analgesics, barbiturates, alcohol). May increase alcohol effects.

PREGNANCY: Not for use in pregnancy or nursing.

MECHANISM OF ACTION: Believed to suppress activity in key regions of subcortical area of CNS; shown to have primary skeletal muscle relaxation, bronchodilator, antihistaminic, and analgesic effects.

PHARMACOKINETICS: Absorption: Rapid (GIT).

HYDROXYZINE PAMOATE   RX
hydroxyzine pamoate (Various)

OTHER BRAND NAME: Vistaril (Pfizer)

THERAPEUTIC CLASS: Piperazine antihistamine

INDICATIONS: Relief of anxiety. Allergic pruritus. For sedation as premedication and following anesthesia.

DOSAGE: *Adults:* Anxiety: 50-100mg qid. Pruritus: 25mg tid-qid. Sedation: 50-100mg. *Pediatrics:* Anxiety/Pruritus: >6 yrs: 50-100mg/day in divided doses. <6 yrs: 50mg/day in divided doses. Sedation: 0.6mg/kg.

HOW SUPPLIED: Cap: 25mg, 50mg, 100mg

CONTRAINDICATIONS: Early pregnancy.

WARNINGS/PRECAUTIONS: Caution in elderly. May impair mental/physical abilities. Effectiveness as an antianxiety agent for long term use (>4 months) has not been established.

ADVERSE REACTIONS: Dry mouth, drowsiness, involuntary motor activity.

INTERACTIONS: Potentiated by CNS depressants (eg, narcotics, non-narcotic analgesics, barbiturates); reduce dose.

PREGNANCY: Safety unknown in pregnancy and is contraindicated in early pregnancy, not for use in nursing.

MECHANISM OF ACTION: Believed to suppress activity in key regions of subcortical area of CNS; shown to have primary skeletal muscle relaxation, bronchodilator, antihistaminic, and analgesic effects.

PHARMACOKINETICS: Absorption: Rapid.

HYOSCYAMINE SULFATE   RX
hyoscyamine sulfate (Various)

THERAPEUTIC CLASS: Anticholinergic

INDICATIONS: Adjunct treatment of peptic ulcer, irritable bowel syndrome, neurogenic bladder, and neurogenic bowel disturbances. To reduce symptoms of functional intestinal disorders (eg, mild dysenteries, diverticulitis). To control gastric secretion, visceral spasm, and hypermotility in spastic colitis, spastic bladder, cystitis, pylorospasm, and associated abdominal cramps. Symptomatic relief of biliary and renal colic with concomitant morphine or other narcotics. "Drying agent" for symptomatic relief of acute rhinitis. To reduce rigidity and tremors of Parkinson's disease and control associated sialorrhea and hyperhidrosis. For anticholinesterase poisoning.

DOSAGE: *Adults:* 0.125-0.25mg q4h or prn. Max: 1.5mg/24hrs. Take with or without water.
Pediatrics: ≥12 yrs: 0.125-0.25mg q4h or prn. Max: 1.5mg/24hrs. 2 to <12 yrs: 0.0625-0.125mg q4h or prn. Max: 0.75mg/24hrs. Take with or without water.

HOW SUPPLIED: Tab, Disintegrating: 0.125mg

CONTRAINDICATIONS: Glaucoma, obstructive uropathy, GI tract obstruction, paralytic ileus; intestinal atony of elderly/debilitated, unstable cardiovascular status in acute hemorrhage, toxic megacolon complicating ulcerative colitis, myasthenia gravis.

WARNINGS/PRECAUTIONS: Risk of heat prostration with high environmental temperature. Avoid activities requiring mental alertness. Psychosis has been reported in sensitive patients. Caution with diarrhea, autonomic neuropathy, hyperthyroidism, coronary heart disease, CHF, arrhythmias/tachycardia, HTN, renal disease, and hiatal hernia associated with reflux esophagitis. Contains phenylalanine.

ADVERSE REACTIONS: Anticholinergic effects, drowsiness, headache, nervousness.

INTERACTIONS: Additive effects with other antimuscarinics, amantadine, haloperidol, phenothiazines, MAOIs, TCAs, and some antihistamines. Antacids interfere with absorption; take ac and antacids pc.

PREGNANCY: Category C, caution in nursing.

MECHANISM OF ACTION: Belladonna alkaloid; inhibits action of acetylcholine on structures innervated by postganglionic cholinergic nerves and on smooth muscle that respond to acetylcholine but lack cholinergic innervation, inhibiting GI propulsive motility, decreasing gastric acid secretion, and controlling excess pharyngeal, tracheal, and bronchial secretions.

PHARMACOKINETICS: Absorption: Complete. **Distribution:** Crosses placenta and BBB. **Metabolism:** Partial hydrolysis; tropic acid, tropine (metabolites). **Elimination:** Urine (primarily unchanged); $T_{1/2}$=2-3.5 hrs.

HYTONE   RX
hydrocortisone (Dermik)

THERAPEUTIC CLASS: Corticosteroid

INDICATIONS: Corticosteroid-responsive dermatoses.

DOSAGE: *Adults:* Apply bid-qid depending on the severity. May use occlusive dressings for psoriasis or recalcitrant conditions. D/C dressings if infection develops.
Pediatrics: Apply bid-qid depending on the severity. May use occlusive dressings for psoriasis or recalcitrant conditions. D/C dressings if infection develops.

HOW SUPPLIED: Cre: 2.5% (30g, 60g); Lot: 2.5% (60mL); Oint: 2.5% (30g)

WARNINGS/PRECAUTIONS: May produce reversible HPA axis suppression, manifestations of Cushing's syndrome, hyperglycemia, and glucosuria. Caution when applied to large surface areas or under occlusive dressings. Use appropriate antifungal or antibacterial agent with dermatological infections; d/c if infection does not clear. Pediatrics may be more susceptible to systemic toxicity. Avoid eyes. D/C if irritation occurs.

ADVERSE REACTIONS: Burning, itching, irritation, dryness, folliculitis, hypertrichosis, acneiform eruptions, hypopigmentation, perioral dermatitis, allergic contact dermatitis, skin maceration, secondary infection, skin atrophy, striae, miliaria.

PREGNANCY: Category C, caution in nursing.

MECHANISM OF ACTION: Corticosteroid; possesses anti-inflammatory, antipruritic, and vasoconstrictive actions. Anti-inflammatory effects not established.

PHARMACOKINETICS: Absorption: Percutaneous; inflammation, other skin diseases, and use of occlusive dressings may increase absorption. **Distribution:** Bound to plasma protein to varying degrees. Systemically administered corticosteroids are found in breast milk. **Metabolism:** Liver. **Elimination:** Kidneys (major), bile.

HYTONE 1%
hydrocortisone (Dermik)

OTC

THERAPEUTIC CLASS: Corticosteroid

INDICATIONS: Relief of itching associated with minor skin irritation, inflammation and rashes due to eczema, insect bites, poison ivy/oak/sumac, soaps/detergents, cosmetics, jewelry, seborrheic dermatitis, psoriasis, and/or external feminine and external anal itching.

DOSAGE: *Adults:* Apply up to tid-qid. External Anal Itching: Clean and dry area before applying.
Pediatrics: ≥2 yrs: Apply up to tid-qid. External Anal Itching: ≥12 yrs: Clean and dry area before applying.

HOW SUPPLIED: Lot: 1% (30mL, 120mL)

WARNINGS/PRECAUTIONS: Avoid eyes. D/C use if condition worsens, if symptoms persist for more than 7 days, or if symptoms recur after clearing up. Not for diaper rash. For external feminine itching, avoid use with vaginal discharge. For external anal itching, do not insert into rectum with fingers or applicator.

PREGNANCY: Safety in pregnancy and nursing is not known.

MECHANISM OF ACTION: Corticosteroid; possesses anti-inflammatory, anti-pruritic, and vasoconstrictive properties. Anti-inflammatory actions not established.

PHARMACOKINETICS: Absorption: Percutaneous; inflammation, other disease states, and the use of occlusive dressings may increase percutaneous absorption. **Distribution:** Bound to plasma proteins to varying degrees. Systemically administered corticosteroids are found in breast milk. **Metabolism:** Liver. **Excretion:** Kidneys (major), bile.

IB-STAT
hyoscyamine sulfate (InKine)

RX

THERAPEUTIC CLASS: Anticholinergic

INDICATIONS: Adjunct treatment of peptic ulcer, irritable bowel syndrome, functional GI disorders, neurogenic bladder, neurogenic bowel disturbances. Management of functional intestinal disorders (eg, mild dysenteries, diverticulitis). To control gastric secretion, visceral spasm, and hypermotility in spastic colitis, spastic bladder, cystitis, pylorospasm, and associated abdominal cramps. Symptomatic relief of biliary and renal colic with concomitant morphine or other narcotics. "Drying agent" for symptomatic relief of acute rhinitis. To reduce rigidity and tremors of Parkinson's disease and control associated sialorrhea and hyperhidrosis. For anticholinesterase poisoning.

DOSAGE: *Adults:* 1-2 sprays q4h or prn. Max: 12 sprays/24hrs.
Pediatrics: ≥12 yrs: 1-2 sprays q4h or prn. Max: 12 sprays/24hrs.

HOW SUPPLIED: Sol: 0.125mg/mL (30mL)

CONTRAINDICATIONS: Glaucoma, obstructive uropathy, GI tract obstructive disease, paralytic ileus, intestinal atony of elderly/debilitated, unstable cardiovascular status in acute hemorrhage, severe ulcerative colitis, toxic megacolon, myasthenia gravis.

WARNINGS/PRECAUTIONS: Risk of heat prostration with high environmental temperature. May impair mental/physical abilities. Psychosis has been reported. Caution with diarrhea, autonomic neuropathy, hyperthyroidism, coronary heart disease, CHF, arrhythmias/tachycardia, HTN, renal disease, hiatal hernia with reflux esophagitis.

ADVERSE REACTIONS: Drowsiness, dizziness, blurred vision, mouth dryness, urinary hesitancy and retention, tachycardia, palpitations.

INTERACTIONS: Additive effects with other antimuscarinics, amantadine, haloperidol, phenothiazines, MAOIs, TCAs, or some antihistamines. Antacids interfere with absorption; take ac and antacids pc.

PREGNANCY: Category C, caution in nursing.

IC-GREEN RX
indocyanine green (Akorn)

THERAPEUTIC CLASS: Diagnostic dye

INDICATIONS: To determine cardiac output, hepatic function and liver blood flow, and for ophthalmic angiography.

DOSAGE: *Adults:* For Dilution Curves: 5mg. Max: 2 mg/kg. Refer to prescribing information for further instructions for dilution curves and administration depending on study being conducted.
Pediatrics: For Dilution Curves: 2.5mg. Infants: 1.25mg. Max: 2 mg/kg. Refer to prescribing information for further instructions for dilution curves and administration depending on study being conducted.

HOW SUPPLIED: Inj: 25mg

CONTRAINDICATIONS: Caution with allergy to iodides.

WARNINGS/PRECAUTIONS: Use solvent provided for dissolution. Use aqueous solution within 6 hrs.

ADVERSE REACTIONS: Anaphylactic or urticarial reactions.

INTERACTIONS: Do not use with heparin preparations containing sodium bisulfate; may reduce absorption. Do not perform radioactive iodine uptake studies for at least 1 week following use.

PREGNANCY: Category C, caution in nursing.

MECHANISM OF ACTION: Diagnostic dye; helpful index of hepatic function.

PHARMACOKINETICS: Distribution: Plasma protein binding (95%).

IMODIUM A-D OTC
loperamide HCl (McNeil Consumer)

THERAPEUTIC CLASS: Anti-peristalsis agent

INDICATIONS: Management of diarrhea and traveler's diarrhea.

DOSAGE: *Adults:* ≥12 yrs: (Tab) Initial: 4mg after the first loose stool then 2mg after each additional loose stool, take with plenty of liquid. Max: 8mg/day for no more than 2 days. (Sol) 30mL after first loose stool then 15mL after each additional loose stool. Max: 60mL/day for no more than 2 days.
Pediatrics: 9-11 yrs (60-95 lbs): (Tab) 2mg after the first loose stool then 1mg after each additional loose stool, take with plenty of liquid. Max: 6mg/day for no more than 2 days. (Sol) 15mL after first loose stool then 7.5mL after each additional loose stool. Max: 45mL/day for no more than 2 days. 6-8 yrs (48-59 lbs): (Tab) 2mg after the first loose stool then 1mg after each additional loose stool. Max: 4mg/day for no more than 2 days. (Sol) 15mL after first loose stool then 7.5mL after each additional loose stool. Max: 30mL/day for no more than 2 days.

HOW SUPPLIED: Sol: 1mg/7.5mL (120mL); Tab: 2mg

WARNINGS/PRECAUTIONS: Do not use if diarrhea is accompanied with high fever, blood, or mucus in stool. Caution with history of liver disease. D/C if diarrhea worsens, lasts more than 2 days, or abdominal swelling or bulging occurs.

PREGNANCY: Safety in pregnancy and nursing is not known.

IMOGAM RABIES-HT RX
rabies immune globulin (Sanofi Pasteur)

THERAPEUTIC CLASS: Immunoglobulin

INDICATIONS: Suspected exposure to rabies, particularly severe exposure, except persons previously immunized with HDCV Rabies Vaccine in a pre- or post-exposure.

DOSAGE: *Adults:* 20IU/kg IM. Infiltrate as much of dose around wound, if feasible, with remaining portion given IM in gluteal region.
Pediatrics: 20IU/kg IM. Infiltrate as much of dose around wound, if feasible, with remaining portion given IM in gluteal region.

HOW SUPPLIED: Inj: 150IU/mL

CONTRAINDICATIONS: Do not repeat dose once vaccine treatment has started.

WARNINGS/PRECAUTIONS: Do not give in same syringe or into same site as vaccine. Made from human plasma, risk of infection. Patients with IgA deficiency could have anaphylactic reaction to IgA containing blood products. Have epinephrine (1:1000) available.

ADVERSE REACTIONS: Local reactions: tenderness, pain, soreness, stiffness. Systemic reactions: headache, malaise.

INTERACTIONS: Wait 3 months before giving live vaccines.

PREGNANCY: Category C, safety in nursing not known.

MECHANISM OF ACTION: Anti-rabies immunoglobulin; provides passive protection from rabies virus exposure.

IMOVAX RABIES VACCINE RX
rabies vaccine (Sanofi Pasteur)

THERAPEUTIC CLASS: Vaccine

INDICATIONS: Pre-exposure immunization and postexposure treatment of rabies.

DOSAGE: *Adults:* Pre-exposure: 3 doses of 1mL IM on days 0, 7, and either 21 or 28. 1mL booster every 2 yrs (see PI for details). Post-exposure: 1mL IM on days 0, 3, 7, 14, 30 (ACIP recommendations; 5 doses) and 90 (WHO recommendations; 6 doses). Give 1st dose with rabies immune globulin (RIG) or antirabies serum (ARS). If possible, infiltrate half of RIG or ARS into wound. Previously Immunized: 2 doses; immediately after exposure and 3 days later (no RIG needed).
Pediatrics: Pre-exposure: 3 doses of 1mL IM on days 0, 7, and either 21 or 28. 1mL booster every 2 yrs (see PI for details). Post-exposure: 1mL IM on days 0, 3, 7, 14, 30 (ACIP recommendations; 5 doses), and 90 (WHO recommendations; 6 doses). Give 1st dose with rabies immune globulin (RIG) or antirabies serum (ARS). If possible, infiltrate half of the RIG or ARS into the wound. Previously Immunized: 2 doses; immediately after exposure and 3 days later (no RIG needed).

HOW SUPPLIED: Inj: 2.5IU

WARNINGS/PRECAUTIONS: Postpone pre-exposure immunization during acute febrile illness. Neurologic illness resembling Guillain-Barre syndrome reported. May give antihistamines with history of hypersensitivity. Have epinepherine (1:1000) available. Suboptimal response may occur in immunocompromised patients.

ADVERSE REACTIONS: Local reactions: pain, erythema, swelling, itching. Systemic reactions: headache, nausea, abdominal pain, muscle aches, dizziness.

INTERACTIONS: Immunosuppressants can interfere with development of active immunity.

PREGNANCY: Category C, safety in nursing not known.

MECHANISM OF ACTION: Stimulates the immune system to produce antibodies that may protect against rabies disease.

INAPSINE RX
droperidol (Akorn)

> QT prolongation, torsade de pointes, arrhythmias reported. Use in patients resistant or intolerant to other therapies. Monitor ECG before and 2-3 hrs after treatment. Extreme caution if at risk for developing prolonged QT syndrome.

THERAPEUTIC CLASS: Neuroleptic butyrophenone

INDICATIONS: To reduce incidence of nausea and vomiting associated with surgical and diagnostic procedures.

DOSAGE: *Adults:* Initial (Max): 2.5mg IM/IV. May give additional 1.25mg cautiously to achieve desired effect. Lower initial doses in elderly, debilitated, poor-risk patients.
Pediatrics: 2-12 yrs: Initial (Max): 0.1 mg/kg IM/IV. May give additional dose cautiously. Lower initial doses in debilitated, poor-risk patients.

HOW SUPPLIED: Inj: 2.5mg/mL

CONTRAINDICATIONS: Known or suspected QT prolongation, including congenital long QT syndrome.

WARNINGS/PRECAUTIONS: Caution with renal/hepatic impairment. HTN, tachycardia reported with pheochromocytoma. Risk of prolonged QT syndrome with CHF, cardiac disease, bradycardia, cardiac hypertrophy, electrolyte imbalances (eg, hypokalemia, hypomagnesemia), >65 yrs, alcohol abuse. NMS reported; give dantrolene with increased temperature, HR, or carbon dioxide production. May decrease pulmonary arterial pressure.

ADVERSE REACTIONS: QT interval prolongation, torsade de pointes, cardiac arrest, hypotension, tachycardia, dysphoria, post-op drowsiness, restlessness, hyperactivity, anxiety, depression, syncope, irregular cardiac rhythm.

INTERACTIONS: Avoid drugs that prolong the QT interval (eg, antimalarials, CCBs, anti-depressants, Class I and III antiarrhythmics, certain antihistamines, neuroleptics). Caution with MAOIs, alcohol, diuretics and drugs that induce hypokalemia, hypomagnesemia. May potentiate and be potentiated by CNS depressants (eg, barbiturates, benzodiazepines, tranquilizers, opioids, general anesthetics); use lower doses. Caution with conduction anesthesia (eg, spinal, peridural). Increased BP with fentanyl citrate or other parenteral analgesics. Epinephrine may paradoxically decrease BP.

PREGNANCY: Category C, caution in nursing.

MECHANISM OF ACTION: Neuroleptic; produces marked tranquilization and sedation, allays apprehension and provides mental detachment and indifference while maintaining reflex alertness, produces mild α-adrenergic blockade, peripheral vascular dilation, reduction of pressor effect, and produces antiemetic effects.

INDERAL
propranolol HCl (Wyeth)

RX

THERAPEUTIC CLASS: Nonselective beta-blocker

INDICATIONS: (Tab) Management of hypertension, angina pectoris, hypertrophic subaortic stenosis. Migraine prophylaxis. (Inj/Tab) For cardiac arrhythmias (supraventricular, ventricular tachycardia, tachyarrhythmia of digitalis intoxication, resistant tachyarrhythmia), reduction of cardiovascular mortality post-MI, essential tremor, and pheochromocytoma.

DOSAGE: *Adults:* HTN: (Tab) Initial: 40mg bid. Titrate: Increase gradually. Maint: 120-240mg/day. Angina: (Tab) 80-320mg/day, given bid-qid. Arrhythmia: (Inj) 1-3mg IV at 1 mg/min. (Tab) 10-30mg tid-qid ac and qhs. MI: (Tab) 180-240mg/day, given bid-tid. Migraine: (Tab) Initial: 80mg/day in divided doses. Usual: 160-240mg/day in divided doses. Tremor: (Tab) Initial: 40mg bid. Maint: 120mg/day. Max: 320mg/day. Hypertrophic Subaortic Stenosis: (Tab) 20-40mg tid-qid, ac and qhs. Pheochromocytoma: (Tab) 60mg/day in divided doses for 3 days before surgery with α-blocker. Inoperable Tumor: (Tab) 30mg/day in divided doses.
Pediatrics: HTN (Tab): Initial: 1mg/kg/day PO. Usual: 1-2mg/kg bid. Max: 16mg/kg/day.

HOW SUPPLIED: Inj: 1mg/mL; Tab: 10mg*, 20mg*, 40mg*, 60mg*, 80mg* *scored

CONTRAINDICATIONS: Cardiogenic shock, sinus bradycardia and >1st-degree block, bronchial asthma, CHF (unless failure is secondary to tachyarrhythmia treatable with propranolol).

WARNINGS/PRECAUTIONS: Caution with well-compensated cardiac failure, nonallergic bronchospasm, Wolff-Parkinson-White (WPW) syndrome, hepatic or renal dysfunction. Withdrawal before surgery is controversial. May mask hypoglycemia or hyperthyroidism symptoms. Avoid abrupt discontinuation. May reduce IOP. Can cause cardiac failure. Both digitalis glycosides and β-blockers slow atrioventricular conduction and decrease HR. Concomitant use can increase risk of bradycardia.

ADVERSE REACTIONS: Bradycardia, CHF, hypotension, lightheadedness, mental depression, nausea, vomiting, allergic reactions, agranulocytosis.

INTERACTIONS: Increased propranolol levels/toxicity with CYP2D6 inhibitors (eg, amiodarone, cimetidine, fluoxetine, paroxetine, quinidine, ritonavir), CYP1A2 inhibitors (eg, imipramine, cimetidine, ciprofloxacin, fluvoxamine, isoniazid, ritonavir, theophylline, zileuton, zolmitriptan, rizatriptan), and CYP2C19 inhibitors (eg, fluconazole, cimetidine, fluoxetine, fluvoxamine, tenioposide, tolbutamide). Decreased blood levels with hepatic enzyme inducers (eg, rifampin, ethanol, phenytoin, phenobarbital, cigarette smoking). Propafenone levels increased with concurrent administration. Lidocaine metabolism is inhibited with coadministration. Increased levels with concurrent nisoldipine and nicardipine. Zolmitriptan and rizatriptan concentrations increased with concurrent administration. Decreased theophylline clearance with concrrent administration. Increased concentrations of diazepam and its metabolites with coadministration. Increased thioridazine plasma concentrations with concurrent administration of doses ≥160mg/day. Increased plasma concentrations with chlorpromazine. Aluminum hydroxide gel may decrease plasma concentrations. Decreased plasma concentrations with coadministration of cholestyramine or colestipol. Concurrent administration increases warfarin levels and PT. Increased risk of bradycardia with concomitant digitalis glycosides.

PREGNANCY: Category C, caution in nursing. Intrauterine growth retardation, small placenta, and congenital abnormalities have been reported in neonates whose mothers received propranolol during pregnancy. Neonates whose mothers received propranolol at parturition have exhibited bradycardia, hypoglycemia, and/or respiratory depression.

MECHANISM OF ACTION: Nonselective β-adrenergic receptor blocker; not established, proposed to decrease cardiac output, inhibit renin, and diminute tonic sympathetic nerve outflow.

PHARMACOKINETICS: Absorption: T_{max}=1-4 hrs. **Distribution:** V_d=4 L/kg; plasma protein binding (90%). Crosses placenta; found in breast milk. **Metabolism:** CYP2D6 (hydroxylation), CYP1A2, 2D6 (oxidation), N-dealkylation, glucuronidation. Propranolol glucuronide, naphthyloxylactic acid, glucuronic acid, sulfate conjugates (major metabolites). **Elimination:** $T_{1/2}$=3-6 hrs.

INDOCIN I.V.
indomethacin sodium trihydrate (Merck)

RX

THERAPEUTIC CLASS: NSAID

INDICATIONS: To close hemodynamically significant patent ductus arteriosus in premature infants weighing between 500-1750g after 48 hrs of ineffective medical management.

DOSAGE: *Pediatrics:* Neonates 500-1750g: Therapy includes 3 doses at 12-24 hr intervals. <48 hrs old: 0.2mg/kg IV followed by 0.1mg/kg IV then 0.1mg/kg IV. 2-7 days old: 0.2mg/kg IV for 3 doses. >7 days old: 0.2mg/kg IV followed by 0.25mg/kg IV then 0.25mg/kg IV. If anuria or marked oliguria (urinary output <0.6mL/kg/hr) occurs at scheduled time of second or third dose, hold doses until renal function normalizes. May repeat course if ductus arteriosus reopens. Surgery may be needed if unresponsive after 2 courses.

HOW SUPPLIED: Inj: 1mg

CONTRAINDICATIONS: Untreated infection, bleeding, thrombocytopenia, coagulation defects, necrotizing enterocolitis, significant renal impairment, congenital heart disease when patency of ductus arteriosus is necessary for pulmonary or systemic blood flow.

WARNINGS/PRECAUTIONS: Risk of minor GI bleeding, intraventricular bleeding. May reduce urine output, CrCl, glomerular filtration rate and may increase serum creatinine, BUN. May cause renal insufficiency, including acute renal failure; caution with extracellular volume depletion, CHF, sepsis, hepatic dysfunction. Monitor renal function and serum electrolytes. May mask signs of infection. D/C if liver disease develops. Avoid extravascular injection or leakage.

ADVERSE REACTIONS: Intracranial bleeding, GI bleeding, hyponatremia, elevated serum potassium, retrolental fibroplasia.

INTERACTIONS: May prolong half-life of digitalis; monitor ECG and serum digitalis levels. May elevate gentamicin and amikacin levels. May decrease natriuretic effect of furosemide. May reduce renal function; consider reducing dosage of medications that rely on adequate renal function for elimination. Increased risk of renal insufficiency with nephrotoxic drugs. Increased risk of bleeding with anticoagulants.

PREGNANCY: Safety in pregnancy or nursing not known.

MECHANISM OF ACTION: NSAID; not fully established, believed to inhibit prostaglandin synthesis.

PHARMACOKINETICS: Elimination: Renal, biliary; half-life varies with age and weight.

INDOMETHACIN RX
indomethacin (Various)

> NSAIDs may cause an increased risk of serious cardiovascular thrombotic events, MI, stroke and serious GI adverse events including bleeding, ulceration, and perforation of the stomach or intestines. Contraindicated for the treatment of perioperative pain in the setting of coronary artery bypass graft (CABG) surgery.

OTHER BRAND NAME: Indocin (Merck)

THERAPEUTIC CLASS: NSAID

INDICATIONS: Management of moderate to severe rheumatoid arthritis (RA), ankylosing spondylitis, osteoarthritis (OA), acute painful shoulder (bursitis and/or tendinitis) and/or acute gouty arthritis.

DOSAGE: *Adults:* RA/Ankylosing Spondylitis/OA: Initial: 25mg PO bid-tid. Titrate: May increase by 25-50mg/day at weekly intervals. Max: 200mg/day. Bursitis/Tendinitis: 75-150mg/day given tid-qid for 7-14 days. Acute Gouty Arthritis: 50mg PO tid until pain is tolerable, then d/c. Take with food.
Pediatrics: ≥14 yrs: RA/Ankylosing Spondylitis/OA: Initial: 25mg PO bid-tid. Titrate: May increase by 25-50mg/day at weekly intervals. Max: 200mg/day. Bursitis/Tendinitis: 75-150mg/day given tid-qid for 7-14 days. Acute Gouty Arthritis: 50mg PO tid until pain is tolerable, then d/c. 2-14 yrs (safety and effectiveness not established): Initial: 1-2mg/kg/day in divided doses. Max: 3mg/kg/day or 150-200mg/day. Take with food.

HOW SUPPLIED: Cap: 25mg, 50mg; Sus: 25mg/5mL (237mL)

CONTRAINDICATIONS: ASA or other NSAID allergy that precipitates acute asthmatic attack, urticaria, or rhinitis. Do not give suppositories with history of proctitis or recent rectal bleeding. Treatment of perioperative pain in the setting of CABG surgery.

WARNINGS/PRECAUTIONS: May lead to onset of new HTN or worsening of pre-existing HTN; monitor BP closely. Fluid retention and edema reported; caution with fluid retention or heart failure. Renal papillary necrosis and other renal injury reported after long-term use. Not recommended for use with advanced renal disease; if therapy must be initiated, monitor renal function. Anaphylactoid reactions may occur. May cause serious skin adverse events (eg, exfoliative dermatitis, Stevens-Johnson syndrome, and toxic epidermal necrolysis). Avoid in late pregnancy; may cause premature closure of ductus arteriosis. May cause elevations of LFTs; d/c if liver disease develops or systemic manifestations occur. Caution in elderly. Anemia may occur; with long-term use, monitor Hgb/Hct if signs or symptoms of anemia develop. May inhibit platelet aggregation and prolong bleeding time; monitor with coagulation disorders. Caution with asthma and avoid with ASA-sensitive asthma. Corneal deposits and retinal disturbances reported with prolonged therapy; perform eye exams at periodic intervals during prolonged therapy. May aggravate depression or other psychiatric disturbances, epilepsy, and parkinsonism; use with caution. D/C if severe CNS adverse reactions develop. May impair mental/physical abilities.

ADVERSE REACTIONS: Headache, dizziness, NV, dyspepsia, diarrhea, abdominal pain, constipation, vertigo, somnolence, depression, fatigue.

INTERACTIONS: Avoid salicylates, diflunisal, other NSAIDs, and triamterene. Potassium-sparing diuretics may cause hyperkalemia. Increase toxicity of methotrexate, cyclosporine, lithium, and digoxin. Probenecid increases levels. Caution with antihypertensives and anticoagulants. May decrease effects of diuretics, β-blockers, captopril.

PREGNANCY: Category C, not for use in nursing.

MECHANISM OF ACTION: NSAID; not established; exhibits antipyretic, analgesic, and anti-inflammatory properties. Potent inhibitor of prostaglandin synthesis; decreases prostaglandins in peripheral tissues, suppresses inflammation in RA, and diminishes basal and CO_2-stimulated cerebral blood flow.

PHARMACOKINETICS: Absorption: Readily absorbed. Bioavailability (100%); C_{max}=1-2mcg/mL; T_{max}=2 hrs. **Distribution:** Plasma protein binding (99%); crosses blood-brain barrier and placenta; found in breast milk. **Metabolism:** Desmethyl, desbenzoyl, desmethyldesbenzoyl (metabolites). **Elimination:** Urine (60% as drug/metabolites), feces (33% as drug); $T_{1/2}$=4.5 hrs.

INFANRIX RX

diphtheria toxoid - pertussis vaccine, acellular - tetanus toxoid (GlaxoSmithKline)

THERAPEUTIC CLASS: Vaccine/toxoid combination

INDICATIONS: Active immunization against diphtheria, tetanus, and pertussis as a 5-dose series in infants and children 6 weeks-7yrs old.

DOSAGE: *Pediatrics:* ≥6 weeks up to 7 yrs: 3 doses of 0.5mL IM at 4-8 week intervals. Start at 2 months or as early as 6 weeks if necessary. 2 Booster doses: Give at 15-20 months and at 4 to 6 years. Do not start series over again, regardless of time elapsed between doses. May use to complete primary series in infants who received 1-2 doses of whole-cell DTP vaccine.

HOW SUPPLIED: Inj: 0.5mL

CONTRAINDICATIONS: Hypersensitivity to any component; serious allergic (eg, anaphylaxis) associated with previous dose. Encephalopathy not due to an identifiable cause within 7 days prior to pertussis immunization and progressive neurologic disorder, uncontrolled epilepsy, or progressive encephalopathy. Not contraindicated in individuals with HIV infection.

WARNINGS/PRECAUTIONS: Caution if within 48 hrs of previous whole-cell DTP or acellular DTP vaccine, fever ≥105°F not due to another identifiable cause, collapse or shock-like state, or inconsolable crying lasting ≥3 hrs occurs, or if convulsions occur within 3 days. For high seizure risk, give APAP at time of vaccination and q4-6h for 24 hrs. Caution with neurologic or CNS disorders. Avoid with coagulation disorders. Have epinephrine available. Suboptimal response may occur in immunocompromised patients.

ADVERSE REACTIONS: Local reactions, fever, irritability, drowsiness, anorexia, vomiting, diarrhea, crying.

INTERACTIONS: Avoid with anticoagulants. Immunosuppressive therapy (eg, irradiation, antimetabolites, alkylating agents, cytotoxic drugs, corticosteroids) may decrease response. Administer tetanus immune globulin, diphtheria antitoxin, hepatitis B vaccine, and *Haemophilus influenzae* type b vaccine at separate site.

PREGNANCY: Category C, safety in nursing not known.

MECHANISM OF ACTION: Vaccine/toxoid combination: provides active immunization by producing antibodies against diphtheria, tetanus, and pertussis.

INFeD RX

iron dextran (Watson)

> Anaphylactic-type reactions and death possible. Only use when indication clearly established and lab investigations confirm iron deficient state not amenable to oral therapy.

THERAPEUTIC CLASS: Iron supplement

INDICATIONS: Treatment of iron deficiency when oral administration is not possible.

DOSAGE: *Adults:* Iron Deficiency Anemia: Dose (mL)=0.0442 (desired Hgb-observed Hgb) x LBW + (0.26 x LBW); LBW=lean body wt (kg). See PI for details. Blood Loss: Replace equivalent amount of iron in blood loss.
Pediatrics: ≥4 months: >15kg: Iron Deficiency Anemia: Dose (mL)=0.0442 (desired Hgb-observed Hgb) x LBW + (0.26 x LBW); LBW=lean body wt (kg). 5-15kg: Dose (mL)=0.0442 (desired Hgb-observed Hgb) x wt + (0.26 x weight). See PI for details. Blood Loss: Replace equivalent amount of iron in blood loss.

HOW SUPPLIED: Inj: 50mg/mL

CONTRAINDICATIONS: Anemia not associated with iron deficiency.

WARNINGS/PRECAUTIONS: Large IV doses associated with increased incidence of adverse effects. Caution with serious hepatic impairment, significant allergies, asthma. Avoid during acute phase of infectious kidney disease. May exacerbate cardiovascular complications in pre-existing cardiovascular disease and joint pain or swelling in rheumatoid arthritis. Hypersensitivity reactions reported after uneventful test doses. Unwarranted therapy can cause exogenous hemosiderosis. Have epinephrine (1:1000) available. Risk of carcinogenesis with IM use. Give 0.5mL test dose before IM/IV administration.

ADVERSE REACTIONS: Anaphylactic reactions, chest pain/tightness, urticaria, pruritus, abdominal pain, nausea, arthralgia, convulsions, respiratory arrest, hematuria, febrile episodes.

INTERACTIONS: Discontinue oral iron before use.

PREGNANCY: Category C, caution in nursing.

PHARMACOKINETICS: Absorption: Capillaries; lymphatic system. **Elimination:** $T_{1/2}$=5-20 hrs.

INTRON A   RX
interferon alfa-2b (Schering)

> May cause or aggravate fatal or life-threatening neuropsychiatric, autoimmune, ischemic, and infectious disorders. Monitor closely with periodic clinical and laboratory evaluations.

THERAPEUTIC CLASS: Biological response modifier

INDICATIONS: Treatment of hairy cell leukemia, malignant melanoma, follicular lymphoma, condylomata acuminata, AIDS-related Kaposi's sarcoma, chronic hepatitis C and B.

DOSAGE: *Adults:* ≥18 yrs: Hairy Cell Leukemia: 2 MIU/m^2 IM/SQ 3x/week up to 6 months. Reduce dose by 50% or stop therapy with severe reactions. Malignant Melanoma: Initial: 20 MIU/m^2 IV for 5 consecutive days/week for 4 weeks. Maint: 10 MIU/m^2 SQ 3x/week for 48 weeks. Follicular Lymphoma: 5 MIU SQ 3x/week up to 18 months. Condylomata Acuminata: 1 MIU into lesion 3x/week alternating days for 3 weeks. Max: 5 lesions/course. Kaposi's Sarcoma: 30 MIU/m^2 3x/week IM/SQ. Hepatitis C: 3 MIU IM/SQ 3x/week for 18-24 months. Hepatitis B: IM/SC: 5 MIU qd or 10 MIU IM/SQ 3x/week for 16 weeks. Dose adjust according to severe adverse reactions and laboratory abnormalities (See PI for more information).
Pediatrics: ≥1 yr: Hepatitis B: 3 MIU/m^2 SQ 3x/week for 1 week, then 6 MIU/m^2 3x/week for total therapy of 16-24 weeks. Max: 10 MIU/m^2 3x/week. Reduce dose by 50% or stop therapy with severe reactions. Adjust based on WBC, granulocyte, and/or platelet counts. Dose adjust according to severe adverse reactions and laboratory abnormalities (See PI for more information).

HOW SUPPLIED: Inj: 10 MIU, 18 MIU, 50 MIU, 10 MIU/mL, 3 MIU/0.2mL, 5 MIU/0.2mL, 10 MIU/0.2mL

CONTRAINDICATIONS: Autoimmune hepatitis, decompensated liver disease.

WARNINGS/PRECAUTIONS: Do not give IM if platelet count is less than 50,000 cells/mm^3. Hepatotoxicity, retinal hemorrhages, autoimmune diseases, pulmonary infiltrates, pneumonitis, thyroid abnormalities and pneumonia reported. Avoid with immunosuppressed transplant, autoimmune disorders, decompensated liver disease. Caution with cardiac disease, coagulation disorders, severe myelosuppression, pulmonary disease, thyroid disorders, or DM prone to ketoacidosis. Avoid with pre-existing psychiatric condition; depression, suicidal behavior, and aggressive behavior; monitor during treatment and in the 6 month follow-up period. D/C if psychiatric symptoms worsen or suicidal ideation is identified. Cases of encephalopathy observed in elderly treated with higher doses. Dental and periodontal disorders have been reported with ribavirin and interferon combination therapy. May exacerbate psoriasis or sarcoidosis. Do not interchange brands.

ADVERSE REACTIONS: Fever, headache, chills, fatigue, myalgia, GI disturbances, alopecia, dyspnea, depression.

INTERACTIONS: Increases theophylline levels by 100%. Caution with myelosuppressive agents (eg, zidovudine). Antidiabetics and thyroid agents may need adjustments. Increased risk of hemolytic anemia when coadministered with ribavirin. Risk of aplastic anemia and pure red cell aplasia with Rebetol.

PREGNANCY: Category C, Category X when used with ribavirin, not for use in nursing.

MECHANISM OF ACTION: α-interferon; binds to specific membrane receptors on cell surface initiating induction of enzymes, suppression of cell proliferation, immunomodulating activities, and inhibition of virus replication.

PHARMACOKINETICS: Absorption: (IM, SQ) C_{max}=18-116 IU/mL, T_{max}=3-12 hrs; (IV) C_{max}=135-273 IU/mL, T_{max}=30 min. **Elimination:** (IM, SQ) $T_{1/2}$=2-3 hrs; (IV) $T_{1/2}$=2 hrs.

INVANZ
ertapenem sodium (Merck)

RX

THERAPEUTIC CLASS: Carbapenem

INDICATIONS: Treatment of complicated intra-abdominal infections; complicated skin and skin structure infections (cSSSI), including diabetic foot infections without osteomyelitis; community-acquired pneumonia (CAP); complicated urinary tract infections (UTI), including pyelonephritis; acute pelvic infections, including postpartum endomyetritis, septic abortion, and post-surgical gynecologic infections caused by susceptible strains of microorganisms. Prophylaxis of surgical site infection following elective colorectal surgery.

DOSAGE: *Adults:* Treatment: 1g IM/IV qd. Duration: Intra-Abdominal Infections: 5-14 days. cSSSI: 7-14 days. CAP/UTI: 10-14 days. Acute Pelvic Infections: 3-10 days. May give IV for up to 14 days and IM for up to 7 days. Prophylaxis Following Colorectal Surgery: 1g IV as single dose given 1 hr prior to surgical incision. CrCl ≤30mL/min/1.73m^2: 500mg IM/IV qd. Hemodialysis: Give 150mg IM/IV after dialysis only if 500mg dose was given within 6 hrs prior to dialysis.
Pediatrics: ≥13 yrs: 1g IM/IV qd. 3 months-12 yrs: 15mg/kg IM/IV bid (Max: 1g/day). Treatment Duration: Intra-Abdominal Infections: 5-14 days. SSSI: 7-14 days. CAP/UTI: 10-14 days. Pelvic Infections: 3-10 days. May administer IV for up to 14 days and IM for up to 7 days.

HOW SUPPLIED: Inj: 1g

CONTRAINDICATIONS: Anaphylactic reactions to β-lactams, hypersensitivity to local anesthetics of the amide type (due to lidocaine diluent).

WARNINGS/PRECAUTIONS: Serious, sometimes fatal, hypersensitivity reported with β-lactam therapy. *Clostridium difficile*-associated diarrhea (CDAD) reported. D/C if CDAD confirmed. Seizures and CNS adverse experiences reported. Increased risk of seizures with CNS disorders and/or compromised renal function. Use lidocaine HCl as diluent for IM use. Monitor renal, hepatic, hematopoietic functions during prolonged therapy. Do not inject into blood vessel.

ADVERSE REACTIONS: Diarrhea, infused vein complication, NV, headache, edema/swelling, fever, abdominal pain, constipation, altered mental status, headache, insomnia, rash, pruritis.

INTERACTIONS: Decreased clearance with probenecid. Do not mix or coinfuse with other drugs. May decrease serum levels of valproic acid when coadministered.

PREGNANCY: Category B, caution in nursing.

MECHANISM OF ACTION: Broad-spectrum carbapenem; penetrates bacterial cells and interferes with synthesis of vital cell wall components, resulting in cell death.

PHARMACOKINETICS: **Absorption:** Administration of different doses resulted in different parameters. (IM): Absolute bioavailability (90%); T_{max}=2.3 hrs. **Distribution:** V_d=0.12L/kg (adult); 0.2L/kg (3 months-12 yrs); 0.16L/kg (13-17 yrs). Plasma protein binding (95%); found in breast milk. **Metabolism:** Liver via hydrolysis of the β-lactam ring. **Elimination:** (Adults, 13-17 yrs old) $T_{1/2}$=4 hrs. (3 months-12 years old) Urine (38% unchanged, 37% metabolite), feces (10%); $T_{1/2}$=2.5 hrs.

INVIRASE
saquinavir mesylate (Roche Labs)

RX

Not interchangeable with Fortovase®.

THERAPEUTIC CLASS: Protease inhibitor

INDICATIONS: Treatment of HIV infection in combination with other antiretrovirals.

DOSAGE: *Adults:* 1000mg bid with ritonavir 100mg bid. Take within 2 hrs after a full meal. *Pediatrics:* >16 yrs: 1000mg bid with ritonavir 100mg bid. Take within 2 hrs after a full meal.

HOW SUPPLIED: Cap: 200mg; Tab: 500mg

CONTRAINDICATIONS: Concomitant amiodarone, bepridil, flecainide, propafenone, quinidine, rifampin, pimozide, terfenadine, cisapride, astemizole, triazolam, midazolam, ergot derivatives.

WARNINGS/PRECAUTIONS: New onset DM, exacerbation of pre-existing DM, hyperglycemia may occur. Exacerbation of chronic liver dysfunction reported with hepatitis or cirrhosis. Spontaneous bleeding may occur with hemophilia A, B. Possible redistribution or accumulation of body fat. Caution with hepatic dysfunction. Interrupt therapy if serious toxicity occurs.

ADVERSE REACTIONS: Diarrhea, abdominal discomfort, NV, dyspepsia, mucosa damage, headache, paresthesia, extremity numbness, asthenia, myalgia, fatigue, pneumonia, lipodystrophy.

INTERACTIONS: See contraindications. Avoid lovastatin, simvastatin, St. John's wort, garlic capsules, tipranavir, trazodone, fluticasone. Decreased plasma levels with nevirapine. Consider alternatives to CYP3A4 inducers (eg, phenobarbital, phenytoin, dexamethasone, carbamazepine). Ritonavir increases adverse effects. Risk of toxicity with substrates of CYP3A4 substrates (eg, calcium CCBs, clindamycin, dapsone, quinidine, triazolam). Delavirdine increases plasma levels; monitor LFTs frequently. Saquinavir/ritonavir increases digoxin levels; monitor digoxin serum concentration and reduce dose if needed.

PREGNANCY: Category B, not for use in nursing.

MECHANISM OF ACTION: HIV protease inhibitor; binds to the protease active site and inhibits activity of the enzyme, preventing cleavage of the viral polyproteins and resulting in formation of immature, noninfectious virus particles.

PHARMACOKINETICS: Absorption: Administration of variable doses and combinations resulted in different parameters. **Distribution:** Plasma protein binding (98%). (IV): V_d=700L. **Metabolism:** Hepatic via CYP3A4. **Elimination:** (PO): Urine (1%), feces (88%). (IV): Urine (3%), feces (81%).

IONAMIN
phentermine (Celltech)   CIV

THERAPEUTIC CLASS: Anorectic sympathomimetic amine

INDICATIONS: Short term adjunct for exogenous obesity if initial BMI ≥30kg/m^2 or ≥27kg/m^2 with other risk factors (eg, HTN, diabetes, hyperlipidemia).

DOSAGE: *Adults:* 15-30mg before breakfast or 10-14 hrs before bedtime. Swallow caps whole.
Pediatrics: ≥16 yrs: 15-30mg prior to breakfast or 10-14 hrs before bedtime. Swallow caps whole.

HOW SUPPLIED: Cap: 15mg, 30mg

CONTRAINDICATIONS: Advanced arteriosclerosis, CVD, moderate to severe HTN, hyperthyroidism, glaucoma, agitated states, history of drug abuse, within 14 days of MAOI use.

WARNINGS/PRECAUTIONS: Primary pulmonary HTN and valvular heart disease reported. D/C if tolerance occurs. Abuse potential. Caution with mild HTN.

ADVERSE REACTIONS: Primary pulmonary HTN, palpitations, tachycardia, BP elevation, restlessness, dizziness, insomnia, headache, diarrhea, constipation, impotence.

INTERACTIONS: See Contraindications. May alter insulin requirements. Avoid with weight loss products including SSRIs. Valvular heart disease and primary pulmonary hypertension reported with fenfluramine and dexfenfluramine. May decrease effects of adrenergic neuron blocking agents.

PREGNANCY: Safety in pregnancy and nursing not known.

MECHANISM OF ACTION: Anorectic sympathomimetic amine; not established as appetite suppressor; causes CNS stimulation and elevation of BP.

IQUIX
levofloxacin (Santen)

RX

THERAPEUTIC CLASS: Fluoroquinolone

INDICATIONS: Bacterial corneal ulcer.

DOSAGE: *Adults:* Days 1-3: 1-2 drops q30min-2h while awake and 4-6 hrs after retiring. Days 4-completion: 1-2 drops q1-4h while awake.
Pediatrics: ≥6 yrs: Days 1-3: 1-2 drops q30min-2h while awake and 4-6 hrs after retiring. Days 4-completion: 1-2 drops q1-4h while awake.

HOW SUPPLIED: Sol: 1.5% (5mL)

WARNINGS/PRECAUTIONS: D/C if hypersensitivity or superinfection occurs. Avoid contact lenses with corneal ulcer.

ADVERSE REACTIONS: Headache, taste disturbance.

INTERACTIONS: Systemic quinolone therapy increases theophylline levels, interferes with caffeine metabolism, enhances warfarin effects, and may elevate SCr with cyclosporine.

PREGNANCY: Category C, caution in nursing.

MECHANISM OF ACTION: Fluoroquinolone; antibacterial active against a broad spectrum of gram-positive and gram-negative ocular pathogens. Responsible for inhibition of bacterial topoisomerase IV and DNA gyrase, enzymes required for DNA replication, transcription, repair, and recombination.

PHARMACOKINETICS: Absorption: C_{max}=3.22ng/mL (initial dose), 10.9ng/mL (multiple doses).

IROFOL
folic acid - polysaccharide iron complex (Dayton)

RX

THERAPEUTIC CLASS: Iron/vitamin

INDICATIONS: Prevention and treatment of iron and folic acid deficiencies.

DOSAGE: *Adults:* 1-2 tabs or 5-10mL qd.
Pediatrics: >12 yrs: 1-2 tabs or 5-10mL qd.

HOW SUPPLIED: (Folic Acid-Polysaccharide Iron Complex) Liquid: 1mg-100mg/5mL; Tab: 1mg-150mg

WARNINGS/PRECAUTIONS: Not for the treatment of pernicious anemia and other megaloblastic anemias. Folic acid >0.1mg/day may obscure pernicious anemia.

ADVERSE REACTIONS: Gastric intolerance, allergic sensitization.

INTERACTIONS: Absorption may be inhibited by eggs, milk, magnesium trisilicate or antacids containing carbonates.

PREGNANCY: Safety in pregnancy and nursing not known.

ISONIAZID
isoniazid (Various)

RX

> **Severe, fatal hepatitis may develop. Monitor LFTs monthly.**

OTHER BRAND NAME: Nydrazid (Sandoz)

THERAPEUTIC CLASS: Isonicotinic acid hydrazide

INDICATIONS: Prevention and treatment of TB.

DOSAGE: *Adults:* Active TB: 5mg/kg as a single dose. Max: 300mg/day or 15mg/kg 2 to 3 times/week. Max: 900mg/day. Use with other antituberculosis agents. Prevention: 300mg qd single dose.
Pediatrics: Active TB: 10-15mg/kg as a single dose. Max: 300mg qd or 20-40mg/kg 2 to 3 times/week. Max: 900mg/day. Use with other antituberculosis agents. Prevention: 10mg/kg qd single dose. Max: 300mg qd.

HOW SUPPLIED: Inj: 100mg/mL; Syrup: 50mg/5mL; Tab: 100mg, 300mg

CONTRAINDICATIONS: Severe hypersensitivity reactions including drug-induced hepatitis, previous INH-associated hepatic injury, severe adverse effects to INH (eg, drug fever, chills, arthritis), acute liver disease.

WARNINGS/PRECAUTIONS: D/C if hypersensitivity occurs. Monitor closely with liver or renal disease. Take with vitamin B$_6$ in malnourished and those predisposed to neuropathy.

ADVERSE REACTIONS: Peripheral neuropathy, NV, epigastric distress, elevated serum transaminases, bilirubinemia, jaundice, hepatitis, skin eruptions, pyridoxine deficiency.

INTERACTIONS: Alcohol is associated with hepatitis. May increase phenytoin, theophylline, and valproate serum levels. Do not take with food. Severe acetaminophen toxicity reported. Decreases carbamazepine metabolism and AUC of ketoconazole. Avoid tyramine- and histamine-containing foods.

PREGNANCY: Category C, caution in nursing.

MECHANISM OF ACTION: Inhibits mycoloic acid synthesis and acts against actively growing tuberculosis bacilli.

PHARMACOKINETICS: Distribution: Passes through placental barrier and into milk. **Metabolism:** Acetylation and dehydrazination. **Elimination:** Urine (50-70%).

KALETRA   RX
lopinavir - ritonavir (Abbott)

THERAPEUTIC CLASS: Protease inhibitor

INDICATIONS: Treatment of HIV infection in combination with other antiretrovirals.

DOSAGE: *Adults:* Therapy-Naive: 400/100mg (2 tabs or 5mL) bid or 800/200mg qd (4 tabs or 10mL). Therapy-Experienced: 400/100mg (2 tabs or 5mL) bid. Once daily administration not recommended. Concomitant Efavirenz, Nevirapine, Fosamprenavir, Nelfinavir: Therapy-Naive: 400/100mg (2 tabs) bid. Concomitant Efavirenz, Nevirapine, Amprenavir or Nelfinavir: 533/133mg (6.5mL) bid. Concomitant Efavirenz, Nevirapine, Fosamprenavir without Ritonavir, or Nelfinavir: Treatment-Experienced with Decreased Susceptibility to Lopinavir: 600/150mg (3 tabs) bid. Tabs can be taken with or without food. Oral solution must be taken with food.
Pediatrics: >12 yrs: Therapy-Naive: 400/100mg (2 tabs or 5mL) bid or 800/200mg qd (4 tabs or 10mL). Therapy-Experienced: 400/100mg (2 tabs or 5mL) bid. Once daily administration not recommended. Concomitant Efavirenz, Nevirapine, Fosamprenavir, Nelfinavir: Therapy-Naive: 400/100mg (2 tabs) bid. Concomitant Efavirenz, Nevirapine, Amprenavir or Nelfinavir: 533/133mg (6.5mL) bid. Concomitant Efavirenz, Nevirapine, Fosamprenavir without Ritonavir, or Nelfinavir: Treatment-Experienced with Decreased Susceptibility to Lopinavir: 600/150mg (3 tabs) bid. 6 months-12 yrs: >40kg: 400/100mg (4 tabs 100/25 mg, 2 tabs 200/50 mg or 5 mL) bid. 15-40kg: (Tab,Sol) 10/2.5mg/kg bid. 7-<15kg: (Sol) 12/3mg/kg bid. Concomitant Efavirenz, Nevirapine, (Fos)amprenavir: >45kg: 533/133mg (4 tabs 100/25 mg, 2 tabs 200/50 mg, or 6.5mL) bid. 15-45kg: (Tab,Sol) 11/2.75mg/kg bid. 7-<15kg: (Sol) 13/3.25mg/kg bid. Tabs can be taken with or without food. Oral solution must be taken with food.

HOW SUPPLIED: Tab: (Lopinavir-Ritonavir) 200mg-50mg, 100mg-25mg; Sol: 80mg-20mg/mL (160mL)

CONTRAINDICATIONS: Concomitant drugs dependent on CYP3A or CYP2D6 for clearance (eg, rifampin, St John's wort, lovastatin, simvastatin, dihydroergotamine, ergonovine, ergotamine, methylergonovine, cisapride, pimozide, midazolam, triazolam).

WARNINGS/PRECAUTIONS: May elevate triglyceride and total cholesterol levels; monitor levels at baseline then periodically. Possible redistribution or accumulation of body fat. D/C if symptoms of pancreatitis occur. May exacerbate DM or cause hyperglycemia. Caution in hepatic impairment. Increased bleeding may occur with hemophilia A and B. Risk of further transaminase elevation or hepatic decompensation in patients with underlying hepatitis B or C or marked transaminase elevation prior to treatment; monitor ALT/AST more frequently during first several months of therapy. Hepatic dysfunction reported.

ADVERSE REACTIONS: Abdominal pain, asthenia, headache, diarrhea, NV, dyspepsia, flatulence, insomnia, hepatotoxicity, pancreatitis.

INTERACTIONS: See Contraindications. Avoid use with rifampin, St. John's wort; may cause loss of virologic response and resistance. Avoid use with lovastatin and simvastatin; risk of myopathy and rhabdomyolysis. May increase levels of antiarrhythmics (eg, amiodarone, bepridil, systemic lidocaine, quinidine), dihydropyridine CCBs (eg, felodipine, nifedipine, nicardipine), immunosuppressants (eg, cyclosporine, tacrolimus, rapamycin); monitoring recommended. May increase levels of trazodone; use with caution and consider lower trazodone dose. May increase levels of fluticasone; coadministration not recommended. CYP3A inducers may decrease lopinavir levels. CYP3A inhibitors may increase lopinavir levels. May increase levels of drugs primarily metabolized by CYP3A. May increase levels of amprenavir, indinavir, saquinavir. May increase levels of clarithromycin with renal impairment; reduce clarithromycin dose by 50% if CrCl 30-60mL/min and by 75% if CrCl <30mL/min. Decreased effect with dexamethasone, carbamazepine, phenobarbital, phenytoin. Monitor PT/INR with warfarin. Space dosing with didanosine; give 1 hr before or 2 hrs after lopinavir/ritonavir. Increased levels with delavirdine. Efavirenz, nevirapine, and tipranavir may decrease levels; adjust dose. May increase levels of ketoconazole or itraconazole; avoid ketoconazole or itraconazole doses >200mg/day. May increase rifabutin levels; reduce usual rifabutin dose by 75%. Decreases atovaquone levels. Oral solution contains alcohol; disulfiram reaction may occur with disulfiram or metronidazole. May increase sildenafil, tadalafil, vardenafil levels; reduce dose of sildenafil (eg, 25mg q48h); reduce dose of tadalafil (eg, 10mg q72h); reduce dose of vardenafil (eg, 2.5mg q72h). May decrease methadone levels; may need to increase methadone dose. May decrease ethinyl estradiol levels; use alternate/additional contraception. Increased atorvastatin levels; use lowest atorvastatin or rosuvastatin dose or consider alternate HMG-CoA reductase inhibitors (eg, pravastatin, fluvastatin). Increases tenofovir levels. May increase nelfinavir levels; dosage adjustments needed. Do not administer with tipranavir coadministered with ritonavir.

PREGNANCY: Category C, not for use in nursing.

MECHANISM OF ACTION: Lopinavir: HIV-1 protease inhibitor; prevents cleavage of the Gag-Pol polyprotein, resulting in the production of immature, noninfectious viral particles. Ritonavir: CYP3A inhibitor; inhibits metabolism of lopinavir, increasing its plasma levels.

PHARMACOKINETICS: Absorption: Lopinavir: C_{max}=9.8mcg/mL, T_{max}=4 hrs, AUC=92.6mcg•h/mL. **Distribution:** Lopinavir: Plasma protein binding (98-99%). **Metabolism:** Lopinavir: Hepatic via CYP3A. Ritonavir: Induces own metabolism. **Elimination:** Urine (2.2%), feces (19.8%).

KAYEXALATE   RX
sodium polystyrene sulfonate (Sanofi-Aventis)

THERAPEUTIC CLASS: Cation-exchange resin

INDICATIONS: Treatment of hyperkalemia.

DOSAGE: *Adults:* PO: 15g qd-qid. Rectal Enema: 30-50g q6h.
Pediatrics: Use 1g per 1mEq of K^+ as basis of calculation. Avoid PO administration in neonates.

HOW SUPPLIED: Sus: 15g/60mL

CONTRAINDICATIONS: Hypokalemia, obstructive bowel disease, neonates with reduced gut motility (post-op or drug-induced), oral administration in neonates.

WARNINGS/PRECAUTIONS: Hypokalemia may occur. May be insufficient for emergency correction of hyperkalemia. Monitor for electrolyte disturbances. Caution in those intolerant to sodium increases (eg, severe CHF or HTN, or marked edema).

ADVERSE REACTIONS: Anorexia, NV, constipation, hypokalemia, hypocalcemia, sodium retention, diarrhea, (elderly) fecal impaction.

INTERACTIONS: Avoid nonabsorbable cation-donating antacids and laxatives; systemic alkalosis may occur (eg, magnesium hydroxide, aluminum carbonate). Hypokalemia exaggerates toxic effects of digitalis. Intestinal obstruction reported with aluminum hydroxide. May decrease absorption of lithium and thyroxine. Avoid sorbitol.

PREGNANCY: Category C, caution in nursing.

MECHANISM OF ACTION: Cation exchange resin; partially releases sodium ions and replaced by K^+ ions.

KEFLEX   RX
cephalexin (Middlebrook)

THERAPEUTIC CLASS: Cephalosporin (1st generation)

INDICATIONS: Treatment of otitis media and skin and skin structure (SSSI), bone, genito-urinary tract, and respiratory tract infections caused by susceptible strains of microorganisms.

DOSAGE: *Adults:* Usual: 250mg q6h. Streptococcal Pharyngitis/SSSI/Uncomplicated Cystitis (>15 yrs): 500mg q12h. Treat cystitis for 7-14 days. Max: 4g/day.
Pediatrics: Usual: 25-50mg/kg/day in divided doses. Streptococcal Pharyngitis (>1 yr)/SSSI: May divide dose and give q12h. Otitis Media: 75-100mg/kg/day in divided doses. Administer for ≥10 days in β-hemolytic streptococcal infections.

HOW SUPPLIED: Cap: 250mg, 500mg, 750mg

WARNINGS/PRECAUTIONS: Caution with markedly impaired renal function, history of GI disease. Cross-sensitivity with cephalosporins and PCNs. *Clostridium difficile*-associated diarrhea reported. Positive direct Coombs' tests reported. False (+) for urine glucose with Benedict's, Fehling's solution, and Clinitest® tabs. May result in overgrowth of nonsusceptible bacteria.

ADVERSE REACTIONS: Diarrhea, allergic reactions, dyspepsia, gastritis, abdominal pain, superinfection (prolonged use).

INTERACTIONS: Probenecid inhibits excretion.

PREGNANCY: Category B, caution in nursing.

MECHANISM OF ACTION: Cephalosporin; bactericidal due to inhibition of cell-wall synthesis.

PHARMACOKINETICS: Absorption: Rapid; oral administration of variable doses resulted in different parameters. T_{max}=1 hr. **Elimination:** Urine (90% unchanged).

KEPPRA   RX
levetiracetam (UCB Pharma)

THERAPEUTIC CLASS: Pyrrolidine derivative

INDICATIONS: (PO) Adjunctive therapy for partial onset seizures in adults and children ≥4 yrs of age. Adjunctive therapy in the treatment of myoclonic seizures in adults and children ≥12 yrs with juvenile myoclonic epilepsy (JME). Adjunctive therapy in the treatment of primary generalized tonic-clonic (PGTC) seizures in adults and children ≥6 yrs with idiopathic generalized epilepsy. (Inj) Adjunctive therapy for partial onset seizures in adults with epilepsy. Adjunctive therapy for myoclonic seizures in adults with JME. Alternative for adults (≥16 yrs) when oral administration is temporarily not feasible.

DOSAGE: *Adults:* Inj/PO: Initial: 500mg bid. Titrate: Increase by 1000mg/day every 2 weeks. Max: 3000mg/day. Inj: Replacement Therapy: Initial total daily dosage and frequency should equal total daily dosage and frequency of oral therapy. Dilute injection in 100mL of compatible diluent and give as 15-min IV infusion. CrCl >80mL/min: 500mg-1500mg q12h. CrCl 50-80mL/min: 500mg-1000mg q12h. CrCl 30-50mL/min: 250mg-750mg q12h. CrCl <30mL/min: 250mg-500mg q12h. ESRD with Dialysis: 500-1000mg q24h. A supplemental dose of 250mg-500mg after dialysis is recommended.
Pediatrics: PO: Partial Onset Seizures/PGTC: ≥16 yrs or JME: ≥12 yrs: Initial: 500mg bid. Titrate: Increase by 1000mg/day every 2 weeks. Max: 3000mg/day. Partial Onset Seizures: 4 to <16 yrs or PGTC: 6-16 yrs: Initial: 10mg/kg bid: Titrate: Increase by 20mg/kg/day every 2 weeks. Max: 60mg/kg/day. Inj: Partial Onset Seizures: Initial: 500mg bid. Titrate: Increase by 1000mg/day every 2 weeks. Max: 3000mg/day. Replacement Therapy: Initial total daily dosage and frequency should equal total daily dosage and frequency of oral therapy. Dilute injection in 100mL of compatible diluent and give as 15-min IV infusion. CrCl >80mL/min: 500mg-1500mg q12h. CrCl 50-80mL/min: 500mg-1000mg q12h. CrCl 30-50mL/min: 250mg-750mg q12h. CrCl <30mL/min: 250mg-500mg q12h. ESRD with Dialysis: 500mg-1000mg q24h. A supplemental dose of 250mg-500mg after dialysis is recommended.

HOW SUPPLIED: Inj: 500mg/5mL; Sol: 100mg/mL; Tab: 250mg*, 500mg*, 750mg*, 1000mg*
*scored

WARNINGS/PRECAUTIONS: Associated with somnolence, fatigue, coordination difficulties, and behavioral abnormalities (eg, psychotic symptoms, suicide ideation, and other abnormalities). Avoid abrupt withdrawal. Hematologic abnormalities reported. Caution in renal dysfunction. Myoclonic seizures reported.

ADVERSE REACTIONS: Somnolence, asthenia, headache, infection, pain, anorexia, dizziness, nervousness, vertigo, ataxia, pharyngitis, rhinitis, irritability, hepatic failure.

PREGNANCY: Category C, caution in nursing.

MECHANISM OF ACTION: Antiepileptic drug; not established, proposed that it inhibits burst firing without affecting normal neuronal excitability, suggesting that it may selectively prevent hypersynchronization of epileptiform burst firing and propagation of seizure activity.

PHARMACOKINETICS: Absorption: Rapid; complete. **Distribution:** Plasma protein binding (<10%); excreted in breast milk. **Metabolism:** Enzymatic hydrolysis (not extensive). Metabolite: Ucb L057. **Elimination:** Renal; urine (66%); $T_{1/2}$=6-8 hrs. Refer to PI for pediatric parameters.

KETAMINE
ketamine HCl (Various)

`CIII`

THERAPEUTIC CLASS: Nonbarbiturate anesthetic

INDICATIONS: Sole anesthetic agent for diagnostic and surgical procedures that do not require skeletal muscle relaxation. Induction of anesthesia prior to the administration of other general anesthetic agents. To supplement low-potency agents (eg, nitrous oxide).

DOSAGE: *Adults:* Initial: IV: 1-4.5mg/kg. Infuse slowly over 60 seconds. May administer with 2-5mg doses of diazepam over 60 seconds. IM: 6.5-13mg/kg. Maint: Adjust according to anesthetic needs. May increase in increments of one-half to full induction dose.
Pediatrics: Initial: IV: 1-4.5mg/kg. Infuse slowly over 60 seconds. IM: 6.5-13mg/kg. Maint: Adjust according to anesthetic needs. May increase in increments of one-half to full induction dose.

HOW SUPPLIED: Inj: 50mg/mL

CONTRAINDICATIONS: Patients in whom a significant elevation in BP would constitute a serious hazard.

WARNINGS/PRECAUTIONS: Monitor cardiac function with HTN or cardiac dysfunction. Postoperative confusional states may occur during recovery. Respiratory depression may occur; maintain airway and respiration. Do not use alone in pharynx, larynx, or bronchial tree procedures. Use with caution in chronic alcoholics and acutely intoxicated patients. May increase CSF pressure; use with extreme caution in patients with preanesthetic CSF pressure. Use with agent that obtunds visceral pain when surgical procedure involving visceral pain.

ADVERSE REACTIONS: Nausea, vomiting, anorexia, elevated blood pressure and pulse, hypotension, bradycardia, arrhythmia, respiratory depression, apnea, airway obstruction, diplopia, nystagmus, slight elevation of IOP, enhanced skeletal muscle tone.

INTERACTIONS: Prolonged recovery time with barbiturates and/or narcotics.

PREGNANCY: Not recommended with pregnancy, use in nursing unknown.

MECHANISM OF ACTION: Nonbarbiturate anesthetic; produces anesthetic state characterized by profound analgesia, normal pharyngeal-laryngeal reflexes, normal or slightly enhanced skeletal muscle tone, cardiovascular and respiratory stimulation, and occasionally a transient and minimal respiratory depression.

PHARMACOKINETICS: Metabolism: Hepatic, via N-dealkylation, hydroxylation, conjugation, and dehydration.. **Elimination:** $T_{1/2}$=10-15 min (α phase), $T_{1/2}$=2.5 hrs (β phase).

KETOROLAC

RX

ketorolac tromethamine (Various)

> For short-term use only (≤5 days). Contraindicated with peptic ulcer disease, GI bleeding/perforation, perioperative pain in coronary artery bypass graft (CABG) surgery, advanced renal impairment, risk of renal failure due to volume depletion, CV bleeding, hemorrhagic diathesis, incomplete hemostasis, high-risk of bleeding, intraoperatively when hemostasis is critical, intrathecal/epidural use, L&D, nursing, and with ASA, NSAIDs, or probenecid. Caution greater risk of GI events with elderly patients. NSAIDs may cause an increased risk of CV thrombotic events (MI, stroke). (PO) Contraindicated in pediatric patients and in minor or chronic painful conditions.

OTHER BRAND NAME: Toradol (Roche Labs)

THERAPEUTIC CLASS: NSAID

INDICATIONS: Short-term (≤5 days) management of moderately severe, acute pain as continuation therapy from IV/IM.

DOSAGE: *Adults:* >16 yrs to <65 yrs: Single-Dose: 60mg IM or 30mg IV. Multiple-Dose: 30mg IM/IV q6h. Max: 120mg/day. Transition from IM/IV to PO: 20mg PO single dose, then 10mg PO q4-6h. Max: 40mg/24 hrs. ≥65 yrs/Renal Impairment/<50kg: Single-Dose: 30mg IM or 15mg IV. Multiple-Dose: 15mg IM/IV q6h. Max: 60mg/day. Transition from IM/IV to PO: 10mg PO q4-6h. Max: 40mg/24 hrs.
Pediatrics: 2-16 yrs: Single-Dose: IM: 1mg/kg. Max: 30mg. IV: 0.5mg/kg. Max: 15mg.

HOW SUPPLIED: Inj: 15mg/mL, 30mg/mL; Tab: 10mg

CONTRAINDICATIONS: Active or history of peptic ulcer, GI bleeding, perioperative pain in CABG surgery, advanced renal impairment or risk of renal failure due to volume depletion, labor/delivery, nursing mothers, ASA or NSAID allergy, preoperatively or intraoperatively when hemostasis is critical, cerebrovascular bleeding, hemorrhagic diathesis, incomplete hemostasis, high risk of bleeding, neuraxial (epidural or intrathecal) administration, and concomitant ASA, NSAIDs, probenecid, or pentoxifylline.

WARNINGS/PRECAUTIONS: Do not exceed 5 days of therapy. Risk of GI ulcerations, bleeding, and perforation. Caution with renal/hepatic dysfunction, dehydration, HTN, CHF, coagulation disorders, debilitated and elderly, pre-existing asthma. Preoperative use prolongs bleeding. CV thrombotic events, fluid retention, edema, NaCl retention, oliguria, anaphylactic reactions, elevated BUN and serum creatinine, anemia reported. Correct hypovolemia before therapy.

ADVERSE REACTIONS: Nausea, dyspepsia, GI pain, diarrhea, edema, headache, drowsiness, dizziness.

INTERACTIONS: May increase risk of bleeding with anticoagulants. May reduce diuretic response to furosemide. Increased serum levels with salicylates. Avoid ASA, NSAIDs, and probenecid. Increased lithium and methotrexate levels. May increase risk of renal impairment with ACE-inhibitors. May increase seizures with phenytoin and carbamazepine. Hallucinations reported with fluoxetine, thiothixene, and alprazolam. Do not mix in the same syringe as morphine. May have adverse effects with nondepolarizing muscle relaxants.

PREGNANCY: Category C, not for use in nursing.

MECHANISM OF ACTION: NSAID; suspected to inhibit prostaglandin synthetase; exerts anti-inflammatory, analgesic, and antipyretic actions.

PHARMACOKINETICS: Absorption: Absolute bioavailability (100%). **Distribution:** V_d=13L; plasma protein binding (99%); enters breast milk. **Metabolism:** Liver; hydroxylation, conjugation. **Elimination:** Urine (92%; 40% metabolites, 60% unchanged), feces (6%); $T_{1/2}$=5-6 hrs.

KLARON

RX

sulfacetamide sodium (Dermik)

THERAPEUTIC CLASS: Sulfonamide

INDICATIONS: Topical treatment of acne vulgaris.

DOSAGE: *Adults:* Apply thin film bid.
Pediatrics: ≥12 yrs: Apply thin film bid.

HOW SUPPLIED: Lot: 10% (118mL)

WARNINGS/PRECAUTIONS: D/C if irritation, rash, or hypersensitivity reaction occurs. Avoid eyes. Contains sulfites. Caution with denuded or abraded skin.

ADVERSE REACTIONS: Erythema, itching, edema, stinging, burning, local irritation.

PREGNANCY: Category C, caution in nursing.

MECHANISM OF ACTION: Sulfonamide; acts as a competitive inhibitor of para-aminobenzoic acid (PABA) utilization, an essential component for bacterial growth.

PHARMACOKINETICS: Absorption: Percutaneous (about 4%). **Distribution:** Small amounts of orally administered sulfonamides reported to be eliminated in breast milk. **Elimination:** Urine; $T_{1/2}$=7-13 hrs.

KLONOPIN
clonazepam (Roche Labs)

OTHER BRAND NAME: Klonopin Wafers (Roche Labs)

THERAPEUTIC CLASS: Benzodiazepine

INDICATIONS: Adjunct or monotherapy in Lennox-Gastaut syndrome, akinetic and myoclonic seizures. Absence seizures refractory to succinimides. Panic disorder with or without agoraphobia.

DOSAGE: *Adults:* Seizure Disorders: Initial: Not to exceed 1.5mg/day given tid. Titrate: May increase by 0.5-1mg every 3 days. Max: 20mg qd. Panic Disorder: Initial: 0.25mg bid. Titrate: Increase to 1mg/day after 3 days, then may increase by 0.125-0.25mg bid every 3 days. Max: 4mg/day. Wafer: Dissolve in mouth with or without water. *Pediatrics:* <10 yrs or 30kg: Seizure Disorders: Initial: 0.01-0.03mg/kg/day up to 0.05mg/kg/day given bid-tid. Titrate: Increase by no more than 0.25-0.5mg every 3 days. Maint: 0.1-0.2mg/kg/day given tid. Wafer: Dissolve in mouth with or without water.

HOW SUPPLIED: Tab: 0.5mg*, 1mg, 2mg; Tab, Disintegrating (Wafer): 0.125mg, 0.25mg, 0.5mg, 1mg, 2mg *scored

CONTRAINDICATIONS: Significant liver disease, acute narrow-angle glaucoma, untreated open-angle glaucoma.

WARNINGS/PRECAUTIONS: May increase incidence of generalized tonic-clonic seizures. Monitor blood counts and LFTs periodically with long-term therapy. Caution with renal dysfunction, chronic respiratory depression. Increased fetal risks during pregnancy. Avoid abrupt withdrawal. Hypersalivation reported.

ADVERSE REACTIONS: Somnolence, depression, ataxia, CNS depression, upper respiratory tract infection, fatigue, dizziness, sinusitis, colpitis.

INTERACTIONS: Decreased serum levels with CYP450 inducers (eg, phenytoin, carbamazepine, phenobarbital). Caution with CYP3A inhibitors (eg, oral antifungals). Alcohol, narcotics, barbiturates, nonbarbiturate hypnotics, antianxiety agents, phenothiazines, thioxanthene and butyrophenone antipsychotics, MAOIs, TCAs and other anticonvulsant drugs potentiate CNS-depressant effects.

PREGNANCY: Category D, not for use in nursing.

MECHANISM OF ACTION: Benzodiazepine; not established, suspected to enhance activity of GABA, the major inhibitory neurotransmitter in the CNS.

PHARMACOKINETICS: Absorption: Rapid and complete. Absolute bioavailability (90%), T_{max}=1-4 hrs. **Distribution:** Plasma protein binding (85%). **Metabolism:** Hepatic via acetylation, hydroxylation, and glucuronidation, CYP450. **Elimination:** Renal. Urine (<2% unchanged); $T_{1/2}$=30-40 hrs.

KOGENATE FS   RX
antihemophilic factor (Bayer Healthcare)

THERAPEUTIC CLASS: Antihemophilic Factor (Recombinant)

INDICATIONS: Treatment of hemophilia A in which there is a deficiency of activity of clotting factor FVIII.

DOSAGE: *Adults:* Minor hemorrhage: 10-20 IU/kg IV; repeat if evidence of further bleeding. Moderate to major hemorrhage/surgery (minor): 15-30 IU/kg IV; repeat one dose at 12-24 hrs if needed. Major to life-threatening hemorrhage/fractures/head trauma: Initial: 40-50 IU/kg IV; repeat dose 20-25 IU/kg IV q 8-12 hrs. Surgery (major): Preoperative dose: 50 IU/kg IV (verify 100% FVIII activity prior to surgery); repeat as necessary after 6-12 hrs initially, and for 10-14 days until healing is complete.
Pediatrics: Minor hemorrhage: 10-20 IU/kg IV; repeat if evidence of further bleeding. Moderate to major hemorrhage/surgery (minor): 15-30 IU/kg IV; repeat one dose at 12-24 hrs if needed. Major to life-threatening hemorrhage/fractures/head trauma: Initial: 40-50 IU/kg IV; repeat dose 20-25 IU/kg IV q 8-12 hrs. Surgery (major): Preoperative dose: 50 IU/kg IV (verify 100% FVIII activity prior to surgery); repeat as necessary after 6-12 hrs initially, and for 10-14 days until healing is complete.

HOW SUPPLIED: Inj: 250 IU, 500 IU, 1000 IU, 2000 IU

CONTRAINDICATIONS: Known hypersensitivity to mouse or hamster protein.

WARNINGS/PRECAUTIONS: Development of circulating neutralizing antibodies to FVIII may occur; monitor by appropriate clinical observation and laboratory tests. Hypotension, urticaria, and chest tightness in association with hypersensitivity reported.

ADVERSE REACTIONS: Local injection site reactions, dizziness, rash, unusual taste, mild increase in BP, pruritus, depersonalization, nausea, rhinitis.

PREGNANCY: Category C, safety not known in nursing.

MECHANISM OF ACTION: Antihemophilic factor.

K-Phos Neutral   RX

dibasic sodium phosphate - monobasic potassium phosphate - monobasic sodium phosphate (Beach)

THERAPEUTIC CLASS: Urinary acidifier

INDICATIONS: To increase urinary phosphate and pyrophosphate.

DOSAGE: *Adults:* 1-2 tabs qid, with meals and hs. Take with full glass of water.
Pediatrics: >4 yrs: 1 tab qid, with meals and hs. Take with full glass of water.

HOW SUPPLIED: Tab: (Monobasic Potassium Phosphate-Dibasic Sodium Phosphate-Monobasic Sodium Phosphate) 155mg-852mg-130mg* (equivalent to 250mg phosphorous/298mg sodium (13mEq)/45mg potassium (1.1mEq)) *scored

CONTRAINDICATIONS: Infected phosphate stones, severely impaired renal function, hyperphosphatemia.

WARNINGS/PRECAUTIONS: May produce mild laxative effects. Caution with cardiac disease/failure, severe adrenal insufficiency, acute dehydration, renal disease/impairment, extensive tissue breakdown, myotonia congenita, cirrhosis, severe hepatic disease, peripheral/pulmonary edema, hypernatremia, HTN, toxemia of pregnancy, hypoparathyroidism, acute pancreatitis, and rickets. Monitor renal function and serum electrolytes periodically. High serum phosphate levels may increase extra-skeletal calcification.

ADVERSE REACTIONS: GI upset, bone and joint pain, headache, dizziness, mental confusion, seizures, weakness, muscle cramps, numbness, tingling, pain, irregular heartbeat, shortness of breath, swelling of feet or lower legs, weight gain, low urine output, thirst.

INTERACTIONS: Antacids containing magnesium, aluminum, or calcium may prevent phosphate absorption. Hypernatremia may occur with antihypertensives (especially diazoxide, guanethidine, hydralazine, methyldopa, rauwolfia alkaloids) or corticosteroids (especially mineralocorticoids or corticotropin). Calcium-containing agents or Vitamin D may antagonize phosphate effects for hypercalcemia treatment. K⁺-containing or K⁺-sparing agents may cause hyperkalemia; monitor K⁺.

PREGNANCY: Category C, caution in nursing.

MECHANISM OF ACTION: Phosphorus supplement; urinary acidifier; plays key role in osteoblastic and osteoclastic activities; plays vital role in metabolism of CHO, lipids, and protein; plays role in modifing steady-state tissue concentrations of calcium and in urinary excretion of hydrogen ion.

KYTRIL

RX

granisetron HCI (Roche Labs)

THERAPEUTIC CLASS: 5-HT$_3$-antagonist

INDICATIONS: (Inj, Sol, Tab) Prevention of nausea and vomiting associated with chemotherapy. (Sol, Tab) Prevention of nausea and vomiting associated with radiation. (Inj) Prevention and treatment of post-op nausea and vomiting.

DOSAGE: *Adults:* Prevention with Chemotherapy: (PO) 2mg qd up to 1 hr before chemotherapy or 1mg bid (up to 1 hr before chemotherapy and 12 hrs later). (IV) 10mcg/kg within 30 min before chemotherapy. Prevention with Radiation: (PO) 2mg within 1 hr of radiation. Post-Op Prevention: (IV) Administer 1mg over 30 sec before induction of anesthesia or immediately before anesthesia reversal. Post-Op Treatment: (IV) Administer 1mg over 30 sec.
Pediatrics: 2-16 yrs: Prevention with Chemotherapy: 10mcg/kg IV within 30 min before chemotherapy.

HOW SUPPLIED: Inj: 0.1mg/mL, 1mg/mL; Sol: 2mg/10mL (30mL); Tab: 1mg

WARNINGS/PRECAUTIONS: (Inj) Does not stimulate gastric or intestinal peristalsis. Do not use instead of nasogastric suction. May mask progressive ileus or gastric distension.

ADVERSE REACTIONS: Headache, asthenia, somnolence, diarrhea, constipation, abdominal pain, dizziness, insomnia, increased hepatic enzymes.

INTERACTIONS: Hepatic CYP450 enzyme inducers or inhibitors may alter clearance.

PREGNANCY: Category B, caution in nursing.

MECHANISM OF ACTION: 5-HT$_3$ receptor antagonist; blocks serotonin stimulation on vagal nerve terminals and in chemoreceptor trigger zone and subsequent vomiting after emetogenic stimuli.

PHARMACOKINETICS: Absorption: (IV, 40mcg/kg) C$_{max}$=63.8 ng/mL. (PO,1mg) C$_{max}$=3.63ng/mL. **Distribution:** Plasma protein binding (65%). (IV) V$_d$=3.07L/kg; (PO) V$_d$=3.94L/kg. **Metabolism:** CYP3A4; N-demethylation, oxidation, conjugation. **Elimination:** PO: Urine (11% unchanged), feces. Inj: Urine (12% unchanged), feces; (IV, PO) T$_{1/2}$=8.95 hrs, 6.23hrs

LAC-HYDRIN

RX

ammonium lactate (Ranbaxy)

THERAPEUTIC CLASS: Emollient

INDICATIONS: Treatment of ichthyosis vulgaris and xerosis.

DOSAGE: *Adults:* Apply bid and rub thoroughly.
Pediatrics: (Lot) Infants/Children: (Cre) ≥2 yrs: Apply bid and rub in thoroughly.

HOW SUPPLIED: Cre: 12% (140g, 385g); Lot: 12% (225g, 400g)

WARNINGS/PRECAUTIONS: Avoid sun exposure to treated skin. Avoid eyes, lips, mucous membranes, intravaginal use and oral use. Caution if used on face; potential for irritation Stinging, burning may occur if applied to fissures, erosions, or abrasions. D/C if hypersensitivity observed.

ADVERSE REACTIONS: Burning, stinging, itching, erythema.

PREGNANCY: Category B, caution in nursing.

LACTULOSE

RX

lactulose (Various)

OTHER BRAND NAMES: Constulose (Actavis) - Enulose (Alpharma) - Generlac (Morton Grove)

THERAPEUTIC CLASS: Osmotic laxative

INDICATIONS: Treatment of constipation. Prevention and treatment of portal-systemic encephalopathy, including stages of hepatic pre-coma and coma.

DOSAGE: *Adults:* Constipation: 15-30mL qd. Max 60mL/day. May mix with fruit juice, water, or milk. Portal-Systemic Encephalopathy: 30-45mL tid-qid. Adjust dose every 1 or

2 days to produce 2-3 soft stools daily. Rectal Use: Reversal of Coma: Mix 300mL with 700mL of water or saline and retain for 30-60 min. May repeat q4-6h. Oral doses should be started before completely stopping enema.

Pediatrics: Portal-Systemic Encephalopathy: Older Children/Adolescents: 40-90mL/day divided tid-qid adjusted to produce 2-3 soft stools daily. *Infants:* 2.5-10mL in divided doses to produce 2-3 soft stools daily.

HOW SUPPLIED: Sol: 10g/15mL

CONTRAINDICATIONS: Patients who require a low galactose diet.

WARNINGS/PRECAUTIONS: Caution in DM due to galactose and lactose content. Monitor electrolytes periodically in elderly or debilitated if used >6 months. Potential for explosive reaction with electrocautery procedures during proctoscopy or colonoscopy.

ADVERSE REACTIONS: Flatulence, intestinal cramps, diarrhea, nausea, vomiting.

INTERACTIONS: Decreased effect with nonabsorbable antacids.

PREGNANCY: Category B, caution in nursing.

MECHANISM OF ACTION: Synthetic disaccharide; broken down primarily to lactic acid, by the action of colonic bacteria, resulting in increased osmotic pressure and slight acidification of colonic content, causing an increase in stool water content and softens the stool. In portal-systemic encephalopathy, acidification of colonic contents results in retention of ammonia in colon as ammonium ion; ammonia then migrates from blood into colon to form ammonium ion, which traps and prevents absorption of ammonia; finally, laxative actions expels trapped ammonium ion from colon.

PHARMACOKINETICS: Absorption: Poor. **Elimination:** Urine (≤3%).

LAMICTAL   RX
lamotrigine (GlaxoSmithKline)

> Serious life-threatening rash, including Stevens-Johnson syndrome and toxic epidermal necrolysis, reported. Occurs more often in pediatrics than adults. D/C at 1st sign of rash.

OTHER BRAND NAME: Lamictal CD (GlaxoSmithKline)

THERAPEUTIC CLASS: Phenyltriazine

INDICATIONS: Adjunctive therapy in patients (≥2 yrs) with partial seizures and for generalized seizures of Lennox-Gastaut syndrome. For conversion to monotherapy in adults (≥16 yrs) with partial seizures receiving a single enzyme-inducing antiepileptic drug (EIAED) or valproate (VPA). Maintenance treatment of bipolar I disorder to delay the time to occurrence of mood episodes (depression, mania, hypomania, mixed episodes) in patients treated for acute mood episodes with standard therapy.

DOSAGE: *Adults:* Epilepsy: Concomitant AEDs with valproate (VPA): Weeks 1 and 2: 25mg every other day. Weeks 3 and 4: 25mg qd. Titrate: Increase every 1-2 weeks by 25-50mg/day. Maint: 100-400mg/day, given qd or bid; 100-200mg/day when added to VPA alone. Concomitant EIAEDs without VPA: Weeks 1 and 2: 50mg qd. Weeks 3 and 4: 50mg bid. Titrate: Increase every 1-2 weeks by 100mg/day. Maint: 150-250mg bid. Conversion to Monotherapy From Single EIAED: ≥16 yrs: Weeks 1 and 2: 50mg qd. Weeks 3 and 4: 50mg bid. Titrate: Increase every 1-2 weeks by 100mg/day. Maint: 250mg bid. Withdraw EIAED over 4 weeks. Conversion to Monotherapy From VPA: ≥16 yrs: Step 1: Follow Concomitant AEDs with VPA dosing regimen to achieve Lamictal dose of 200mg/day. Maintain previous VPA dose. Step 2: Maintain Lamictal 200mg/day. Decrease VPA to 500mg/day by decrements of ≤500mg/day per week. Maintain VPA 500mg/day for 1 week. Step 3: Increase to Lamictal 300mg/day for 1 week. Decrease VPA simultaneously to 250mg/day for 1 week. Step 4: D/C VPA. Increase Lamictal 100mg/day every week to maint dose of 500mg/day. Bipolar Disorder: Patients not taking carbamazepine, other enzyme-inducing drugs (EIDs) or VPA: Weeks 1 and 2: 25mg qd. Weeks 3 and 4: 50mg qd. Week 5: 100mg qd. Weeks 6 and 7: 200mg qd. Patients taking VPA: Weeks 1 and 2: 25mg every other day. Weeks 3 and 4: 25mg qd. Week 5: 50mg qd. Weeks 6 and 7: 100mg qd. Patients taking carbamazepine (or other EIDs) and not taking VPA: Weeks 1 and 2: 50mg qd. Weeks 3 and 4: 100mg qd (divided doses). Week 5: 200mg qd (divided doses). Week 6: 300mg qd (divided doses). Week 7: up to 400mg qd (divided doses). After d/c of psychotropic drugs excluding VPA, carbamazepine, or other EIDs: Maintain current dose. After d/c of VPA and current lamotrigine dose of 100mg qd: Week 1: 150mg qd. Week 2 and onward: 200mg qd.

After d/c of carbamazepine or other EIDs and current lamotrigine dose of 400mg qd: Week 1: 400mg qd. Week 2: 300mg qd. Week 3 and Onward: 200mg qd. Concomitant or starting estrogen-containing oral contraceptives: not taking carbamazepine, phenytoin, phenobarbital, primidone, or rifampin, lamictal should be increased by as much as 2-fold over the recommended target maintenance dose; the dose increase should start at the same time as the initiation and continuation of contraceptives. Stopping estrogen-containing oral contraceptives: may decrease lamictal by as much as 50%. Hepatic Impairment: Initial/Titrate/Maint: Reduce by 50% for moderate (Child-Pugh Grade B) and 75% for severe (Child-Pugh Grade C) impairment. Significant Renal Impairment: Maint: Reduce dose. Elderly: Start at low end of dosing range. *Pediatrics:* Round dose down to nearest whole tab. 2-12 yrs: ≥6.7kg: Lennox-Gastaut/ Partial Seizures: Concomitant AEDs with VPA: Weeks 1 and 2: 0.15mg/kg/day given qd-bid. Weeks 3 and 4: 0.3mg/kg/day given qd or bid. Titrate: Increase every 1-2 weeks by 0.3mg/kg/day. Maint: 1-5mg/kg/day given qd or bid; 1-3mg/kg/day when added to VPA alone. Max: 200mg/day. Concomitant EIAEDs without VPA: Weeks 1 and 2: 0.3mg/kg bid. Weeks 3 and 4: 0.6mg/kg bid. Titrate: Increase every 1-2 weeks by 1.2mg/kg/day. Maint: 2.5-7.5mg/kg bid. Max: 400mg/day. >12 yrs: Concomitant AEDs with VPA: Weeks 1 and 2: 25mg every other day. Weeks 3 and 4: 25mg qd. Titrate: Increase every 1-2 weeks by 25-50mg/day. Maint: 100-400mg/day, given qd or bid; 100-200mg/day when added to VPA alone. Concomitant EIAEDs without VPA: Weeks 1 and 2: 50mg qd. Weeks 3 and 4: 50mg bid. Titrate: Increase every 1-2 weeks by 100mg/day. Maint: 150-250mg bid. Hepatic Impairment: Initial/Titrate/Maint: Reduce by 50% for moderate (Child-Pugh Grade B) and 75% for severe (Child-Pugh Grade C) impairment. Significant Renal Impairment: Maint: Reduce dose.

HOW SUPPLIED: Tab: 25mg*, 100mg*, 150mg*, 200mg*; Tab, Chewable: (Lamictal CD) 2mg, 5mg, 25mg *scored

WARNINGS/PRECAUTIONS: Risk of serious life-threatening rash; d/c if rash occurs. Multiorgan failure, sudden unexplained death, hypersensitivity reactions, and pure red cell aplasia reported. Avoid abrupt withdrawal. Caution with renal, hepatic, or cardiac functional impairment. May cause ophthalmic toxicity. Do not exceed recommended initial dose and dose escalations. Caution in elderly. Chewable tabs may be swallowed whole, chewed (with water/diluted fruit juice) or dispersed in water/diluted fruit juice; do administer partial quantities.

ADVERSE REACTIONS: Serious rash, dizziness, ataxia, somnolence, headache, diplopia, blurred vision, nausea, vomiting, insomnia, back/abdominal pain, fatigue, xerostomia, rhinitis.

INTERACTIONS: Decreased levels with phenytoin, carbamazepine, phenobarbital, primidone, rifampin, estrogen-containing oral contraceptives. Risk of life-threatening rash with valproic acid. Lamotrigine decreases valproic acid levels; valproic acid increases lamotrigine levels. Inhibits dihydrofolate reductase; may potentiate folate inhibitors.

PREGNANCY: Category C, not for use in nursing.

MECHANISM OF ACTION: Phenyltriazine; not established. Suspected to inhibit voltage-sensitive sodium channels, thereby stabilizing neuronal membranes and consequently modulating presynaptic transmitter release of excitatory amino acids.

PHARMACOKINETICS: Absorption: Rapid and complete. Absolute bioavailability (98%), T_{max}=1.4-4.8 hrs. **Distribution:** V_d=0.9-1.3L/kg; plasma protein binding (55%); Found in breast milk. **Metabolism:** Liver via glucuronic acid conjugation, 2-N-glucuronide conjugate (major metabolite, inactive). **Elimination:** Renal, urine (94%), feces (2%). Refer to full PI for pediatric parameters.

L<small>AMISIL</small>
terbinafine HCl (Novartis)

RX

THERAPEUTIC CLASS: Allylamine antifungal

INDICATIONS: (Granules) Treatment of tinea capitis in patients ≥4 yrs. (Tabs) Treatment of onychomycosis of toenail or fingernail due to dermatophytes (tinea unguium).

DOSAGE: *Adults:* Tabs: Fingernail: 250mg qd for 6 weeks. Toenail: 250mg qd for 12 weeks. Granules: Take qd with food for 6 weeks. <25 kg: 125mg/day. 25-35kg:

187.5mg/day. >35kg: 250mg/day.
Pediatrics: ≥4 yrs: Granules: Take qd with food for 6 weeks. <25 kg: 125mg/day.
25-35kg: 187.5mg/day. >35kg: 250mg/day.

HOW SUPPLIED: Granules: 125mg/pkt, 187.5mg/pkt; Tab: 250mg

WARNINGS/PRECAUTIONS: Liver disease and serious skin reactions reported; d/c therapy if these develop. Avoid with liver disease or renal impairment (CrCl ≤50 mL/min). Check serum transaminases before therapy. Monitor CBC if immunocompromised and taking terbinafine >6 weeks. Severe neutropenia reported; d/c therapy if neutrophil count ≤1,000 cells/mm^3. Changes in ocular lens and retina reported (unknown significance).

ADVERSE REACTIONS: (Granules) Nasopharyngitis, headache, pyrexia, cough, vomiting, upper respiratory tract infection, upper abdominal pain, diarrhea, liver enzyme abnormalities, rash. (Tabs) Headache, diarrhea, dyspepsia, abdominal pain, liver enzyme abnormalities, rash.

INTERACTIONS: Increased clearance of cyclosporine. May potentiate levels of drugs metabolized by CYP2D6 (eg, TCAs, β-blockers, SSRIs, MAOIs-type B). Decreased clearance of IV caffeine. Clearance increased by rifampin and decreased by cimetidine.

PREGNANCY: Category B, not for use in nursing.

MECHANISM OF ACTION: Allylamine antifungal; acts by inhibiting squalene epoxidase, thus blocking biosynthesis of ergosterol, an essential component of fungal-cell membranes.

PHARMACOKINETICS: Absorption: (Tab) Well-absorbed (>70%), absolute bioavailability (40%); (250mg) C_{max}=1mcg/mL; T_{max}=2 hrs; AUC =4.56mcg.h/mL. **Distribution:** Plasma protein binding (>99%). **Metabolism:** Extensive, CYP2D6. **Elimination:** Urine (70%); $T_{1/2}$=200-400 hrs.

LAMISIL AT OTC
terbinafine HCl (Novartis Consumer)

THERAPEUTIC CLASS: Allylamine antifungal

INDICATIONS: Treatment of t.pedis, t.cruris, t.corporis.

DOSAGE: *Adults:* Wash and dry area. Tinea pedis: Apply bid for 1 week (interdigital) or for 2 weeks (bottom or sides of foot). Tinea cruris/corporis: Apply qd for 1 week. *Pediatrics:* ≥12 yrs: Wash and dry area. Tinea pedis: Apply bid for 1 week (interdigital) or for 2 weeks (bottom or sides of foot). Tinea cruris/corporis: Apply qd for 1 week.

HOW SUPPLIED: Cre: 1% (12g, 24g); Spray: 1% (30mL)

WARNINGS/PRECAUTIONS: Do not use on nails, scalp, in or near the mouth or eyes, or for vaginal yeast infections.

PREGNANCY: Not rated in pregnancy or nursing.

MECHANISM OF ACTION: Allylamine antifungal; acts by inhibiting squalene epoxidase, thus blocking the biosynthesis of ergosterol, an essential component of fungal cell membranes.

PHARMACOKINETICS: Distribution: Plasma protein binding (>99%). **Metabolism:** Rapidly and extensively metabolized by CYP450:2C9, 1A2, 3A4,2C8, and 2C19. **Elimination:** Urine (approximately 70%).

LANOXIN RX
digoxin (GlaxoSmithKline)

OTHER BRAND NAMES: Digitek (Mylan Bertek) - Lanoxicaps (GlaxoSmithKline)

THERAPEUTIC CLASS: Cardiac glycoside

INDICATIONS: Treatment of mild to moderate heart failure and to control ventricular response rate with chronic atrial fibrillation.

DOSAGE: *Adults:* Rapid Digitalization: LD: (Cap/Inj) 0.4-0.6mg PO/IV or (Tab) 0.5-0.75mg PO, may give additional (Cap/Inj) 0.1-0.3mg or (Tab) 0.125-0.375mg at 6-8 hr intervals until clinical effect. Maint: (Tab) 0.125-0.5mg qd. Elderly (>70 yrs)/Renal Dysfunction: Initial: 0.125mg qd. Marked Renal Dysfunction: Initial: 0.0625mg qd. Titrate: Increase every 2 weeks based on response. A-Fib: Titrate to minimum effective dose for desired response.

Pediatrics: (Ped Sol) Oral Digitalizing Dose: Premature Infants: 20-30mcg/kg. Full-Term Infants: 25-35mcg/kg. 1-24 months: 35-60mcg/kg. 2-5 yrs: 30-40mcg/kg. 5-10 yrs: 20-35mcg/kg. >10 yrs: 10-15mcg/kg. Maint: Premature Infants: 20-30% of PO digitalizing dose/day. Full-Term Infants to >10 yrs: 25-35% of PO digitalizing dose. (Ped Inj) IV Digitalizing Dose: Premature Infants: 15-25mcg/kg. Full-Term Infants: 20-30mcg/kg. 1-24 months: 30-50mcg/kg. 2-5 yrs: 25-35mcg/kg. 5-10 yrs: 15-30mcg/kg. >10 yrs: 8-12mcg/kg. Maint: Premature Infants: 20-30% of IV digitalizing dose. Full-Term Infants to >10 yrs: 25-35% of IV digitalizing dose/day. (Cap) Oral Digitalizing Dose: 2-5 yrs: 25-35mcg/kg. 5-10 yrs: 15-30mcg/kg. >10 yrs: 8-12mcg/kg. Maint: ≥2 yrs: 25-25% of PO or IV digitalizing dose. (Tab) Maint: 2-5 yrs: 10-15mcg/kg. 5-10 yrs: 7-10mcg/kg. >10 yrs: 3-5mcg/kg. A-Fib: Titrate to minimum effective dose for desired response.

HOW SUPPLIED: Cap: (Lanoxicaps) 0.1mg, 0.2mg; Inj: (Pediatric Inj) 0.1mg/mL, 0.25mg/mL; Sol: (Pediatric Sol) 0.05mg/mL (60mL); Tab: 0.125mg*, 0.25mg* *scored

CONTRAINDICATIONS: Ventricular fibrillation, digitalis hypersensitivity.

WARNINGS/PRECAUTIONS: May cause severe sinus bradycardia or sinoatrial block with pre-existing sinus node disease. May cause advanced or complete heart block with pre-existing incomplete AV block. May cause very rapid ventricular response or ventricular fibrillation. Caution with thyroid disorders, AMI, hypermetabolic states, restrictive cardiomyopathy, constrictive pericarditis, amyloid heart disease, elderly, acute cor pulmonale, and idiopathic hypertrophic subaortic stenosis. Caution with renal dysfunction; high risk for toxicity. Caution with hypokalemia, hypomagnesemia, or hypercalcemia; toxicity may occur. Hypocalcemia can nullify effects of digoxin. Monitor electrolytes and renal function periodically. Risk of ventricular arrhythmia with electrical cardioversion. Bioavailability is different between dosage forms.

ADVERSE REACTIONS: Heart block, rhythm disturbances, anorexia, NV, diarrhea, visual disturbances, headache, weakness, dizziness, mental disturbances.

INTERACTIONS: Risk of toxicity with K⁺-depleting diuretics. Increased risk of arrhythmias with calcium, sympathomimetics, and succinylcholine. Increased serum levels with quinidine, verapamil, amiodarone, propafenone, indomethacin, itraconazole, alprazolam, and spironolactone; monitor for toxicity. Increased absorption with propantheline, diphenoxylate, macrolides, and tetracycline; monitor for toxicity. Decreased intestinal absorption with antacids, kaolin-pectin, sulfasalazine, neomycin, cholestyramine, certain anticancer drugs, and metoclopramide. Decreased serum levels with rifampin. Increased digoxin dose requirement with thyroid supplements. Additive effects on AV node conduction with β-blockers or CCBs. Caution with drugs that deteriorate renal function.

PREGNANCY: Category C, caution in nursing.

MECHANISM OF ACTION: Cardiac glycoside; inhibits Na⁺-K⁺ ATPase, leading to increase in intracellular concentration of Ca⁺.

PHARMACOKINETICS: Absorption: (Tab) Absolute bioavailability (60%-80%), T_{max}=1-3 hrs. (Sol) Absolute bioavailability (70-85%). (Lanoxicaps) Absolute bioavailability (90-100%). (Inj) Absolute bioavailability (100%). **Distribution:** Plasma protein binding (25%), crosses placenta. **Metabolism:** Hydrolysis, oxidation, and conjugation. **Elimination:** Urine (50%-70%); $T_{1/2}$=1.5-2 days.

LANTUS

RX

insulin glargine, human (Sanofi-Aventis)

THERAPEUTIC CLASS: Insulin

INDICATIONS: Treatment of adults and pediatrics with type 1 diabetes mellitus. Treatment of adults with type 2 diabetes mellitus who require basal (long-acting) insulin.

DOSAGE: *Adults:* Individualize dose. For SQ injection only. Administer qd at same time each day. Insulin naive patients on oral antidiabetic drugs, start with 10 U qd. Switching from once-daily NPH or Ultralente does not require initial dose change. Switching from bid NPH, reduce initial dose by 20%. Maint: 2-100 U/day.

Pediatrics: ≥6 yrs: Individualize dose. For SQ injection only. Administer qd at same time each day. Insulin naive patients on oral antidiabetic drugs, start with 10 U qd. Switching from once-daily NPH or Ultralente does not require initial dose change. Switching from bid NPH, reduce initial dose by 20%. Maint: 2-100 U/day.

HOW SUPPLIED: Inj: 100 U/mL; OptiClik: 100 U/mL

WARNINGS/PRECAUTIONS: Human insulin differs from animal source insulin. Any change of insulin should be made cautiously. Changes in strength, manufacturer, type or method of manufacture may result in the need for a change in dosage. Hypoglycemia may occur with taking too much insulin, missing or delaying meals, exercising or working more than usual. An infection or illness (especially with diarrhea or vomiting) may change insulin requirements. Administration of insulin SQ can result in lipodystrophy. Not for IV use. Do not mix with other insulins. May cause sodium retention and edema. Caution in patients with renal and hepatic dysfunction.

ADVERSE REACTIONS: Hypoglycemia, allergic reactions, injection site reactions, lipodystrophy, pruritus, rash.

INTERACTIONS: Increased glucose lowering effects with ACE inhibitors, disopyramide, fibrates, fluoxetine, MAOIs, propoxyphene, salicylates, somatostatin analog, sulfonamide antibiotics, and other antidiabetic agents. Decreased blood glucose lowering effects with corticosteroids, danazol, diuretics, sympathomimetic amines, isoniazid, phenothiazine derivatives, somatropin, thyroid hormones, estrogens, progestogens, protease inhibitors and atypical antipsychotics. Pentamidine may cause hypoglycemia, followed by hyperglycemia. β-blockers, clonidine, lithium salts, and alcohol may potentiate or weaken glucose lowering effect. β-blockers, clonidine, guanethidine, and reserpine may reduce or mask signs of hypoglycemia.

PREGNANCY: Category C, caution in nursing.

MECHANISM OF ACTION: Insulin glargine (rDNA origin); regulates glucose metabolism by stimulating peripheral glucose uptake by skeletal muscle and fat, inhibits hepatic glucose production, lipolysis in the adipocyte, proteolysis, and enhances protein synthesis.

PHARMACOKINETICS: Absorption: Slow, prolonged, and relatively constant. **Metabolism:** Partly metabolized into 2 active metabolites (M1 (21^A-Gly-insulin) and M2 (21^A-Gly-des-30^B-Thr-insulin)).

LARIAM RX
mefloquine HCl (Roche Labs)

THERAPEUTIC CLASS: Quinolinemethanol derivative

INDICATIONS: Treatment and prophylaxis of mild to moderate acute malaria caused by *P.falciparum* or *P.vivax*.

DOSAGE: *Adults:* Treatment: 1250mg single dose. Prophylaxis: 250mg/week. Start 1 week before arrival in endemic area and continue weekly (same day of week) while in area. Continue for 4 weeks after leaving the area. Take with food and 8 oz of water. *Pediatrics:* ≥6 months: Treatment: Usual: 20-25mg/kg, split in 2 doses. Take 6-8 hrs apart. If vomiting occurs <30 min after dose, give a 2nd full dose. If vomiting occurs 30-60 min after dose, give additional half-dose. Prophylaxis: ≥3 months: 3-5mg/kg/week. >45kg: 250mg/week. 31-45kg: 3/4 tab/week. 21-30kg: 125mg/week. 5-20kg: 1/4 tab/week. Take with food and water. May crush and mix with water.

HOW SUPPLIED: Tab: 250mg* *scored

CONTRAINDICATIONS: Hypersensitivity to related compounds (eg, quinine, quinidine). Use as prophylaxis with active or recent history of depression, generalized anxiety disorder, psychosis or schizophrenia, or other major psychiatric disorder, or with a history of convulsions.

WARNINGS/PRECAUTIONS: In life-threatening malaria infection due to *P.falciparum*, use IV antimalarials. High risk of relapse seen with acute *P.vivax*; after initial treatment, subsequently treat with 8-aminoquinoline (eg, primaquine). May cause psychiatric symptoms. During prophylaxis, d/c if symptoms of acute anxiety, depression, restlessness, or confusion occur. In long-term therapy, monitor LFTs and perform ophthalmic exams. May impair mental/physical abilities. Increase risk of convulsions in epileptic patients. Caution with cardiac disease, hepatic dysfunction and elderly.

ADVERSE REACTIONS: NV, myalgia, fever, dizziness, headache, somnolence, sleep disorders, loss of balance, chills, diarrhea, abdominal pain, fatigue, tinnitus, pruritus, skin rash.

INTERACTIONS: Avoid halofantrine; may prolong QTc interval. Concomitant administration with other related compounds (eg, quinine, quinidine, chloroquine) may cause

ECG abnormalities and increased risk of convulsions; delay mefloquine dose for 12 hrs after last dose of these drugs. Avoid propranolol; cardiopulmonary arrest reported. Drugs that may alter cardiac conduction (eg, anti-arrhythmic or β-blockers, CCBs, antihistamines, H_1-blockers, TCAs, and phenothiazines) may prolong QT_c interval. May lower plasma levels of anticonvulsants (eg, valproic acid, carbamazepine, phenobarbital, phenytoin); monitor blood levels and adjust dosage accordingly. Complete vaccinations with live, attenuated vaccines (eg, typhoid vaccine) at least 3 days before mefloquine therapy. Caution with anticoagulants, antidiabetic agents.

PREGNANCY: Category C, not for use in nursing.

MECHANISM OF ACTION: Quinolinemethanol derivative; suspected to act as blood schizonticide.

PHARMACOKINETICS: Absorption: Mefloquine: C_{max}=1000 mcg/L, T_{max}=6-24 hrs; 2,8-bis-trifluoromethyl-4-quinoline carboxylic acid: T_{max}=2 weeks. **Distribution:** V_d=20l/kg; plasma protein binding (80%); crosses placenta; found in breast milk. **Metabolism:** Active metabolite: 2,8-bis-trifluoromethyl-4-quinoline carboxylic acid. **Elimination:** Bile, feces; $T_{1/2}$=2-4 weeks. Hepatic excretion.

LESCOL **XL**
fluvastatin sodium (Novartis)

RX

OTHER BRAND NAME: Lescol (Novartis)

THERAPEUTIC CLASS: HMG-CoA reductase inhibitor

INDICATIONS: Adjunct to diet, to reduce elevated total cholesterol (Total-C), LDL-C, TG, and Apo B levels, and to increase HDL-C in primary hypercholesterolemia and mixed dyslipidemia (Types IIa and IIb) when response to nonpharmacological measures is inadequate. To slow coronary atherosclerosis progression in coronary heart disease by lowering Total-C and LDL-C. To reduce risk of undergoing coronary revascularization procedures in patients with coronary heart disease. Adjunct to diet, to reduce Total-C, LDL-C, and Apo B levels in adolescent boys and girls who are at least 1 yr post-menarche, 10-16 yrs of age, with heterozygous familial hypercholesterolemia when response to dietary restriction is inadequate and LDL-C remains ≥190mg/dL or if LDL-C remains ≥160mg/dL and there is positive family history of premature CV disease or 2 or more other CV disease risk factors are present.

DOSAGE: *Adults:* ≥18 yrs: (For LDL-C reduction of ≥25%) Initial: 40mg cap qpm or 80mg XL tab at any time of day or 40mg cap bid. (For LDL-C reduction of <25%) Initial: 20mg cap qpm. Range: 20-80mg/day. Severe Renal Impairment: Caution with dose >40mg/day. Take 2 hrs after bile-acid resins qhs.
Pediatrics: Heterozygous Familial Hypercholesterolemia: 10-16 yrs (≥1 yr post-menarche): Individualize dose: Initial: One 20mg cap. Titrate: Adjust dose at 6-week intervals. Max: 40mg cap bid or 80mg XL tab qd.

HOW SUPPLIED: Cap: (Lescol) 20mg, 40mg; Tab, Extended-Release: (Lescol XL) 80mg

CONTRAINDICATIONS: Active liver disease or unexplained, persistent elevations of serum transaminases, pregnancy, nursing mothers.

WARNINGS/PRECAUTIONS: Monitor LFTs prior to therapy, at 12 weeks, or with dose elevation. D/C if AST or ALT ≥3x ULN on 2 consecutive occasions. Risk of myopathy and/or rhabdomyolysis reported. D/C if markedly elevated CPK levels occur, if myopathy is diagnosed or suspected, or if predisposition to renal failure secondary to rhabdomyolysis. Less effective with homozygous familial hypercholesterolemia. Caution with heavy alcohol use and/or history of hepatic disease. Evaluate if endocrine dysfunction develops.

ADVERSE REACTIONS: Dyspepsia, abdominal pain, headache, nausea, diarrhea, abnormal LFTs, myalgia, flu-like symptoms.

INTERACTIONS: Rifampicin significantly decreases serum levels. Increases levels of glyburide, diclofenac, and phenytoin. Increased serum levels with glyburide, phenytoin, cimetidine, ranitidine, and omeprazole. Caution with drugs that decrease levels of endogenous steroid hormones (eg, ketoconazole, spironolactone, cimetidine). Avoid fibrates. Cyclosporine, colchicine, gemfibrozil, erythromycin, or niacin may increase risk of myopathy/rhabdomyolysis. Cholestyramine given within 4 hrs decreases serum levels but has additive effects when given 4 hrs after fluvastatin (immediate-release). Monitor digoxin, anticoagulants.

PREGNANCY: Category X, not for use in nursing.

MECHANISM OF ACTION: Competitive inhibition of HMG-CoA reductase; inhibits conversion of HMG-CoA to mevalonate (precursor of sterols, including cholesterol). Inhibition of cholesterol biosynsthesis reduces cholesterol in hepatic cells, which stimulates the synthesis of LDL receptors, thereby increasing uptake of LDL particles, resulting in reduction of plasma cholesterol concentration.

PHARMACOKINETICS: Absorption: Rapid and complete, bioavailability (29%); T_{max}=3 hrs (fasting). **Distribution:** V_d=0.35L/kg, plasma protein binding (98%); found in breast milk. **Metabolism:** Liver via CYP2C9, 2C8 and 3A4 through N-dealkylation, β-oxidation pathways. **Elimination:** Feces, (90% metabolites, <2% unchanged), urine (5%); $T_{1/2}$=9 hrs.

LEVBID   RX
hyoscyamine sulfate (Alaven)

OTHER BRAND NAMES: Levsin (Alaven) - Levsinex (Alaven)

THERAPEUTIC CLASS: Anticholinergic

INDICATIONS: Adjunct treatment of peptic ulcer, irritable bowel syndrome, neurogenic bladder, and neurogenic bowel disturbances. Management of functional intestinal disorders (eg, mild dysenteries, diverticulitis). To control gastric secretion, visceral spasm, and hypermotility in spastic colitis, spastic bladder, cystitis, pylorospasm, and associated abdominal cramps. Symptomatic relief of biliary and renal colic with concomitant morphine or other narcotics. Drying agent for symptomatic relief of acute rhinitis. To reduce rigidity and tremors of Parkinson's disease and control associated sialorrhea and hyperhidrosis. For anticholinesterase poisoning. To reduce pain and hypersecretion in pancreatitis. For certain cases of partial heart block associated with vagal activity. (Elixir, Drops) Treatment of infant colic. (Inj) Facilitates GI diagnostic procedures. Reduces pain and hypersecretion in pancreatitis, in cases of partial heart block associated with vagal activity, and as antidote for anticholinesterase poisoning. In anesthesia as a pre-op antimuscarinic. In urology to improve radiologic visibility of kidneys.

DOSAGE: *Adults:* May also chew or swallow SL tab. (Drops, Elixir, Tab, and Tab, SL) 0.125-0.25mg q4h or prn. Max: 1.5mg/24 hrs. (Cap and Tab, Extended-Release) 0.375-0.75mg q12h; or 1 cap q8h. Max: 1.5mg/24 hrs. Do not crush or chew. (Inj) GI Disorders: 0.25-0.5mg IM/IV/SQ as single dose or up to qid at 4-hr intervals. Diagnostic Procedures: 0.25-0.5mg IV 5-10 min before procedure. Anesthesia: 5mcg/kg IM/IV/SQ 30-60 min before anesthesia or with narcotic/sedative administration. GI Disorders: 0.25-0.5mg IM/IV/SQ as single dose; may require bid-qid administration at 4-hr intervals. Diagnostic Procedures: 0.25-0.5mg IV 5-10 min prior. Drug-Induced Bradycardia (Surgery): Increments of 0.25mL IV; repeat prn. Neuromuscular Blockade Reversal: 0.2mg for every 1mg neostigmine or equal dose of physostigmine or pyridostigmine.
Pediatrics: May also chew or swallow SL tab. ≥12 yrs: (Drops, Elixir, Tab, and Tab, SL) 0.125-0.25mg q4h or prn. Max: 1.5mg/24 hrs. (Cap and Tab, Extended-Release) 0.375-0.75mg q12h; or 1 cap may be given q8h. Max: 1.5mg/24 hrs. Do not crush or chew. 2 to <12 yrs: (Tab and Tab, SL) 0.0625-0.125mg q4h or prn. Max: 0.75mg/24 hrs. (Elixir) Give q4h or prn. 10kg: 1.25mL. 20kg: 2.5mL. 40kg: 3.75mL. 50kg: 5mL. Max: 30mL/24 hrs. (Drops) 0.25-1mL q4h or prn. Max: 6mL/24 hrs. <2 yrs: (Drops) Give q4h or prn. 3.4kg: 4 drops. Max: 24 drops/24 hrs. 5kg: 5 drops. Max: 30 drops/24 hrs. 7kg: 6 drops. Max: 36 drops/24 hrs. 10kg: 8 drops. Max: 48 drops/24 hrs. >2 yrs: Anesthesia: (Inj) 5mcg/kg IM/IV/SQ 30-60 min before anesthesia or with narcotic/sedative administration.

HOW SUPPLIED: (Levbid) Tab, Extended-Release: 0.375mg. (Levsin) Drops: 0.125mg/mL (15mL); Elixir: 0.125mg/5mL (473mL); Inj: 0.5mg/mL; Tab: 0.125mg*; Tab, SL: 0.125mg*. (Levsinex) Cap, Extended-Release: 0.375mg *scored

CONTRAINDICATIONS: Glaucoma, obstructive uropathy, GI tract obstruction, paralytic ileus; intestinal atony of elderly/debilitated, unstable CV status in acute hemorrhage, toxic megacolon complicating ulcerative colitis, myasthenia gravis.

WARNINGS/PRECAUTIONS: Risk of heat prostration with high environmental temperature. Avoid activities requiring mental alertness. Psychosis has been reported. Caution with diarrhea, autonomic neuropathy, hyperthyroidism, coronary heart disease, CHF, arrhythmias/tachycardia, HTN, renal disease, and hiatal hernia associated with reflux esophagitis. D/C if diarrhea occurs.

ADVERSE REACTIONS: Anticholinergic effects, drowsiness, headache, nervousness.

INTERACTIONS: Additive effects with other antimuscarinics, amantadine, haloperidol, phenothiazines, MAOIs, TCAs, and some antihistamines. Antacids interfere with absorption; take ac and antacids pc.

PREGNANCY: Category C, caution in nursing.

MECHANISM OF ACTION: Anticholinergic/antispasmodic; inhibits specifically the actions of acetylcholine on structures innervated by postganglionic cholinergic nerves and on smooth muscles that respond to acetylcholine but lack cholinergic innervation.

PHARMACOKINETICS: Absorption: Complete. **Distribution:** Crosses blood-brain barrier and placental barrier. **Metabolism:** Hydrolyzed partially to tropic acid. **Elimination:** Urine (unchanged); $T_{1/2}$=2-3.5 hrs.

LEVEMIR RX
insulin detemir, rDNA origin (Novo Nordisk)

THERAPEUTIC CLASS: Insulin

INDICATIONS: Treatment of adults and pediatrics with type 1 diabetes or adults with type 2 diabetes who require basal (long acting) insulin for the control of hyperglycemia.

DOSAGE: *Adults:* Individualize dose. Administer SQ qd or bid. Once-Daily Dosing: Administer with evening meal or bedtime. Twice-Daily Dosing: Administer evening dose with evening meal, at bedtime, or 12 hrs after morning dose. Type 1/Type 2 Diabetes on Basal-Bolus Treatment or Patients Only on Basal Insulin: Change on a unit-to-unit basis. Insulin-Naive with Type 2 Diabetes Inadequately Controlled on Oral Antidiabetics: Initial: 0.1-0.2 U/kg in evening or 10 U qd or bid.
Pediatrics: Individualize dose. Administer SQ qd or bid. Once-Daily Dosing: Administer with evening meal or bedtime. Twice-Daily Dosing: Administer evening dose with evening meal, at bedtime, or 12 hrs after morning dose. Type 1 Diabetes on Basal-Bolus Treatment or Patients Only on Basal Insulin: Change on a unit-to-unit basis.

HOW SUPPLIED: Inj: 100 U/mL (3mL, 10mL)

WARNINGS/PRECAUTIONS: Monitor glucose; may cause hypoglycemia. Not for use in an insulin infusion pump. Should not be diluted or mixed with any other insulin preparations. May cause lipodystrophy or hypersensitivity. Dose adjustment may be needed in renal or hepatic impairment and during intercurrent conditions such as illness, emotional distrubances, or other stresses.

ADVERSE REACTIONS: Allergic reactions, injection site reactions, lipodystrophy, pruritus, rash, hypoglycemia, weight gain.

INTERACTIONS: Avoid mixing with other insulins. Increased glucose lowering effects with ACE inhibitors, disopyramide, fibrates, fluoxetine, MAOIs, propoxyphene, salicylates, somatostatin analog, sulfonamide antibiotics, and other antidiabetic agents. Decreased blood glucose lowering effects with corticosteroids, danazol, diuretics, sympathomimetic agents, isoniazid, phenothiazine derivates, somatotropin, thyroid hormones, estrogens, progestogens. Pentamidine may cause hypoglycemia, followed by hyperglycemia. β-blockers, clonidine, lithium salts, and alcohol may potentiate or weaken glucose lowering effect. β-blockers, clonidine, guanethidine, and reserpine may reduce or mask signs of hypoglycemia.

PREGNANCY: Category C, caution in nursing.

MECHANISM OF ACTION: Insulin detemir (rDNA origin); regulates glucose metabolism and lowers blood glucose by facilitating cellular uptake and inhibiting the glucose output from the liver.

PHARMACOKINETICS: Absorption: Slow, prolonged; absolute bioavailability (60%); T_{max}=6-8 hrs. **Distribution:** V_d=0.1L/kg; plasma protein binding (≥98%). **Metabolism:** Liver. **Elimination:** $T_{1/2}$=5-7 hrs.

LEVOTHROID

RX

levothyroxine sodium (Forest)

THERAPEUTIC CLASS: Thyroid replacement hormone

INDICATIONS: Hypothyroidism. As a pituitary TSH suppressant for nonendemic goiter and for chronic lymphocytic thyroiditis. Diagnostic agent in suppression tests to differentiate mild hyperthyroidism or thyroid gland autonomy. Adjunct therapy with antithyroid drugs to treat thyrotoxicosis. Adjunct to surgery and radioiodine therapy for TSH-dependent thyroid cancer.

DOSAGE: *Adults:* Hypothyroidism: Usual: 100-200mcg/day. Endocrine/Cardiovascular Complications: Initial: 50mcg/day. Titrate: Increase by 50mcg/day every 2-4 weeks until euthyroid. Hypothyroid with Angina: Initial: 25mcg/day. Titrate: Increase by 25-50mcg every 2-4 weeks until euthyroid.
Pediatrics: Hypothyroidism: >12 yrs: Usual: 100-200mcg/day. 6-12 yrs: 4-5mcg/kg/day. 1-5 yrs: 5-6mcg/kg/day. 6-12 months: 6-8mcg/kg/day. 0-6 months: 10-15mcg/kg/day. May crush tab and sprinkle over food (applesauce) or mix with 5-10mL water, formula (non-soy), or breast milk.

HOW SUPPLIED: Tab: 25mcg*, 50mcg*, 75mcg*, 88mcg*, 100mcg*, 112mcg*, 125mcg*, 137mcg*, 150mcg*, 175mcg*, 200mcg*, 300mcg* *scored

CONTRAINDICATIONS: Untreated thyrotoxicosis, acute MI, and uncorrected adrenal insufficiency.

WARNINGS/PRECAUTIONS: Do not use in the treatment of obesity; larger doses in euthyroid patients can cause serious or even life threatening toxicity. Caution with cardiovascular disease, HTN. May aggravate diabetes mellitus or insipidus and adrenal cortical insufficiency. Excessive doses in infants may produce craniosynostosis. Add glucocorticoid with myxedema coma.

ADVERSE REACTIONS: Lactose hypersensitivity, transient partial hair loss in children.

INTERACTIONS: Monitor insulin and oral hypoglycemic requirements. May potentiate anticoagulant effects of warfarin; adjust warfarin dose and monitor PT/INR. Increased adrenergic effects of catecholamines; caution with CAD. Decreased absorption with cholestyramine and colestipol; space dosing by 4-5 hrs. Estrogens increase thyroxine-binding globulin; increase in thyroid dose may be needed. Large dose may cause life-threatening toxicities with sympathomimetic amines. Avoid mixing crushed tabs with foods/formula with large amounts of iron, soybean or fiber.

PREGNANCY: Category A, caution in nursing.

MECHANISM OF ACTION: Thyroid hormone; not understood, suspected to control DNA transcription and protein synthesis. Regulates multiple metabolic processes.

PHARMACOKINETICS: Distribution: Plasma protein binding (99%). **Metabolism:** Deiodination (major pathway), conjugation (minor pathway) in liver (mainly), kidneys, and other tissues. **Elimination:** Urine; T_4 (feces; 20% unchanged); $T_{1/2}$= 6-7 days; $T_{1/2} \le 2$ days (T_3).

LEVOXYL

RX

levothyroxine sodium (King)

THERAPEUTIC CLASS: Thyroid replacement hormone

INDICATIONS: Hypothyroidism. As a pituitary TSH suppressant in the treatment and prevention of euthyroid goiters, including thyroid nodules, lymphocytic thyroiditis, and multinodular goiter. Adjunct to surgery and radioiodine therapy for thyrotropin-dependent well-differentiated thyroid cancer.

DOSAGE: *Adults:* Take in the AM at least one-half hour before food. Hypothyroid: Usual: 1.7mcg/kg/day. >200mcg/day (seldom). >50 yrs/<50 yrs with Cardiac Disease: Initial: 25-50mcg/day. Titrate: Increase by 12.5-25mcg/day every 6-8 weeks until euthyroid. Elderly with Cardiac Disease: Initial: 12.5-25mcg/day. Titrate: Increase by 12.5-25mcg/day every 4-6 weeks until euthyroid. Severe Hypothyroidism: Initial: 12.5-25mcg/day. Titrate: Increase by 25mcg/day every 2-4 weeks until euthyroid. Pregnancy: May increase dose requirements. Subclinical Hypothyroidism: Lower doses required.
Pediatrics: Take in the AM at least one-half hour before food. Hypothyroidism: 0-3 months: 10-15mcg/kg/day. 3-6 months: 8-10mcg/kg/day. 6-12 months: 6-8mcg/kg/day.

1-5 yrs: 5-6mcg/kg/day. 6-12 yrs: 4-5mcg/kg/day. >12 yrs: 2-3mcg/kg/day. Growth/ Puberty Complete: 1.7mcg/kg/day. Cardiac Risk: Initial: Use lower dose. Titrate: Increase dose every 4-6 weeks until euthyroid. Infants with Serum T_4 <5mcg/dL: Initial: 50mcg/day. Chronic/Severe Hypothyroidism: Children: Initial: 25mcg/day. Titrate: Increase by 25mcg/day every 2-4 weeks until desired effect. Minimize Hyperactivity in Older Children: Initial: Give 1/4 of full replacement dose. Titrate: Increase by same amount weekly until full dose achieved. May crush tab and mix with 5-10mL water.

HOW SUPPLIED: Tab: 25mcg*, 50mcg*, 75mcg*, 88mcg*, 100mcg*, 112mcg*, 125mcg*, 137mcg*, 150mcg*, 175mcg*, 200mcg* *scored

CONTRAINDICATIONS: Untreated thyrotoxicosis, acute MI, and uncorrected adrenal insufficiency.

WARNINGS/PRECAUTIONS: Do not use in the treatment of obesity; larger doses in euthyroid patients can cause serious or even life threatening toxicity. Caution with cardiovascular disease, CAD, adrenal insufficiency, and the elderly with risk of occult cardiac disease. Carefully titrate dose to avoid over or under treatment. Decreased bone mineral density with long term use. Caution with nontoxic diffuse goiter or nodular thyroid disease. With adrenal insufficiency supplement with glucocorticoids before therapy.

ADVERSE REACTIONS: Pseudotumor cerebri in children reported. Seizures (rare), hypersensitivity reactions, dysphagia, choking, gagging, hyperthyroidism (increased appetite, weight loss, heat intolerance, hyperactivity, tremors, palpitations, tachycardia, diarrhea, vomiting, hair loss).

INTERACTIONS: Sympathomimetics may increase risk of coronary insufficiency with CAD. Upward dose adjustments needed for insulin and oral hypoglycemic agents. Decreased absorption with soybean flour (infant formula), cottonseed meal, walnuts, and fiber. May potentiate oral anticoagulant effects; adjust dose and monitor PT/INR. May decrease levels and effects of digitalis glycosides. Cholestyramine, colestipol, ferrous sulfate, aluminum hydroxide, sodium polystyrene, soybean flour, sucralfate may decrease absorption. Reduced TSH secretion with dopamine/dopamine agonists, glucocorticoids, octreotide. Decreased thyroid hormone secretion with aminoglutethimide, amiodarone, iodine (including iodine-containing radiographic contrast agents), lithium, methimazole, PTU, sulfonamides, tolbutamide. Increased thyroid hormone secretion with amiodarone, iodide (including iodine-containing radiographic contrast agents). Decreased T_4 absorption with antacids (aluminum & magnesium hydroxides), simethicone, bile acid sequestrants (cholestyramine, colestipol), calcium carbonate, cation exchange resins (kayexalate), ferrous sulfate, sucralfate. Increased serum TBG concentration with clofibrate, estrogens, heroin/methadone, 5-FU, mitotane, tamoxifen. Decreased serum TBG concentration with androgens/anabolic steroids, asparaginase, glucocorticoids, nicotinic acid (slow-release). Protein-binding site displacement with furosemide, heparin, hydantoins, NSAIDs, salicylates. Increased hepatic metabolism with carbamazepine, hydantoins, phenobarbital, rifampin. Decreased conversion of T_4 to T_3 levels with amiodarone, β-adrenergic antagonists (propranolol >160mg/day), glucocorticoids (dexamethasone >4mg/day), PTU. Additive effects of both agents with antidepressants. Interferon-(alpha) may cause development of antithyroid microsomal antibodies causing transient hypothyroidism, hyperthyroidism, or both. Interleukin-2 has been associated with transient painless thyroiditis. Excessive use with growth hormones may accelerate epiphyseal closure. Ketamine use may produce marked HTN and tachycardia. May reduce uptake of iodine-containing radiographic contrast agents. Altered levels of thyroid hormone and/or TSH level with choral hydrate, diazepam, ethionamide, lovastatin, metoclopramide, 6-mercaptopurine, nitroprusside, paraaminosalicylate sodium, perphenazine, resorcinol (excessive topical use), thiazide diuretics.

PREGNANCY: Category A, caution in nursing.

MECHANISM OF ACTION: Thyroid hormone; not understood, suspected to control DNA transcription and protein synthesis.

PHARMACOKINETICS: Distribution: Plasma protein binding (99%); found in breast milk. **Metabolism:** Deiodination (major pathway) and conjugation in liver (mainly), kidneys, other tissues. **Elimination:** Urine, feces (20% unchanged); (T_4) $T_{1/2}$=6-7days; (T_3) $T_{1/2}$≤2 days.

LEXIVA   RX
fosamprenavir calcium (GlaxoSmithKline)

THERAPEUTIC CLASS: Protease inhibitor

INDICATIONS: Treatment of HIV infection in combination with other antiretrovirals.

DOSAGE: *Adults:* Therapy-naive: 1400mg bid OR 1400mg qd + ritonavir 200mg qd OR 700mg bid + ritonavir 100mg bid. PI-Experienced: 700mg bid + ritonavir 100mg bid. Mild/Moderate Hepatic Impairment (without ritonavir): 700mg bid. Mild Hepatic Impairment: 700mg bid + ritonavir 100mg qd. Moderate Hepatic Impairment: 450mg bid + ritonavir 100mg qd. Severe Hepatic Impairment: 350mg bid (without ritonavir). *Pediatrics:* 2-5 yrs: Therapy-naive: 30mg/kg bid, do not exceed 1,400mg bid; Therapy-naive ≥6 yrs: : 30mg/kg bid, not to exceed 1,400mg bid. or 18mg/kg + ritonavir 3mg/kg bid, not to exceed 700mg + ritonavir 100mg bid. Therapy-experienced: ≥6 yrs: 18 mg/kg + ritonavir 3 mg/kg, not to exceed 700 mg + ritonavir 100 mg bid. For patients weighing >47 kg use adult Lexiva monotherapy. When administered in combination with ritonavir, Lexiva tabs may be used in patients weighing >39 kg and ritonavir caps for patients weighing >33 kg.

HOW SUPPLIED: Tab: 700mg; Sus: 50mg/mL (225mL)

CONTRAINDICATIONS: Concomitant drugs dependent on CYP3A4 for clearance (eg, flecainide, propafenone, rifampin, delavirdine, lovastatin, simvastatin, dihydroergotamine, ergonovine, ergotamine, methylergonovine, cisapride, pimozide, midazolam, triazolam). If used with ritonavir, refer to ritonavir monograph.

WARNINGS/PRECAUTIONS: Severe and life-threatening skin reactions (including Stevens-Johnson syndrome), hemolytic anemia, new onset, or exacerbation of, DM, hyperglycemia, diabetic ketoacidosis, and immune reconstitution syndrome reported. Caution with known sulfonamide allergy. Reduce dose and use caution in hepatic impairment. Caution with underlying hepatitis B or C or marked elevations in transaminases; monitor LFTs prior to and during therapy. Spontaneous bleeding reported with hemophilia A and B. Redistribution/accumulation of body fat observed. Increased triglycerides may occur.

ADVERSE REACTIONS: Diarrhea, NV, headache, rash, severe skin reactions, AST increased, ALT increased.

INTERACTIONS: See Contraindications. Concurrent nevirapine without ritonavir not recommended. Indinavir and nelfinavir may increase levels. Decreased levels with efavirenz (add additional 100mg/day ritonavir), nevirapine, lopinavir/ritonavir (also decreases lopinavir), saquinavir, carbamazepine, phenobarbital, phenytoin, dexamethasone, H_2 antagonists. May decrease levels of methadone (consider dose increase) and paroxetine. May increase levels of oral contraceptives (use alternate non-hormonal methods), amiodarone, lidocaine (systemic), quinidine, bepridil, ketoconazole/itraconazole (reduce dose with >400mg/day; avoid >200mg/day with concurrent ritonavir), rifabutin (reduce dose by at least 50% or 75% with ritonavir; monitor CBCs weekly), benzodiazepines, CCBs, atorvastatin, rosuvastatin (use lowest possible dose), cyclosporine, tacrolimus, rapamycin, fluticasone (use with caution and avoid with ritonavir), sildenafil/tadalafil/vardenafil (reduce dose), amitriptyline, imipramine, trazodone. May affect warfarin levels; monitor INR.

PREGNANCY: Category C, not for use in nursing.

MECHANISM OF ACTION: HIV protease inhibitor; hydrolyzed to prodrug (amprenavir) which binds to HIV-1 protease active site and prevents the processing of viral Gag and Gag-Pol polyprotein precursors; forms immature infectious viral particles.

PHARMACOKINETICS: Absorption: Oral administration of variable doses resulted in different parameters. **Distribution:** Amprenavir: Plasma protein binding (90%). **Metabolism:** Fosamprenavir: Hepatic (hydrolyzation). Amprenavir: Hepatic via CYP3A4. **Elimination:** Amprenavir: Urine (1%); $T_{1/2}$=7.7 hrs.

LIBRIUM
chlordiazepoxide HCl (Valeant) `CIV`

THERAPEUTIC CLASS: Benzodiazepine

INDICATIONS: Management of anxiety disorders and short-term relief of anxiety symptoms, withdrawal symptoms of acute alcoholism, and preoperative apprehension and anxiety.

DOSAGE: *Adults:* Mild-Moderate Anxiety: 5-10mg tid-qid. Severe Anxiety: 20-25mg tid-qid. Alcohol Withdrawal: 50-100mg; repeat until agitation controlled. Max: 300mg/day. Preoperative Anxiety: 5-10mg PO tid-qid on days prior to surgery. Elderly/Debilitated: 5mg bid-qid.
Pediatrics: ≥6 yrs: 5mg bid-qid. May increase to 10mg bid-tid.

HOW SUPPLIED: Cap: 5mg, 10mg, 25mg

WARNINGS/PRECAUTIONS: Avoid in pregnancy. Paradoxical reactions reported in psychiatric patients and in hyperactive aggressive pediatrics. Caution with porphyria, renal or hepatic dysfunction. Reduce dose in elderly, debilitated. Avoid abrupt withdrawal after extended therapy. May impair mental/physical abilities.

ADVERSE REACTIONS: Drowsiness, ataxia, confusion, skin eruptions, edema, nausea, constipation, extrapyramidal symptoms, libido changes, EEG changes.

INTERACTIONS: Additive effects with CNS depressants and alcohol. Avoid other psychotropic agents.

PREGNANCY: Not for use in pregnancy, safety in nursing not known.

MECHANISM OF ACTION: MOA not established; has antianxiety, sedative, appetite stimulating, and weak analgesic actions; suspected to block EEG arousal from stimulation of brain stem reticular formation.

PHARMACOKINETICS: Elimination: Urine (1-2% unchaged, 3-6% as conjugates); $T_{1/2}$=24-48 hrs.

LIDOCAINE OINTMENT
lidocaine (Fougera) RX

THERAPEUTIC CLASS: Acetamide local anesthetic

INDICATIONS: Topical anesthesia of the oropharynx. Anesthetic lubricant for intubation. Temporary relief of pain associated with minor burns, abrasions, and insect bites.

DOSAGE: *Adults:* Apply up to 5g (6 inches)/application. Max: 17-20g/day.
Pediatrics: Determine dose by age and weight. Max: 4.5mg/kg.

HOW SUPPLIED: Oint: 5% (35g)

WARNINGS/PRECAUTIONS: Reduce dose in elderly, debilitated, acutely ill, and children. Avoid excessive dosage or too frequent administration; may result in serious adverse effects requiring resuscitative measures. Caution with heart block and severe shock. Extreme caution if mucosa is traumatized or sepsis is present in the area of application; risk of rapid systemic absorption.

ADVERSE REACTIONS: Lightheadedness, nervousness, confusion, euphoria, dizziness, drowsiness, blurred vision, tremors, convulsions, respiratory depression, bradycardia, hypotension, urticaria, edema, anaphylactoid reactions.

PREGNANCY: Category B, caution in nursing.

MECHANISM OF ACTION: Local anesthetic; stabilizes neuronal membrane by inhibiting ionic fluxes required for the initiation and conduction of impulses.

PHARMACOKINETICS: Absorption: Rapid (after intratracheal administration). **Distribution:** Plasma protein binding (60-80%); crosses placenta. **Metabolism:** Hepatic (biotransformation). **Elimination:** Urine. (IV) $T_{1/2}$=1.5-2 hrs.

LINCOCIN
RX
lincomycin HCl (Pharmacia & Upjohn)

> Diarrhea, colitis, pseudomembranous colitis reported; may begin up to several weeks after discontinuation. Reserve for serious infections where less toxic antimicrobials are inappropriate.

THERAPEUTIC CLASS: *Streptomyces lincolnensis* derivative

INDICATIONS: Treatment of serious infections due to streptococci, pneumococci, and staphylococci. Reserve for PCN allergy or if PCN is inappropriate.

DOSAGE: *Adults:* IM: Serious Infection: 600mg q24h. More Severe Infection: 600mg q12h or more often. IV: Dose depends on severity. Serious Infection: 600mg-1g q8-12h. More Severe Infection: Increase dose. Infuse over ≥1 hr. Life-Threatening Situation: Up to 8g/day has been given. Max: 8g/day. Severe Renal Dysfunction: 25-30% of normal dose.
Pediatrics: >1 month: IM: Serious Infection: 10mg/kg q24h. More Severe Infection: 10mg/kg q12h or more often. IV: 10-20mg/kg/day, depending on severity infused in divided doses as described for adults. Severe Renal Dysfunction: 25-30% of normal dose.

HOW SUPPLIED: Inj: 300mg/mL

CONTRAINDICATIONS: Clindamycin hypersensitivity.

WARNINGS/PRECAUTIONS: See Black Box Warning. May be inadequate for meningitis treatment. Contains benzyl alcohol. Monitor elderly for change in bowel frequency. Caution with severe renal/hepatic dysfunction, or with history of GI disease (eg, colitis), asthma, significant allergies. Superinfections may occur. Perform periodic CBC, LFTs, and renal function tests with prolonged therapy. Do not administer undiluted as IV bolus. Cardiopulmonary arrest and hypotension with too rapid IV administration.

ADVERSE REACTIONS: Glossitis, stomatitis, NV, diarrhea, colitis, pruritus, blood dyscrasias, hypersensitivity reactions, rash, urticaria, vaginitis, tinnitus, vertigo.

INTERACTIONS: Caution with neuromuscular blockers; may enhance effects. Possible antagonism with erythromycin; avoid concomitant use. Kaolin-pectin inhibits oral lincomycin.

PREGNANCY: Category C, not for use in nursing.

MECHANISM OF ACTION: Streptomyces lincolnensis derivative; possess antibacterial activity.

PHARMACOKINETICS: Absorption: C_{max}(600mg, IM, IV)=11.6, 15.9 mcg/mL. **Elimination:** Urine, bile; $T_{1/2}$=5.4 hrs.

LINDANE
RX
lindane (Alpharma)

> Only for patients who are intolerant or have failed first-line therapy with safer agents. Seizures and deaths reported with repeat or prolonged use. Caution in infants, children, elderly, those with other skin conditions, and those <50kg due to increased risk of neurotoxicity. Contraindicated in premature infants or those with uncontrolled seizure disorders. Instruct patients on proper use and inform that itching occurs after successful killing of scabies or lice.

THERAPEUTIC CLASS: Ectoparasiticide/ovicide

INDICATIONS: (Lot) Treatment of *Sarcoptes scabiei* (scabies) resistant to other therapies. (Shampoo) Treatment of head and pubic lice resistant to or if intolerant to other therapies.

DOSAGE: *Adults:* (Lot) Apply 1-2oz to dry skin; rub in thoroughly. Apply to whole body from neck down. Wash off after 8-12 hrs. Apply only once. (Shampoo) Wash and dry hair with regular shampoo. Apply lindane to hair without water. Add water after 4 min; lather then rinse immediately. Towel briskly. Remove nits with comb or tweezers. Use 1oz for short hair, 1.5oz for medium length hair, and 2oz for long hair. Max: 2oz/application. Retreat if lice remain after 7 days.
Pediatrics: (Lot) Apply (≥6 yrs) 1-2oz or 1oz (<6 yrs) to dry skin; rub in thoroughly. Apply to whole body from neck down. Wash off after 8-12 hrs. Apply only once. (Shampoo) Wash and dry hair with regular shampoo. Apply lindane to hair without water. Add

water after 4 min; lather then rinse immediately. Towel briskly. Remove nits with comb or tweezers. Use 1oz for short hair, 1.5oz for medium length hair, and 2oz for long hair. Max: 2oz/application. Retreat if lice remain after 7 days.

HOW SUPPLIED: Lot, Shampoo: 1% (60mL, 480mL)

CONTRAINDICATIONS: Premature infants, Norwegian (crusted) scabies, skin conditions (eg, atopic dermatitis, psoriasis) that increase systemic absorption of the drug, uncontrolled seizure disorders.

WARNINGS/PRECAUTIONS: Adverse events with serious outcomes reported. Caution in those at increased risk of seizure (eg, HIV, head trauma, prior seizure, CNS tumor, severe hepatic cirrhosis, excessive alcohol use, abrupt alchol or sedative withdrawal). Give Medication Guide to each patient when dispensing. Avoid eyes and mouth. Do not use with open wounds, cuts, or scores. Use rubber gloves to apply.

ADVERSE REACTIONS: CNS stimulation, dizziness, convulsions.

INTERACTIONS: Avoid creams, ointments, oils, oil-based hair dressings or conditioners; may enhance absorption. Caution with drugs that may lower seizure threshold (eg, antipsychotics, antidepressants, theophylline, cyclosporine, mycophenolate, tacrolimus, penicillins, imipenem, quinolones, chloroquine sulfate, pyrimethamine, isoniazid, meperidine, radiographic contrast agents, centrally active anticholinesterases, methocarbamol).

PREGNANCY: Category C, not for use in nursing.

MECHANISM OF ACTION: Ectoparasiticide/ovicide; exerts action by being directly absorbed into parasites and their ova.

PHARMACOKINETICS: Absorption: C_{max}=28ng/mL, T_{max}=6 hrs (infants and children). **Distribution:** Found in breast milk.

LIPITOR
atorvastatin calcium (Parke-Davis/Pfizer)

RX

THERAPEUTIC CLASS: HMG-CoA reductase inhibitor

INDICATIONS: Adjunct to diet, to reduce total cholesterol (total-C), LDL-C, TG, and Apo B levels, and to increase HDL-C in primary hypercholesterolemia (heterozygous familial and nonfamilial) and mixed dyslipidemia (Types IIa and IIb). Adjunct to diet for elevated serum TG levels (Type IV). Treatment of primary dysbetalipoproteinemia (Type III) inadequately responding to diet. Adjunct to other lipid-lowering treatments or if treatments are unavailable, to reduce total-C and LDL-C in homozygous familial hypercholesterolemia. Adjunct to diet to lower total-C, LDL-C and apolipoprotein B in postmenarchal adolescents with heterozygous familial hypercholesterolemia. To reduce the risk of MI, revascularization procedures, and angina in adults without clinically evident CHD but with multiple risk factors for CHD. To reduce the risk of MI and stroke in patients with Type II DM, and without clinically evident CHD, but with multiple risk factors for CHD. In patients with clinically evident CHD to reduce the risk of non-fatal MI, fatal and non-fatal stroke, revascularization procedures, hospitalization for CHF, and angina.

DOSAGE: *Adults:* Hypercholesterolemia/Mixed Dyslipidemia: Initial: 10-20mg qd (or 40mg qd for LDL-C reduction >45%). Titrate: Adjust dose if needed at 2-4 week intervals. Usual: 10-80mg qd. Homozygous Familial Hypercholesterolemia: 10-80mg qd. *Pediatrics:* Heterozygous Familial Hypercholesterolemia: 10-17 yrs (postmenarchal): Initial: 10mg/day. Titrate: Adjust dose if needed at intervals of ≥4 weeks. Max: 20mg/day.

HOW SUPPLIED: Tab: 10mg, 20mg, 40mg, 80mg

CONTRAINDICATIONS: Active liver disease, unexplained persistent elevations of serum transaminases, pregnancy, nursing mothers.

WARNINGS/PRECAUTIONS: Monitor LFTs prior to therapy, at 12 weeks or with dose elevation, and periodically thereafter. Reduce dose or withdraw if AST or ALT ≥3x ULN persist. Caution with heavy alcohol use and/or history of hepatic disease. D/C if markedly elevated CPK levels occur, if myopathy is diagnosed or suspected, or if predisposition to renal failure secondary to rhabdomyolysis. Caution in patients with recent stroke or TIA. Rare cases of rhabdomyolysis reported.

ADVERSE REACTIONS: Constipation, flatulence, dyspepsia, abdominal pain, transaminase and CK elevation in higher doses.

INTERACTIONS: Increases levels with erythromycin. Increases levels of oral contraceptives (norethindrone, ethinyl estradiol), digoxin. Monitor digoxin. Cyclosporine, fibric acid derivatives, niacin, erythromycin, and azole antifungals may increase risk of myopathy. Caution with drugs that decrease levels or activity of endogenous steroid hormones (eg, ketoconazole, spironolactone, cimetidine). Decreases levels with Maalox® TC, but LDL-C reduction not altered. Colestipol decreases levels when coadministered, but greater LDL-C reduction with coadministration than when each given alone. Avoid fibrates.

PREGNANCY: Category X, not for use in nursing.

MECHANISM OF ACTION: Competitive inhibitor of HMG-CoA reductase; inhibits conversion of HMG-CoA to mevalonate (precursor of sterols, including cholesterol).

PHARMACOKINETICS: Absorption: Rapid; absolute bioavailability (14%); T_{max}=1-2 hrs. **Distribution:** V_d=381L; plasma protein binding (≥98%); found in breast milk. **Metabolism:** Extensive; via CYP3A4 to ortho- and parahydroxylated derivatives, and various β-oxidation products. **Elimination:** Bile (drug, metabolites), urine (<2%); $T_{1/2}$=14 hrs.

LITHIUM CARBONATE   RX
lithium carbonate (Roxane)

> Lithium toxicity is related to serum lithium levels and can occur at doses close to therapeutic levels.

THERAPEUTIC CLASS: Antimanic agent

INDICATIONS: Treatment of manic episodes of bipolar disorder and maintenance treatment of bipolar disorder.

DOSAGE: *Adults:* Acute Mania: 600mg tid to achieve effective serum levels of 1-1.5mEq/L; monitor levels twice a week until stabilized. Maint: 300mg tid-qid to maintain serum levels of 0.6-1.2 mEq/L; monitor levels every 2 months. Elderly: Reduce dose. *Pediatrics:* ≥12 yrs: Acute Mania: 600mg tid. Effective serum levels are 1-1.5mEq/L; monitor levels twice a week until stabilized. Maint: 300mg tid-qid to maintain serum levels of 0.6-1.2mEq/L; monitor levels every 2 months.

HOW SUPPLIED: Cap: 150mg, 300mg, 600mg; Tab: 300mg

CONTRAINDICATIONS: Renal or cardiovascular disease, severe debilitation or dehydration, sodium depletion, and diuretic use.

WARNINGS/PRECAUTIONS: May cause fetal harm; if possible withdraw for at least the 1st trimester of pregnancy. Caution in the elderly. Maintain normal diet, adequate salt/fluid intake. Assess kidney function prior to and during therapy. May impair mental/physical abilities. Reduce dose or d/c with sweating, diarrhea, infection with elevated temperatures. Caution with thyroid disorders; monitor thyroid function. Chronic therapy associated with diminution of renal concentrating ability (eg, diabetes insipidus), glomerular and interstitial fibrosis, and nephron atrophy.

ADVERSE REACTIONS: Fine hand tremor, polyuria, mild thirst, nausea, incoordination, diarrhea, vomiting, drowsiness, muscular weakness.

INTERACTIONS: Risk of encephalopathic syndrome (eg, weakness, lethargy, fever, tremulousness, confusion, EPS) with haloperidol and other antipsychotics; discontinue therapy if such signs occur. May prolong effects of neuromuscular blockers. Increased levels with indomethacin, piroxicam and other NSAIDs. Increased risk of toxicity due to decreased clearance with diuretics and ACE inhibitors; contraindicated with diuretics.

PREGNANCY: Category D, not for use in nursing.

MECHANISM OF ACTION: Mood-stabilizing agent; mechanism not established. Suspected to alter sodium transport in nerve and muscle cells and effect a shift toward intraneuronal metabolism of catecholamines.

PHARMACOKINETICS: Distribution: Found in breast milk. **Elimination:** Urine (primary), feces; $T_{1/2}$=24 hrs.

LITHOBID   RX
lithium carbonate (JDS)

| **Lithium toxicity is related to serum levels, and can occur at doses close to therapeutic levels.** |

THERAPEUTIC CLASS: Antimanic agent

INDICATIONS: Treatment of manic episodes of manic-depressive illness.

DOSAGE: *Adults:* Acute Mania: Initial: 900mg bid or 600mg tid to achieve effective serum levels of 1-1.5mEq/L; monitor levels twice weekly until stabilized. Maint: 900-1200mg/day, given bid-tid to maintain serum levels of 0.6-1.2mEq/L; monitor levels every 2 months.
Pediatrics: ≥12 yrs: Acute Mania: Initial: 900mg bid or 600mg tid to achieve effective serum levels of 1-1.5mEq/L; monitor levels twice weekly until stabilized. Maint: 900-1200mg/day, given bid-tid to maintain serum levels of 0.6-1.2 mEq/L; monitor levels every 2 months.

HOW SUPPLIED: Tab, Extended-Release: 300mg

WARNINGS/PRECAUTIONS: Avoid with significant renal or cardiovascular disease, severe debilitation, dehydration, or sodium depletion. Assess kidney function prior to and during therapy. Risk of encephalopathic syndrome (eg, weakness, lethargy, fever, tremulousness, confusion, EPS); d/c therapy. May impair mental/physical abilities. Reduce dose or d/c with sweating, diarrhea, infection with elevated temperatures. Caution with hypothyroidism; may need supplemental therapy. Chronic therapy associated with diminution of renal concentrating ability, glomerular and interstitial fibrosis, and nephron atrophy.

ADVERSE REACTIONS: Fine hand tremor, polyuria, mild thirst, nausea, general discomfort, diarrhea, vomiting, drowsiness, muscular weakness.

INTERACTIONS: Avoid diuretics and ACE inhibitors; risk of lithium toxicity due to reduced renal clearance. May prolong effects of neuromuscular blockers. Decreased levels with acetazolamide, urea, xanthine preparations, and alkalinizing agents. May produce hypothyroidism with iodide preparations. Increased plasma levels with indomethacin, piroxicam, other NSAIDs. Increased risk of neurotoxic effects with carbamazepine and CCBs. Reduced renal clearance with metronidazole. Fluoxetine may increase and/or decrease lithium levels.

PREGNANCY: Category D, not for use in nursing.

MECHANISM OF ACTION: Not established; suspected to alter sodium transport in nerve and muscle cells and effects a shift toward intraneuronal metabolism of catecholamines.

PHARMACOKINETICS: Elimination: Urine (primary), feces (insignificant); $T_{1/2}$=24 hrs.

LOCOID   RX
hydrocortisone butyrate (Ferndale)

THERAPEUTIC CLASS: Corticosteroid

INDICATIONS: (Cre, Oint) Corticosteroid responsive dermatoses. (Sol) Seborrheic dermatitis.

DOSAGE: *Adults:* (Cre, Oint) Apply bid-tid. May use occlusive dressings for psoriasis or recalcitrant conditions. D/C dressings if infection develops. (Sol) Apply bid-tid.
Pediatrics: (Cre, Oint) Apply bid-tid. May use occlusive dressings for psoriasis or recalcitrant conditions. D/C dressings if infection develops. (Sol) Apply bid-tid.

HOW SUPPLIED: Cre, Oint: 0.1% (15g, 45g); Sol: 0.1% (20mL, 60mL)

WARNINGS/PRECAUTIONS: May produce reversible HPA axis suppression, manifestations of Cushing's syndrome, hyperglycemia, and glucosuria. D/C if irritation occurs. Use appropriate antifungal or antibacterial agent with dermatological infections. Peds may be more susceptible to systemic toxicity. Caution when applied to large surface areas. Avoid contact with eyes. Limit to least amount compatible with an effective therapeutic regimen. Chronic corticosteroid therapy may interfere with the growth and development of children.

ADVERSE REACTIONS: Burning, itching, irritation, dryness, folliculitis, hypertrichosis, acneiform eruptions, hypopigmentation, perioral dermatitis, allergic dermatitis, skin maceration, secondary infection, skin atrophy, striae, miliaria.

PREGNANCY: Category C, caution in nursing.

MECHANISM OF ACTION: Corticosteroid; possesses anti-inflammatory, anti-pruritic, and vasoconstrictive properties. Anti-inflammatory actions not established.

PHARMACOKINETICS: Absorption: Percutaneous; inflammation, other disease states, and occlusive dressings may increase absorption. **Distribution:** Bound to plasma proteins to varying degrees. Systemically administered corticosteroids found in breast milk. **Metabolism:** Liver. **Elimination:** Renal (major), bile.

LODRANE 24   RX
brompheniramine maleate (ECR)

THERAPEUTIC CLASS: Antihistamine

INDICATIONS: Temporary relief of seasonal and perennial allergic rhinitis and vasomotor rhinitis.

DOSAGE: *Adults:* 12-24mg qd.
Pediatrics: ≥12 yrs: 12-24mg qd. 6-12 yrs: 12mg qd.

HOW SUPPLIED: Cap, Extended-Release: 12mg

CONTRAINDICATIONS: Nursing mothers, patients taking MAOIs, narrow angle glaucoma, urinary retention, peptic ulcer, and during an asthmatic attack.

WARNINGS/PRECAUTIONS: Caution with HTN, DM, ischemic heart disease, hyperthyroidism, bronchial asthma, increased IOP, prostatic hypertrophy, CVD, and elderly. May impair mental/physical abilities.

ADVERSE REACTIONS: Drowsiness, confusion, restlessness, nausea, vomiting, rash, vertigo, palpitation, anorexia, dizziness, headache, insomnia, anxiety, tension, excitability.

INTERACTIONS: See Contraindications. MAOIs and TCA's may prolong and intensify the anticholinergic effects of antihistamines. Concomitant use of antihistamines with alcohol, TCA's, barbiturates, other CNS depressants may have an additive effect.

PREGNANCY: Category C, not for use in nursing.

LOMOTIL
atropine sulfate - diphenoxylate HCl (Pharmacia & Upjohn)

OTHER BRAND NAME: Lonox (Sandoz)

THERAPEUTIC CLASS: Opioid/anticholinergic

INDICATIONS: Adjunctive therapy for management of diarrhea.

DOSAGE: *Adults:* Initial: 2 tabs or 10mL qid. Titrate: Reduce dose after symptoms are controlled. Maint: 2 tabs or 10mL qd. Max: 20mg/day diphenoxylate. D/C if symptoms not controlled after 10 days at max dose of 20mg/day (diphenoxylate).
Pediatrics: 2-12 yrs: Initial: 0.3-0.4mg/kg/day of solution given qid. 13-16 yrs: Initial: 2 tabs or 10mL tid. Titrate: Reduce dose after symptoms are controlled. Maint: 25% of initial dose. D/C if no improvement within 48 hrs.

HOW SUPPLIED: (Diphenoxylate-Atropine) Sol: 2.5mg-0.025/5mL (60mL); Tab: 2.5mg-0.025mg

CONTRAINDICATIONS: Obstructive jaundice, diarrhea associated with pseudomembranous enterocolitis or enterotoxin-producing bacteria.

WARNINGS/PRECAUTIONS: May induce toxic megacolon in ulcerative colitis; d/c if abdominal distention occurs. May cause intestinal fluid retention. Avoid with diarrhea associated with organisms that penetrate the intestinal mucosa, and with pseudomembranous enterocolitis. Caution in pediatrics, especially with Down's syndrome. Extreme caution advanced hepatorenal disease and liver dysfunction. Do not use with severe dehydration or electrolyte imbalance until corrective therapy is initiated.

ADVERSE REACTIONS: Numbness of extremities, dizziness, anaphylaxis, hyperthermia, tachycardia, urinary retention, flushing, drowsiness, toxic megacolon, nausea, vomiting.

INTERACTIONS: May potentiate barbiturates, tranquilizers and alcohol. MAOIs may precipitate hypertensive crisis.

PREGNANCY: Category C, caution in nursing.

MECHANISM OF ACTION: Diphenoxylate: Antidiarrheal. Atropine: Anticholinergic.

PHARMACOKINETICS: Absorption: (4 tabs): C_{max} =163ng/mL. T_{max}=2 hrs. **Metabolism:** Rapid and extensive metabolism through ester hydrolysis to diphenoxylic acid (major metabolite). **Elimination:** $T_{1/2}$=12-14 hrs (diphenoxylic acid). Urine (14%, 6% conjugate), feces (49%).

LOPROX   RX
ciclopirox (Medicis)

OTHER BRAND NAME: Loprox TS (Medicis)

THERAPEUTIC CLASS: Broad-spectrum antifungal

INDICATIONS: (Cre/Sus) Treatment of dermal infections of tinea pedis, tinea cruris, tinea corporis, cutaneous candidiasis and tinea versicolor. (Gel) Treatment of interdigital tinea pedis and tinea corporis. (Gel/Shampoo) Treatment of seborrheic dermatitis of the scalp.

DOSAGE: *Adults:* (Cre/Gel/Sus) Massage affected and surrounding areas bid (am and pm) up to 4 weeks. (Shampoo) Apply about 5mL (up to 10mL for long hair) to wet scalp. Lather and rinse off after 3 min. Repeat twice weekly for 4 weeks, at least 3 days apart.
Pediatrics: ≥10 yrs: (Cre/Sus) Massage affected and surrounding areas bid (am and pm) up to 4 weeks. Gel or shampoo not recommended in pediatrics <16 yrs.

HOW SUPPLIED: Cre: 0.77% (15g, 30g, 90g); Gel: 0.77% (30g, 45g, 100g); Shampoo: 1% (120mL); Sus: (Loprox TS) 0.77% (30mL, 60mL)

WARNINGS/PRECAUTIONS: Avoid eyes, mucous membranes, occlusive wrappings or dressings. D/C if sensitization or chemical irritation occurs. Hair discoloration reported in patients with lighter hair color.

ADVERSE REACTIONS: Contact dermatitis, pruritus, burning.

PREGNANCY: Pregnancy B, caution in nursing.

MECHANISM OF ACTION: Broad-spectrum antifungal; acts by chelation of polyvalent cations (Fe^{3+}or Al^{3+}) resulting in the inhibition of the metal-dependent enzymes that are responsible for degradation of peroxides in the fungal cell wall. Inhibits the growth of pathogenic dermatophytes, yeasts, and and *Malassezia furfur*.

PHARMACOKINETICS: Elimination: Renal and feces; $T_{1/2}$= 5.5 hrs.

LORTAB
acetaminophen - hydrocodone bitartrate (UCB Pharma)

THERAPEUTIC CLASS: Opioid analgesic

INDICATIONS: Relief of moderate to moderately severe pain.

DOSAGE: *Adults:* (2.5/500, 5/500) 1-2 tabs q4-6h prn. Max: 8 tabs/day. (7.5/500, 10/500) 1 tab q4-6h prn. Max: 6 tabs/day. (Sol) 15mL q4-6h prn. Max: 90mL/day.
Pediatrics: ≥2 yrs: (Sol) 12-15kg: 3.75mL. 16-22kg: 5mL. 23-31kg: 7.5mL. 32-45kg: 10mL. ≥46kg: 15mL. May repeat q4-6h prn.

HOW SUPPLIED: (Hydrocodone-APAP) Sol: 7.5mg-500mg/15mL; Tab: 2.5mg-500mg*, 5mg-500mg*, 7.5mg-500mg*, 10mg-500mg* *scored

WARNINGS/PRECAUTIONS: May produce dose-related respiratory depression. May obscure acute abdominal conditions or head injuries. Caution in elderly, debilitated, severe hepatic or renal dysfunction, hypothyroidism, Addison's disease, prostatic hypertrophy, urethral stricture, pulmonary disease, postoperative use. May be habit-forming. Suppresses cough reflex.

ADVERSE REACTIONS: Lightheadedness, dizziness, sedation, NV.

INTERACTIONS: Additive CNS depression with other narcotics, antihistamines, antipsychotics, antianxiety agents, alcohol, CNS depressants. Increased effect of antidepressant or hydrocodone with MAOIs or TCAs.

PREGNANCY: Category C, not for use in nursing.

MECHANISM OF ACTION: Hydrocodone: Narcotic analgesic and antitussive; not established. Suspected to be related to existence of opiate receptors in CNS. APAP: Nonopioid, nonsalicylate analgesic, and antipyretic. Analgesic action involves peripheral influences; specific mechanism not established. Antipyretic activity is mediated through hypothalamic heat-regulating centers. Inhibits prostaglandin synthetase.

PHARMACOKINETICS: Administration: Hydrocodone: C_{max}=23.6ng/mL; T_{max}=1.3 hrs. APAP: Rapidly absorbed. **Distribution:** Hydrocodone: Crosses placental barrier. APAP: Found in breast milk. **Metabolism:** Hydrocodone: O-demethylation, N-demethylation and 6-keto reduction. APAP: Liver (conjugation). **Elimination:** Hydrocodone: $T_{1/2}$=3.8 hrs; APAP: Urine (85%); $T_{1/2}$=1.25-3 hrs.

LOTENSIN RX
benazepril HCl (Novartis)

> When used in pregnancy, ACE inhibitors can cause injury and even death to the developing fetus. D/C therapy when pregnancy detected.

THERAPEUTIC CLASS: ACE inhibitor

INDICATIONS: Treatment of hypertension. May be used alone or with thiazide diuretics.

DOSAGE: *Adults:* If possible, d/c diuretic 2-3 days prior to initiation of therapy. Initial: 10mg qd or 5mg with concomitant diuretic. Maint: 20-40mg/day given qd-bid. Resume diuretic if BP not controlled. Max: 80mg/day. CrCl <30mL/min/1.73m²: Initial: 5mg qd. Max: 40mg/day.
Pediatrics: ≥6 yrs: Initial: 0.2mg/kg qd. Max: 0.6mg/kg.

HOW SUPPLIED: Tab: 5mg, 10mg, 20mg, 40mg

WARNINGS/PRECAUTIONS: D/C if angioedema, jaundice, or if marked LFT elevation occurs. Risk of hyperkalemia with DM, renal dysfunction. Persistent nonproductive cough reported. Monitor WBCs in renal and collagen vascular disease. Anaphylactoid reactions reported. Fetal/neonatal morbidity and death reported. Monitor for hypotension in high risk patients (eg, surgery/anesthesia, prolonged diuretic therapy, heart failure, volume and/or salt depletion, etc). Caution with CHF, renal dysfunction, and renal artery stenosis. Less effective on BP in blacks and more reports of angioedema than nonblacks.

ADVERSE REACTIONS: Cough, dizziness, headache, fatigue, somnolence, postural dizziness, nausea.

INTERACTIONS: May increase lithium levels. Hypotension risk with diuretics. Increased risk of hyperkalemia with K⁺-sparing diuretics, K⁺-containing salt substitutes, or K⁺ supplements.

PREGNANCY: Category D, not for use in nursing.

MECHANISM OF ACTION: ACE inhibitor; not established, effects appear to result from suppression of renin-angiotensin-aldosterone system.

PHARMACOKINETICS: Absorption: Absolute bioavailability (≥37%); T_{max}=0.5-1 hr, 1-4 hrs (metabolite). **Distribution:** Parent, metabolite: Plasma protein binding (96.7%, 95.3%). **Metabolism:** Cleavage of ester group; benazeprilat (active metabolite). **Elimination:** Urine (7%). Benazeprilat: Urine (20%), biliary (11-12%); $T_{1/2}$=10-11 hrs (adults), 5 hrs (pediatrics).

LOTRIMIN AF OTC
clotrimazole (Schering)

THERAPEUTIC CLASS: Azole antifungal

INDICATIONS: Tinea pedis, t.cruris, t.corporis.

DOSAGE: *Adults:* Cleanse skin with soap and water and dry thoroughly. Apply to affected area am and pm. Athlete's Foot and Ringworm: Treat for 4 weeks. Jock Itch: Treat for 2 weeks.
Pediatrics: ≥2 yrs: Cleanse skin with soap and water and dry thoroughly. Apply to affected area am and pm. Athlete's Foot and Ringworm: Treat for 4 weeks. Jock Itch: Treat for 2 weeks.

HOW SUPPLIED: Cre: 1% (24g); Lot: 1% (20mL); Sol: 1% (10mL)

WARNINGS/PRECAUTIONS: D/C if irritation occurs or no improvement in 4 weeks (t.pedis or t. corporis) or 2 weeks (t. cruris). Avoid eye contact. Not effective on scalp or nails.

PREGNANCY: Safety in pregnancy and nursing not known.

LOTRIMIN AF SPRAY & POWDER   OTC
miconazole nitrate (Schering)

THERAPEUTIC CLASS: Azole antifungal

INDICATIONS: To treat and relieve the itching, cracking, burning, and scaling of athlete's foot (tinea pedis), jock itch, (tinea cruris), and ringworm (tinea corporis). Powder aids in the drying of moist areas.

DOSAGE: *Adults:* Cleanse skin with soap and water and dry thoroughly. (Powder) Sprinkle thin layer over affected area am and pm. (Spray) Spray thin layer over affected area am and pm. Athlete's Foot and Ringworm: Treat for 4 weeks. Jock Itch: Treat for 2 weeks.
Pediatrics: ≥2 yrs: Cleanse skin with soap and water and dry thoroughly. (Powder) Sprinkle thin layer over affected area am and pm. (Spray) Spray thin layer over affected area am and pm. Athlete's Foot and Ringworm: Treat for 4 weeks. Jock Itch: Treat for 2 weeks.

HOW SUPPLIED: Powder: 2% (90g); Spray, Powder: 2% (100g); Spray: 2% (113g)

WARNINGS/PRECAUTIONS: Avoid eye contact. D/C if irritation occurs or no improvement in 4 weeks (athlete's foot or ringworm) or 2 weeks (jock itch). Avoid while smoking or near heat/flame.

PREGNANCY: Safety in pregnancy and nursing not known.

LOTRIMIN ULTRA   OTC
butenafine HCl (Schering)

THERAPEUTIC CLASS: Benzylamine antifungal

INDICATIONS: To cure and relieve itching, cracking, burning, and scaling of athlete's foot (tinea pedis), jock itch, (tinea cruris), and ringworm (tinea corporis).

DOSAGE: *Adults:* Wash and dry area. Tinea Pedis: Apply between toes bid (am and pm) for 1 week, or qd for 4 weeks. Tinea Cruris/Corporis: Apply qd for 2 weeks.
Pediatrics: ≥12 yrs: Wash and dry area. Tinea Pedis: Apply between toes bid (am and pm) for 1 week, or qd for 4 weeks. Tinea Cruris/Corporis: Apply qd for 2 weeks.

HOW SUPPLIED: Cre: 1% (12g)

WARNINGS/PRECAUTIONS: Avoid nails, scalp, mouth, and eyes. D/C if too much irritation occurs. Not for vaginal yeast infections. Effectiveness on bottom of foot unknown.

PREGNANCY: Safety in pregnancy and nursing not known.

LUPRON PEDIATRIC   RX
leuprolide acetate (TAP)

OTHER BRAND NAME: Lupron Depot-Ped (TAP)

THERAPEUTIC CLASS: Synthetic gonadotropin releasing hormone analog

INDICATIONS: Treatment of central precocious puberty.

DOSAGE: *Pediatrics:* Initial: 50mcg/kg/d as single SQ dose or (depot) 0.3mg/kg every 4 weeks (minimum 7.5mg) as single IM dose. Depot Start Dose: ≤25kg: 7.5mg; >25-37.5kg: 11.25mg; >37.5kg: 15mg. Titrate: Increase by 10 mcg/kg/day SQ or (depot) 3.75mg IM every 4 weeks if downregulation not achieved. Maint: Dose that produces adequate downregulation. Verify adequate downregulation with significant weight increase.

HOW SUPPLIED: Inj: 5mg/mL, (Depot) 7.5mg, 11.25mg, 15mg

CONTRAINDICATIONS: Pregnancy.

WARNINGS/PRECAUTIONS: Monitor hormonal effects after 1-2 months of therapy. Measure bone age every 6-12 months. Increase in clinical signs and symptoms may occur in early phase of therapy due to rise in gonadotropins and sex steroids. D/C before age 11 in females and age 12 in males.

ADVERSE REACTIONS: Initial exacerbation of signs and symptoms, injection site reactions, pain, acne/seborrhea, rash, urogenital bleeding/discharge, vaginitis.

PREGNANCY: Category X, not for use in nursing.

MECHANISM OF ACTION: A GnRH agonist; initially stimulates gonadotropins. Chronic stimulation results in reversible suppression of ovarian and testicular steroidogenesis.

PHARMACOKINETICS: Absorption: C_{max}=20ng/mL, T_{max}=4 hrs. **Distribution:** V_d=27L, plasma protein binding (43-49%). **Metabolism:** M-I (major metabolite). **Elimination:** Urine (<5% parent and metabolite). $T_{1/2}$=3 hrs.

LURIDE   RX
sodium fluoride (Colgate Oral)

THERAPEUTIC CLASS: Fluoride supplement

INDICATIONS: To prevent dental caries in areas where drinking water fluoride content is <0.6ppm.

DOSAGE: *Pediatrics:* (Drops) <0.3ppm: 6 months-3 yrs: 0.5mL qd. 3-6 yrs: 1mL qd. 6-16 yrs: 2mL qd. 0.3-0.6ppm: 3-6 yrs: 0.5mL qd. 6-16 yrs: 1mL qd. (Tab) <0.3ppm: 6 months-<3 yrs: 0.25mg qd. 3-6 yrs: 0.5mg qd. 6-16 yrs: 1mg qd. 0.3-0.6ppm: 3-6 yrs: 0.25mg qd. 6-16 yrs: 0.5mg qd. Dissolve tab in mouth or chew tab before swallowing. Take at bedtime after brushing teeth.

HOW SUPPLIED: Drops: 0.5mg/mL (50mL); Tab, Chewable: 0.25mg, 0.5mg, 1mg

CONTRAINDICATIONS: (Drips) Areas where drinking water fluoride is >0.6 ppm, pediatrics <6 months. (Tab) 1mg: Water fluoride is >0.3ppm, pediatrics <6 yrs. 0.5mg: Water fluoride is >0.6ppm, pediatrics <6 yrs. 0.25mg: Water fluoride is >0.6ppm.

WARNINGS/PRECAUTIONS: Dental fluorosis may result from daily ingestion of excessive fluoride in pediatrics <6 yrs especially if water fluoride is >0.6ppm.

ADVERSE REACTIONS: Allergic rash.

INTERACTIONS: Do not eat or drink dairy products within 1 hour of administration.

PREGNANCY: Safety in pregnancy not known. Caution in nursing.

MECHANISM OF ACTION: Fluoride supplement; increases tooth resistance to acid dissolution by promoting remineralization and inhibiting cariogenic microbial process.

LUSTRA   RX
hydroquinone (Taro)

OTHER BRAND NAME: Lustra-AF (Taro)

THERAPEUTIC CLASS: Depigmenting agent

INDICATIONS: Gradual treatment of UV-induced dyschromia and discoloration resulting from use of oral contraceptives, pregnancy, hormone replacement therapy, or skin trauma.

DOSAGE: *Adults:* Apply bid (am and hs). Use with sunscreen.
Pediatrics: ≥12 yrs: Apply bid (am and hs). Use with sunscreen.

HOW SUPPLIED: Cre: 4% (56.8g)

WARNINGS/PRECAUTIONS: Avoid sun exposure on bleached skin. Lustra-AF contains sunscreen; use sunscreen with Lustra. May produce unwanted cosmetic effects if not used as directed. Test for skin sensitivity. D/C if no lightening effect after 2 months of therapy, if blue-black darkening of the skin occurs, or if itching, vesicle formation, or excessive inflammatory reactions occur. Contains sodium metabisulfite, may cause serious allergic type reactions. Avoid contact wtih eyes.

ADVERSE REACTIONS: Cutaneous hypersensitivity (contact dermatitis).

PREGNANCY: Category C, caution in nursing.

MECHANISM OF ACTION: Produces reversible depigmentation of skin; inhibits enzymatic oxidation of tyrosine to 3-(3,4-dihydroxyphenyl) alanine (dopa) and suppresses other melanocyte metabolic processes.

MACROBID   RX
nitrofurantoin monohydrate (Procter & Gamble)

THERAPEUTIC CLASS: Imidazolidinedione antibacterial

INDICATIONS: Treatment of acute uncomplicated urinary tract infections (acute cystitis).

DOSAGE: *Adults:* 100mg q12h for 7 days. Take with food.
Pediatrics: >12 yrs: 100mg q12h for 7 days. Take with food.

HOW SUPPLIED: Cap: 100mg

CONTRAINDICATIONS: Anuria, oliguria, CrCl <60mL/min, pregnancy at term (38-42 weeks gestation), labor and delivery, and neonates <1 month of age.

WARNINGS/PRECAUTIONS: Acute, subacute, or chronic pulmonary reactions have occurred. Anemia, diabetes mellitus, renal dysfunction, electrolyte imbalance, vitamin B deficiency, and debilitating disease enhance occurrence of peripheral neuropathy. Stop therapy with acute and chronic pulmonary reactions, hepatic disorders, hemolysis, or peripheral neuropathy. Monitor renal function, LFTs and pulmonary function periodically during long-term therapy. Optic neuritis and hepatic reactions reported. *Clostridium difficile*- associated diarrhea has been reported.

ADVERSE REACTIONS: Pulmonary disorders, hepatic damage, peripheral neuropathy, nausea, headache, flatulence, anorexia, diarrhea, dizziness, alopecia, exfoliative dermatitis, Stevens-Johnson syndrome, anaphylaxis, blood dyscrasias, aplastic anemia.

INTERACTIONS: Antacids, especially magnesium trisilicate, decrease rate and extent of absorption. Uricosuric drugs (eg, probenecid and sulfinpyrazone) increase nitrofurantoin levels.

PREGNANCY: Category B, not for use in nursing.

MECHANISM OF ACTION: Imidazolidinedione antibacterial; inhibits protein synthesis, aerobic energy metabolism, DNA, RNA, and cell-wall synthesis.

PHARMACOKINETICS: Absorption: C_{max} ≤1mcg/mL. **Elimination:** Urine (20-25% unchanged).

MACRODANTIN   RX
nitrofurantoin macrocrystals (Procter & Gamble)

THERAPEUTIC CLASS: Imidazolidinedione antibacterial

INDICATIONS: Treatment of urinary tract infection.

DOSAGE: *Adults:* 50-100mg qid for at least 7 days. Take with food. Long-term Suppressive Use: 50-100mg at bedtime.
Pediatrics: ≥1 month: 5-7mg/kg/day given qid for at least 7 days. Take with food. Long-term Suppressive Use: 1mg/kg/day given qd-bid.

HOW SUPPLIED: Cap: 25mg, 50mg, 100mg

CONTRAINDICATIONS: Anuria, oliguria, CrCl <60mL/min, pregnancy at term (38-42 weeks gestation), labor and delivery, neonates <1 month of age.

WARNINGS/PRECAUTIONS: Acute, subacute or chronic pulmonary reactions have occurred. Anemia, diabetes mellitus, renal dysfunction, electrolyte imbalance, vitamin B deficiency, and debilitating disease enhance occurrence of peripheral neuropathy. Stop therapy with acute and chronic pulmonary reactions, hepatic disorders, hemolysis, or peripheral neuropathy. Monitor renal function, LFTs and pulmonary function periodically during long-term therapy. Optic neuritis and hepatic reactions reported. False (+) reaction for glucose in urine may occur with Benedict's and Fehling's solution.

ADVERSE REACTIONS: Pulmonary disorders, hepatic damage, peripheral neuropathy, nausea, emesis, anorexia, dizziness, alopecia, exfoliative dermatitis, Stevens-Johnson syndrome, anaphylaxis, headache, drowsiness, asthenia, vertigo.

INTERACTIONS: Antacids, especially magnesium trisilicate, decrease rate and extent of absorption. Uricosuric drugs (eg, probenecid and sulfinpyrazone) increase nitrofurantoin levels.

PREGNANCY: Category B, not for use in nursing

MECHANISM OF ACTION: Imidazolidinedione antibacterial; inhibits protein synthesis, aerobic energy metabolism, DNA, RNA, and cell-wall synthesis.

MALARONE RX
atovaquone - proguanil HCl (GlaxoSmithKline)

OTHER BRAND NAME: Malarone Pediatric (GlaxoSmithKline)

THERAPEUTIC CLASS: Pyrimidine synthesis inhibitor

INDICATIONS: Prophylaxis or treatment of malaria caused by *P.falciparum.*

DOSAGE: *Adults:* Prevention: Begin 1-2 days before entering endemic area, continue during stay and for 7 days after return. 1 tab qd. Treatment: 4 tabs qd for 3 days. Repeat dose if vomiting occurs within 1 hr after dosing. Take as single dose with food or milky drink.
Pediatrics: Prevention: Begin 1-2 days before entering endemic area, continue during stay and for 7 days after return. 11-20kg: 1 pediatric tab qd. 21-30kg: 2 pediatric tabs qd. 31-40kg: 3 pediatric tabs qd. >40kg: Dose as adult. Treatment: Treat for 3 consecutive days. 5-8kg: 2 pediatric tabs qd. 9-10kg: 3 pediatric tabs. 11-20kg: 1 tab qd. 21-30kg: 2 tabs qd. 31-40kg: 3 tabs. >40kg: Dose as adult. Repeat dose if vomiting occurs within 1 hr after dosing. Take as single dose with food or milky drink.

HOW SUPPLIED: (Atovaquone-Proguanil) Tab: 250mg-100mg; Tab, Pediatric: 62.5mg-25mg

CONTRAINDICATIONS: For prophylaxis in severe renal impairment (CrCl <30mL/min).

WARNINGS/PRECAUTIONS: Not for cerebral malaria. Patients with severe malaria are not candidates for PO therapy. Rare cases of anaphylaxis reported.

ADVERSE REACTIONS: Vomiting, pruritus, elevation of LFTs.

INTERACTIONS: Rifampin, rifabutin may decrease levels; concomitant use is not recommended. Reduced bioavailability with metoclopramide and tetracycline.

PREGNANCY: Category C, caution in nursing.

MECHANISM OF ACTION: Pyramidine synthesis inhibitor. Atovaquone: Antiparasitic agent that acts as a selective inhibitor of parasite mitochondrial electron transport. Proguanil: Antiparasitic agent that acts on the metabolite cycloguanil, which inhibits dihydrofolate reductase in the malaria parasite, resulting in disruption of deoxythymidylate synthesis.

PHARMACOKINETICS: Absorption: Atovaquone: Absolute bioavailability (23%). Proguanil: Extensively absorbed. **Distribution:** Atovaquone: V_d=8.8L/kg; plasma protein binding (≥99%). Proguanil: V_d=1617-2502L (adult and pediatric patients ≥15 yrs with body weight 31-110kg), V_d=462-966L (pediatric patients ≤15 yrs with body weight 11-56kg). Plasma protein binding (75%). **Metabolism:** Proguanil: CYP2C19. **Elimination:** Atovaquone: Feces (unchanged), urine (≤0.6%). $T_{1/2}$=2-3 days (adult). Proguanil: Via hepatic biotransformation and renal excretion; urine (40-60%); $T_{1/2}$=12-21 hrs (adult and pediatric patients).

MARCAINE RX
bupivacaine HCl (Hospira)

THERAPEUTIC CLASS: Local anesthetic

INDICATIONS: Production of local or regional anesthesia for surgery, dental or oral surgery procedures, diagnostic and therapeutic procedures, and for obstetrical procedures. Only 0.25% and 0.5% are indicated for obstetrical anesthesia.

DOSAGE: *Adults:* Individualize dose. Dosage varies depending on procedure, area to be anesthetized, vascularity of tissues, number of neural segments to be blocked, depth and duration of anesthesia, degree of muscle relaxation required, and patient tolerance and physical condition. Single Dose Max: 175mg. May repeat once every 3 hrs. Total Daily Dose Max: 400mg. Epidural Anesthesia: 0.5% or 0.75% in 3-5mL increments. In obstetrics, use only 0.25% or 0.5%. Use 3-5mL increments of 0.5% solution not to exceed 50-100mg at any dosing interval. Test dose using 0.5% with 1:200,000 epinephrine recommended prior to caudal and lumbar epidural blocks. Elderly/Debilitated/Cardiac or Liver Disease: Reduce dose.

Pediatrics: ≥12 yrs: Individualize dose. Dosage varies depending on procedure, area to be anesthetized, vascularity of tissues, number of neural segments to be blocked, depth and duration of anesthesia, degree of muscle relaxation required, and patient tolerance and physical condition. Single Dose Max: 175mg. May repeat once every 3 hrs. Total Daily Dose Max: 400mg. Epidural Anesthesia: 0.5% or 0.75% in 3-5mL increments. In obstetrics, use only 0.25% or 0.5%. Use 3-5mL increments of 0.5% solution not to exceed 50-100mg at any dosing interval. Test dose using 0.5% with 1:200,000 epinephrine recommended prior to caudal and lumbar epidural blocks.

HOW SUPPLIED: Inj: 0.25%, 0.5%, 0.75%

CONTRAINDICATIONS: Obstetrical paracervical block anesthesia.

WARNINGS/PRECAUTIONS: The 0.75% strength is not recommended for obstetrical anesthesia. Acidosis, cardiac arrest, death reported from delay in toxicity management. Local anesthetic solutions containing antimicrobial preservatives should not be used for epidural or caudal anesthesia. Not recommended for IV regional anesthesia. Monitor cardiovascular and respiratory vital signs and state of consciousness after each injection. Caution with hepatic disease and impaired cardiovascular function. Monitor circulation and respiration with injections into head and neck area. Respiratory arrest following local anesthetic injection during retrobulbar blocks has been reported.

ADVERSE REACTIONS: Restlessness, anxiety, dizziness, tinnitus, blurred vision, tremors, convulsions, nausea, vomiting, chills, hypotension, bradycardia, ventricular arrhythmias, urticaria, pruritus, erythema, edema.

INTERACTIONS: Avoid use with any other local anesthetics.

PREGNANCY: Category C, not for use in nursing.

MECHANISM OF ACTION: Aminoacyl local anesthetic; blocks the generation and conduction of nerve impulses, presumably by increasing the threshold for electrical excitation in the nerve by slowing the propagation of nerve impulse and by reducing rate of rise of the action potential.

PHARMACOKINETICS: Distribution: Crosses placenta, founf in breast milk. Plasma protein binding (95%). **Excretion:** Urine 6% (unchanged).

MARCAINE WITH EPINEPHRINE   RX
bupivacaine HCl - epinephrine (Hospira)

THERAPEUTIC CLASS: Local anesthetic

INDICATIONS: Production of local or regional anesthesia for surgery, dental, or oral surgery procedures, diagnostic and therapeutic procedures, and for obstetrical procedures. Only 0.25% and 0.5% are indicated for obstetrical anesthesia.

DOSAGE: *Adults:* Individualize dose. Dosage varies depending on procedure, area to be anesthetized, vascularity of tissues, number of neural segments to be blocked, depth and duration of anesthesia, degree of muscle relaxation required, and patient tolerance and physical condition. Single Dose Max: 225mg. May repeat once every 3 hrs. Total Daily Dose Max: 400mg. Epidural Anesthesia: 0.5% or 0.75% in 3-5mL increments. In obstetrics, use only 0.25% or 0.5%. Use 3-5mL increments of 0.5% solution not to exceed 50-100mg at any dosing interval. Test dose using 0.5% with 1:200,000 epinephrine recommended prior to caudal and lumbar epidural blocks. Dentistry: 0.5% with epinephrine. Average Dose: 1.8mL (9mg) per inj site. May repeat after 2-10 min if necessary. Max: 90mg total dose for all sites. Elderly/Debilitated/Cardiac or Liver Disease: Reduce dose.

Pediatrics: ≥12 yrs: Individualize dose. Dosage varies depending on procedure, area to be anesthetized, vascularity of tissues, number of neural segments to be blocked, depth and duration of anesthesia, degree of muscle relaxation required, and patient tolerance and physical condition. Single Dose Max: 225mg. May repeat once every 3 hrs. Total Daily Dose Max: 400mg. Epidural Anesthesia: 0.5% or 0.75% in 3-5mL increments. In obstetrics, use only 0.25% or 0.5%. Use 3-5mL increments of 0.5% solution not to exceed 50-100mg at any dosing interval. Test dose using 0.5% with 1:200,000 epineph-

rine recommended prior to caudal and lumbar epidural blocks. Dentistry: 0.5% with epinephrine. Average Dose: 1.8mL (9mg) per inj site. May repeat after 2-10 min if
necessary. Max: 90mg total dose for all sites.

HOW SUPPLIED: Inj: (Bupivacaine-Epinephrine) 0.25%/1:200,000, 0.5%/1:200,000.

CONTRAINDICATIONS: Obstetrical paracervical block anesthesia.

WARNINGS/PRECAUTIONS: The 0.75% strength is not recommended for obstetrical anesthesia. Acidosis, cardiac arrest, death reported from delay in toxicity management.
Local anesthetic solutions containing antimicrobial preservatives should not be used for
epidural or caudal anesthesia. Not recommended for IV regional anesthesia.
Bupivacaine with epinephrine solutions contain sodium metabisulfite which may cause
allergic-type reactions in susceptible people. Monitor cardiovascular and respiratory
vital signs and state of consciousness after each injection. Caution when local anesthetic solutions containing a vasoconstrictor are used in areas of the body supplied by
end arteries or having otherwise compromised blood supply; ischemic injury or necrosis
may result with hypertensive vascular disease. Caution with hepatic disease and
impaired cardiovascular function. Monitor circulation and respiration with injections into
head and neck area. Respiratory arrest following local anesthetic injection during retrobulbar blocks has been reported.

ADVERSE REACTIONS: Restlessness, anxiety, dizziness, tinnitus, blurred vision, tremors, convulsions, nausea, vomiting, chills, hypotension, bradycardia, ventricular arrhythmias, urticaria, pruritus, erythema, edema.

INTERACTIONS: Avoid use with any other local anesthetics. Anesthetic solutions containing epinephrine or norepinephrine with MAOIs or TCAs may produce severe, prolonged
HTN; avoid concurrent use or monitor closely if concurrent use is necessary. Concurrent
administration of vasopressors and ergot-type oxytocic drugs may cause severe, persistent HTN or CVA. Phenothiazines and butyrophenones may reduce or reverse the pressor effect of epinephrine. Serious dose-related cardiac arrhythmias may occur with use
during or following administration of potent inhalation anesthetics.

PREGNANCY: Category C, not for use in nursing.

MECHANISM OF ACTION: Aminoacyl local anesthetic; blocks generation and conduction of nerve impulses, presumably by increasing threshold for electrical excitation in
the nerve by slowing propagation of nerve impulse and by reducing rate of rise of
action potential.

PHARMACOKINETICS: Distribution: Crosses placenta; found in breast milk. Plasma protein
binding (95%). **Excretion:** Urine 6% (unchanged).

MATULANE   RX
procarbazine HCl (Sigma-Tau)

> To be given only by or under supervision of experienced physician in use of potent
> antineoplastics. Proper monitoring with adequate clinical and laboratory facilities should be
> conducted.

THERAPEUTIC CLASS: Hydrazine derivative

INDICATIONS: In combination with other antineoplastics for the treatment of Stage III/IV
Hodgkin's disease. Used part of MOPP regimen.

DOSAGE: *Adults:* 2-4mg/kg/day as single or divided doses for first week then increase to
4-6mg/kg/day until maximum response or WBC <4000/mm³ or platelets <100,000/mm³.
Maint: 1-2mg/kg/day. In MOPP: 100mg/m² qd for 14 days. Adjust dose for combination
regimens.
Pediatrics: 50mg/m²/day for first week then increase to 100mg/m²/day until response is
obtained or leukopenia or thrombocytopenia occurs. Maint: 50mg/m²/day. Adjust
dose for combination regimens.

HOW SUPPLIED: Cap: 50mg

CONTRAINDICATIONS: Inadequate marrow reserve.

WARNINGS/PRECAUTIONS: Toxicity may occur in renal or hepatic impairment. Wait one
month or longer with prior use of bone marrow suppressing radiation or chemotherapy.
D/C if CNS symptoms (paresthesias, neuropathies, confusion), leukopenia, thrombocy-

topenia, hypersensitivity, stomatitis, diarrhea, hemorrhage or bleeding tendencies occur. Bone marrow depression often occurs 2-8 weeks after initiation. Monitor urinalysis, transaminases, LFTs weekly, hematologic status every 3-4 days.

ADVERSE REACTIONS: Leukopenia, anemia, thrombopenia, nausea, vomiting.

INTERACTIONS: Avoid sympathomimetics, TCAs, tyramine-containing drugs/foods, alcohol (may cause disulfiram-type reaction), tobacco. Caution with barbiturates, antihistamines, narcotics, hypotensives, phenothiazines.

PREGNANCY: Category D, not for use in nursing.

MECHANISM OF ACTION: Hydrazine derivative; inhibits protein, RNA, and DNA synthesis.

PHARMACOKINETICS: Absorption: Rapid and complete; T_{max}=60 min. **Metabolism:** Liver and kidney. **Elimination:** Urine (70%); $T_{1/2}$=10 min (IV).

MAXAIR
pirbuterol acetate (Graceway)

RX

OTHER BRAND NAME: Maxair Autohaler (Graceway)

THERAPEUTIC CLASS: Beta$_2$ -agonist

INDICATIONS: Prevention and reversal of bronchospasm in reversible bronchospasm (eg, asthma).

DOSAGE: *Adults:* 1-2 inh q4-6h. Max: 12 inh/day.
Pediatrics: ≥12 yrs: 1-2 inh q4-6h. Max: 12 inh/day.

HOW SUPPLIED: Autohaler: 0.2mg/inh (14g, 25.6g); MDI: 0.2mg/inh (14g)

WARNINGS/PRECAUTIONS: Caution with cardiovascular disorders, (eg, ischemic heart disease, HTN, arrhythmias), hyperthyroidism, diabetes, convulsive disorders. Fatalities reported with excessive use. Can produce paradoxical bronchospasm. Monitor BP.

ADVERSE REACTIONS: Nervousness, tremor, headache, dizziness, palpitations, tachycardia, cough, nausea.

INTERACTIONS: Avoid other aerosol β$_2$ agonists. Vascular effects may be potentiated by MAOIs, TCAs, and sympathomimetics. ECG changes and/or hypokalemia may occur with non-potassium sparing diuretics. Decreased effect with β-blockers.

PREGNANCY: Category C, caution in nursing.

MECHANISM OF ACTION: β$_2$-adrenergic bronchodilator; activates adenyl cyclase on airway smooth muscles and increases intracellular concentration of cyclic AMP. Increased cAMP levels are associated with relaxation of bronchial smooth muscle and inhibition of release of mediators of immediate hypersensitivity.

PHARMACOKINETICS: Elimination: Urine, $T_{1/2}$=2 hrs.

MAXIPIME
cefepime HCl (Elan)

RX

THERAPEUTIC CLASS: Cephalosporin (4th generation)

INDICATIONS: Treatment of uncomplicated/complicated urinary tract (UTI), uncomplicated skin and skin structure (SSSI), and complicated intra-abdominal infections, and pneumonia caused by susceptible strains of microorganisms. Emperic therapy for febrile neutropenia.

DOSAGE: *Adults:* Moderate-Severe Pneumonia: 1-2g IV q12h for 10 days. Febrile Neutropenia Emperic Therapy: 2g IV q8h for 7 days or until neutropenia resolved. Mild-Moderate UTI: 0.5-1g IM/IV q12h for 7-10 days. Severe UTI/Moderate-Severe SSSI: 2g IV q12h for 10 days. Complicated Intra-Abdominal Infections: 2g IV q12h for 7-10 days. Renal Impairment: Initial: Normal dose. Maint: CrCl >60mL/min: Normal dose. CrCl 30-60mL/min: 500mg-2g q24h or 2g q12h. CrCl 11-29mL/min: 500mg-2g q24h. CrCl <11mL/min: 250mg-1g q24h. CAPD: 500mg-2g q48h. Hemodialysis: 1g on Day 1, then 500mg q24h.
Pediatrics: 2 months-16 yrs: ≤40kg: UTI/SSSI/Pneumonia: 50mg/kg IV q12h. Febrile Neutropenia: 50mg/kg IV q8h. Max: Do not exceed adult dose.

HOW SUPPLIED: Inj: 500mg, 1g, 2g

WARNINGS/PRECAUTIONS: Caution with PCN sensitivity; cross hypersensitivity may occur. *Clostridium difficile*-associated diarrhea reported. Treatment may result in overgrowth of nonsusceptible organisms. Caution with renal impairment or history of GI disease especially colitis. Encephalopathy, myoclonus, seizures, and/or renal failure reported. D/C if seizure occurs. Associated with a fall in PT; monitor PT with renal or hepatic impairment, poor nutritional state, and protracted course of antimicrobials; give vitamin K as indicated. Associated with (+) direct Coombs' test.

ADVERSE REACTIONS: Local reactions (eg, phlebitis) rash, diarrhea.

INTERACTIONS: Increased risk of nephrotoxicity and ototoxicity with aminoglycosides. Risk of nephrotoxicity with potent diuretics (eg, furosemide).

PREGNANCY: Category B, caution in nursing.

MECHANISM OF ACTION: Cephalosporin; bactericidal due to inhibition of cell-wall synthesis.

PHARMACOKINETICS: Absorption: IV administration of variable doses resulted in different parameters. **Distribution:** V_d=18L; plasma protein binding (20%). **Metabolism:** Metabolized to N-methylpyrrolidine, which is rapidly converted to N-oxide. **Elimination:** Urine; $T_{1/2}$=2hrs.

MEBARAL   CIV
mephobarbital (Ovation)

THERAPEUTIC CLASS: Barbiturate

INDICATIONS: As a sedative for relief of anxiety, tension, and apprehension. Treatment of grand mal and petit mal epilepsy.

DOSAGE: *Adults:* Epilepsy: 400-600mg/day. Start with small dose, gradually increase over 4-5 days until optimum dose. Elderly/Debilitated/Renal or Hepatic Dysfunction: Reduce dose. Concomitant Phenobarbital: Give 50% of each drug. Concomitant Phenytoin: Reduce phenytoin dose. Sedation: 32-100mg tid-qid. Optimum Dose: 50mg tid-qid.
Pediatrics: Epilepsy: >5 yrs: 32-64mg tid-qid. <5 yrs: 16-32mg tid-qid. Start with small dose, gradually increase over 4-5 days until optimum dose. Sedation: 16-32mg tid-qid.

HOW SUPPLIED: Tab: 32mg*, 50mg*, 100mg *scored

CONTRAINDICATIONS: Manifest or latent porphyria.

WARNINGS/PRECAUTIONS: May be habit forming; tolerance and dependence may occur with continued use. Avoid abrupt withdrawal. Caution in acute/chronic pain; paradoxical excitement may occur or symptoms masked. Can cause fetal damage. May cause marked excitement, depression, and confusion in elderly or debilitated. Reduce initial dose with hepatic damage. Careful adjustment in impaired renal, cardiac, or respiratory function, myasthenia gravis, and myxedema. May increase vitamin D requirements. Caution with depression, suicidal tendencies, and history of drug abuse.

ADVERSE REACTIONS: Somnolence, agitation, confusion, hyperkinesia, ataxia, CNS depression, hypoventilation, apnea, bradycardia, hypotension, syncope, nausea, vomiting, headache.

INTERACTIONS: MAOIs may prolong effects. Additive CNS depression with alcohol and other CNS depressants. Decreases effects of oral anticoagulants, oral contraceptives. Increases corticosteroid metabolism. Interferes with griseofulvin absorption. Decreases half-life of doxycycline. May alter phenytoin metabolism. Sodium valproate and valproic acid decrease metabolism.

PREGNANCY: Category D, caution with nursing.

MECHANISM OF ACTION: Barbiturate; depresses the sensory cortex, decreases motor activity, alters cerebellar function, and produces drowsiness, sedation, and hypnosis. Produces significant anticonvulsant activity.

PHARMACOKINETICS: Absorption: Rapid. **Distribution:** Crosses placenta, excreted in breast milk. **Metabolism:** Hepatic via N-demethylation. Phenobarbital (major metabolite). **Elimination:** Urine.

MEBENDAZOLE RX

mebendazole (Various)

THERAPEUTIC CLASS: Broad-spectrum anthelmintic

INDICATIONS: Treatment of Enterobiasis (pinworm), Trichuriasis (whipworm), Ascariasis (common roundworm), *Ancylostoma duodenale* (common hookworm), *Necator americanus* (American hookworm).

DOSAGE: *Adults:* Pinworm: 100mg single dose. Other Parasites: 100mg bid for 3 days. May repeat in 3 weeks if needed. Chew, swallow, crush or mix tab with food. *Pediatrics:* ≥2 yrs: Pinworm: 100mg single dose. Other Parasites: 100mg bid for 3 days. May repeat in 3 weeks if needed. Chew, swallow, crush or mix tab with food.

HOW SUPPLIED: Tab, Chewable: 100mg

WARNINGS/PRECAUTIONS: Neutropenia, agranulocytosis reported with prolonged use. Periodically assess organ system functions with prolonged use. Not effective for hydatid disease.

ADVERSE REACTIONS: Abdominal pain, diarrhea.

INTERACTIONS: Cimetidine may increase plasma levels.

PREGNANCY: Category C, caution in nursing.

MECHANISM OF ACTION: Broad-spectrum anthelmintic; inhibits formation of worms' microtubules and causes worms' glucose depletion.

PHARMACOKINETICS: Metabolism: 2-amine (primary metabolite). **Elimination:** Urine (approximately 2%), feces (unchanged drug or primary metabolite).

MECLOFENAMATE RX

meclofenamate sodium (Various)

THERAPEUTIC CLASS: NSAID

INDICATIONS: Relief of mild to moderate pain, primary dysmenorrhea, and idiopathic heavy menstrual blood loss. Symptomatic treatment of acute and chronic rheumatoid arthritis (RA) and osteoarthritis (OA).

DOSAGE: *Adults:* Mild to Moderate Pain: 50mg q4-6h. Max: 400mg/day. Excessive Menstrual Blood Loss/Primary Dysmenorrhea: 100mg tid for up to 6 days starting at onset of menstrual flow. RA/OA: 200-400mg/day in 3-4 divided doses. Max: 400mg/day. *Pediatrics:* ≥14 yrs: Mild to Moderate Pain: 50mg q4-6h. Max: 400mg/day. Excessive Menstrual Blood Loss/Primary Dysmenorrhea: 100mg tid for up to 6 days starting at onset of menstrual flow. RA/OA: 200-400mg/day in 3-4 divided doses. Max: 400mg/day.

HOW SUPPLIED: Cap: 50mg, 100mg

CONTRAINDICATIONS: ASA or other NSAID allergy that precipitates bronchospasm, allergic rhinitis or urticaria.

WARNINGS/PRECAUTIONS: Risk of GI ulcerations, bleeding, and perforation. Borderline LFT elevations may occur. Renal and hepatic toxicity. Extreme caution in the elderly. D/C if visual symptoms occur.

ADVERSE REACTIONS: Diarrhea, nausea, vomiting, abdominal pain, edema, urticaria, pruritus, headache, dizziness, tinnitus, pyrosis, flatulence, anorexia, constipation, peptic ulcer.

INTERACTIONS: Enhanced effects of warfarin. ASA may lower levels.

PREGNANCY: Safety in pregnancy is not known. Not for use in nursing.

MECHANISM OF ACTION: NSAID; not established; suspected to inhibit prostaglandin synthesis and compete for binding at prostaglandin receptor site (animal studies); inhibits human leukocyte 5-lipoxygenase activity (in vitro).

PHARMACOKINETICS: Absorption: Rapid; C_{max}=4.8mcg/mL; T_{max}=0.9 hrs. Metabolite: C_{max}=1mcg/mL; T_{max}=2.4 hrs. **Distribution:** V_d=23.3L; plasma protein binding (>99%). Found in breast milk. **Metabolism:** 3-Hydroxymethyl metabolite (major metabolite). **Elimination:** Urine, feces; $T_{1/2}$=1.3 hrs. Metabolite: Urine (0.5%), feces; $T_{1/2}$=15.3 hrs.

MEDROL   RX
methylprednisolone (Pharmacia & Upjohn)

OTHER BRAND NAME: Medrol Dose Pack (Pharmacia & Upjohn)

THERAPEUTIC CLASS: Glucocorticoid

INDICATIONS: Steroid-responsive disorders.

DOSAGE: *Adults:* Initial: 4-48mg/day depending on disease and response. Maint: Decrease dose by small amounts to lowest effective dose. MS: Initial: 160mg/day for 1 week. Maint: 64mg every other day for 1 month. Alternate Day Therapy: Twice the usual dose every other day for long-term therapy.
Pediatrics: Initial: 4-48mg/day depending on disease and response. Maint: Decrease dose by small amounts to lowest effective dose. MS: Initial: 160mg/day for 1 week. Maint: 64mg every other day for 1 month. Alternate Day Therapy: Twice the usual dose every other day for long-term therapy.

HOW SUPPLIED: Tab: 2mg*, 4mg*, 8mg*, 16mg*, 32mg*; (Dose-Pak) 4mg* (21⁵) *scored

CONTRAINDICATIONS: Systemic fungal infections.

WARNINGS/PRECAUTIONS: May need to increase dose before, during, and after stressful situations. May mask signs of infection or or cause new infections. Prolonged use may produce glaucoma, optic nerve damage, secondary ocular infections. Increases BP, salt/water retention, potassium excretion. More severe/fatal course of infections reported with chickenpox, measles. Caution with Strongyloides, latent TB, hypothyroidism, cirrhosis, ocular herpes simplex, HTN, diverticulitis, fresh intestinal anastomoses, ulcerative colitis, osteoporosis, myasthenia gravis, renal insufficiency, peptic ulcer disease. Kaposi's sarcoma reported. Growth and development of children on prolonged therapy should be monitored. Monitor for psychic disturbances. Avoid abrupt withdrawal. The 24mg tabs contain tartrazine; caution with tartrazine sensitivity.

ADVERSE REACTIONS: Fluid and electrolyte disturbances, HTN, osteoporosis, muscle weakness, cushingoid state, menstrual irregularities, nervousness, insomnia, impaired wound healing, DM, ulcerative esophagitis, excessive sweating, increases intracranial pressure, carbohydrate intolerance, glaucoma, cataracts, weight gain, nausea, malaise.

INTERACTIONS: Reduced efficacy with hepatic enzyme inducers (eg, phenobarbital, phenytoin, and rifampin). Increases clearance of chronic high dose ASA. Caution with ASA in hypoprothrombinemia. Effects on oral anticoagulants are variable; monitor PT. Increased insulin and oral hypoglycemic requirements in DM. Avoid live vaccines with immunosuppressive doses. Possible decreased vaccine response with killed or inactivated vaccines with immunosuppressive doses. Mutual inhibition of metabolism with cyclosporine; convulsions reported. Potentiated by ketoconazole and troleandomycin.

PREGNANCY: Safety in pregnancy and nursing not known.

MECHANISM OF ACTION: Anti-inflammatory glucocorticoid; causes profound and varied metabolic effects and modifies the body's immune responses to diverse stimuli.

PHARMACOKINETICS: Absorption: Readily absorbed from GI tract.

MENACTRA   RX
meningococcal polysaccharide diptheria toxoid conjugate vaccine (Sanofi Pasteur)

THERAPEUTIC CLASS: Vaccine

INDICATIONS: Active immunization of adolescents and adults 2-55 yrs of age for the prevention of invasive meningococcal disease caused by *N.meningitidis* serogroups A, C, Y and W-135. Not indicated for prevention of meningitis caused by other microorganisms; prevention of invasive meningococcal disease caused by *N.meningitidis* serogroups B; treatment of meningococcal infections; or immunization against diphtheria.

DOSAGE: *Adults:* ≤55 yo: 0.5 mL IM into deltoid region.
Pediatrics: ≥2 yo: 0.5mL IM into deltoid region.

HOW SUPPLIED: Inj: 0.5mL

CONTRAINDICATIONS: Life-threatening reaction after previous administration of vaccine with similar contents. Known hypersensitivity to dry natural rubber latex.

WARNINGS/PRECAUTIONS: Guillain-Barre syndrome (GBS) has been reported. Avoid with bleeding disorders (eg. hemophilia, thrombocytopenia, anticoagulant therapy). Do not administer IV, SC, or intradermally. Have epinephrine injection (1:1000) available, in case of anaphylatic reaction.

ADVERSE REACTIONS: Redness, swelling, induration, pain, headache, fatigue, malaise, arthralgia, anorexia, chills, fever.

INTERACTIONS: Caution with anticoagulants. Immunosuppressive therapies may reduce immune response to vaccines.

PREGNANCY: Category C, caution in nursing.

MECHANISM OF ACTION: Stimulates immune system to produce bactericidal anticapsular meningococcal antibodies (specific to capsular polysaccharides of serogroups A, C, Y and W-135) that may protect against invasive meningococcal disease.

Mentax
butenafine HCl (Mylan Bertek)

RX

THERAPEUTIC CLASS: Benzylamine antifungal

INDICATIONS: Interdigital tinea pedis, tinea corporis, tinea cruris, and tinea versicolor.

DOSAGE: *Adults:* T.pedis: Apply bid for 7 days or qd for 4 weeks. T.corporis/T.cruris/T.versicolor: Apply qd for 2 weeks.
Pediatrics: ≥12 yrs: T.pedis: Apply bid for 7 days or qd for 4 weeks. T.corporis/T.cruris/T.versicolor: Apply qd for 2 weeks.

HOW SUPPLIED: Cre: 1% (15g, 30g)

WARNINGS/PRECAUTIONS: Avoid eyes, nose, mouth, and other mucous membranes. D/C if irritation or sensitivity develops. Confirm diagnosis. Caution if sensitive to other allylamine antifungals.

ADVERSE REACTIONS: Burning, stinging, itching, contact dermatitis, irritation, erythema, worsening of condition.

PREGNANCY: Category B, caution in nursing.

MECHANISM OF ACTION: Benzylamine antifungal; inhibits epoxidation of squalene, thus blocking the biosynthesis of ergosterol, which is an essential component of fungal cell membranes.

PHARMACOKINETICS: Absorption: Topical administration of variable doses result in different parameters.

Meprobamate
meprobamate (Various)

CIV

THERAPEUTIC CLASS: Carbamate derivative

INDICATIONS: Management of anxiety disorders or short-term relief of symptoms of anxiety.

DOSAGE: *Adults:* Usual: 1200-1600mg/day given tid-qid. Max: 2400mg/day. Elderly: >65 yrs: Start at low end of dosing range.
Pediatrics: 6-12 yrs: 200-600mg/day given bid-tid.

HOW SUPPLIED: Tab: 200mg, 400mg

CONTRAINDICATIONS: Porphyria, allergic or idiosyncratic reactions to carisoprodol, mebutamate, tybamate, carbromal.

WARNINGS/PRECAUTIONS: Physical and psychological dependence reported. Avoid abrupt withdrawal after prolonged or excessive use. Increased risk of congenital malformations with use during 1st trimester of pregnancy. Caution with liver or renal dysfunction, and in elderly. May precipitate seizures in epileptic patients. Prescribe small quantities in suicidal patients.

ADVERSE REACTIONS: Drowsiness, ataxia, slurred speech, vertigo, weakness, nausea, vomiting, diarrhea, tachycardia, transient ECG changes, rash, leukopenia, petechiae.

INTERACTIONS: Administration with other CNS depressants, alcohol, psychotropics have additive effects.

PREGNANCY: Safety in pregnancy and nursing not known.

MECHANISM OF ACTION: Anxiolytic agent; acts on the thalamus and limbic system.

PHARMACOKINETICS: Distribution: Passes placental barrier; found in umbilical cord blood and breast milk. **Metabolism:** Liver. **Elimination:** Renal excretion.

MEPRON   RX
atovaquone (GlaxoSmithKline)

THERAPEUTIC CLASS: Napthoquinone antiprotozoal

INDICATIONS: Prevention and treatment of mild to moderate *Pneumocystis carinii* pneumonia (PCP) in those intolerant to trimethoprim-sulfamethoxazole.

DOSAGE: *Adults:* Take with food. Prevention: 1500mg qd. Treatment: 750mg bid for 21 days.
Pediatrics: 13-16 yrs: Take with food. Prevention: 1500mg qd. Treatment: 750mg bid for 21 days.

HOW SUPPLIED: Sus: 750mg/5mL (5mL, 42^s; 210mL)

WARNINGS/PRECAUTIONS: Monitor with severe hepatic impairment. Absorption significantly increased with food.

ADVERSE REACTIONS: Rash, nausea, GI effects, cough increased, rhinitis, asthenia, infection, dyspnea, insomnia, asthenia, pruritus.

INTERACTIONS: Significantly decreased plasma levels with rifampin. Caution with other highly protein-bound drugs.

PREGNANCY: Category C, caution in nursing.

MECHANISM OF ACTION: Naphthoquinone antiprotozoal; site of action appears to be cytochrome bc_1 complex which is linked to mitochondrial electron transport. Inhibition of electron transport by atovaquone will result in indirect inhibition of these enzymes, resulting in nucleic acid and ATP synthesis inhibition.

PHARMACOKINETICS: Absorption: Absolute bioavailability (47%); PO administration of variable doses resulted in different parameters. **Distribution:** V_d =0.6L/kg; plasma protein binding (99.9%). **Elimination:** Feces (≥94%, unchanged), urine (≤0.6%).

MERIDIA   CIV
sibutramine HCl monohydrate (Abbott)

THERAPEUTIC CLASS: Dopamine/norepinephrine/serotonin reuptake inhibitor

INDICATIONS: To induce and maintain weight loss in obese patients with an initial BMI ≥30kg/m^2 or ≥27kg/m^2 with risk factors (eg, HTN, diabetes, dyslipidemia).

DOSAGE: *Adults:* Initial: 10mg qd. Titrate: May increase after 4 weeks to 15mg qd. Max: 15mg/day. Use 5mg/day in patients unable to tolerate 10mg/day. May continue for up to 2 yrs.
Pediatrics: ≥16 yrs: Initial: 10mg qd. Titrate: May increase after 4 weeks to 15mg qd. Use 5mg/day in patients unable to tolerate 10mg/day. Max: 15mg/day. May continue for up to 2 yrs.

HOW SUPPLIED: Cap: 5mg, 10mg, 15mg

CONTRAINDICATIONS: Concomitant MAOIs or centrally acting appetite suppressants, eating disorders (eg, anorexia/bulimia nervosa).

WARNINGS/PRECAUTIONS: May increase BP and/or pulse. Avoid with uncontrolled or poorly controlled HTN, CAD, CHF, arrhythmias, stroke, severe hepatic or renal dysfunction. Monitor BP and pulse before therapy and regularly thereafter. Caution with narrow angle glaucoma, mild to moderate renal impairment, seizures and if predisposed to bleeding. Exclude organic causes of obesity. Gallstones precipitated with weight loss.

ADVERSE REACTIONS: Anorexia, constipation, increased appetite, nausea, dyspepsia, dry mouth, insomnia, dizziness, nervousness, HTN, tachycardia, dysmenorrhea, headache.

INTERACTIONS: Avoid excess alcohol, CNS-active drugs, other serotonergic agents (eg, SSRIs, migraine therapy agents, certain opioids), within 14 days of MAOI use. Caution with drugs affecting hemostasis or platelet function; ephedrine, pseudoephedrine; and other agents that increase BP, heart rate. Possible decreased metabolism with ketoconazole and erythromycin.

PREGNANCY: Category C, not for use in nursing.

MECHANISM OF ACTION: Inhibits norepinephrine, serotonin, and dopamine reuptake.

PHARMACOKINETICS: Absorption: Rapid; T_{max}=1.2 hrs; (15mg Dose, M_1, M_2) C_{max}=4ng/mL, 6.4ng/mL; T_{max}=3.6 hrs, 3.5 hrs; AUC=25.5ng•h/mL, 92.1ng•h/mL. **Distribution:** Plasma protein binding (97%); M_1, M_2 (94%). **Metabolism:** Liver via CYP3A4; M_1 and M_2 (active metabolites). **Elimination:** Urine (77%), feces; $T_{1/2}$=1.1 hrs, 14 hrs (M_1), 16 hrs (M_2).

MERREM
meropenem (AstraZeneca)

RX

THERAPEUTIC CLASS: Carbapenem

INDICATIONS: Treatment of intra-abdominal infections, bacterial meningitis, and complicated skin and skin structure infections (cSSSI) caused by susceptible strains of microorganisms.

DOSAGE: *Adults;* IV: Intra-Abdominal: 1g q8h. CrCl 26-50mL/min: 1g q12h. CrCl 10-25mL/min: 500mg q12h. CrCl <10mL/min: 500mg q24h. cSSSI: 500mg q8h. CrCl 26-50mL/min: 500mg q12h. CrCl 10-25mL/min: 250mg q12h. CrCl <10mL/min: 250mg q24h.
Pediatrics: IV: ≥3 months: >50kg: Intra-Abdominal: 1g q8h. Meningitis: 2g q8h. cSSSI: 500mg q8h. ≤50kg: Intra-Abdominal: 20mg/kg q8h. Max: 1g q8h. Meningitis: 40mg/kg q8h. Max: 2g q8h. cSSSI: 10mg/kg q8h. Max: 500mg q8h.

HOW SUPPLIED: Inj: 500mg, 1g

CONTRAINDICATIONS: Hypersensitivity to β-lactams.

WARNINGS/PRECAUTIONS: Severe and fatal hypersensitivity reported; increased risk with allergens and/or PCN sensitivity. *Clostridium difficile*-associated diarrhea reported. Seizures and other CNS effects reported particularly with pre-existing CNS disorders, bacterial meningitis, and renal dysfunction. Thrombocytopenia reported with severe renal impairment. Prolonged use may result in superinfection. Use as monotherapy for meningitis caused by penicillin nonsusceptible strains of *Streptococcus pneumoniae* has not been established.

ADVERSE REACTIONS: Headache, rash, local reactions, diarrhea, NV, constipation.

INTERACTIONS: Probenecid inhibits renal excretion; avoid concomitant use. May reduce valproic acid levels.

PREGNANCY: Category B, caution in nursing.

MECHANISM OF ACTION: Broad-spectrum carbapenem; penetrates bacterial cells and interferes with synthesis of vital cell wall components, resulting in cell death.

PHARMACOKINETICS: Absorption: 30 min infusion: C_{max}=23µg/mL (500mg); 49µg/mL (1g). 5-min bolus injection: C_{max}=45µg/mL (500mg); 112µg/mL (1g). **Distribution:** Plasma protein binding (2%). **Elimination:** Urine (70%); $T_{1/2}$=1 hr, 1.5 hrs (3mo-2yrs).

MERUVAX II
rubella vaccine live (Merck)

RX

THERAPEUTIC CLASS: Vaccine

INDICATIONS: Vaccination against rubella.

DOSAGE: *Adults:* 0.5mL SQ in outer aspect of upper arm.
Pediatrics: Primary Vaccination at 12-15 months: 0.5mL SQ in outer aspect of upper arm. Revaccinate with MMR II prior to elementary school entry.

HOW SUPPLIED: Inj: 1000 $TCID_{50}$

CONTRAINDICATIONS: Avoid pregnancy for 3 months after vaccine, anaphylactic reaction to neomycin, febrile/active respiratory illness, immunosuppressive therapy (except corticosteroids as replacement therapy), blood dyscrasias, leukemia, lymphoma, malignant neoplasms affecting bone marrow or lymphatic system, immunodeficiency states.

WARNINGS/PRECAUTIONS: May worsen thrombocytopenia. Defer vaccination for at least 3 months after blood or plasma transfusions, immune globulin (except susceptible postpartum patients with follow-up HI titer after 6-8 weeks). Do not vaccinate with active untreated TB. Temperature elevation may occur after vaccination. Contains albumin, remote risk of viral infection transmission. Have epinephrine (1:1000) available.

ADVERSE REACTIONS: Fever, syncope, headache, dizziness, malaise, irritability, thrombocytopenia, arthritis, vasculitis, diarrhea, local reactions.

INTERACTIONS: Do not give with immune globulin. May depress TB skin sensitivity, administer test either simultaneously or before. Do not give <1 month before or after other live viral vaccines. Do not give simultaneously with DTP or oral poliovirus vaccine.

PREGNANCY: Category C, contraindicated in pregnancy and caution in nursing.

MECHANISM OF ACTION: Induces a broader profile of circulating antibodies, including anti-theta and anti-iota antibodies against RA 27/3 rubella virus.

METADATE CD   `CII`
methylphenidate HCl (UCB)

THERAPEUTIC CLASS: Sympathomimetic amine

INDICATIONS: Treatment of attention deficit hyperactivity disorder (ADHD).

DOSAGE: *Pediatrics:* ≥6 yrs: Usual: 20mg qam before breakfast. Titrate: Increase weekly by 20mg depending on tolerability/efficacy. Max: 60mg/day. Reduce dose or discontinue if paradoxical aggravation of symptoms occur. D/C if no improvement after appropriate dose adjustments over 1 month. Swallow whole with liquids or open and sprinkle on 1 tbs applesauce followed by water. Do not crush, chew, or divide.

HOW SUPPLIED: Cap, Extended-Release: 10mg, 20mg, 30mg, 40mg, 50mg, 60mg

CONTRAINDICATIONS: Marked anxiety, tension, and agitation; glaucoma; motor tics, family history or diagnosis of Tourette's syndrome, severe HTN, angina pectoris, cardiac arrhythmias, heart failure, recent MI, hyperthyroidism or thyrotoxicosis; during or within 14 days of MAOI use.

WARNINGS/PRECAUTIONS: Monitor growth in children. Not for severe depression or fatigue. May exacerbate symptoms of behavior disturbance and thought disorder in psychotic patients. Caution when using stimulants to treat patients with comorbid bipolar disorder because of concern for possible induction of mixed/manic episode in such patients. Stimulants at usual doses can cause treatment emergent psychotic or manic symptoms (eg, hallucinations, delusional thinking, mania) in children and adolescents without prior history of psychotic illness. Aggressive behavior or hostility reported in clinical trials and postmarketing experience of some medications indicated for the treatment of ADHD. May lower seizure threshold, especially in known EEG abnormalities. Caution with HTN, conditions affected by BP or HR elevation, history of drug abuse or alcoholism. Monitor during withdrawal from abusive use. Visual disturbances may occur (rare). Monitor CBC, differential, and platelets with prolonged use. Avoid with serious structural cardiac abnormalities, cardiomyopathy, serious heart rhythm abnormalities, CAD, or other serious cardiac problems.

ADVERSE REACTIONS: Headache, abdominal pain, anorexia, insomnia.

INTERACTIONS: See Contraindications. Potentiates anticoagulants, anticonvulsants (eg, phenobarbital, phenytoin, primidone), TCAs, and SSRIs. Caution with α_2-agonist (eg, clonidine) and pressor agents.

PREGNANCY: Category C, caution in nursing.

MECHANISM OF ACTION: CNS stimulant; not established, thought to block reuptake of norepinephrine and dopamine into presynaptic neuron and increase release of these monoamines into extraneuronal space.

PHARMACOKINETICS: Absorption: (PO) Readily absorbed. Administration of variable doses resulted in different parameters. **Metabolism:** Via de-esterification. Metabolite: Alpha-phenyl-piperidine acetic acid (ritalinic acid). **Elimination:** $T_{1/2}$=6.8 hrs.

Metadate ER
methylphenidate HCl (UCB)

THERAPEUTIC CLASS: Sympathomimetic amine

INDICATIONS: Treatment of attention deficit disorder and narcolepsy.

DOSAGE: *Adults:* (Immediate-Release Methylphenidate) 10-60mg/day given bid-tid 30-45 min ac. Take last dose before 6 pm if insomnia occurs. (Tab, Extended-Release) May use in place of immediate release tabs when the 8 hr dose corresponds to the titrated 8 hr immediate release dose. Swallow whole; do not chew or crush.
Pediatrics: ≥6 yrs: (Immediate-Release Methylphenidate) Initial: 5mg bid before breakfast and lunch. Titrate: Increase gradually by 5-10mg weekly. Max: 60mg/day. (Tab, Extended-Release) May use in place of immediate release tabs when the 8 hr dose corresponds to the titrated 8hr immediate release dose. Swallow whole; do not chew or crush. Reduce dose or discontinue if paradoxical aggravation of symptoms occur. Discontinue if no improvement after appropriate dose adjustment over 1 month.

HOW SUPPLIED: Tab, Extended-Release: 10mg, 20mg

CONTRAINDICATIONS: Marked anxiety, tension, and agitation; glaucoma; motor tics or family history or diagnosis of Tourette's syndrome; during or within 14 days of MAOI use.

WARNINGS/PRECAUTIONS: Caution with comorbid bipolar disorder. Monitor growth in children. Not for severe depression or fatigue. May exacerbate symptoms of behavior disturbance and thought disorder in psychotic children. Treatment emergent psychotic/manic symptoms in children and adolescents may occur. Aggressive behavior or hostility observed. May lower seizure threshold, especially in known EEG abnormalities. Caution with HTN, emotionally-unstable patients. Monitor during withdrawal. Visual disturbances may occur (rare). Monitor CBC, differential, and platelets with prolonged use. Periodically d/c to assess condition.

ADVERSE REACTIONS: Nervousness, insomnia, hypersensitivity reactions, anorexia, nausea, dizziness, palpitations, headache, dyskinesia, drowsiness, BP and pulse changes, tachycardia, angina, arrhythmia, abdominal pain.

INTERACTIONS: See Contraindications. May decrease hypotensive effect of guanethidine. Caution with pressor agents. Potentiates anticoagulants, anticonvulsants (eg, phenobarbital, phenytoin, primidone), phenylbutazone, TCAs (eg, imipramine, clomipramine, desipramine).

PREGNANCY: Safety in pregnancy and nursing not known.

MECHANISM OF ACTION: Not established, suspected to have sympathomimetic activity in the brain stem arousal system and cortex.

PHARMACOKINETICS: Absorption: Slowly absorbed. T_{max}=1.3-8.2 hrs (sustained-release tab), 0.3-4.4 hrs (immediate release tab).

Metaproterenol
metaproterenol sulfate (Various)

RX

OTHER BRAND NAME: Alupent (Boehringer Ingelheim)

THERAPEUTIC CLASS: Beta$_2$ -agonist

INDICATIONS: For bronchial asthma and reversible bronchospasm.

DOSAGE: *Adults:* (MDI) 2-3 inh q3-4h. Max: 12 inh/day. (Sol 0.4%, 0.6%) 2.5mL by IPPB tid-qid, up to q4h. (Syr, Tab) 20mg tid-qid.
Pediatrics: (MDI) ≥12 yrs: 2-3 inh q3-4h. Max: 12 inh/day. (Sol 0.4%, 0.6%) ≥12 yrs: 2.5mL by IPPB tid-qid, up to q4h. (Syr, Tab) >9 yrs or >60 lbs: 20mg tid-qid. 6-9 yrs or <60 lbs: 10mg tid-qid.

HOW SUPPLIED: MDI: 0.65mg/inh (14g); Sol, Inhalation: 0.4% (2.5mL), 0.6% (2.5mL); Syrup: 10mg/5mL (480mL); Tab: 10mg, 20mg

CONTRAINDICATIONS: Cardiac arrhythmias associated with tachycardia.

WARNINGS/PRECAUTIONS: Caution with cardiovascular disorders, (eg, ischemic heart disease, HTN, arrhythmias), hyperthyroidism, diabetes, convulsive disorders. Fatalities reported with excessive use. Can produce paradoxical bronchospasm. Monitor BP. Nebulized solution single dose may not abort an asthma attack.

ADVERSE REACTIONS: Headache, dizziness, HTN, GI distress, throat irritation, cough, asthma exacerbation, nervousness, tremor, nausea, vomiting.

INTERACTIONS: Avoid other aerosol β_2 agonists. Vascular effects may be potentiated by MAOIs, TCAs, and sympathomimetics.

PREGNANCY: Category C, caution in nursing.

MECHANISM OF ACTION: β-adrenergic stimulator (bronchodilator); activates adenyl cylase, the enzyme that catalyzes the formation of cAMP from ATP. Increased cAMP levels are associated with relaxation of bronchial smooth muscle and inhibition of release of mediators of immediate hypersensitivity.

PHARMACOKINETICS: Absorption: 40% absorbed after oral dosing.

METHOTREXATE
methotrexate (Various)

RX

> Should only be used by physicians whose knowledge and experience includes the use of anti-metabolite therapy. Only for life-threatening neoplastic diseases, or with severe, recalcitrant, disabling disease not adequately responsive to other forms of therapy. Fetal death/congenital anomalies reported. Elimination reduced with impaired renal function, ascites, or pleural effusions; monitor carefully. Severe, sometimes fatal, bone marrow suppression and GI toxicity reported with concomitant NSAIDs. May cause hepatotoxicity, fibrosis, and cirrhosis (usually after prolonged use). Lung disease, malignant melanomas, and potentially fatal opportunistic infections may occur. Interrupt therapy if diarrhea or ulcerative colitis occur. May induce tumor lysis syndrome. Severe, occasionally fatal, skin reactions reported. Concomitant radiotherapy may increase risk of soft tissue necrosis and osteonecrosis.

OTHER BRAND NAME: Rheumatrex (Stada)

THERAPEUTIC CLASS: Dihydrofolic acid reductase inhibitor

INDICATIONS: (Inj/PO) Treatment of neoplastic diseases (eg, acute lymphocytic leukemia, gestational choriocarcinoma, chorioadenoma destruens, hydatidiform mole, breast cancer, epidermoid cancer of the head and neck, advanced mycosis fungoides, lung cancer, advanced stage non-Hodgkin's lymphomas). Prophylaxis and treatment of meningeal leukemia, and maintenance with other chemotherapeutics. For prolonging relapse-free survival in non-metastatic osteosarcoma followed by leucovorin. Symptomatic control of severe, recalcitrant, disabling psoriasis. (PO) Management of rheumatoid arthritis (RA) or polyarticular-course juvenile rheumatoid arthritis (JRA) unresponsive to other therapies.

DOSAGE: *Adults:* Choriocarcinoma/Trophoblastic Disease: 15-30mg qd PO/IM for 5 days. May repeat 3-5 times as required with rest period of ≥1 week. Leukemia: Induction: 3.3mg/m^2 with prednisone 60mg/m^2 qd. Remission Maintenance: 15mg/m^2 PO/IM twice weekly or 2.5mg/kg IV every 14 days. Burkitt's Tumor: Stages I-II: 10-25mg/day PO for 4-8 days. Administer several courses with rest periods of 7-10 days in between. Lymphosarcoma: Stage III: 0.625-2.5mg/kg/day with other antitumor agents. Mycosis Fungoides: 5-50mg once weekly. If poor response, give 15-37.5mg twice weekly. Adjust dose based on response and hematologic monitoring. Osteosarcoma: Initial: 12g/m^2 IV, increase to 15g/m^2 if peak serum levels of 1000 micromolar not reached at end of infusion. Meningeal Leukemia: Dilute preservative free MTX to 1mg/mL. Give 12mg intrathecally at 2-5 day intervals. Psoriasis: Initial: 10-25mg PO/IM/IV weekly until response or use divided oral dose schedule, 2.5mg at 12 hr intervals for 3 doses. Titrate: Increase gradually until optimal response. Maint: Reduce to lowest effective dose. Max: 30mg/week. Rheumatoid Arthritis: Initial: 7.5mg PO once weekly, or 2.5mg q12h for 3 doses given as a course once weekly. Titrate: Gradual increase. Max: 20mg weekly. After response, reduce dose to lowest effective amount of drug.
Pediatrics: Meningeal Leukemia: Dilute preservative free MTX to 1mg/mL. <1 yr: 6mg. 1 yr: 8mg. 2 yrs: 10mg. ≥3yrs: 12mg. Give intrathecally at 2-5 day intervals. JRA: 2-16 yrs: Initial: 10mg/m^2 once weekly. Adjust dose gradually to achieve optimal response.

HOW SUPPLIED: Inj: (Generic) (Methotrexate Sodium) 25mg/mL, 1g; Tab: (Generic) (Methotrexate) 2.5mg*; Tab: (Rheumatrex) (Methotrexate) 2.5mg* (Dose Pack 15mg, 4 x 6 tabs; 12.5mg, 4 x 5 tabs; 10mg, 4 x 4 tabs; 7.5mg, 4 x 3 tabs; 5mg, 4 x 2 tabs) *scored

CONTRAINDICATIONS: Pregnant women with psoriasis or RA (should be used in treatment of pregnant women with neoplastic diseases only when potential benefit outweighs risk), nursing mothers. Psoriasis or RA patients with alcoholism, alcoholic liver disease, chronic liver disease, immunodeficiency syndromes, and pre-existing blood dyscrasias (eg, bone marrow hypoplasia, leukopenia, thrombocytopenia, significant anemia).

WARNINGS/PRECAUTIONS: Monitor closely; toxicity may be related to dose and frequency of administration. When reactions do occur, doses should be reduced or discontinued and corrective measures should be taken. Avoid pregnancy if either partner is receiving therapy. Avoid intrathecal administration or high-dose therapy. Injection contains benzyl alcohol; avoid use in neonates (<1 month), may cause gasping syndrome.

ADVERSE REACTIONS: Ulcerative stomatitis, leukopenia, nausea, abdominal distress, malaise, fatigue, chills, fever, dizziness, decreased resistance to infection, anemia, photosensitivity, rash, pruritus, hepatotoxicity.

INTERACTIONS: See Black Box Warning. Avoid NSAIDs with high doses. Caution with nephrotoxic agents (eg, cisplatin), NSAIDs, probenecid, and highly protein bound drugs (eg, sulfonamides, phenytoin, phenylbutazone, salicylates). Oral antibiotics (eg, tetracycline, chloramphenicol) may decrease absorption or interfere with enterohepatic circulation. Penicillins may decrease clearance. Closely monitor with hepatotoxins (eg, azathioprine, retinoids, sulfasalazine). Folic acid may decrease response to MTX. TMP/SMZ may increase bone marrow suppression. May decrease theophylline clearance.

PREGNANCY: Category X, contraindicated in nursing.

MECHANISM OF ACTION: Dihydrofolic acid reductase inhibitor; interferes with DNA synthesis, repair, and cellular replication. MOA in rheumatoid arthritis not established; may affect immune function.

PHARMACOKINETICS: Absorption: (PO, Healthy) T_{max}=1-2 hrs. (IM) T_{max}=30-60 min. Oral administration resulted in different parameters according to disease state and dosing; refer to PI for further information. **Distribution:** (IV, Initial) V_d=0.18L/kg; (Steady state) V_d=0.4-0.8L/kg; plasma protein binding (50%); found in breast milk. **Metabolism:** Hepatic and intracellular; 7-hydroxymethotrexate (metabolite). **Elimination:** Renal (primary route), bile (≤10%). (Psoriasis, rheumatoid arthritis, low-dose chemotherapy at <30mg/m^2) $T_{1/2}$=3-10 hrs; (High dose) $T_{1/2}$=8-15 hrs.

METHYLDOPA
methyldopa (Various)

RX

THERAPEUTIC CLASS: Central alpha-adrenergic agonist

INDICATIONS: Treatment of hypertension.

DOSAGE: *Adults:* Initial: 250mg bid-tid for 48 hrs. Adjust dose at intervals of not less than 2 days. Maint: 500mg-2g/day given bid-qid. Max: 3g/day. Concomitant Antihypertensives (other than thiazides): Initial: Limit to 500mg/day. Renal Impairment: May respond to lower doses.
Pediatrics: Initial: 10mg/kg/day given bid-qid. Max: 65mg/kg/day or 3g/day, whichever is less.

HOW SUPPLIED: Tab: 125mg, 250mg, 500mg

CONTRAINDICATIONS: Active hepatic disease, history of methyldopa associated liver disorder, concomitant MAOIs.

WARNINGS/PRECAUTIONS: Positive Coombs test, hemolytic anemia, and liver disorders may occur. Fever reported within the first 3 weeks of therapy. HTN has recurred after dialysis. Caution with liver disease or dysfunction. D/C if signs of heart failure, or involuntary choreoathetotic movements develop. Edema and weight gain reported. Blood count, Coombs test and LFTs prior to therapy and periodically thereafter.

ADVERSE REACTIONS: Sedation, headache, asthenia, edema/weight gain, hepatic disorders, vomiting, diarrhea, nausea, sore or "black" tongue, blood dyscrasias, BUN increase, gynecomastia, impotence.

INTERACTIONS: See Contraindications. May potentiate other antihypertensives. Anesthetics may need dose reduction. Monitor for lithium toxicity. Ferrous sulfate and ferrous gluconate may decrease bioavailability; avoid coadministration.

PREGNANCY: Category B, caution in nursing.

METHYLDOPA HCL

MECHANISM OF ACTION: Aromatic-aminoacid decarboxylase inhibitor; not established, antihypertensive effect probably due to metabolism to α-methylnorepinephrine, which lowers arterial pressure by stimulation of central inhibitory α-adrenergic receptors, false neurotransmission, and reduction of plasma renin activity.

PHARMACOKINETICS: Distribution: Crosses placenta, found in breast milk. **Metabolism:** Extensive. **Elimination:** Urine; $T_{1/2}$=105 min.

METHYLDOPATE HCL
methyldopate HCl (American Regent)

RX

THERAPEUTIC CLASS: Central alpha-adrenergic agonist

INDICATIONS: Treatment of hypertension and hypertensive crises.

DOSAGE: *Adults:* 250-500mg IV q6h as needed. Max: 1gm q6h. Elderly/Renal Dysfunction: May reduce dose. Switch to oral therapy once BP is controlled.
Pediatrics: 20-40mg/kg/day IV given q6h. Max: 65mg/kg/day or 3 g/day, whichever is less. Switch to oral therapy once BP is controlled.

HOW SUPPLIED: Inj: 50mg/mL

CONTRAINDICATIONS: Hypersensitivity to sulfites, active hepatic disease, liver disorders previously associated with methyldopa therapy, concomitant MAOIs.

WARNINGS/PRECAUTIONS: Positive Coombs test, hemolytic anemia, and liver disorders may occur. Fever reported within the first 3 weeks of therapy. HTN has recurred after dialysis. Caution with liver disease or dysfunction. D/C if signs of heart failure develop. Edema and weight gain reported. Blood count, Coombs test and LFTs prior to therapy and periodically thereafter. Caution with cerebrovascular disease.

ADVERSE REACTIONS: Sedation, headache, asthenia, weakness, edema, weight gain, liver disorders, NV, diarrhea, sore or "black" tongue, blood dyscrasias, BUN increase, gynecomastia, impotence.

INTERACTIONS: See Contraindications. May potentiate other antihypertensives. Anesthetics may need dose reduction. May increase lithium levels. Ferrous sulfate and ferrous gluconate may decrease bioavailability; avoid coadministration.

PREGNANCY: Category C, caution in nursing.

MECHANISM OF ACTION: Aromatic-amino-acid decarboxylase inhibitor; not established, antihypertensive effect probably due to metabolism to α-methyl-norepinephrine, which lowers arterial pressure by stimulating central inhibitory α-adrenergic receptors, false neurotransmission, and/or reduction of plasma renin activity.

PHARMACOKINETICS: Distribution: Crosses placental barrier; appears in breast milk and cord blood. **Metabolism:** Extensive. **Elimination:** Urine (49%); $T_{1/2}$=90-127 min.

METHYLIN
methylphenidate HCl (Mallinckrodt)

CII

OTHER BRAND NAME: Methylin ER (Mallinckrodt)

THERAPEUTIC CLASS: Sympathomimetic amine

INDICATIONS: Treatment of attention deficit disorder and narcolepsy.

DOSAGE: *Adults:* (Sol/Tab/Tab, Chewable) 10-60mg/day given bid-tid 30-45 min ac. Take last dose before 6 pm if insomnia occurs. (Tab, Extended-Release) May use in place of immediate release tabs when 8 hr dose corresponds to titrated 8 hr immediate release dose. Swallow whole; do not chew or crush.
Pediatrics: ≥ 6 yrs: (Sol/Tab/Tab, Chewable) Initial: 5mg bid before breakfast and lunch. Titrate: Increase gradually by 5-10mg weekly. Max: 60mg/day. (Tab, Extended-Release) May be use in place of immediate release tabs when 8 hr dose corresponds to titrated or immediate release dose. Swallow whole; do not chew or crush. Reduce dose or if paradoxical aggravation of symptoms occur. D/C if no improvement after appropriate dose adjustment over 1 month.

HOW SUPPLIED: Sol: 5mg/5mL (500mL), 10mg/5mL (500mL); Tab: 5mg, 10mg, 20mg; Tab, Chewable: 2.5mg, 5mg, 10mg; Tab, Extended-Release: 10mg, 20mg

CONTRAINDICATIONS: Marked anxiety, tension, and agitation; glaucoma; motor tics or history or diagnosis of Tourette's syndrome; during or within 14 days of MAOI use.

WARNINGS/PRECAUTIONS: Monitor growth in children. Not for severe depression or fatigue. May exacerbate symptoms of behavior disturbance or thought disorder in psychotic children. Caution when using stimulants to treat patients with comorbid bipolar disorder because of concern for possible induction of mixed/manic episode in such patients. Stimulants at usual doses can cause treatment emergent psychotic or manic symptoms (hallucinations, delusional thinking, mania) in children and adolescents without prior history of psychotic illness. Aggressive behavior or hostility has been reported in clinical trials and the postmarketing experience of some medications indicated for the treatment of ADHD. May lower seizure threshold, especially in known EEG abnormalities. Caution with HTN, heart failure, recent MI, ventricular arrhythmia, or emotionally-unstable patients. Monitor during withdrawal. Visual disturbances may occur (rare). Monitor CBC, differential, and platelets with prolonged use. Periodically d/c to assess condition. Avoid with serious structural cardiac abnormalities, cardiomyopathy, serious heart rhythm abnormalities, CAD, or other serious cardiac problems. Caution in emotionally unstable patients with history of drug dependence or alcoholism.

ADVERSE REACTIONS: Nervousness, insomnia, hypersensitivity reactions, anorexia, nausea, dizziness, palpitations, headache, dyskinesia, drowsiness, BP and pulse changes, tachycardia, angina, arrhythmia, abdominal pain.

INTERACTIONS: May decrease hypotensive effect of guanethidine. Caution with pressor agents. Avoid during or within 14 days of MAOI use. Potentiates anticoagulants, anticonvulsants (phenobarbital, diphenylhydantoin, primidone), phenylbutazone, TCAs (imipramine, clomipramine, desipramine). Caution with α_2 agonists (eg, clonidine); serious adverse reactions reported with concurrent use.

PREGNANCY: Category C, caution in nursing.

MECHANISM OF ACTION: CNS stimulant; activates the brain-stem arousal system and cortex to produce its stimulant effect. Blocks the reuptake of norepinephrine and dopamine into the presynaptic neuron and increases the release of monoamines into the extraneuronal space.

PHARMACOKINETICS: Absorption: (20mg, Sol) C_{max}=9ng/mL, T_{max}=1-2 hrs. **Metabolism:** Deesterification to α-phenyl-piperidine acetic acid. **Elimination:** Urine (90%), $T_{1/2}$=2.7 hrs (sol), 3 hrs (chewable).

METOCLOPRAMIDE   RX
metoclopramide HCl (Various)

OTHER BRAND NAMES: Reglan (Schwarz) - Reglan Injection (Baxter)

THERAPEUTIC CLASS: Dopamine antagonist/prokinetic

INDICATIONS: (PO) Symptomatic treatment of gastroesophageal reflux in patients who fail to respond to conventional therapy. (Inj, PO) Symptomatic relief of diabetic gastroparesis. (Inj) Prevention of post-op or chemo-induced nausea/vomiting. Diagnostic aid during radiological examination and facilitates intubation of small intestine.

DOSAGE: *Adults:* GERD: PO: 10-15mg qid 30 min ac and hs. Elderly: 5 mg qid. Max: 12 weeks of therapy. Intermittent Symptoms: Up to 20mg as single dose prior to provoking situation. Gastroparesis: 10mg PO 30 min ac and hs for 2-8 weeks. Severe Gastroparesis: May give same doses IV/IM for up to 10 days if needed. Antiemetic: (Post-op) 10-20mg IM near end of surgery. (Chemotherapy-Induced) 1-2mg/kg 30 min before chemotherapy then q2h for 2 doses, then q3h for 3 doses. Give 2mg/kg for highly emetogenic drugs for initial 2 doses. Small Bowel Intubation/Radiological Exam: 10mg IV as single dose. CrCl <40mL/min: 50% of normal dose.
Pediatrics: Small Bowel Intubation: 6-14 yrs: 2.5-5mg IV single dose. <6 yrs: 0.1mg/kg IV single dose. CrCl <40mL/min: 50% of normal dose.

HOW SUPPLIED: Inj: 5mg/mL; Syr: 5mg/5mL; Tab: 5mg, 10mg* *scored

CONTRAINDICATIONS: Where GI mobility stimulation is dangerous (eg, perforation, obstruction, hemorrhage), pheochromocytoma, seizure disorder, concomitant drugs that cause EPS effects.

WARNINGS/PRECAUTIONS: Caution with HTN, Parkinson's disease, depression. EPS, tardive dyskinesia, Parkinsonian-like symptoms, neuroleptic malignant syndrome reported. Administer IV injection slowly. Risk of developing fluid retention and volume overload especially with cirrhosis or CHF; d/c if these occur. May increase pressure of suture lines.

ADVERSE REACTIONS: Restlessness, drowsiness, fatigue, EPS effects (acute dystonic reactions), galactorrhea, hyperprolactinemia, hypotension, arrhythmia, diarrhea, dizziness, urinary frequency.

INTERACTIONS: See Contraindications. May decrease gastric absorption of drugs (eg, digoxin) and increase intestinal absorption of drugs (eg, APAP, tetracycline, levodopa, ethanol, and cyclosporine). Additive sedation with alcohol, hypnotics, narcotics, or tranquilizers. Caution with MAOIs. Antagonized by anticholinergics, narcotics. Insulin dose or timing of dose may need adjustment to prevent hypoglycemia.

PREGNANCY: Category B, caution with nursing.

MECHANISM OF ACTION: Dopamine antagonist/promotility agent; not established, stimulates motility of upper GI tract, increases tone of gastric contractions, relaxes pyloric sphincter and duodenal bulb, increases peristalsis of duodenum and jejunum resulting in increased gastric emptying and intestinal transit, increases resting tone of LES, antagonizes central and peripheral dopamine receptors blocking stimulation of CTZ.

PHARMACOKINETICS: Absorption: Rapid; absolute bioavailability (80%). (Peds) C_{max} at tenth dose =56.8mcg/L. T_{max} =2.5 hrs. (Adults) T_{max}=1-2 hrs. **Distribution:** Plasma protein binding (30%); (adults)V_d=3.5L/kg; (peds) V_d =4.4L/kg. **Elimination:** Urine; (adults) $T_{1/2}$=5-6 hrs; (peds) $T_{1/2}$=4.1 hrs.

MEVACOR

RX

lovastatin (Merck)

THERAPEUTIC CLASS: HMG-CoA reductase inhibitor

INDICATIONS: To reduce risk of MI, unstable angina, and coronary revascularization procedures in patients without symptomatic coronary disease, average to moderately elevated total-C and LDL-C, and below average HDL-C. To slow coronary atherosclerosis progression in patients with coronary heart disease to reduce total-C and LDL-C. Adjunct to diet to lower total-C and LDL-C in primary hypercholesterolemia (Types IIa and IIb). Adjunct to diet to lower total-C, LDL-C and apolipoprotein B in adolescents at least 1-yr postmenarchal with heterozygous familial hypercholesterolemia.

DOSAGE: *Adults:* Initial: 20mg qd at dinner (10mg/day if need LDL-C reduction <20%). Usual: 10-80mg/day given qd or bid. May adjust every 4 weeks. Max: 80mg/day. Concomitant Cyclosporine: Initial: 10mg/day. Max: 20mg/day. Fibrates/Niacin (≥1g/day): Max: 20mg/day. Concomitant Amiodarone/Verapamil: Max: 40mg/day. CrCl <30mL/min: Consider dose increase of >20mg/day carefully and implement cautiously. *Pediatrics:* Heterozygous Familial Hypercholesterolemia: 10-17 yrs (at least 1-yr postmenarchal): Initial: If <20% LDL-C Reduction Needed: 10mg qd. If ≥20% LDL-C Reduction Needed: 20mg qd. May adjust every 4 weeks. Max: 40mg/day. Concomitant Cyclosporine: Initial: 10mg/day. Max: 20mg/day. Fibrates/Niacin (≥1g/day): Max: 20mg/day. Concomitant Amiodarone/Verapamil: Max: 40mg/day. CrCl <30mL/min: Consider dose increase of >20mg/day carefully and implement cautiously.

HOW SUPPLIED: Tab: 20mg, 40mg

CONTRAINDICATIONS: Active liver disease, unexplained persistent elevations of serum transaminases, pregnancy, nursing mothers.

WARNINGS/PRECAUTIONS: May increase serum transaminases and CPK levels; consider in differential diagnosis of chest pain. D/C if AST or ALT ≥3x ULN persist, or if myopathy diagnosed or suspected. Monitor LFTs prior to therapy, at 6 weeks, 12 weeks, then periodically or with dose elevation. Caution with heavy alcohol use and/or history of hepatic disease. Caution with dose escalation in renal insufficiency. Less effective with homozygous familial hypercholesterolemia. Rhabdomyolysis (rare), myopathy reported. D/C a few days before elective major surgery and when any major acute medical or surgical condition supervenes.

ADVERSE REACTIONS: Headache, constipation, flatulence, dizziness, rash, elevated transaminases or CK levels, GI upset, blurred vision.

INTERACTIONS: Increased risk of myopathy with CYP3A4 inhibitors (eg, cyclosporine, itraconazole, ketoconazole, erythromycin, clarithromycin, telithromycin, protease inhibitors, nefazodone, >1 quart/day of grapefruit juice), verapamil, amiodarone, fibrates (eg, gemfibrozil), danazol, and ≥1g/day of niacin. Monitor anticoagulants. Caution with drugs that diminish levels or activity of steroid hormones (eg, ketoconazole, spironolactone, cimetidine).

PREGNANCY: Category X, not for use in nursing.

MECHANISM OF ACTION: HMG-CoA reductase inhibitor; causes reduction of VLDL-C concentration and induction of LDL-receptor, leading to reduced production and/or increased catabolism of LDL-C. Also causes lowering of apolipoprotein B, component of LDL particles, consequently leading to reduction in concentration of circulating LDL.

PHARMACOKINETICS: Absorption: T_{max}=2-4 hrs. **Distribution:** Plasma protein binding (>95%). **Metabolism:** Liver (first pass); CYP450 3A4, β-hydroxyacid, 6´-hydroxy derivative (major active metabolites). **Elimination:** Urine (10%), feces (83%).

MIDAZOLAM INJECTION   CIV
midazolam HCl (Various)

> Associated with respiratory depression and respiratory arrest especially when used for sedation in noncritical care settings. Do not administer by rapid injection to neonates. Continuous monitoring required.

THERAPEUTIC CLASS: Benzodiazepine

INDICATIONS: For sedation, anxiolysis, and amnesia induction pre-op, prior to or during diagnostic, therapeutic, or endoscopic procedures, either alone or in combination with other CNS depressants. For induction of general anesthesia. For sedation of intubated and ventilated patients.

DOSAGE: *Adults:* IV: Sedation/Anxiolysis/Amnesia Induction: <60 yrs: Initial: 1-2.5mg IV over 2 min. Max: 5mg. Titrate: In small increments at 2 min intervals if needed. Concomitant Narcotics/Other CNS Depressants: Reduce by 30%. ≥60 yrs/Debilitated/Chronically Ill: Initial: 1-1.5mg IV over 2 min. Max: 3.5mg. Titrate: In small increments at 2 min intervals if needed. Concomitant Narcotics/Other CNS Depressants. Reduce by 50%. Maint: 25% of sedation dose by slow titration. IM: Preoperative Sedation/Anxiolysis/Amnesia: <60 yrs: 0.07-0.08mg/kg IM up to 1 hr before surgery. ≥60 yrs/Debilitated: 1-3mg IM. Anesthesia Induction: Unpremedicated: <55 yrs: Initially: 0.3-0.35mg/kg IV over 20-30 seconds. May give additional doses of 25% of initial dose to complete induction. ≥55 yrs: Initial: 0.3mg/kg IV. Debilitated: Initial: 0.15-0.25mg/kg IV. Premedicated: <55 yrs: Initial: 0.25mg/kg IV over 20-30 seconds. ≥55 yrs: Initial: 0.2mg/kg IV. Debilitated: 0.15mg/kg IV. Maintenance Sedation: LD: May repeat dose at 10-15 min intervals until adequate sedation. Maint: 0.02-0.1mg/kg/hr. Titrate to desired level of sedation using 25-50% adjustments. Infusion rate should be decreased 10-25% every few hrs to find minimum effective infusion rate.
Pediatrics: Sedation/Anxiolysis/Amnesia Induction: IV: <6 months: Limited information; titrate with small increments and monitor. 6 months-5 yrs: Initial: 0.05-0.1mg/kg IV over 2-3 min, up to 0.6mg/kg if needed. Max: 6mg. 6-12 yrs: Initial: 0.025-0.05mg/kg IV over 2-3 min, up to 0.4mg/kg if needed. Max: 10mg. 12-16 yrs: 1-2.5mg IV over 2 min. Titrate: In small increments at 2 min intervals if needed. Max: 10mg. IM: 0.1-0.15mg/kg IM, up to 0.5mg/kg if needed. Max: 10mg. Sedation: LD: 0.05-0.2mg/kg IV infusion over 2-3 min. Maint: 0.06-0.12mg/kg/hr IV infusion. May adjust dose by 25%. Sedation in Critical Care: Neonatal Dose: <32 weeks: Initial: 0.03mg/kg/hr IV infusion. >32 weeks: Initial: 0.06mg/kg/hr IV infusion. Adjust to lowest effective dose.

HOW SUPPLIED: Inj: 1mg/mL, 5mg/mL

CONTRAINDICATIONS: Acute narrow-angle glaucoma, untreated open-angle glaucoma, intrathecal or epidural use.

WARNINGS/PRECAUTIONS: Agitation, involuntary movements, hyperactivity, and combativeness reported. Caution with CHF, chronic renal failure, pulmonary disease, uncompensated acute illnesses (eg, severe fluid or electrolyte disturbances), elderly or debilitated. Avoid use with shock or coma, or in acute alcohol intoxication with depression of vital signs. Contains benzyl alcohol. Administer IM or IV only.

ADVERSE REACTIONS: Decreased tidal volume and/or respiratory rate, BP/HR variations, apnea, hypotension, pain and local reactions at injection site, hiccoughs, nausea, vomiting.

INTERACTIONS: Prolonged sedation with CYP450 3A4 inhibitors (eg, erythromycin, diltiazem, verapamil, ketoconazole, itraconazole, saquinavir, cimetidine). Increased sedative effects with morphine, meperidine, fentanyl, secobarbital, droperidol or other CNS depressants. Avoid use with acute alcohol intoxication. May decrease concentration of halothane and thiopental required for anesthesia. May cause severe hypotension with concomitant use of fentanyl in neonates.

PREGNANCY: Category D, caution in nursing.

MECHANISM OF ACTION: Benzodiazepine; short-acting CNS depressant.

PHARMACOKINETICS: Absorption: (IM) Absolute bioavailability (>90%), C_{max}=90ng/mL, T_{max}=0.5 hr; (1-hydroxy-midazolam) C_{max}=8 ng/ml, T_{max}=1 hr. **Distribution:** Crosses placenta, found in breast milk and CSF. V_d=1.0-3.1L/kg; plasma protein binding (97%). **Metabolism:** Liver via CYP450-3A4;1-hydroxy-midazolam (major metabolite). **Elimination:** Urine; (0.5% unchanged, 45%-57% as 4-hydroxy-midazolam); $T_{1/2}$= approximately 3 hrs.

MIDAZOLAM SYRUP   CIV
midazolam HCl (Various)

> **Associated with respiratory depression and respiratory arrest especially when used for sedation in noncritical care settings. Reports of airway obstruction, desaturation, hypoxia, and apnea especially with other CNS depressants. Continuous monitoring required.**

THERAPEUTIC CLASS: Benzodiazepine

INDICATIONS: Use in pediatric patients for sedation, anxiolysis and amnesia prior to diagnostic procedures or before induction of anesthesia.

DOSAGE: *Pediatrics:* single dose of 0.25-1mg/kg. 6 months-5 yrs or less cooperative patients: 1mg/kg. Max: 20mg. 6-15 yrs or cooperative patients: 0.25mg/kg. Max 20mg. Cardiac/respiratory compromised, higher risk surgical patients, or patients who have received concomitant narcotics or other CNS depressants: 0.25mg/kg. Max: 20mg.

HOW SUPPLIED: Syrup: 2mg/mL (118mL)

CONTRAINDICATIONS: Acute narrow-angle glaucoma.

WARNINGS/PRECAUTIONS: Monitor for respiratory adverse events and paradoxical reactions. Agitation, involuntary movements, hyperactivity, and combativeness reported. Caution with CHF, chronic renal failure, chronic hepatic disease, pulmonary disease, cardiac or respiratory compromised patients. Avoid use with shock or coma, or in acute alcohol intoxication with depression of vital signs.

ADVERSE REACTIONS: Emesis, nausea, agitation, hypoxia, laryngospasm, agitation.

INTERACTIONS: Decreased levels with CYP3A4 inducers (eg, rifampin, carbamazepine, phenytoin). Increased levels with CYP3A4 inhibitors (eg, azole antimycotics, protease inhibitors, CCBs, macrolide antibiotics, cimetidine). Increased sedative and respiratory effects with narcotics, propofol, ketamine, nitrous oxide, droperidol, barbiturates, alcohol and other CNS depressants. Caution with anesthetics.

PREGNANCY: Category D, caution in nursing.

MECHANISM OF ACTION: Benzodiazepine; short-acting CNS depressant.

PHARMACOKINETICS: Absorption: Rapidly absorbed; T_{max}=0.17-2.65 hrs (0.25, 0.5, 1 mg/kg). **Distribution:** V_d=1.24-2.02L/kg; plasma protein binding (97% midazolam), (89% α-hydroxymidazolam). **Metabolism:** Liver and gut via CYP3A4 and glucuronidation; α-hydroxymidazolam (major metabolite), 4-hydroxy metabolite and 1,4-dihydroxy metabolite (minor metabolites). **Elimination:** Urine (63%-80% as α-hydroxymidazolam glucuronide); $T_{1/2}$=2.2-6.8 hrs.

MINOCIN   RX
minocycline HCl (Triax)

THERAPEUTIC CLASS: Tetracycline derivative

INDICATIONS: Treatment of inclusion conjunctivitis, nongonococcal urethritis, and other infections (eg, respiratory tract, endocervical, rectal, urinary tract, skin and skin structure) caused by susceptible strains of microorganisms. Alternative treatment, when penicillin is contraindicated, in certain other infections (eg, urethritis, gonococcal, syphilis, anthrax). Adjunctive therapy in acute intestinal amebiasis and severe acne. Treatment of *Mycobacterium marinum* and asymptomatic carriers of *Neisseria meningitidis*.

DOSAGE: *Adults:* Usual: 200mg initially, then 100mg q12h; alternative is 100-200mg initially, then 50mg qid. Uncomplicated Gonococcal Infection (Men, other than urethritis and anorectal infections): 200mg initially, then 100mg q12h for minimum 4 days. Uncomplicated Gonococcal Urethritis (Men): 100mg q12h for 5 days. Syphilis: Administer usual dose for 10-15 days. Meningococcal Carrier State: 100mg q12h for 5 days. *Mycobacterium marinum:* 100mg q12h for 6-8 weeks. Uncomplicated Urethral, Endocervical, or Rectal Infection Caused by *Chlamydia trachomatis* or *Ureaplasma urealyticum:* 100mg q12h for at least 7 days. Gonorrhea in Patients Sensitive to PCN: 200mg initially, then 100mg q12h for at least 4 days, with post-therapy cultures within 2-3 days. Take with plenty of fluids. Renal Dysfunction: Max: 200mg/24 hrs.
Pediatrics: >8 yrs: 4mg/kg initially followed by 2mg/kg q12h, not to exceed adult dose. Take with plenty of fluids. Renal Dysfunction: Max: 200mg/24 hrs.

HOW SUPPLIED: Cap: 50mg, 100mg; Inj: 100mg; Sus: 50mg/5mL (60mL)

WARNINGS/PRECAUTIONS: May cause fetal harm during pregnancy. Use during tooth development (last half of pregnancy, infancy, <8 yrs) may cause permanent discoloration of the teeth or enamel hypoplasia; avoid use during this period. Renal toxicity, hepatotoxicity, photosensitivity, increased BUN, superinfection, pseudotumor cerebri may occur; perform hematopoietic, renal, and hepatic monitoring. Caution with hepatic dysfunction. Caution in renal impairment; may lead to azotemia, hyperphosphatemia, and acidosis. Use alternate form of contraception other than oral contraceptives. May decrease bone growth in premature infants. If *Clostridium difficile*-associated diarrhea (CDAD) develops, appropriate therapy should be initiated.

ADVERSE REACTIONS: Anorexia, NV, diarrhea, dysphagia, enterocolitis, pancreatitis, increased LFTs, renal toxicity, rash, exfoliative dermatitis, Stevens-Johnson syndrome, skin and mucous membrane pigmentation, blood dyscrasias, headache, tooth discoloration.

INTERACTIONS: May require downward adjustments of anticoagulant dosage. May interfere with bactericidal action of penicillin; avoid concurrent use when possible. May decrease efficacy of oral contraceptives. Impaired absorption with antacids containing aluminum, calcium, or magnesium- and iron-containing products. Fatal renal toxicity with methoxyflurane has been reported. Avoid isotretinoin shortly before, during and after therapy. Caution with other hepatotoxic drugs. Risk of ergotism with ergot alkaloids.

PREGNANCY: Category D, not for use in nursing.

MECHANISM OF ACTION: Tetracycline; bacteriostatic, thought to inhibit protein synthesis.

PHARMACOKINETICS: Absorption: Rapid; C_{max}=3.5mcg/mL; T_{max}=2.1 hrs. **Elimination:** Urine, feces; $T_{1/2}$=15.5 hrs.

MINOXIDIL RX
minoxidil (Par)

> May cause pericardial effusion, occasionally progressing to tamponade, and angina pectoris may be exacerbated. Only for nonresponders to maximum therapeutic doses of two other antihypertensives and a diuretic. Administer under supervision with a β-blocker and diuretic. Monitor in hospital for a decrease in BP in those receiving guanethidine with malignant hypertension.

THERAPEUTIC CLASS: Peripheral vasodilator

INDICATIONS: Treatment of hypertension that is symptomatic or associated with target organ damage and is not manageable with maximum therapeutic doses of diuretic plus 2 other antihypertensive drugs.

DOSAGE: *Adults:* Initial: 5mg qd. Titrate: Increase by no less than 3 days; may increase every 6 hrs if closely monitored. Usual: 10-40mg/day. Max: 100mg/day. Frequency: Give qd if diastolic BP is reduced to <30mmHg and if reduced to >30mmHg give bid. Give with a diuretic (eg, HCTZ 50mg bid, furosemide 40mg bid) and a β-blocker (equivalent to propranolol 80-160mg/day) or methyldopa (250-750mg bid starting 24 hrs before therapy). Renal Failure/Dialysis: Reduce dose.
Pediatrics: >12 yrs: Initial: 5mg qd. Titrate: Increase by no less than 3 days; may increase every 6 hrs if closely monitored. Usual: 10-40mg/day. Max: 100mg/day. Fre-

quency: Give qd if diastolic BP is reduced to <30mmHg and if reduced to >30mmHg give bid. Give with a diuretic (eg, HCTZ 50mg bid, furosemide 40mg bid) and a β-blocker (equivalent to propranolol 80-160mg/day) or methyldopa (250-750mg bid starting 24 hrs before therapy). <12 yrs: 0.2mg/kg qd. Titrate: May increase by 50-100% increments. Usual: 0.25-1mg/kg/day. Max: 50mg/day. Renal Failure/Dialysis: Reduce dose.

HOW SUPPLIED: Tab: 2.5mg*, 10mg* *scored

CONTRAINDICATIONS: Pheochromocytoma.

WARNINGS/PRECAUTIONS: Administer with a diuretic and β-blocker. Pericarditis, pericardial effusion and tamponade reported. With renal failure or dialysis, reduce dose to prevent renal failure exacerbation and precipitation of cardiac failure. Avoid rapid control with severe HTN. Monitor body weight, fluid and electrolyte balance. Extreme caution with post-MI. Hypersensitivity reactions reported.

ADVERSE REACTIONS: Salt and water retention, pericarditis, pericardial effusion, tamponade, hypertrichosis, nausea, vomiting, rash, ECG changes, hemodilution effects.

INTERACTIONS: Severe orthostatic hypotension with guanethidine.

PREGNANCY: Category C, not for use in nursing.

MECHANISM OF ACTION: Antihypertensive peripheral vasodilator; reduces systolic and diastolic blood pressure by decreasing peripheral vascular resistance.

PHARMACOKINETICS: Absorption: Almost complete (90%); T_{max}=1 hr. **Metabolism:** Glucuronide conjugation. **Elimination:** Urine; $T_{1/2}$=4.2 hrs.

MINTEZOL   RX
thiabendazole (Merck)

THERAPEUTIC CLASS: Vermicidal and/or vermifugal agent

INDICATIONS: Treatment of strongyloidiasis (threadworm), cutaneous larva migrans (creeping eruption), visceral larva migrans, and trichinosis. Second line or adjunct treatment for uncinariasis, trichuriasis, ascariasis (intestinal roundworms).

DOSAGE: *Adults:* 100 lbs: 1g or 10mL bid. 125 lbs: 1.25g or 12.5mL bid. ≥150 lbs: 1.5g or 15mL bid. Max: 3g/day. Take with meals. Treatment Duration: Strongyloidiasis/Cutaneous Larva Migrans/Intestinal Roundworms: 2 days. Trichinosis: 2-4 days. Visceral Larva Migrans: 7 days.
Pediatrics: 30 lbs: 250mg or 2.5mL bid. 50 lbs: 500mg or 5mL bid. 75 lbs: 750mg or 7.5mL bid. Max: 3g/day. Take with meals. Treatment Duration: Strongyloidiasis/Cutaneous Larva Migrans/Intestinal Roundworms: 2 days. Trichinosis: 2-4 days. Visceral Larva Migrans: 7 days.

HOW SUPPLIED: Sus: 500mg/5mL (120mL); Tab, Chewable: 500mg* *scored

CONTRAINDICATIONS: Prophylactic treatment for pinworm infestation.

WARNINGS/PRECAUTIONS: D/C if hypersensitivity reactions occurs. Erythema multiforme and Stevens-Johnson syndrome, jaundice, cholestasis, and parenchymal hepatic damage reported. Prolonged use may cause abnormal sensation in eyes, xanthopsia, and blurred vision. Not for mixed infections with ascaris, prophylaxis, or first line treatment of enterobiasis. Monitor with hepatic or renal dysfunction. CNS side effects may occur; avoid activities requiring mental alertness.

ADVERSE REACTIONS: Anorexia, NV, diarrhea, weariness, drowsiness, dizziness, abnormal sensation in eyes, xanthopsia, hypotension, hyperglycemia, leukopenia, hematuria, pruritus, fever.

INTERACTIONS: Decreases metabolism of xanthine derivatives; monitor blood levels and/or reduce dose.

PREGNANCY: Category C, not for use in nursing.

MECHANISM OF ACTION: Vermicidal agent; suspected to inhibit helminth-specific enzyme fumarate reductase.

PHARMACOKINETICS: Absorption: Rapidly absorbed; T_{max}=1-2 hrs. **Metabolism:** Almost completely metabolized in liver to 5-hydroxy form. **Elimination:** Urine (90%), feces (5%).

MiraLax
polyethylene glycol 3350 (Schering-Plough)
OTC

THERAPEUTIC CLASS: Osmotic laxative

INDICATIONS: Treatment of occasional constipation.

DOSAGE: *Adults:* Stir and dissolve 17g in 4-8 oz of beverage and drink qd. Use no more than 7 days.
Pediatrics: ≥17 yrs: Stir and dissolve 17g in 4-8 oz of beverage and drink qd. Use no more than 7 days.

HOW SUPPLIED: Powder: 17g/dose (119g, 238g)

WARNINGS/PRECAUTIONS: Avoid in kidney disease.

M-M-R II
measles vaccine live - mumps vaccine live - rubella vaccine live (Merck)
RX

THERAPEUTIC CLASS: Vaccine

INDICATIONS: Vaccination against measles, mumps, and rubella.

DOSAGE: *Adults:* 0.5mL SQ into outer aspect of upper arm.
Pediatrics: 12-15 months: 0.5mL SQ into outer aspect of upper arm. Repeat before elementary school entry. If vaccinated at 6-12 months due to measles outbreak, give another dose between 12-15 months and then before elementary school entry.

HOW SUPPLIED: Inj: 0.5mL

CONTRAINDICATIONS: Avoid pregnancy for 3 months after vaccine, anaphylactic reaction to neomycin, febrile/active respiratory illness, immunosuppressive therapy (except corticosteroids as replacement therapy), blood dyscrasias, leukemia, lymphoma, malignant neoplasms affecting bone marrow or lymphatic system, immunodeficiency states.

WARNINGS/PRECAUTIONS: Caution with egg allergy, cerebral injury, and individual/family history of convulsions. Defer vaccination for 3 months after blood or plasma transfusions or administration of human immune globulin. Avoid pregnancy for 3 months after vaccination. May worsen thrombocytopenia. Contains albumin, remote risk of viral infection transmission. Have epinephrine (1:1000) available.

ADVERSE REACTIONS: Atypical measles, fever, syncope, headache, dizziness, malaise, diarrhea, local reactions, vomiting, nausea, arthralgia, pneumonitis, sore throat, Stevens-Johnson Syndrome.

INTERACTIONS: Do not give with immune globulin. May depress TB skin sensitivity, administer test either simultaneously or before. Do not give <1 month before or after other live viral vaccines. Do not give simultaneously with DTP or oral poliovirus vaccine.

PREGNANCY: Category C, caution in nursing.

MECHANISM OF ACTION: May induce antibodies that may protect against measles, mumps, and rubella.

MOBAN
molindone HCl (Endo)
RX

THERAPEUTIC CLASS: Dihydroindolone

INDICATIONS: Management of schizophrenia.

DOSAGE: *Adults:* Initial: 50-75mg/day. Titrate: Increase to 100mg/day in 3-4 days; adjust to patient response. Maint: Mild: 5-15mg tid-qid. Moderate: 10-25mg tid-qid. Severe: 225mg/day.
Pediatrics: ≥12 yrs: Initial: 50-75mg/day. Titrate: Increase to 100mg/day in 3-4 days; adjust to patient response. Maint: Mild: 5-15mg tid-qid. Moderate: 10-25mg tid-qid. Severe: 225mg/day.

HOW SUPPLIED: Tab: 5mg, 10mg, 25mg*, 50mg* *scored

CONTRAINDICATIONS: Severe CNS depression (alcohol, barbiturates, narcotics), comatose states.

WARNINGS/PRECAUTIONS: Tardive dyskinesia, NMS may occur. Concentrate contains sulfites. Caution with activities requiring alertness. Convulsions, increased activity reported. May obscure signs of intestinal obstruction or brain tumor. May elevate prolactin levels.

ADVERSE REACTIONS: Drowsiness, depression, hyperactivity, euphoria, extrapyramidal reactions, akathisia, Parkinson's syndrome, blurred vision, nausea, dry mouth.

INTERACTIONS: Tabs contain calcium sulfate; may interfere with phenytoin sodium and tetracycline absorption.

PREGNANCY: Safety in pregnancy and nursing not known.

MECHANISM OF ACTION: Dihydroindolone compound; exerts effect on the ascending reticular activating system. Causes reduction of spontaneous locomotion and aggressiveness, suppression of a conditioned response, and antagonism of hyperactivity induced by amphetamines in lab animals.

PHARMACOKINETICS: Absorption: Rapidly absorbed, T_{max}=1.5 hrs. **Elimination:** Urine; feces (unchanged).

MOBIC

RX

meloxicam (Boehringer Ingelheim)

> NSAIDs may cause an increased risk of serious cardiovascular thrombotic events, MI, stroke and serious GI adverse events including bleeding, ulceration, and perforation of the stomach or intestines. Contraindicated for the treatment of perioperative pain in the setting of coronary artery bypass graft (CABG) surgery.

THERAPEUTIC CLASS: NSAID

INDICATIONS: Relief of signs and symptoms of osteoarthritis (OA) and rheumatoid arthritis (RA). Relief of the signs and symptoms of pauciarticular or polyarticular course juvenile rheumatoid arthritis (JRA) in patients ≥2 yrs.

DOSAGE: *Adults:* ≥18 yrs: OA/RA: Initial/Maint: 7.5mg qd. Max: 15mg/day. *Pediatrics:* >2 yrs: JRA: 0.125mg/kg qd. Max: 7.5mg/day.

HOW SUPPLIED: Sus: 7.5mg/5mL; Tab: 7.5mg, 15mg

CONTRAINDICATIONS: ASA or other NSAID allergy that precipitates asthma, urticaria, or allergic-type reactions. Treatment of perioperative pain in the setting of CABG surgery.

WARNINGS/PRECAUTIONS: May lead to onset of new HTN or worsening of pre-existing HTN; monitor BP closely. Fluid retention and edema reported; caution with fluid retention, HTN, or heart failure. Renal papillary necrosis, renal insufficiency, acute renal failure, and other renal injury reported after long-term use. Not recommended for use with advanced renal disease; if therapy must be initiated, monitor renal function. Anaphylactoid reactions may occur. May cause serious skin adverse events (eg, exfoliative dermatitis, Stevens-Johnson syndrome, and toxic epidermal necrolysis). Avoid in late pregnancy; may cause premature closure of ductus arteriosis. May cause elevations of LFTs; d/c if liver disease develops or systemic manifestations occur. Caution with considerable dehydration and in elderly. Anemia may occur; with long-term use, monitor Hgb/Hct if signs or symptoms of anemia develop. May inhibit platelet aggregation and prolong bleeding time; monitor with coagulation disorders. Caution with asthma and avoid with ASA-sensitive asthma.

ADVERSE REACTIONS: Abdominal pain, constipation, diarrhea, dyspepsia, NV, headache, anemia, arthralgia, insomnia, upper respiratory tract infection, UTI.

INTERACTIONS: May decrease antihypertensive effects of ACE inhibitors. Potentiates GI bleeds with ASA; avoid concomitant use. Increased clearance with cholestyramine. May decrease natriuretic effects of furosemide, thiazides. Decreased lithium clearance/ increased serum levels. Monitor PT/INR with warfarin. Caution with methotrexate.

PREGNANCY: Category C, not for use in nursing.

MECHANISM OF ACTION: NSAIDs; unknown, may inhibit prostaglandin synthetase.

PHARMACOKINETICS: Absorption: Absolute bioavailability (89%), C_{max}=1.05mcg/mL, T_{max}=4.9 hrs. **Distribution:** V_d=10 L/kg, plasma protein binding (99.4%). **Metabolism:** Hepatic (oxidation) via CYP2C9 (major), CYP3A4 (minor). **Elimination:** Urine (0.2%), feces (1.6%); $T_{1/2}$=20.1 hrs. Significant biliary and/or enteral secretion.

MONISTAT

OTC

miconazole nitrate (Personal Products Company)

OTHER BRAND NAMES: Monistat 3 (Personal Products Company) - Monistat 7 (Personal Products Company)

THERAPEUTIC CLASS: Azole antifungal

INDICATIONS: Treatment of vaginal yeast infections.

DOSAGE: *Adults:* 100mg sup or 2% cream intravaginaIly qhs for 7 days or 200mg sup or 4% cream intravaginally qhs for 3 days.
Pediatrics: ≥12 yrs: 100mg sup or 2% cream intravaginally qhs for 7 days or 200mg sup or 4% cream intravaginally qhs for 3 days.

HOW SUPPLIED: (Monistat 3) Cre: 4% (15g, 25g); Sup: 200mg (3s); (Monistat 7) Cre: 2% (35g, 45g); Sup: 100mg (7s)

WARNINGS/PRECAUTIONS: Avoid or d/c if abdominal pain, fever (>100°F), shoulder pain, back pain, or foul smelling discharge occurs. Do not use with tampons. Do not rely on condoms or diaphragm to prevent STDs or pregnancy.

ADVERSE REACTIONS: Vulvovaginal burning.

PREGNANCY: Safety in pregnancy and nursing not known.

MONISTAT 1 COMBINATION PACK

OTC

miconazole nitrate (Personal Products Company)

THERAPEUTIC CLASS: Azole antifungal

INDICATIONS: (Cre) Relief of external vulvular itching and irritation associated with a yeast infection. (Sup) Topical treatment of vulvovaginal candidiasis.

DOSAGE: *Adults:* 1200mg intravaginally qhs for 1 day. Apply 2% cream bid for up to 7 days for external itching.
Pediatrics: ≥12 yrs: 1200mg intravaginally qhs for 1 day. Apply 2% cream bid for up to 7 days for external itching.

HOW SUPPLIED: Cre: 2% (9g); Sup: 1200mg

WARNINGS/PRECAUTIONS: Do not rely on condoms or diaphragm to prevent STDs or pregnancy until 3 days after last use. Do not use tampons, douches, or spermicides until 7 days after last use. Confirm diagnosis by KOH smears and/or cultures; reconfirm if no response.

ADVERSE REACTIONS: Female genitalia burning and irritation, external female genitalia pruritus, female genitalia discharge.

PREGNANCY: Category C, caution in nursing.

MONODOX

RX

doxycycline monohydrate (Watson)

THERAPEUTIC CLASS: Tetracycline derivative

INDICATIONS: Treatment of rocky mountain spotted fever, typhus fever and the typhus group, Q fever, rickettsialpox, and ticks fever, respiratory tract, urinary tract, skin and skin structure, inclusion conjunctivitis, uncomplicated urethral/endocervical/rectal infection caused by *C.trachomatis*, nongonococcal urethritis caused by *C.trachomatis* and *U.urealyticum*, lymphogranuloma, psittacosis, trachoma, tularemia, campylobacter fetus, yaws, vincent's infection, actinomycosis, chancroid, plague, cholera, brucellosis. Treatment of uncomplicated gonorrhea, syphilis, listeriosis, anthrax, *Clostridium* species when PCN is contraindicated. Adjunct therapy for amebicides and severe acne.

DOSAGE: *Adults:* Usual: 100mg q12h or 50mg q6h for 1 day, then 100mg/day. Severe Infection: 100mg q12h. Uncomplicated Gonococcal Infections (except anorectal infections in men): 100mg bid for 7 days or 300mg stat, then repeat in 1 hr. Acute Epididymo-Orchitis caused by *N.gonorrhea* or *C.trachomatis:* 100mg bid for at least 10 days. Primary/Secondary Syphilis: 300mg/day in divided dose for at least 10 days. Uncomplicated Urethral/Endocervical/Rectal Infection caused by *C.trachomatis:* 100mg bid for at least 7 days. Nongonococcal Urethritis caused by *C.trachomatis* and

U.urealyticum: 100mg bid for at least 7 days. Take with full glass of water. Take with food if GI upset occurs. Inhalational Anthrax (post-exposure): 100mg bid for 60 days. *Pediatrics:* >8 yrs: ≤100 lbs: 2mg/lb divided in 2 doses for 1 day, then 1mg/lb daily in single or 2 divided doses. Severe Infection: May use up to 2mg/lb/day. >100 lbs: 100mg q12h or 50mg q6h for 1 day, then 100mg/day. Severe Infection: 100mg q12h. Take with full glass of water. Take with food if GI upset occurs.

HOW SUPPLIED: Cap: 50mg, 75mg, 100mg

WARNINGS/PRECAUTIONS: Avoid direct sunlight or UV light. May cause permanent tooth discoloration during tooth development (last half of pregnancy and children <8 years). Enamel hypoplasia reported. Monitor renal/hepatic function, and blood with long-term therapy. May increase BUN. Photosensitivity, pseudotumor cerebri reported. D/C if superinfection occurs. Bulging fontanels in infants and intracranial HTN in adults reported. *Clostridium difficile*-associated diarrhea reported.

ADVERSE REACTIONS: GI effects, photosensitivity, rash, blood dyscrasias, hypersensitivity reactions.

INTERACTIONS: Carbamazepine, barbiturates, phenytoin decrease half-life of doxycycline. May decrease PT; adjust anticoagulants. May decrease bactericidal agents (eg, penicillin). May decrease effects of oral contraceptives. Take 1 hr before or 2 hrs after dairy products. Aluminum-, calcium-, iron-, and magnesium-containing products and bismuth subsalicylate impair absorption. Fatal renal toxicity may occur with methoxyflurane.

PREGNANCY: Category D, not for use in nursing.

MECHANISM OF ACTION: Tetracycline; bacteriostatic, thought to inhibit protein synthesis.

PHARMACOKINETICS: Absorption: C_{max}=3.61mcg/mL; T_{max}=2.6 hrs. **Elimination:** Urine, feces; $T_{1/2}$=16.33 hrs.

MOTRIN   RX
ibuprofen (Pharmacia & Upjohn)

> NSAIDs may cause an increased risk of serious cardiovascular thrombotic events, MI, stroke and serious GI adverse events including bleeding, ulceration, and perforation of the stomach or intestines. Contraindicated for the treatment of perioperative pain in the setting of coronary artery bypass graft (CABG) surgery.

THERAPEUTIC CLASS: NSAID

INDICATIONS: *Adults:* Relief of mild-to-moderate pain. Dysmenorrhea. Rheumatoid arthritis (RA). Osteoarthritis (OA). *Pediatrics:* Fever. Relief of mild to moderate pain. Juvenile arthritis (JA).

DOSAGE: *Adults:* Pain: 400mg q4-6h prn. Max: 2400mg/day. Dysmenorrhea: 400mg q4-6h prn. Max: 2400mg/day. RA/OA: 300mg qid or 400mg, 600mg or 800mg tid-qid. Max: 3200mg/day. Fever: 200-400mg q4-6h. Max: 1200mg/day. Take with meals/milk. Renal Impairment: Reduce dose.
Pediatrics: Fever: 6 months-12 yrs: 5mg/kg for temp <102.5°F; 10mg/kg if temp ≥102.5°F q6-8h. Max: 40mg/kg/day. Pain: 6 months-12 yrs: 10mg/kg q6-8h. Max: 40mg/kg/day. JA: 30-40mg/kg/day divided into 3 or 4 doses. Milder disease may use 20mg/kg/day.

HOW SUPPLIED: Sus: 100mg/5mL; Tab: 400mg, 600mg, 800mg

CONTRAINDICATIONS: Syndrome of nasal polyps, angioedema, and bronchospastic reactions to ASA or other NSAIDs. Treatment of perioperative pain in the setting of CABG surgery.

WARNINGS/PRECAUTIONS: May lead to onset of new HTN or worsening of pre-existing HTN; monitor BP closely. Fluid retention and edema reported; caution with fluid retention or heart failure. Renal papillary necrosis and other renal injury reported after long-term use. Not recommended for use with advanced renal disease; if therapy must be initiated, monitor renal function. Anaphylactoid reactions may occur. May cause serious skin adverse events (eg, exfoliative dermatitis, Stevens-Johnson syndrome, and toxic epidermal necrolysis). Avoid in late pregnancy; may cause premature closure of ductus arteriosis. May cause elevations of LFTs; d/c if liver disease develops or systemic manifestations occur. Caution in elderly. Anemia may occur; with long-term use, monitor Hgb/Hct if signs or symptoms of anemia develop. May inhibit platelet aggregation and prolong bleeding time; monitor with coagulation disorders. Caution with asthma and avoid with ASA-sensitive asthma. D/C if visual disturbances occur. Aseptic meningitis with fever and coma reported.

ADVERSE REACTIONS: Nausea, epigastric pain, heartburn, dizziness, rash.

INTERACTIONS: Use caution with anticoagulants. May enhance methotrexate toxicity. May decrease natriuretic effects of furosemide or thiazides. Avoid use with ASA. May decrease lithium clearance; monitor for toxicity. May diminish antihypertensive effect of ACE inhibitors. Caution with concomitant warfarin use.

PREGNANCY: Category C, not for use in nursing.

MECHANISM OF ACTION: NSAIDs; unknown, suspected to inhibit prostaglandin synthetase.

PHARMACOKINETICS: Absorption: (Tab) Rapid. (Susp) *Adults:* C_{max}=19µg/mL; T_{max}=0.79 hrs; AUC=64µg•h/mL. Febrile children: C_{max}= 55µg/mL; T_{max}=0.97 hrs; AUC=155µg•h/mL. **Distribution:** (Susp) Plasma protein binding (>99%). *Adults:* V_d=0.12L/kg; febrile children: V_d=0.2L/kg. **Metabolism:** Hepatic. **Elimination:** (Tab): $T_{1/2}$=1.8-2 hrs. (Sus): Urine (1%); $T_{1/2}$=2 hrs.

MOTRIN IB
ibuprofen (McNeil Consumer)
OTC

THERAPEUTIC CLASS: NSAID

INDICATIONS: Temporarily relieves minor aches and pains due to headache, muscular aches, arthritis, toothache, backache, the common cold, menstrual cramps. Temporarily reduces fever.

DOSAGE: *Adults:* 200mg q4-6h. 400mg if symptoms do not respond. Max: 1200mg/24 hrs.
Pediatrics: ≥12 yrs: 200mg q4-6h. 400mg if symptoms do not respond. Max: 1200mg/24 hrs.

HOW SUPPLIED: Tab: 200mg

WARNINGS/PRECAUTIONS: Do not take for >10 days for pain or >3 days for fever. May cause severe allergic reaction, especially in people allergic to ASA. Do not use if history of allergic reaction to other pain relievers/fever reducers or right before or after heart surgery. May cause stomach bleeding; increased risk ≥60 yrs; stomach ulcers or bleeding problems; concomitant blood thinning or steroid drug, and other NSAIDs; ≥3 alcoholic drinks every day; longer course of therapy. Caution if taking ASA for heart attack or stroke, it may decrease this benefit of ASA.

INTERACTIONS: Avoid other ibuprofen-containing products.

PREGNANCY: Safety in pregnancy and nursing not known.

MOTRIN, CHILDREN'S
ibuprofen (McNeil Consumer)
OTC

OTHER BRAND NAMES: Motrin, Infants (McNeil Consumer) - Motrin, Junior (McNeil Consumer)

THERAPEUTIC CLASS: NSAID

INDICATIONS: To temporarily reduce fever, relief of minor aches and pains associated with the common cold, flu, sore throat, headaches, and toothaches.

DOSAGE: *Pediatrics:* Infant Drops: 6-11 months (12-17 lbs): 1.25mL q6-8h. 12-23 months (18-23 lbs): 1.875mL q6-8h. Use only with enclosed dropper. Sus: 2-3 yrs (24-35 lbs): 5mL q6-8h. 4-5 yrs (36-47 lbs): 7.5mL q6-8h. 6-8 yrs (48-59 lbs): 10mL q6-8h. 9-10 yrs (60-71 lbs): 12.5mL q6-8h. 11 yrs (72-95 lbs): 15mL q6-8h. Use only with enclosed measuring cup. Children's Chewable Tab: 4-5 yrs (36-47 lbs): 150mg q6-8h. 6-8 yrs (48-59 lbs): 200mg q6-8h. 9-10 yrs (60-71 lbs): 250mg q6-8h. 11 yrs (72-95 lbs): 300mg q6-8h. Junior Tab/Chewable Tab: 6-8 yrs (48-59 lbs): 200mg q6-8h. 9-10 yrs (60-71 lbs): 250mg q6-8h. 11 yrs (72-95 lbs): 300mg q6-8h. Max: 4 doses/24 hrs. Take with food/milk to avoid upset stomach. Take chewable tabs with food/water to avoid mouth/throat burning.

HOW SUPPLIED: Infant Drops: 50mg/1.25mL (15mL, 30mL); Children's Sus: 100mg/5mL (60mL, 120mL); Children's Tab, Chewable: 50mg; Junior Tab/Tab, Chewable: 100mg

WARNINGS/PRECAUTIONS: May cause severe allergic reaction (eg, hives, facial swelling, wheezing, shock). Avoid with history of allergic reaction to any other pain reliever/fever reducer. Not for use >10 days; or >2 days if severe/persistent sore throat or sore throat accompanied by high fever, headache, nausea/vomiting; or >3 days if fever/pain persists or gets worse.

INTERACTIONS: Caution with other products that contain ibuprofen or any other pain reliever/fever reducer.

PREGNANCY: Safety in pregnancy and nursing not known.

MECHANISM OF ACTION: Unknown; suspected to inhibit prostaglandin synthetase; has anti-inflammatory, analgesic, and antipyretic activities.

PHARMACOKINETICS: Absorption: C_{max}=55µg/mL; T_{max}=0.97hrs; AUC=155µg.h/mL. **Distribution:** Plasma protein binding (99%). **Elimination:** Urine (1%-unchanged), hydroxyphenylpropionic acid (25%), carboxypropylphenylpropionic acid (37%), free ibuprofen (1%), conjugated ibuprofen (14%), feces (metabolites and unabsorbed drug); $T_{1/2}$=2 hrs.

MUCINEX OTC
guaifenesin (Adams)

THERAPEUTIC CLASS: Expectorant

INDICATIONS: To help loosen phlegm, thin bronchial secretions and make coughs more productive.

DOSAGE: *Adults:* 1-2 tabs every 12hrs. Max: 4 tabs/24hrs. Take with full glass of water. Do not crush, chew or break.
Pediatrics: ≥12 yrs: 1-2 tabs every 12hrs. Max: 4 tabs/24hrs. Take with full glass of water. Do not crush, chew or break.

HOW SUPPLIED: Tab, Extended-Release: 600mg

WARNINGS/PRECAUTIONS: D/C if cough lasts >7 days, recurs, or occurs with fever, rash, or persistent headache.

PREGNANCY: Safety in pregnancy or nursing not known.

MUCINEX D OTC
guaifenesin - pseudoephedrine HCl (Adams)

THERAPEUTIC CLASS: Expectorant/decongestant

INDICATIONS: Help loosen phlegm and thin bronchial secretions. Temporarily relieves nasal congestion due to common cold, hay fever, or upper respiratory allergies. Temporarily restores freer breathing through the nose. Promotes nasal and sinus drainage. Temporarily relieves sinus congestion and pressure.

DOSAGE: *Adults:* 2 tabs every 12hrs. Max: 4 tabs/24hrs. Take with full glass of water. Do not crush, chew or break.
Pediatrics: ≥12 yrs: 2 tabs every 12hrs. Max: 4 tabs/24hrs. Take with full glass of water. Do not crush, chew or break.

HOW SUPPLIED: Tab, Extended-Release: (Guaifenesin-Pseudoephedrine HCl) 600mg-60mg

WARNINGS/PRECAUTIONS: Avoid use during or for 2 weeks after stopping MAOI therapy. Caution with heart disease, high BP, thyroid disease, diabetes, difficulty urinating due to enlarged prostate, persistent or chronic cough. D/C if cough lasts >7 days, or occurs with fever, rash or persistent headache.

INTERACTIONS: See Warnings and Precautions.

PREGNANCY: Safety in pregnancy and nursing not known.

MUCINEX DM   OTC
dextromethorphan hydrobromide - guaifenesin (Adams)

THERAPEUTIC CLASS: Cough suppressant/expectorant

INDICATIONS: To help loosen phlegm, thin bronchial secretions and make coughs more productive. Temporarily relieves cough due to minor throat and bronchial irritations, intensity of coughing, and impulse to cough.

DOSAGE: *Adults:* 1-2 tabs q12hrs. Max: 4 tabs/24hrs. Take with full glass of water. Do not crush, chew or break.
Pediatrics: ≥12 yrs: 1-2 tabs q12hrs. Max: 4 tabs/24hrs. Take with full glass of water. Do not crush, chew or break.

HOW SUPPLIED: Tab: (Dextromethorphan-Guaifenesin) 30mg-600mg

WARNINGS/PRECAUTIONS: D/C if cough lasts >7 days, recurs, or occurs with fever, rash, or persistent headache. Avoid during or within 14 days of MAOIs.

INTERACTIONS: See Warnings and Precautions.

PREGNANCY: Safety in pregnancy or nursing not known.

MUMPSVAX   RX
mumps virus vaccine live (Merck)

THERAPEUTIC CLASS: Vaccine

INDICATIONS: Vaccination against mumps.

DOSAGE: *Adults:* 0.5mL SQ into outer aspect of upper arm.
Pediatrics: ≥12 mos: 0.5mL SQ in outer aspect of upper arm. Give primary vaccine at 12-15 months. Revaccinate prior to elementary school.

HOW SUPPLIED: Inj: 20,000 $TCID_{50}$

CONTRAINDICATIONS: Avoid pregnancy for 3 months after vaccine, anaphylactic reaction to neomycin, febrile/active respiratory illness, immunosuppressive therapy (except corticosteroids as replacement therapy), blood dyscrasias, leukemia, lymphoma, malignant neoplasms affecting bone marrow or lymphatic system, immunodeficiency states.

WARNINGS/PRECAUTIONS: Caution with hypersensitivity to eggs and neomycin. May worsen thrombocytopenia. Defer vaccine for at least 3 months after blood or plasma transfusion and immune globulin. Do not revaccinate with active untreated TB. Monitor for temperature elevation after administration. Contains albumin, remote risk of viral infection transmission. Have epinephrine (1:1000) available.

ADVERSE REACTIONS: Fever, syncope, irritability, diarrhea, diabetes, purpura, cough, febrile seizures, local site reactions.

INTERACTIONS: Do not give with immune globulin. May depress TB skin sensitivity, administer test either simultaneously or before. Do not give <1 month before or after other live viral vaccines. Do not give simultaneously with DTP or oral poliovirus vaccine.

PREGNANCY: Category C, caution in nursing.

MECHANISM OF ACTION: Induces the immune system to produce antibodies that may protect against mumps.

MYAMBUTOL   RX
ethambutol HCl (X-Gen)

THERAPEUTIC CLASS: Cell metabolism inhibitor

INDICATIONS: Adjunct treatment of pulmonary TB with at least 1 other anti-TB drug.

DOSAGE: *Adults:* Initial: 15mg/kg q24h. Retreatment: 25mg/kg q24h. After 60 days, decrease to 15mg/kg q24h. Renal Dysfunction: Reduce dose.
Pediatric: ≥13 yrs: Initial: 15mg/kg q24h. Retreatment: 25mg/kg q24h. After 60 days, decrease to 15mg/kg q24h. Renal Dysfunction: Reduce dose.

HOW SUPPLIED: Tab: 100mg, 400mg* *scored

CONTRAINDICATIONS: Optic neuritis. Patients unable to appreciate and report visual side effects or changes in vision.

WARNINGS/PRECAUTIONS: Test visual acuity before and periodically during therapy; monthly with dose >15mg/kg/day. Liver toxicity reported; monitor hepatic function at baseline and periodically. Evaluate renal and hematopoietic functions periodically.

ADVERSE REACTIONS: Decreased visual acuity, optic neuropathy, anaphylactic reactions, dermatitis, pruritus, joint pain, GI effects, malaise, dizziness, elevated uric acid levels, pulmonary infiltrates, abnormal LFTs, eosinophilia.

INTERACTIONS: Avoid concurrent administration with aluminum hydroxide containing antacids.

PREGNANCY: Category C, safety in nursing not known.

MECHANISM OF ACTION: Antitubercular agent; inhibits synthesis of one or more metabolites, thus causing impairment of cell metabolism, arrest of multiplication, and cell death.

PHARMACOKINETICS: Absorption: C_{max}=2-5mcg/mL; T_{max}=2-4 hrs. **Distribution:** Excreted in breast milk. **Metabolism:** Initial oxidation of alcohol to aldehydic metabolite, followed by conversion to dicarboxylic acid. **Elimination:** Urine (50% unchanged), (8-15% metabolites), feces (20-22% unchanged).

MYCELEX TROCHE   RX
clotrimazole (Ortho-McNeil)

THERAPEUTIC CLASS: Azole antifungal

INDICATIONS: Local treatment of oropharyngeal candidiasis. Prophylactically to reduce the incidence of oropharyngeal candidiasis in immunocompromised conditions (eg, chemotherapy, radiotherapy, steroid therapy).

DOSAGE: *Adults:* Treatment: Slowly dissolve 1 troche in mouth 5 times/day for 14 days. Prophylaxis: Slowly dissolve 1 troche in mouth tid for duration of chemotherapy or until steroids reduced to maint levels.
Pediatrics: ≥3 yrs: Treatment: Slowly dissolve 1 troche in mouth 5 times/day for 14 days. Prophylaxis: Slowly dissolve 1 troche in mouth tid for duration of chemotherapy or until steroids reduced to maint levels.

HOW SUPPLIED: Tab: 10mg

WARNINGS/PRECAUTIONS: Not for systemic mycoses. May cause abnormal LFTs; monitor hepatic function. Only use in patients mentally and physically able to dissolve the troche. Confirm diagnosis by KOH smear and/or culture.

ADVERSE REACTIONS: Abnormal LFTs, NV, unpleasant mouth sensations, pruritus.

PREGNANCY: Category C, safety in nursing is not known.

MECHANISM OF ACTION: Broad-spectrum antifungal agent; inhibits growth of pathogenic yeasts by altering cell membrane permeability.

PHARMACOKINETICS: Absorption: C_{max}=4.98ng/mL (30 min), 3.23ng/mL (60 min).

MYCELEX-3   OTC
butoconazole nitrate (Bayer Healthcare)

THERAPEUTIC CLASS: Azole antifungal

INDICATIONS: Treatment of vaginal yeast infection.

DOSAGE: *Adults:* Insert 1 applicatorful vaginally qhs for 3 days.
Pediatrics: ≥12 yrs: Insert 1 applicatorful vaginally qhs for 3 days.

HOW SUPPLIED: Cre: 2% (5g, 20g)

WARNINGS/PRECAUTIONS: Do not use if abdominal pain, fever, foul smelling discharge, pregnancy, diabetes, HIV positive and AIDS patients. Avoid tampons. Do not rely on condoms or diaphragms to prevent STDs or pregnancy while on therapy; use alternate birth control method.

PREGNANCY: Safety in pregnancy or nursing not known.

MYCELEX-7

OTC

clotrimazole (Bayer Healthcare)

THERAPEUTIC CLASS: Azole antifungal

INDICATIONS: (Cre, Combination Pack) Treatment of vaginal yeast infection. (Combination Pack) For relief of external vulvar itching and irritation associated with vaginal yeast infections.

DOSAGE: *Adults:* (Cre) Insert 1 applicatorful vaginally qhs for 7 days. (Combination Pack) 1 insert vaginally qhs for 7 days. Apply small amount of cream onto irritated area of vulva qd-bid for up to 7 days.
Pediatrics: ≥12 yrs: (Cre) Insert 1 applicatorful vaginally qhs for 7 days. (Combination Pack) 1 insert vaginally qhs for 7 days. Apply small amount of cream onto irritated area of vulva qd-bid for up to 7 days.

HOW SUPPLIED: Cre: 1% (45g); (Combination Pack) Cre: 1% (7g), Vaginal Insert: 100 mg (7^s)

WARNINGS/PRECAUTIONS: Do not use if abdominal pain, fever, foul smelling discharge, during pregnancy. Avoid tampons. May reduce effectiveness of condoms, diaphragm or vaginal spermicides.

PREGNANCY: Safety in pregnancy or nursing not known.

MYFORTIC

RX

mycophenolic acid (Novartis)

> Increased susceptibility to infection. Possible development of lymphoma and other neoplasms. Female users of childbearing potential must use contraception. Increased risk of pregnancy loss and congenital malformations.

THERAPEUTIC CLASS: Inosine monophosphate dehydrogenase inhibitor

INDICATIONS: Prophylaxis of organ rejection in patients receiving allogeneic renal transplants, administered in combination with cyclosporine and corticosteroids.

DOSAGE: *Adults:* 720mg bid on empty stomach, 1 hr before or 2 hrs after food intake. *Pediatrics:* 400mg/m^2 bid. Max: 720mg bid. BSA 1.19-1.58m^2; 540mg bid. BSA >1.58m^2; 720mg bid. BSA <1.19m^2 cannot be accurately adminsitered with current formulations.

HOW SUPPLIED: Tab, Delayed-Release: 180mg, 360mg

WARNINGS/PRECAUTIONS: Risk of lymphomas and other malignancies, especially of the skin. Avoid sunlight to decrease risk of skin cancer. May cause fetal harm during pregnancy. Must have negative serum/urine pregnancy test within 1 week before therapy. Two reliable forms of contraception required before and during therapy, and 6 weeks following discontinuation. Monitor for bone marrow suppression. Risk of GI ulceration, hemorrhage, and perforation; caution with active digestive system disease. Caution with delayed renal graft function post-transplant. Oral suspension contains phenylalanine; caution with phenylketonurics. Monitor CBC weekly during the 1st month, twice monthly for the 2nd and 3rd months, and then monthly through 1st year. Avoid with rare hereditary deficiency of hypoxanthine-guanine phosphoribosyl-transferase (eg, Lesch-Nyhan and Kelley-Seegmiller syndrome). Female users of childbearing potential must use contraception. Increased risk of pregnancy loss and congenital malformations.

ADVERSE REACTIONS: Infections, diarrhea, leukopenia, sepsis, vomiting, GI bleeding, pain, abdominal pain, fever, headache, asthenia, chest pain, back pain, anemia, leukopenia, thrombocytopenia.

INTERACTIONS: Additive bone marrow suppression with azathioprine; avoid use. Reduced efficacy with drugs that interfere with enterohepatic recirculation (eg, cholestyramine). Efficacy/safety with other immunosuppressive agents not determined. Avoid live attenuated vaccines. Increased levels of both drugs with acyclovir, ganciclovir. Decreased levels with magnesium- and aluminum-containing antacids; space dosing. Decreased effects of oral contraceptives. Increased levels with probenecid. Other drugs that compete for renal tubular secretion may raise levels of both drugs.

PREGNANCY: Category D, not for use in nursing.

MECHANISM OF ACTION: Inosine monophosphate dehydrogenase inhibitor; inhibits the de novo pathway of guanosine nucleotide synthesis without incorporation to DNA.

PHARMACOKINETICS: Absorption: Absolute bioavailability (72%); T_{max}=1.5-2.75 hrs. **Distribution:** V_d=54L (steady state). Plasma protein binding: ≥98% (mycophenolic acid (MPA), 82% (mycophenolic acid glucuronide (MPAG). **Metabolism:** (MPA) metabolized by glucuronyl transferase to MPAG (major metabolite). **Elimination:** Urine: >60% (MPAG), 3% (unchanged), and bile; $T_{1/2}$=8-16 hrs (MPA), 13-17 hrs (MPAG).

MYLANTA MAXIMUM STRENGTH LIQUID   OTC
aluminum hydroxide - magnesium hydroxide - simethicone (J&J -- Merck)

OTHER BRAND NAME: Mylanta Regular Strength Liquid (J&J -- Merck)

THERAPEUTIC CLASS: Antacid/antigas

INDICATIONS: For the relief of heartburn, acid indigestion, sour stomach, upset stomach, pressure and bloating.

DOSAGE: *Adults:* ≥12 yrs: 2-4 tsp between meals or at bedtime. Max: 24 tsp/day for 2 weeks. Shake well.
Pediatrics: ≥12 yrs: 2-4 tsp between meals or at bedtime. Max: 24 tsp/day for 2 weeks. Shake well.

HOW SUPPLIED: Liq: (Aluminum Hydroxide-Magnesium Hydroxide-Simethicone) Maximum Strength: 400mg/5mL-400mg/5mL-40mg/5mL. Regular Strength: 200mg/5mL-200mg/5mL-20mg/5mL

MYLERAN   RX
busulfan (GlaxoSmithKline)

> Do not use unless CML diagnosis is established. May induce severe bone marrow hypoplasia; reduce dose or d/c if unusual depression of bone marrow function occurs.

THERAPEUTIC CLASS: Alkylating agent

INDICATIONS: Palliative treatment of chronic myelogenous leukemia (CML).

DOSAGE: *Adults:* 60mcg/kg/day or 1.8mg/m^2/day. Range: 4-8mg/day. Reserve dose >4mg/day for the most compelling symptoms.
Pediatrics: 60mcg/kg/day or 1.8mg/m^2/day. Range: 4-8mg/day. Reserve dose >4mg/day for the most compelling symptoms.

HOW SUPPLIED: Tab: 2mg* *scored

CONTRAINDICATIONS: Lack of definitive diagnosis of CML.

WARNINGS/PRECAUTIONS: Induction of bone marrow failure resulting in severe pancytopenia reported. Bronchopulmonary dysplasia with pulmonary fibrosis, cellular dysplasia, malignant tumors, acute leukemias, hepatic veno-occlusive disease reported. Ovarian suppression and amenorrhea with menopausal symptoms have occurred. Cardiac tamponade in patients with thalassemia and seizures reported. Caution with compromised bone marrow reserve from prior irradiation/chemotherapy. Seizures reported.

ADVERSE REACTIONS: Myelosuppression, pulmonary fibrosis, cardiac tamponade, hyperpigmentation, weakness, fatigue, weight loss, nausea, vomiting, melanoderma, hyperuricemia, myasthenia gravis, hepatic veno-occlusive disease.

INTERACTIONS: Additive myelosuppression with myelosuppressive drugs. Additive pulmonary toxicity with myelotoxic drugs. Increased clearance of cyclophosphamide and busulfan with phenytoin pretreatment. Decreased clearance with concomitant cyclophosphamide alone. Reduced clearance with itraconazole; monitor for signs of toxicity. Concurrent thioguanine was associated with portal HTN and esophageal varices with abnormal LFTs; caution with long-term therapy.

PREGNANCY: Category D, not for use in nursing.

MECHANISM OF ACTION: Bifunctional alkylating agent.

PHARMACOKINETICS: Absorption: (IV, PO) Absolute bioavailability (adults 80%, children 68%); C_{max}(2mg, 4mg)=30ng/mL, 68ng/mL; T_{max}=0.9 hrs; AUC (4mg) =269ng•hr/mL Dis-

tribution: Crosses blood-brain barrier; plasma protein binding (32%). **Metabolism**: Liver (extensive); 3-hydroxytetrahydrothiopene-1, 1-dioxide (major metabolite). **Elimination**: Urine (>2%, unchanged); $T_{1/2}$=2.69 hrs.

MYOZYME   RX
alglucosidase alfa (Genzyme)

> Risk of hypersensitivity reactions. Life-threatening anaphylactic reactions, including anaphylactic shock observed during infusion. Appropriate medical support should be readily available when administered.

THERAPEUTIC CLASS: Enzyme

INDICATIONS: Treatment of Pompe Disease.

DOSAGE: *Adults:* 20 mg/kg IV every 2 weeks. Administer over 4 hrs.
Pediatrics: 20 mg/kg IV every 2 weeks. Administer over 4 hrs.

HOW SUPPLIED: Inj: 50 mg

WARNINGS/PRECAUTIONS: See Black Box Warning. Risk of cardiac arrhythmia, sudden cardiac death during general anesthesia for central venous catheter placement, and acute cardiorespiratory failure. Infusion reactions observed. Caution with acutely ill patients.

ADVERSE REACTIONS: Pyrexia, cough, respiratory distress/failure, pneumonia, otitis media, upper respiratory tract infection, gastroenteritis, pharyngitis, diarrhea, vomiting, rash, decreased oxygen saturation, anemia, oral candidiasis.

PREGNANCY: Category B, caution in nursing.

MECHANISM OF ACTION: Enzyme; provides exogenous source of human enzyme α-glucosidase (GAA). Binds to mannose-6-phosphate receptors on cell surface via carbohydrate groups on GAA molecule. It is then internalized and transported into lysosomes where it undergoes proteolytic cleavage, producing an increase in enzymatic activity (cleaving glycogen).

PHARMACOKINETICS: Absorption: (20mg/kg single dose) C_{max}=162mcg/mL, AUC=811mcg-hr/mL; (40mg/kg single Dose) C_{max}=276mcg/mL, AUC=1781mcg-hr/mL. **Distribution:** (20mg/kg single dose) V_d=69ml/kg; (40mg/kg single dose) V_d=119mL/kg. **Elimination:** (20mg/kg Single Dose) $T_{1/2}$=2.6 hrs; (40mg/kg Single Dose) $T_{1/2}$=2.9 hrs.

MYSOLINE   RX
primidone (Valeant)

THERAPEUTIC CLASS: Pyrimidinedione derivative

INDICATIONS: For control of grand mal, psychomotor, and focal epileptic seizures.

DOSAGE: *Adults:* Initial: Day 1-3: 100-125mg qhs. Day 4-6: 100-125mg bid. Day 7-9: 100-125mg tid. Day 10-Maint: 250mg tid. Max: 500mg qid. Effective serum level is 5-12mcg/mL. Prior Anticonvulsant Therapy: Initial: 100-125mg qhs. Titrate: Increase gradually to maintenance dose as other drug is discontinued over 2 weeks.
Pediatrics: ≥8 yrs: Initial: Day 1-3: 100-125mg qhs. Day 4-6: 100-125mg bid. Day 7-9: 100-125mg tid. Day 10-Maint: 250mg tid. Max: 500mg qid. <8 yrs: Day 1-3: 50mg qhs. Day 4-6: 50mg bid. Day 7-9: 100mg bid. Day 10-Maint: 125-250mg tid or 10-25mg/kg/day in divided doses. Effective serum level is 5-12mcg/mL. Prior Anticonvulsant Therapy: Initial: 100-125mg qhs. Titrate: Increase gradually to maintenance dose as other drug is discontinued over 2 weeks.

HOW SUPPLIED: Tab: 50mg*, 250mg* *scored

CONTRAINDICATIONS: Porphyria, phenobarbital hypersensitivity.

WARNINGS/PRECAUTIONS: Avoid abrupt withdrawal. May take several weeks to assess therapeutic efficacy. Pregnant women should receive prophylactic vitamin K_1 therapy for one month prior to, and during, delivery. Perform CBC and a SMA-12 test every 6 months. Phenobarbital is a metabolite of primidone.

ADVERSE REACTIONS: Ataxia, vertigo, nausea, anorexia, vomiting, fatigue, hyperirritability, emotional disturbances, sexual impotency, diplopia, nystagmus, drowsiness, morbilliform skin eruptions.

PREGNANCY: Safety in pregnancy not known, caution in nursing.

MECHANISM OF ACTION: Pyrimidinedione. Not established; suspected to raise electro- or chemoshock seizure thresholds or alter seizure patterns. Has anticonvulsant activity.

PHARMACOKINETICS: Distribution: Found in breast milk. **Metabolism:** Metabolites: Phenobarbital and phenylethylmalonamide (PEMA) (Both active).

NALOXONE RX
naloxone HCl (Various)

OTHER BRAND NAME: Narcan (Endo)

THERAPEUTIC CLASS: Opioid antagonist

INDICATIONS: For complete or partial opioid depression reversal induced by natural and synthetic opioids. Diagnosis of suspected opioid tolerance or acute opioid overdose. Adjunct in management of septic shock to increase blood pressure.

DOSAGE: *Adults:* Opioid Overdose: Initial: 0.4-2mg IV every 2-3 minutes up to 10mg. IM/SQ if IV route not available. Post-op Opioid Depression: 0.1-0.2mg IV every 2-3 minutes to desired response. May repeat in 1-2 hr intervals. Supplemental IM doses last longer. Narcan Challenge Test: IV: 0.1-0.2mg, observe 30 secs for signs of withdrawal, then 0.6mg, observe for 20 min. SQ: 0.8mg, observe for 20 min.
Pediatrics: Opioid Overdose: Initial: 0.01mg/kg IV. Inadequate Response: repeat 0.1mg/kg once. IM/SQ in divided doses if IV route not available. Post-op Opioid Depression: 0.005-0.01mg IV every 2-3 min to desired response. May repeat in 1-2 hr intervals. Supplemental IM doses last longer. Neonates: Opioid-induced Depression: 0.01mg/kg IV/IM/SQ, may repeat every 2-3 min until desired response.

HOW SUPPLIED: Inj: 0.4mg/mL, 1mg/mL

WARNINGS/PRECAUTIONS: Caution in patients including newborns of mothers known or suspected of opioid physical dependence. May precipitate acute withdrawal syndrome. Have other resuscitative measures available. Caution with cardiac, renal, or hepatic disease. Monitor patients satisfactorily responding due to extended opioid duration of action. Abrupt postoperative opioid depression reversal may result in serious adverse effects leading to death.

ADVERSE REACTIONS: HTN, hypotension, ventricular tachycardia and fibrillation, dyspnea, pulmonary edema, cardiac arrest, nausea, vomiting, sweating, seizures, body aches, fever, nervousness.

INTERACTIONS: Caution using drugs with potential adverse cardiac effects. Reversal of buprenorphine-induced respiratory depression may be incomplete.

PREGNANCY: Category B, caution in nursing.

MECHANISM OF ACTION: Narcotic antagonist; prevents or reverses effects of opioids, including respiratory depression, sedation, and hypotension, by competing for same receptor sites. Also reverses psychotomimetic and dysphoric effects of agonist-antagonists (eg, pentazocine).

PHARMACOKINETICS: Distribution: Rapid; plasma protein binding (weak). **Metabolism:** Liver; via glucuronide conjugation; naloxone-3-glucuronide (major metabolite). **Elimination:** Urine (25-40%); $T_{1/2}$=30-80 min (adults), 3.1 hrs (neonates).

NAPHCON-A OTC
naphazoline HCl - pheniramine maleate (Alcon)

THERAPEUTIC CLASS: H_1-antagonist/alpha-agonist (imidazoline)

INDICATIONS: Temporary relief of ocular itching and redness caused by ragweed, pollen, grass, animal hair and dander.

DOSAGE: *Adults:* 1-2 drops up to 4 times daily.
Pediatrics: ≥6 yrs: 1-2 drops up to 4 times daily.

HOW SUPPLIED: Sol: (Pheniramine-Naphazoline) 0.3%-0.025% (15mL)

CONTRAINDICATIONS: Heart disease, high BP, enlargement of the prostate, narrow-angle glaucoma.

WARNINGS/PRECAUTIONS: Do not use if solution changes color or becomes cloudy. D/C with eye pain, changes in vision, continued redness or irritation, and if the condition worsens or persists for more than 72 hrs. Remove contact lenses before use. Supervision required with heart disease, high BP, difficulty in urination due to prostate enlargement or narrow angle glaucoma.

PREGNANCY: Safety in pregnancy and nursing not known.

NAPROSYN   RX

naproxen (Roche Labs)

> NSAIDs may cause an increased risk of serious cardiovascular thrombotic events, MI, stroke and serious GI adverse events including bleeding, ulceration, and perforation of the stomach or intestines. Contraindicated for the treatment of perioperative pain in the setting of coronary artery bypass graft (CABG) surgery.

OTHER BRAND NAME: EC-Naprosyn (Roche Labs)

THERAPEUTIC CLASS: NSAID

INDICATIONS: (Naprosyn, EC-Naprosyn) Relief of signs and symptoms of rheumatoid arthritis (RA), osteoarthritis (OA), ankylosing spondylitis, and juvenile arthritis (JA). (Naprosyn) Relief of signs and symtoms of tendinitis, bursitis, and acute gout. Management of pain and primary dysmenorrhea. EC-Naprosyn not recommended for initial treatment of acute pain.

DOSAGE: *Adults:* RA/OA/Ankylosing Spondylitis: Naprosyn: 250, 375, or 500mg bid; EC-Naprosyn: 375 or 500mg bid. Max: 1500mg/day. Acute Gout: Naprosyn: 750mg followed by 250mg q8h until attack subsides. Pain/Dysmenorrhea/Tendinitis/Bursitis: Naprosyn: 500mg followed by 500mg q12h or 250mg q6-8h prn. Max: 1250mg on Day 1, then 1000mg/day. EC-Naprosyn should not be chewed, crushed, or broken. *Pediatrics:* ≥2 yrs: JA: (Sus) 5mg/kg bid. Max: 15mg/kg/day.

HOW SUPPLIED: (Naproxen) Sus: 25mg/mL; Tab: 250mg*, 375mg, 500mg*; Tab, Delayed-Release: (EC-Naprosyn) 375mg, 500mg *scored

CONTRAINDICATIONS: History of ASA or NSAID allergy that cause symptoms of asthma, rhinitis, nasal polyps, and hypotension. Treatment of peri-operative pain in the setting of CABG surgery.

WARNINGS/PRECAUTIONS: May lead to onset of new HTN or worsening of pre-existing HTN; monitor BP closely. Fluid retention, edema, and peripheral edema reported; caution with fluid retention, HTN, or heart failure. Renal papillary necrosis and other renal injury reported after long-term use. Not recommended for use with advanced renal disease; if therapy must be initiated, monitor renal function. Anaphylactoid reactions may occur. May cause serious skin adverse events (eg, exfoliative dermatitis, Stevens-Johnson syndrome, and toxic epidermal necrolysis). Avoid in late pregnancy; may cause premature closure of ductus arteriosis. Monitor Hgb levels with long-term therapy if initial Hgb ≤10g. Monitor for visual changes or disturbances. May cause elevations of LFTs; d/c if liver disease develops or systemic manifestations occur. Caution with high doses in chronic alcoholic liver disease and elderly. Anemia may occur; with long-term use, monitor Hgb/Hct if signs or symptoms of anemia develop. May inhibit platelet aggregation and prolong bleeding time; monitor with coagulation disorders. Caution with asthma and avoid with ASA-sensitive asthma.

ADVERSE REACTIONS: Edema, drowsiness, dizziness, constipation, heartburn, abdominal pain, nausea, headache, tinnitus, dyspnea, pruritus, skin eruptions, ecchymoses.

INTERACTIONS: (Naprosyn, EC-Naprosyn) Avoid with other products containing naproxen. Decreased plasma levels with ASA. May reduce tubular secretion of methotrexate; monitor for toxicity. May increase nephrotoxicity of cyclosporine; caution when coadministering. May diminish antihypertensive effect and potentiate renal disease with ACE inhibitors. May reduce natriuretic effect of furosemide and thiazides; monitor for renal failure. May increase lithium levels; monitor for toxicity. Synergistic effects on GI bleeding with warfarin. Observe for dose adjustment with hydantoins, sulfonamides, or sulfonylureas. May reduce antihypertensive effects of propranolol and other β-blockers. Probenecid may increase half-life. (EC-Naprosyn) Avoid with H_2-blockers, sucralfate, or intensive antacid therapy.

PREGNANCY: Category C, not for use in nursing.

MECHANISM OF ACTION: NSAIDs; unknown, suspected to inhibit prostaglandin synthetase.

PHARMACOKINETICS: Absorption: Rapid and complete. Bioavailability (95%), C_{max}=97.4mcg/mL; T_{max}=1.9 hrs; AUC_{0-12h}=767mcg•hr/mL. (Tab, Delayed-Release) C_{max}=94.9mcg/mL; T_{max}=4 hrs; AUC_{0-12h}=845mcg•hr/mL. (Sus) T_{max}=1-4 hrs. **Distribution:** V_d=0.16L/kg; plasma protein binding (>99%); excreted in breast milk. **Metabolism:** Hepatic. Metabolite (6-O-desmethyl naproxen). **Elimination:** Urine (95%), feces (≤3%); $T_{1/2}$=12-17 hrs.

NASACORT AQ   RX
triamcinolone acetonide (Sanofi-Aventis)

THERAPEUTIC CLASS: Corticosteroid

INDICATIONS: Nasal treatment of seasonal and perennial allergic rhinitis symptoms.

DOSAGE: *Adults:* Initial/Max: 2 sprays per nostril qd. With improvement, may reduce dose to 1 spray per nostril qd.
Pediatrics: ≥12 yrs: Initial/Max: 2 sprays per nostril qd. With improvement, may reduce dose to 1 spray per nostril qd. 6-12 yrs: Initial: 1 spray per nostril qd. Max: 2 sprays per nostril qd.

HOW SUPPLIED: AQ Spray: 55mcg/spray (16.5g)

WARNINGS/PRECAUTIONS: Risk of adrenal insufficiency and withdrawal symptoms when replacing systemic corticosteroid with a topical corticosteroids. Caution with active or quiescent TB, ocular herpes simplex, or untreated bacterial, fungal and systemic viral infections. Avoid with recent nasal trauma, surgery or septum ulcers. Risk for more severe/fatal course of infections (eg, chickenpox, measles) and for *Candida* infections of the nose and pharynx. Potential for growth velocity reduction in pediatrics.

ADVERSE REACTIONS: Pharyngitis, epistaxis, infection, otitis media, headache, sneezing, rhinitis, nasal irritation, cough, sinusitis, vomiting.

PREGNANCY: Category C, caution in nursing.

MECHANISM OF ACTION: Corticosteroid; not established; anti-inflammatory action.

PHARMACOKINETICS: Absorption: C_{max}=0.5ng/mL; T_{max}=1.5 hrs; AUC (110mcg, 400mcg)=1.4ng•hr/mL, 4.7ng•hr/mL. **Elimination:** $T_{1/2}$=3.1 hrs.

NASAREL   RX
flunisolide (Ivax)

THERAPEUTIC CLASS: Corticosteroid

INDICATIONS: Relief of seasonal or perennial rhinitis.

DOSAGE: *Adults:* Initial: 2 sprays per nostril bid. Titrate: May increase to 2 sprays per nostril tid. Max: 8 sprays per nostril/day.
Pediatrics: 6-14 yrs: Initial: 1 spray per nostril tid or 2 sprays per nostril bid. Max: 4 sprays per nostril/day.

HOW SUPPLIED: Spray: 29mcg/spray (25mL)

CONTRAINDICATIONS: Untreated localized infection of the nasal mucosa.

WARNINGS/PRECAUTIONS: Risk of adrenal insufficiency and withdrawal symptoms when replacing systemic corticosteroids with a topical corticosteroids. Caution with active or quiescent TB, ocular herpes simplex, or untreated bacterial, fungal and systemic viral infections. Avoid with recent nasal trauma, surgery or septum ulcers. Risk for more severe/fatal course of infections (eg, chickenpox, measles) and for *Candida* infections of the nose and pharynx. Potential for growth velocity reduction in pediatrics.

ADVERSE REACTIONS: Aftertaste, nasal burning/stinging, cough, epistaxis, nasal dryness, pharyngitis, sinusitis.

INTERACTIONS: Concomitant systemic corticosteroids increases risk of hypercorticism and/or HPA axis suppression.

PREGNANCY: Category C, caution in nursing.

MECHANISM OF ACTION: Glucocorticosteroid; anti-inflammatory agent with potent glucucorticoid and weak mineralocorticoid activity.

PHARMACOKINETICS: Absorption: Well absorbed. **Metabolism:** Liver (rapidly). **Elimination:** Urine (65-70%) primary metabolite, feces.

NASONEX
mometasone furoate monohydrate (Schering)

THERAPEUTIC CLASS: Corticosteroid

INDICATIONS: Treatment of the nasal symptoms of seasonal and perennial allergic rhinitis. Prophylaxis of the nasal symptoms of seasonal allergic rhinitis. Treatment of nasal polyps in patients 18 years of age and older.

DOSAGE: *Adults:* Allergic Rhinitis: Treatment/Prophylaxis: 2 sprays per nostril qd. For prophylaxis, start 2-4 weeks before allergy season. Nasal Polyps: 2 sprays per nostril bid. *Pediatrics:* ≥12 yrs: Treatment/Prophylaxis: 2 sprays per nostril qd. For prophylaxis, start 2-4 weeks before allergy season. 2-11 yrs: Treatment: 1 spray per nostril qd.

HOW SUPPLIED: Spray: 50mcg/spray (17g)

WARNINGS/PRECAUTIONS: Risk of adrenal insufficiency and withdrawal symptoms when replacing systemic corticosteroids with a topical corticosteroids. Caution with active or quiescent TB, ocular herpes simplex, or untreated bacterial, fungal and systemic viral infections. Avoid with recent nasal trauma, surgery or septum ulcers. Risk for more severe/fatal course of infections (eg, chickenpox, measles) and for *Candida* infections of the nose and pharynx. Potential for growth velocity reduction in pediatrics.

ADVERSE REACTIONS: Headache, viral infection, pharyngitis, epistaxis, cough, upper respiratory tract infection, dysmenorrhea, myalgia, sinusitis.

PREGNANCY: Category C, caution with nursing.

MECHANISM OF ACTION: Corticosteroid; not established; demonstrates anti-inflammatory properties, shown to have a wide range of effects on multiple cell types (eg, mast cells, eosinophils, neutrophils, macrophages, lymphocytes) and mediators (eg, histamine, eicosanoids, leukotrienes, cytokines) involved in inflammation.

PHARMACOKINETICS: Distribution: Plasma protein binding (98-99%). **Metabolism**: Liver (extensive) via CYP3A4. **Elimination**: Bile (as metabolites), $T_{1/2}$=5.8 hrs.

NAVANE
thiothixene (Pfizer)

THERAPEUTIC CLASS: Thioxanthene

INDICATIONS: Management of schizophrenia.

DOSAGE: *Adults:* Mild Condition: Initial: 2mg tid. Titrate: May increase to 15mg/day. Severe Condition: Initial: 5mg bid. Usual: 20-30mg/day. Max: 60mg/day. *Pediatrics:* ≥12 yrs: Mild Condition: Initial: 2mg tid. Titrate: May increase to 15mg/day. Severe Condition: Initial: 5mg bid. Usual: 20-30mg/day. Max: 60mg/day.

HOW SUPPLIED: Cap: 1mg, 2mg, 5mg, 10mg, 20mg

CONTRAINDICATIONS: Circulatory collapse, comatose states, CNS depression, blood dyscrasias.

WARNINGS/PRECAUTIONS: May develop tardive dyskinesia, NMS. May mask symptoms of overdose of toxic drugs. May obscure conditions such as intestinal obstruction and brain tumor. May lower seizure threshold. Monitor for pigmentary retinopathy and lenticular pigmentation. Caution with cardiovascular disease, extreme heat exposure, activities requiring alertness. May elevate prolactin levels.

ADVERSE REACTIONS: Tachycardia, hypotension, lightheadedness, syncope, drowsiness, agitation, insomnia, hyperreflexia, cerebral edema, pseudoparkinsonism, LFT elevation, blood dyscrasias, rash, photosensitivity, dry mouth, blurred vision.

INTERACTIONS: Possible additive effects including hypotension with CNS depressants, alcohol. Caution with atropine or related drugs. Paradoxical effects with pressor agents.

PREGNANCY: Safety in pregnancy and nursing not known.

MECHANISM OF ACTION: Thioxanthene derivative.

NEMBUTAL SODIUM SOLUTION　　CII
pentobarbital sodium (Ovation)

THERAPEUTIC CLASS: Barbiturate

INDICATIONS: Short-term treatment of insomnia; sedation; preoperative anesthesia; anticonvulsant in the emergency control of certain acute convulsive episodes.

DOSAGE: *Adults:* Usual: 150-200mg as a single IM injection. IV: 100mg (commonly used initial dose for 70kg adult); if needed additional small increments may be given up to 200-500mg total dose. Rate of IV injection should not exceed 50mg/min. Elderly/ Debilitated/Renal or Hepatic Impairment: Reduce dose.
Pediatrics: 2-6mg/kg as a single IM injection. Max: 100mg. IV: Proportional reduction in dosage. Slow IV injection is essential.

HOW SUPPLIED: Inj: 50mg/mL

CONTRAINDICATIONS: History of manifest or latent porphyria.

WARNINGS/PRECAUTIONS: May be habit forming; avoid abrupt cessation after prolonged use. Avoid rapid administration. Tolerance to hypnotic effect can occur. Prehepatic coma use not recommended. Use with caution in patients with chronic or acute pain, mental depression, suicidal tendencies, history of drug abuse or hepatic impairment. Monitor blood, liver and renal function. May impair mental/physical abilities. Avoid alcohol.

ADVERSE REACTIONS: Agitation, confusion, hyperkinesia, ataxia, CNS depression, somnolence, bradycardia, hypotension, nausea, vomiting, constipation, headache, hypersensitivity reactions, liver damage.

INTERACTIONS: May produce additive CNS depression with other CNS depressants (eg, other sedatives/hypnotics, antihistamines, tranquilizers, alcohol). May decrease levels of oral anticoagulants, corticosteroids, griseofulvin, and doxycycline. Dosage adjustments may be required for anticoagulants and corticosteroids. Variable effects on phenytoin and increased levels with valproic acid, sodium valproate; monitor blood levels and adjust dose appropriately. May decrease effects of estradiol; alternative contraceptive method should be suggested. Prolonged effect with MAOIs.

PREGNANCY: Category D, caution with nursing.

MECHANISM OF ACTION: Not established; barbiturates are nonslective CNS depressants; depress the sensory cortex, decrease motor activity, alter cerebellar function, and produce drowsiness, sedation, and hypnosis.

PHARMACOKINETICS: Distribution: Found in breast milk, crosses placental barrier. **Metabolism:** Liver. **Elimination:** Urine (25-50%, unchanged), feces; $T_{1/2}$=15-50 hrs.

NEOMYCIN/POLY B/HYDROCORTISONE OTIC
RX

hydrocortisone - neomycin - polymyxin B Sulfate (Various)

THERAPEUTIC CLASS: Antibacterial/corticosteroid combination

INDICATIONS: (Sol/Sus) Treatment of superficial bacterial infections of the external auditory canal. (Sus) Treatment of infections of mastoidectomy and fenestration cavities.

DOSAGE: *Adults:* Clean and dry ear canal. Dropper: 4 drops tid-qid for up to 10 days. Alternate Regimen: Insert cotton wick into ear canal, then saturate cotton. Repeat q4h to keep cotton moist. Replace wick q24h.
Pediatrics: Clean and dry ear canal. Dropper: 3 drops tid-qid for up to 10 days. Alternate Regimen: Insert cotton wick into ear canal, then saturate cotton. Repeat q4h to keep cotton moist. Replace wick q24h.

HOW SUPPLIED: Sol, Sus: (Neomycin-Hydrocortisone-Polymyxin B) 0.35%-1%-10,000 U/mL (10mL)

CONTRAINDICATIONS: Herpes simplex, vaccinia, and varicella infections.

WARNINGS/PRECAUTIONS: Caution with perforated eardrum, chronic otitis media. Prolonged use may result in secondary infection. Re-evaluate if no improvement after 1 week. D/C after 10 days. Solution contains sulfites. May cause cutaneous sensitization.

ADVERSE REACTIONS: Skin sensitization, burning, itching, irritation, dryness, folliculitis, hypertrichosis, acneiform eruptions, secondary infection.

PREGNANCY: Category C, caution in nursing.

MECHANISM OF ACTION: Neomycin, Polymyxin B: Anti-infective agents; provide anti-bacterial activity against susceptible organsims. Hydrocortisone: Corticosteroid; possesses anti-inflammatory activity and inhibits body's defense mechanism against infection.

NEOSPORIN + PAIN RELIEF MAXIMUM STRENGTH
OTC
bacitracin - neomycin - polymyxin B - pramoxine HCl (McNeil)

THERAPEUTIC CLASS: Antibacterial/analgesic

INDICATIONS: To help prevent infection and provide temporary relief of pain or discomfort in minor cuts, scrapes, and burns.

DOSAGE: *Adults:* Clean area and apply a small amount qd-tid. May cover with sterile bandage.
Pediatrics: ≥2 yrs: Clean area and apply a small amount qd-tid. May cover with sterile bandage.

HOW SUPPLIED: Cre: (Neomycin-Polymyxin-Pramoxine) 3.5mg-10,000 U-10mg/g (15g); Oint: (Bacitracin-Neomycin-Polymyxin-Pramoxine) 500 U-3.5mg-10,000 U-10mg/g (15g, 30g)

WARNINGS/PRECAUTIONS: Avoid eyes. Do not use over large areas. D/C if needed longer than 1 week, condition persists, worsens, or if a rash or other allergic reaction develops.

NEOSPORIN OINTMENT
OTC
bacitracin zinc - neomycin - polymyxin B Sulfate (McNeil)

THERAPEUTIC CLASS: Antibacterial combination

INDICATIONS: To help prevent infection in minor cuts, scrapes, and burns.

DOSAGE: *Adults:* Clean area and apply a small amount qd-tid. May cover with sterile bandage.
Pediatrics: Clean area and apply a small amount qd-tid. May cover with sterile bandage.

HOW SUPPLIED: Oint: (Neomycin-Polymyxin-Bacitracin) 3.5mg-5000 U-400 U/g (15g, 30g), (Neo To Go, 10 x 0.9g pkts)

WARNINGS/PRECAUTIONS: Avoid eyes. Do not use over large areas. D/C if condition persists, worsens, or if a rash or other allergic reaction develops, or if needed longer than 1 week.

PREGNANCY: Safety in pregnancy and nursing not known.

NESACAINE
RX
chloroprocaine HCl (Abraxis)

OTHER BRAND NAME: Nesacaine-MPF (Abraxis)

THERAPEUTIC CLASS: Local anesthetic

INDICATIONS: (Nesacaine) Production of local anesthesia by infiltration and peripheral nerve block. (Nesacaine-MPF) Production of local anesthesia by infiltration, peripheral and central nerve block, including lumbar and caudal epidural blocks.

DOSAGE: *Adults:* Dosage varies depending on procedure, vascularity of tissues, depth and duration of anesthesia, degree of muscle relaxation required, and patient physical condition. Max: 11mg/kg (800mg total dose) without epinephrine or 14mg/kg (1000mg total dose) with epinephrine. MPF: Caudal/Lumbar Epidural Block: Test dose: 3mL of 3% or 5mL of 2% prior to complete block. Caudal Epidural: 15-25mL of 2% or 3% solution. Repeat dose may be given at 40-60 min intervals. Lumbar Epidural: 2-2.5mL/segment of 2% or 3% solution. Usual: 15-25mL. Repeat doses of 2-6mL less than original dose at

40-50 min intervals. Elderly/Debilitated/Acutely Ill/Cardiac or Liver Disease: Reduce dose.

Pediatrics: >3 yrs: Max: 11mg/kg. Use 0.5-1% for infiltration and 1-1.5% for nerve block.

HOW SUPPLIED: Inj: 1%, 2%; (MPF) 2%, 3%

CONTRAINDICATIONS: Extreme caution with lumbar and caudal epidural anesthesia in existing neurological disease, spinal deformities, septicemia, severe HTN.

WARNINGS/PRECAUTIONS: Acidosis, cardiac arrest, death reported from delay in toxicity management. Nesacaine contains methylparaben and should not be used for lumbar or caudal epidural anesthesia. MPF formulation contains no preservative; discard any unused injection after initial use. Use lowest effective dose. Perform syringe aspiration to avoid intravascular injection. Caution with hepatic disease or impaired cardiovascular function. Monitor cardiovascular and respiratory vital signs and state of consciousness after each injection. Caution when local anesthetic injections containing a vasoconstrictor are used in areas of the body supplied by end arteries or having otherwise compromised blood supply; ischemic injury or necrosis may result with peripheral or hypertensive vascular disease due to exaggerated vasoconstrictor response. Do not rely on lack of corneal sensation after retrobulbar block to determine if patient is ready for surgery.

ADVERSE REACTIONS: Restlessness, anxiety, dizziness, tinnitus, blurred vision, tremors, convulsions, drowsiness, hypotension, bradycardia, ventricular arrhythmias, urticaria, pruritus, nausea, vomiting, loss of bladder/bowel control, loss of sexual function.

INTERACTIONS: Caution regarding toxic equivalence when using local anesthetic mixtures. Vasopressors, ergot-type oxytocic drugs may cause severe, persistent HTN or CVA. Anesthetic solutions containing epinephrine or norepinephrine with MAOIs, TCAs, or phenothiazines may produce severe, prolonged hypotension or HTN. Avoid sulfonamides.

PREGNANCY: Category C, caution in nursing.

MECHANISM OF ACTION: Local anesthetic agent; blocks the generation and conduction of nerve impulses, presumably by increasing the threshold for electrical excitation in the nerve by slowing the propagation of the nerve impulse and by reducing the rate of rise of the action potential.

PHARMACOKINETICS: Absorption: Rapid absorption. **Distribution:** Crosses placenta. **Metabolism:** (Rapid) by hydrolysis of the ester linkage by pseudocholinesterase. **Elimination:** Urine.

NEURONTIN   RX
gabapentin (Parke-Davis)

THERAPEUTIC CLASS: GABA analog

INDICATIONS: Adjunct therapy for partial seizures with or without secondary generalization in patients ≥12 yrs. Adjunct therapy for partial seizures in pediatrics 3-12 yrs. Management of postherpetic neuralgia (PHN).

DOSAGE: *Adults:* Epilepsy: Initial: 300mg tid. Titrate: Increase up to 1800mg/day. Max: 3600mg/day. PHN: 300mg single dose on Day 1, then 300mg bid on Day 2, and 300mg tid on Day 3. Increase further prn for pain. Max: 600mg tid. Renal Impairment: CrCl 30-59mL/min: 400-1400 mg/day. CrCl 15-29mL/min: 200-700 mg/day. CrCl 15mL/min: 100-300mg/day. CrCl <15 mL/min: Reduce dose in proportion to CrCl. Hemodialysis: Maint: Base on CrCl. Give supplemental dose (125-350mg) after 4 hrs of hemodialysis. Refer to prescribing information for dose-adjustment.

Pediatrics: Epilepsy: >12 yrs: Initial: 300mg tid. Titrate: Increase up to 1800mg/day. Max: 3600mg/day. 3-12 yrs: Initial: 10-15mg/kg/day given tid. Titrate: Increase over 3 days. Usual: 3-4 yrs: 40mg/kg/day given tid. ≥5 yrs: 25-35mg/kg/day given tid. Max: 50mg/kg/day. Renal Impairment: ≥12 yrs: CrCl 30-59mL/min: 400-1400 mg/day. CrCl 15-29mL/min: 200-700 mg/day. CrCl 15mL/min: 100-300mg/day. CrCl <15 mL/min: Reduce dose in proportion to CrCl. Hemodialysis: Maint: Base on CrCl. Give supplemental dose (125-350 mg) after 4 hrs of hemodialysis. Refer to prescribing information for dose-adjustment.

HOW SUPPLIED: Cap: 100mg, 300mg, 400mg; Sol: 250mg/5mL; Tab: 600mg*, 800mg*
*scored

WARNINGS/PRECAUTIONS: Avoid abrupt withdrawal. Possible tumorigenic potential. Sudden and unexplained deaths reported. Neuropsychiatric adverse events in pediatrics (3-12 yrs).

ADVERSE REACTIONS: Somnolence, dizziness, ataxia, nystagmus, fatigue, tremor, rhinitis, weight gain, nausea, vomiting, viral infection, fever, dysarthria, diplopia.

INTERACTIONS: Take 2 hrs after antacids. Increased levels with controlled-release morphine.

PREGNANCY: Category C, caution in nursing.

MECHANISM OF ACTION: Anticonvulsant; not established. Anticonvulsant activity: Suspected to bind to different areas of the brain including neocortex and hippocampus. Analgesic effects: Prevents allodynia and hyperalgesia.

PHARMACOKINETICS: Absorption: PO administration of variable doses resulted in different parameters. **Distribution:** V_d =58L; plasma protein binding (<3%); found in breast milk. **Metabolism:** Not appreciably metabolized. **Elimination:** Renal excretion (unchanged); $T_{1/2}$=5-7 hrs. Refer to PI for pediatric parameters.

NEXIUM RX
esomeprazole magnesium (AstraZeneca)

THERAPEUTIC CLASS: Proton pump inhibitor

INDICATIONS: Symptomatic treatment of GERD; healing and maintenance treatment of erosive esophagitis. Reduction in occurrence of gastric ulcers associated with continuous NSAID therapy in patients at risk for developing gastric ulcers. Adjunct therapy (with amoxicillin and clarithromycin) for *H.pylori* eradication to reduce the risk of duodenal ulcer recurrence. Long-term treatment of pathological hypersecretory conditions including Zollinger-Ellison syndrome.

DOSAGE: *Adults:* Erosive Esophagitis: Healing: 20mg or 40mg qd for 4-8 weeks; may extend treatment for 4-8 weeks if not healed. Maint: 20mg qd for up to 6 months. Risk Reduction of NSAID-Associated Gastric Ulcer: 20mg or 40mg qd for up to 6 months. Symptomatic GERD: 20mg qd for 4 weeks; may extend treatment for 4 weeks if symptoms do not resolve. *H.pylori:* Triple Therapy: 40mg qd + amoxicillin 1000mg bid + clarithromycin 500mg bid, all for 10 days. Zollinger-Ellison Syndrome: 40mg bid. Severe Hepatic Dysfunction: Max: 20mg/day. Take 1 hr before meals. Swallow capsule whole. Contents may be mixed with soft food (eg, applesauce, yogurt) that does not require chewing.
Pediatrics: GERD: 12-17 yrs: 20mg or 40mg qd for up to 8 weeks. 1-11 yrs: 10mg qd for up to 8 weeks. Erosive Esophagitis: 1-11 yrs: ≥20kg: 10mg or 20mg qd for 8 weeks. <20kg: 10mg qd for 8 weeks. Severe Hepatic Dysfunction: Max: 20mg/day. Take 1 hr before meals. Swallow capsule whole. Contents may be mixed with soft food (eg, applesauce, yogurt) that does not require chewing.

HOW SUPPLIED: Cap, Delayed-Release: 20mg, 40mg; Sus, Delayed-Release: 20mg, 40mg (granules/pkt).

CONTRAINDICATIONS: Hypersensitivity to substituted benzimidazoles. Clarithromycin is contraindicated with pimozide.

WARNINGS/PRECAUTIONS: Atrophic gastritis may occur. Symptomatic response does not preclude gastric malignancy.

ADVERSE REACTIONS: Headache, diarrhea, abdominal pain, constipation, nausea, flatulence, dry mouth.

INTERACTIONS: Potentiates diazepam. May alter absorption of pH-dependent drugs (eg, ketoconazole, digoxin, iron salts). May reduce levels of atazanavir when used concomitantly. Increased levels with amoxicillin and clarithromycin. Clarithromycin is contraindicated with pimozide. Concomitant use with warfarin may increase INR and PT.

PREGNANCY: Category B, not for use in nursing.

MECHANISM OF ACTION: Proton pump inhibitor; suppresses gastric acid secretion by specific inhibition of the H^+/K^+-ATPase in the gastric parietal cell.

PHARMACOKINETICS: Absorption: (40 mg) C_{max}=4.7µmol/L; T_{max}=1.6 hrs; AUC=12.6µmol•hr/L. (20mg) C_{max}=2.1µmol/L; T_{max}=1.6 hrs; AUC=4.2µmol•hr/L. **Distribu-**

tion: V_d=16L; plasma protein binding (97%). **Metabolism:** Liver (extensive) via CYP2C19, CYP3A4. **Elimination:** Urine (80%), feces; $T_{1/2}$=1-1.5 hrs. For pediatric parameters, refer to full PI.

NIFEREX
iron (Ther-Rx)
OTC

THERAPEUTIC CLASS: Iron supplement

INDICATIONS: Treatment of uncomplicated iron deficiency anemias.

DOSAGE: *Adults:* 1-2 tabs bid or 5-10mL qd.
Pediatrics: ≥6 yrs: 1-2 tabs qd or 5mL qd. <6 yrs: (Sol): Individualize dose.

HOW SUPPLIED: Cap: 60mg; Sol: 100mg/5mL

WARNINGS/PRECAUTIONS: Fatal poisoning reported in children <6 yrs with accidental overdose of iron-containing products.

PREGNANCY: Safety in pregnancy and nursing not known.

NIMBEX
cisatracurium besylate (Abbott)
RX

THERAPEUTIC CLASS: Skeletal muscle relaxant (nondepolarizing)

INDICATIONS: Adjunct to general anesthesia, to facilitate tracheal intubation, and to provide skeletal muscle relaxation during surgery/mechanical ventilation.

DOSAGE: *Adults:* Initial: 0.15mg/kg (3 x ED$_{95}$) or 0.20mg/kg (4 x ED$_{95}$) IV. Serious Cardiovascular Disease: Up to 8 x ED$_{95}$. Maint/Prolonged Surgical Procedures: 0.03mg/kg IV (for 20 min blockade) 40-50 min after initial 0.15mg/kg, and 50-60 min after initial 0.20mg/kg. Operating Room Infusion: After initial bolus dose, give 3mcg/kg/min to counteract recovery from bolus, then 1-2mcg/kg/min. ICU: 3mcg/kg/min IV; dose requirements may increase/decrease with time.
Pediatrics: >12 yrs: Initial: 0.15mg/kg (3 x ED$_{95}$) or 0.20mg/kg (4 x ED$_{95}$) IV. Serious Cardiovascular Disease: Up to 8 x ED$_{95}$. Maint/Prolonged Surgical Procedures: 0.03mg/kg IV (for 20 min blockade) 40-50 min after initial 0.15mg/kg, and 50-60 min after initial 0.20mg/kg. 2-12 yrs: Initial: 0.10-0.15mg/kg over 5-10 seconds during halothane or opioid anesthesia. (1-23 months): Initial: 0.15mg/kg over 5-10 sec during halothane or opioid anesthesia. (≥ 2 yrs): Operating Room Infusion: After initial bolus dose, give 3mcg/kg/min to counteract recovery from bolus, then 1-2mcg/kg/min.

HOW SUPPLIED: Inj: 2mg/mL, 10mg/mL

CONTRAINDICATIONS: Hypersensitivity to bisbenzylisoquinolinium agents and benzyl alcohol.

WARNINGS/PRECAUTIONS: Avoid administration before unconsciousness has been induced. Use in facility with resuscitation and life support, and have antagonist available. Monitor neuromuscular function with peripheral nerve stimulator during administration. Multi-dose vials contain benzyl alcohol. Not for rapid sequence endotracheal intubation. May have profound effect with neuromuscular diseases (eg, myasthenia gravis, carcinomatosis); monitor neuromuscular function with peripheral nerve stimulator. Resistance may develop in burn victims; consider increasing dose. Resistance with hemiparesis or paraparesis. Acid-base and/or serum electrolyte abnormalities may potentiate or antagonize effect. Monitor for malignant hyperthermia.

ADVERSE REACTIONS: Bradycardia, hypotension, flushing, bronchospasm, rash, muscle weakness, myopathy, prolonged/inadequate neuromuscular blockade.

INTERACTIONS: Prolonged duration of action and required infusion rate decreased with isoflurane or enflurane with nitrous oxide/oxygen. Enhanced neuromuscular blocking action with certain antibiotics (eg, aminoglycosides, tetracyclines, bacitracin, polymyxins, lincomycin, clindamycin, colistin, sodium colistimethate), magnesium salts, lithium, local anesthetics, procainamide, and quinidine. Antagonized effect with phenytoin and carbamazepine. May not be compatible with pH >8.5 alkaline solutions (eg, barbiturate solutions).

PREGNANCY: Category B, caution in nursing.

MECHANISM OF ACTION: Non depolarizing skeletal muscle relaxant; binds competitively to cholinergic receptors on the motor end-plate to antagonize the action of acetylcholine, resulting in block of neuromuscular transmission.

PHARMACOKINETICS: Distribution: V_d=145mL/kg. **Metabolism:** Laudanosine (major active metabolite). **Elimination:** Hoffmann elimination (80%); hepatic/renal elemination (20%). Urine (95% metabolites), (<10% unchanged), feces (4%); $T_{1/2}$=22-29 min.

NIX
OTC
permethrin (Insight Pharmaceuticals)

THERAPEUTIC CLASS: Pyrethroid pediculicide

INDICATIONS: (Liquid) Treatment of head lice and prophylactic use during epidemics (at least 20% of population are infested). (Spray) To kill lice on bedding and furniture. Not for use in humans.

DOSAGE: *Adults:* (Liquid) Treatment: Wash then towel dry hair. Apply liquid and saturate hair and scalp. Rinse with water after 10 min. Remove nits with comb provided. Repeat after 7 days if live lice is observed. Prophylaxis: Same as treatment. Repeat therapy after 2 weeks in epidemic setting. (Spray) Use from an 8-10 inch distance. Treat only garments, bedding, and furniture that cannot be washed or dry cleaned. Allow area to dry completely.
Pediatrics: ≥2 months: (Liquid) Treatment: Wash and dry hair, then saturate hair and scalp. Rinse with water after 10 min. Remove nits with comb provided. Repeat after 7 days if observe lice. Prophylaxis: Same as treatment. Do not use nit comb.

HOW SUPPLIED: Liq: (Creme Rinse) 1% (60mL); Spray: 0.25% (148mL)

WARNINGS/PRECAUTIONS: (Liquid) Protect from getting into eyes, inside nose, mouth, or vagina. May cause breathing difficulty or asthmatic episodes in susceptible persons. D/C if skin irritation persists or infection develops. (Spray) Do not use in food serving areas or while food is exposed. Do not apply in classrooms while in use.

ADVERSE REACTIONS: Itching, redness, swelling of the scalp.

PREGNANCY: Safety in pregnancy and nursing not known.

NIZORAL
RX
ketoconazole (Janssen)

> Risk of fatal hepatotoxicity. Concomitant terfenadine, astemizole and cisapride are contraindicated due to serious cardiovascular adverse events.

THERAPEUTIC CLASS: Azole antifungal

INDICATIONS: Treatment of the following systemic fungal infections: candidiasis, chronic mucocutaneous candidiasis, oral thrush, candiduria, blastomycosis, coccidioidomycosis, histoplasmosis, chromomycosis, and paracoccidioidomycosis. Treatment of severe recalcitrant cutaneous dermatophyte infections not responsive to topical therapy or oral griseofulvin. Not for treatment of fungal meningitis.

DOSAGE: *Adults:* Initial: 200mg qd. Max: 400mg qd.
Pediatrics: >2 yrs: 3.3-6.6mg/kg/day.

HOW SUPPLIED: Tab: 200mg* *scored

CONTRAINDICATIONS: Concomitant terfenadine, astemizole, cisapride or oral triazolam.

WARNINGS/PRECAUTIONS: Hepatotoxicity reported. Monitor LFTs prior to therapy and periodically thereafter. Serum testosterone levels may be lowered. Hypersensitivity reactions reported. Tablets require acidity for dissolution. Not for use in children unless benefit outweighs risk.

ADVERSE REACTIONS: NV, abdominal pain, pruritus.

INTERACTIONS: See Contraindications. Give antacids, anticholinergics, and H_2 blockers 2 hrs after ketoconazole. May potentiate midazolam, triazolam, oral hypoglycemics. May enhance anticoagulant effect of coumarin-like drugs. Avoid rifampin, isoniazid. Monitor digoxin, phenytoin. May alter metabolism of cyclosporine, tacrolimus, methylprednisolone and drugs metabolized by CYP3A4.

PREGNANCY: Category C, not for use in nursing.

MECHANISM OF ACTION: Azole antifungal; impairs synthesis of ergosterol, a vital component of fungal cell membranes.

PHARMACOKINETICS: Absorption: C_{max}=3.5µg/mL; T_{max}=1-2 hrs. **Distribution:** Plasma protein binding (99%). **Metabolism:** Via oxidation, degradation of imidazole and piperazine rings, oxidative dealkylation and aromatic hydroxylation. CYP3A4 inhibitor. **Elimination:** Biphasic. $T_{1/2}$=2 hrs (during first 10 hrs); $T_{1/2}$=8 hrs (thereafter); bile (major), urine (13%).

NIZORAL A-D

OTC

ketoconazole (McNeil Consumer)

THERAPEUTIC CLASS: Azole antifungal

INDICATIONS: Controls flaking, scaling and itching associated with dandruff.

DOSAGE: *Adults:* Wet hair. Apply and lather. Rinse thoroughly and repeat. Apply every 3-4 days up to 8 weeks if needed.
Pediatrics: >12 yrs: Wet hair. Apply and lather. Rinse thoroughly and repeat. Apply every 3-4 days up to 8 weeks if needed.

HOW SUPPLIED: Shampoo: 1% (4oz, 7oz)

CONTRAINDICATIONS: Scalp that is broken or inflamed.

WARNINGS/PRECAUTIONS: Avoid eyes. D/C if rash appears, or if condition worsens or does not improve in 2-4 weeks.

PREGNANCY: Use in pregnancy and nursing not known.

NORDITROPIN

RX

somatropin (Novo Nordisk)

OTHER BRAND NAME: Norditropin Nordiflex (Novo Nordisk)

THERAPEUTIC CLASS: Human growth hormone

INDICATIONS: (Adults) Replacement of endogenous growth hormone deficiency who meet either of the following criteria: (1) adult onset-patients with growth hormone deficiency, either alone or associated with multiple hormone deficiencies (hypopituitarism), as a result of pituitary disease, hypothalamic disease, surgery, radiation therapy, or trauma; or (2) childhood onset-patients who were growth hormone deficient during childhood should have growth hormone deficiency confirmed as an adult before replacement therapy is started. (Pediatrics) Long-term treatment of children with growth failure due to inadequate growth hormone secretion. Treatment of children with short stature associated with Noonan syndrome and Turner syndrome.

DOSAGE: *Adults: Initial:* No more than 0.004mg/kg/day. Increase to no more than 0.016mg/kg/day after 6 weeks.
Pediatrics: Growth Hormone Deficiency: 0.024-0.034mg/kg SQ 6-7x/week. Noonan Syndrome: Dose up to 0.066mg/kg/day. Turner Syndrome: Dose up to 0.067mg/kg/day.

HOW SUPPLIED: Inj: (Norditropin (cartridge) and Norditropin Nordiflex (prefilled pen)) 5mg/1.5mL, 10mg/1.5ml, 15mg/1.5mL

CONTRAINDICATIONS: Presence of active neoplasia; acute critical illness due to complications following open heart or abdominal surgery, multiple accidental trauma or acute respiratory failure; proliferative or preproliferative diabetic retinopathy; closed epiphyses; and Prader-Willi syndrome with severe obesity or severe respiratory impairment.

WARNINGS/PRECAUTIONS: Monitor for recurrence or progression of underlying disease in growth hormone deficiency secondary to intracranial lesions. Hypothyroidism reported. May develop slipped capital epiphyses. Intracranial HTN with papilledema, visual changes, headache, nausea, and vomiting reported. Progression of scoliosis may occur in rapid growth. Monitor for any form of malignant skin lesion prior to and during therapy. May decrease insulin sensitivity; monitor blood sugar. Dose dependent/transient fluid retention may occur. Increased occurrence of otitis media in patients with Turner syndrome. Monitor closely for cardiovascular disorders (e.g., stroke, aortic aneurysm/dissection, hypertension).

ADVERSE REACTIONS: (Pediatrics) Headache, injection site reaction, localized muscle pain, rash, weakness, mild hyperglycemia, glucosuria, arthralgia, leukemia. (Adults) Edema, arthralgia, myalgia, infection, parasthesia, skeletal pain, headache, bronchitis.

INTERACTIONS: Diminished effects with glucocorticoid therapy. Insulin resistance reported. May reduce plasma levels of oral estrogens.

PREGNANCY: Category C, caution in nursing.

MECHANISM OF ACTION: Human growth hormone; binds to dimeric GH receptor in cell membrane of target cells resulting in intracellular signal transduction.

PHARMACOKINETICS: Absorption: T_{max}=4-5 hrs; (4mg) C_{max}=13.8ng/mL; (8mg) C_{max}=17.1ng/mL. **Elimination:** $T_{1/2}$=7-10 hrs.

NORPACE
RX

disopyramide phosphate (Pharmacia & Upjohn)

OTHER BRAND NAME: Norpace CR (Pharmacia & Upjohn)

THERAPEUTIC CLASS: Class I antiarrhythmic

INDICATIONS: Treatment of documented life-threatening ventricular arrhythmias.

DOSAGE: *Adults:* Usual: 400-800mg/day in divided dose. Recommended: 150mg q6h immediate-release (IR) or 300mg q12h extended-release (CR). Adjust dose with anticholinergic effects. Weight <110lbs/Moderate Hepatic or Renal Insufficiency (CrCl >40mL/min): 100mg q6h IR or 200mg q12h CR. Severe Renal Insufficiency (with or without initial 150mg LD): CrCl 30-40mL/min: 100mg q8h IR. CrCl 30-15mL/min: 100mg q12h IR. CrCl <15mL/min: 100mg q24h IR. Rapid Control of Ventricular Arrhythmia: LD: 300mg IR (200mg if <110lbs). Follow with maint dose. Cardiomyopathy/Cardiac Decompensation: Initial: 100mg q6-8h IR. Adjust gradually. See PI if no response or toxicity occurs. Elderly: Start at low end of dosing range.
Pediatrics: <1 yr: 10-30mg/kg/day. 1-4 yrs: 10-20mg/kg/day. 4-12 yrs: 10-15mg/kg/day. 12-18 yrs: 6-15mg/kg/day. Give in equally divided doses q6h. Hospitalize patient during initial therapy. Start dose titration at lower end of range.

HOW SUPPLIED: Cap: (Norpace) 100mg, 150mg; Cap, Extended-Release: (Norpace CR) 100mg, 150mg

CONTRAINDICATIONS: Cardiogenic shock, 2nd- or 3rd-degree AV block (if no pacemaker present), congenital QT prolongation.

WARNINGS/PRECAUTIONS: Proarrhythmic; reserve for life-threatening ventricular arrhythmias. May cause or worsen CHF and produce hypotension due to negative inotropic properties. Reduce dose if 1st-degree heart block occurs. Avoid with urinary retention, glaucoma, and myasthenia gravis unless adequate overriding measures taken. Atrial flutter/fibrillation; digitalize first. Monitor closely or withdraw if QT prolongation >25% occurs and ectopy continues. D/C if QRS widening >25% occurs. Avoid LD with cardiomyopathy or cardiac decompensation. Correct K⁺ abnormalities before therapy. Reduce dose with renal/hepatic dysfunction; monitor ECG. Avoid CR formulation with CrCl ≤40mL/min. Caution with sick sinus syndrome, Wolff-Parkinson-White syndrome, bundle branch block, or elderly. May significantly lower blood glucose.

ADVERSE REACTIONS: Dry mouth, urinary retention/frequency/urgency, constipation, blurred vision, GI effects, dizziness, fatigue, headache.

INTERACTIONS: Avoid type IA and IC antiarrhythmics, and propranolol except in unresponsive, life-threatening arrhythmias. Hepatic enzyme inducers may lower levels. Avoid within 48 hrs before or 24 hrs after verapamil. Possible fatal interactions with CYP3A4 inhibitors. Monitor blood glucose with β-blockers, alcohol.

PREGNANCY: Category C, not for use in nursing.

MECHANISM OF ACTION: Type I antiarrhythmic; decreases rate of diastolic depolarization in cells with augmented automaticity, decreases upstroke velocity, and increases action potential duration of normal cardiac cells. Decreases disparity in refractoriness between infracted and adjacent normally perfused myocardium and has no effect on α- or β-adrenergic receptors.

PHARMACOKINETICS: Absorption: Rapid and complete; C_{max}=2.22mcg/mL, T_{max}=4.5 hrs. **Distribution:** Plasma protein binding (50-65%). **Metabolism:** Liver. **Elimination:** Urine (50% unchanged), (20% mono-N-dealkylated metabolite), (10% other metabolite); $T_{1/2}$=11.65 hrs.

NORVASC

RX

amlodipine besylate (Pfizer)

THERAPEUTIC CLASS: Calcium channel blocker (dihydropyridine)

INDICATIONS: Treatment of hypertension and Coronary Artery Disease (CAD) including chronic stable or vasospastic angina (Prinzmetal's or Variant Angina).

DOSAGE: *Adults:* HTN: Initial: 5mg qd. Titrate over 7-14 days. Max: 10mg qd. Small, Fragile, or Elderly/Hepatic Dysfunction/Concomitant Antihypertensive: Initial: 2.5mg qd. Angina: 5-10mg qd. Elderly/Hepatic Dysfunction: 5mg qd. CAD: 5-10mg qd.
Pediatrics: 6-17 yrs: HTN: 2.5-5mg qd.

HOW SUPPLIED: Tab: 2.5mg, 5mg, 10mg

WARNINGS/PRECAUTIONS: May increase angina or MI with severe obstructive CAD. Caution with severe aortic stenosis, CHF, severe hepatic impairment, and in elderly.

ADVERSE REACTIONS: Edema, flushing, palpitation, dizziness, headache, fatigue.

PREGNANCY: Category C, not for use in nursing.

MECHANISM OF ACTION: A dihydropyridine calcium antagonist (calcium ion antagonist or slow-channel blocker) that inhibits transmembrane influx or calcium ions into vascular smooth muscle and cardiac muscle. Binds to both dihydropyridine and nondihydropyridine binding sites which results in peripheral arterial vasodilation and reduction in BP.

PHARMACOKINETICS: **Absorption:** Absolute bioavailability (64-90%); T_{max}=6-12 hrs. **Distribution:** Plasma protein binding (93%). **Metabolism:** Hepatic. **Elimination:** Urine, $T_{1/2}$=30-50 hrs.

NORVIR

RX

ritonavir (Abbott)

> **Use with certain non-sedating antihistamines, sedative hypnotics, antiarrhythmics, or ergot alkaloids may result in life-threatening adverse events.**

THERAPEUTIC CLASS: Protease inhibitor

INDICATIONS: Treatment of HIV infection in combination with other antiretrovirals.

DOSAGE: *Adults:* Initial: 300mg bid. Titrate: Increase every 2-3 days by 100mg bid. Maint: 600mg bid. If combined with saquinavir, adjust dose to 400mg bid. Elderly: Start at low end of dosing range. Take with meals if possible.
Pediatrics: >1 month: Initial: 250mg/m² po bid. Titrate: Increase by 50mg/m² every 2-3 days. Maint: 350-400mg/m² po bid or highest tolerated dose. Max: 600mg bid.

HOW SUPPLIED: Cap: 100mg; Sol: 80mg/mL (240mL)

CONTRAINDICATIONS: Alfuzosin, amiodarone, bepridil, flecainide, propafenone, quinidine, voriconazole, astemizole, terfenadine, ergot derivatives, midazolam, triazolam, cisapride, pimozide, dihydroergotamine, ergonovine, ergotamine, methylergonovine, midazolam, triazolam.

WARNINGS/PRECAUTIONS: Allergic reactions (eg, urticaria, mild skin eruptions, bronchospasm, and angioedema), pancreatitis, new onset/exacerbation of pre-existing diabetes mellitus, hyperglycemia, immune reconstitution syndrome, hepatic transaminase elevations and hepatic dysfunction reported. Caution with moderate to severe hepatic impairment and in elderly. Monitor LFTs, especially 1st three months. Increased bleeding may occur with hemophilia A and B. Possible redistribution or accumulation of body fat. May increase total triglyceride and cholesterol levels.

ADVERSE REACTIONS: Diarrhea, anorexia, NV, abdominal pain, asthenia, headache, malaise, vasodilation, constipation, dizziness, taste perversion, peripheral paresthesia.

INTERACTIONS: See Contraindications. Avoid use with rifampin, St. John's wort; may cause loss of virologic response and resistance. Avoid use with lovastatin and simvastatin; risk of myopathy and rhabdomyolysis. Neurologic and cardiac events reported with disopyramide, mexiletine, nefazodone, fluoxetine, and β-blockers. Concomitant use with tipranavir may cause hepatitis and hepatic decompensation. May increase levels of saquinavir, atazanavir, darunavir, fosamprenavir, desipramine, indinavir, rifabutin. May increase levels of clarithromycin with renal impairment; reduce clarithromycin dose by 50% if CrCl 30-60mL/min and by 75% if CrCl<30mL/min. May increase ketoconazole levels; avoid ketoconazole doses >200mg/day. May increase sildenafil levels; do not exceed sildenafil 25mg/48 hrs. May increase levels of tramadol, propoxyphene, disopyramide, lidocaine, mexiletine, carbamazepine, clonazepam, eth-osuximide, bupropion, nefazodone, SSRIs, TCAs, dronabinol, itraconazole, quinine, metoprolol, timolol, diltiazem, nifedipine, verapamil, atorvastatin, rosuvastatin, cyclo-sporine, tacrolimus, sirolimus, perphenazine, risperidone, thioridazine, clorazepate, diaz-epam, estazolam, flurazepam, zolpidem, dexamethasone, fluticasone, prednisone, methamphetamine. May increase levels of trazodone; use with caution and consider lower trazodone dose. Decreases levels of theophylline, meperidine, methadone. May decrease levels of phenytoin, divalproex, lamotrigine, and atovaquone. Separate dos-ing with didanosine by 2.5 hrs. May increase plasma levels of drugs metabolized by CYP3A or CYP2D6. May decrease ethinyl estradiol levels; use alternative contraceptive measures. Monitor PT/INR with warfarin. Contains alcohol; may produce disulfiram-like reactions with disulfiram, metronidazole.

PREGNANCY: Category B, not for use in nursing.

MECHANISM OF ACTION: HIV protease inhibitor; renders enzyme incapable of process-ing *gag-pol* polyprotein precursor, which leads to production of non-infectious imma-ture HIV particles.

PHARMACOKINETICS: Absorption: C_{max}=11.2mcg/mL; T_{max}=2 hrs (fasting), 4 hrs (fed); AUC=121.7mcg•h/mL (Cap), 129mcg•hr/mL (Sol). **Metabolism:** CYP3A, 2D6 (oxidation); isopropylthiazole (major metabolite). **Elimination:** Urine (3.5%), feces (33.8%); $T_{1/2}$=3-5 hrs.

NOVACORT RX
hydrocortisone acetate - pramoxine HCl (Primus)

THERAPEUTIC CLASS: Corticosteroid/anesthetic

INDICATIONS: Relief of the inflammatory and pruritic manifestations of corticosteroid-responsive dermatoses.

DOSAGE: *Adults:* Apply to affected area(s) tid-qid. May use occlusive dressings for pso-riasis or recalcitrant conditions. D/C dressings if infection develops.
Pediatrics: Apply to affected area(s) tid-qid. May use occlusive dressings for psoriasis or recalcitrant conditions. D/C dressings if infection develops.

HOW SUPPLIED: Gel: (Hydrocortisone-Pramoxine) 2%-1% (29g)

WARNINGS/PRECAUTIONS: May produce reversible HPA axis suppression, manifestations of Cushing's syndrome, hyperglycemia, and glucosuria. Caution when applied to large surface areas, under occlusive dressings, or with prolonged use. Use appropriate anti-fungal or antibacterial agent with dermatological infections; d/c if infection does not clear. Pediatrics may be more susceptible to systemic toxicity. D/C if irritation develops. Avoid eyes.

ADVERSE REACTIONS: Burning, itching, irritation, dryness, folliculitis, hypertrichosis, acnei-form eruptions, hypopigmentation, perioral dermatitis, allergic dermatitis, skin macera-tion, secondary infection, skin atrophy, striae, miliaria.

PREGNANCY: Category C, caution in nursing.

MECHANISM OF ACTION: Topical corticosteroid/anesthetic. Hydrocortisone: Possesses anti-inflammatory, anti-pruritic, and vasoconstrictive properties. Anti-inflammatory mechanism not established. Pramoxine: Stabilizes neuronal membrane of nerve end-ings with which it comes into contact.

PHARMACOKINETICS: Absorption: Percutaneous; occlusion, inflammation, other disease states may increase absorption. **Distribution:** Bound to plasma protein in varying degrees. Systemically administered corticosteroids found in breast milk. **Metabolism:** Liver. **Elimination:** Kidney (major), bile.

NOVAREL RX
chorionic gonadotropin (Ferring)

THERAPEUTIC CLASS: Human chorionic gonadotropin

INDICATIONS: For prepubertal cryptorchidism not due to anatomic obstruction. For hypogonadotropic hypogonadism (secondary to a pituitary deficiency) in males. To induce ovulation (OI) and pregnancy in anovulatory, infertile women in whom anovulation is not due to primary ovarian failure and pretreated with human menotropins.

DOSAGE: *Adults:* Hypogonadism: 500-1000 U IM 3x/week (TIW) for 3 weeks, then twice weekly for 3 weeks; or 4000 U IM TIW for 6-9 months, then reduce to 2000 U TIW for 3 months. OI: 5000-10,000 U IM 1 day after last dose of menotropins.
Pediatrics: ≥4 yrs: Cryptorchidism: 4000 U IM TIW for 3 weeks; or 5000 U IM every 2nd day for 4 doses; or 15 doses of 500-1000 U over 6 weeks; or 500 U TIW for 4-6 weeks (if treatment fails, give 1000 U/injection starting 1 month later). Initiate therapy between 4-9 yrs. Hypogonadism: 500-1000 U IM TIW for 3 weeks, then twice weekly for 3 weeks; or 4000 U IM TIW for 6-9 months, then reduce to 2000 U TIW for 3 months.

HOW SUPPLIED: Inj: 10,000 U

CONTRAINDICATIONS: Precocious puberty, prostatic carcinoma or other androgen-dependent neoplasms, pregnancy.

WARNINGS/PRECAUTIONS: Potential ovarian hyperstimulation, enlargement or rupture of ovarian cysts, multiple births, and arterial thromboembolism with infertility treatment. D/C if precocious puberty occurs in cryptorchidism patients. Caution with cardiac or renal disease, epilepsy, migraine, asthma. Not effective treatment for obesity.

ADVERSE REACTIONS: Headache, irritability, restlessness, depression, fatigue, edema, precocious puberty, gynecomastia, injection site pain.

PREGNANCY: Category C, caution in nursing.

MECHANISM OF ACTION: Human chorionic gonadotropin; stimulates production of gonadal steriod hormones by stimulating the interstitial cells (leydig cells) of testis to produce androgens and the corpus luteum of the ovary to produce progesterone.

NOVOLIN OTC
insulin human, rDNA origin - insulin, human isophane - insulin, human regular (Novo Nordisk)

OTHER BRAND NAMES: Novolin N (Novo Nordisk) - Novolin R (Novo Nordisk)
THERAPEUTIC CLASS: Insulin

INDICATIONS: To control hyperglycemia in diabetes.

DOSAGE: *Adults:* Individualize dose.
Pediatrics: Individualize dose.

HOW SUPPLIED: Inj: 100 U/mL (Novolin N, Novolin R); PenFill: 100 U/mL (Novolin N, Novolin R); Prefilled: 100 U/mL (Novolin N, Novolin R)

WARNINGS/PRECAUTIONS: Human insulin differs from animal source insulin. Any change in insulin should be made cautiously. Changes in strength, manufacturer, type or method of manufacture may result in the need for a change in dosage. Hypoglycemia may occur with taking too much insulin, missing or delaying meals, exercising or working more than usual. An infection or illness (especially if accompanied by diarrhea or vomiting) may change insulin requirements. Administration of insulin SQ can result in lipoatrophy. Novolin R is not recommended for use in insulin pumps.

ADVERSE REACTIONS: Hypoglycemia, sweating, dizziness, palpitations, tremor, hunger, restlessness, lightheadedness, inability to concentrate, headache, injection-site reaction, allergic reaction.

INTERACTIONS: Increased insulin requirements with oral contraceptives, corticosteroids, or thyroid replacement therapy. Reduced insulin requirements with oral hypoglycemics, salicylates, sulfa antibiotics, and certain antidepressants. Alcoholic beverages may change insulin requirements. β-blockers may mask symptoms of hypoglycemia.

PREGNANCY: Pregnancy category is not known.

MECHANISM OF ACTION: Insulin (rDNA origin); regulates glucose metabolism, lowers blood glucose by facilitating cellular uptake of glucose and simultaneously inhibiting the glucose output from the liver.

NOVOLOG

RX

insulin aspart (Novo Nordisk)

THERAPEUTIC CLASS: Insulin

INDICATIONS: To control hyperglycemia in diabetes.

DOSAGE: *Adults:* Individualize dose. Inject SQ within 5-10 min before a meal. Draw first when mixing with NPH human insulin; inject immediately. Do not mix with crystalline zinc insulins, animal source insulins, or other manufacturer insulins. (External Pump) Do not use or mix with any other insulin or diluent in pump.
Pediatrics: ≥4 yrs: Individualize dose. Inject SQ within 5-10 min before a meal. Draw first when mixing with NPH human insulin; inject immediately. Do not mix with crystalline zinc insulins, animal source insulins, or other manufacturer insulins. (External Pump) Do not use or mix with any other insulin or diluent in pump.

HOW SUPPLIED: Inj: 100 U/mL; PenFill: 100 U/mL; Prefilled: 100 U/mL

CONTRAINDICATIONS: Hypoglycemia.

WARNINGS/PRECAUTIONS: Any change of insulin should be made cautiously. Changes in strength, manufacturer, type or method of manufacture may result in the need for a change in dosage. Hypoglycemia may occur with taking too much insulin, missing or delaying meals, exercising or working more than usual, diseases of adrenal, pituitary, or thyroid glands, or progression of kidney or liver disease. May cause hypokalemia. Dosage adjustments may be needed with hepatic or renal dysfunction, during any infection, illness (especially with diarrhea or vomiting) or pregnancy. A longer-acting insulin is usually required to maintain adequate glucose control. Infusion sets and the insulin in the infusion sets should be changed q48h or sooner. Do not use in quick-release infusion sets or cartridge adapters.

ADVERSE REACTIONS: Hypoglycemia, hypokalemia, lipodystrophy, hypersensitivity reaction, injection site reactions, pruritus, rash.

INTERACTIONS: Increased glucose lowering effects with ACE inhibitors, disopyramide, fibrates, fluoxetine, MAOIs, propoxyphene, salicylates, somatostatin analog, sulfonamide antibiotics and other antidiabetic agents. Decreased blood glucose lowering effects with corticosteroids, niacin, danazol, diuretics, sympathomimetic agents, isoniazid, phenothiazine derivatives, somatropin, thyroid hormones, estrogens, progesterones. Pentamidine may cause hypoglycemia followed by hyperglycemia. β-blockers, clonidine, lithium salts, and alcohol may potentiate or weaken glucose lowering effect. Masked or reduced hypoglycemic symptoms with β-blockers, clonidine, guanethidine, and reserpine.

PREGNANCY: Category B, caution in nursing.

MECHANISM OF ACTION: Insulin aspart (rDNAorigin); regulates glucose metabolism, lowers blood glucose by facilitating cellular uptake of glucose and simultaneously inhibiting glucose output from the liver.

PHARMACOKINETICS: Absorption: C_{max}=82.1 mU/L; T_{max}=40-50 min. **Distribution:** Plasma protein binding (0-9%). **Elimination:** $T_{1/2}$=81 min.

NOXAFIL

RX

posaconazole (Schering)

THERAPEUTIC CLASS: Azole antifungal

INDICATIONS: Prophylaxis of invasive *Aspergillus* and *Candida* infections in patients, ≥13 yrs, who are at high risk of developing these infections due to being severely immunocompromised. Treatment of oropharyngeal candidiasis, including oropharyngeal candidiasis refractory to itraconazole and/or fluconazole.

DOSAGE: *Adults:* Prophylaxis of Invasive Fungal Infections: 200mg (5mL) tid. Base duration of therapy on recovery from neutropenia or immunosuppression. Oropharyngeal Candidiasis: LD: 100mg (2.5mL) bid on 1st day, then 100mg qd for 13 days. Oropharyngeal Candidiasis Refractory to Itraconazole and/or Fluconazole: 400mg (10mL) bid.

Base duration of therapy on severity of underlying disease and clinical response. Give each dose with full meal or nutritional supplement.
Pediatrics: ≥13 yrs: Prophylaxis of Invasive Fungal Infections: 200mg (5mL) tid. Base duration of therapy on recovery from neutropenia or immunosuppression. Oropharyngeal Candidiasis: LD: 100mg (2.5mL) bid on 1st day, then 100mg qd for 13 days. Oropharyngeal Candidiasis Refractory to Itraconazole and/or Fluconazole: 400mg (10mL) bid. Base duration of therapy on severity of underlying disease and clinical response. Give each dose with full meal or nutritional supplement.

HOW SUPPLIED: Susp: 40mg/mL

CONTRAINDICATIONS: Concomitant ergot alkaloids, terfenadine, astemizole, cisapride, pimozide, halofantrine, or quinidine.

WARNINGS/PRECAUTIONS: Hepatic reactions (eg, mild to moderate elevations in ALT, AST, alkaline phosphatase, total bilirubin, and/or clinical hepatitis) reported; monitor LFTs at start of and during therapy. Caution with hepatic impairment. Monitor closely with severe renal impairment. Prolongation of QT interval reported; caution with potentially proarrhythmic conditions.

ADVERSE REACTIONS: Fever, headache, rigors, HTN, anemia, neutropenia, diarrhea, NV, abdominal pain, constipation, hypokalemia, thrombocytopenia, coughing, dyspnea.

INTERACTIONS: See Contraindications. May elevate cyclosporine and tacrolimus levels; consider dose reduction and more frequent clinical monitoring of cyclosporine, tacrolimus, and sirolimus when therapy is initiated. Avoid use with drugs that are known to prolong the QTc interval and are metabolized through CYP3A4. Avoid concurrent use of cimetidine, rifabutin, and phenytoin unless benefits outweigh risks. If concomitant phenytoin is required, monitor closely and consider phenytoin dose reduction. If concomitant rifabutin is required, monitor CBC and adverse events. Monitor adverse events with concomitant benzodiazepines metabolized by CYP3A4; consider dose reduction of these benzodiazepines during coadministration. May increase levels of vinca alkaloids; consider dose adjustment of vinca alkaloid. Consider dose reduction of concomitant HMG-CoA reductase inhibitors (statins). Monitor for adverse events and toxicity with concomitant CCBs; dose reduction of CCBs may be needed.

PREGNANCY: Category C, not for use in nursing.

MECHANISM OF ACTION: Antifungal agent; blocks synthesis of ergosterol, a key component of fungal cell membrane, through inhibition of the enzyme lanosterol 14α-demethylase and accumulation of methylated sterol precursors.

PHARMACOKINETICS: Administration: Oral administration of variable doses resulted in different parameters. **Distribution:** V_d=1774L, plasma protein binding (≥98%). **Metabolism:** Via UDP glucuronidation; CYP3A4 enzyme. **Elimination:** Feces (71%), urine (13%); $T_{1/2}$=35 hrs.

NUCOFED

codeine phosphate - pseudoephedrine HCl (King)

THERAPEUTIC CLASS: Antitussive/decongestant

INDICATIONS: Relief of cough and congestion associated with respiratory infections, bronchitis, influenza, and sinusitis.

DOSAGE: *Adults:* 1 cap q6h. Max: 4 caps/24 hrs.
Pediatrics: ≥12 yrs: 1 cap q6h. Max: 4 caps/24 hrs.

HOW SUPPLIED: (Codeine-Pseudoephedrine) Cap: 20mg-60mg; Syrup: 20mg-60mg/5mL

WARNINGS/PRECAUTIONS: Not for cough associated with smoking, emphysema, asthma, or excessive secretions. May cause constipation. Caution with pulmonary disease, shortness of breath, HTN, heart disease, DM, thyroid disease, prostatic hypertrophy, Addison's disease, children, ulcerative colitis, drug dependence, liver or kidney dysfunction. May impair alertness.

ADVERSE REACTIONS: Nervousness, restlessness, insomnia, drowsiness, dysuria, dizziness, headache, nausea, vomiting, constipation, trembling, dyspnea, sweating, paleness, weakness, heart rate changes.

INTERACTIONS: β-blockers, MAOIs, sympathomimetics may increase the effects of pseudoephedrine. Avoid within 14 days of MAOI use. TCAs may antagonize effects of pseudoephedrine. Caution with CNS depressants, general anesthetics, alcohol. Anticholinergics may cause paralytic ileus. Digitalis glycosides may cause cardiac arrhythmias. Decreases effects of antihypertensive agents.

PREGNANCY: Category C, caution in nursing.

MECHANISM OF ACTION: Codeine: Antitussive-decongestant; causes cough suppression by direct effect on the cough center in the medulla oblongata, exerts a drying effect on respiratory tract mucosa, increases viscosity of bronchial secretions. Pseudoephedrine: Directly stimulates α-adrenergic receptors, causing vasoconstriction. Directly stimulates β-adrenergic receptors to a lesser degree, causing bronchial smooth muscle relaxation.

PHARMACOKINETICS: Absorption: Codeine: GIT (well-absorbed). T_{max}=1-2 hrs. Pseudoephedrine: T_{max}=4-6 hrs. **Distribution:** Codeine: Found in breast milk; crosses placenta. Pseudoephedrine: Crosses placenta and enters CSF. **Metabolism**: Codeine: Liver (O-demethylation, N-demethylation, and partial conjugation with glucuronic acid). Pseudoephedrine: Liver (incomplete). N-demethylation. **Elimination**: Both in urine; pseudoephedrine (55-75% unchanged).

NUCOFED PEDIATRIC EXPECTORANT   `CV`
codeine phosphate - guaifenesin - pseudoephedrine HCI (King)

OTHER BRAND NAME: Mytussin DAC (Morton Grove)

THERAPEUTIC CLASS: Antitussive/expectorant/decongestant

INDICATIONS: Relief of cough and congestion associated with respiratory infections, bronchitis, influenza, and sinusitis.

DOSAGE: *Adults:* 10mL q6h. Max: 40mL/24 hrs.
Pediatrics: ≥12 yrs: 10mL q6h. Max: 40mL/24hrs. 6 to <12 yrs: 5mL q6h. Max: 20mL/24hrs. 2 to <6 yrs: 2.5mL q6h. Max: 10mL/24hrs.

HOW SUPPLIED: (Codeine-Guaifenesin-Pseudoephedrine) Syrup: 10mg-100mg-30mg/5mL

WARNINGS/PRECAUTIONS: Not for cough associated with smoking, emphysema, asthma, or excessive secretions. May cause constipation. Caution with pulmonary disease, shortness of breath, HTN, heart disease, DM, thyroid disease, prostatic hypertrophy, Addison's disease, children, ulcerative colitis, drug dependence, liver or kidney dysfunction. May impair alertness.

ADVERSE REACTIONS: Nervousness, restlessness, insomnia, drowsiness, dysuria, dizziness, headache, nausea, vomiting, constipation, trembling, dyspnea, sweating, paleness, weakness, heart rate changes.

INTERACTIONS: β-blockers, MAOIs, sympathomimetics may increase the effects of pseudoephedrine. Avoid within 14 days of MAOI use. TCAs may antagonize effects of pseudoephedrine. Caution with CNS depressants, general anesthetics, alcohol. Anticholinergics may cause paralytic ileus. Digitalis glycosides may cause cardiac arrhythmias. Decreases effects of antihypertensive agents.

PREGNANCY: Category C, caution in nursing.

NULYTELY   RX
polyethylene glycol 3350 - potassium chloride - sodium bicarbonate - sodium chloride (Braintree)

OTHER BRAND NAME: Trilyte (Schwarz Pharma)

THERAPEUTIC CLASS: Bowel cleanser

INDICATIONS: Bowel cleansing prior to colonoscopy.

DOSAGE: *Adults:* Oral: 240mL every 10 min until fecal discharge is clear or 4L is consumed. NG Tube: 20-30mL/min (1.2-1.8L/hr). Patient should fast at least 3-4 hours before administration.
Pediatrics: ≥6 months: Oral/Nasogastric Tube: 25mL/kg/hr until fecal discharge is clear. Patient should fast at least 3-4 hours before administration.

HOW SUPPLIED: Sol: (Polyethylene Glycol-Potassium Chloride-Sodium Bicarbonate-Sodium Chloride) 420g-1.48g-5.72g-11.2g (4000mL)

CONTRAINDICATIONS: GI obstruction, gastric retention, bowel perforation, toxic colitis, toxic megacolon, ileus.

WARNINGS/PRECAUTIONS: Do not add additional ingredients (eg, flavorings). Caution with severe ulcerative colitis. Monitor therapy with impaired gag reflex, unconsciousness/semiconsciousness and patients prone to regurgitation and aspiration. Temporarily d/c if develop severe bloating, distention, or abdominal pain. Monitor for hypoglycemia in pediatrics <2 yrs of age.

ADVERSE REACTIONS: Nausea, abdominal fullness/cramps, bloating, vomiting, anal irritation.

INTERACTIONS: Oral medications taken within 1 hr of start of administration may not be absorbed from GI tract.

PREGNANCY: Category C, caution in nursing.

MECHANISM OF ACTION: Osmotic laxative which induces diarrhea..

NUTROPIN   RX
somatropin (Genentech)

OTHER BRAND NAME: Nutropin AQ (Genentech)

THERAPEUTIC CLASS: Human growth hormone

INDICATIONS: (Adults) Replacement of endogenous growth hormone (GH) in GH deficiency (GHD). (Pediatrics) Long-term treatment of growth failure due to lack of adequate endogenous GH secretion, in short stature associated with Turner Syndrome, and in idiopathic short stature (ISS). Treatment of growth failure associated with chronic renal insufficiency (CRI) up to the time of renal transplantation.

DOSAGE: *Adults:* GHD: Initial: Up to 0.006mg/kg/day SQ. Max: <35 yrs: 0.025mg/kg/day. ≥35 yrs: 0.0125mg/kg/day. Alternatively may use 0.2mg/day (range: 0.15-0.30mg/day). Increase every 1-2 months by increments of 0.1-0.2mg/day.
Pediatrics: GHD: Usual: 0.3mg/kg/week divided into daily SQ doses. Pubertal Patients: Up to 0.7mg/kg/week divided into daily SQ doses. CRI: 0.35mg/kg/week divided into daily SQ doses. Continue until renal transplantation. Hemodialysis: Give qhs or 3-4 hrs post dialysis. Chronic Cycling Peritoneal Dialysis: Give in am after dialysis. Chronic Ambulatory Peritoneal Dialysis: Give qhs during overnight exchange. Turner Syndrome: Up to 0.375mg/kg/week SQ in divided doses 3-7x/week. ISS: 0.3mg/kg/week divided into daily SQ doses.

HOW SUPPLIED: Inj: 5mg, 10mg, (AQ) 5mg/mL

CONTRAINDICATIONS: Acute critical illness after serious surgeries (eg, open heart or abdominal surgery, accidental trauma, acute respiratory failure), closed epiphyses in pediatrics, active proliferative or severe non-proliferative diabetic retinopathy, active neoplasia, evidence of recurrence or progression of an intracranial tumor. Prader-Willi syndrome (unless also diagnosed with GH deficiency) with severe obesity or respiratory impairment.

WARNINGS/PRECAUTIONS: Caution with epiphyseal closure in adults treated with GH-replacement therapy in childhood. Recurrence/progression reported with intracranial lesions. Renal osteodystrophy may occur with growth failure secondary to renal impairment. Scoliosis and slipped capital femoral epiphysis may develop in rapid growth. Caution with Turner syndrome and ISS. Intracranial hypertension with papilledema, visual changes, headache, nausea, and/or vomiting has been reported. Funduscopic exam should be done before and during treatment. Monitor for malignant transformation of skin lesions. Injecting SQ in same site over long period of time may cause tissue atrophy. May decrease insulin sensitivity; monitor blood sugar.

ADVERSE REACTIONS: Antibodies to the protein, leukemia, transient peripheral edema, arthralgia, carpal tunnel syndrome, malignant transformations, gynecomastia, pancreatitis.

INTERACTIONS: Decreased effects with glucocorticoids. May reduce insulin sensitivity; may need insulin adjustment. May need to increase dose in adult women on estrogen replacement.

PREGNANCY: Category C, caution in nursing.

MECHANISM OF ACTION: Human growth hormone; increases growth rate and serum insulin-like growth factor-I levels.

PHARMACOKINETICS: Absorption: (SQ) Absolute bioavailability (81%), C_{max}=71.1mcg/L T_{max}=3.9 hrs, AUC=677 mcg•hr/L. **Distribution:** V_d=50mL/kg. **Metabolism:** Liver and kidneys. **Elimination:** (SQ): $T_{1/2}$=2.3 hrs. (IV): $T_{1/2}$=19.5 min.

NYSTATIN ORAL

RX

nystatin (Various)

THERAPEUTIC CLASS: Polyene antifungal

INDICATIONS: (Sus) Treatment of oral candidiasis. (Tab) Treatment of non-esophageal mucous membrane GI candidiasis.

DOSAGE: *Adults:* Oral Candidiasis: (Sus) 4-6mL qid. Retain in mouth as long as possible before swallowing. GI Candidiasis: (Tab) 500,000-1,000,000 U tid.
Pediatrics: Oral Candidiasis: (Sus) 4-6mL qid. Infants: 2mL qid. Retain in mouth as long as possible before swallowing.

HOW SUPPLIED: Sus: 100,000 U/mL (60mL, 480mL); Tab: 500,000 U

WARNINGS/PRECAUTIONS: Not for systemic mycoses. D/C if irritation/hypersensitivity occurs. Confirm diagnosis with KOH smear and/or cultures if symptoms persist after course of therapy. Continue at least 48 hrs after clinical response.

ADVERSE REACTIONS: Diarrhea, NV, GI distress, rash, urticaria, Stevens-Johnson syndrome, oral irritation.

PREGNANCY: Category C, caution in nursing.

MECHANISM OF ACTION: Fungistatic and fungicidal agent; acts by binding to sterols in the cell membrane of susceptible *Candida* species with a resultant change in membrane permeability, allowing leakage of intracellular components.

PHARMACOKINETICS: Absorption: GI (insignificant). **Elimination:** Stool (unchanged).

NYSTATIN TOPICAL

RX

nystatin (Various)

THERAPEUTIC CLASS: Polyene antifungal

INDICATIONS: Treatment of cutaneous or mucocutaneous mycotic infections caused by susceptible *Candida* species.

DOSAGE: *Adults:* (Cre) Apply to affected area bid until healing is complete. (Powder) Apply to lesions bid-tid until healing is complete. For fungal infections of the feet, dust powder on feet and in shoes also.
Pediatrics: Neonates and Older: (Cre) Apply to affected area bid until healing is complete. (Powder) Apply to lesions bid-tid until healing is complete. For fungal infections of the feet, dust powder on feet and in shoes also.

HOW SUPPLIED: Cre: 100,000 U/g (30g); Powder, Topical: 100,000 U/g (15g)

WARNINGS/PRECAUTIONS: D/C if irritation or sensitization occurs. Confirm diagnosis. Not for systemic, oral, intravaginal, or ophthalmic use. For fungal infections of the feet, dust powder on feet as well as in all footwear. Moist lesions are best treated with topical dusting powder.

ADVERSE REACTIONS: Allergic reactions, burning, itching, rash, eczema, pain at application site.

PREGNANCY: Category C, caution in nursing.

MECHANISM OF ACTION: Polyene antifungal; binds sterols in the cell membrane of susceptible species, causing a change in membrane permeability and subsequent leakage of intracellular components. Fungistatic and fungicidal.

PHARMACOKINETICS: Absorption: Not absorbed from intact skin or mucous membranes.

NYSTATIN/TRIAMCINOLONE

RX

nystatin - triamcinolone acetonide (Various)

THERAPEUTIC CLASS: Polyene antifungal/corticosteroid

INDICATIONS: Topical treatment of cutaneous candidiasis.

DOSAGE: *Adults:* Apply bid (am and pm). Max: 25 days of treatment.
Pediatrics: Apply bid (am and pm). Max: 25 days of treatment.

HOW SUPPLIED: Cre, Oint: (Nystatin-Triamcinolone) 100,000 U/g-0.1% (15g, 30g, 60g)

WARNINGS/PRECAUTIONS: Avoid occlusive dressing. Monitor periodically for HPA axis suppression with prolonged use or when applied over a large area. D/C if hypersensitivity or irritation develops. Systemic absorption with topical corticosteroids reported; children are more prone to systemic toxicity. May cause Cushing's syndrome, hyperglycemia, and glucosuria.

ADVERSE REACTIONS: Acneiform eruption, burning, itching, irritation, secondary infection.

PREGNANCY: Category C, caution in nursing.

MECHANISM OF ACTION: Nystatin: Polyene antifungal; binds to sterols in cell membrane, which renders cell membrane incapable of functioning as selective barrier. Triamcinolone: Synthetic corticosteroid; produces anti-inflammatory, antipruritic, and vasoconstrictive actions. Dermatological effects not established.

PHARMACOKINETICS: Absorption: Triamcinolone: Percutaneous; inflammation, other disease states, and the use of occlusive dressings may increase absorption. **Metabolism:** Triamcinolone: Liver. **Excretion:** Triamcinolone: Urine (primary); bile.

NYSTOP

RX

nystatin (Paddock)

THERAPEUTIC CLASS: Polyene antifungal

INDICATIONS: Treatment of cutaneous and mucocutaneous mycotic infections caused by susceptible *Candida* species.

DOSAGE: *Adults:* Apply to lesions bid-tid until healing is complete. For fungal infections of the feet, dust powder on feet and also in shoes.
Pediatrics: Neonates and Older: Apply to lesions bid-tid until healing is complete. For fungal infections of the feet, dust powder on feet and in shoes also.

HOW SUPPLIED: Powder, Topical: 100,000 U/g (15g, 30g, 60g)

WARNINGS/PRECAUTIONS: D/C if irritation or sensitization occurs. Confirm diagnosis. Not for systemic, oral, intravaginal, or ophthalmic use.

ADVERSE REACTIONS: Allergic reactions, burning, itching, rash, eczema, pain at application site.

PREGNANCY: Category C, caution in nursing.

MECHANISM OF ACTION: Polyene antifungal; binds sterols in the cell membrane of susceptible species, causing a change in membrane permeability and subsequent leakage of intracellular components. Fungistatic and fungicidal.

PHARMACOKINETICS: Absorption: Not absorbed from intact skin or mucous membranes.

OCUFLOX

RX

ofloxacin (Allergan)

THERAPEUTIC CLASS: Fluoroquinolone

INDICATIONS: Management of bacterial infections in conjunctivitis and corneal ulcers.

DOSAGE: *Adults:* Conjunctivitis: 1-2 drops q2-4h for 2 days, then 1-2 drops qid for 5 days. Corneal Ulcer: 1-2 drops every 30 min while awake and 1-2 drops 4-6 hrs after retiring for 2 days, then 1-2 drops q1h while awake for 5-7 days, then 1-2 drops qid for 2 days or until treatment completion.
Pediatrics: ≥1 yr: Conjunctivitis: 1-2 drops q2-4h for 2 days, then 1-2 drops qid for 5

days. Corneal Ulcer: 1-2 drops every 30 min while awake and 1-2 drops 4-6 hrs after retiring for 2 days, then 1-2 drops q1h while awake for 5-7 days, then 1-2 drops qid for 2 days or until treatment completion.

HOW SUPPLIED: Sol: 0.3% (5mL, 10mL)

WARNINGS/PRECAUTIONS: Not for injection into eye. Do not inject subconjunctivally nor into the eye's anterior chamber. Superinfection may result with prolonged use. Fatal hypersensitivity reactions reported after 1st dose of systemic quinolone therapy. Avoid allowing tip of container to contact fingers, eye or surrounding structures.

ADVERSE REACTIONS: Transient ocular burning or discomfort, stinging, redness, itching, keratitis, ocular periocular/facial edema, photophobia, blurred vision, tearing, dryness, eye pain.

INTERACTIONS: Systemic quinolone therapy may increase theophylline levels, interfere with caffeine metabolism, enhance warfarin effects, and elevate SrCr with cyclosporine.

PREGNANCY: Category C, not for use in nursing.

MECHANISM OF ACTION: Fluoroquinolone: exerts bactericidal effect on susceptible bacteria by inhibiting DNA gyrase, an essential bacterial enzyme that is a critical catalyst in duplication, transcription, and repair of bacterial DNA.

PHARMACOKINETICS: Absorption: C_{max}=1.1 ng/mL (Day 1, qid dosing), 1.9 ng/mL (Day 11, qid dosing). **Excretion:** Urine.

OLUX
clobetasol propionate (Stiefel)

RX

THERAPEUTIC CLASS: Corticosteroid

INDICATIONS: Short-term treatment of inflammatory and pruritic manifestations of moderate to severe corticosteroid responsive dermatoses of the scalp. Short-term treatment of mild to moderate plaque-type psoriasis of non-scalp regions excluding the face and intertriginous areas.

DOSAGE: *Adults:* Apply to affected area bid (am and pm). No more than 1.5 capfuls/application. Limit to 2 consecutive weeks. Avoid with occlusive dressings. Max 50g/week.
Pediatrics: ≥12 yrs: Apply to affected area bid (am and pm). No more than 1.5 capfuls/application. Limit to 2 consecutive weeks. Avoid with occlusive dressings. Max 50g/week.

HOW SUPPLIED: Foam: 0.05% (50g, 100g)

WARNINGS/PRECAUTIONS: May produce reversible HPA axis suppression, manifestations of Cushing's syndrome, hyperglycemia, and glucosuria. Caution when applied to large surface areas or under occlusive dressings. Use appropriate antifungal or antibacterial agent with dermatological infections; d/c if infection does not clear. Pediatrics may be more susceptible to systemic toxicity. Avoid eyes. D/C if irritation occurs.

ADVERSE REACTIONS: Burning/stinging, pruritus, irritation, erythema, folliculitis, cracking/fissuring of skin, numbness of fingers, telangiectasia, skin atrophy.

PREGNANCY: Category C, caution in nursing.

MECHANISM OF ACTION: Corticosteroid; possesses anti-inflammatory, antipruritic, and vasoconstrictive properties. Anti-inflammatory effects not established; suspected to act by induction of phospholipase A_2 inhibitory proteins, lipocortins. Lipocortins control biosynthesis of inflammation mediators (prostaglandins and leukotrienes) by inhibiting release of their common precursor, arachidonic acid.

PHARMACOKINETICS: Absorption: Percutaneous; occlusion, inflammation, and other disease states may increase absorption. **Distribution:** Systemically administered corticosteroids are found in breast milk. **Metabolism:** Liver. **Elimination:** Kidney (major), bile.

OLUX-E
clobetasol propionate (Stiefel)

RX

THERAPEUTIC CLASS: Corticosteroid

INDICATIONS: Treatment of inflammatory and pruritic manifestations of corticosteroid-responsive dermatoses.

DOSAGE: *Adults:* Apply thin layer to affected area bid (am and pm). Limit to 2 consecutive weeks. Avoid with occlusive dressings. Max: 50g/week.
Pediatrics: ≥12 yrs: Apply thin layer to affected area bid (am and pm). Limit to 2 consecutive weeks. Avoid with occlusive dressings. Max: 50g/week.

HOW SUPPLIED: Foam: 0.05% (50g, 100g)

WARNINGS/PRECAUTIONS: May produce reversible HPA axis suppression, manifestations of Cushing's syndrome, hyperglycemia, and glucosuria. Caution when applied to large surface area or under occlusive dressings. Use appropriate antifungal or antibacterial agent with dermatological infections; d/c if infection does not clear. Pediatrics may be more susceptible to systemic toxicity. D/C if irritation occurs. Should not be used to treat rosacea or perioral dermatitis. Avoid use on face, groin, axillae, or other intertriginous areas.

ADVERSE REACTIONS: Folliculitits, acneiform eruptions, hypopigmentation, perioral dermatitis, allergic contact dermatitis, secondary infection, irritation, striae, miliaria.

PREGNANCY: Category C, caution in nursing.

MECHANISM OF ACTION: Corticosteroid; possesses anti-inflammatory, antipruritic, and vasoconstrictive properties. Anti-inflammatory effect not established; suspected to act by induction of phospholipase A_2 inhibitory proteins called lipocortins. Lipocortins control biosynthesis of inflammation mediators (prostaglandins and leukotrienesn) by inhibiting release of their common precursor, arachidonic acid.

PHARMACOKINETICS: Absorption: Percutaneous; occlusion, inflammation, and other disease states may increase absorption; C_{max}=59pg/mL; T_{max}=5 hrs. **Distribution:** Systemically administered corticosteroids are found in breast milk. **Metabolism:** Liver. **Elimination:** Kidneys, bile.

OMNARIS
ciclesonide (Sepracor)

RX

THERAPEUTIC CLASS: Non-halogenated glucocorticoid

INDICATIONS: Treatment of nasal symptoms associated with seasonal allergic rhinitis in adults and children ≥6 yrs of age. Treatment of nasal symptoms associated with perennial allergic rhinitis in adults and adolescents ≥12 yrs of age.

DOSAGE: *Adults:* Seasonal Allergic Rhinitis/Perennial Allergic Rhinitis: 2 sprays (50mcg/spray) each nostril qd.
Pediatrics: Seasonal Allergic Rhinitis: ≥6 yrs: 2 sprays (50mcg/spray) each nostril qd. Perennial Allergic Rhinitis: ≥12 yrs: 2 sprays (50mcg/spray) each nostril qd.

HOW SUPPLIED: Spray: 50mcg/spray (12.5g)

WARNINGS/PRECAUTIONS: Risk of acute adrenal insufficiency and withdrawal symptoms when replacing systemic corticosteroids with a topical corticosteroids; monitor closely. Risk for more severe/fatal course of infections (eg, chickenpox, measles); avoid exposure in patients who have not had the disease or been properly immunized. May cause growth velocity reduction in pediatrics. Monitor routinely the growth of pediatrics. May impair wound healing; avoid in recent nasal septal ulcers, nasal surgery, or nasal trauma until healed. Candida infections of the nose or pharynx may occur; examine periodically and treat accordingly. Caution in patients with active or quiescent tuberculosis infections, untreated local or systemic fungal or bacterial infections, systemic viral or parasitic infections, or ocular herpes simplex. Taper dose if symptoms of hypercorticism occur. Caution in patients with history of glaucoma and/or cataracts; monitor IOP accordingly.

ADVERSE REACTIONS: Headache, epistaxis, nasopharyngitis, ear pain, pharyngolaryngeal pain.

INTERACTIONS: Ketoconazole may increase levels of the pharmacologically active metabolite des-ciclesonide; co-administer with caution.

PREGNANCY: Category C, caution in nursing.

MECHANISM OF ACTION: Not established; glucocorticoid has an anti-inflammatory effect and other effects on multiple cell types (eg, mast cells, eosinophils, macrophages, and lymphocytes) and mediators (eg, histamine, eicosanoids, leukotrienes, and cytokines) involved in allergic inflammation.

PHARMACOKINETICS: Absorption: (50-800mcg) C_{max}<30pg/mL (adults); (25-200mcg) C_{max}<45pg/mL (pediatrics). **Metabolism:** Nasal mucosa estrases to des-ciclesonide (active metabolite) followed by liver CYP3A4, 2D6.

OMNICEF
cefdinir (Abbott)

RX

THERAPEUTIC CLASS: Cephalosporin (3rd generation)

INDICATIONS: Community-acquired pneumonia (CAP), acute exacerbations of chronic bronchitis (AECB), acute maxillary sinusitis, pharyngitis/tonsillitis, uncomplicated skin and skin structure infections (SSSI), and acute bacterial otitis media.

DOSAGE: *Adults:* (Cap) SSSI/CAP: 300mg q12h for 10 days. AECB/Pharyngitis/Tonsillitis: 300mg q12h for 5-10 days or 600mg q24h for 10 days. Sinusitis: 300mg q12h or 600mg q24h for 10 days. CrCl <30mL/min: 300mg qd.
Pediatrics: (Sus) 6 months-12 yrs: Otitis Media/Pharyngitis/Tonsillitis: 7mg/kg q12h for 5-10 days or 14mg/kg q24h for 10 days. Sinusitis: 7mg/kg q12h or 14mg/kg q24h for 10 days. SSSI: 7mg/kg q12h or 14mg/kg q24h for 10 days. (Cap) ≥13 yrs: CAP/SSSI: 300mg q12h for 10 days. AECB/Pharyngitis/Tonsillitis: 300mg q12h for 5-10 days or 600mg q24h for 10 days. Sinusitis: 300mg q12h or 600mg q24h for 10 days. CrCl <30mL/min/1.73m²: 7mg/kg qd. Max: 300mg qd.

HOW SUPPLIED: Cap: 300mg; Sus: 125mg/5mL, 250mg/5mL (60mL, 100mL)

WARNINGS/PRECAUTIONS: Cross-sensitivity to PCNs and other cephalosporins may occur. *Clostridium difficile*-associated diarrhea has been reported. Positive direct Coombs' tests may occur. Caution with renal dysfunction, history of colitis. Suspension contains 2.86g/5mL of sucrose; caution in diabetes. False (+) for urine glucose with Clinitest and Benedict's or Fehling's solution.

ADVERSE REACTIONS: Diarrhea, vaginal moniliasis, nausea, headache, abdominal pain, superinfection (prolonged use).

INTERACTIONS: Iron-fortified foods, iron supplements, and aluminum- or magnesium-containing antacids reduce absorption; separate doses by 2 hrs. Probenecid inhibits the renal excretion. Reddish stools reported with iron-containing products.

PREGNANCY: Category B, safe in nursing.

MECHANISM OF ACTION: Extended-spectrum cephalosporin; bactericidal activity from inhibition of cell-wall synthesis.

PHARMACOKINETICS: Absorption: Cap: (300mg) Bioavailability (21%), C_{max}=1.6µg/mL, T_{max}=2.9 hrs, AUC=7.05µg•h/mL. (600mg) Bioavailability (16%), C_{max}=2.87µg/mL, T_{max}=3 hrs, AUC=11.1µg•h/mL. Sus: (7mg/kg) Bioavailability (25%), C_{max}=2.3µg/mL, T_{max}=2.2 hrs, AUC=8.31µg•h/mL. (14mg/kg) C_{max}=3.86µg/mL, T_{max}=1.8 hrs, AUC=13.4µg•h/mL. **Distribution:** V_d=0.35L/kg (adults), 0.67L/kg (pediatrics); plasma protein binding (60-70%). **Elimination:** (300mg) Urine (18.4%); (600mg) Urine (11.6%); $T_{1/2}$=1.7 hrs.

OMNITROPE
somatropin (Sandoz)

RX

THERAPEUTIC CLASS: Human growth hormone

INDICATIONS: Long-term treatment of pediatric patients who have growth failure due to an inadequate secretion of endogenous growth hormone. Long-term replacement therapy in adults with growth hormone deficiency (GHD) of either childhood- or adult-onset etiology.

DOSAGE: *Adults:* Individualize dose. GHD: ≤0.04mg/kg/week. May increase at 4-8 week intervals. Max: 0.08mg/kg/week. Divide dose into daily SQ injections (give preferably in

the evening).
Pediatrics: Individualize dose. GHD: 0.16-0.24mg/kg/week. Divide dose into daily SQ injections (give preferably in the evening).

HOW SUPPLIED: Inj: 1.5mg, 5.8mg

CONTRAINDICATIONS: Evidence of neoplastic activity. Pediatrics with fused epiphyses. Acute critical illness due to complications after open heart or abdominal surgery, multiple accidental trauma, or with acute respiratory failure. Patients with Prader-Willi syndrome who are severely obese or have severe respiratory impairment.

WARNINGS/PRECAUTIONS: Contains benzyl alcohol; avoid use in newborns. Patients with GHD secondary to an intracranial lesion should be monitored closely for progression or recurrence of underlying disease process. Monitor closely for any malignant transformation of skin lesions, scoliosis progression, or gait abnormalities. Monitor closely with DM, glucose intolerance, hypopituitarism. Intracranial HTN reported. Funduscopic exam recomended at initiation, and periodically during course of therapy.

ADVERSE REACTIONS: Hypothyroidism, elevated HbA_{1c}, eosinophilia, hematoma, headache, hypertriglyceridemia, leg pain.

INTERACTIONS: Growth promoting effects may be inhibited by glucocorticoids. May alter clearance of CYP450 substrates (eg, corticosteroids, sex steroids, anticonvulsants, cyclosporine); monitor closely. May need insulin dose adjustment.

PREGNANCY: Category B, caution in nursing.

MECHANISM OF ACTION: Human growth hormone; binds to dimeric GH receptor in cell membrane of target cells resulting in intracellular signal transduction.

PHARMACOKINETICS: Absorption: C_{max}=72mcg/mL, T_{max}=4 hrs. **Elimination:** $T_{1/2}$=2.8 hrs.

ONCASPAR   RX
pegaspargase (Enzon)

THERAPEUTIC CLASS: Protein synthesis inhibitor

INDICATIONS: Acute lymphoblastic leukemia in patients who have developed hypersensitivity to the native forms of L-asparaginase. May be given as monotherapy if multiagent therapy is inappropriate.

DOSAGE: *Adults:* Usual: 2500 IU/m^2 IM or IV every 14 days.
Pediatrics: 1-9 yrs: 2500 IU/m^2 IM on Day 3 of 4-Week induction phase and on Day 3 of each of two 8-Week delayed intensifications phases.

HOW SUPPLIED: Inj: 750 IU/mL (5mL)

CONTRAINDICATIONS: Pancreatitis. History of pancreatitis, significant hemorrhagic events, or serious thrombosis with prior L-asparaginase therapy.

WARNINGS/PRECAUTIONS: May be a contact irritant. Avoid inhalation or contact with skin or mucous membranes. Serious allergic reaction, pancreatitis, or glucose intolerance can occur. Increased prothrombin time, partial thromboplastin time, and hypofibrinogenemia can occur; monitor coagulation parameters. May predispose to infections, bleeding, thrombosis. D/C in patients with serious thrombotic event including sagittal sinus thrombosis.

ADVERSE REACTIONS: Allergic reactions (including anaphylaxis), CNS thrombosis, coagulopathy, elevated transaminases, hyperbilirubinemia, hyperglycemia, pancreatitis.

INTERACTIONS: May increase toxicity of protein bound drugs. May interfere with the action of drugs that require cell replication for their lethal effects (eg, methotrexate), and the enzymatic detoxification of other drugs, particularly in the liver. Caution with concomitant anticoagulants (eg, coumadin, heparin, dipyridamole, ASA, or NSAIDs), hepatotoxic agents.

PREGNANCY: Category C, not for use in nursing.

MECHANISM OF ACTION: Protein synthesis inhibitor; selectively kills leukemic cells due to depletion of plasma asparagine.

PHARMACOKINETICS: Elimination: $T_{1/2}$=5.8 days.

OPCON-A
naphazoline HCl - pheniramine maleate (Bausch & Lomb)

OTC

THERAPEUTIC CLASS: H₁-antagonist/alpha-agonist (imidazoline)

INDICATIONS: Temporary relief of redness and itching of the eye due to various allergens.

DOSAGE: *Adults:* 1-2 drops up to qid.
Pediatrics: ≥6 yrs: 1-2 drops up to qid.

HOW SUPPLIED: Sol: (Pheniramine-Naphazoline) 0.3%-0.027% (15mL)

CONTRAINDICATIONS: Cardiovascular disease, HTN, narrow angle glaucoma, BPH.

WARNINGS/PRECAUTIONS: D/C if pain, vision changes, no improvement, condition worsens or persists >72 hrs. Remove contact lens before use. Overuse may produce increased redness of eye. Temporary pupil enlargement may occur. Supervision required with heart disease, high BP, difficulty in urination due to prostate enlargement, or narrow angle glaucoma.

ADVERSE REACTIONS: Brief tingling sensation.

PREGNANCY: Safety in pregnancy and nursing not known.

OPHTHETIC
proparacaine HCl (Allergan)

RX

THERAPEUTIC CLASS: Anesthetic agent

INDICATIONS: For procedures in which topical ophthalmic anesthesia are indicated: corneal anesthesia of short duration (eg, tonometry, gonioscopy, corneal foreign body removal, short corneal and conjunctival procedures).

DOSAGE: *Adults:* Tonometry/Removal of Foreign Bodies or Sutures: 1-2 drops in each eye before procedure. Short Corneal/Conjunctival Procedures: 1 drop in each eye every 5-10 min for 5-7 doses.
Pediatrics: >12 yrs: Tonometry/Removal of Foreign Bodies or Sutures: 1-2 drops in each eye before procedure. Short Corneal/Conjunctival Procedures: 1 drop in each eye every 5-10 min for 5-7 doses.

HOW SUPPLIED: Sol: 0.5% (15mL)

WARNINGS/PRECAUTIONS: Not for prolonged use. May produce permanent corneal opacification with accompanying visual loss.

ADVERSE REACTIONS: Temporary stinging, burning or conjunctival redness, allergic contact dermatitis.

PREGNANCY: Category C, caution in nursing.

OPTIVAR
azelastine HCl (MedPointe)

RX

THERAPEUTIC CLASS: H₁-antagonist

INDICATIONS: Treatment of itching of the eye associated with allergic conjunctivitis.

DOSAGE: *Adults:* 1 drop bid.
Pediatrics: ≥3 yrs: 1 drop bid.

HOW SUPPLIED: Sol: 0.05% (6mL)

WARNINGS/PRECAUTIONS: Not for injection or oral use. Do not wear contact lens if the eye is red. Not for treatment of contact-lens irritation. Wait 10 min after instilling drops to insert contact lens.

ADVERSE REACTIONS: Transient eye burning/stinging, headaches, asthma, conjunctivitis, dyspnea, eye pain, fatigue, influenza-like symptoms, pharyngitis, pruritus, rhinitis, temporary blurring.

PREGNANCY: Category C, caution in nursing.

MECHANISM OF ACTION: Antihistaminic agent; relatively selective H$_1$-receptor antagonist; inhibits release of histamine and other mediators from cells (eg, mast cells) involved in the allergic response and decreases chemotaxis and activation of eosinophils.

PHARMACOKINETICS: Metabolism: N-desmethylazelastine (principle metabolite).

ORAP
RX
pimozide (Gate)

THERAPEUTIC CLASS: Diphenylbutylperidine

INDICATIONS: Suppression of motor and phonic tics in Tourette's syndrome in patients that failed standard therapy.

DOSAGE: *Adults:* Initial: 1-2mg/day in divided doses. May increase every other day. Maint: <0.2mg/kg/day or 10mg/day, whichever is less. Max: 0.2mg/kg/day or 10mg/day.
Pediatrics: >12 yrs: Initial: 0.05mg/kg qhs. Titrate: May increase every 3 days. Max: 0.2mg/kg/day or 10mg/day.

HOW SUPPLIED: Tab: 1mg*, 2mg* *scored

CONTRAINDICATIONS: Severe CNS depression, comatose states, congenital long QT syndrome, history of cardiac arrhythmias, hypokalemia, hypomagnesemia, simple tics or tics not associated with Tourette's syndrome. CYP3A4 inhibitors (eg, nefazodone, macrolide antibiotics, azole antifungals, protease inhibitors), sertraline, and drugs that cause motor and phonic tics (eg, pemoline, methylphenidate, amphetamines) or prolong the QT interval.

WARNINGS/PRECAUTIONS: May cause tardive dyskinesia, NMS, hyperpyrexia. Caution with history of seizures, EEG abnormalities, severe hepatic/renal impairment. Perform ECG before therapy, periodically thereafter, with dose adjustment. Produces anticholinergic effects. Sudden death reported. May impair mental/physical abilities.

ADVERSE REACTIONS: Akinesia, QT prolongation, tardive dyskinesia, sedation, loss of libido, constipation, dry mouth, visual disturbances, headache, asthenia, increased salivation.

INTERACTIONS: May potentiate CNS depressants (eg, analgesics, sedatives, anxiolytics, alcohol). Bradycardia reported with fluoxetine. Avoid grapefruit juice, CYP3A4 inhibitors (eg, azole antifungal drugs, macrolides, protease inhibitors, zileuton, fluvoxamine), sertraline. May interact with CYP1A2 inhibitors. Avoid other drugs that may potentiate QT prolongation such as phenothiazines, TCAs, antiarrhythmics, sparfloxacin, gatifloxacin, moxifloxacin, halofantrine, mefloquine, pentamidine, arsenic trioxide, levomethadyl acetate, dolasetron mesylate, probucol, tacrolimus, ziprasidone.

PREGNANCY: Category C, not for use in nursing.

MECHANISM OF ACTION: Antipsychotic agent; not established. Blocks dopaminergic receptors on neurons in the CNS.

PHARMACOKINETICS: Absorption: T$_{max}$=6-8 hrs. **Metabolism:** Liver (extensive) through N-dealkylation mediated CYP 3A4. Metabolites: 1-(4-piperidyl)-2-benzimidazoline and 4,4-bis (4-fluorophenyl) butyric acid. **Elimination:** Urine; T$_{1/2}$=55 hrs.

ORAPRED
RX
prednisolone sodium phosphate (Biomarin)

OTHER BRAND NAME: Orapred ODT (Alliant)

THERAPEUTIC CLASS: Glucocorticoid

INDICATIONS: Steroid-responsive disorders.

DOSAGE: *Adults:* (Sol) Initial: 5-60mg/day depending on disease and response. (Tab) Initial: 10-60mg/day depending on disease and response. Maint: Decrease dose by small amounts to lowest effective dose. (Sol/Tab) MS Exacerbations: 200mg qd for 1 week, then 80mg every other day for 1 month.
Pediatrics: (Sol/Tab) Initial: 0.14-2mg/kg/day, depending on disease and response,

given tid-qid. Nephrotic Syndrome: 20mg/m² tid for 4 weeks, then 40mg/m² every other day for 4 weeks. Uncontrolled Asthma: 1-2mg/kg/day in single or divided doses until peak expiratory flow rate of 80% is achieved (usually 3-10 days).

HOW SUPPLIED: Sol: 15mg/5mL (237mL); Tab, Orally Disintegrating: 10mg, 15mg, 30mg

CONTRAINDICATIONS: Systemic fungal infections.

WARNINGS/PRECAUTIONS: May produce reversible HPA axis suppression. Adjust dose during stress or change in thyroid status. May mask signs of infection or cause new infections. May activate latent amebiasis. Avoid with cerebral malaria. Avoid exposure to chickenpox or measles. Not for treatment of optic neuritis or active ocular herpes simplex. May cause elevation of BP or IOP, cataracts, glaucoma, optic nerve damage, Kaposi's sarcoma, psychic derangements, salt/water retention, increased excretion of potassium and/or calcium, osteoporosis, growth suppression in children, secondary ocular infections. Caution with Strongyloides, CHF, diverticulitis, HTN, renal insufficiency, fresh intestinal anastomoses, active or latent peptic ulcer, ulcerative colitis. Enhanced effect in hypothyroidism or cirrhosis. Avoid abrupt withdrawal.

ADVERSE REACTIONS: Edema, fluid/electrolyte disturbances, osteoporosis, muscle weakness, pancreatitis, peptic ulcer, impaired wound healing, increased intracranial pressure, cushingoid state, hirsutism, menstrual irregularities, growth suppression in children, glaucoma, nausea, weight gain.

INTERACTIONS: Enhanced metabolism with barbiturates, phenytoin, ephedrine, and rifampin. Use with cyclosporine may increase activity of both drugs; convulsions reported with concomitant use. Decreased metabolism with estrogens or ketoconazole. May inhibit response to warfarin. Increased risk of GI side effects with ASA or other NSAIDs. May increase clearance of salicylates. High doses or concurrent neuromuscular drugs may cause acute myopathy. Enhanced possibility of hypokalemia when given with potassium-depleting agents. May produce severe weakness in myasthenia gravis patients on anticholinesterase agents. Avoid live vaccines with immunosuppressive doses. Possible diminished response with killed or inactivated vaccines. May increase blood glucose; adjust antidiabetic agents. May suppress reactions to skin tests.

PREGNANCY: Category C, caution in nursing.

MECHANISM OF ACTION: Synthetic adrenocorticoid steroid; promotes gluconeogenesis, increases deposition of glycogen in the liver, inhibits glucose utilization, increases catabolism of protein, lipolysis, glomerular filtration that leads to increased urinary excretion of urate and calcium.

PHARMACOKINETICS: Absorption: Readily absorbed from GI tract. **Distribution:** Plasma protein binding (70-90%), found in breast milk. **Metabolism:** Liver. **Elimination:** Urine (as sulfate and glucuronide conjugates), T $_{1/2}$=2-4 hrs.

ORENCIA

RX

abatacept (Bristol-Myers Squibb)

THERAPEUTIC CLASS: Selective costimulation modulator

INDICATIONS: To reduce signs and symptoms, inducing major clinical response, inhibiting the progression of structural damage, and improving physical function in adult patients with moderately to severely active rheumatoid arthritis who have had an inadequate response to one or more disease-modifying, anti-rheumatic drugs (DMARDs) (eg, MTX, TNF antagonists). May be used as monotherapy or concomitantly with DMARDs other than TNF-antagonists. For reducing signs and symptoms in pediatric patients ≥6 yrs with moderately to severely active polyarticular juvenile idiopathic arthritis. May be used as monotherapy or concomitantly with MTX.

DOSAGE: *Adults:* Initial: <60kg: 500mg; 60-100kg: 750mg; >100kg: 1g IV over 30 min. Maint: Give at 2 and 4 weeks after initial infusion, then every 4 weeks thereafter. *Pediatrics:* 6-17 yrs: >75 kg: Follow adult dosing regimen. Max: 1000mg; <75kg: Initial: 10mg/kg IV over 30 min. Maint: Give at 2 and 4 weeks after initial infusion, then every 4 weeks thereafter.

HOW SUPPLIED: Inj: 250mg

WARNINGS/PRECAUTIONS: Increased risk of infections and serious infections with concomitant TNF-antagonist therapy; concurrent use not recommended. Anaphylaxis or anaphylactoid reactions reported. Caution with history of recurrent infections; d/c if

319

serious infections develop. Screen for latent TB prior to initiation. Avoid live vaccines. Caution with COPD. Concurrent use with anakinra is not recommended. Cases of lung cancer and lymphoma reported. Screening for viral hepatitis is recommended before initiation of therapy. Juvenile idiopathic arthritis patients should be brought up to date with all immunizations prior to therapy.

ADVERSE REACTIONS: Headache, nasopharyngitis, dizziness, cough, back pain, HTN, dyspepsia, UTI, rash, pain in extremities.

INTERACTIONS: See Warnings/Precautions.

PREGNANCY: Category C, not for use in nursing.

MECHANISM OF ACTION: Selective costimulation modulator; inhibits T cell activation by binding to CD80 and CD86, thereby blocking interaction with CD28.

PHARMACOKINETICS: Absorption: C_{max}=292mcg/mL. **Distribution:** V_d=0.09L/Kg. **Elimination:** $T_{1/2}$=16.7 days.

ORFADIN RX
nitisinone (Rare Disease Therapeutics)

THERAPEUTIC CLASS: Nitisinone

INDICATIONS: Adjunct to dietary restriction of tyrosine and phenylalanine in the treatment of hereditary tyrosinemia type I.

DOSAGE: *Adults:* Initial: 1mg/kg/day in divided doses, qam and qpm. Titrate: Increase to 1.5mg/kg/day if biochemical parameters (except plasma succinylacetone) are not normalized within 1 month. Max: 2mg/kg/day. Take at least 1 hr before a meal. May sprinkle contents of capsule in small amount of water, formula, or applesauce immediately before use.
Pediatrics: Initial: 1mg/kg/day in divided doses, qam and qpm. Titrate: Increase to 1.5mg/kg/day if biochemical parameters (except plasma succinylacetone) are not normalized within 1 month. Max: 2mg/kg/day. Take at least 1 hr before a meal. May sprinkle contents of capsule in small amount of water, formula, or applesauce immediately before use.

HOW SUPPLIED: Cap: 2mg, 5mg, 10mg

WARNINGS/PRECAUTIONS: Inadequate restriction of tyrosine and phenylalanine can result in elevated tyrosine levels. Maintain tyrosine levels <500µmol/L to avoid toxicity. Transient thrombocytopenia and leucopenia reported; monitor platelet and WBC count. Perform slit-lamp eye examination before initiation and if patient develops photophobia, eye pain or inflammation. Do not adjust dose further to lower tyrosine levels; may deteriorate patient's condition; use diet restriction instead. Increased risk of porphyric crises, liver failure, or hepatic neoplasms; monitor liver by imaging and lab tests including serum alpha-fetoprotein. Monitor urine succinylacetone levels to guide dose adjustment. Monitor serum phosphate to screen for renal involvement.

ADVERSE REACTIONS: Hepatic neoplasm, liver failure, conjunctivitis, corneal opacity, keratitis, photophobia, thrombocytopenia, leucopenia.

PREGNANCY: Category C, caution in nursing.

MECHANISM OF ACTION: Competitively inhibits 4-hydroxyphenyl-pyruvate dioxygenase, an enzyme upstream of FAH in the tyrosine catabolic pathways, thereby preventing accumulation of the catabolic intermediates maleylacetoacetate and fumarylacetoacetate, which is converted to the toxic metabolite succinylacetone and succinylacetoacetate.

PHARMACOKINETICS: Absorption: T_{max}=3 hrs. **Elimination:** $T_{1/2}$=54 hrs.

ORTHO TRI-CYCLEN RX
ethinyl estradiol - norgestimate (Ortho-McNeil)

OTHER BRAND NAMES: Tri-Previfem (Teva) - Tri-Sprintec (Barr)

THERAPEUTIC CLASS: Estrogen/progestogen combination

INDICATIONS: Prevention of pregnancy. Treatment of acne vulgaris in females ≥15 yrs who want contraception, have achieved menarche and are unresponsive to topical acne agents.

DOSAGE: *Adults:* Contraception/Acne: 28-day: 1 tab qd for 28 days, then repeat. Start 1st Sunday after menses begin or 1st day of menses.
Pediatrics: Contraception (postpubertal adolescents)/Acne: 28-day: 1 tab qd for 28 days, then repeat. Start 1st Sunday after menses begin or 1st day of menses.

HOW SUPPLIED: Tab: (Ethinyl Estradiol-Norgestimate) 0.035mg-0.18mg, 0.035mg-0.215mg, 0.035mg-0.25mg

CONTRAINDICATIONS: Thrombophlebitis, deep vein thrombophlebitis, thromboembolic disorders, pregnancy, cerbrovascular or coronary artery disease, migraine with focal aura, acute or chronic hepatocellular disease with abnormal liver function, undiagnosed abnormal genital bleeding, cholestatic jaundice of pregnancy or jaundice with prior pill use, hepatic adenomas or carcinomas, breast cancer, endometrium carcinoma, or other estrogen-dependent neoplasia.

WARNINGS/PRECAUTIONS: Cigarette smoking increases risk of serious cardiovascular side effects. This risk increases with age (especially >35 yrs) and heavy smoking. Increased risk of MI, vascular disease, thromboembolism, stroke, and gallbladder disease. Retinal thrombosis, hepatic neoplasia, carcinoma of breast and reproductive organs reported. May cause glucose intolerance, fluid retention, breakthrough bleeding, and spotting. May increase BP, elevate LDL levels, or cause other lipid changes. May cause or exacerbate migraine. May develop visual changes with contact lens. Increased risk of morbidity and mortality with HTN, hyperlipidemia, obesity, and diabetes. D/C if jaundice, significant depression, or ophthalmic irregularities develop. Perform annual physical exam. Use before menarche is not indicated. May affect certain endocrine, LFTs, and blood components.

ADVERSE REACTIONS: Nausea, vomiting, breakthrough bleeding, spotting, amenorrhea, migraine, depression, vaginal candidiasis, edema, weight changes.

INTERACTIONS: Reduced effects, increased breakthrough bleeding, and menstrual irregularities with rifampin, barbiturates, phenylbutazone, phenytoin, carbamazepine, griseofulvin, topiramate, St. John's wort, and possibly with ampicillin and tetracyclines.

PREGNANCY: Category X, not for use in nursing.

MECHANISM OF ACTION: Estrogen/progestogen oral contraceptive; acts by suppressing gonadotropin, inhibiting ovulation, and causing other alterations, including changes in cervical mucus, (which increases difficulty of sperm entry into uterus) and endometrium (which reduces likelihood of implantation).

PHARMACOKINETICS: Absorption: Rapid. Oral administration on various days during dosing led to altered parameters. **Distribution:** Norgestimate: Albumin binding (>97%). Ethinyl estradiol: Albumin binding (>97%). **Metabolism:** Norgestimate: GI tract and/or liver (1st pass mechanism). Norelgestromin (primary active metabolite): Hepatic, norgestrel (active metabolite). Ethinyl estradiol: Hydroxylated, glucuronide, sulfate conjugates. **Elimination:** Norgestimate: Urine (47%), feces (37%).

OVIDE
malathion (Taro)

RX

THERAPEUTIC CLASS: Organophosphate/cholinesterase inhibitor

INDICATIONS: For infections of *Pediculus humanus capitis* (head lice and their ova) of scalp hair.

DOSAGE: *Adults:* Apply sufficient amount on dry hair to thoroughly wet hair and scalp. Allow hair to dry naturally. Shampoo after 8-12 hrs. Rinse and use a fine-toothed comb to remove dead lice and eggs. Repeat with 2nd application if lice present after 7-9 days.
Pediatrics: ≥6 yrs: Apply sufficient amount on dry hair to thoroughly wet hair and scalp. Allow hair to dry naturally. Shampoo after 8-12 hrs. Rinse and use a fine-toothed comb to remove dead lice and eggs. Repeat with 2nd application if lice present after 7-9 days.

HOW SUPPLIED: Lot: 0.5% (59mL)

CONTRAINDICATIONS: Neonates, infants.

WARNINGS/PRECAUTIONS: Lotion is flammable; do not expose lotion or wet hair to open flames or electric heat sources (eg, hair dryers, electric curlers). If contact with eyes, flush immediately with water. If skin irritation develops, d/c until irritation clears. Slight stinging sensations reported. Adult supervision is required with use in children.

ADVERSE REACTIONS: Skin and scalp irritation, mild conjunctivitis (with eye contact).

PREGNANCY: Category B, caution in nursing.

MECHANISM OF ACTION: Organophosphate/cholinesterase inhibitor; acts as a pediculocide by inhibiting cholinesterase activity.

OXANDRIN
oxandrolone (Savient)

THERAPEUTIC CLASS: Anabolic steroid

INDICATIONS: Adjunctive therapy to promote weight gain after weight loss following extensive surgery, chronic infections, severe trauma, and for those who fail to gain or maintain normal weight without pathophysiologic reasons, to offset protein catabolism associated with prolonged administration of corticosteroids, for the relief of osteoporotic bone pain.

DOSAGE: *Adults:* Usual: 2.5-20mg/day given bid-qid for 2-4 weeks. May repeat course intermittently as indicated. Elderly: 5mg bid.
Pediatrics: ≤0.1mg/kg/day. May repeat intermittently as indicated.

HOW SUPPLIED: Tab: 2.5mg*, 10mg *scored

CONTRAINDICATIONS: Carcinoma of the prostate or breast, carcinoma of the breast in females with hypercalcemia, pregnancy, nephrosis, hypercalcemia.

WARNINGS/PRECAUTIONS: D/C if peliosis hepatis, liver cell tumors, cholestatic hepatitis, jaundice, LFT abnormalities, hypercalcemia or signs of virilization (females) occur. Edema, with or without CHF, may occur with pre-existing cardiac, renal, or hepatic disease. Monitor bone growth in children every 6 months. Increased risk of prostatic hypertrophy/carcinoma in the elderly. May decrease levels of thyroxine-binding globulin, suppress clotting factors II, V, VII, and X and increase PT. Caution with CAD and history of MI. Lower dose recommended in elderly.

ADVERSE REACTIONS: Cholestatic jaundice, gynecomastia, edema, CNS effects, acne, phallic enlargement, increased frequency/persistence of erections, inhibition of testicular function, chronic priapism, epididymitis, impotence, testicular atrophy, oligospermia, bladder irritability, menstrual irregularities, virilization.

INTERACTIONS: Increased sensitivity to oral anticoagulants (eg, warfarin). May increase edema with adrenal cortical steroids or ACTH. May inhibit metabolism of oral hypoglycemics.

PREGNANCY: Category X, not for use in nursing.

MECHANISM OF ACTION: Anabolic steroid; inhibits endogenous testosterone release through inhibition of pituitary luteinizing hormone.

PHARMACOKINETICS: Elimination: $T_{1/2}$=13.3 hrs (elderly), 10.4 hrs (young).

OXISTAT RX
oxiconazole nitrate (GlaxoSmithKline)

THERAPEUTIC CLASS: Azole antifungal

INDICATIONS: (Cre/Lot) Topical treatment of tinea pedis, tinea cruris and tinea corporis due to *Trichophyton rubrum*, *Trichophyton mentagrophytes* , or *Epidermophyton floccosum*. (Cre) Topical treatment of tinea versicolor due to *Malassezia furfur*.

DOSAGE: *Adults:* (Cre/Lot) T.pedis/T.corporis/T.cruris: Apply qd-bid. (Cre) T.versicolor: Apply qd. Treat t.pedis for 1 month and other infections for 2 weeks.
Pediatrics: ≥12 yrs: (Cream) T.pedis/T.corporis/T.cruris: Apply qd-bid. T.versicolor: Apply qd. Treat t.pedis for 1 month and other infections for 2 weeks.

HOW SUPPLIED: Cre: 1% (15g, 30g, 60g); Lot: 1% (30mL)

WARNINGS/PRECAUTIONS: Not for ophthalmic or intravaginal use. D/C if irritation or sensitivity occurs.

ADVERSE REACTIONS: Pruritus, burning/stinging.

PREGNANCY: Category B, caution in nursing.

MECHANISM OF ACTION: Azole antifungal; acts by inhibition of ergosterol biosynthesis, which is critical for cellular membrane integrity.

PHARMACOKINETICS: **Distribution**: Excreted in breast milk. **Elimination**: Urine (<0.3%).

OXSORALEN RX
methoxsalen (Valeant)

THERAPEUTIC CLASS: Psoralen

INDICATIONS: As a topical repigmenting agent in vitiligo with controlled doses of UVA (320-400nm) or sunlight.

DOSAGE: *Adults:* Apply to small well defined lesions before UVA exposure. Determine treatment intervals by erythema response; generally 1 week or less often.
Pediatrics: ≥12 yrs: Apply to small well defined lesions before UVA exposure. Determine treatment intervals by erythema response; generally 1 week or less often.

HOW SUPPLIED: Lot: 1% (30mL)

CONTRAINDICATIONS: Current or history of melanoma, invasive skin carcinoma, photosensitive diseases (eg, acute lupus erythematosus, porphyria, xeroderma pigmentosum), patients <12 yrs.

WARNINGS/PRECAUTIONS: May develop serious burns if exceed recommended dose or exposure. Protect treated areas from sunlight. Increased risk of skin cancer in fair-skinned patients or prior coal tar UVA treatment, ionizing radiation, or taken arsenical compounds. Protect treated areas from light by using protective clothing or sunscreen.

ADVERSE REACTIONS: Minor blistering, severe burns (from overexposure to UVA).

INTERACTIONS: Caution with photosensitizers such as anthralin, coal tar and its derivatives, griseofulvin, phenothiazines, nalidixic acid, halogenated salicylanilides, sulfonamides, tetracyclines, thiazides, and certain organic staining dyes (eg, methylene blue, toluidine blue, rose bengal, methyl orange).

PREGNANCY: Category C, caution in nursing.

MECHANISM OF ACTION: Antipsoriatic agent; not established. Believed that upon photoactivation, conjugates and forms covalent bonds with DNA, which leads to formation of monofunctional and bifunctional adducts.

PALGIC RX
carbinoxamine maleate (PamLab)

THERAPEUTIC CLASS: H$_1$-antagonist

INDICATIONS: Seasonal and perennial allergic rhinitis, vasomotor rhinitis, allergic conjunctivitis, urticaria, angioedema, dermatographism, allergic reactions to blood or plasma. Adjunct in anaphylaxis.

DOSAGE: *Adults:* Usual: 4mg prn. Max: 24mg/day given q6-8h.
Pediatrics: ≥6 yrs: Usual: 4mg prn. Max: 24mg/day given q6-8h. 1-6 yrs: Usual: 2mg prn. May increase to 0.2-0.4mg/kg/day given q6-8h.

HOW SUPPLIED: Sol: 4mg/5mL; Tab: 4mg* *scored

CONTRAINDICATIONS: Concomitant MAOIs, newborns, premature infants, lower respiratory tract disorders (eg, asthma), nursing mothers.

WARNINGS/PRECAUTIONS: Caution in narrow angle glaucoma, stenosing peptic ulcer, symptomatic prostatic hypertrophy, bladder neck or pyloroduodenal obstruction, history of bronchial asthma, increased IOP, hyperthyroidism, CVD, HTN, and elderly. May impair mental/physical abilities.

ADVERSE REACTIONS: Sedation, sleepiness, dizziness, disturbed coordination, epigastric distress, thickening of bronchial secretions, excitation, diminished mental alertness.

INTERACTIONS: See Contraindications. Intensified anticholinergic effects with MAOIs; avoid concurrent use. Additive effects with alcohol, other CNS depressants (eg, hypnotics, sedatives, tranquilizers).

PREGNANCY: Category C, not for use in nursing.

MECHANISM OF ACTION: H$_1$ receptor blocking agent; competes with histamine for receptor sites on effector cells. Also has anticholinergic and sedative properties.

PANCREASE MT
amylase - lipase - protease (McNeil Consumer)

RX

THERAPEUTIC CLASS: Pancreatic enzyme supplement

INDICATIONS: Treatment of steatorrhea secondary to pancreatic insufficiency such as cystic fibrosis (CF) and chronic alcoholic pancreatitis.

DOSAGE: *Adults:* Initial: 400 U lipase/kg/meal. Max: 2500 U lipase/kg/meal. Adjust dose based on 3-day fecal fat studies. Take with plenty of water. Do not chew/crush caps. May add capsule contents to soft food (pH <7.3) and swallow immediately without chewing.
Pediatrics: ≤12 months: 2000-4000 U lipase/120mL formula or per breast feeding. 13 months-3 yrs: Initial: 1000 U lipase/kg/meal. Max: 2500 U lipase/kg/meal. ≥4 yrs: Initial: 400U lipase/kg/meal. Max: 2500 U lipase/kg/meal. Adjust dose based on 3-day fecal fat studies. Take with plenty of water. Do not chew/crush caps. May add capsule contents to soft food (pH <7.3) and swallow immediately without chewing.

HOW SUPPLIED: Cap: (Amylase-Lipase-Protease) (MT 4) 12,000 U-4000 U-12,000 U, (MT 10) 30,000 U-10,000 U-30,000 U, (MT 16) 48,000 U-16,000 U-48,000 U, (MT 20) 56,000 U-20,000 U-44,000 U

CONTRAINDICATIONS: Pork protein hypersensitivity.

WARNINGS/PRECAUTIONS: May cause fibrotic strictures in colon of primarily CF patients. Caution when changing dose or brand of medication.

ADVERSE REACTIONS: Diarrhea, abdominal pain, intestinal obstruction, vomiting, flatulence, nausea, constipation, melena, perianal irritation, weight loss, pain.

PREGNANCY: Category B, safety in nursing not known.

PANCURONIUM
pancuronium bromide (Various)

RX

> Administer by adequately trained individuals familiar with actions, characteristics, and hazards.

THERAPEUTIC CLASS: Skeletal muscle relaxant (nondepolarizing)

INDICATIONS: Adjunct to general anesthesia, to facilitate endotracheal intubation, and to provide skeletal muscle relaxation during surgery or mechanical ventilation.

DOSAGE: *Adults:* Individualize dose. Initial: 0.04-0.1mg/kg IV. Late incremental doses of 0.01mg/kg may be used. Skeletal Muscle Relaxation For Endotracheal Intubation: 0.06-0.1mg/kg bolus.
Pediatrics: Individualize dose. Initial: 0.04-0.1mg/kg IV. Late incremental doses of 0.01mg/kg may be used. Skeletal Muscle Relaxation For Endotracheal Intubation: 0.06-0.1mg/kg bolus. Neonates: Use test dose of 0.02mg/kg.

HOW SUPPLIED: Inj: 1mg/mL, 2mg/mL

WARNINGS/PRECAUTIONS: May have profound effect in myasthenia gravis or myasthenic (Eaton Lambert) syndrome; use small test dose and monitor closely. Contains benzyl alcohol; caution in neonates. Use peripheral nerve stimulator to monitor neuromuscular blocking effect. Caution with pre-existing pulmonary, hepatic, or renal disease. Conditions associated with slower circulation time in cardiovascular disease, old age, and edematous states may delay onset time; dosage should not be increased. Possible slower onset, higher total dosage, and prolongation of neuromuscular blockade with hepatic and/or biliary tract disease. In ICU, long-term use may be associated with prolonged paralysis and/or skeletal muscle weakness; monitor closely. Severe obesity and neuromuscular disease may pose airway or ventilatory problems. Electrolyte imbalances may alter neuromuscular blockade.

ADVERSE REACTIONS: Skeletal muscle weakness and paralysis, salivation, rash.

INTERACTIONS: Prior administration of succinylcholine may enhance neuromuscular blocking effect. Avoid use with vercuronium, atracurium, d-tubocurarine, metocurine, gallamine. Enhanced neuromuscular blockade with enflurane, isoflurane, halothane, aminoglycosides, tetracyclines, bacitracin, polymyxin B, colistin, sodium colistimethate, and magnesium salts. Quinidine injection during recovery from use of other muscle relaxants suggests that recurrent paralysis may occur.

PREGNANCY: Category C, safety in nursing not known.

MECHANISM OF ACTION: Nondepolarizing neuromuscular blocking agent; competes for cholinergic receptors at the motor-end plate.

PHARMACOKINETICS: Distribution: V_d=241-280mL/kg; plasma protein unbound (13%). **Metabolism:** 17-hydroxy and 3,17-dihydroxy (metabolites). **Elimination:** Urine (40% unchanged and metabolites), bile (11%); $T_{1/2}$=89-161 min.

PANIXINE
RX
cephalexin (Ranbaxy)

THERAPEUTIC CLASS: Cephalosporin (1st generation)

INDICATIONS: Skin and skin structure (SSSI), bone, genitourinary and respiratory tract infections, otitis media, acute prostatitis.

DOSAGE: *Adults*: ≥15 yrs: Usual: 250mg q6h. Streptococcal pharyngitis/SSSI: 500mg q12h. Cystitis: 500mg q12h for minimum of 7-14 days. Max: 4g/day. Do not crush, cut, or chew tab. Treat β-hemolytic streptococcal infections for ≥10 days.
Pediatrics: Usual: 25-50mg/kg/day in divided doses. Streptococcal Pharyngitis (>1 yr)/SSSI: May divide into 2 doses, give q12h. Otitis Media: 75-100mg/kg/day given qid. Treat β-hemolytic streptococcal infections for ≥10 days.

HOW SUPPLIED: Tab, Dispersible: 125mg, 250mg

WARNINGS/PRECAUTIONS: Caution with PCN sensitivity. Caution with markedly impaired renal function, history of GI disease. Cross-sensitivity with cephalosporins and penicillins. Pseudomembranous colitis reported. False (+) direct Coombs' tests reported. False (+) for urine glucose with Benedict's, Fehling's solution, and Clinitest® tablets.

ADVERSE REACTIONS: Diarrhea, dyspepsia, gastritis, abdominal pain, allergic reactions, genital and anal pruritus, moniliasis, vaginitis, dizziness, fatigue, headache, superinfection (prolonged use).

INTERACTIONS: Probenecid inhibits excretion. Concomitant usage with metformin may require monitoring and dose adjustment.

PREGNANCY: Category B, caution in nursing.

MECHANISM OF ACTION: Cephalosporin; bactericidal due to inhibition of cell-wall synthesis.

PHARMACOKINETICS: Absorption: Rapid; C_{max}=15.25 mcg/mL; T_{max}=1 hr. **Elimination:** Urine (>90%).

PARLODEL
RX
bromocriptine mesylate (Novartis)

THERAPEUTIC CLASS: Dopamine receptor agonist

INDICATIONS: Management of hyperprolactinemia including amenorrhea with or without galactorrhea, infertility, or hypogonadism. Treatment of prolactin-secreting adenomas, acromegaly, and symptoms of Parkinson's disease.

DOSAGE: *Adults:* Take with food. Parkinson's Disease: Initial: 1.25mg bid. Titrate: if needed, increase by 2.5mg/day every 2-4 weeks. Max: 100mg/day.
Hyperprolactinemia: Initial: 1.25mg-2.5mg qd. Titrate: If needed, increase by 2.5mg every 2-7 days. Usual: 2.5-15mg/day. Acromegaly: Initial: 1.25-2.5mg qhs for 3 days. Titrate: Increase by 1.25-2.5mg every 3-7 days until optimal response. Usual: 20-30mg/day. Max: 100mg/day. Withdraw for 4-8 weeks every year in patients treated with pituitary irradiation.
Pediatrics: Take with food. 11-15 yrs: Prolactin-Secreting Pituitary Adenomas: Initial: 1.25-2.5mg/day. Titrate: Increase as tolerated. Usual: 2.5-10mg/day.

HOW SUPPLIED: Cap: 5mg; Tab: 2.5mg* *scored

CONTRAINDICATIONS: Uncontrolled HTN, ergot alkaloid sensitivity, postpartum with CVD unless withdrawal is medically contraindicated, pregnancy if treating hyperprolactinemia, HTN in pregnancy.

WARNINGS/PRECAUTIONS: Caution with renal or hepatic dysfunction, psychosis, CVD, peptic ulcer, dementia. D/C with macroadenomas associated with rapid regrowth of tumor and increased prolactin levels and if severe headache or HTN develops. Risk of pulmonary infiltrates, pleural effusion, thickening of pleura, and retroperitoneal fibrosis with long-term use. Not for prevention of physiological lactation. Monitor BP for symptomatic hypotension and HTN.

ADVERSE REACTIONS: Headache, dizziness, GI effects, orthostatic hypotension, fatigue, arrhythmia, insomnia, hallucinations, abnormal involuntary movements, depression, syncope.

INTERACTIONS: Decreased effects with dopamine antagonists (eg, butyrophenones, haloperidol, phenothiazines, pimozide, metoclopramide). Levodopa may cause hallucinations. Caution with antihypertensives. Alcohol may potentiate side effects. Not for use with other ergot alkaloids.

PREGNANCY: Category B, not for use in nursing.

MECHANISM OF ACTION: Dopamine receptor agonist; activates post-synaptic dopamine receptors and modulates prolactin secretion from anterior pituitary by secreting prolactin inhibitory factor.

PHARMACOKINETICS: Absorption: GI tract (28%); C_{max} =0.4652ng/mL (5mg); T_{max}=1-3 hrs. **Distribution:** Serum albumin binding (90-96%). **Metabolism:** Liver, via CYP3A and hydroxylation. **Elimination:** Liver and kidneys (6%); $T_{1/2}$=8-20 hrs.

PASER RX
aminosalicylic acid (Jacobus)

THERAPEUTIC CLASS: Hydroxybenzoic acid derivative

INDICATIONS: Treatment of TB in combination with other agents.

DOSAGE: *Adults:* 4g tid. Sprinkle on apple sauce, yogurt, or mix with tomato or orange juice.
Pediatrics: Use correspondingly smaller doses to the adult dose. Sprinkle on apple sauce, yogurt, or mix with tomato or orange juice.

HOW SUPPLIED: Pkt: 4g

CONTRAINDICATIONS: Severe renal disease.

WARNINGS/PRECAUTIONS: Monitor for rash, or signs of intolerance during 1st 3 months. D/C if hypersensitivity occurs. Can desensitize by administering small, gradually increasing doses.

ADVERSE REACTIONS: Diarrhea, NV, abdominal pain, fever, dermatitis, lymphoma-like syndrome, agranulocytosis, thrombocytopenia, anemia, jaundice, hepatitis, hypoglycemia.

INTERACTIONS: Reduces acetylation of isoniazid, especially in rapid acetylators. Decreases vitamin B_{12} absorption; consider vitamin B_{12} maintenance treatment. Decreases digoxin levels.

PREGNANCY: Category C, safety in nursing not known.

MECHANISM OF ACTION: Bacteriostatic agent; believed to inhibit folic acid synthesis and/or inhibition of synthesis of the cell-wall component, mycobactin, thus reducing iron uptake by *M.tuberculosis*.

PHARMACOKINETICS: Absorption: C_{max}=20mcg/mL; T_{max}=6 hrs. **Distribution:** Plasma protein binding (50-60%), CSF penetration occurs only if the meninges is inflamed. **Metabolism:** Via acetylation. **Excretion:** Urine (80%); aminosalicylic acid (metabolite); $T_{1/2}$=26.4 min.

PATANOL RX
olopatadine HCl (Alcon)

THERAPEUTIC CLASS: H_1-antagonist and mast cell stabilizer

INDICATIONS: Allergic conjunctivitis.

DOSAGE: *Adults:* 1 drop bid, q6-8h.
Pediatrics: ≥3 yrs: 1 drop bid, q6-8h.

HOW SUPPLIED: Sol: 0.1% (5mL)

WARNINGS/PRECAUTIONS: May re-insert contact lens 10 min after dosing if eye is not red.

ADVERSE REACTIONS: Headache, asthenia, blurred vision, burning, stinging, cold syndrome, dry eye, foreign body sensation, hyperemia, hypersensitivity, keratitis, lid edema, nausea, pharyngitis, pruritus, rhinitis, sinusitis, taste perversion.

PREGNANCY: Category C, caution in nursing.

MECHANISM OF ACTION: Antihistaminic drug; relatively selective histamine H_1-antagonist; inhibits the type 1 immediate hypersensitivity reaction, including inhibition of histamine induced effects on human conjunctival epithelial cells.

PHARMACOKINETICS: Absorption: C_{max}=0.5-1.3ng/mL; T_{max}=2 hrs. **Metabolism:** Metabolites: Mono-desmethyl and N-oxide. **Elimination:** Urine (60-70% parent drug).

PCE
erythromycin (Abbott)

RX

THERAPEUTIC CLASS: Macrolide

INDICATIONS: Treatment of mild to moderate upper/lower respiratory tract and skin and skin structure infections, listeriosis, pertussis, diphtheria, erythrasma, intestinal amebiasis, acute pelvic inflammatory disease (PID) (N.gonorrhea), primary syphilis (if PCN allergy), Legionnaires' disease, chlamydial infections (eg, newborn conjunctivitis, pneumonia of infancy, urogential infections during pregnancy or urethral, endocervical, or rectal infections when tetracyclines are contraindicated or not tolerated), and nongonococcal urethritis caused by susceptible strains of microorganisms. Prophylaxis of initial and recurrent attacks of rheumatic fever if PCN allergy.

DOSAGE: *Adults:* Usual: 333mg q8h or 500mg q12h without food. Max: 4g/day. Do not take bid when dose is ≥1g/day. Treat strep infections for at least 10 days. Streptococcal Infection Long-Term Prophylaxis of Rheumatic Fever: 250mg bid. Chlamydial Urogenital Infection During Pregnancy: 500mg qid or 666mg q8h for at least 7 days, or 500mg q12h, 333mg q8h, or 250mg qid for at least 14 days. Urethral/Endocervical/Rectal Chlamydial Infections and Nongonococcal Urethritis: 500mg qid or 666mg q8h for at least 7 days. Primary Syphilis: 30-40g in divided doses over 10-15 days. Acute PID: 500mg (erythromycin lactobionate) IV q6h for 3 days, then 500mg PO q12h or 333mg PO q8h for 7 days. Intestinal Amebiasis: 500mg q12h, 333mg q8h, or 250mg q6h for 10-14 days. Pertussis: 40-50mg/kg/day in divided doses for 5-14 days. Legionnaires' Disease: 1-4g/day in divided doses.
Pediatrics: Usual: 30-50mg/kg/day in divided doses without food. Severe Infections: May double dose. Max: 4g/day. Treat strep infections for at least 10 days. Streptococcal Infection Long-Term Prophylaxis of Rheumatic Fever: 250mg bid. Chlamydial Conjunctivitis of Newborns/Chlamydial Pneumonia in Infancy: (Sus) 12.5mg/kg qid for 2 weeks and 3 weeks, respectively. Intestinal Amebiasis: 30-50mg/kg/day in divided doses for 10-14 days.

HOW SUPPLIED: Tab, Extended-Release: 333mg, 500mg

CONTRAINDICATIONS: Concomitant terfenadine, astemizole, pimozide, or cisapride.

WARNINGS/PRECAUTIONS: *Clostridium difficile*-associated diarrhea, hepatic dysfunction reported. Caution with impaired hepatic function. May aggravate weakness of patients with myasthenia gravis. Erythromycin does not reach adequate concentrations in fetus to prevent congenital syphilis.

ADVERSE REACTIONS: NV, abdominal pain, diarrhea, anorexia, hepatic dysfunction, abnormal LFTs, allergic reactions, superinfection (prolonged use).

INTERACTIONS: See Contraindications. Rhabdomyolysis reported with lovastatin. May increase levels of theophylline, digoxin, drugs metabolized by CYP450 (eg, carbamazepine, cyclosporine, phenytoin, alfentanil, disopyramide, lovastatin, bromocriptine, valproate, etc). Increases effects of oral anticoagulants, triazolam, midazolam. Risk of acute ergot toxicity with ergotamine and dihydroergotamine. May increase AUC of sildenafil; consider dose reduction of sildenafil.

PREGNANCY: Category B, caution in nursing.

MECHANISM OF ACTION: Macrolide; inhibits protein synthesis by binding 50S ribosomal subunits of susceptible organisms.

PHARMACOKINETICS: Distribution: Crosses placenta, found in breast milk. **Elimination:** Biliary excretion, urine (<5%).

PEDIALYTE
electrolyte maintenance solution (Ross)

OTC

THERAPEUTIC CLASS: Electrolyte replacement

INDICATIONS: To quickly replace fluids and electrolytes, and help prevent dehydration from diarrhea and vomiting. To maintain water and electrolytes following corrective parenteral therapy for severe diarrhea.

DOSAGE: *Pediatrics:* Adjust total daily intake to meet individual needs; base on thirst and response to therapy. See PI for administration guide.

HOW SUPPLIED: Pops: (Chloride-Citrate-Dextrose-Potassium-Sodium) 3.5mEq-3mEq-2.5g-2mEq-4.5mEq/100mL; Sol: (Chloride-Citrate-Dextrose-Fructose-Potassium-Sodium) 3.5mEq-3mEq-2g-0.5g-2mEq-4.5mEq/100mL

WARNINGS/PRECAUTIONS: No mixing or diluting necessary or recommended. Use under medical supervision.

PREGNANCY: Safety in pregnancy and nursing not known.

MECHANISM OF ACTION: Electrolyte replacement.

PEDIAPRED
prednisolone sodium phosphate (Celltech)

RX

THERAPEUTIC CLASS: Glucocorticoid

INDICATIONS: Steroid-responsive dermatoses.

DOSAGE: *Adults:* Initial: 5-60mg/day depending on disease and response. Maint: Decrease dose by small amounts to lowest effective dose. MS Exacerbations: 200mg qd for 1 week, then 80mg every other day for 1 month.
Pediatrics: Initial: 0.14-2mg/kg/day given tid-qid. Nephrotic Syndrome: 20mg/m^2 tid for 4 weeks, then 40mg/m^2 every other day for 4 weeks. Uncontrolled Asthma: 1-2mg/kg/day in single or divided doses peak expiratory rate of 80% is achieved (usually 3-10 days).

HOW SUPPLIED: Sol: 5mg/5mL (120mL)

CONTRAINDICATIONS: Systemic fungal infections.

WARNINGS/PRECAUTIONS: May produce reversible HPA axis suppression. Adjust dose during stress or change in thyroid status. May mask signs of infection or cause new infections. May activate latent amebiasis. Avoid with cerebral malaria. Avoid exposure to chickenpox or measles. Not for treatment of optic neuritis or active ocular herpes simplex. May cause elevation of BP or IOP, cataracts, glaucoma, optic nerve damage, Kaposi's sarcoma, psychic derangements, salt/water retention, increased excretion of potassium and/or calcium, osteoporosis, growth suppression in children, secondary ocular infections. Caution with Strongyloides, CHF, diverticulitis, HTN, renal insufficiency, fresh intestinal anastomoses, active or latent peptic ulcer, ulcerative colitis. Enhanced effect in hypothyroidism or cirrhosis. Avoid abrupt withdrawal. Use with caution in elderly, increased risk of corticosteroid-induced side effects; start at low end of dosing range; monitor bone mineral density.

ADVERSE REACTIONS: Edema, fluid/electrolyte disturbances, osteoporosis, muscle weakness, pancreatitis, peptic ulcer, impaired wound healing, increased intracranial pressure, cushingoid state, hirsutism, menstrual irregularities, growth suppression in children, glaucoma, nausea, weight gain.

INTERACTIONS: Enhanced metabolism with barbiturates, phenytoin, ephedrine, and rifampin. Use with cyclosporine may increase activity of both drugs; convulsions reported with concomitant use. Decreased metabolism with estrogens or ketoconazole. May inhibit response to warfarin. Increased risk of GI side effects with ASA or other NSAIDs. May increase clearance of salicylates. High doses or concurrent neuromuscular drugs may cause acute myopathy. Enhanced possibility of hypokalemia when given with potassium-depleting agents. May produce severe weakness in myasthenia gravis patients on anticholinesterase agents. Avoid live vaccines with immunosuppressive doses. Possible diminished response with killed or inactivated vaccines. May increase blood glucose; adjust antidiabetic agents. May suppress reactions to skin tests.

PREGNANCY: Category C, caution in nursing.

MECHANISM OF ACTION: Synthetic adrenocorticoid steroid; promotes gluconeogenesis, increases deposition of glycogen in the liver, inhibits glucose utilization, increases catabolism of protein, lipolysis, glomerular filtration that leads to increased urinary excretion of urate and calcium.

PHARMACOKINETICS: Absorption: Rapidly absorbed from GI tract. **Distribution:** Plasma protein binding (70-90%), found in breast milk. **Metabolism:** Liver. **Elimination:** Urine (as sulfate and glucuronide congugates). $T_{1/2}$=2-4 hrs.

PEDIARIX   RX

diphtheria toxoid - hepatitis B (Recombinant) - pertussis vaccine, acellular - poliovirus vaccine, inactivated - tetanus toxoid (GlaxoSmithKline)

THERAPEUTIC CLASS: Vaccine/toxoid combination

INDICATIONS: Active immunization against diphtheria, tetanus, pertussis, hepatitis B, and poliomyelitis (polioviruses Types 1, 2, and 3).

DOSAGE: *Pediatrics:* ≥6 weeks-up to 7 yrs: 3 doses of 0.5mL IM at 6-8 week intervals. Start at 2 months old or as early as 6 weeks old if necessary. May use to complete primary series in infants who have received 1 or 2 doses of Infanrix® or IPV or to complete a hepatitis B vaccine (Recombinant) series. Not recommended for completion of the first 3 doses of the DTaP vaccination series initiated with a DTaP vaccine from a different manufacturer.

HOW SUPPLIED: Inj: 0.5mL

CONTRAINDICATIONS: Hypersensitivity to yeast, neomycin, and polymyxin B. Anaphylaxis associated with previous dose or encephalopathy within 7 days of previous vaccine, progressive neurologic disorder (including infantile spasms, uncontrolled epilepsy, progressive encephalopathy).

WARNINGS/PRECAUTIONS: Higher rates of fever reported. Tip cap and plunger contains latex. Caution if within 48 hrs of previous whole-cell DTP or vaccine containing an acellular pertussis component, fever ≥105°F not due to another identifiable cause, collapse or shock-like state, or inconsolable crying lasting ≥3 hrs occurs, or if seizures occur within 3 days. Re-evaluate need if Guillain-Barre syndrome occurs within 6 weeks of receipt of tetanus toxoid-containing vaccine. Defer vaccination with moderate or severe illness, with or without fever. Administer antipyretic for initial 24 hours for those with higher risk for seizures. Caution with bleeding disorders (eg, hemophilia, thrombocytopenia). Have epinephrine available. Suboptimal response may occur in immunocompromised patients.

ADVERSE REACTIONS: Local injection-site reactions, fever, fussiness.

INTERACTIONS: Avoid with anticoagulants unless benefit outweighs risk. Immunosuppressive therapy (eg, irradiation, antimetabolites, alkylating agents, cytotoxic drugs, large doses of corticosteroids) may decrease response. Do not mix with other vaccines in same syringe/vial. Tetanus immune globulin or diphtheria antitoxin should be given at separate site with separate needle/syringe.

PREGNANCY: Category C, safety in nursing not known.

MECHANISM OF ACTION: Vaccine/toxoid combination: stimulates immune system to elicit immune response which produces antibodies that may protect against diphtheria, tetanus, pertussis, hepatitis B, and poliovirus infections.

PEDIAZOLE   RX

erythromycin ethylsuccinate - sulfisoxazole acetyl (Ross)

THERAPEUTIC CLASS: Macrolide/sulfonamide

INDICATIONS: Acute otitis media caused by *H.influenzae*.

DOSAGE: *Pediatrics:* ≥2 months: Dose based on 50mg/kg/day erythromycin or 150mg/kg/day sulfisoxazole given tid-qid for 10 days. Max: 6g/day sulfisoxazole.

HOW SUPPLIED: Sus: (Erythromycin Ethylsuccinate-Sulfisoxazole Acetyl) 200mg-600mg/5mL (100mL, 150mL, 200mL)

CONTRAINDICATIONS: Pediatrics <2 months old, pregnant women at term, mothers nursing infants <2 months old, concomitant terfenadine.

WARNINGS/PRECAUTIONS: Pseudomembranous colitis, hepatic dysfunction reported. Severe, fatal allergic reactions reported with sulfonamides. Caution with hepatic or renal dysfunction, bronchial asthma, and severe allergies. May aggravate myasthenia gravis. Erythromycin does not reach adequate concentrations in fetus' to prevent congenital syphilis. Hemolysis may occur in G6P-deficiency patients. Sulfonamides not for treatment of group A β-hemolytic infections.

ADVERSE REACTIONS: NV, abdominal pain, diarrhea, anorexia, hepatic dysfunction, abnormal LFTs, allergic reactions, tachycardia, syncope, blood dyscrasias, BUN elevation, edema, superinfection.

INTERACTIONS: Rhabdomyolysis reported with lovastatin. May increase levels of theophylline, digoxin, methotrexate, drugs metabolized by CYP450 (eg, carbamazepine, cyclosporine, tacrolimus, phenytoin, alfentanil, disopyramide, lovastatin, bromocriptine, valproate, etc). Increases effects of oral anticoagulants, triazolam, midazolam, sulfonylureas. Risk of acute ergot toxicity with ergotamine or dihydroergotamine. Avoid terfenadine. May require less thiopental for anesthesia. May have cross-sensitivity with thiazides, acetazolamide, and oral hypoglycemics.

PREGNANCY: Category C, not for use in nursing.

PEDIOTIC RX
hydrocortisone - neomycin sulfate - polymyxin B Sulfate (King)

THERAPEUTIC CLASS: Antibacterial/corticosteroid combination

INDICATIONS: Superficial bacterial infections of the external auditory canal. Infections of mastoidectomy and fenestration cavities.

DOSAGE: *Adults:* Clean and dry ear canal. Instill 4 drops tid-qid. Max: 10 days. *Pediatrics:* Clean and dry ear canal. Instill 4 drops tid-qid. Max: 10 days.

HOW SUPPLIED: Sus: (Neomycin-Hydrocortisone-Polymyxin B) 0.35%-1%-10,000 U/mL (7.5mL)

CONTRAINDICATIONS: Herpes simplex, vaccinia, and varicella infections.

WARNINGS/PRECAUTIONS: Caution with perforated eardrum or chronic otitis media; ototoxicity may develop. Re-evaluate if no improvement after 10 days.

ADVERSE REACTIONS: Allergic sensitization, superinfection.

INTERACTIONS: Cross-reactivity with kanamycin, paromomycin, streptomycin, and gentamycin.

PREGNANCY: Category C, caution in nursing.

MECHANISM OF ACTION: Antibacterial and anti-inflammatory otic suspension.

PHARMACOKINETICS: Distribution: Found in breast milk.

PEDVAXHIB RX
haemophilus B Conjugate (Merck)

THERAPEUTIC CLASS: Vaccine

INDICATIONS: Vaccination against *Haemophilus influenzae* type b.

DOSAGE: *Pediatrics:* 2-14 months: 0.5mL IM. Repeat 2 months later. If 2 doses given before 12 months of age, give booster dose (0.5mL) at 12-15 months ≥2 months after 2nd dose. 15-71 months (Not Previously Vaccinated): 0.5mL IM single dose.

HOW SUPPLIED: Inj: 7.5mcg/0.5mL

WARNINGS/PRECAUTIONS: Suboptimal response may occur in immunocompromised patients. Have epinephrine (1:1000) available.

ADVERSE REACTIONS: Fever, injection site pain/soreness and erythema, irritability, sleepiness, crying, diarrhea, vomiting.

INTERACTIONS: May not obtain immune response with immunosuppressive therapy.

PREGNANCY: Category C, safety in nursing not known.

MECHANISM OF ACTION: PRP-conjugate vaccine; produces antigen that is postulated to convert T-independent antigen into T-dependent antigen, resulting in enhanced antibody response and immunologic memory.

PENICILLIN VK   RX
penicillin V Potassium (Various)

OTHER BRAND NAME: Veetids (Sandoz)

THERAPEUTIC CLASS: Penicillin

INDICATIONS: Treatment of mild to moderately severe bacterial infections including conditions of the respiratory tract, oropharynx, skin and soft tissue caused by susceptible strains of microorganisms. Prevention of recurrence following rheumatic fever and/or chorea.

DOSAGE: *Adults:* Usual: Streptococcal Infections (Scarlet Fever/Erysipelas/Upper Respiratory Tract): 125-250mg q6-8h for 10 days. Pneumococcal Infections (Otitis Media/ Respiratory Tract): 250-500mg q6h until afebrile for at least 2 days. Staphylococcus Infections (Skin/Soft Tissue): 250-500mg q6-8h. Fusospirochetosis Infections (Oropharnyx): 250-500mg q6-8h. Rheumatic Fever/Chorea Prevention: 125-250mg bid.
Pediatrics: ≥12 yrs: Usual: Streptococcal Infections (Scarlet Fever/Erysipelas/Upper Respiratory Tract): 125-250mg q6-8h for 10 days. Pneumococcal Infections (Otitis Media/ Respiratory Tract): 250-500mg q6h until afebrile for at least 2 days. Staphylococcus Infections (Skin/Soft Tissue): 250-500mg q6-8h. Fusospirochetosis Infections (Oropharnyx): 250-500mg q6-8h. Rheumatic Fever/Chorea Prevention: 125-250mg bid.

HOW SUPPLIED: Sus: 125mg/5mL, 250mg/5mL (100mL, 200mL); Tab: 250mg, 500mg

WARNINGS/PRECAUTIONS: Not for severe pneumonia, empyema, bacteremia, pericarditis, meningitis and arthritis during the acute stage. Serious, fatal anaphylactic reactions reported. Pseudomembranous colitis reported. Oral administration may not be effective with severe illnesses, nausea, vomiting, gastric dilation, cardiospasm, intestinal hypermotility. Cross-sensitivity with cephalosporins. Caution with asthma and allergies.

ADVERSE REACTIONS: NV, epigastric distress, diarrhea, hypersensitivity reactions, black hairy tongue, anaphylaxis, superinfection (prolonged use).

PREGNANCY: Category B, caution in nursing.

MECHANISM OF ACTION: Phenoxymethyl analog of penicillin G; exerts bactericidal action during stage of active multiplication by inhibiting biosynthesis of cell-wall mucopeptide.

PHARMACOKINETICS: Distribution: Plasma protein binding (80%). **Elimination:** Urine.

PENTACEL   RX
acellular pertussis, adsorbed - diphtheria toxoid - haemophilus B Conjugate - poliovirus vaccine, inactivated - tetanus toxoid (Sanofi Pasteur)

THERAPEUTIC CLASS: Vaccine/toxoid combination

INDICATIONS: Active immunization against diphtheria, tetanus, pertussis, poliomyelitis, and invasive disease due to *Haemophilus influenzae* type b in children 6 weeks through 4 yrs of age (prior to 5th dirthday).

DOSAGE: *Pediatrics:* ≥6 weeks up to 4 yrs: 0.5mL IM into anterolateral aspect of thigh (<1 yr) or deltoid muscle (older children). 4-Dose Series: Administer at 2, 4 and 6, and 15-18 months of age. First dose may be given as early as 6 weeks of age. Children who have completed 4-dose series should receive a 5th dose of DTaP vaccine at 4-6 yrs of age; these children should receive Daptacel vaccine as their 5th dose of DTaP. Children Previously Vaccinated With 1 or More Doses of Daptacel Vaccine: Pentacel vaccine may be used to complete first 4 doses of DTaP series in infants/children who have received 1 or more doses of Daptacel and are also scheduled to receive the other antigens of Pentacel vaccine. Children Previously Vaccinated With 1 or More Doses of IPV: Pentacel vaccine may be used to complete the 4-dose IPV series in infants/ children who have received 1 or more doses of another IPV vaccine and are also scheduled to receive the other antigens of Pentacel vaccine. Previously Vaccinated With 1 or More Doses of Haemophilus b Conjugate Vaccine: Pentacel vaccine may be used to complete the vaccination series in infants/children previously vaccinated with 1 or more doses of Haemophilus b Conjugate Vaccine who are also scheduled to receive the other antigens of Pentacel vaccine.

HOW SUPPLIED: Inj: 0.5mL

CONTRAINDICATIONS: Severe allergic reaction (eg, anaphylaxis) to any component; encephalopathy within 7 days of administration of a previous pertussis-containing vaccine; progressive neurologic disorders.

WARNINGS/PRECAUTIONS: Not for IV or SQ use. Re-evaluate need if Guillain-Barre syndrome occurs within 6 weeks of receipt of tetanus toxoid-containing vaccine. Weigh benefits vs risks if any of the following occur within specified period after administration of whole-cell pertussis or acellular pertussis-containing vaccine: fever ≥105°F within 48 hrs not due to another identifiable cause; collapse or shock-like state within 48 hrs; persistent, inconsolable crying lasting ≥3 hrs within 48 hrs; or if seizures (with or without fever) occur within 3 days. May administer antipyretic for initial 24 hrs for children with higher risk for seizures. Have epinephrine available.

ADVERSE REACTIONS: Local injection-site reactions (redness, swelling, tenderness), fever, decreased activity/lethargy, inconsolable crying, fussiness/irritability.

INTERACTIONS: Immunosuppressive therapies, including irradiation, antimetabolites, alkylating agents, cytotoxic drugs, and corticosteroids (used in greater than physiologic doses), may reduce immune response. Do not mix with any other vaccine in the same syringe.

PREGNANCY: Category C, safety in nursing not known.

MECHANISM OF ACTION: Vaccine/toxoid combination:

PEPCID
famotidine (Merck)

RX

OTHER BRAND NAME: Pepcid RPD (Merck)

THERAPEUTIC CLASS: H₂-blocker

INDICATIONS: (PO/Inj) Short term treatment of active duodenal ulcer (DU), active benign gastric ulcer (GU), gastroesophageal reflux disease (GERD) and esophagitis due to GERD. Maintenance therapy for DU. Treatment of hypersecretory conditions (eg, Zollinger-Ellison syndrome). (Inj) For hospitalized patients with hypersecretory conditions or intractable ulcers. As an alternative in patients unable to take oral forms.

DOSAGE: *Adults:* (PO) Acute DU: 40mg qhs or 20mg bid for 4-8 weeks. Maint DU: 20mg qhs. GU: 40mg qhs. GERD: 20mg bid up to 6 weeks. GERD with Esophagitis: 20-40mg bid up to 12 weeks. Hypersecretory Conditions: Initial: 20mg q6h. Max: 160mg q6h. (Inj) 20mg IV q12h, hypersecretory conditions may require higher doses. CrCl <50mL/min: Reduce to 1/2 dose, or increase interval to q36-48h.
Pediatrics: 1-16 yrs: (PO) DU/GU: Usual: 0.5mg/kg/day qhs or divided bid. Max: 40mg/day. GERD With or Without Esophagitis: 0.5mg/kg PO bid. Max: 40mg bid. (Inj) 0.25mg/kg IV q12h up to 40mg/day. Base duration of therapy on clinical response, and/or pH, and endoscopy. (PO) GERD: 3 months-1yr: 0.5mg/kg bid for up to 8 weeks. <3 months: 0.5mg/kg qd for up to 8 weeks. CrCl <50mL/min: Reduce to 1/2 dose, or increase interval to q36-48h.

HOW SUPPLIED: Inj: 0.4mg/mL, 10mg/mL; Sus: 40mg/5mL (50mL); Tab: 20mg, 40mg; Tab, Disintegrating: (RPD) 20mg, 40mg

CONTRAINDICATIONS: Hypersensitivity to other H₂ antagonists.

WARNINGS/PRECAUTIONS: CNS adverse effects reported with moderate to severe renal insufficiency; adjust dose. Disintegrating tabs contain phenylalanine; caution in phenylketonurics. Symptomatic response does not preclude the presence of gastric malignancy.

ADVERSE REACTIONS: Headache, dizziness, constipation, diarrhea, convulsions, interstitial pneumonia, Stevens-Johnson syndrome.

INTERACTIONS: May give with antacids.

PREGNANCY: Category B, not for use in nursing.

MECHANISM OF ACTION: Histamine H₂-receptor antagonist; inhibits both acid concentration and volume of gastric secretion.

PHARMACOKINETICS: Absorption: (Adults PO): Incompletely absorbed; $T_{max}=1.3$ hrs. (Adults, IV): $T_{max}=20$-30 min. **Distribution:** (Adult) Plasma protein binding (15-20%); excreted in breast milk. **Metabolism:** S-oxide (metabolite). **Elimination:** Renal (65-70%), (PO) 25-30% unchanged; (IV) 65-70% unchanged. Metabolic (65-70%); (Adults) $T_{1/2}=2.5$-3.5 hrs. Refer to package insert for pediatric parameters.

PEPCID AC

OTC

famotidine (J&J - Merck)

THERAPEUTIC CLASS: H_2-blocker

INDICATIONS: Relief and prevention of heartburn, acid indigestion, and sour stomach.

DOSAGE: *Adults:* Relief: 1 tab/cap prn. Max: 2 doses/24 hrs. Prevention: 1 tab/cap 15-60 min before food or beverages that cause heartburn. Max: 2 doses/24 hrs. *Pediatrics:* ≥12yrs: 1 tab/cap prn. Max: 2 doses/24 hrs. Prevention: 1 tab/cap 15-60 min before food or beverages that cause heartburn. Max: 2 doses/24 hrs.

HOW SUPPLIED: Cap: 10mg; Tab: 10mg, 20mg; Tab, Chewable: 10mg

INTERACTIONS: Avoid with other acid reducers.

PEPCID COMPLETE

OTC

calcium carbonate - famotidine - magnesium hydroxide (J&J - Merck)

THERAPEUTIC CLASS: H_2-blocker/antacid

INDICATIONS: To relieve heartburn associated with acid indigestion and sour stomach.

DOSAGE: *Adults:* Chew 1 tab to relieve symptoms. Max: 2 tabs/24hrs. *Pediatrics:* ≥12 yrs: Chew 1 tab to relieve symptoms. Max: 2 tabs/24hrs.

HOW SUPPLIED: Tab, Chewable: (Famotidine-Calcium Carbonate-Magnesium Hydroxide) 10mg-800mg-165mg

WARNINGS/PRECAUTIONS: Not for use in those with trouble swallowing. Avoid with other acid reducers.

PREGNANCY: Safety in pregnancy and nursing not known.

PEPTO-BISMOL

OTC

bismuth subsalicylate (Procter & Gamble)

OTHER BRAND NAME: Pepto-Bismol Maximum Strength (Procter & Gamble)

THERAPEUTIC CLASS: Antimicrobial

INDICATIONS: To control diarrhea within 24 hrs, relieving associated abdominal cramps; soothes heartburn, and indigestion without constipation; and relieves nausea and upset stomach.

DOSAGE: *Adults:* (Sus) 30mL every 0.5-1 hr prn. Max: 8 doses/24hrs. (Sus, Max Strength) 30mL hourly prn. Max: 4 doses/24 hrs. (Tab; Tab, Chewable) 2 tabs every 0.5-1 hr prn. Max: 8 doses/24hrs. Drink plenty of clear fluids. *Pediatrics:* (Sus) 9-12 yrs: 15mL every 0.5-1 hr prn. 6-9 yrs: 10mL every 0.5-1 hr prn. 3-6 yrs: 5mL every 0.5-1 hr. Max: 8 doses/24hrs. (Sus, Max Strength) 9-12 yrs: 15mL hourly prn. 6-9 yrs: 10mL hourly prn. 3-6 yrs: 5mL hourly prn. Max: 4 doses/24hrs. (Tab; Tab, Chewable) 9-12 yrs: 1 tab every 0.5-1 hr prn. 6-9 yrs: 2/3 tab every 0.5-1 hr prn. 3-6 yrs: 1/3 tab every 0.5-1 hr prn. Max: 8 doses/24 hrs. Drink plenty of clear fluids.

HOW SUPPLIED: Sus: 262mg/15mL; Sus, Maximum Strength: 525mg/15mL; Tab: 262mg; Tab, Chewable: 262mg

WARNINGS/PRECAUTIONS: Avoid in children and teenagers with or recovering from chickenpox or flu. Do not give with ASA or non-ASA salicylate allergy. May cause temporary darkening of tongue or stool. Product may contain small amounts of naturally occurring lead.

INTERACTIONS: May cause ringing in ears with ASA; d/c if this occurs. Caution with anticoagulants, antidiabetic, and antigout agents.

PREGNANCY: Safety in pregnancy and nursing not known.

PERI-COLACE
docusate sodium - senna (Purdue Products)

OTC

THERAPEUTIC CLASS: Stool softener/laxative combination

INDICATIONS: Management of constipation.

DOSAGE: *Adults:* 2-4 tabs daily
Pediatrics: ≥12yrs: 2-4 tabs daily. 6-<12yrs: 1-2 tabs daily. 2-<6yrs: Max of 1 tab daily.

HOW SUPPLIED: (Docusate Sodium-Sennosides) Tab: 50mg-8.6mg

WARNINGS/PRECAUTIONS: Caution with use >1 week.

INTERACTIONS: Caution with mineral oil.

PREGNANCY: Safety in pregnancy and nursing not known.

PERMAPEN
penicillin G Benzathine (Pfizer)

RX

THERAPEUTIC CLASS: Penicillin

INDICATIONS: Treatment of microorganisms susceptible to low and very prolonged serum levels in upper respiratory tract infections (streptococci group A - without bacteremia), syphilis, yaws, bejel, and pinta. Prophylaxis for rheumatic fever and/or chorea. Follow-up prophylactic therapy for rheumatic heart disease and acute glomerulonephritis.

DOSAGE: *Adults:* Streptococcal Infection: 1.2 MU IM single dose. Primary/Secondary/Latent Syphilis: 1 MU IM single dose. Late (Tertiary/Neurosyphilis) Syphilis: 3 MU IM every 7 days for total of 6-9 MU. Yaws/Bejel/Pinta: 1.2 MU IM single dose. Rheumatic Fever/Glomerulonephritis Prophylaxis: 1.2 MU IM once monthly or 600,000 U IM twice monthly. Use upper outer quadrant of buttock. Rotate injection site.
Pediatrics: ≤12 yrs: Adjust dose according to age and weight and severity of infection. Streptococcal Infection: 900,000 U IM single dose in older children. Congenital Syphilis: <2 yrs: 50,000 U/kg IM single dose. 2-12 yrs: Adjust dose based on adult schedule. Use midlateral aspect of thigh in infants and small children. May divide dose between 2 buttocks in peds <2 yrs. Rotate injection site.

HOW SUPPLIED: Inj: 600,000 U/mL

WARNINGS/PRECAUTIONS: Caution in newborns; evaluate organ system function frequently. Evaluate renal, hepatic and hematopoietic systems with prolonged therapy. Serious, fatal anaphylactic reactions reported; increased risk with hypersensitivity to PCNs, cephalosporins, and other allergens. Avoid IV, intra-arterial administration, or injection into/near major peripheral nerves or blood vessels may cause severe neurovascular damage. May result in overgrowth of nonsusceptible organisms. Avoid subcutaneous and fat-layer injections. Take culture after therapy completion to determine streptococci eradication.

ADVERSE REACTIONS: Skin eruptions, urticaria, laryngeal edema, anaphylaxis, fever, eosinophilia.

INTERACTIONS: Bacteriostatic agents (eg, tetracycline, erythromycin) may diminish effects. Prolonged levels with probenecid.

PREGNANCY: Category B, caution in nursing.

MECHANISM OF ACTION: Penicillin; exerts bactericidal action during stage of multiplication by inhibiting biosynthesis of cell-wall mucopeptide.

PHARMACOKINETICS: Absorption: Slow. **Distribution:** Plasma protein binding (60%). **Metabolism:** Hydrolysis. **Elimination:** Kidneys, bile.

PERPHENAZINE
perphenazine (Various)

RX

THERAPEUTIC CLASS: Phenothiazine

INDICATIONS: Treatment of schizophrenia. To control severe nausea and vomiting.

DOSAGE: *Adults:* Moderately Disturbed Non-Hospitalized With Schizophrenia: Initial: 4-8mg tid. Maint: Reduce to minimum effective dose. Hospitalized Psychotic Patients With Schizophrenia: 8-16mg bid-qid. Max: 64mg/day. Severe Nausea/Vomiting: 8-16mg/day in divided doses. Max: 24mg/day. Elderly: Lower dosages recommended. *Pediatrics:* ≥12 yrs: Use lowest limits of adult dose.

HOW SUPPLIED: Tab: 2mg, 4mg, 8mg, 16mg

CONTRAINDICATIONS: Comatose or greatly obtunded patients, large doses of CNS depressants (eg, barbiturates, alcohol, narcotics, analgesics, or antihistamines), blood dyscrasias, bone marrow depression, liver damage, subcortical brain damage with or without hypothalamic involvement.

WARNINGS/PRECAUTIONS: Tardive dyskinesia may develop. NMS, photosensitivity reported. May lower convulsive threshold; caution with alcohol withdrawal. Caution with psychic depression, renal impairment, respiratory impairment. May impair mental/physical abilities. May mask signs of overdosage to other drugs. May obsure diagnosis of intestinal obstruction, brain tumor. Severe hypotension may occur in surgery. May elevate prolactin levels. Monitor hepatic/renal functions, blood counts. Increased risk of liver damage, jaundice, corneal and lenticular deposits, and irreversible dyskinesias with long-term use.

ADVERSE REACTIONS: Extrapyramidal reactions, tardive dyskinesia, cerebral edema, seizures, drowsiness, dry mouth, salivation, nausea, vomiting, diarrhea, anorexia, constipation, urticaria, erythema, eczema, postural hypotension, tachycardia.

INTERACTIONS: See Contraindications. Additive effects with CNS depressants and phenothiazine; use reduced amount of added drug. Additive anticholinergic effects with atropine/atropine-like drugs, exposure to phosphorous insecticide. Additive effects and hypotension may occur with alcohol. Cytochrome P450 2D6 inhibitors (TCAs, SSRIs) may increase levels; lower doses may be required.

PREGNANCY: Safety in pregnancy and nursing not known.

MECHANISM OF ACTION: Piperazinyl phenothiazine; mechanism not known, has actions at all levels of the CNS, particularly the hypothalamus.

PHARMACOKINETICS: Absorption: C_{max}=984(43)pg/mL; T_{max}=1-3 hrs. **Metabolism:** Liver (extensive) via sulfoxidation, hydroxylation mediated by CYP450 (2D6), dealkylation, and glucoronidation. **Elimination:** Urine (primarily), feces, bile; $T_{1/2}$=9-12 hrs.

PFIZERPEN
penicillin G Potassium (Pfizer)

RX

THERAPEUTIC CLASS: Penicillin

INDICATIONS: For therapy of severe infections when rapid and high blood levels of penicillin required. Management of streptococcal, pneumococcal, staphylococcal, clostridial, fusospirochetal, listeria, and gram negative bacillary, and pasteurella infections. For anthrax, actinomycosis, diphtheria, erysipeloid, meningitis, endocarditis, bacteremia, rat-bite fever, syphilis, and gonorrheal endocarditis and arthritis. With combined oral therapy, prophylaxis against endocarditis in patients with congenital heart disease, rheumatic, or other acquired valvular heart disease undergoing dental procedures or surgical procedures of upper respiratory tract.

DOSAGE: *Adults:* Anthrax/Gonorrheal Endocarditis/Severe Infections (Streptococci, Pneumococci, Staphylococci): Minimum of 5MU/day. Syphilis: Administer in hospital. Determine dose and duration based on age and weight. Meningococcic Meningitis: 1-2MU IM q2h or 20-30MU/day continuous IV. Actinomycosis: 1-6MU/day for cervicofacial cases; 10-20MU/day for thoracic and abdominal disease. Clostridial Infections: 20MU/day (adjunct to antitoxin). Fusospirochetal Severe Infections: 5-10MU/day for oropharynx, lower respiratory tract, and genital area infection. Rat-bite Fever: 12-15MU/day for 3-4 weeks. Listeria Endocarditis: 15-20MU/day for 4 weeks. Pasteurella Bacteremia/Meningitis: 4-6MU/day for 2 weeks. Erysipeloid Endocarditis: 2-20MU/day for 4-6 weeks. Gram Negative Bacillary Bacteremia: 20-80MU/day. Diphtheria (carrier state): 0.3-0.4MU/day in divided doses for 10-12 days. Endocarditis Prophylaxis: 1MU IM mixed with 0.6MU procaine penicillin G 0.5-1 hr before procedure. Renal/Cardiac/Vascular Dysfunction: Consider dose reduction. For streptococcal infection, treat for minimum 10 days.
Pediatrics: Listeria Infections: Neonates: 0.5-1MU/day. Congenital Syphilis: Administer in

335

hospital. Determine dose and duration based on age and weight. Endocarditis Prophylaxis: 30,000U/kg IM mixed with 0.6MU procaine penicillin G 0.5-1 hr before procedure. For streptococcal infection, treat for minimum 10 days.

HOW SUPPLIED: Inj: 1MU, 5MU, 20MU

WARNINGS/PRECAUTIONS: Serious, fatal anaphylactic reactions reported; increased risk with hypersensitivity to PCNs, cephalosporins, and other allergens. Avoid IV, intra-arterial administration, or injection into/near major peripheral nerves or blood vessels; may cause severe neurovascular damage. Take culture after therapy completion to determine streptococci eradication. Caution with history of significant allergies or asthma. May result in overgrowth of nonsusceptible organisms. Evaluate renal, hepatic and hematopoietic systems with prolonged therapy. Administer slowly to avoid electrolyte imbalance from potassium or sodium content; monitor electrolytes and consider dose reductions with renal, cardiac, or vascular dysfunction. Caution in newborns; evaluate organ system function frequently.

ADVERSE REACTIONS: Skin rash (eg, maculopapular eruption, exfoliative dermatitis) urticaria, chills, fever, edema, arthralgia, prostration, anaphylaxis, arrhythmias, cardiac arrest, Jarisch-Herxheimer reaction.

INTERACTIONS: Bacteriostatic agents (eg, tetracycline, erythromycin) may diminish effects. Prolonged levels with probenecid.

PREGNANCY: Category B, caution in nursing.

MECHANISM OF ACTION: Penicillin; exerts bactericidal action during stage of active multiplication by inhibiting biosynthesis of cell-wall mucopeptide.

PHARMACOKINETICS: Absorption: Rapid. **Distribution:** Found in breast milk. **Elimination:** Urine.

PHENERGAN INJECTION RX
promethazine HCl (Baxter)

THERAPEUTIC CLASS: Phenothiazine derivative

INDICATIONS: For blood or plasma allergic reactions, allergic reactions where oral therapy is not possible, sedation, and special surgical situations (eg, repeated bronchoscopy). Adjunct for anaphylactic reactions and postoperative pain. Treatment of motion sickness. Prevention and control of nausea and vomiting in surgery.

DOSAGE: *Adults:* (IM/IV) IM is preferred. Allergy: Initial: 25mg, may repeat within 2 hrs. Sedation: 25-50mg qhs. Nausea/Vomiting: 12.5-25mg q4h. Preoperative/Postoperative: 25-50mg. Obstetrics: 50mg in early labor, 25-75mg in established labor, may repeat once or twice q4h. Max: 100mg/24 hrs of labor. Do not give IV administration >25mg/mL and at a rate >25mg/min.
Pediatrics: ≥2 yrs: Dose should not exceed half of adult dose. Premedication: Usual: 0.5mg/lb. Do not give IV administration >25mg/mL and at a rate >25mg/min.

HOW SUPPLIED: Inj: 25mg/mL, 50mg/mL

CONTRAINDICATIONS: Comatose states, intra-arterial or subcutaneous injection. Hypersensitivity to other phenothiazines.

WARNINGS/PRECAUTIONS: Caution in patients ≥2 yrs. Not recommended for uncomplicated vomiting in pediatrics. May cause marked drowsiness; caution with operating machinery. Fatal respiratory depression reported; avoid with respiratory dysfunction (eg, COPD, sleep apnea). Avoid prolonged sun exposure. May lower seizure threshold. Caution with bone marrow depression. NMS reported. Caution in acutely ill pediatric patients. Avoid in pediatrics with Reye's syndrome or hepatic disease. Avoid perivascular extravasation or inadvertent intra-arterial injection. Caution with narrow-angle glaucoma, prostatic hypertrophy, stenosing peptic ulcer, bladder-neck or pyloroduodenal obstruction, cardiovascular disease, hepatic dysfunction. Cholestatic jaundice reported. Alters HCG pregnancy test reading. May increase blood glucose.

ADVERSE REACTIONS: Drowsiness, dizziness, tinnitus, blurred vision, dry mouth, increased or decreased blood pressure, urticaria, nausea, vomiting, blood dyscrasia.

INTERACTIONS: Added sedative effects with CNS depressants (eg, alcohol, narcotics, narcotic analgesics, sedatives, hypnotics, general anesthetics, tranquilizers, TCAs); reduce dose or eliminate these agents. Reduce barbiturate dose by one-half and analgesic depressant dose by one-quarter to one-half. Caution with drugs that alter seizure threshold (eg, narcotics, local anesthetics). Do not use epinephrine for promethazine injection overdose. Caution with anticholinergics. Possible adverse reactions with MAOIs.

PREGNANCY: Category C, caution in nursing.

MECHANISM OF ACTION: Phenothiazine derivative/H_1 receptor antagonist; possesses antihistamine (does not block release of histamine), sedative, anti-motion sickness, antiemetic, and anticholinergic effects.

PHARMACOKINETICS: Metabolism: Liver; sulfoxides, N-desmethylpromethazine (metabolites). **Elimination:** Urine; $T_{1/2}$=9-16 hrs (IV), 9.8 hrs (IM).

PHENOBARBITAL
phenobarbital (Various)   `CIV`

THERAPEUTIC CLASS: Barbiturate

INDICATIONS: Treatment of generalized, tonic-clonic and cortical focal seizures. For relief of anxiety, tension and apprehension. Short-term treatment of insomnia.

DOSAGE: *Adults:* Sedation: 30-120mg/day given bid-tid. Max: 400mg/24h. Hypnotic: 100-200mg. Seizures: 60-200mg/day. Elderly/Debilitated/Renal or Hepatic Dysfunction: Reduce dosage.
Pediatrics: Seizures: 3-6mg/kg/day.

HOW SUPPLIED: Elixir: 20mg/5mL; Tab: 15mg, 30mg, 32.4mg, 60mg, 64.8mg, 100mg

CONTRAINDICATIONS: Respiratory disease with dyspnea or obstruction, porphyria, severe liver dysfunction. Large doses with nephritic patients.

WARNINGS/PRECAUTIONS: May be habit forming. Avoid abrupt withdrawal. Caution with acute or chronic pain; may mask symptoms or paradoxical excitement may occur. Cognitive deficits reported in children with febrile seizures. May cause excitement in children and excitement, depression or confusion in elderly, debilitated. Caution with hepatic dysfunction, borderline hypoadrenal function, depression.

ADVERSE REACTIONS: Drowsiness, residual sedation, lethargy, vertigo, somnolence, respiratory depression, hypersensitivity reactions, nausea, vomiting, headache.

INTERACTIONS: May be potentiated by MAOIs, antihistamines, alcohol, tranquilizers, sedative/hypnotics, other CNS depressants. Decreases effects of oral anticoagulants. Increases corticosteroid metabolism. Decreases effects of oral contraceptives. Decreases absorption of griseofulvin. Decreases half-life of doxycycline. May alter phenytoin metabolism. Increased levels with sodium valproate and valproic acid.

PREGNANCY: Category D, caution in nursing.

MECHANISM OF ACTION: Barbiturate; nonselective CNS depressant. Capable of producing all levels of CNS mood alteration. Responsible for depressing the sensory cortex, decreasing motor activity, altering cerebellar function, causing sedation and hypnosis.

PHARMACOKINETICS: Distribution: Distributed to all tissues and fluids. High concentrations found in the brain, liver, and kidneys. Found in breast milk. **Metabolism:** Hepatic. **Elimination:** Urine (primary), feces; $T_{1/2}$=79 hrs (adults), 110 hrs (children and newborns less than 48 hrs old).

PHENYTEK
phenytoin sodium (Mylan Bertek)   RX

THERAPEUTIC CLASS: Hydantoin

INDICATIONS: Control of generalized tonic-clonic (grand mal) and complex partial (psychomotor, temporal lobe) seizures. Prevention and treatment of neurosurgically induced seizures.

DOSAGE: *Adults:* No Previous Treatment: Initial: 100mg extended phenytoin sodium capsule tid. Titrate: May increase at 7-10 day intervals. Usual: 100mg tid-qid. May increase up to 200mg Phenytek tid. Once Daily Dosing: 300mg Phenytek qd may replace 100mg extended phenytoin sodium capsule tid if seizures are controlled. LD (clinic/hospital): 1g in 3 divided doses (400mg, 300mg, 300mg) given 2 hrs apart. Start maintenance 24 hrs later. Avoid LD with renal and hepatic disease.

Pediatrics: Initial: 5mg/kg/day given bid-tid. Titrate: May increase at 7-10 day intervals. Maint: 4-8mg/kg/day. Max: 300mg/day. >6 yrs: May require the minimum adult dose (300mg/day).

HOW SUPPLIED: Cap, Extended-Release: 200mg, 300mg

WARNINGS/PRECAUTIONS: Avoid abrupt discontinuation. Caution with porphyria, hepatic dysfunction, elderly, diabetes, debilitated. D/C if rash occurs. Lymphadenopathy reported. Serum sickness may occur with lymph node involvement. Gingival hyperplasia reported; maintain proper dental hygiene. Hyperglycemia, birth defects, and osteomalacia reported. Monitor levels. Confusional states reported with toxic levels. Increased seizure frequency during pregnancy. Neonatal coagulation defects reported within first 24 hrs of birth; give vitamin K to mother before delivery and to neonate after birth. Avoid use with seizures due to hypoglycemia or other metabolic causes. Hemopoietic complications reported.

ADVERSE REACTIONS: Nystagmus, ataxia, slurred speech, decreased coordination, confusion, dizziness, insomnia, transient nervousness, motor twitchings, headaches, nausea, vomiting, constipation, rash, hypersensitivity reactions.

INTERACTIONS: Increased levels with acute alcohol intake, amiodarone, chloramphenicol, chlordiazepoxide, diazepam, dicumarol, disulfiram, estrogens, H_2-antagonists, halothane, isoniazid, methylphenidate, phenothiazines, phenylbutazone, salicylates, succinamides, sulfonamides, tolbutamide, trazodone. Decreased levels with chronic alcohol abuse, carbamazepine, reserpine, sucralfate. Decreases effects of corticosteroids, coumarin anticoagulants, digitoxin, doxycycline, estrogens, furosemide, oral contraceptives, quinidine, rifampin, theophylline, vitamin D. Phenobarbital, sodium valproate, valproic acid may increase or decrease levels. May increase or decrease levels of phenobarbital, sodium valproate, valproic acid. Calcium antacids decrease absorption; space dosing. Moban® contains calcium ions that interfere with absorption. TCAs may precipitate seizures. Increased risk of phenytoin hypersensitivity with barbiturates, succinamides, oxazolidinediones.

PREGNANCY: Possibly teratogenic, weigh benefits versus risk; not for use in nursing.

MECHANISM OF ACTION: Inhibits spread of seizure activity; primary site of action appears to be the motor cortex. Possibly promotes sodium efflux from neurons, stabilizing the threshold against hyperexcitability caused by excessive stimulation or environmental changes capable of reducing membrane sodium gradient. Also reduces the posttetanic potentiation at synapses, which prevents cortical seizure foci from detonating adjacent cortical areas.

PHARMACOKINETICS: Absorption: T_{max}=4-12 hrs. **Metabolism:** Hepatic via hydroxylation. **Elimination:** Renal; bile (inactive metabolite) and urine; $T_{1/2}$=22 hrs.

pHisoHex   RX
hexachlorophene (Sanofi-Aventis)

THERAPEUTIC CLASS: Detergent cleanser

INDICATIONS: As a surgical scrub and a bacteriostatic skin cleanser. Also to control outbreak of gram-positive infection, when other infection control methods failed.

DOSAGE: *Adults:* Surgical Scrub: Apply 5mL with water and lather over hands and forearms. Scrub well with a wet brush for 3 min, including nails and interdigital spaces. Rinse thoroughly then repeat. Bacteriostatic Cleansing: Apply 5mL with water and lather, apply to areas that need cleansing. Rinse thoroughly.
Pediatrics: Bacteriostatic Cleansing: Apply 5mL with water and lather, apply to areas that need cleansing. Rinse thoroughly. Do not use routinely for bathing infants.

HOW SUPPLIED: Liq: 3% (150mL, 480mL, 3840mL)

CONTRAINDICATIONS: Burned/denuded skin. Should not use as wet pack, vaginal pack, tampon, occlusive dressing, lotion, on mucous membranes, or as a routine prophylactic bath. Light sensitivity to halogenated phenol derivatives.

WARNINGS/PRECAUTIONS: D/C promptly if cerebral irritability occurs. Infants are more susceptible to CNS toxicity. Avoid skin lesions; may cause toxic blood levels. Do not apply to burns; may cause neurotoxicity and death. Avoid eye contact.

ADVERSE REACTIONS: Dermatitis, photosensitivity, redness, mild scaling, dryness.

INTERACTIONS: Skin products containing alcohol may decrease efficacy.

PREGNANCY: Category C, not for use in nursing.

MECHANISM OF ACTION: Bacteriostatic cleansing agent; cleanses the skin thoroughly and has bacteriostatic action against staphylococci and other gram-positive bacteria.

PHOSPHOLINE IODIDE   RX
echothiophate iodide (Wyeth)

THERAPEUTIC CLASS: Cholinesterase inhibitor

INDICATIONS: Treatment of glaucoma and accommodative esotropias.

DOSAGE: *Adults:* Early Chronic Simple Glaucoma: (0.3%) 1 drop bid, am and hs. Advanced Chronic Simple Glaucoma/Glaucoma Secondary to Cataract Surgery: Initial: (0.3%) 1 drop bid, am and hs. Titrate: May increase to higher strengths prn. *Pediatrics:* Accommodative Esotropia: Diagnosis: (0.125%) 1 drop qhs for 2-3 weeks. Treatment: Decrease dose to 1 drop (0.125%) every other day or (0.6%) 1 drop qd. Titrate: Decrease strength gradually. Max: (0.125%) 1 drop qd.

HOW SUPPLIED: Sol: 0.03%, 0.06%, 0.125%, 0.25% (5mL)

CONTRAINDICATIONS: Active uveal inflammation, angle-closure glaucoma.

WARNINGS/PRECAUTIONS: Avoid with quiescent uveitis. Should hold nose for 1-2 min to prevent absorption. D/C with cardiac irregularities, salivation, urinary incontinence, diarrhea, profuse sweating, muscle weakness, or respiratory difficulties. Caution with vagotonia, bronchial asthma, spastic GI disturbance, peptic ulcer, bradycardia, hypotension, recent MI, epilepsy, parkinsonism, retinal detachment. Tolerance may develop.

ADVERSE REACTIONS: Stinging, burning, lacrimation, lid muscle twitching, conjunctival and ciliary redness, browache, induced myopia, visual blurring.

INTERACTIONS: Risk of respiratory or cardiovascular collapse with succinylcholine during general anesthesia. May potentiate effects of other cholinesterase inhibitors (eg, succinylcholine, organophosphate, carbamate insecticides, myasthenia gravis drugs).

PREGNANCY: Category C, not for use in nursing.

MECHANISM OF ACTION: Long-acting cholinesterase inhibitor; enhances effect of endogenously liberated acetylcholine in the iris, ciliary muscle, and other parasympathetically innervated structures of eye. Responsible for causing miosis, an increase in aqueous humor outflow, decrease in IOP, and potentiation of accomodation.

PHRENILIN FORTE   RX
acetaminophen - butalbital (Amarin)

OTHER BRAND NAME: Phrenilin (Amarin)

THERAPEUTIC CLASS: Barbiturate/analgesic

INDICATIONS: Tension or muscle contraction headaches.

DOSAGE: *Adults:* (Phrenilin Forte) 1 cap q4h. (Phrenilin) 1-2 tabs q4h. Max: 6 caps/tabs/day.
Pediatrics: ≥12 yrs: (Phrenilin Forte) 1 cap q4h. (Phrenilin) 1-2 tabs q4h. Max: 6 caps/tabs/day.

HOW SUPPLIED: (Butalbital-APAP) Cap: (Phrenilin Forte) 50mg-650mg; Tab: (Phrenilin)50mg-325mg.

CONTRAINDICATIONS: Porphyria.

WARNINGS/PRECAUTIONS: Abuse potential. Caution in elderly/debilitated, severe renal/hepatic impairment, and acute abdominal conditions.

ADVERSE REACTIONS: Drowsiness, lightheadedness, dizziness, sedation, SOB, NV, abdominal pain, intoxicated feeling.

INTERACTIONS: Enhanced CNS effects with MAOIs. May enhance CNS depression effects of narcotic analgesics, alcohol, general anesthetics, tranquilizers (eg, chlordiazepoxide, sedative hypnotics, CNS depressants).

PREGNANCY: Category C, not for use in nursing.

MECHANISM OF ACTION: Butalbital: Short to intermediate acting barbiturate; not established. Acetaminophen (APAP): Nonopiate, nonsalicylate analgesic, and antipyretic; not established.

PHARMACOKINETICS: Absorption: APAP: Rapid; GIT. Butalbital: GIT. **Metabolism:** APAP: Liver (conjugation). **Distribution:** Butalbital: Crosses placental barrier, found in breast milk. **Elimination:** Butalbital: Urine (3.6%). $T_{1/2}$=35 hrs. APAP: $T_{1/2}$=1.25-3 hrs.

PHYTONADIONE   RX
phytonadione (Various)

> Severe, fatal reactions reported during or immediately after IV or IM use. Only use IV or IM route when SC route is not feasible.

THERAPEUTIC CLASS: Vitamin K derivative

INDICATIONS: For coagulation disorders caused by vitamin K deficiency or interference with vitamin K activity, including prophylaxis and therapy of hemorrhagic disease of the newborn; anticoagulant-induced prothrombin deficiency caused by coumarin and indanedione derivatives; and hypoprothrombinemia caused by antibacterials, secondary factors that limit absorption or synthesis of vitamin K (obstructive jaundice, biliary fistula), or by drugs that interfere with vitamin K metabolism (eg, salicylates).

DOSAGE: *Adults:* Administer SQ when possible. Anticoagulant-Induced PT Deficiency: Initial: 2.5-10mg up to 25mg (rarely 50mg). May repeat if PT is still elevated 6-8 hrs after initial dose. Hypoprothrombinemia Due to Other Causes: 2.5-25mg or more (rarely up to 50mg); route depends on severity of condition and response.
Pediatrics: Prophylaxis of Hemorrhagic Disease in Newborn: 0.5-1mg IM within 1 hr of birth. Treatment of Hemorrhagic Disease in Newborn: 1mg SQ/IM (may need higher dose if mother has received oral anticoagulants).

HOW SUPPLIED: Inj: 1mg/0.5 mL, 10mg/mL

WARNINGS/PRECAUTIONS: Contains benzyl alcohol; toxicity in newborns may occur. Takes 1-2 hrs to observe improvement in PT. Maintain lowest possible dose to prevent original thromboembolic events. Avoid repeated large doses with hepatic disease. Failure to respond may indicate a congenital coagulation defect or a condition unresponsive to vitamin K. Monitor PT regularly.

ADVERSE REACTIONS: Anaphylactoid reactions, flushing, peculiar taste sensations, dizziness, rapid and weak pulse, profuse sweating, hypotension, dyspnea, cyanosis, injection site tenderness or swelling, hyperbilirubinemia (in newborns).

INTERACTIONS: Does not counteract anticoagulant effects of heparin. Temporary resistance to prothrombin-depressing anticoagulants, especially with large doses.

PREGNANCY: Category C, caution in nursing.

MECHANISM OF ACTION: Vitamin K derivative; works in the liver as a necessary component in the production of active clotting factors: prothrombin (factor II), proconvertin (factor VII), plasma thromboplastin component (factor IX), and Stuart factor (factor X).

PHARMACOKINETICS: Absorption: (IM) Readily absorbed. **Metabolism:** Liver.

PIPERACILLIN   RX
piperacillin sodium (Various)

THERAPEUTIC CLASS: Broad-spectrum penicillin

INDICATIONS: Treatment of serious infections caused by susceptible strains of microorganisms in the following conditions: intra-abdominal, urinary tract, gynecologic, lower respiratory tract, skin and skin structure, bone/joint, and uncomplicated gonococcal urethritis, and septicemia. Perioperative surgical prophylaxis during certain procedures.

DOSAGE: *Adults:* Usual: 3-4g IM/IV q4-6h. Max: 24g/day; IM: 2g/site. Serious Infections: 200-300mg/kg/day IV divided q4-6h. Complicated UTI: 125-200mg/kg/day IV divided q6-8h. Uncomplicated UTI/CAP: 100-125mg/kg/day IM/IV divided q6-12h. Uncomplicated Gonorrhea: 2g IM single dose with 1g PO probenecid 1/2 hr before injection. Surgical Prophylaxis: 2g IV 20-30 min just prior to anesthesia (See PI for follow-up dosing). Renal Impairment: Uncomplicated/Complicated UTI: CrCl <20mL/min: 3g q12h. Complicated UTI: CrCl 20-40mL/min: 3g q8h. Serious Infection: CrCl 20-40mL/min: 4g q8h. CrCl <20mL/min: 4g q12h. Hemodialysis: Give 1g additional dose after each dialysis. Max: 2g q8h. Usual treatment is for 7-10 days; treat gynecologic infections for 3-10 days; treat *S.pyogenes* infections for at least 10 days.

Pediatrics: ≥12 yrs: Usual: 3-4g IM/IV q4-6h. Max: 24g/day; IM: 2g/site. Serious Infections: 200-300mg/kg/day IV divided q4-6h. Complicated UTI: 125-200mg/kg/day IV divided q6-8h. Uncomplicated UTI/CAP: 100-125mg/kg/day IM/IV divided q6-12h. Uncomplicated Gonorrhea: 2g IM single dose with 1g PO probenecid 1/2 hr before injection. Surgical Prophylaxis: 2g IV 20-30 min just prior to anesthesia (See PI for follow-up dosing). Renal Impairment: Uncomplicated/Complicated UTI: CrCl <20mL/min: 3g q12h. Complicated UTI: CrCl 20-40mL/min: 3g q8h. Serious Infection: CrCl 20-40mL/min: 4g q8h. CrCl <20mL/min: 4g q12h. Hemodialysis: Give 1g additional dose after each dialysis. Max: 2g q8h. Usual treatment is for 7-10 days; treat gynecologic infections for 3-10 days; treat *S.pyogenes* infections for at least 10 days.

HOW SUPPLIED: Inj: 2g, 3g, 4g

CONTRAINDICATIONS: Hypersensitivity to cephalosporins.

WARNINGS/PRECAUTIONS: Serious, sometimes fatal, hypersensitivity reactions reported with PCN therapy. *Clostridium difficile*-associated diarrhea reported. Cross-sensitivity to cephalosporins. Monitor renal, hepatic and hematopoietic functions with prolonged use. D/C if bleeding manifestations occur; increased risk with renal failure. Prolonged use may cause superinfections. May experience neuromuscular excitability or convulsions with higher than recommended doses. Contains 1.85mEq/g sodium; caution with salt restriction. Monitor electrolytes periodically with low potassium levels. Increased incidence of rash and fever in cystic fibrosis. Continue treatment for at least 48-72 hrs after patient becomes asymptomatic.

ADVERSE REACTIONS: Thrombophlebitis, erythema and pain at injection site, diarrhea, headache, dizziness, anaphylaxis, rash, superinfections.

INTERACTIONS: Do not mix with aminoglycoside in a syringe or infusion bottle; may cause inactivation of aminoglycoside. May prolong neuromuscular blockade of nondepolarizing muscle relaxants (eg, vecuronium). Increased risk of hypokalemia with cytotoxic therapy or diuretics. May reduce methotrexate clearance. Probenecid may increase levels. Monitor coagulation parameters closely with concomitant anticoagulants.

PREGNANCY: Category B, caution in nursing.

MECHANISM OF ACTION: Broad-spectrum penicillin; exerts bacterial activity by inhibiting both septum and cell wall synthesis; active against a variety of gram-positive and gram-negative aerobic and anaerobic bacteria.

PHARMACOKINETICS: Absorption: (2g) Rapid; C_{max}=36mcg/mL, T_{max}=30 min. **Distribution:** Plasma protein binding (16%). **Elimination:** Urine (60%-80%); (2g) $T_{1/2}$=54 min., (6g) 63 min.

PLAQUENIL

RX

hydroxychloroquine sulfate (Sanofi-Aventis)

> Be familiar with complete prescribing information before prescribing hydroxychloroquine.

THERAPEUTIC CLASS: Quinine derivative

INDICATIONS: Suppression and treatment of acute attacks of malaria in adults and children. Treatment of discoid and systemic lupus erythematosus and rheumatoid arthritis (RA) in adults.

DOSAGE: *Adults:* Malaria Suppression: 400mg weekly. Begin 2 weeks before exposure and continue for 8 weeks after leaving endemic area. Give 400mg q6h for 2 doses if therapy is not begun before exposure. Acute Attack: 800mg, then 400mg 6-8 hrs later, then 400mg for 2 more days. RA: Initial: 400-600mg qd with food or milk; increase until optimum response. Maint: After 4-12 weeks, 200-400mg qd with food or milk. Lupus Erythematosus: Initial: 400mg qd-bid for several weeks depending on response. Maint: 200-400mg/day.

Pediatrics: Malaria Suppression: 5mg/kg (base) weekly, max 400mg/dose. Begin 2 weeks before exposure and continue for 8 weeks after leaving endemic area. q6h for 2 doses if therapy is not begun before exposure. Acute Attack: 10mg base/kg, max 800mg/dose; then 5mg base/kg, max 400mg/dose at 6, 24 and 48 hrs after 1st dose.

HOW SUPPLIED: Tab: 200mg (200mg tab=155mg base)

CONTRAINDICATIONS: Long term therapy in children or if retinal/visual field changes due to 4-aminoquinoline compounds.

WARNINGS/PRECAUTIONS: Caution with hepatic disease, G6PD deficiency, alcoholism, psoriasis, and porphyria. Perform baseline and periodic (3 months) ophthalmologic exams and blood cell counts with prolonged therapy. Test periodically for muscle weakness. D/C if blood disorders occur. Avoid if possible in pregnancy. D/C after 6 months if no improvement in RA.

ADVERSE REACTIONS: Headache, dizziness, diarrhea, loss of appetite, muscle weakness, nausea, abdominal cramps, bleaching of hair, dermatitis, ocular toxicity, visual field defects.

INTERACTIONS: Caution with hepatotoxic drugs.

PREGNANCY: Safety in pregnancy and nursing not known.

MECHANISM OF ACTION: Quinine derivative; has antimalarial action. Precise mechanism not established.

PLEXION   RX
sulfacetamide sodium - sulfur (Medicis)

OTHER BRAND NAMES: Plexion SCT (Medicis) - Plexion TS (Medicis)

THERAPEUTIC CLASS: Sulfonamide/sulfur combination

INDICATIONS: Topical treatment of acne vulgaris, acne rosacea, and seborrheic dermatitis.

DOSAGE: *Adults:* (Cleanser) Wash qd-bid. Massage into skin for 10-20 sec, then rinse and dry. (TS) Apply qd-tid. (Cre) Apply to wet skin. Rinse off with water after 10 min or if dry.
Pediatrics: ≥12 yrs: (Cleanser) Wash qd-bid. Massage into skin for 10-20 sec, then rinse and dry. (TS) Apply qd-tid. (Cre) Apply to wet skin. Rinse off with water after 10 min or if dry.

HOW SUPPLIED: Cleanser: (Sulfacetamide-Sulfur) 10%-5% (170.3g, 340.2g); Cre: (SCT) 10%-5% (120g); Lot: (TS) 10%-5% (30g); Pads: 10%-5% (30s)

CONTRAINDICATIONS: Kidney disease.

WARNINGS/PRECAUTIONS: D/C if irritation occurs. Avoid eye contact or mucous membranes. Caution with denuded or abraded skin, patients prone to topical sulfonamide hypersensitivity. Can cause reddening and scaling of epidermis.

ADVERSE REACTIONS: Local irritation.

PREGNANCY: Category C, caution in nursing.

MECHANISM OF ACTION: Sulfonamide/sulfur combination. Sodium sulfacetamide: Acts as a competitive antagonist to para-aminobenzoic acid (PABA), Sulfur: Not established. Responsible for inhibiting the growth of *Propionibacterium acnes* and the formation of free fatty acids.

PHARMACOKINETICS: Absorption: (PO) Readily absorbed **Excretion:** (PO) Urine (unchanged).

PNEUMOVAX 23   RX
pneumococcal vaccine (Merck)

THERAPEUTIC CLASS: Vaccine

INDICATIONS: Immunization against pneumococcal disease caused by those pneumococcal types included in the vaccine.

DOSAGE: *Adults:* Usual: 0.5mL SQ/IM in deltoid muscle or lateral mid-thigh.
Pediatrics: ≥2 yrs: 0.5mL SQ/IM in deltoid muscle or lateral mid-thigh.

HOW SUPPLIED: Inj: 575mcg/0.5mL

WARNINGS/PRECAUTIONS: Vaccination timing is critical for chemotherapy or immunosuppressive therapy. Suboptimal response may occur in immunocompromised patients. Caution with severely compromised cardiovascular or pulmonary function where systemic reaction would be a significant risk. Delay vaccine with febrile respiratory illness or other active infection. Do not revaccinate immunocompetent patients. Continue prophylaxis pneumococcal antibiotics. May not prevent pneumococcal meningitis with chronic CSF leakage.

ADVERSE REACTIONS: Local injection site reactions (eg, soreness, warmth, erythema, swelling, induration), fever (≤102°F).

PREGNANCY: Category C, caution use in nursing.

MECHANISM OF ACTION: Active immunization that may protect against pneumococcal infection.

POLYTRIM   RX
polymyxin B Sulfate - trimethoprim sulfate (Allergan)

THERAPEUTIC CLASS: Dihydrofolate reductase inhibitor/antibiotic

INDICATIONS: Surface ocular bacterial infections, including blepharoconjunctivitis, acute bacterial conjunctivitis.

DOSAGE: *Adults:* Mild-Moderate Infections: 1 drop q3h for 7-10 days. Max: 6 doses/day. *Pediatrics:* ≥2 months: Mild-Moderate Infections: 1 drop q3h for 7-10 days. Max: 6 doses/day.

HOW SUPPLIED: Sol: (Trimethoprim-Polymyxin B) 1mg-10,000U/mL (10mL)

WARNINGS/PRECAUTIONS: Not indicated for the prophylaxis or treatment of ophthalmia neonatorum.

ADVERSE REACTIONS: Local irritation, lid edema, itching, increased redness, tearing, burning, stinging, circumocular rash, superinfection (prolonged use).

PREGNANCY: Category C, caution in nursing.

MECHANISM OF ACTION: Dihydrofolate reductase inhibitor/antibiotic. Polymyxin B: increases permeability of bacterial cell membrane by interacting with phospholipid components of membrane. Trimethoprim: blocks production of tetrahydrofolic acid from dihydrofolic acid by binding to and reversibly inhibiting the enzyme dihydrofolate reductase. Binding is stronger for bacterial enzyme than for corresponding mammalian enzyme, and therefore selectively interferes with bacterial biosynthesis of nucleic acids and proteins.

PHARMACOKINETICS: Absorption: C_{max}=0.03mcg/mL (trimethoprim), 1 unit/mL (polymyxin B) (following two-time dosing of 2 drops of ophthalmic solution containing 1mg of trimethoprim and 10,000 units of polymyxin B).

POLY-VI-FLOR   RX
multiple vitamin - sodium fluoride (Mead Johnson)

THERAPEUTIC CLASS: Multiple vitamin/fluoride supplement

INDICATIONS: Vitamin supplement. Fluoride supplement for caries prophylaxis in areas where water contains less than optimal fluoride levels.

DOSAGE: *Pediatrics:* (Sol) 6 months-3 yrs and <0.3 ppm Fluoride or 3-6 yrs and 0.3-0.6 ppm Fluoride: 1mL (0.25mg) qd. 3-6 yrs and <0.3 ppm Fluoride or >6 yrs and 0.3-0.6 ppm Fluoride: 1mL (0.5mg) qd. (Tab) 4-6 yrs and 0.3-0.6 ppm Fluoride: 0.25mg qd. 4-6 yrs and <0.3 ppm Fluoride or ≥6 yrs and 0.3-0.6 ppm Fluoride: 0.5mg qd. 6-16 yrs and <0.3 ppm Fluoride: 1mg qd.

HOW SUPPLIED: Sol: Vitamin A 1500 IU-Vitamin C 35mg-Vitamin D 400 IU-Vitamin E 5 IU-Thiamin 0.5mg-Riboflavin 0.6mg-Niacin 8mg-Vitamin B_6 0.4mg-Vitamin B_{12} 2mcg. 0.25mg drops contains 0.25mg Fluoride (50mL), 0.5mg drops contain 0.5mg Fluoride (50mL); Tab, Chewable: Vitamin A 2500 IU-Vitamin C 60mg-Vitamin D 400 IU-Vitamin E 15 IU-Thiamin 1.05mg-Riboflavin 1.2mg-Niacin 13.5mg-Vitamin B_6 1.05mg-Folate 0.3mg-Vitamin B_{12} 4.5mcg. 0.25mg tabs contain 0.25mg Fluoride; 0.5mg tabs contain 0.5mg Fluoride; 1mg tabs contain 1mg Fluoride

WARNINGS/PRECAUTIONS: Must chew tab; not for pediatrics <4yrs. Risk of dental fluorosis from ingestion of large amounts of fluoride. Children up to 16 yrs, in areas where water contains less than optimal fluoride levels, should receive daily fluoride supplementation.

ADVERSE REACTIONS: Allergic rash.

PREGNANCY: Safety in pregnancy and nursing not known.

PONSTEL   RX
mefenamic acid (Sciele)

> NSAIDs may cause an increased risk of serious cardiovascular thrombotic events, MI, stroke, and serious GI adverse events including bleeding, ulceration, and perforation of the stomach or intestines. Contraindicated for the treatment of perioperative pain in the setting of coronary artery bypass graft (CABG) surgery.

THERAPEUTIC CLASS: NSAID

INDICATIONS: Relief of mild to moderate pain in patients ≥14 yrs, when therapy will not exceed 7 days. Treatment of primary dysmenorrhea.

DOSAGE: *Adults:* Acute Pain: Usual: 500mg, then 250mg q6h prn up to 1 week. Primary Dysmenorrhea: Usual: 500mg, then 250mg q6h up to 3 days. Take with food.
Pediatrics: ≥14 yrs: Acute Pain: Usual: 500mg, then 250mg q6h prn up to 1 week. Primary Dysmenorrhea: Usual: 500mg, then 250mg q6h up to 3 days. Take with food.

HOW SUPPLIED: Cap: 250mg

CONTRAINDICATIONS: Pre-existing renal disease, active ulceration or chronic inflammation of the GI tract. Allergic-type reactions, including asthma and urticaria, after taking ASA or other NSAIDs. Treatment of perioperative pain in the setting of CABG surgery.

WARNINGS/PRECAUTIONS: May lead to onset of new HTN or worsening of pre-existing HTN; monitor BP closely. Fluid retention and edema reported; caution with fluid retention or heart failure. Renal papillary necrosis and other renal injury reported after long-term use. Not recommended for use with advanced renal disease. Anaphylactoid reactions may occur. May cause serious skin adverse events (eg, exfoliative dermatitis, Stevens-Johnson syndrome, and toxic epidermal necrolysis). Avoid in late pregnancy; may cause premature closure of ductus arteriosis. May cause elevations of LFTs; d/c if liver disease develops or systemic manifestations occur. Caution in elderly. Anemia may occur; with long-term use, monitor Hgb/Hct if signs or symptoms of anemia develop. May inhibit platelet aggregation and prolong bleeding time; monitor with coagulation disorders. Caution with asthma and avoid with ASA-sensitive asthma.

ADVERSE REACTIONS: Abdominal pain, constipation, diarrhea, dyspepsia, flatulence, gross bleeding/perforation, heartburn, nausea, GI ulcers, vomiting, abnormal renal function, anemia, dizziness, edema, elevated liver enzymes, headache, increased bleeding time, pruritus, rash, tinnitus.

INTERACTIONS: Caution with CYP2C9 inhibitors. ASA may increase adverse effects; avoid use. Warfarin may increase GI bleeding. May prolong PT with oral anticoagulants. May enhance methotrexate toxicity. Decreases effects of ACE inhibitors, furosemide, and thiazides; monitor for renal toxicity. Increases lithium levels. Magnesium hydroxide may increase mefenamic acid levels. Enhances methotrexate toxicity; caution with concomitant use.

PREGNANCY: Category C, not for use in nursing.

MECHANISM OF ACTION: NSAID (fenamate derivative); suspected to inhibit prostaglandin synthetase, exerts anti-inflammatory, analgesic, and antipyretic actions.

PHARMACOKINETICS: Absorption: Rapid; C_{max}=10-20mcg/mL^3, T_{max}=2-4 hrs. Distribution: V_d=1.06L/kg^2; plasma protein binding (90%). Metabolism: Via CYP2C9. Elimination: Urine (52%), feces (20%); $T_{1/2}$=2 hrs.

POTABA   RX
potassium p-Aminobenzoate (Glenwood)

THERAPEUTIC CLASS: Vitamin B complex

INDICATIONS: Possibly effective for the treatment of Peyronie's disease, dermatomyositis, linear scleroderma, pemphigus.

DOSAGE: *Adults:* Usual: 12g/day, in 4 to 6 divided doses. Take with meals or snacks. Tabs should be taken with plenty of liquid. Dissolve powder in water or juice.
Pediatrics: 1g/day for each 10 lbs of body weight given in divided doses. Dissolve powder in water or juice. Take with food and plenty of liquid.

HOW SUPPLIED: Cap: 0.5g; Pow: 2g/envule (50⁹); Tab: 0.5g

CONTRAINDICATIONS: Concomitant sulfonamides.

WARNINGS/PRECAUTIONS: Suspend therapy if anorexia, nausea, occurs. D/C if hypersensitivity reaction develops. Caution with renal disease.

ADVERSE REACTIONS: Anorexia, nausea, fever, rash.

PREGNANCY: Safety in pregnancy or nursing not known.

MECHANISM OF ACTION: Vitamin B complex; anti-fibrosis action due to its mediation of increased oxygen uptake at tissue level.

PRAMOSONE
RX
hydrocortisone acetate - pramoxine HCl (Ferndale)

THERAPEUTIC CLASS: Corticosteroid/anesthetic

INDICATIONS: Relief of the inflammatory and pruritic manifestations of corticosteroid-responsive dermatoses.

DOSAGE: *Adults:* Apply tid-qid. May use occlusive dressings for psoriasis or recalcitrant conditions. D/C dressings if infection develops.
Pediatrics: Apply tid-qid. May use occlusive dressings for psoriasis or recalcitrant conditions. D/C dressings if infection develops.

HOW SUPPLIED: (Pramoxine-Hydrocortisone) Cre: 1%-1%, 1%-2.5% (30g, 60g); Lot: 1%-1% (60mL, 120mL, 240mL), 1%-2.5% (60mL, 120mL); Oint: 1%-1%, 1%-2.5% (30g)

WARNINGS/PRECAUTIONS: May produce reversible HPA axis suppression, manifestations of Cushing's syndrome, hyperglycemia, and glucosuria. Caution when applied to large surface areas or under occlusive dressings. Use appropriate antifungal or antibacterial agent with dermatological infections; d/c if infection does not clear. Peds may be more susceptible to systemic toxicity. Avoid eyes. D/C if irritation occurs.

ADVERSE REACTIONS: Burning, itching, irritation, dryness, folliculitis, hypertrichosis, acneiform eruptions, hypopigmentation, perioral dermatitis, allergic dermatitis, skin maceration, secondary infection, skin atrophy, striae, miliaria.

PREGNANCY: Category C, caution in nursing.

MECHANISM OF ACTION: Corticosteroid/anesthetic. Hydrocortisone: Possesses anti-inflammatory, anti-pruritic, and vasoconstrictive properties. Anti-inflammatory action not established. Pramoxine: Provides temporary relief from itching and pain. Stabilizes neuronal membrane of nerve endings with which it comes into contact.

PHARMACOKINETICS: Absorption: Percutaneous; occlusion, inflammation, and other disease states may increase absorption. **Distribution:** Bound to plasma proteins in varying degrees. Systemically administered corticosteroids found in breast milk. **Metabolism:** Liver. **Excretion:** Kidneys (major), bile.

PRAVACHOL
RX
pravastatin sodium (Bristol-Myers Squibb)

THERAPEUTIC CLASS: HMG-CoA reductase inhibitor

INDICATIONS: As adjunct to diet, to reduce elevated total-C, LDL-C, Apo B, TG levels, and to increase HDL-C in primary hypercholesterolemia and mixed dyslipidemia (Type IIa and IIb). Treatment of primary dysbetalipoproteinemia (Type III) and heterozygous familial hypercholesterolemia. To reduce elevated serum TG levels (Type IV). In hypercholesterolemic patients without coronary heart disease, to reduce risk of: MI, undergoing myocardial revascularization procedures, and cardiovascular mortality with no increase in death from non-cardiovascular causes. In patients with coronary heart disease, to reduce risk of: mortality by reducing coronary death, undergoing myocardial revascularization procedures, MI, stroke, and TIA; and to slow progression of coronary atherosclerosis.

DOSAGE: *Adults:* ≥18 yrs: Initial: 40mg qd. Perform lipid tests within 4 weeks and adjust according to response and guidelines. Titrate: May increase to 80mg qd if needed. Significant Renal/Hepatic Dysfunction: Initial: 10mg qd. Concomitant Immunosuppressives (eg, cyclosporine): Initial:10mg qhs. Max: 20mg/day.

Pediatrics: Heterozygous Familial Hypercholesterolemia: 14-18 yrs: Initial: 40mg qd. 8-13 yrs: 20mg qd. Concomitant Immunosuppressives (eg, cyclosporine): Initial: 10mg qhs. Max: 20mg/day.

HOW SUPPLIED: Tab: 10mg, 20mg, 40mg, 80mg

CONTRAINDICATIONS: Active liver disease, unexplained persistent elevations of LFTs, pregnancy, nursing mothers.

WARNINGS/PRECAUTIONS: Perform LFTs before therapy, before dose increases, and if clinically indicated. Risk of myopathy, myalgia, and rhabdomyolysis. D/C if AST or ALT ≥3x ULN persists, if elevated CPK levels occur, or if myopathy diagnosed or suspected. Less effective with homozygous familial hypercholesterolemia. Monitor for endocrine dysfunction. Closely monitor with heavy alcohol use, recent history or signs of hepatic disease, or renal dysfunction.

ADVERSE REACTIONS: Rash, NV, diarrhea, headache, chest pain, influenza, abdominal pain, dizziness, increases ALT, AST, CPK.

INTERACTIONS: Risk of myopathy with fibrates, niacin, cyclosporine, erythromycin. Increased levels with gemfibrozil, itraconazole. Avoid fibrates unless benefit outweighs drug combination risk. Decreased levels with concomitant cholestyramine/colestipol; take 1 hr before or 4 hrs after resins. Caution with drugs that diminish levels or activity of steroid hormones (eg, ketoconazole, spironolactone, cimetidine).

PREGNANCY: Category X, not for use in nursing.

MECHANISM OF ACTION: HMG-CoA reductase inhibitor; causes increased number of LDL-receptors on cell surfaces and enhanced receptor mediated catabolism and clearance of circulating LDL. Inhibits LDL production by inhibiting hepatic synthesis of VLDL, LDL precursor.

PHARMACOKINETICS: Absorption: Rapid. Absolute bioavailability (17%); T_{max}=1-1.5 hrs. **Distribution:** Plasma protein binding (50%). **Metabolism:** Liver. **Elimination:** Feces (70%), urine (20%); $T_{1/2}$=77 hrs.

PREDNISONE   RX
prednisone (Roxane)

OTHER BRAND NAME: Deltasone (Pharmacia & Upjohn)

THERAPEUTIC CLASS: Glucocorticoid

INDICATIONS: Steroid-responsive disorders.

DOSAGE: *Adults:* Initial: 5-60mg/day depending on disease and response. Maint: Decrease dose by small amounts to lowest effective dose.
Pediatrics: Initial: 5-60mg/day depending on disease and response. Maint: Decrease dose by small amounts to lowest effective dose.

HOW SUPPLIED: Sol: 5mg/mL, 5mg/5mL; Tab: 1mg, 2.5mg*, 5mg*, 10mg*, 20mg*, 50mg* *scored

CONTRAINDICATIONS: Systemic fungal infections.

WARNINGS/PRECAUTIONS: May need to increase dose before, during, and after stressful situations. May mask signs of infection or cause new infections. Prolonged use may produce glaucoma, optic nerve damage, secondary ocular infections. Increases BP, salt/water retention, potassium excretion. More severe/fatal course of infections reported with chickenpox, measles. Caution with latent TB, hypothyroidism, cirrhosis, ocular herpes simplex, HTN, diverticulitis, fresh intestinal anastomosis, ulcerative colitis, osteoporosis, myasthenia gravis, renal insufficiency, peptic ulcer disease. Growth and development of children on prolonged therapy should be monitored. Monitor for psychic disturbances. Avoid abrupt withdrawal.

ADVERSE REACTIONS: Fluid and electrolyte disturbances, HTN, osteoporosis, muscle weakness, cushingoid state, menstrual irregularities, nervousness, insomnia, impaired wound healing, DM, ulcerative esophagitis, excessive sweating, increases intracranial pressure, carbohydrate intolerance, glaucoma, cataracts, weight gain, nausea, malaise.

INTERACTIONS: Increases clearance of high dose ASA; caution in hypoprothrombinemia. Increased insulin and oral hypoglycemic requirements in DM. Avoid small pox vaccine, and live vaccines with immunosuppressive doses. Possible decreased vaccine response with killed or inactivated vaccines with immunosuppressive doses. Increased clearance with hepatic enzyme inducers. Decreased metabolism with troleandomycin, ketoconazole. Variable effect on oral anticoagulants.

PREGNANCY: Safety in pregnancy and nursing not known.

MECHANISM OF ACTION: Anti-inflammatory glucocorticoid; causes profound and varied metabolic effects and modifies the body's immune responses to diverse stimuli.

PHARMACOKINETICS: Absorption: Readily absorbed (GI tract).

PREGNYL   RX
chorionic gonadotropin (Organon)

THERAPEUTIC CLASS: Human chorionic gonadotropin

INDICATIONS: For prepubertal cryptorchidism not due to anatomic obstruction. For hypogonadotropic hypogonadism (secondary to a pituitary deficiency) in males. To induce ovulation (OI) and pregnancy in anovulatory, infertile women in whom anovulation is not due to primary ovarian failure and pretreated with human menotropins.

DOSAGE: *Adults:* Hypogonadism: 500-1000 U IM 3x/week (TIW) for 3 weeks, then twice weekly for 3 weeks; or 4000 U IM TIW for 6-9 months, then reduce to 2000 U TIW for 3 months. OI: 5000-10,000 U IM 1 day after last dose of menotropins.
Pediatrics: Cryptorchidism: 4000 U IM TIW for 3 weeks; or 5000 U IM every 2nd day for 4 doses; or 15 doses of 500-1000 U over 6 weeks; or 500 U TIW for 4-6 weeks (if treatment fails, give 1000 U/injection starting 1 month later). Initiate therapy between 4-9 yrs. Hypogonadism: 500-1000 U IM TIW for 3 weeks, then twice weekly for 3 weeks; or 4000 U IM TIW for 6-9 months, then reduce to 2000 U TIW for 3 months.

HOW SUPPLIED: Inj: 10,000 U

CONTRAINDICATIONS: Precocious puberty, prostatic carcinoma or other androgen-dependent neoplasms, pregnancy.

WARNINGS/PRECAUTIONS: Potential ovarian hyperstimulation, enlargement or rupture of ovarian cysts, multiple births, and arterial thromboembolism with infertility treatment. D/C if precocious puberty occurs in cryptorchidism patients. Caution with cardiac or renal disease, epilepsy, migraine, asthma. Not effective treatment for obesity.

ADVERSE REACTIONS: Headache, irritability, restlessness, depression, fatigue, edema, precocious puberty, gynecomastia, injection site pain.

PREGNANCY: Safety in pregnancy and nursing not known.

MECHANISM OF ACTION: Human chorionic gonadotropin; stimulates production of gonadal steriod hormones by stimulating interstitial cells (leydig cells) of testis to produce androgens and the ovary's corpus luteum to produce progesterone.

PRELONE   RX
prednisolone (Muro)

THERAPEUTIC CLASS: Glucocorticoid

INDICATIONS: Treatment of steroid-responsive disorders.

DOSAGE: *Adults:* Initial: 5-60mg/day depending on disease and response. Maint: Decrease dose by small amounts to lowest effective dose.
Pediatrics: Initial: 5-60mg/day depending on disease and response. Maint: Decrease dose by small amounts to lowest effective dose.

HOW SUPPLIED: Syrup: 5mg/5mL (120mL), 15mg/5mL (240mL, 480mL)

CONTRAINDICATIONS: Systemic fungal infections.

WARNINGS/PRECAUTIONS: Adjust dose during stress or change in thyroid status. May mask signs of infection or or cause new infections. Prolonged use may produce glaucoma, optic nerve damage, secondary ocular infections. Increases BP, salt/water retention, potassium excretion. Avoid exposure to chickenpox, measles. Caution with latent TB, hypothyroidism, cirrhosis, ocular herpes simplex, HTN, diverticulitis, fresh intestinal anastomosis, ulcerative colitis, osteoporosis, myasthenia gravis, renal insufficiency, peptic ulcer disease. Growth and development of children on prolonged therapy should be monitored. Monitor for psychic disturbances. Avoid abrupt withdrawal.

ADVERSE REACTIONS: Fluid and electrolyte disturbances, osteoporosis, muscle weakness, cushingoid state, menstrual irregularities, nervousness, insomnia, impaired wound healing, excessive sweating, carbohydrate intolerance, glaucoma, cataracts, weight gain, nausea, malaise.

INTERACTIONS: Avoid ASA with hypoprothrombinemia. May increase blood glucose; adjust antidiabetic agents. Avoid smallpox vaccination, and live vaccines with immunosuppressive doses. Possible decreased vaccine response with killed or inactivated vaccines with immunosuppressive doses.

PREGNANCY: Safety in pregnancy and nursing not known.

MECHANISM OF ACTION: Systemic corticosteroid. Unkown, suspected to cause profound and varied metabolic effects.

PREVACID
lansoprazole (TAP)

RX

OTHER BRAND NAMES: Prevacid IV (TAP) - Prevacid Solutab (TAP)

THERAPEUTIC CLASS: Proton pump inhibitor

INDICATIONS: (PO) Treatment of active duodenal ulcer (DU), active benign gastric ulcer (GU), erosive esophagitis, symptomatic GERD. Maintain healing of erosive esophagitis and duodenal ulcers. Treatment of pathological hypersecretory conditions (eg, Zollinger-Ellison syndrome). Combination therapy with amoxicillin +/- clarithromycin for H.pylori eradication in duodenal ulcer disease, to reduce risk of ulcer recurrence. Treatment and risk reduction in NSAID induced gastric ulcer. (Inj) Short-term treatment of erosive esophagitis.

DOSAGE: Adults: >17 yrs: (PO) DU: 15mg qd for 4 weeks. Maint: 15mg qd. GU: 30mg qd up to 8 weeks. GERD: 15mg qd up to 8 weeks. Erosive Esophagitis: 30mg qd up to 8 weeks. May repeat for 8 weeks if needed. Maint: 15mg qd. NSAID-Induced GU: 30mg qd for 8 weeks. Reduce Risk of NSAID Induced GU: 15mg qd for 12 weeks. Hypersecretory Conditions: Initial: 60mg qd, then adjust. Max: 90mg bid. Divide dose if >120mg/day. H.pylori: Triple Therapy: 30mg + clarithromycin 500mg + amoxicillin 1000mg, all bid (q12h) for 10-14 days. Dual Therapy: 30mg + amoxicillin 1000mg both tid (q8h) for 14 days. Take before eating. Caps: Swallow whole or sprinkle cap contents on 1 tbsp of applesauce, ENSURE® pudding, cottage cheese, yogurt, strained pears, or in 60mL orange juice or tomato juice; swallow immediately. Sus: Do not chew or crush. Mix pkt with 30mL of water; stir well and drink immediately; not for use with NG tube. Solutab: Place on tongue with or without water. Oral Syringe: (SoluTab) Place 15mg tab in oral syringe and draw up 4mL of water, or 30mg tab in oral syringe and draw up 10mL of water. Shake contents and administer after tablet has dispersed within 15 mins. Refill syringe with 2mL (5mL for 30mg tab) of water, shake, and give any remaining contents. NG Tube: (Cap) Mix cap contents with 40mL apple juice and inject into NG tube; flush with additional juice to clear tube. (SoluTab) Place 15mg tab and draw up 4mL of water, or 30mg tab and draw up 10mL of water. Shake contents and after tablet has dispersed, inject through NG tube into stomach within 15 mins. Refill syringe with 5mL of water, shake, and flush NG tube. (Inj) Erosive Esophagitis: 30mg IV qd over 30 mins for 7 days. May switch to PO formulation for total of 6 to 8 weeks of therapy once patient is able to take oral medications. Severe Hepatic Impairment: Adjust dose.
Pediatrics: 12-17 yrs: Short-Term Symptomatic GERD: 15mg qd for up to 8 weeks. Erosive Esophagitis: 30mg qd for up to 8 weeks. 1-11 yrs: Short-Term Symptomatic GERD/Erosive Esophagitis: ≤30kg: 15mg qd for up to 12 weeks. >30kg: 30mg qd for up to 12 weeks. Titrate: May increase up to 30mg bid after 2 weeks if symptomatic. Severe Hepatic Impairment: Adjust dose. Take before eating. Caps: Swallow whole or sprinkle contents on 1 tbsp of applesauce, ENSURE® pudding, cottage cheese, yogurt, strained pears, or in 60mL orange juice or tomato juice; swallow immediately. Sus: Do not chew or crush. Mix pkt with 30mL water; stir well and drink immediately; not for use with NG tube. Solutab: Place on tongue with or without water. Oral Syringe: (SoluTab) Place 15mg tab in oral syringe and draw up 4mL of water, or 30mg tab in oral syringe and draw up 10mL of water. Shake contents and administer after tablet has dispersed within 15 mins. Refill syringe with 2mL (5mL for 30mg tab) of water, shake, and give any remaining contents. NG Tube: (Cap) Mix cap contents with 40mL apple juice and inject into NG tube; flush with additional juice to clear tube. (SoluTab) Place 15mg tab and draw up 4mL of

water, or 30mg tab and draw up 10mL of water. Shake contents and after tablet has dispersed, inject through NG tube into stomach within 15 mins. Refill syringe with 5mL of water, shake, and flush NG tube.

HOW SUPPLIED: Cap, Delayed-Release: 15mg, 30mg; Inj: 30mg; Sus, Delayed-Release: 15mg, 30mg (granules/pkt); Tab, Disintegrating (SoluTab): 15mg, 30mg.

WARNINGS/PRECAUTIONS: Symptomatic response does not preclude the presence of gastric malignancy. Adjust dose with hepatic impairment.

ADVERSE REACTIONS: Abdominal pain, constipation, diarrhea, nausea, myositis, interstitial nephritis

INTERACTIONS: May alter absorption of pH-dependent drugs (eg, ketoconazole, ampicillin esters, digoxin, and iron salts). Give at least 30 minutes prior to sucralfate. Theophylline may need dose adjustment. Concomitant use with warfarin may increase INR and prothrombin time.

PREGNANCY: Category B, not for use in nursing.

MECHANISM OF ACTION: Proton pump inhibitor; suppresses gastric acid secretion by specific inhibition of the (H^+, K^+)-ATPase enzyme system at the secretory surface of the gastric parietal cell.

PHARMACOKINETICS: Absorption: (PO, adult) absolute bioavailability (>80%); T_{max}=1.7 hrs. (IV, adult) C_{max}=1705ng/mL; AUC=3192ng•hr/mL. **Distribution:** V_d=15.7L; plasma protein binding (97%). **Metabolism:** Liver (extensive) via CYP3A4 and CYP2C19. **Elimination:** Urine, feces; $T_{1/2}$≤2 hrs. Refer to package insert for pediatric parameters.

PREVIDENT
sodium fluoride (Colgate Oral)

RX

OTHER BRAND NAME: PreviDent 5000 Plus (Colgate Oral)

THERAPEUTIC CLASS: Fluoride preparation

INDICATIONS: Prevention of dental caries.

DOSAGE: *Adults:* Apply thin ribbon to teeth with toothbrush or mouth tray qhs for at least 1 min with gel and 2 min with cream after regular brushing. Expectorate after use. Do not eat, drink, or rinse for 30 min.
Pediatrics: 6-16 yrs: Apply thin ribbon to teeth with toothbrush or mouth tray qhs for at least 1 min with gel and 2 min with cream after regular brushing. Expectorate and rinse mouth thoroughly after use.

HOW SUPPLIED: Gel: (PreviDent) 1.1%; Cre: (PreviDent 5000 Plus) 1.1%

CONTRAINDICATIONS: Not for children <6 years of age, unless recommended by dentist or physician.

WARNINGS/PRECAUTIONS: Prolonged ingestion may lead to dental fluorosis in children <6 years of age. Not for systemic treatment. Do not swallow.

ADVERSE REACTIONS: Allergic reactions.

PREGNANCY: Category B, caution in nursing.

MECHANISM OF ACTION: Fluoride preparation; increases tooth resistance to acid dissolution and enhances penetration of fluoride ion into tooth enamel.

PREVNAR
pneumococcal vaccine, diphtheria conjugate (Wyeth)

RX

THERAPEUTIC CLASS: Vaccine

INDICATIONS: Active immunization of children against invasive disease caused by S.pneumoniae. Active immunization of children against otitis media caused by serotypes included in the vaccine.

DOSAGE: *Pediatrics:* 6 weeks-2 months: 4 doses of 0.5mL IM. Give 3 doses at 2 month intervals and 4th dose at 12-15 months old. Unvaccinated Children: 7-11 months: 3 doses of 0.5mL IM. Give 1st 2 doses at least 4 weeks apart and 3rd dose after 1yr birthday; separate from 2nd dose by at least 2 months. 12-23 months: 2 doses of 0.5mL IM at least 2 months apart. ≥24 months-9 yrs: 0.5mL IM single dose.

HOW SUPPLIED: Inj: 16mcg/0.5mL

CONTRAINDICATIONS: Severe or moderate febrile illness.

WARNINGS/PRECAUTIONS: Avoid with thrombocytopenia or coagulation disorder. Impaired immune responses may cause reduced response to active immunization. Not a substitute for diphtheria or 23-valent pneumococcal vaccinations. Do not give IV. Have epinephrine (1:1000) available. Caution with latex sensitivity; packaging contains dry natural rubber. Fever and rarely febrile seizures reported.

ADVERSE REACTIONS: Injection site reactions, irritability, drowsiness, restless sleep, decreased appetite, vomiting, diarrhea, fever.

INTERACTIONS: Suboptimal response with immunosuppressants. Caution with anticoagulants.

PREGNANCY: Category C, not for use in nursing.

MECHANISM OF ACTION: Immunostimulant; elicits formation of antibodies that may protect against invasive pneumococcal disease and otitis media.

PRIFTIN   RX
rifapentine (Sanofi-Aventis)

THERAPEUTIC CLASS: Rifamycin derivative

INDICATIONS: Treatment of pulmonary TB. Do not use alone, as initial or retreatment.

DOSAGE: *Adults:* Intensive Phase: Initial: 600mg twice weekly with an interval of not <3 days (72 hrs) between doses. Continue for 2 months. Maint: 600mg once weekly for 4 months. Elderly: Start at low end of dosing range.
Pediatrics: ≥12 yrs: Intensive Phase: Initial: 600mg twice weekly with an interval of not <3 days (72 hrs) between doses. Continue for 2 months. Maint: 600mg once weekly for 4 months.

HOW SUPPLIED: Tab: 150mg

WARNINGS/PRECAUTIONS: Give with pyridoxine in the malnourished, if predisposed to neuropathy (eg, alcoholics, diabetics), and adolescents. Caution with hepatic impairment; monitor LFTs before and every 2-4 weeks during therapy. May cause postnatal hemorrhages in mother and infant during last weeks of pregnancy; monitor clotting parameters; may need vitamin K. May produce a red-orange discoloration of body tissues, fluids. May stain/discolor contact lenses, breast milk, or dentures. Pseudomembranous colitis reported. Avoid with porphyria. Caution in elderly.

ADVERSE REACTIONS: Hyperuricemia, increased ALT/AST, neutropenia, pyuria, proteinuria, lymphopenia, urinary casts, rash, pruritus, acne, anorexia, anemia.

INTERACTIONS: Antagonizes drugs metabolized by CYP3A4, CYP2C8, and CYP2C9 due to enzyme induction (eg, anticonvulsants, antiarrhythmics, oral anticoagulants, antibiotics, antifungals, barbiturates, benzodiazepines, β-blockers, CCB, corticosteroids, cardiac glycosides, clofibrate, hormonal contraceptives, oral hypoglycemics, haloperidol, immunosuppressants, levothyroxine, narcotic analgesics, progestins, quinine, reverse transcriptase inhibitors, sildenafil, theophylline, TCAs). Increases indinavir metabolism; extreme caution with protease inhibitors. Avoid hormonal contraceptives. Consider hepatotoxic effects of other antituberculosis drug therapies (eg, isoniazid, pyrazinamide).

PREGNANCY: Category C, not for use in nursing.

MECHANISM OF ACTION: Cyclopentyl rifamycin; inhibits DNA-dependent RNA polymerase in susceptible strains of *Mycobacterium tuberculosis* (but not in mammalian cells). It also exhibits bactericidal activity against both intracellular and extracellular *M. tuberculosis* organisms.

PHARMACOKINETICS: Absorption: Relative bioavailabilty (70%); C_{max}=15.05±4.62µg/mL; AUC=319.54±91.52µg•hr/mL; T_{max}=4.83±1.8 hrs. **Distribution:** V_d=70.2±9.1L; Plasma protein binding: 97.7% (rifapentine), 93.2% (metabolite). **Metabolism:** Metabolite: 25-desacetyl rifapentine. **Elimination:** Urine (17%), feces (70%).

PRILOSEC
omeprazole (AstraZeneca)

RX

THERAPEUTIC CLASS: Proton pump inhibitor

INDICATIONS: Short-term treatment of active duodenal ulcer and active benign gastric ulcer in adults. Treatment of heartburn and other symptoms associated with GERD in adults and pediatrics. Short-term treatment of erosive esophagitis and to maintain healing of erosive esophagitis in adults and pediatrics. Long-term treatment of pathological hypersecretory conditions (eg, Zollinger-Ellison syndrome, multiple endocrine adenomas, systemic mastocytosis) in adults. Combination therapy with clarithromycin +/- amoxicillin for *H.pylori* eradication in duodenal ulcer disease, and to reduce risk of ulcer recurrence, in adults.

DOSAGE: *Adults:* Duodenal Ulcer: 20mg qd for 4-8 weeks. Gastric Ulcer: 40mg qd for 4-8 weeks. GERD: 20mg qd up to 4 weeks without esophageal lesions. Treatment Erosive Esophagitis with GERD: 20mg qd for 4-8 weeks. Maint: 20mg qd. Hypersecretory Conditions: Initial: 60mg qd, then adjust if needed. Divide dose if >80mg/day. Doses up to 120mg tid have been given. *H.pylori* Triple Therapy: 20mg + clarithromycin 500mg + amoxicillin 1g, all bid for 10 days. Give additional 18 days of omeprazole 20mg every morning if ulcer present initially. Dual Therapy: 40mg qd + clarithromycin 500mg tid for 14 days. Give additional 14 days of omeprazole 20mg every morning if ulcer present initially. Do not crush or chew. Take before eating. Can add contents of caps to applesauce if difficulty swallowing; swallow immediately without chewing.
Pediatrics: 1-16 yrs: GERD/Erosive Esophagitis: ≥20kg: 20mg qd. 10 to <20kg: 10mg qd. 5 to <10kg: 5mg qd. Do not crush or chew. Take before eating. Can add contents of caps to applesauce if difficulty swallowing; swallow immediately without chewing.

HOW SUPPLIED: Cap, Delayed-Release: 10mg, 20mg, 40mg; Sus, Delayed-Release: 2.5mg, 10mg granules/packet

WARNINGS/PRECAUTIONS: Atrophic gastritis reported with long-term use. Symptomatic response does not preclude the presence of gastric malignancy.

ADVERSE REACTIONS: Headache, diarrhea, abdominal pain, asthenia, nausea, vomiting.

INTERACTIONS: May potentiate diazepam, warfarin, phenytoin and drugs metabolized by oxidation. May alter absorption of pH-dependent drugs (eg, ketoconazole, ampicillin esters, iron salts). Monitor drugs metabolized by CYP450 (eg, cyclosporine, disulfiram, benzodiazepines). Increased levels with clarithromycin. Increases levels of clarithromycin. Voriconazole may increase levels. May reduce plasma levels of atazanavir. May increase levels of tacrolimus.

PREGNANCY: Category C, not for use in nursing.

MECHANISM OF ACTION: Proton pump inhibitor; suppresses gastric acid secretion by specific inhibition of the H^+/K^+ ATPase enzyme system at the secretory surface of the gastric parietal cell.

PHARMACOKINETICS: Absorption: Rapid; Absolute bioavailability (30-40%); T_{max}=0.5-3.5 hrs. (Adult, single dose) C_{max}=668ng/mL; AUC=1220ng•hr/mL. (Children<20 kg, 2-5yrs, 10 mg single dose) C_{max}=288ng/mL; AUC=511ng•hr/mL. (Children >20kg, 6-16yrs, 20 mg single dose) C_{max}=495ng/mL; AUC=1140ng•hr/mL. **Distribution:** Plasma protein binding (95%); found in breast milk. **Metabolism:** Hydroxyomeprazole and corresponding carboxylic acid (metabolites). **Elimination:** Urine (77%), feces; $T_{1/2}$=0.5-1 hr.

PRIMAXIN I.M.
cilastatin - imipenem (Merck)

RX

THERAPEUTIC CLASS: Thienamycin/dehydropeptidase I inhibitor

INDICATIONS: Treatment of lower respiratory tract (LRTI), skin and skin structure (SSSI), intra-abdominal, and gynecologic infections caused by susceptible strains of microorganisms. Not for severe or life-threatening infections.

DOSAGE: *Adults:* Dose according to imipenem. Mild to Moderate LRTI/SSSI/Gynecologic Infection: 500mg or 750mg IM q12h depending on severity. Intra-Abdominal Infection: 750mg IM q12h. Continue for at least 2 days after symptoms resolve. Elderly: Start at low end of dosing range. Continue for at least 2 days after symptoms resolve; do not treat >14 days. Max: 1500mg/day. Avoid if CrCl <20mL/min.

Pediatrics: ≥12 yrs: Dose according to imipenem. Mild to Moderate LRTI/SSSI/ Gynecologic Infections: 500mg or 750mg IM q12h depending on severity. Intra-Abdominal Infection: 750mg IM q12h. Continue for at least 2 days after symptoms resolve; do not treat >14 days. Max: 1500mg/day. Avoid if CrCl <20mL/min.

HOW SUPPLIED: Inj: (Imipenem-Cilastatin) 500mg-500mg, 750mg-750mg

CONTRAINDICATIONS: Severe shock, heart block, hypersensitivity to local anesthetics of amide type (due to lidocaine diluent).

WARNINGS/PRECAUTIONS: Serious, sometimes fatal, hypersensitivity reactions reported with β-lactam therapy. *Clostridium difficile*-associated diarrhea reported. Prolonged use may result in overgrowth of nonsusceptible organisms. Avoid injection into blood vessel. Caution in elderly. CNS adverse events (eg, myoclonic activity, confusion, seizures) reported most commonly with CNS disorders and renal dysfunction; d/c if any occur. Positive Coombs test reported.

ADVERSE REACTIONS: Injection site pain, NV, diarrhea, fever, rash, hypotension, seizures, dizziness, pruritus, urticaria, somnolence.

INTERACTIONS: Avoid probenecid. Do not mix or physically add with other antibiotics. May give concomitantly with other antibiotics. May decrease levels of valproic acid.

PREGNANCY: Category C, caution in nursing.

MECHANISM OF ACTION: Imipenem: Thienamycin; inhibits cell-wall synthesis. Cilastatin: Dehydropeptidase I inhibitor; prevents renal metabolism of parent drug.

PHARMACOKINETICS: Absorption: Imipenem: C_{max}=10mcg/mL (500mg), 12mcg/mL (750mg); T_{max}=2 hrs. Cilastatin: C_{max}=24mcg/mL (500mg), 33mcg/mL (750mg); T_{max}=1 hr. **Distribution:** Imipenem: Plasma protein binding (20%). Cilastatin: Plasma protein binding (40%). **Metabolism:** Imipenem: Kidneys. **Elimination:** Imipenem: Urine. Cilastatin: Urine.

PRIMAXIN I.V.   RX
cilastatin - imipenem (Merck)

THERAPEUTIC CLASS: Thienamycin/dehydropeptidase I inhibitor

INDICATIONS: Treatment of serious lower respiratory tract, urinary tract (UTI), intra-abdominal, gynecologic, skin and skin structure, bone and joint, septicemia, endocarditis, and polymicrobic infections caused by susceptible strains of microorganisms.

DOSAGE: *Adults:* ≥70kg and CrCl >70mL/min: Dose based on imipenem component. Uncomplicated UTI: 250mg q6h. Complicated UTI: 500mg q6h. Mild Infection: 250-500mg q6h. Moderate Infection: 500mg q6-8h or 1g q8h. Severe, Life-Threatening Infection: 500mg-1g q6h or 1g q8h. Max: 50mg/kg/day or 4g/day, whichever lower. Renal Impairment and/or <70kg: Refer to PI. CrCl 6-20mL/min: 125-250mg q12h. CrCl ≤5mL/min: Administer hemodialysis within 48 hrs of dose.

Pediatrics: ≥3 months: Dose based on imipenem component. Non-CNS Infections: 15-25mg/kg q6h. Max: 2g/day if susceptible or 4g/day if moderately susceptible. May use up to 90mg/kg/day in older cystic fibrosis children. 4 weeks-3 months and ≥1500g: 25mg/kg q6h. 1-4 weeks and ≥1500g: 25mg/kg q8h. <1 week and ≥1500g: 25mg/kg q12h. Not recommended with CNS infection, and <30kg with impaired renal function.

HOW SUPPLIED: Inj: (Imipenem-Cilastatin) 250mg-250mg, 500mg-500mg

WARNINGS/PRECAUTIONS: Serious, sometimes fatal, hypersensitivity reactions reported with β-lactam therapy. *Clostridium difficile*-associated diarrhea reported. Prolonged use may result in overgrowth of nonsusceptible organisms. CNS adverse events (eg, myoclonic activity, confusion, seizures) reported most commonly with CNS disorders and renal dysfunction.

ADVERSE REACTIONS: Phlebitis/thrombophlebitis, NV, diarrhea, rash, fever, hypotension, seizures, dizziness, pruritus, urticaria, somnolence, hepatitis (including fulminant hepatitis), hepatic failure.

INTERACTIONS: Seizures reported with ganciclovir; avoid concomitant use. Avoid probenecid. Do not mix or physically add to other antibiotics. May give concomitantly with other antibiotics. May decrease levels of valproic acid.

PREGNANCY: Category C, caution in nursing.

MECHANISM OF ACTION: Imipenem: Thienamycin; inhibits cell-wall synthesis. Cilastatin: Dehydropeptidase I inhibitor; prevents renal metabolism of parent drug.

PHARMACOKINETICS: Absorption: Variable doses resulted in different parameters. **Distribution:** Imipenem: Plasma protein binding (20%). Cilastatin: Plasma protein binding (40%). **Metabolism:** Imipenem: Kidneys. **Elimination:** Imipenem: Urine (70%). Cilastatin: Urine (70%).

PRIMSOL
trimethoprim HCl (FSC Laboratories)

RX

THERAPEUTIC CLASS: Tetrahydrofolic acid inhibitor

INDICATIONS: Treatment of acute otitis media in pediatrics and urinary tract infection (UTI) in adults due to susceptible microorganisms.

DOSAGE: *Adults:* UTI: Usual: 100mg q12h or 200mg q24h for 10 days. CrCl: 15-30mL/min: Give 50% of usual dose.
Pediatrics: Otitis Media: ≥6 months: 5mg/kg q12h for 10 days. CrCl: 15-30mL/min: Give 50% of usual dose.

HOW SUPPLIED: Sol: 50mg/5mL

CONTRAINDICATIONS: Megaloblastic anemia due to folate deficiency.

WARNINGS/PRECAUTIONS: May interfere with hematopoiesis. Serious blood disorders; monitor for sore throat, fever, pallor, and purpura. Caution with folate deficiency and renal/hepatic impairment, diarrhea, rash.

ADVERSE REACTIONS: Epigastric distress, NV, anemia, methemoglobinemia, hyperkalemia, hyponatremia, fever, elevation of serum transaminases and bilirubin, increases BUN and serum creatinine.

INTERACTIONS: May inhibit phenytoin metabolism.

PREGNANCY: Category C, caution in nursing.

MECHANISM OF ACTION: Dihydrofolate reductase inhibitor; blocks production of tetrahydrofolic acid from dihydrofolic acid by binding to and reversibly inhibiting dihydrofolate reductase.

PHARMACOKINETICS: Absorption: Rapid; C_{max}=1mcg/mL; T_{max}=1-4 hrs. **Distribution:** Crosses placenta; found in breast milk. **Metabolism:** Liver; 1- and 3-oxide, 3'- and 4'-hydroxy derivative (principal metabolites). **Elimination:** Urine; $T_{1/2}$=9 hrs.

PRINIVIL
lisinopril (Merck)

RX

> ACE inhibitors can cause death/injury to developing fetus during 2nd and 3rd trimesters. Stop therapy if pregnancy detected.

THERAPEUTIC CLASS: ACE inhibitor

INDICATIONS: Treatment of hypertension. Adjunct therapy in heart failure if inadequately controlled by diuretics and digitalis. Adjunct therapy in stable patients within 24 hrs of AMI to improve survival.

DOSAGE: *Adults:* HTN: If possible, d/c diuretic 2-3 days prior to therapy. Initial: 10mg qd; 5mg qd with diuretic. Usual: 20-40mg qd. Resume diuretic if BP not controlled. Max: 80mg/day. CrCl 10-30mL/min: Initial: 5mg/day. Max: 40mg/day. CrCl <10mL/min: Initial: 2.5mg/day. Max: 40mg/day. Heart Failure: Initial: 5mg qd. Usual: 5-20mg qd. Hyponatremia or CrCl ≤30mL/min: Initial: 2.5mg qd. AMI: Initial: 5mg within 24 hrs, then 5mg after 24 hrs, then 10mg after 48 hrs, then daily. Use 2.5mg during first 3 days with low systolic BP. Maint: 10mg qd for 6 weeks, 2.5-5mg with hypotension. D/C with prolonged hypotension. Elderly: Caution with dose adjustment.
Pediatrics: ≥6 yrs: HTN: Initial: 0.07mg/kg qd (up to 5mg total). Adjust dose based on BP response. Max: 0.61mg/kg qd (40mg/day).

HOW SUPPLIED: Tab: 5mg*, 10mg*, 20mg* *scored

CONTRAINDICATIONS: History of ACE inhibitor-associated angioedema and hereditary or idiopathic angioedema.

WARNINGS/PRECAUTIONS: Intestinal/head/neck angioedema reported. D/C if angioedema, jaundice, or if marked LFT elevation occurs. Risk of hyperkalemia with DM, renal dysfunction. Persistent nonproductive cough reported. Monitor WBCs in renal and collagen vascular disease. Anaphylactoid reactions reported. Fetal/neonatal morbidity and death reported. Monitor for hypotension in high-risk patients (eg, heart failure with systolic BP <100mmHg, surgery/anesthesia, hyponatremia, high dose diuretic therapy, severe volume and/or salt depletion). Caution with renal artery stenosis, CHF, renal dysfunction, or if obstruction to left ventricle outflow tract. Less effective on BP in blacks and more reports of angioedema than nonblacks. Caution in hypoglycemia and leukopenia/neutropenia. Patients should report any indication of infection which may be sign of leukopenia/neutropenia.

ADVERSE REACTIONS: Hypotension, diarrhea, headache, dizziness, cough, chest pain.

INTERACTIONS: May increase lithium levels. Hypotension risk with diuretics. May further decrease renal dysfunction with NSAIDs. Hyperkalemia with K^+-sparing diuretics, K^+-containing salt substitutes, or K^+ supplements. Nitroid reactions have been reported rarely in patients on therapy with injectable gold and concomitant ACE inhibitor therapy. NSAIDs may diminish antihypertensive effects.

PREGNANCY: Category C (1st trimester) and D (2nd and 3rd trimesters), not for use in nursing.

MECHANISM OF ACTION: ACE inhibitor; inhibition results in decreased plasma angiotensin II, which leads to decreased vasopressor activity and aldosterone secretion.

PHARMACOKINETICS: Absorption: 25%; T_{max}=7 hrs. **Elimination:** Urine (unchanged); $T_{1/2}$=12 hrs.

PROAIR HFA   RX
albuterol sulfate (Ivax)

THERAPEUTIC CLASS: Beta$_2$-agonist

INDICATIONS: Prevention and treatment of bronchospasm with reversible obstructive airway disease; prevention of exercise-induced bronchospasm (EIB) in patients ≥12 yrs.

DOSAGE: *Adults:* Bronchospasm or Asthmatic Symptoms: 2 inh q4-6h or 1 inh q4h. EIB: 2 inh 15-30 min before activity.
Pediatrics: ≥12 yrs: Bronchospasm or Asthmatic Symptoms: 2 inh q4-6h or 1 inh q4h. EIB: 2 inh 15-30 min before activity.

HOW SUPPLIED: MDI: 90mcg/inh (8.5g)

WARNINGS/PRECAUTIONS: Hypersensitivity reactions reported. Monitor for worsening asthma. Fatalities reported with excessive use. Caution with cardiovascular disorders, especially coronary insufficiency, arrhythmias and HTN. May need concomitant corticosteroids. Can produce paradoxical bronchospasm. Caution with DM, hyperthyroidism, and seizures. May cause transient hypokalemia.

ADVERSE REACTIONS: Pharyngitis, headache, rhinitis, dizziness, pain, tachycardia, tremor, nervousness.

INTERACTIONS: Avoid other sympathomimetic agents. Extreme caution with MAOIs and TCAs, and β-blockers. Monitor digoxin. May worsen ECG changes and/or hypokalemia with nonpotassium-sparing diuretics.

PREGNANCY: Category C, not for use in nursing.

MECHANISM OF ACTION: β$_2$-adrenergic bronchodilator; stimulates adenyl cylase, the enzyme that catalyzes the formation of cAMP from ATP. Increased cAMP levels are associated with relaxation of bronchial smooth muscle and inhibition of release of mediators of immediate hypersensitivity.

PHARMACOKINETICS: Absorption: C_{max}=4100pg/mL; AUC=28,426pg•hr/mL. **Metabolism:** GI tract by SULTIA3. **Elimination:** Renal excretion (80-100%), urine (unchanged), feces (≤20%); $T_{1/2}$=6 hrs.

PROBENECID   RX
probenecid (Various)

THERAPEUTIC CLASS: Uricosuric

INDICATIONS: Treatment of hyperuricemia associated with gout and gouty arthritis. Adjunct to penicillin, ampicillin, methicillin, oxacillin, cloxacillin, or nafcillin for elevation and prolongation of plasma levels.

DOSAGE: *Adults:* Gout: Initial: 250mg bid for 1 week. Titrate: May increase by 500mg every 4 weeks. Maint: 500mg bid. Max: 2g/day. May reduce by 500mg every 6 months if acute attack has been absent ≥6 months and serum urate levels are normal. Renal Impairment: Usual: 1g/day. Adjunct Antibiotic Therapy: 500mg qid. Elderly/Renal Impairment: Reduce dose. Decrease dose with gastric intolerance. May not be effective if CrCl ≤30mL/min.
Pediatrics: 2-14 yrs: Adjunct Antibiotic Therapy: Initial: 25mg/kg. Maint: 10mg/kg qid. ≥50kg: 500mg qid.

HOW SUPPLIED: Tab: 500mg

CONTRAINDICATIONS: Blood dyscrasias, uric acid kidney stones and children <2 yrs. Do not use in acute gout attack.

WARNINGS/PRECAUTIONS: Initiate therapy when acute gout attack subsides. Exacerbation of gout may occur; treat with colchicine. Use APAP if analgesic needed. Severe allergic reactions and anaphylaxis reported. D/C if hypersensitivity occurs. Caution with peptic ulcer. Monitor for glycosuria. Maintain liberal fluid intake and alkalization of urine.

ADVERSE REACTIONS: Headache, acute gouty arthritis, dizziness, hepatic necrosis, vomiting, nausea, anorexia, sore gums, nephrotic syndrome, uric acid stones, renal colic, costovertebral pain, urinary frequency, anaphylaxis, fever, urticaria, pruritus, blood dyscrasias, dermatitis, alopecia, flushing.

INTERACTIONS: Probenecid increases plasma levels of penicillin and other β-lactams; psychic disturbances reported. Avoid use with penicillin in the presence of renal impairment. Salicylates and pyrazinamide antagonize uricosuric effects. Increased plasma levels of methotrexate, sulfonamides, sulfonylureas, thiopental or ketamine-induced anesthesia, some NSAIDs (eg, indomethacin, naproxen), lorazepam, APAP, and rifampin. Possible false high plasma levels of theophylline.

PREGNANCY: Safety in pregnancy and nursing is not known.

MECHANISM OF ACTION: Uricosuric/renal tubular blocking agent; inhibits tubular reabsorption of urate, increasing urinary excretion of uric acid and decreasing serum urate levels.

PROCHLORPERAZINE   RX
prochlorperazine (Various)

THERAPEUTIC CLASS: Phenothiazine derivative

INDICATIONS: Control of severe nausea and vomiting. Management of psychotic disorders (eg, schizophrenia). Short-term treatment of generalized non-psychotic anxiety.

DOSAGE: *Adults:* Nausea/Vomiting: (Tab) Usual: 5-10mg tid-qid. Max: 40mg/day. (IM) 5-10mg IM q3-4h prn. Max: 40mg/day. (IV) 2.5-10mg IV (not bolus). Max: 10mg single dose and 40mg/day. Nausea/Vomiting with Surgery: 5-10mg IM 1-2 hrs or 5-10mg IV 15-30 min before anesthesia, or during or after surgery; repeat once if needed. Non-Psychotic Anxiety: (Tab) 5mg tid-qid. Psychosis: Mild/Outpatient: 5-10mg PO tid-qid. Moderate-Severe/Hospitalized: Initial: 10mg PO tid-qid. May increase in small increments every 2-3 days. Severe: (PO) 100-150mg/day. (IM) 10-20mg, may repeat q2-4 hrs if needed. Switch to oral after obtain control or if needed, 10-20mg IM q4-6h. Elderly: use lower dosing range and titrate more gradually.
Pediatrics: Nausea/Vomiting: >2 yrs and >20 lbs: (PO/PR) 20-29 lbs: Usual: 2.5mg qd-bid. Max: 7.5mg/day. 30-39 lbs: 2.5mg bid-tid. Max: 10mg/day. 40-85 lbs: 2.5mg tid or 5mg bid. Max: 15mg/day. (IM) 0.06mg/lb, usually single dose for control. Psychosis: (PO/PR) 2-12 yrs: Initial: 2.5mg bid-tid, up to 10mg/day on 1st day. Max: 2-5 yrs: 20mg/day. 6-12 yrs: 25mg/day. (IM) <12 yrs: 0.06mg/lb single dose. Switch to oral after obtain control.

HOW SUPPLIED: Inj: (Edisylate) 5mg/mL; Supp: 5mg, 25mg; Tab: (Maleate) 5mg, 10mg

CONTRAINDICATIONS: Comatose states, concomitant large dose CNS depressants (alcohol, barbiturates, narcotics), pediatric surgery, pediatrics <2 yrs or <20lbs.

WARNINGS/PRECAUTIONS: Secondary extrapyramidal symptoms can occur. Tardive dyskinesia, NMS may develop. Caution with activities requiring alertness. May mask symptoms of overdose of other drugs. May obscure diagnosis of intestinal obstruction, brain tumor, and Reye's syndrome. May interfere with thermoregulation. Caution with glaucoma, cardiac disorders. Caution in children with dehydration or acute illness and the elderly. D/C 48 hrs before myelography and may resume after 24 hrs post-procedure.

ADVERSE REACTIONS: Drowsiness, dizziness, amenorrhea, blurred vision, skin reactions, hypotension, NMS, cholestatic jaundice.

INTERACTIONS: May decrease oral anticoagulant effects. May potentiate α-adrenergic blockade. Thiazide diuretics potentiate orthostatic hypotension. Increased levels of both drugs with propranolol. Anticonvulsants may need adjustment. Risk of encephalopathic syndrome with lithium. May antagonize antihypertensive effects of guanethidine and related compounds.

PREGNANCY: Safety in pregnancy is not known; caution in nursing.

MECHANISM OF ACTION: Phenothiazine derivative; anti-emetic and antipsychotic.

PROCRIT   RX
epoetin alfa (Ortho Biotech)

> Increased mortality, serious cardiovascular/thromboembolic events, and tumor progression. (Renal Failure) Patients experienced greater risks for death and serious cardiovascular events when administered erythropoiesis-stimulating agents (ESAs) to target higher vs lower Hgb levels (13.5 vs 11.3 g/dL; 14 vs 10 g/dL) in 2 clinical studies. Individualize dosing to achieve and maintain Hgb levels within range of 10-12g/dL. (Cancer) ESAs shortened overall survival and/or time-to-tumor progression in clinical studies in patients with breast, head and neck, lymphoid, non-small cell lung, and cervical cancers when dosed to target Hgb ≥12g/dL. The risks of shortened survival and tumor progression have not been excluded when ESAs are dosed to target Hgb <12g/dL. To minimize these risks, as well as the risk of serious cardio- and thrombovascular events, use lowest dose needed to avoid RBC transfusions. Use only for treatment of anemia due to concomitant myelosuppressive chemotherapy. D/C following completion of a chemotherapy course. (Perisurgery) Epoetin alfa increased the rate of DVT in patients not receiving prophylactic anticoagulation. Consider DVT prophylaxis.

THERAPEUTIC CLASS: Erythropoiesis stimulator

INDICATIONS: Treatment of anemia due to chronic renal failure (CRF), anemia related to zidovudine treatment of HIV, chemotherapy-induced anemia in non-myeloid malignancies, and reduction of allogeneic blood transfusions in anemic patients (>10 to ≤13g/dL) scheduled for elective, noncardiac, nonvascular surgery.

DOSAGE: *Adults:* CRF: Initial: 50-100 U/kg IV/SQ 3x/week. IV is preferred route in dialysis patients. Maint: Individually titrate. Reduce if Hgb approaches 12g/dL or if Hgb increases >1g/dL in any 2-week period. Increase when Hgb does not increase by 2g/dL after 8 weeks of therapy and Hgb is below target range (10-12g/dL). Zidovudine-Treated HIV Patients: If serum erythropoietin levels ≤500 mU/mL and zidovudine ≤4200mg/week, give 100 U/kg IV/SQ 3x/week for 8 weeks. Titrate: Increase by 50-100 U/kg 3x/week after 8 weeks if necessary. Max: 300 U/kg 3x/week. Maint: If Hgb >13g/dL, d/c until Hgb <12g/dL, then reduce dose by 25% when therapy resumes. Chemotherapy-Induced Anemia: Initial: 150 U/kg SQ 3x/week. Titrate: Reduce by 25% when Hgb approaches 12g/dL or Hgb increases >1g/dL in any 2-week period. If Hgb >13g/dL, withhold until Hgb <12g/dL then restart at 25% below previous dose. May increase to 300 U/kg 3x/week if no response after 8 weeks of therapy. Max: 300 U/kg 3x/week. Weekly Dosing: 40,000 U SQ weekly. Titrate: If Hgb not increased by ≥1g/dL after 4 weeks, increase to 60,000 U weekly. If Hgb >13g/dL, withhold until Hgb <12g/dL then restart with 25% dose reduction. Reduce dose by 25% if very rapid Hgb response (eg, increase >1g/dL in any 2-week period). Max: 60,000 U weekly. Surgery: 300 U/kg/day SQ for 10 days before surgery, on surgery day, and 4 days post-op or 600 U/kg SQ once weekly on 21, 14, and 7 days before surgery and a 4th dose on surgery day, with adequate iron supplement.
Pediatrics: CRF: Initial: 50 U/kg 3x/week IV/SQ. Titrate: Reduce if Hgb approaches 12g/dL or if Hgb increases by >1g/dL in any 2-week period. Increase if Hgb does not increase by 2g/dL after 8 weeks of therapy and Hgb is below target range (10-12g/dL). Maint: Individually titrate. Chemotherapy Induced Anemia: Initial: 600 U/kg IV weekly. Titrate: If Hgb not increased by ≥1g/dL after 4 weeks, increase to 900 U/kg IV weekly. If Hgb >13g/dL, withhold until Hgb <12g/dL then restart with 25% dose reduction. Reduce dose by 25% if very rapid Hgb response (eg, increase >1g/dL in any 2-week period). Max: 60,000 U weekly.

HOW SUPPLIED: Inj: 2000 U/mL, 3000 U/mL, 4000 U/mL, 10,000 U/mL, 20,000 U/mL, 40,000 U/mL

CONTRAINDICATIONS: Uncontrolled HTN. Hypersensitivity to mammalian cell-derived products and albumin (human).

WARNINGS/PRECAUTIONS: Pure red cell aplasia and severe anemia (with or without other cytopenias) may occur. Caution with porphyria, HTN, or history of seizures. Monitor patients with pre-existing CV disease closely. Evaluate iron stores before and during therapy; most patients need iron supplementation. Monitor Hgb, BP, iron levels, serum chemistry, and CBC. Multidose formulation contains benzyl alcohol, which has been associated with an increased incidence of neurological and other complications in premature infants; these complications are sometimes fatal.

ADVERSE REACTIONS: HTN, headache, fatigue, arthralgias, nausea, vomiting, diarrhea, edema, rash, pyrexia, constipation, respiratory congestion, dyspnea, asthenia, skin reaction.

INTERACTIONS: Adjust anticoagulant dose in dialysis patients.

PREGNANCY: Category C, caution in nursing.

MECHANISM OF ACTION: Erythropoiesis stimulator.

PHARMACOKINETICS: Absorption: (SQ) T_{max}=5-24 hrs. **Elimination:** (IV) $T_{1/2}$=4-13 hrs.

PROCTOCORT CREAM
hydrocortisone (Salix)

RX

THERAPEUTIC CLASS: Corticosteroid

INDICATIONS: Corticosteroid responsive dermatoses.

DOSAGE: *Adults:* Apply bid-qid. May use occlusive dressings for psoriasis or recalcitrant conditions; d/c dressings if infection develops.
Pediatrics: Apply bid-qid. May use occlusive dressings for psoriasis or recalcitrant conditions; d/c dressings if infection develops.

HOW SUPPLIED: Cre: 1% (30g)

WARNINGS/PRECAUTIONS: May produce reversible HPA axis suppression, manifestations of Cushing's syndrome, hyperglycemia, and glucosuria. Caution when applied to large surface areas or under occlusive dressings. Use appropriate therapy with infections. Pediatrics may be more susceptible to systemic toxicity. D/C if irritation occurs. Avoid eyes.

ADVERSE REACTIONS: Burning, itching, irritation, dryness, folliculitis, hypertrichosis, acneiform eruptions, hypopigmentation, perioral dermatitis, allergic contact dermatitis, maceration skin, secondary infection, skin atrophy, striae, miliaria.

PREGNANCY: Category C, caution in nursing.

MECHANISM OF ACTION: Topical corticosteroid; not established. Suspected to have anti-inflammatory, antipruritic, and vasoconstrictive activities.

PHARMACOKINETICS: Absorption: Skin. **Metabolism:** Liver. **Elimination:** Kidneys (major); bile (minor).

PROCTOFOAM-HC
hydrocortisone acetate - pramoxine HCl (Schwarz Pharma)

RX

THERAPEUTIC CLASS: Corticosteroid/anesthetic

INDICATIONS: Corticosteroid responsive dermatoses of the anal region.

DOSAGE: *Adults:* Apply to anal/perianal area tid-qid.
Pediatrics: Apply to anal/perianal area tid-qid.

HOW SUPPLIED: Foam: (Hydrocortisone-Pramoxine) 1%-1% (10g)

WARNINGS/PRECAUTIONS: D/C if no improvement in 2-3 weeks. May produce reversible HPA axis suppression, manifestations of Cushing's syndrome, hyperglycemia, and glucosuria. Caution when applied to large surface areas or under occlusive dressings. Use appropriate therapy if infections develop; d/c steroid if favorable response does not occur promptly. D/C if irritation develops. Pediatrics may be more susceptible to systemic toxicity. Avoid eyes.

PROGRAF

ADVERSE REACTIONS: Burning, itching, irritation, dryness, folliculitis, hypertrichosis, acneiform eruptions, hypopigmentation, perioral dermatitis, allergic contact dermatitis, skin maceration, secondary infection, skin atrophy, striae, miliaria.

PREGNANCY: Category C, caution in nursing.

PROGRAF

RX

tacrolimus (Astellas)

> Increased susceptibility to infection and development of lymphoma.

THERAPEUTIC CLASS: Macrolide immunosuppressant

INDICATIONS: Prophylaxis of organ rejection in allogenic liver, kidney, or heart transplants with concomitant adrenal corticosteroids. In heart transplant patients, azathioprine or mycophenolate mofetil co-administration is recommended.

DOSAGE: *Adults:* Initial (6h after transplantation): 0.03-0.05mg/kg/day (liver, kidney) or 0.01mg/kg/day (heart) IV infusion if cannot tolerate PO. Hepatic Transplant: 0.05-0.075mg/kg PO q12h with grapefruit juice; start 8-12 hrs after last IV dose. Kidney Transplant: 0.1mg/kg PO q12h, 24 hrs after transplant or until renal function recovered. Heart Transplant: 0.0375mg/kg PO q12h; start 8-12 hrs after last IV dose. Renal/Hepatic Impairment: Give lowest recommended dose. Severe Hepatic Impairment (Pugh ≥10): May require lower doses. Wait at least 48 hrs with post-op oliguria.
Pediatrics: Liver Transplant: Initial: 0.03-0.05mg/kg/day IV or 0.15-0.2mg/kg/day PO. Severe Hepatic Impairment (Pugh ≥10): May require lower doses.

HOW SUPPLIED: Cap: 0.5mg, 1mg, 5mg; Inj: 5mg/mL

CONTRAINDICATIONS: Hypersensitivity to HCO-60.

WARNINGS/PRECAUTIONS: Insulin-dependent post-transplant DM, HTN, myocardial hypertrophy, neurotoxicity, hyperkalemia, nephrotoxicity reported. Monitor drug levels frequently to prevent organ rejection and/or reduce potential toxicity. Monitor for anaphylaxis with infusion. Monitor levels closely with hepatic impairment.

ADVERSE REACTIONS: HTN, headache, insomnia, fever, pruritus, hyperglycemia, hyperkalemia, hypomagnesemia, diarrhea, nausea, vomiting, increased BUN, anorexia, constipation, tremor, rash, pleural effusion, gastroenteritis.

INTERACTIONS: CYP450 3A inducers (eg, carbamazepine, phenobarbital, phenytoin, rifabutin, rifampin, St. John's wort, etc.) may decrease plasma levels. Caution with other nephrotoxic drugs (eg. aminoglycosides, amphotericin B, cisplatin). May affect drugs metabolized by CYP450 3A. Avoid grapefruit juice. CYP450 3A inhibitors (eg, diltiazem, nicardipine, nifedipine, verapamil, azole antifungal, macrolides, cisapride, metoclopramide, etc) may increase plasma levels. Vaccination may be less effective. Avoid live vaccines, cyclosporine (when switching to tacrolimus, wait at least 24 hrs. after last cyclosporine dose), and K⁺ sparing diuretics.

PREGNANCY: Category C, not for use in nursing.

MECHANISM OF ACTION: Macrolide immunosuppressant; not established. Suspected to inhibit T-lymphocyte activation. Binds to intracellular protein (FKBP-12). Complex of tacrolimus-FKBP-12, calcium, calmodulin, and calcineurin is then formed and phosphatase activity of calcineurin inhibited. Effect may prevent dephosphorylation and translocation of nuclear factor of activated T cells (NF-AT), a nuclear component responsible for initiating gene transcription for the formation of lymphokines. Results in inhibition of T-lymphocyte activation.

PHARMACOKINETICS: Absorption: (PO) Incomplete and variable, absolute bioavailability (18%), C_{max}=29.7ng/mL, T_{max}=1.6 hrs, AUC=243ng•hr/mL; (IV) AUC=598ng•hr/mL. **Distribution:** Plasma protein binding (99%), appears in breast milk; (PO) V_d=1.94L/kg; (IV) V_d=1.91 L/kg. **Metabolism:** Hepatic, via CYP3A (demethylation and hydroxylation); 13-methyl tacrolimus (major metabolite); 31-demethyl (active metabolite). **Elimination:** (PO) Feces (92%), urine (2.3%); $T_{1/2}$=34.8 hrs. (IV) Feces (92.4%); $T_{1/2}$=34.2 hrs. Refer to PI for parameters in patients with renal, hepatic, and cardiac transplants.

PROMETHAZINE

RX

promethazine HCl (Various)

OTHER BRAND NAMES: Phenergan (Wyeth) - Promethegan (G & W Labs)

THERAPEUTIC CLASS: Phenothiazine derivative

INDICATIONS: Allergic and vasomotor rhinitis, allergic conjunctivitis, blood or plasma allergic reactions, dermographism, urticaria, angioedema. Pre- and postoperative sedation. Adjunct in anaphylaxis, postoperative pain. Prevention and control of nausea, vomiting, and motion sickness.

DOSAGE: *Adults:* Allergy: 25mg qhs or 12.5mg ac and hs. Motion Sickness: Initial: 25mg 30-60 min before travel, then 25mg 8-12 hrs later if needed. Maint: 25mg bid. Prevention/Control of Nausea/Vomiting: 25mg initially, then 12.5-25mg q4-6h prn. Sedation: 25-50mg qhs. Preoperative: 50mg night before surgery, then 50mg preoperatively. Postoperative: 25-50mg.
Pediatrics: ≥2 yrs: Allergy: 25mg or 0.5mg/lb qhs or 6.25-12.5 tid. Motion Sickness: 12.5-25mg bid. Prevention/Control of Nausea/Vomiting: 25mg or 0.5mg/lb initially then 12.5-25mg or 0.5mg/lb q4-6h prn. Sedation: 12.5-25mg hs. Preoperative: 12.5-25mg night before surgery, then 0.5mg/lb preoperatively. Postoperative: 12.5-25mg.

HOW SUPPLIED: Sup: (Promethegan, Phenergan, Promethazine)12.5mg, 25mg, 50mg; Tab: (Phenergan, Promethazine)12.5mg*, 25mg*, 50mg *scored

CONTRAINDICATIONS: Treatment of lower respiratory tract symptoms (eg, asthma). Pediatric patients <2 yrs.

WARNINGS/PRECAUTIONS: Potential for fatal respiratory depression in pediatric patients <2 yrs. Caution in patients ≥2 yrs. Avoid with compromised respiratory function (eg, COPD, sleep apnea). Caution with bone marrow depression, narrow-angle glaucoma, stenosing peptic ulcer, bladder or pyloroduodenal obstruction, prostatic hypertrophy, CVD, hepatic dysfunction. Cholestatic jaundice reported. Alters HCG pregnancy tests. May lower seizure threshold, increase blood glucose, cause sun sensitivity. May impair mental/physical abilities.

ADVERSE REACTIONS: Drowsiness, sedation, blurred vision, dizziness, increased or decreased blood pressure, urticaria, dry mouth, nausea, vomiting.

INTERACTIONS: Additive sedative effects with CNS depressants (eg, alcohol, narcotic analgesics, sedatives, hypnotics, tranquilizers); reduce dose or eliminate these agents. Reduce barbiturate dose by one-half and analgesic depressant dose by one-quarter to one-half. Caution with drugs that alter seizure threshold (eg, narcotics, local anesthetics). Avoid sedatives and CNS depressants with sleep apnea.

PREGNANCY: Category C, not for use in nursing.

MECHANISM OF ACTION: Phenothiazine derivative; H_1 receptor-blocking agent. Also has sedative and antiemetic properties.

PHARMACOKINETICS: Absorption: GI tract (well absorbed). **Metabolism:** Liver. **Elimination:** Urine.

PROMETHAZINE DM

RX

dextromethorphan HBr - promethazine HCl (Various)

THERAPEUTIC CLASS: Phenothiazine derivative/antitussive

INDICATIONS: Temporary relief of coughs and upper respiratory symptoms associated with allergy or the common cold.

DOSAGE: *Adults:* 5mL q4-6h. Max: 30mL/24 hr.
Pediatrics: ≥12 yrs: 5mL q4-6h. Max: 30mL/24hr. 6-11 yrs: 2.5-5mL q4-6h. Max: 20mL/24hr. 2-5 yrs: 1.25-2.5mL q4-6h. Max: 10mL/24hr.

HOW SUPPLIED: Syrup: (Promethazine-Dextromethorphan) 6.25mg-15mg/5mL

CONTRAINDICATIONS: Concomitant MAOIs, comatose states, treatment of lower respiratory tract symptoms (eg, asthma), pediatric patients <2 yrs.

WARNINGS/PRECAUTIONS: Caution in pediatrics ≥2 yrs. Avoid in pediatric patients whose signs and symptoms may suggest Reye's syndrome or other hepatic diseases. May impair mental/physical abilities. May lower seizure threshold; caution with seizure disorders. May lead to potentially fatal respiratory depression; avoid with compromised respiratory function (eg, COPD, sleep apnea). Caution with bone marrow depression; leukopenia and agranulocytosis reported. Neuroleptic malignant syndrome reported. Caution with narrow-angle glaucoma, prostatic hypertrophy, stenosing peptic ulcer, bladder neck or pyloroduodenal obstruction, cardiovascular disease, hepatic impairment, atopic children, sedated, elderly, or debilitated patients, and patients confined to supine position. Cholestatic jaundice reported. May alter HCG pregnancy test reading. May increase blood glucose. Avoid prolonged exposure to sunlight.

ADVERSE REACTIONS: Drowsiness, dizziness, sedation, GI disturbance, blurred vision, dry mouth, increased or decreased BP, rash, nausea, vomiting.

INTERACTIONS: See Contraindications. Hyperpyrexia, hypotension and death associated with MAOIs. May increase, prolong, or intensify sedative action of other CNS depressants, such as alcohol, sedatives/hypnotics (including barbiturates), narcotics, narcotic analgesics, general anesthetics, TCAs, and tranquilizers; avoid such agents or administer in reduced dosages. Reduce barbiturate dose by at least one-half and narcotic analgesics by one-quarter to one-half. May reverse epinephrine's vasopressor effect. May lower seizure threshold; caution with concomitant medications which may also affect seizure threshold (eg, narcotics, local anesthetics). Avoid concomitant administration with other respiratory depressants in pediatrics. Caution with concomitant use of other agents with anticholinergic properties.

PREGNANCY: Category C, caution in nursing.

MECHANISM OF ACTION: Dextromethorphan: Antitussive agent; acts centrally and elevates the threshold for coughing. Promethazine: Phenothiazine derivative, (antihistaminic); H_1 receptor blocking agent and provides clinically useful sedative and antiemetic effects.

PHARMACOKINETICS: Absorption: Dextromethorphan (rapid); Promethazine (well-absorbed). **Metabolism:** Promethazine: Liver. Dextromethorphan: Liver via O-demethylation, N-demethylation, and partial conjugation with glucuronic acid and sulfate. **Elimination:** Promethazine: Urine (sulfoxides and N-demethylpromethazine). Dextromethorphan: Urine.

PROMETHAZINE VC   RX
phenylephrine HCl - promethazine HCl (Various)

THERAPEUTIC CLASS: Phenothiazine derivative/ sympathomimetic

INDICATIONS: Temporary relief of upper respiratory symptoms (eg, nasal congestion) associated with allergy or the common cold.

DOSAGE: *Adults:* 5mL q4-6h. Max: 30mL/24 hr.
Pediatrics: ≥12 yrs: 5mL q4-6h. Max: 30mL/24 hr. 6-11 yrs: 2.5-5mL q4-6h. Max: 30mL/24 hr. 2-5 yrs: 1.25-2.5mL q4-6h.

HOW SUPPLIED: Syrup: (Promethazine-Phenylephrine) 6.25mg-5mg/5mL

CONTRAINDICATIONS: Concomitant MAOIs, comatose states, treatment of lower respiratory tract symptoms (eg, asthma), HTN, peripheral vascular insufficiency, pediatric patients <2 yrs.

WARNINGS/PRECAUTIONS: Caution in pediatrics ≥2 yrs. Avoid in pediatric patients whose signs and symptoms may suggest Reye's syndrome or other hepatic diseases. May impair mental/physical abilities. May lower seizure threshold; caution with seizure disorders. May lead to potentially fatal respiratory depression; avoid with compromised respiratory function (eg, COPD, sleep apnea). Caution with bone marrow depression; leukopenia and agranulocytosis reported. Neuroleptic malignant syndrome reported. Caution with narrow-angle glaucoma, prostatic hypertrophy, stenosing peptic ulcer, bladder neck or pyloroduodenal obstruction, cardiovascular disease, and elderly patients. Cholestatic jaundice reported. May alter HCG pregnancy test reading. May increase blood glucose. Avoid prolonged exposure to sunlight.

ADVERSE REACTIONS: Drowsiness, dizziness, anxiety, tremor, sedation, blurred vision, dry mouth, increased or decreased blood pressure, rash, nausea, vomiting.

INTERACTIONS: See Contraindications. May increase, prolong, or intensify the sedative action of other CNS depressants, such as alcohol, sedatives/hypnotics (including barbiturates), narcotics, narcotic analgesics, general anesthetics, TCAs, and tranquilizers. avoid such agents or administer in reduced dosages. Reduce barbiturate dose by at least one-half and narcotic analgesics by one-quarter to one-half. Cardiac pressor response potentiated and possible hypertensive crisis with MAOIs. Pressor response increased with TCAs. Excessive rise in BP with ergot alkaloids. Tachycardia or other arrhythmias may occur with sympathomimetics. Reflex bradycardia blocked and pressor response enhanced with atropine. Cardiostimulating effects blocked with β-blockers. Pressor response decreased with α-adrenergic blockers. Synergistic adrenergic response with amphetamines or phenylpropanolamine. Avoid concomitant administration with other respiratory depressants in pediatrics. May lower seizure threshold; caution with concomitant medications which may also affect seizure threshold (eg, narcotics, local anesthetics). Relex bradycardia blocked; pressor response enhanced with atropine.

PREGNANCY: Category C, caution in nursing.

MECHANISM OF ACTION: Promethazine: Phenothiazine derivative; H₁-receptor blocking agent. Phenylephrine: Sympathomimetic; α-receptor agonist with little effect on β-receptors of heart; increases resistance and decreases capacitance of blood vessels; has mild central stimulant effect.

PHARMACOKINETICS: Absorption: Promethazine: Well-absorbed (GI tract). Phenylephrine: Irregularly absorbed. **Metabolism:** Promethazine: Liver, sulfoxides and N-demethylpromethazine (metabolites). Phenylephrine: Liver and intestine via monoamine oxidase. **Elimination:** Promethazine: Urine (sulfoxides and N-demethylpromethazine).

PROMETHAZINE VC/CODEINE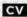

codeine phosphate - phenylephrine HCl - promethazine HCl (Various)

THERAPEUTIC CLASS: Phenothiazine derivative/antitussive/sympathomimetic

INDICATIONS: Temporary relief of cough and upper respiratory symptoms (eg, nasal congestion) associated with allergy or the common cold.

DOSAGE: *Adults:* 5mL q4-6h. Max: 30mL/24hr.
Pediatrics: ≥16 yrs: 5mL q4-6h. Max: 30mL/24hr.

HOW SUPPLIED: Syrup: (Promethazine-Codeine-Phenylephrine) 6.25mg-10mg-5mg/5mL

CONTRAINDICATIONS: Concomitant MAOIs, comatose states, treatment of lower respiratory tract symptoms (eg, asthma), HTN, peripheral vascular insufficiency, pediatric patients <16 yrs.

WARNINGS/PRECAUTIONS: May cause or aggravate constipation. May lead to potentially fatal respiratory depression; avoid with compromised respiratory function (eg, COPD, sleep apnea). Caution in atopic children. May elevate CSF pressure; caution with head injury, intracranial lesions, or pre-existing increase in ICP. Avoid with asthma, acute febrile illness with chronic cough, or with chronic respiratory disease where interference with ability to clear tracheobronchial tree of secretions would have a deleterious effect on patient's respiratory function. May cause orthostatic hypotension. May impair mental/physical abilities. May lower seizure threshold; caution with seizure disorders. Caution with bone marrow depression; leukopenia and agranulocytosis reported. Neuroleptic malignant syndrome reported. Hallucinations and convulsions have occurred in pediatrics. Cholestatic jaundice reported. Caution with acute abdominal conditions, convulsive disorders, significant hepatic/renal impairment, fever, hypothyroidism, Addison's disease, ulcerative colitis, prostatic hypertrophy, recent GI or urinary tract surgery, elderly, debilitated, narrow-angle glaucoma, stenosing peptic ulcer, pyloroduodenal or bladder-neck obstruction, cardiovascular disease, thyroid disease, DM, heart disease. Urinary retention may occur with BPH. May decrease cardiac output; use extreme caution with arteriosclerosis, elderly, and patients with initially poor cerebral or coronary circulation. May alter HCG pregnancy test reading. May increase blood glucose. Avoid prolonged exposure to sunlight.

ADVERSE REACTIONS: Drowsiness, dizziness, sedation, tremor, anxiety, blurred vision, dry mouth, increased or decreased blood pressure, rash, nausea, vomiting, constipation, urinary retention.

INTERACTIONS: See Contraindications. May increase, prolong, or intensify the sedative action of other CNS depressants such as alcohol, sedatives/hypnotics (including barbiturates), narcotics, narcotic analgesics, general anesthetics, TCAs, and tranquilizers. Reduce barbiturate dose by at least one-half and narcotic analgesics by one-quarter to one-half. Cardiac pressor response potentiated and acute hypertensive crisis may occur with MAOIs; consider small test dose. May reverse epinephrine's vasopressor effect. Caution with concomitant use of other agents with anticholinergic properties. Pressor response increased with TCAs. Excessive rise in BP with ergot alkaloids. Tachycardia or other arrhythmias may occur with other sympathomimetics. Cardiostimulating effects blocked with β-blockers. Reflex bradycardia blocked and pressor response enhanced with atropine. Pressor response decreased with α-adrenergic blockers. Synergistic adrenergic response with diet preparations (eg, amphetamines or phenylpropanolamine). Avoid concomitant administration with other respiratory agents in pediatrics. May lower seizure threshold; caution with concomitant medications which may also affect seizure threshold (eg, narcotics, local anesthetics).

PREGNANCY: Category C, caution in nursing.

MECHANISM OF ACTION: Promethazine: phenothiazine derivative. Blocks H$_1$-receptor. Phenylephrine; sympathomimetic. Potent postsynaptic-α-receptor agonist with little effect on β-receptors of heart; increases resistance and decreases capacitance of blood vessels. Codeine: narcotic analgesic/antitussive. Primary effects on central CNS and GI tract.

PHARMACOKINETICS: Absorption: Codeine: Well-absorbed. Promethazine: Well-absorbed (GI tract). Phenylephrine: Irregularly-absorbed. **Distribution:** Codeine: Found in breast milk. **Metabolism:** Promethazine: Liver. Phenylephrine: Liver and intestine, via monoamine oxidase. Codeine: Liver, via O-demethylation, N-demethylation, and partial conjugation with glucuronic acid. **Elimination:** Promethazine: Urine (sulfoxides and N-demethylpromethazine). Codeine: Urine (inactive metabolite and free/conjugated morphine), feces.

PROMETHAZINE W/CODEINE
codeine phosphate - promethazine HCl (Various)

THERAPEUTIC CLASS: Phenothiazine derivative/antitussive

INDICATIONS: Temporary relief of coughs and upper respiratory symptoms associated with allergy or the common cold.

DOSAGE: *Adults:* 5mL q4-6h. Max: 30mL/24 hr.
Pediatrics: ≥16 yrs: 5mL q4-6h. Max: 30mL/24 hr.

HOW SUPPLIED: Syrup: (Promethazine-Codeine) 6.25mg-10mg/5mL

CONTRAINDICATIONS: Comatose states, reatment of lower respiratory tract symptoms (eg, asthma), pediatric patients <16 yrs.

WARNINGS/PRECAUTIONS: May cause or aggravate constipation. May lead to potentially fatal respiratory depression; avoid with compromised respiratory function (eg, COPD, sleep apnea). Caution in atopic children. May elevate CSF pressure; caution with head injury, intracranial lesions, or pre-existing increase in ICP. Avoid with asthma, acute febrile illness with chronic cough, or with chronic respiratory disease where interference with ability to clear tracheobronchial tree of secretions would have a deleterious effect on patient's respiratory function. May cause orthostatic hypotension. May impair mental/physical abilities. May lower seizure threshold; caution with seizure disorders. Caution with bone marrow depression; leukopenia and agranulocytosis reported. Neuroleptic malignant syndrome reported. Hallucinations and convulsions have occurred in pediatrics. Cholestatic jaundice reported. Caution with acute abdominal conditions, convulsive disorders, significant hepatic/renal impairment, fever, hypothyroidism, Addison's disease, ulcerative colitis, prostatic hypertrophy, recent GI or urinary tract surgery, elderly, debilitated, narrow-angle glaucoma, stenosing peptic ulcer, pyloroduodenal or bladder-neck obstruction, or cardiovascular disease. May alter HCG pregnancy test reading. May increase blood glucose. Avoid prolonged exposure to sunlight.

ADVERSE REACTIONS: Drowsiness, dizziness, sedation, blurred vision, dry mouth, increased or decreased blood pressure, rash, nausea, vomiting, constipation, urinary retention.

INTERACTIONS: May increase, prolong, or intensify the sedative action of other CNS depressants such as alcohol, sedative/hypnotics (including barbiturates), narcotics, narcotic analgesics, general anesthetics, TCAs, and tranquilizers; avoid such agents or administer in reduced dosages. Reduce barbiturate dose by at least one-half and narcotic analgesics by one-quarter to one-half. May reverse epinehrine's vasopressor effect. Caution with concomitant use of other agents with anticholinergic properties. May lower seizure threshold; caution with concomitant medications which may also affect seizure threshold (eg, narcotics, local anesthetics). Avoid concomitant administration with other respiratory depressants in pediatrics. Possible interaction with MAOIs; consider small test dose.

PREGNANCY: Category C, caution in nursing.

MECHANISM OF ACTION: Promethazine: phenothiazine derivative; blocks H_1 receptor (antihistaminic action) and provides sedative and antiemetic effects. Codeine: Narcotic analgesic and antitussive; primary effects are on CNS and GI tract.

PHARMACOKINETICS: Absorption: Promethazine and codeine (well absorbed). **Distribution:** Codeine: Found in breast milk. **Metabolism:** Promethazine: Liver. Codeine: Liver via O-demethylation, N-demethylation, and partial conjugation with glucuronic acid. **Elimination:** Promethazine: Urine (sulfoxides and N-demethylpromethazine). Codeine: Urine (inactive metabolites and free/conjugated morphine), feces (codeine and metabolites).

PROPYLTHIOURACIL   RX
propylthiouracil (Various)

THERAPEUTIC CLASS: Thiourea-derivative antithyroid agent

INDICATIONS: Treatment of hyperthyroidism.

DOSAGE: *Adults:* Initial: 300mg/day in 3 divided doses, q8h. Severe Hyperthyroidism/ Very Large Goiters: Initial: 400mg/day in 3 divided doses; may give up to 600-900mg/ day if needed. Maint: 100-150mg/day.
Pediatrics: 6-10 yrs: Initial: 50-150mg/day. ≥10 yrs: Initial: 150-300mg/day. Maint: Determine by patient response.

HOW SUPPLIED: Tab: 50mg

CONTRAINDICATIONS: Nursing mothers.

WARNINGS/PRECAUTIONS: D/C with agranulocytosis, aplastic anemia, hepatitis, fever, or exfoliative dermatitis. Rare reports of severe hepatic reactions exist. D/C with significant hepatic abnormality, including transaminases >3x ULN. Caution with pregnancy, may cause fetal harm. Monitor PT and TFTs.

ADVERSE REACTIONS: Agranulocytosis, granulopenia, thrombocytopenia, aplastic anemia, drug fever, hepatitis, periarteritis, hypoprothrombinemia, skin rash, urticaria, nausea, vomiting, epigastric distress, arthralgia, paresthesias.

INTERACTIONS: May potentiate anticoagulant effects. Hyperthyroidism increases clearance of β-blockers; reduce β-blocker dose when patient becomes euthyroid. Increased digitalis glycoside levels when patient becomes euthyroid; reduce digitalis dose. Decreased theophylline clearance when patient becomes euthyroid; reduce theophylline dose. Caution with other drugs that cause agranulocytosis.

PREGNANCY: Category D, contraindicated in nursing.

MECHANISM OF ACTION: Antithyroid agent; inhibits synthesis of thyroid hormones.

PHARMACOKINETICS: Absorption: GI tract (readily absorbed). **Distribution:** Found in breast milk, crosses the placental membranes. **Elimination:** Urine (35%); $T_{1/2}$= 24 hrs.

PROQUAD   RX
measles vaccine live - mumps vaccine live - rubella vaccine live - varicella virus vaccine live (Merck)

THERAPEUTIC CLASS: Vaccine

INDICATIONS: Vaccination against measles, mumps, rubella, and varicella in children 12 months to 12 yrs of age.

DOSAGE: *Pediatrics:* 12 months-12 yrs: 0.5mL SQ. At least 1 month should elapse between dose of measles-containing vaccine and dose of ProQuad. If for any reason a 2nd dose of varicella-containing vaccine is required, at least 3 months should elapse between doses.

HOW SUPPLIED: Inj: 0.5mL

CONTRAINDICATIONS: Anaphylactic reactions to neomycin; hypsensitivity to gelatin; blood dyscrasias, leukemia, lymphomas, or other malignant neoplasms affecting the bone marrow or lymphatic system; immunosuppressive therapy; primary and acquired immunodeficiency states (e.g., AIDS/HIV); congenital or hereditary immunodeficiency; active untreated tuberculosis; active afebrile illness with fever >101.3°F; pregnant. Disseminated varicella vaccine virus infection has been reported in children with underlying immunodeficiency disorders who were inadvertently vaccinated with a varicella-containing vaccine.

WARNINGS/PRECAUTIONS: Caution with egg allergy. May cause thrombocytopenia. Contains albumin, remote risk of viral infection transmission. Have epinephrine (1:1000) available.

ADVERSE REACTIONS: Injection Site: Pain/tenderness/soreness, erythema, swelling. Systemic: Fever, irritability, measles-like rash, herpes zoster and varicella infection, anaphylactic reaction, ataxia, convulsion, febrile seizure, pruritus.

INTERACTIONS: Do not give with immune globulin. Avoid use of salicylates for 6 weeks after vaccination. Avoid use of immunosuppressive doses of corticosteriods or other immunosuppressive drugs.

PREGNANCY: Category C, not for use in nursing.

MECHANISM OF ACTION: Vaccine; stimulates immune system to elicit immune response to produce antibodies that may protect against measles, mumps, rubella, and varicella disease.

PROSED EC
RX

atropine sulfate - benzoic acid - hyoscyamine sulfate - methenamine - methylene blue - phenyl salicylate (Esprit)

OTHER BRAND NAME: Prosed DS (Star)

THERAPEUTIC CLASS: Urinary tract analgesic

INDICATIONS: Relief of lower urinary tract discomfort due to hypermotility. Treatment of formaldehyde-susceptible cystitis, urethritis, trigonitis.

DOSAGE: Adults: 1 tab qid with plenty of fluid.
Pediatrics: >12 yrs: Individualize dose. Take with plenty of fluid.

HOW SUPPLIED: Tab, Enteric Coated: Atropine 0.06mg-Benzoic Acid 9mg-Hyoscyamine 0.06mg-Methenamine 81.6mg-Methylene Blue 10.8mg-Phenyl Salicylate 36.2mg

CONTRAINDICATIONS: Risk-benefit assessment in glaucoma, urinary bladder neck obstruction, pyloric or duodenal obstruction, cardiospasm.

WARNINGS/PRECAUTIONS: D/C if tachycardia, dizziness, or blurred vision occurs. Delay in gastric emptying time may obscure gastric ulcer therapy.

ADVERSE REACTIONS: Rapid pulse, flushing, blurred vision, dizziness, shortness of breath, difficult micturition, acute urinary retention, dry mouth, nausea, vomiting.

INTERACTIONS: May decrease absorption of other oral agents (dose 2 hrs after ketoconazole). Reduced effectiveness with urinary alkaliners, thiazide diuretics, antacids/antidiarrheals (space dosing by 1 hr). Antimuscarinic effects potentiated with other antimuscarinics, MAOIs. Caution with antimyasthenics. Increased risk of constipation with opioids. Increased risk of crystalluria with sulfonamides.

PREGNANCY: Category C, caution in nursing.

MECHANISM OF ACTION: Methenamine: Degrades in an acidic urine environment, releasing formaldehyde, which provides bactericidal or bacteriostatic action. Phenyl salicylate: Releases salicylate, a mild analgesic for pain. Methylene blue: Possesses weak antiseptic properties. Benzoic acid: Has mild antibacterial and antifungal action; helps maintain an acid pH in the urine, necessary for the degradation of methenamine. Hyoscyamine sulfate: Parasympathetic drug which relaxes smooth muscles.

PHARMACOKINETICS: Absorption: Well (methenamine, methylene blue, and hyoscyamine). **Distribution:** Methenamine and hyoscyamine, crosses placenta; found in breast milk. **Metabolism:** Methenamine: Hydrolizes in acidic urine to formaldehyde. Methylene blue: Reduced to leukomethylene blue (metabolite). Hyoscyamine: Hepatic biotransformation. **Elimination:** Methenamine: Urine (70-90% unchanged). Methylene blue: Urine (75% unchanged). Hyoscyamine: Unchanged.

PROSTIN VR PEDIATRIC

RX

alprostadil (Pharmacia & Upjohn)

> **Apnea occurs in about 10-12% of neonates, usually appearing during the 1st hr of drug infusion. Monitor respiratory status throughout treatment.**

THERAPEUTIC CLASS: Prostaglandin E$_1$

INDICATIONS: Palliative therapy to maintain patency of the ductus arteriosus until corrective surgery in neonates with congenital heart defects.

DOSAGE: *Pediatrics:* Initial: 0.05-0.1mcg/kg/min IV. Maint: 0.025-0.01mcg/kg/min IV. Max: 0.4mcg/kg/min.

HOW SUPPLIED: Inj: 0.5mg/mL

WARNINGS/PRECAUTIONS: May cause gastric outlet obstruction secondary to antral hyperplasia, monitor closely after 120 hrs of therapy. Limit infusion to minimum effective dose and time. May inhibit platelet aggregation; caution with bleeding tendencies. Cortical proliferation of long bones, localized and aneurysmal dilatations, vessel wall edema, intimal lacerations, decrease in medial muscularity and disruption of medial and internal lamina reported. Avoid in respiratory distress syndrome. Monitor arterial pressure intermittently; decrease rate of infusion with significant fall in pressure.

ADVERSE REACTIONS: Apnea, fever, seizures, bradycardia, flushing, diarrhea, hypotension, tachycardia.

PREGNANCY: Safety in pregnancy and nursing not known.

MECHANISM OF ACTION: Prostaglandin; causes vasodilation, inhibits platelet aggregation, stimulates intestinal and uterine smooth muscles.

PHARMACOKINETICS: Metabolism: Rapid. Lungs (β- and omega oxidation). **Elimination:** Kidneys.

PROTOPIC

RX

tacrolimus (Astellas)

THERAPEUTIC CLASS: Macrolide immunosuppressant

INDICATIONS: Short-term and intermittent long-term therapy of moderate to severe atopic dermatitis intolerant or unresponsive to conventional therapy.

DOSAGE: *Adults:* (0.03% or 0.1%) Apply thin layer bid. Rub in gently. Stop use when signs and symptoms resolve.
Pediatrics: ≥16 yrs: (0.03% or 0.1%) Apply thin layer bid. Rub in gently. 2-15 yrs: (0.03%) Apply thin layer bid. Rub in gently. Stop use when signs and symptoms resolve.

HOW SUPPLIED: Oint: 0.03%, 0.1% (30g, 60g, 100g)

WARNINGS/PRECAUTIONS: Do not use with occlusive dressings. Increased risk of varicella zoster, herpes simplex, or eczema herpeticum. Lymphadenopathy reported; monitor closely. D/C if unknown etiology of lymphadenopathy or presence of acute infectious mononucleosis. Avoid in Netherton's syndrome. Minimize or avoid exposure to natural or artificial sunlight. Long-term safety not established. Rare cases of malignancy (eg, skin and lymphoma) reported with topical calcineurin inhibitors; therefore, continuous long-term use should be avoided and application limited to areas of involvement. Should not use in immunocompromised adults and children. Caution in patients predisposed to renal impairment. Not indicated for use in children <2 yrs. Only 0.03% oint is indicated for use in children 2-15 yrs.

ADVERSE REACTIONS: Skin burning, pruritus, flu-like symptoms, allergic reaction, skin erythema, headache, skin infection, fever, herpes simplex, rhinitis.

INTERACTIONS: Caution with CYP3A4 inhibitors (eg, erythromycin, itraconazole, ketoconazole, fluconazole, CCBs, cimetidine) in widespread and/or erythrodermic disease. Increased risk for lymphomas in transplant patients receiving other immunosuppressive therapy.

PREGNANCY: Category C, not for use in nursing.

MECHANISM OF ACTION: Macrolide immunosuppressant; not known in atopic dermatitis. Inhibits T-lymphocyte activation by first binding to an intracellular protein, FKBP-12. A

365

complex of tacrolimus-FKBP-12, calcium, calmodulin, and calcineurin is then formed and the phosphate activity of calcineurin is inhibited. This has been shown to prevent the dephosphorylation and translocation of nuclear factor of activated T-cells.

PHARMACOKINETICS: Absorption: Absolute bioavailability (0.5%), C_{max}<2ng/mL (90% of population). **Distribution:** V_d=99%. **Metabolism:** CYP3A (extensive); demethylation and hydroxylation; 13-demethyl tacrolimus (major metabolite). **Elimination:** Feces (major).

PROVENTIL HFA RX
albuterol sulfate (Schering)

THERAPEUTIC CLASS: Beta$_2$-agonist

INDICATIONS: Prevention and treatment of bronchospasm with reversible obstructive airway disease; prevention of exercise-induced bronchospasm (EIB) in patients ≥4 yrs old.

DOSAGE: *Adults:* Bronchospasm: 2 inh q4-6h or 1 inh q4h. EIB: 2 inh 15-30 min before activity.
Pediatrics: ≥4 yrs: Bronchospasm: 2 inh q4-6h or 1 inh q4h. EIB: 2 inh 15-30 min before activity.

HOW SUPPLIED: MDI: 90mcg/inh (6.7g)

WARNINGS/PRECAUTIONS: Hypersensitivity reactions reported. Monitor for worsening asthma. Fatalities reported with excessive use. Caution with cardiovascular disorders, especially coronary insufficiency, arrhythmias and HTN. May need concomitant corticosteroids. Can produce paradoxical bronchospasm. Caution with DM, hyperthyroidism, and seizures. May cause transient hypokalemia.

ADVERSE REACTIONS: Tachycardia, tremor, dizziness, nausea/vomiting, palpitations, rihinitis, upper respiratory tract infection, fever, inhalation site and taste sensation, back pain, and nervousness.

INTERACTIONS: Avoid other sympathomimetic agents. Extreme caution wtih MAOIs and TCAs. Monitor digoxin. May worsen ECG changes and/or hypokalemia with nonpotassium-sparing diuretics. Antagonized by β-blockers.

PREGNANCY: Category C, not for use in nursing.

MECHANISM OF ACTION: β$_2$-adrenergic bronchodilator; stimulates adenyl cylase, the enzyme that catalyzes the formation of cAMP from ATP. Increased cAMP levels are associated with relaxation of bronchial smooth muscle and inhibition of release of mediators of immediate hypersensitivity.

PROZAC RX

fluoxetine HCl (Lilly)

> Antidepressants increased the risk of suicidal thinking and behavior (suicidality) in short-term studies of children, adolescents, and young adults with Major Depressive Disorder (MDD) and other psychiatric disorders. Fluoxetine is approved for use in pediatric patients with MDD and obsessive compulsive disorder (OCD).

THERAPEUTIC CLASS: Selective serotonin reuptake inhibitor

INDICATIONS: Treatment of MDD, OCD, bulimia nervosa, panic disorder with or without agoraphobia.

DOSAGE: *Adults:* MDD: Daily Dosing: Initial: 20mg qam; increase dose if no improvement after several weeks. Doses >20mg/day, give qam or bid (am and noon). Max: 80mg/day. OCD: Initial: 20mg qam; may increase dose if no significant improvement after several weeks. Maint: 20-60mg/day given qd-bid, am and noon. Max: 80mg/day. Bulimia Nervosa: 60mg qam. Max: 60mg/day. Panic Disorder: Initial: 10mg/day. May increase to 20mg/day after 1 week. May increase further after several weeks if no clinical improvement. Max: 60mg/day. Hepatic Impairment/Elderly: Use lower or less frequent dosage.
Pediatrics: MDD: ≥8 yrs: Higher Weight Peds: Initial: 10 or 20mg/day. After 1 week at 10mg/day, may increase to 20mg/day. Lower Weight Peds: Initial: 10mg/day. Titrate: May increase to 20mg/day after several weeks if clinical improvement is not observed. OCD: ≥7 yrs: Adolescents and Higher Weight Peds: Initial: 10mg/day. Titrate: Increase

to 20mg/day after 2 weeks. Consider additional dose increases after several more weeks if clinical improvement is not observed. Usual: 20-60mg/day. **Lower Weight Peds:** Initial: 10mg/day. Titrate: Consider additional dose increases after several weeks if clinical improvement is not observed. Usual: 20-30mg/day. Max: 60mg/day.

HOW SUPPLIED: Cap: 10mg, 20mg, 40mg; Sol: 20mg/5mL (120mL)

CONTRAINDICATIONS: During or within 14 days of MAOI therapy. Thioridazine during or within 5 weeks of discontinuation. Concomitant use of pimozide.

WARNINGS/PRECAUTIONS: D/C if unexplained allergic reaction occurs. Monitor for symptoms of mania/hypomania. Caution with diseases or conditions that could affect metabolism or hemodynamic responses, diabetes, history of seizures, suicidal tendencies. Altered platelet function, hyponatremia reported. Periodically monitor height and weight in pediatrics. Monitor for clinical worsening and/or suicidality, especially at initiation of therapy or dose changes. Avoid abrupt withdrawal. Monitor for discontinuation symptoms. Caution in third trimester of pregnancy due to risk of serious neonatal complications. May interfere with cognitive and motor performance.

ADVERSE REACTIONS: Nausea, diarrhea, insomnia, anxiety, nervousness, dizziness, somnolence, tremor, decreased libido, sweating, anorexia, asthenia, dry mouth, dyspepsia, headache.

INTERACTIONS: See Contraindications. Antidiabetic drugs may need adjustment. May shift concentrations with plasma-bound drugs (eg, coumadin, digitoxin). May alter warfarin effects. May increase benzodiazepine, phenytoin, carbamazepine levels. Increased adverse effects with tryptophan. Caution with CNS drugs. Lithium levels may increase/decrease; monitor lithium levels. May potentiate drugs metabolized by CYP2D6, antipsychotics (eg, haloperidol, clozapine), other antidepressants. Avoid alcohol. Caution with drugs that interfere with hemostasis (eg, non-selective NSAIDs, ASA, warfarin) due to increased risk of bleeding. Serotonin syndrome reported with use of an SSRI and a triptan; monitor closely. Altered appetite and weight loss reported.

PREGNANCY: Category C, not for use in nursing.

MECHANISM OF ACTION: SSRI; inhibits CNS neuronal reuptake of serotonin.

PHARMACOKINETICS: Absorption: C_{max}=15-55ng/mL, T_{max}=6-8 hrs. **Distribution:** Plasma protein binding (94.5%); excreted in breast milk. **Metabolism:** Liver (extensive) via demethylation, norfluoxetine (active metabolite). **Elimination:** Urine; $T_{1/2}$=1-3 days (fluoxetine), 4-16 days (norfluoxetine).

PULMICORT

RX

budesonide (AstraZeneca)

OTHER BRAND NAMES: Pulmicort Flexhaler (AstraZeneca) - Pulmicort Respules (AstraZeneca)

THERAPEUTIC CLASS: Corticosteroid

INDICATIONS: (Respules) Treatment of asthma and as prophylactic therapy in children 12 months to 8 yrs. (Flexhaler) Maintenance treatment of asthma as prophylactic therapy in patients ≥6 yrs and to reduce or eliminate the need for oral systemic corticosteroidal therapy.

DOSAGE: *Adults:* (Flexhaler) Initial: 180-360mcg bid. Max: 720mcg bid. Individualize dose.

Pediatrics: (Flexhaler) ≥6 yrs: Initial: 180-360mcg bid. Max: 360mcg bid. Individualize dose. (Respules) 1-8 yrs: Previous Bronchodilator Only: Initial: 0.5mg qd or 0.25mg bid. Administer via jet nebulizer. Max: 0.5mg/day. Previous Inhaled Corticosteroid: 0.5mg qd or 0.25mg bid. Max: 1mg/day. Previous Oral Corticosteroid: 1mg qd or 0.5mg bid. Max: 1mg/day. Gradually reduce PO corticosteroid after 1 week of budesonide.

HOW SUPPLIED: Powder, Inhalation: (Flexhaler) 90mcg/dose, 180mcg/dose; Sus, Inhalation: (Respules) 0.25mg/2mL; 0.5mg/2mL (2mL, 30s)

CONTRAINDICATIONS: Primary treatment of status asthmaticus or other acute episodes of asthma where intensive measures are required.

WARNINGS/PRECAUTIONS: Deaths due to adrenal insufficiency have occurred with transfer from systemic corticosteroids to inhaled corticosteroids. Resume oral corticosteroids during stress or severe asthma attack. Transferring from oral to inhalation therapy may unmask allergic conditions (eg, rhinitis, conjunctivitis, arthritis, eosinophilic conditions, eczema). Observe for adrenal insufficiency, systemic corticosteroid withdrawal effects, and growth suppression (children). More susceptible to infections. Not for acute bronchospasm. D/C if bronchospasm occurs after dosing. Caution with TB of respiratory tract; untreated systemic fungal, bacterial, viral or parasitic infections; or ocular herpes simplex. *Candida* infection of mouth and pharynx reported. Patients requiring oral corticosteroids should be weaned slowly from systemic corticosteroid use.

ADVERSE REACTIONS: Nasopharyngitis, pharyngitis, headache, fever, sinusitis, pain, bronchospasm, bronchitis, respiratory infection, monoliasis.

INTERACTIONS: Oral ketoconazole increases plasma levels. CYP3A4 inhibitors (eg, itraconazole, clarithromycin, erythromycin) may inhibit metabolism and increase systemic exposure. (Respules) Slight decrease in clearance and increase in oral bioavailabilty with cimetidine.

PREGNANCY: (Respules) Category B, caution in nursing; (Flexhaler) Category B, caution in nursing.

MECHANISM OF ACTION: Corticosteroid; not established. Shown to have inhibitory effects on multiple cell types (mast cells, eosinophils, neutrophils, macrophages and lymphocytes) and mediators (histamine, eicosanoids, leukotrienes and cytokines) involved in inflammatory and asthmatic response.

PHARMACOKINETICS: Absorption: Respules: (4-6 yrs) Absolute bioavailability (6%); C_{max}=2.6nmol/L, T_{max}=20 min. Turbuhaler: T_{max}=30 min. Flexhaler: (Adults) T_{max}=10 min, (180mg qd) C_{max}=0.6nmol/L. (360mg bid) C_{max}=1.6nmol/L. (Peds) T_{max}=15-30 mins, (180mg qd) C_{max}=0.4nmol/L. (360mg bid) C_{max}=1.5nmol/L. **Distribution:** V_d=3L/kg; Plasma protein binding (85-90%). **Metabolism:** Liver (biotransformation), via CYP3A4. **Elimination:** (Respules) $T_{1/2}$=2.3 hrs. (Turbuhaler, Flexhaler) $T_{1/2}$=2-3 hrs.

PULMOZYME

RX

dornase alfa (Genentech)

THERAPEUTIC CLASS: Protein

INDICATIONS: Adjunct therapy in cystic fibrosis to improve pulmonary function.

DOSAGE: *Adults:* 2.5mg qd-bid via nebulizer.
Pediatrics: ≥5 yrs: 2.5mg qd-bid via nebulizer.

HOW SUPPLIED: Sol: 2.5mg/2.5mL (2.5mL: 1⁵, 30⁶)

CONTRAINDICATIONS: Hypersensitivity to chinese hamster ovary cell products.

WARNINGS/PRECAUTIONS: Use with standard therapies for cystic fibrosis.

ADVERSE REACTIONS: Voice alteration, pharyngitis, rash, laryngitis, chest pain, conjunctivitis, rhinitis, fever, dyspnea.

PREGNANCY: Category B, caution in nursing.

MECHANISM OF ACTION: Protein; hydrolyzes the DNA in sputum and reduces sputum viscoelasticity.

PURINETHOL

RX

mercaptopurine (Gate)

THERAPEUTIC CLASS: Purine analog

INDICATIONS: Remission induction and maintenance therapy of acute lymphatic leukemia (ALL).

DOSAGE: *Adults:* Maint: 1.5-2.5mg/kg/day as single dose. Renal/Hepatic Impairment: Reduce dose. Concomitant Allopurinol: Reduce mercaptopurine dose by 1/3-1/4 of usual dose. TPMT Deficiency: Consider dose reduction.
Pediatrics: Maint: 1.5-2.5mg/kg/day as single dose. Renal/Hepatic Impairment: Reduce dose. Concomitant Allopurinol: Reduce mercaptopurine dose by 1/3-1/4 of usual dose. TPMT Deficiency: Consider dose reduction.

HOW SUPPLIED: Tab: 50mg* *scored

CONTRAINDICATIONS: Lack of definitive diagnosis of ALL. Prior resistance to mercaptopurine or thioguanine.

WARNINGS/PRECAUTIONS: Risk of dose-related bone marrow suppression. Monitor weekly platelet counts, Hgb, Hct, total WBC with differential; increase frequency during induction phase. Monitor closely for life-threatening infection or bleeding. Risk of hepatotoxicity, anorexia, diarrhea, jaundice, and ascites (especially with >2.5mg/kg dose). Perform LFTs weekly initially, then monthly; monitor more frequently with hepatotoxic drugs or pre-existing liver disease. Increased sensitivity to myelosuppressive effects with thiopurine-S-methyltransferase (TPMT) gene deficiency; consider TPMT testing with evidence of severe toxicity.

ADVERSE REACTIONS: Bone marrow toxicity, hepatotoxicity, hyperuricemia (reduce incidence by prehydration, urine alkalinization, prophylactic allopurinol), intestinal ulceration, rash, hyperpigmentation, alopecia, transient oligospermia.

INTERACTIONS: Reduce to 1/3-1/4 of usual dose with allopurinol to avoid toxicity. Reduce dose with myelosuppressants. Bone marrow suppression reported with trimethoprim-sulfamethoxazole. Cross-resistance with thioguanine. Increased bone marrow toxicity with concomitant TPMT inhibitors (eg, olsalazine, mesalazine, sulphasalazine). Inhibition of anticoagulant effect of warfarin with concomitant administration.

PREGNANCY: Category D, not for use in nursing.

MECHANISM OF ACTION: Purine analog; competes with hypoxanthine and guanine for hypoxanthine-guanine phosphoribosyltransferase and gets converted to thiosinic acid, which then inhibits glutamine-5-phosphoribosylpyrophosphate amidotransferase of de novo pathway for purine ribonucleotide synthesis.

PHARMACOKINETICS: Absorption: Incomplete. **Distribution:** Plasma protein binding (19%). **Elimination:** $T_{1/2}$=21 min (pediatric); 47 min (adult).

PYRAZINAMIDE
pyrazinamide (Various)

RX

THERAPEUTIC CLASS: Nicotinamide analogue

INDICATIONS: Adjunctive initial treatment of active TB. For use after treatment failure with other primary drugs.

DOSAGE: *Adults:* Usual: 15-30mg/kg qd. Max: 3g/day. (CDC recommends Max: 2g/day). Alternate Regimen: 50-75mg/kg twice weekly. Dose based on lean body weight. Take initial 2 months of 6 month or longer regimen.
Pediatrics: Usual: 15-30mg/kg qd. Max: 3g/day. (CDC recommends Max: 2g/day). Alternate Regimen: 50-75mg/kg twice weekly. Dose based on lean body weight. Take initial 2 months of 6 month or longer regimen.

HOW SUPPLIED: Tab: 500mg* *scored

CONTRAINDICATIONS: Severe hepatic damage and active gout.

WARNINGS/PRECAUTIONS: Obtain baseline serum uric acid and LFTs before therapy. Caution with hepatic dysfunction or those at risk for drug-related hepatitis (eg, alcoholics) and DM. D/C if hyperuricemia with gouty arthritis or hepatocellular damage occurs. Inhibits renal excretion of urates.

ADVERSE REACTIONS: Gout, hepatotoxicity, NV, anorexia, arthralgia, myalgia, rash, urticaria, pruritus.

PREGNANCY: Category C, caution in nursing.

MECHANISM OF ACTION: Nicotinamide analogue; suspected to act as bacteriostatic and bactericidal against *Mycobacterium* tuberculosis.

PHARMACOKINETICS: Absorption: GI tract (well-absorbed); T_{max}=2hrs. **Distribution:** Plasma protein binding (10%); distributed in liver, lungs, and CSF; found in breast milk. **Metabolism:** Liver, via hydroxylation; pyrazinoic acid (major active metabolite). **Elimination:** Urine (70%); $T_{1/2}$=9-10 hrs.

QUESTRAN
cholestyramine (Par)

RX

OTHER BRAND NAME: Questran Light (Par)
THERAPEUTIC CLASS: Bile acid sequestrant

INDICATIONS: Adjunct to reduce elevated cholesterol in primary hypercholesterolemia not responding to diet or to reduce LDL in hypertriglyceridemia. Relief of pruritus associated with partial biliary obstruction.

DOSAGE: *Adults:* Initial: 1 pkt or scoopful qd or bid. Maint: 2-4 pkts or scoopfuls/day, given bid. Titrate: Adjust at no less than 4 week intervals. Max: 6 pkts/day or 6 scoopfuls/day. May also give as 1-6 doses/day. Mix with fluid or highly fluid food. *Pediatrics:* Usual: 240mg/kg/day of anhydrous cholestyramine resin in 2-3 divided doses. Max: 8g/day.

HOW SUPPLIED: Powder: 4g/pkt (60s, 378g), (Light) 4g/scoopful (60s, 268g)

CONTRAINDICATIONS: Complete biliary obstruction.

WARNINGS/PRECAUTIONS: May produce hyperchloremic acidosis with prolonged use. Caution in renal insufficiency, volume depletion, and with concomitant spironolactone. Chronic use may produce or worsen constipation. Avoid constipation with symptomatic CAD. May increase bleeding tendency due to vitamin K deficiency. Serum or red cell folate reduced with chronic use. Constipation may aggravate hemorrhoids. Light formulation contains phenylalanine. Measure cholesterol during 1st few months; periodically thereafter. Measure TG periodically.

ADVERSE REACTIONS: Constipation, heartburn, nausea, vomiting, abdominal pain, flatulence, diarrhea, anorexia, osteoporosis, rash, hyperchloremic acidosis (children), vitamin A and D deficiency, steatorrhea, hypoprothrombinemia (vitamin K deficiency).

INTERACTIONS: May interfere with absorption of fat-soluble vitamins (A, D, E, K), drugs that undergo enterohepatic circulation, and oral phosphate supplements. Take concomitant drugs 1hr before or 4-6 hrs after. Additive effects with HMG-CoA reductase inhibitors and nicotinic acid. Caution with spironolactone. May reduce or delay absorption of phenylbutazone, warfarin, thiazide diuretics, propranolol, tetracycline, penicillin G, phenobarbital, thyroid and thyroxine agents, estrogens, progestins, digitalis.

PREGNANCY: Category C, caution in nursing.

MECHANISM OF ACTION: Bile acid sequestrant; absorbs and combines with bile acids in intestine to form insoluble complex excreted in the feces, resulting in partial removal of bile acids from enterohepatic circulation by preventing their absorption. This leads to increased oxidation of cholesterol to bile acids and decreased plasma LDL and serum cholesterol levels.

PHARMACOKINETICS: Elimination: Feces.

QUINIDINE GLUCONATE INJECTION RX
quinidine gluconate (Various)

THERAPEUTIC CLASS: Class IA antiarrhythmic/schizonticide antimalarial

INDICATIONS: Treatment of life-threatening *Plasmodium falciparum* malaria. Conversion of atrial fibrillation/flutter (A-Fib/Flutter) to normal sinus rhythm. Treatment of ventricular arrhythmias.

DOSAGE: *Adults:* Malaria: LD: 15mg/kg base (24mg/kg gluconate) over 4 hrs. Maint: After 8 hrs, 7.5mg/kg (12mg/kg gluconate) IV q8h for 7 days. Alternate: Initial: 6.25mg/kg base (10mg/kg/min gluconate) IV over 1-2 hrs. Maint: 12.5mcg/kg/min base (20mcg/kg/min gluconate) for 72h. Switch to PO therapy when possible. A-Fib/Flutter and Ventricular Arrhythmia: 0.25mg/kg/min. Max: 5-10mg/kg. Consider alternate therapy if conversion to sinus rhythm not achieved. Renal/Hepatic Impairment or CHF: Reduce dose. Elderly: Start at low end of dosing range. *Pediatrics:* Malaria: LD: 15mg/kg base (24mg/kg gluconate) over 4 hrs. Maint: After 8 hrs, 7.5mg/kg (12mg/kg gluconate) IV q8h for 7 days. Alternate: Initial: 6.25mg/kg base (10mg/kg/min gluconate) IV over 1-2 hrs. Maint: 12.5mcg/kg/min base (20mcg/kg/min gluconate) for 72h. Switch to PO therapy when possible.

HOW SUPPLIED: Inj: 80mg/mL

CONTRAINDICATIONS: Cardiac rhythm dependent upon a junctional or idioventricular pacemaker (absent of functioning pacemaker), thrombocytopenic purpura with previous treatment, patients adversely affected by anticholinergics (eg, myasthenia gravis).

WARNINGS/PRECAUTIONS: Rapid infusion can cause peripheral vascular collapse and hypotension. May prolong QTc interval. Paradoxical increase in ventricular rate in A-Fib/Flutter. Caution in those at risk of complete AV block without implanted pacemakers, renal/hepatic dysfunction, elderly, and CHF. Physical/pharmacologic maneuvers to terminate paroxysmal supraventricular tachycardia may be ineffective. Exacerbated bradycardia in sick sinus syndrome.

ADVERSE REACTIONS: GI distress, lightheadedness, fatigue, palpitations, weakness, visual problems, NV, diarrhea, sleep disturbances, rash, headache, cinchonism, hepatotoxicity, autoimmune/inflammatory syndromes.

INTERACTIONS: Urine alkalinizers (eg, carbonic anhydrase inhibitors, sodium bicarbonate, thiazide diuretics) reduce renal elimination. CYP3A4 inducers (eg, phenobarbital, phenytoin, rifampin) may accelerate elimination. Verapamil, diltiazem decrease clearance. Caution with drugs metabolized by CYP2D6 (eg, mexiletine, phenothiazines, polycyclic antidepressants, codeine, hydrocodone) or by CYP3A4 (eg, nifedipine, felodipine, nicardipine, nimodipine). β-blockers may decrease clearance. May slow metabolism of nifedipine. Increases levels of digoxin, digitoxin, procainamide and haloperidol. Increased levels with ketoconazole, amiodarone, cimetidine. Potentiates warfarin, depolarizing and nondepolarizing neuromuscular blockers. Additive effects with anticholinergics, vasodilators, and negative inotropes. Antagonistic effects with cholinergics, vasoconstrictors, and positive inotropes.

PREGNANCY: Category C, not for use in nursing.

MECHANISM OF ACTION: Antimalarial schizonticide and antiarrhythmic agent with class 1a activity. Slows phase-0 depolarization by depressing the inward depolarizing Na+ current, which slows conduction, prolongs effective refractory period, and reduces automaticity in the heart. Also has anticholinergic activity, negative ionotropic activity, and acts peripherally as an α-adrenergic antagonist.

PHARMACOKINETICS: Absorption: T_{max} ≤2 hrs. **Distribution:** V_d=2-3 L/kg; plasma protein binding (80-88%), (50-70%) in pregnant women, infants and neonates; found in breast milk. **Metabolism:** Liver, via CYP3A4 pathway. 3-hydroxy-quinidine (3HQ); major metabolite. **Elimination:** Urine (20% unchanged); $T_{1/2}$=6-8 hrs (adults), 3-4 hrs (pediatrics), and 12 hrs (3HQ).

QUINIDINE SULFATE RX
quinidine sulfate (Watson)

THERAPEUTIC CLASS: Class IA antiarrhythmic/schizonticide antimalarial

INDICATIONS: Conversion of symptomatic A-fib/flutter to normal sinus rhythm, reduction of relapse frequency into A-fib/flutter, and suppression of ventricular arrhythmias. Treatment of life-threatening *Plasmodium falciparum* malaria.

DOSAGE: *Adults:* A-Fib/Flutter Conversion: Initial: 400mg q6h. Titrate: Increase cautiously if no effect after 4-5 doses. A-Fib/Flutter Relapse Reduction: 200mg q6h. Titrate: Increase cautiously if needed. Ventricular Arrhythmia: Dosing regimens not adequately studied. Malaria: After LD of quinidine gluconate, 300mg q8h for 7 days. Alternate: After LD of quinidine gluconate, 300mg q8h for 72h or until parasitemia had decreased to ≤1%.
Pediatrics: Malaria: After LD of quinidine gluconate, 300mg q8h for 7 days. Alternate: After LD of quinidine gluconate, 300mg q8h for 72h or until parasitemia had decreased to ≤1%.

HOW SUPPLIED: Tab: 200mg, 300mg

CONTRAINDICATIONS: Cardiac rhythm dependent upon a junctional or idioventricular pacemaker (in the absence of functioning pacemaker), thrombocytopenic purpura with previous treatment, patients adversely affected by anticholinergics (eg, myasthenia gravis).

WARNINGS/PRECAUTIONS: Increases risk of mortality, especially with structural heart disease. May prolong QTc interval. Paradoxical increase in ventricular rate in A-fib/flutter. Adjust dose in renal/hepatic dysfunction and CHF. Caution if at risk of complete AV-block in those without implanted pacemakers or in elderly. Physical/pharmacologic maneuvers to terminate paroxysmal supraventricular tachycardia may be ineffective. Exacerbated bradycardia in sick sinus syndrome. Monitor blood counts, hepatic, and renal function periodically with long-term therapy. D/C if blood dyscrasia or hepatic/renal dysfunction occurs.

ADVERSE REACTIONS: Diarrhea, NV, headache, esophagitis, lightheadedness, fatigue, palpitations, angina-like pain, weakness, rash, visual problems, cinchonism, hepatotoxicity, autoimmune/inflammatory syndromes.

INTERACTIONS: Urine alkalinizers (eg, carbonic anhydrase inhibitors, sodium bicarbonate, thiazide diuretics) reduce renal elimination. CYP3A4 inducers (eg, phenobarbital, phenytoin, rifampin) may accelerate hepatic elimination. Verapamil, diltiazem, β-blockers decrease clearance. Caution with drugs metabolized by CYP3A4 and 2D6. Increases levels of procainamide and haloperidol. Increased levels with ketoconazole, amiodarone, cimetidine. Decreased levels with nifedipine. Potentiates warfarin, depolarizing (eg, succinylcholine, decamethonium) and nondepolarizing (eg, d-tubocurarine, pancuronium) neuromuscular blockers. Additive effects with anticholinergics, vasodilators, and negative inotropics. Avoid grapefruit juice. Dietary salt may affect absorption. Digoxin may need dose reduction.

PREGNANCY: Category C, not for use in nursing.

MECHANISM OF ACTION: An antimalarial schizonticide and an antiarrhythmic agent with class 1a activity. Quinidine depresses rapid inward depolarizing Na current, thereby slowing phase-0 depolarization and reducing the amplitude of action potentials without affecting resting potentials resulting in slowed conduction and reduced automaticity in all parts of the heart, with increase in effective refractory period relative to the duration of action potentials in the atria, ventricles, and Purkinje tissues. Also raises fibrillation thresholds of the atria and ventricles, and raises ventricular defibrillation threshold. It can interrupt or prevent reentrant arrhythmias and arrhythmias due to increased automaticity, including atrial flutter, AF, and PST. It has anticholinergic activity, negative inotropic activity, and acts peripherally as an α-adrenergic antagonist.

PHARMACOKINETICS: Absorption: Absolute bioavailability (70%), T_{max}=6 hrs. **Distribution:** Vd=2-3 L/kg; plasma protein binding (80-88%), (50-70%) in pregnant women, infants and neonates. Found in breast milk. **Metabolism:** Liver via CYP3A4 pathway; 3-hydroxyquinidine (3HQ) major metabolite. **Elimination:** Urine (70% unchanged); $T_{1/2}$=6-8 hrs (adults), 3-4 hrs (pediatrics), and 12 hrs (3HQ).

QUIXIN RX
levofloxacin (Vistakon)

THERAPEUTIC CLASS: Fluoroquinolone

INDICATIONS: Treatment of bacterial conjunctivitis.

DOSAGE: *Adults:* Days 1-2: 1-2 drops q2h while awake, up to 8x/day. Days 3-7: 1-2 drops q4h while awake, up to qid.
Pediatrics: ≥1 yr: Days 1-2: 1-2 drops q2h while awake, up to 8x/day. Days 3-7: 1-2 drops q4h while awake, up to qid.

HOW SUPPLIED: Sol: 0.5% (5mL)

WARNINGS/PRECAUTIONS: D/C if hypersensitivity or superinfection occurs. Avoid contact lenses with conjunctivitis.

ADVERSE REACTIONS: Transient ocular burning, decreased vision, fever, foreign body sensation, headache, ocular pain, pharyngitis, photophobia.

INTERACTIONS: Systemic quinolone therapy may increase theophylline levels, interfere with caffeine metabolism, enhance warfarin effects, and elevate serum creatinine with cyclosporine.

PREGNANCY: Category C, caution in nursing.

MECHANISM OF ACTION: Fluroquinolone; antibacterial active against broad spectrum of gram-positive and gram-negative organisms. Responsible for inhibition of bacterial topoisomerase IV and DNA gyrase, enzymes required for DNA replication, transcription, repair, and recombination.

PHARMACOKINETICS: Absorption: C_{max}=0.94ng/mL (single dose), 2.15ng/mL (multiple doses).

QVAR

RX

beclomethasone dipropionate (Ivax)

THERAPEUTIC CLASS: Corticosteroid

INDICATIONS: Maintenance treatment of asthma as prophylactic therapy in patients ≥5 tears; to reduce or eliminate the need for oral corticosteroidal therapy.

DOSAGE: *Adults:* Previous Bronchodilator Only: 40-80mcg bid. Max: 320mcg bid. Previous Inhaled Corticosteroid (CS) Therapy: 40-160mcg bid. Max: 320mcg bid. Maint With Oral CS: May attempt gradual reduction of oral dose after 1 week on inhaled therapy. *Pediatrics:* Adolescents: Previous Bronchodilator Only: 40-80mcg bid. Max: 320mcg bid. Previous Inhaled Corticosteroid (CS) Therapy: 40-160mcg bid. Max: 320mcg bid. 5-11 yrs: Previous Bronchodilator Only or Inhaled CS Therapy: 40mcg bid. Max: 80mcg bid. ≥5 yrs: Maint With Oral CS: May attempt gradual reduction of oral dose after 1 week on inhaled therapy.

HOW SUPPLIED: MDI: 40mcg/inh, 80mcg/inh (7.3g)

CONTRAINDICATIONS: Status asthmaticus, acute asthmatic attacks.

WARNINGS/PRECAUTIONS: Deaths due to adrenal insufficiency have occurred with transfer from systemic corticosteroids to inhaled corticosteroids. Resume oral corticosteroids during stress or severe asthma attack. Risk of adrenal insufficiency and withdrawal symptoms when replacing systemic corticosteroids. May unmask allergic conditions previously suppressed by systemic steroid therapy. Caution with TB, ocular herpes simplex, or untreated systemic bacterial, fungal, parasitic or viral infections. May suppress growth in children. Exposure to chickenpox or measles requires prophylaxis treatment. Not for rapid relief of bronchospasm.

ADVERSE REACTIONS: Headache, pharyngitis, upper respiratory tract infection, rhinitis, increased asthma symptoms, sinusitis.

PREGNANCY: Category C, not for use in nursing.

MECHANISM OF ACTION: Corticosteroid; inhibits both inflammatory cells and release of inflammatory mediators.

PHARMACOKINETICS: Absorption: C_{max}=88pg/mL: T_{max}=0.5 hr. (17-BMP) C_{max}=1419pg/mL, T_{max}=0.7hr. **Metabolism:** Biotransformation, via CYP3A. (Metabolites) beclomethasone-17-monopropionate (17-BMP), beclonethasone-21-monopropionate (21-BMP) and beclomethasone (BOH). **Elimination:** Feces (major). (17-BMP) $T_{1/2}$=2.8 hrs.

RabAvert

RX

rabies vaccine (Chiron)

THERAPEUTIC CLASS: Vaccine

INDICATIONS: Pre-exposure immunization and post-exposure prophylaxis against rabies.

DOSAGE: *Adults:* Pre-exposure: Primary: 1mL IM on Day 0, 7, either 21 or 28. Booster: 1mL IM in high-risk patients to maintain >1:5 serum dilution by RFFIT. Post-exposure: 1mL IM on days 0, 3, 7, 14, and 28 with rabies immune globulin 20 IU/kg on Day 0. Post-exposure if Previously Immunized: 1mL IM on Day 0 and Day 3.
Pediatrics: Pre-exposure: Primary: 1mL IM on Day 0, 7, either 21 or 28. Booster: 1mL IM in high-risk patients to maintain >1:5 serum dilution by RFFIT. Post-exposure: 1mL IM on days 0, 3, 7, 14, and 28 with rabies immune globulin 20 IU/kg on Day 0. Post-exposure if Previously Immunized: 1mL IM on Day 0 and Day 3.

HOW SUPPLIED: Inj: 2.5 IU

CONTRAINDICATIONS: Caution in sensitivity to bovine gelatin, chicken protein, neomycin, chlortetracycline, and amphotericin B in preexposure vaccination. There is no contraindication to postexposure prophylaxis, including pregnancy.

WARNINGS/PRECAUTIONS: Do not use SQ, intradermally, or IV. Postpone pre-exposure vaccination in the sick, convalescent, or during the incubation period of an infectious disease. Avoid in patients with egg-sensitivity. Active immunity can be impaired in immunocompromised patients. Have epinephrine available.

ADVERSE REACTIONS: Local reactions (eg, induration, swelling, reddening), lymphadenopathy, headache, dizziness, flu-like symptoms (asthenia, fatigue, fever, myalgia, malaise), nausea, rash, arthralgia.

INTERACTIONS: Active immunity can be impaired with corticosteroids, immunosuppressants, and antimalarials. Do not give immunosuppressants during post-exposure unless essential. Do not give rabies immune globulin at greater than the recommended dose.

PREGNANCY: Category C, safety in nursing not known.

MECHANISM OF ACTION: Stimulates the immune system to produce antibodies that may protect against rabies.

RAPAMUNE RX
sirolimus (Wyeth)

> **Increased susceptibility to infection and development of lymphoma.**

THERAPEUTIC CLASS: Macrocyclic lactone immunosuppressant

INDICATIONS: Prophylaxis of organ rejection in renal transplant patients. Recommended to be used initially with cyclosporine and corticosteroids. In low-moderate risk patients, withdraw cyclosporine 2-4 months after transplantation and increase sirolimus dose to reach recommended blood levels.

DOSAGE: *Adults:* LD: 6mg. Maint: 2mg qd. Hepatic Impairment: Reduce maintenance dose by one-third.
Pediatrics: ≥13 yrs and <40kg: LD: 3mg/m² Maint: 1mg/m²/day. Hepatic Impairment: Reduce maintenance dose by one-third. Take 4 hrs after cyclosporine.

HOW SUPPLIED: Sol: 1mg/mL (60mL); Tab: 1mg, 2mg

WARNINGS/PRECAUTIONS: Increased cholesterol and triglycerides that may require treatment. Reduction in renal function due to long-term concomitant cyclosporine. Proteinuria observed in maintenance renal transplant patients, periodic monitoring recommended. May delay recovery of renal function in patients with delayed graft function. Increased risk of lymphocele. Provide 1 year prophylaxis for *Pneumocystis carinii* pneumonia and 3 months for cytomegalovirus after transplant. Limit exposure to sunlight and UV light. Not for use in liver or lung transplants. Interstitial lung disease reported. Increased susceptibility to infection and the possible development of lymphoma and malignancy, especially of the skin, may result from immunosupression. Avoid in liver or lung transplant patients. Increased risk of angioedema, caution with concomitant use of angioedema-causing drugs, such as ACEI. Impaired wound healing and fat accumulation reported.

ADVERSE REACTIONS: Hypercholesterolemia, hyperlipemia, HTN, rash, acne, anemia, leukopenia, arthralgia, diarrhea, hypokalemia, thrombocytopenia, fever, abdominal pain, headache, constipation, creatinine increase, arthralgia, insomnia, dyspnea, upper respiratory infection, anaphylactic/anaphylactoid reactions, angioedema, hypersensitivity vasculitis, incisional hernia, azoospermia, pericardial effusion, tuberculosis.

INTERACTIONS: Increased levels with diltiazem. CYP3A4 inhibitors (eg, CCBs, antifungals, macrolide antibiotics) may increase levels of sirolimus, while CYP3A4 inducers (eg, anticonvulsants, rifabutin, St. John's wort) may decrease levels. Avoid live vaccines, grapefruit juice, rifampin, ketoconazole. Caution with other nephrotoxic drugs (eg, aminoglycosides, amphotericin B). Hepatic artery thrombosis reported with cyclosporine or tacrolimus, and increased death rate and graft loss with tacrolimus in liver transplant patients. Bronchial anastomotic dehiscence reported with immunosupressives in lung transplant patients. Cyclosporine is a substrate and inhibitor of CYP3A4 and P-gp. Caution with dosing. Monitor for rhabdomyolysis with cyclosporine and HMG Co-A reductase inhibitors/fibrates. Monitor renal function with cyclosporine. Grapefruit juice reduces CYP3A4 medicated drug metabolism, should not be administered with rapamune or used for dilution. Increased risk of deterioration of renal function, serum lipid abnormalities, and urinary tract infections with calcineurin inhibitors and corticosteriods.

PREGNANCY: Category C, not for use in nursing.

MECHANISM OF ACTION: Immunosuppressant; inhibits T-lymphocyte activation and proliferation that occurs in response to antigenic and cytokine (interleukin (IL)-2, IL-4, and IL-15) stimulation by a mechanism that is distinct from that of other immunosuppressants. Also inhibits antibody production. Prolongs allograft survival and suppresses immune-mediated events (animal study).

PHARMACOKINETICS: Absorption: T_{max}=1-2 hrs. **Distribution:** V_d=12L/kg; plasma protein binding (approximately 92%). **Metabolism:** CYP3A4 and P-gp, intestinal wall, liver (extensive) via O-demethylation and hydroxylation; hydroxy, demethyl and hydroxymethyl (major metabolites). **Elimination:** Feces (91%), urine (2.2%), $T_{1/2}$=62 hrs. Different pharmacokinetic data resulted from concentration-controlled trials of pediatric renal transplants.

REBETOL

RX

ribavirin (Schering)

> **Not for monotherapy treatment of chronic hepatitis C. Primary toxicity is hemolytic anemia. Avoid with significant or unstable cardiac disease. Contraindicated in pregnancy and male partners of pregnant women. Use 2 forms of contraception during therapy and for 6 months after discontinuation.**

THERAPEUTIC CLASS: Nucleoside analogue

INDICATIONS: In combination with Intron A® for treatment of chronic hepatitis C in patients ≥3 yrs with compensated liver disease previously untreated with alpha interferon or in patients ≥18 yrs who relapsed after alpha interferon therapy. In combination with Peg-Intron™ for treatment of chronic hepatitis C in patients ≥18 yrs with compensated liver disease previously untreated with alpha interferon.

DOSAGE: *Adults:* ≥18 yrs: With Intron A: ≤75kg: 400mg qam and 600mg qpm. >75kg: 600mg qam and 600mg qpm. Treat for 24-48 weeks interferon-naive; 24 weeks in relapse. With Peg-Intron: 400mg bid, qam and qpm with food. Reduce to 600mg qd if Hgb <10g/dL with no cardiac history, or if Hgb decreases by ≥2g/dL during a 4 week-period with a cardiac history. D/C if Hgb <8.5g/dL with no cardiac history or if Hgb <12g/dL after 4 weeks of dose reduction with a cardiac history. CrCl <50mL/min: Avoid use.
Pediatrics: ≥3 yrs: 15mg/kg/day in divided doses qam and qpm. Use sol if ≤25kg or cannot swallow caps. With Intron A: 25-36kg: 200mg bid, qam and qpm. 37-49kg: 200mg qam and 400mg qpm. 50-61kg: 400mg bid, qam and qpm. >61kg: Dose as adult. Genotype 1: Treat for 48 weeks. Genotype 2/3: Treat for 24 weeks. Reduce to 7.5mg/day if Hgb <10g/dL with no cardiac history, or if Hgb decreases by ≥2g/dL during a 4 week-period with a cardiac history. D/C if Hgb <8.5g/dL with no cardiac history or if Hgb <12g/dL after 4 weeks of dose reduction with a cardiac history.

HOW SUPPLIED: Cap: 200mg; Sol: 40mg/mL (100mL)

CONTRAINDICATIONS: Pregnancy, male partners of pregnant women, hemoglobinopathies (eg, thalassemia major, sickle cell anemia). When used with Intron A or PEG-Intron, refer to individual monograph.

WARNINGS/PRECAUTIONS: Severe depression, suicidal ideation, bone marrow suppression, autoimmune and infectious disorders, pulmonary dysfunction, pancreatitis, and DM reported. Assess for underlying cardiac disease (obtain EKG); fatal and nonfatal MI reported with anemia. Hemolytic anemia reported; monitor Hgb or Hct initially then at Week 2 and 4 (or more if needed) of therapy. Suspend therapy if symptoms of pancreatitis arise. Avoid if CrCl <50mL/min. Obtain negative pregnancy test prior to initiation then monthly, and for 6 months post-therapy.

ADVERSE REACTIONS: Hemolytic anemia, headache, fatigue, rigors, fever, nausea, anorexia, myalgia, arthralgia, insomnia, irritability, depression, dyspnea, alopecia.

INTERACTIONS: Dental and periodontal disorders reported with interferon or peginterferon combination therapy. Coadministration not recommended with didanosine. Caution with stavudine and zidovudine.

PREGNANCY: Category X, not for use in nursing.

MECHANISM OF ACTION: Nucleoside analog; not established.

PHARMACOKINETICS: Absorption: Rapid; (Sol) C_{max}=872ng/mL, T_{max}=1 hr, AUC=14098ng•h/mL. (Cap) C_{max}=782ng/mL, T_{max}=1.7 hrs, AUC=13400ng•h/mL; absolute bioavailability (64%). **Distribution:** (Cap) V_d=2825L. **Metabolism:** Nucleated cells (phosphorylation); deribosylation and amide hydrolysis. **Elimination:** Urine (61%), feces (12%). (Cap) $T_{1/2}$=43.6 hrs.

RECOMBIVAX HB
hepatitis B (Recombinant) (Merck)

RX

OTHER BRAND NAMES: Recombivax HB Adult (Merck) - Recombivax HB Dialysis (Merck) - Recombivax HB Pediatric/Adolescent (Merck)

THERAPEUTIC CLASS: Vaccine

INDICATIONS: Vaccination against hepatitis B virus.

DOSAGE: *Adults:* Give IM into deltoid muscle. Give SQ if risk of hemorrhage. ≥20 yrs: 3-Dose Regimen: 10mcg at 0,1,6 months. Predialysis/Dialysis (Dialysis Formulation): 40mcg at 0,1,6, months; consider booster if anti-HBs level <10MIU/mL.
Pediatrics: Give IM into anterolateral thigh in infants/young children. Give SQ if risk of hemorrhage. 0-19 yrs: 3-Dose Regimen (Pediatric/Adolescent Formulation) 5mcg at 0,1,6 months. 11-15 yrs: 2-Dose Regimen (Adult Formulation): 10mcg 1st dose, 10mcg 4-6 months later. Infants Born to HBsAg Positive/Unknown Status Mothers: Give 3-dose regimen vaccine and 0.5mL HBIG in opposite anterolateral thigh.

HOW SUPPLIED: Inj: (Pediatric/Adolescent-Preservative Free) 5mcg/0.5mL, (Adult) 10mcg/mL, (Dialysis) 40mcg/mL

CONTRAINDICATIONS: Yeast hypersensitivity.

WARNINGS/PRECAUTIONS: Do not continue therapy if hypersensitivity occurs after injection. May not prevent hepatitis B with unrecognized infection. Caution with severely compromised cardiopulmonary status and those where febrile or systemic reaction is a significant risk. May delay use with serious active infection (eg, febrile illness). Have epinephrine available. Do not give intradermally or IV.

ADVERSE REACTIONS: Irritability, fever, diarrhea, fatigue/weakness, diminished appetite, rhinitis, injection site reactions.

PREGNANCY: Category C, caution in nursing.

MECHANISM OF ACTION: Stimulation of immune response to produce antibodies that may protect against all subtypes of hepatitis B virus infection.

REGRANEX
becaplermin (Ortho-McNeil)

RX

> Increased rate of mortality secondary to malignancy in patients treated with 3 or more tubes of regranex gel reported in a post-marketing study. Should only be used when the benefits can be expected to outweigh the risks. Use with caution in patients with known malignancy.

THERAPEUTIC CLASS: Platelet-derived growth factor (recombinant human)

INDICATIONS: Treatment of lower extremity diabetic neuropathic ulcers that extend into the subcutaneous tissue or beyond and have an adequate blood supply.

DOSAGE: *Adults:* Amount applied will vary depending on ulcer size. Measure the greatest length by the greatest width of the ulcer to determine amount of gel to apply. To calculate in inches: (For 15g tube) length x width x 0.6; (For 2g tube) length x width x 1.3. To calculate in centimeters: (For 15g tube) length x width/4; (For 2g tube) length x width/2. Adjust amount weekly or biweekly depending on the change in ulcer area. Squeeze gel onto clean measuring surface (eg, wax paper), then apply to ulcer with an application aid. Apply 1/16 of an inch thickness over entire ulcer area qd, then cover with moist saline dressing for 12 hrs. Remove dressing, rinse off residual gel with saline or water and cover again with moist saline dressing for 12 hrs and repeat. Reassess if ulcer does not decrease by 30% after 10 weeks or is not completely healed in 20 weeks.
Pediatrics: ≥16 yrs: Amount applied will vary depending on ulcer size. Measure the greatest length by the greatest width of the ulcer to determine amount of gel to apply. To calculate in inches: (For 15g tube) length x width x 0.6; (For 2g tube) length x width x 1.3. To calculate in centimeters: (For 15g tube) length x width/4; (For 2g tube) length x width/2. Adjust amount weekly or biweekly depending on the change in ulcer area. Squeeze gel onto clean measuring surface (eg, wax paper), then apply to ulcer with an application aid. Apply 1/16 of an inch thickness over entire ulcer area qd, then cover with moist saline dressing for 12 hrs. Remove dressing, rinse off residual gel with

saline or water and cover again with moist saline dressing for 12 hrs and repeat. Reassess if ulcer does not decrease by 30% after 10 weeks or is not completely healed in 20 weeks.

HOW SUPPLIED: Gel: 0.01% (2g, 15g)

CONTRAINDICATIONS: Known neoplasm at application site.

WARNINGS/PRECAUTIONS: Do not use in wounds that close by primary intention. For external use only. May cause application site reactions; consider the possibility of sensitization or irritation caused by parabens or m-cresol.

ADVERSE REACTIONS: Erythematous rash.

PREGNANCY: Category C, caution in nursing.

MECHANISM OF ACTION: Recombinant human platelet-derived growth factor; promotes chemotactic recruitment and proliferation of cells involved in wound repair. Enhances formation of granulation tissue.

RELENZA
zanamivir (GlaxoSmithKline)

RX

THERAPEUTIC CLASS: Neuraminidase inhibitor

INDICATIONS: Treatment of uncomplicated acute illness due to influenza A and B virus in patients symptomatic for ≤2 days. Prophylaxis of influenza.

DOSAGE: *Adults:* Treatment: Usual: 2 inh (10mg) q12h for 5 days. Take 2 doses at least 2 hrs apart on 1st day. Prophylaxis: Household Setting: 2 inh (10mg) qd for 10 days. Community Setting: 2 inh (10mg) qd for 28 days. Administer at same time every day. *Pediatrics:* Treatment: ≥7 yrs: Usual: 2 inh (10mg) q12h for 5 days. Take 2 doses at least 2 hrs apart on 1st day. Prophylaxis: ≥5 yrs: Household Setting: 2 inh (10mg) qd for 10 days. Community Setting: ≥12 yrs: 2 inh (10mg) qd for 28 days. Administer at same time every day.

HOW SUPPLIED: Inh: 5mg/inh (20 blisters)

WARNINGS/PRECAUTIONS: Not recommended for use with underlying airways disease (eg, asthma, COPD). Serious cases of bronchospasm reported during treatment; d/c if bronchospasm or decline in respiratory function develops. D/C if allergic reaction occurs. Postmarketing neuropsychiatric events (seizures, delerium, hallucinations) reported.

ADVERSE REACTIONS: Dizziness, headaches, diarrhea, nausea, sinusitis, bronchitis, cough, ear/nose/throat infections, nasal symptoms.

INTERACTIONS: Use inhaled bronchodilator before zanamivir. Avoid administration of live attenuated influenza vaccine within 2 weeks before or 48 hours after.

PREGNANCY: Category C, caution in nursing

MECHANISM OF ACTION: Neuraminidase inhibitor; inhibits influenza virus neuraminidase, affecting release of particles.

PHARMACOKINETICS: Absorption: Absolute bioavailability (4-17%); C_{max}=17-142ng/mL; T_{max}=1-2 hrs; AUC=111-1364ng•hr/mL. **Distribution:** Plasma protein binding (<10%). **Elimination:** Renal; $T_{1/2}$=2.5-5.1 hrs.

REMICADE
infliximab (Centocor)

RX

> **Reports of TB, invasive fungal infections, and other opportunistic infections. Evaluate for latent TB and treat if necessary prior to initiation of therapy.**

THERAPEUTIC CLASS: Monoclonal antibody/TNF-alpha receptor blocker

INDICATIONS: In combination with methotrexate (MTX), for reducing signs/symptoms, inhibiting structural damage progression and improving physical function in moderately to severely active rheumatoid arthritis (RA). For reducing signs/symptoms and inducing and maintaining clinical remission of moderately to severely active Crohn's disease, when response to conventional therapy is inadequate. For reducing the number of draining enterocutaneous and rectovaginal fistulas and maintaining fistula closure in fistulizing Crohn's disease. For reducing signs/symptoms in patients with active ankylosing spondylitis (AS). For reducing signs/symptoms of active arthritis, inhibiting structural damage progression, and improving physical function in patients with psoriatic arthritis. For reducing signs/symptoms, inducing and maintaining clinical remission and mucosal healing, and eliminating corticosteroid use in patients with moderately to severely active ulcerative colitis (UC) who have inadequate response to conventional therapy. Treatment of patients with chronic, severe plaque psoriasis who are candidates for systemic therapy and when other systemic therapies are medically less appropriate.

DOSAGE: *Adults:* RA (Combo with MTX): 3mg/kg as IV infusion; repeat at 2 and 6 weeks. Maint: 3mg/kg every 8 weeks. Incomplete Response: May increase to 10mg/kg or give every 4 weeks. Crohn's Disease/Fistulizing Crohn's Disease: Induction Regimen: 5mg/kg IV at 0, 2, and 6 weeks. Maint: 5mg/kg every 8 weeks. For patients who respond then lose their response, may increase to 10mg/kg. Consider discontinuing therapy if no response to by Week 14. Alkylosing Spondylitis: 5mg/kg as IV infusion; repeat at 2 and 6 weeks. Maint: 5mg/kg every 6 weeks. Psoriatic Arthritis: 5mg/kg as IV infusion; repeat at 2 and 6 weeks. Maint: 5mg/kg every 8 weeks. May be used with or without MTX. Ulcerative Colitis: 5mg/kg at 0, 2, and 6 weeks. Maint: 5mg/kg every 8 weeks. Plaque Psoriasis: 5mg/kg IV infusion; repeat at 2 and 6 weeks. Maint: 5mg/kg every 8 weeks.
Pediatrics: ≥6 yrs: Crohn's Disease: Induction Regimen: 5mg/kg IV at 0, 2, and 6 weeks. Maint: 5mg/kg every 8 weeks.

HOW SUPPLIED: Inj: 100mg

CONTRAINDICATIONS: Hypersensitivity to murine proteins. Moderate or severe CHF (NYHA Class III/IV) with doses >5mg/kg.

WARNINGS/PRECAUTIONS: Leukopenia, neutropenia, thrombocytopenia, and pancytopenia reported. Serious infections, including sepsis and pneumonia, reported. Avoid with active infection. Monitor for signs of infection during and after therapy; d/c if serious infection develops. Caution in patients who have resided in areas where histoplasmosis or coccidioidomycosis are endemic. Hypersensitivity reactions reported. Caution with optic neuritis, chronic and recurrent infections, CNS demyelinating disease (eg, MS) and seizure disorder. May result in autoantibody formation; d/c if lupus-like syndrome develops. Monitor closely and d/c if new or worsening symptoms of heart failure appear. Lymphoma reported; caution with malignancies. Severe hepatic reactions, including acute liver failure, jaundice, hepatitis and cholestasis reported rarely. Caution in elderly.

ADVERSE REACTIONS: Nausea, infections, infusion reactions, headache, sinusitis, pharyngitis, coughing, abdominal pain, diarrhea, bronchitis, dyspepsia, fatigue, rhinitis, pain, arthralgia, hepatotoxicity.

INTERACTIONS: Do not give concurrently with live vaccines. May increase risk of serious infections and neutropenia with anakinra.

PREGNANCY: Category B, not for use in nursing.

MECHANISM OF ACTION: Monoclonal antibody; neutralizes biological activity of TNF-α by binding with high affinity to the soluble and transmembrane forms of TNF-α and inhibiting binding of TNF-α with its receptors.

PHARMACOKINETICS: Elimination: $T_{1/2}$=7.7-9.5 days.

RESCRIPTOR   RX
delavirdine mesylate (Pfizer)

THERAPEUTIC CLASS: Non-nucleoside reverse transcriptase inhibitor

INDICATIONS: Treatment of HIV-1 infection in combination with other antiretrovirals.

DOSAGE: *Adults:* Usual: 400mg tid. May disperse 100mg tab in ≥3 oz of water (200mg tab is not dispersible). Take with acidic beverage (eg, orange juice) if achlorhydria. *Pediatrics:* ≥16yrs: Usual: 400mg tid. May disperse 100mg tab in ≥3 oz of water (200mg tab is not dispersible). Take with acidic beverage (eg, orange juice) if achlorhydria.

HOW SUPPLIED: Tab: 100mg, 200mg

CONTRAINDICATIONS: Contraindicated with drugs that are highly dependent on CYP3A for clearance (eg, astemizole, terfenadine, dihdroergotamine, egonovine, ergotamine, methylergonovine, cisapride, pimozide, alprazolam, midazolam, triazolam).

WARNINGS/PRECAUTIONS: Caution with hepatic dysfunction. D/C if severe rash develops. May cause immune reconstitution syndrome. May confer cross-resistance to other NNRTIs. May cause body fat redistribution/accumulation.

ADVERSE REACTIONS: Headache, fatigue, NV, diarrhea, increased ALT and AST, rash, maculopapular rash, pruritus, erythema, insomnia, upper respiratory infection.

INTERACTIONS: See Contraindications. Antacids decrease absorption; separate doses by 1 hr. H_2 antagonists reduce absorption; avoid chronic use. CYP3A inducers (eg, carbamazepine, phenobarbital, phenytoin, rifabutin, rifampin) may decrease plasma levels; avoid concomitant use. Increased plasma levels of drugs metabolized by CYP3A and 2C9 and amprenavir. Certain nonsedating antihistamines, sedative hypnotics, antiarrhythmics, CCBs, ergot agents, amphetamines, cisapride, and sildenafil (max of 25mg/48hrs of sildenafil) may result in potentially serious and/or life-threatening adverse events. Reduced effects of both delavirdine and didanosine; separate doses by 1 hr. Monitor LFTs with saquinavir. Increases indinavir plasma levels; reduce indinavir dose to 600mg tid.

PREGNANCY: Category C, not for use in nursing.

MECHANISM OF ACTION: HIV-1 non-nucleoside reverse transcriptase inhibitor (NNRTI). Binds directly to reverse transcriptase (RT) and blocks RNA-dependent and DNA-dependent DNA polymerase activities.

PHARMACOKINETICS: Absorption: Rapid; C_{max}=35µM, T_{max}=1 hr, AUC=180µM•hr. Bioavailability (85%). **Distribution:** Plasma protein binding (98%). **Metabolism:** Hepatic (N-desalkylation, pyridine hydroxylation) via CYP3A (major), 2D6. **Elimination:** Urine (<5%). $T_{1/2}$=5.8 hrs.

RESTASIS

RX

cyclosporine (Allergan)

THERAPEUTIC CLASS: Topical immunomodulator

INDICATIONS: To increase tear production in patients with suppressed tear production due to ocular inflammation associated with keratoconjunctivitis sicca.

DOSAGE: *Adults:* 1 drop bid, q12h. Concomitant Artificial Tears: Space by 15 min. *Pediatrics:* ≥16 yrs: 1 drop bid, q12h. Concomitant Artificial Tears: Space by 15 min.

HOW SUPPLIED: Emul: 0.05% (0.4mL 32⁹)

CONTRAINDICATIONS: Active ocular infections.

WARNINGS/PRECAUTIONS: Not studied in patients with a history of herpes keratitis. Not to be given while wearing contact lenses; lenses may be reinserted 15 minutes following administration.

ADVERSE REACTIONS: Ocular burning, conjunctival hyperemia, discharge, epiphora, eye pain, foreign body sensation, pruritus, stinging, visual disturbance (eg, blurring).

PREGNANCY: Category C, caution in nursing

MECHANISM OF ACTION: Topical immunomodulator; not established. Systemically acts as an immunosuppressive agent.

PHARMACOKINETICS: Distribution: Following systemic administration, found in human breast milk.

RETIN-A

RX

tretinoin (Ortho Neutrogena)

OTHER BRAND NAME: Retin-A Micro (Ortho Neutrogena)

THERAPEUTIC CLASS: Retinoid

INDICATIONS: Topical treatment of acne vulgaris.

DOSAGE: *Adults:* Cleanse area thoroughly, then apply qhs. May temporarily d/c or reduce dosing frequency if irritation occurs.
Pediatrics: ≥12 yrs: (Gel: 0.04%, 0.1%) Cleanse area thoroughly, then apply qhs. May temporarily d/c or reduce dosing frequency if irritation occurs.

HOW SUPPLIED: (Retin-A) Cre: 0.025%, 0.05%, 0.1% (20g, 45g); Gel: 0.01%, 0.025% (15g, 45g); Sol: 0.05% (28mL); (Retin-A Micro) Gel: 0.04%, 0.1% (20g, 45g)

WARNINGS/PRECAUTIONS: Avoid eyes, lips, paranasal creases, mucous membranes, and sunburned skin. Acne exacerbation during 1st weeks of therapy may occur. D/C if sensitivity or irritation occurs. Severe irritation with eczematous skin. Causes photosensitivity. Extreme weather (eg, cold, wind) may irritate skin.

ADVERSE REACTIONS: Local skin reactions (red, edematous, blistered, crusted), photosensitivity, temporary skin pigmentation changes.

INTERACTIONS: Caution with topical agents with strong drying effects, high concentration of alcohol, astringents, spices, or lime. Caution with sulfur, resorcinol, or salicylic acid; allow effects of these agents to subside before application of tretinoin.

PREGNANCY: Category C, caution in nursing.

MECHANISM OF ACTION: Retinoic acid derivative; not established. Responsible for decreasing cohesiveness of follicular epithelial cells with decreased microcomedo formation. Also stimulates mitotic activity and increases turnover of follicular epithelial cells, causing extrusion of the comedones.

RETROVIR

RX

zidovudine (GlaxoSmithKline)

> Associated with hematologic toxicity (eg, neutropenia, severe anemia), especially with advanced HIV disease. Prolonged use associated with symptomatic myopathy. Lactic acidosis and severe, possibly fatal hepatomegaly with steatosis reported.

THERAPEUTIC CLASS: Nucleoside analogue

INDICATIONS: Treatment of HIV infection in combination with other antiretrovirals. Prevention of maternal-fetal HIV transmission.

DOSAGE: *Adults:* (Tab) 600mg/day in divided doses. (Inj) 1mg/kg IV over 1 hr 5-6 times/day. Prevention of Maternal-Fetal HIV Transmission: >14 weeks pregnancy: 100mg PO five times/day until start of labor. During labor and delivery: 2mg/kg IV over 1 hr followed by 1mg/kg/hr IV infusion until clamping of umbilical cord. End-Stage Renal Disease/Dialysis: 100mg PO q6-8h or 1mg/kg IV q6-8h. Significant Anemia/Neutropenia: May require dose interruption and adjunctive epoetin therapy. Less Severe Anemia/Neutropenia: Reduce daily dose.
Pediatrics: 6 weeks-12 yrs: 160mg/m² PO q8h. Max: 200mg PO q8h. Prevention of Maternal-Fetal HIV Transmission: Neonates: 2mg/kg PO q6h (or 1.5mg/kg IV over 30 min q6h) starting within 12 hrs after birth and continue through 6 weeks of age. End-Stage Renal Disease/Dialysis: 100mg PO q6-8h or 1mg/kg IV q6-8h. Significant Anemia/Neutropenia: May require dose interruption and adjunctive epoetin therapy. Pronounced Anemia: Reduce daily dose. Mild to Moderate Hepatic Impairment: Monitor for hematologic toxicity and reduce dose if needed.

HOW SUPPLIED: Cap: 100mg; Inj: 10mg/mL; Syrup: 50mg/5mL (240mL); Tab: 300mg

WARNINGS/PRECAUTIONS: Adverse reactions increase with disease progression. Caution with compromised bone marrow or in elderly. Monitor for hematologic toxicity; reduce dose or stop therapy. Myopathy and myositis with pathological changes associated with prolonged use. Caution with obesity and liver disease; increased risk of lactic acidosis and hepatomegaly with steatosis. Increased risk of toxicity with prolonged exposure to nucleosides, in women, obesity, advanced HIV disease, severe hepatic impairment. Possible redistribution or accumulation of body fat. Hepatic decompensation has occurred in HIV/HCV co-infected patients receiving combination antiretroviral therapy for HIV and interferon alfa with or without ribavirin; monitor for treatment associated toxicities. Immune reconstitution syndrome has been reported with combination antiretroviral therapy.

ADVERSE REACTIONS: Headache, NV, malaise, anorexia, asthenia, constipation, anemia, neutropenia.

INTERACTIONS: Increased risk of hematologic toxicities with ganciclovir, interferon-alpha, bone marrow suppressives and cytotoxic drugs. Possible increased levels with phenytoin, atovaquone, fluconazole, methadone, probenecid, valproic acid. Possible decreased levels with nelfinavir, ritonavir, rifampin. Avoid with stavudine, ribavirin, doxorubicin, other combination products containing zidovudine. Prolonged exposure to antiretroviral nucleoside analogues increases risk of lactic acidosis and hepatomegaly with steatosis. May decrease phenytoin levels.

PREGNANCY: Category C, not for use in nursing.

MECHANISM OF ACTION: Pyrimidine nucleoside analogue; inhibits reverse transcriptase via DNA chain termination.

PHARMACOKINETICS: Absorption: (Tab, Cap, Syrup): Rapid. Bioavailability (64%). T_{max}=0.5-1.5 hrs. (IV) C_{max}=1.06mcg/mL. **Distribution:** V_d=1.6L/kg; plasma protein binding (<38%). **Metabolism:** Hepatic. Metabolite (3'-azido-3'-deoxy-5'-O-β-D-glucopyranuronosylthymidine (GZDV). **Elimination:** (Tab, Cap, Syrup): Zidovudine: Urine (14%). GZDV: Urine (74%); $T_{1/2}$=0.5-3 hrs. (IV): Zidovudine: Urine (18%). GZDV: Urine (60%); $T_{1/2}$=1.1 hrs.

RHINOCORT AQUA

RX

budesonide (AstraZeneca)

THERAPEUTIC CLASS: Corticosteroid

INDICATIONS: Management of seasonal or perennial allergic rhinitis.

DOSAGE: *Adults*: 1 spray per nostril qd. Max: 4 sprays/nostril/day.
Pediatrics: >12 yrs: 1 spray per nostril qd. Max: 4 sprays/nostril/day. 6-12 yrs: 1 spray per nostril qd. Max: 2 sprays/nostril/day.

HOW SUPPLIED: Spray: 32mcg/spray (8.6g)

WARNINGS/PRECAUTIONS: Risk of adrenal insufficiency and withdrawal symptoms when replacing systemic corticosteroids with a topical corticosteroids. Caution with active or quiescent TB, ocular herpes simplex, or untreated bacterial, fungal and systemic viral infections. Avoid with recent nasal trauma, surgery or septum ulcers. Risk of more severe/fatal course of infections (eg, chickenpox, measles) and for *Candida* infections of the nose and pharynx. Potential for growth velocity reduction in pediatrics. Should not delay or interfere infant feeding.

ADVERSE REACTIONS: Nasal irritation, pharyngitis, cough, epistaxis.

INTERACTIONS: Oral ketoconazole and cimetidine increase plasma levels. CYP3A inhibitors (eg, itraconazole, clarithromycin, erythromycin) may decrease metabolism and increase systemic exposure. Concomitant systemic corticosteroids increases risk of hypercorticism and/or HPA axis suppression.

PREGNANCY: Category B, caution in nursing.

MECHANISM OF ACTION: Glucocorticosteroid; not established, suspected to have a wide range of inhibitory activities against multiple cell types (eg, mast cells, eosinophils, neutrophils, macrophages, lymphocyte) and mediators (eg, histamine, leukotrienes, ecosanoids, cytokines) involved in allergic mediated inflammation.

PHARMACOKINETICS: Absorption: Well absorbed, T_{max}=0.7 hr. **Distribution:** V_d=approximately 2-3L/Kg, plasma protein binding (85-90%). **Metabolism:** Liver (extensive), 16α-hydroxyprednisolone and 6β-hydroxybudesonide (major metabolites) via CYP3A4-catalyzed biotransformation. **Elimination:** Urine and feces, $T_{1/2}$(the 22R form)=2-3 hrs.

RIFADIN
rifampin (Sanofi-Aventis)

RX

THERAPEUTIC CLASS: Rifamycin derivative

INDICATIONS: Treatment of all forms of TB. Treatment of asymptomatic carriers of *Neisseria meningitidis* to eliminate meningococci from nasopharynx.

DOSAGE: *Adults:* TB: 10mg/kg PO/IV qd. Max: 600mg/day. Meningococcal Carriers: 600mg bid for 2 days. Take 1 hr before or 2 hrs after a meal with a full glass of water. *Pediatrics:* TB: 10-20mg/kg PO/IV qd. Max: 600mg/day. Meningococcal Carriers: ≥1 month: 10mg/kg q12h for 2 days. Max: 600mg/dose. <1 month: 5mg/kg q12h for 2 days. Take 1 hr before or 2 hrs after a meal with a full glass of water.

HOW SUPPLIED: Cap: 150mg, 300mg; Inj: 600mg

WARNINGS/PRECAUTIONS: May produce liver dysfunction. May cause hyperbilirubinemia. Not for treatment of meningococcal disease. May produce reddish coloration of the urine, sweat, sputum, and tears. May permanently stain soft contact lenses.

ADVERSE REACTIONS: GI distress, thrombocytopenia, visual disturbances, menstrual disturbances, edema of face and extremities, elevated BUN and serum uric acid levels.

INTERACTIONS: May accelerate elimination of drugs metabolized by CYP450 (eg, anticonvulsants, antiarrhythmics, anticoagulants, azole antifungals, barbiturates, β-blockers, CCBs, chloramphenicol, clarithromycin, corticosteroids, cyclosporine, cardiac glycosides, clofibrate, oral or systemic contraceptives, dapsone, diazepam, doxycycline, fluoroquinolones, haloperidol, oral hypoglycemics, levothyroxine, methadone, narcotics, nortriptyline, progestins, quinine, tacrolimus, theophylline, TCAs, and zidovudine). Give antacids at least 1 hr before rifampin. Increased hepatotoxicity with halothane or isoniazid. Increased serum levels with probenecid and cotrimoxazole. Caution with other hepatotoxic agents. Concomitant ketoconazole decreases both drug serum levels. Decreased levels of enalapril, atovaquone. Increased levels with atovaquone.

PREGNANCY: Category C, not for use in nursing.

MECHANISM OF ACTION: Rifamycin derivative; has bacterial activity against intracellular and extracellular *Mycobacterium tuberculosis*. Inhibits DNA-dependent RNA polymerase activity in susceptible cells. Interacts with bacterial RNA polymerase; does not inhibit the mammalian enzyme.

PHARMACOKINETICS: Absorption: Readily absorbed from GI tract. (PO, 600mg) C_{max}=7mcg/mL. (IV, 300mg, 600mg) C_{max} =9.0mcg/mL, 17.5mcg/mL. **Distribution:** (IV, 300mg, 600mg): V_d=0.66L/kg, 0.64L/kg; distributed in body fluids and cerebrospinal fluid; plasma protein binding 80%. **Metabolism:** Via deacetylation; 25-desacetyl-rifampin (major metabolite). **Elimination:** Urine (30%), bile; (600mg, 900mg) $T_{1/2}$=3.35 hrs, 5.08hrs.

RIFATER
isoniazid - pyrazinamide - rifampin (Sanofi-Aventis)

RX

> Isoniazid associated with severe and sometimes fatal hepatitis. Monitor LFTs on a monthly basis.

THERAPEUTIC CLASS: Isonicotinic acid hydrazide/rifamycin derivative/nicotinamide analogue

INDICATIONS: For initial phase of pulmonary TB treatment.

DOSAGE: *Adults:* ≤44kg: 4 tabs single dose qd. 45-54kg: 5 tabs single dose. ≥55kg: 6 tabs single dose. Give pyridoxine in malnourished, if predisposed to neuropathy (eg, alcoholics, diabetics), and adolescents. Take 1 hr before or 2 hrs after meals with full glass of water. Treatment usually lasts 2 months.
Pediatrics: ≥15 yrs: ≤44kg: 4 tabs single dose qd. 45-54kg: 5 tabs qd single dose. ≥55kg: 6 tabs qd single dose. Give pyridoxine in malnourished, if predisposed to neuropathy (eg, alcoholics, diabetics), and adolescents. Take 1 hr before or 2 hrs after meals with full glass of water. Treatment usually lasts 2 months.

HOW SUPPLIED: Tab: (Isoniazid-Pyrazinamide-Rifampin) 50mg-300mg-120mg

CONTRAINDICATIONS: Severe hepatic damage, adverse reactions to isoniazid (eg, drug fever, chills, arthritis), acute liver disease, acute gout.

WARNINGS/PRECAUTIONS: Liver dysfunction, hyperbilirubinemia, and hyperuricemia with acute gouty arthritis reported. Monitor LFTs (every 2-4 weeks), serum uric acid. Perform regular ophthalmologic exams. Caution with DM, severe renal dysfunction. May produce reddish coloration of urine, sweat, sputum, and tears. May permanently stain soft contact lenses.

ADVERSE REACTIONS: GI effects, cutaneous reactions, musculoskeletal pain, hepatitis, CNS and cardiorespiratory effects.

INTERACTIONS: Rifampin may accelerate metabolism of anticonvulsants (eg, phenytoin), antiarrhythmics (eg, disopyramide, mexiletine, quinidine, tocainide), anticoagulants, antifungals (eg, fluconazole, itraconazole, ketoconazole), barbiturates, β-blockers, CCBs, (eg, diltiazem, nifedipine, verapamil), chloramphenicol, ciprofloxacin, corticosteroids, cyclosporine, cardiac glycosides, clofibrate, oral contraceptives, dapsone, diazepam, haloperidol, oral hypoglycemics (eg, sulfonylureas), methadone, narcotic analgesics, nortriptyline, progestins, theophylline. Antacids may reduce rifampin absorption. Avoid foods containing tyramine and histamine (eg, cheese, red wine, tuna). Anticoagulants may need dose increase. Higher incidence of isoniazid hepatitis with daily alcohol ingestion. Avoid halothane. INH inhibits certain CYP450 enzymes; monitor with anticonvulsants, benzodiazepines, haloperidol, ketoconazole, warfarin. Decreased levels with corticosteroids. Exaggerates CNS effects of meperidine, cycloserine, disulfiram. Excess catecholamine stimulation with L-dopa.

PREGNANCY: Category C, not for use in nursing.

MECHANISM OF ACTION: Rifampin: Inhibits DNA-dependent RNA polymerase activity in susceptible *Mycobacterium tuberculosis* organism. Interacts with bacterial RNA polymerase, but does not inhibit the mammalian enzyme. Isoniazid: Kills growing tubercle bacilli by inhibiting the biosynthesis of mycolic acids which are major component of the cell wall of *Mycobacterium tuberculosis*. Pyrazinamide: Inhibits growth of *Mycobacterial tuberculosis*.

PHARMACOKINETICS: Absorption: Isoniazid: Bioavailability (100.6%), C_{max}=3.09mcg/mL, T_{max}=1-2 hrs. Rifampin: Bioavailability (88.8 %), C_{max}=11.04mcg/mL. Pyrazinamide: Bioavailability (96.8%), C_{max}=28.02mcg/mL. **Distribution:** Isoniazid: Passes through placental barrier and into milk. Pyrazinamide: Plasma protein binding (10%), distributed in liver, lungs, and CSF; found in breast milk. Rifampin: Protein binding (80%). **Metabolism:** Isoniazid: Acetylation and dehydrazination. Pyrazinamide: Liver, via hydroxylation; pyrazinoic acid (major active metabolite). Rifampin: Via deacetylation; 25-desacetyl-rifampin (major metabolite). **Elimination:** Rifampin: Urine (30%), bile; $T_{1/2}$=3.35 hrs. Pyrazinamide: Urine (70%), (4-14% unchanged); $T_{1/2}$=9-10 hrs. Isoniazid: Urine (50-70%); $T_{1/2}$=1-4 hrs.

RISPERDAL
RX

risperidone (Janssen)

> Elderly patients with dementia-related psychosis treated with atypical antipsychotic drugs are at an increased risk of death; most appeared to be cardiovascular (eg, heart failure, sudden death) or infectious (eg, pneumonia) in nature. Risperidone is not approved for the treatment of patients with dementia-related psychosis.

OTHER BRAND NAME: Risperdal M-Tab (Janssen)

THERAPEUTIC CLASS: Benzisoxazole derivative

INDICATIONS: Acute and maintenance treatment of schizophrenia in adults. Treatment of schizophrenia in adolescents 13-17 yrs. Short-term treatment of acute manic or mixed episodes associated with bipolar I disorder as monotherapy (adults and adolescents 10-17 yrs) or in combination with lithium or valproate (adults). Treatment of irritability associated with autistic disorder in children and adolescents 5-16 yrs, including symptoms of aggression towards others, deliberate self-injuriousness, temper tantrums, and quickly changing moods.

DOSAGE: *Adults:* Schizophrenia: Initial: 2mg/day given once or twice daily. Titrate: Adjust dose at intervals not <24 hrs, in increments of 1-2mg/day, as tolerated, to recommended dose of 4-8mg/day. Range: 4-16mg/day. Max: 16mg/day. Bipolar Disorder: Initial: 2-3mg qd. Titrate: Adjust dose at intervals not <24 hrs and in increments/

decrements of 1mg/day. Range: 1-6mg/day. Max: 6mg/day. Elderly/Debilitated/
Hypotension/Severe Renal or Hepatic Impairment: Initial: 0.5mg bid. Titrate: Adjust dose
in increments not >0.5mg bid. Increases to doses >1.5mg bid should occur at intervals
of ≥1 week. Periodically reassess to determine maintenance treatment.
Pediatrics: Schizophrenia: 13-17 yrs: Initial: 0.5mg qd in morning or evening. Titrate:
Adjust dose, if needed, in increments of 0.5 or 1mg/day and at intervals not <24 hrs, as
tolerated, to recommended dose of 3mg/day. Max: 6mg/day. Bipolar Disorder: 10-17
yrs: Initial: 0.5mg qd in morning or evening. Titrate: Adjust dose, if needed, in increments of 0.5 or 1mg/day and at intervals not <24 hrs, as tolerated, to recommended
dose of 2.5mg/day. Max: 6mg/day. Irritability with Autistic Disorder: 5-16 yrs: Initial:
<20kg: 0.25mg/day; ≥20kg: 0.5mg/day. Titrate: After at least 4 days, may increase
dose by 0.5mg/day (<20kg) or 1mg/day (≥20kg). Maint: Minimum of 14 days. Inadequate Response: Increase at ≥2-wk intervals: <20kg: Increase by 0.25mg/day; ≥20kg:
Increase by 0.5mg/day. Caution in patients <15kg. Max: <20kg: 1mg/day; ≥20kg:
2.5mg/day; >45kg: 3mg/day.

HOW SUPPLIED: Sol: 1mg/mL (30mL); Tab: 0.25mg, 0.5mg, 1mg, 2mg, 3mg, 4mg; Tab, Disintegrating: (M-Tab) 0.5mg, 1mg, 2mg, 3mg, 4mg

CONTRAINDICATIONS: Anaphylactic reactions and angioedema.

WARNINGS/PRECAUTIONS: Neuroleptic malignant syndrome and/or tardive dyskinesia
may occur. Monitor for hyperglycemia; perform fasting blood glucose testing if symptoms develop or with risk factors for DM. Cerebrovascular events (eg, stroke, TIA)
reported in elderly with dementia-related psychosis. Not approved for the treatment of
dementia-related psychosis. May induce orthostatic hypotension, elevate prolactin levels, have an antiemetic effect. Caution in elderly, renal/hepatic impairment, history of
seizures, cardio- or cerebrovascular disease, suicidal tendencies, risk of aspiration pneumonia, conditions predisposing to hypotension (eg, hypovolemia, dehydration) or
affecting metabolism or hemodynamic responses. May impair judgement, thinking, or
motor skills; caution when operating hazardous machinery. May disrupt body temperature regulation; caution in patients exposed to temperature extremes. Re-evaluate
periodically. Patients with Parkinson's disease or dementia with Lewy bodies who
receive antipsychotics are reported to have an increased sensitivity to antipsychotic
medications.

ADVERSE REACTIONS: Somnolence, increased appetite, fatigue, vomiting, coughing,
urinary incontinence, constipation, fever, parkinsonism, abdominal pain, anxiety, nausea, dizziness, tremor, dyspepsia.

INTERACTIONS: Caution with other CNS drugs or alcohol. May potentiate antihypertensives, antagonize levodopa and dopamine agonists, or increase valproate levels.
Cimetidine and ranitidine may increase bioavailability. CYP3A4 inducers (eg, carbamazepine, phenytoin, rifampin, phenobarbital) may decrease levels. Clozapine, fluoxetine, and paroxetine may increase levels. Increased mortality with furosemide in elderly
patients.

PREGNANCY: Category C, not for use in nursing.

MECHANISM OF ACTION: Benzisoxazole derivatives; suspected to inhibit both dopamine
Type 2(D_2) and serotonin Type 2 (5HT$_2$).

PHARMACOKINETICS: Absorption: Absolute bioavailability (70%). T_{max}=1 hr; (risperidone)
T_{max}=3hrs; 9-hydroxyrisperidone (extensive metabolizers). **Distribution**: V_d=1-2L/kg;
plasma protein binding (risperidone: 90%) (9-hydroxyrisperidone: 77%); found in breast
milk. **Metabolism**: Liver (extensive). Hydroxylation, N-dealkylation; CYP 2D6:
9-hydroxyrisperidone (major metabolite). **Elimination**: Urine (70%), feces (14%); $T_{1/2}$=20
hrs.

RITALIN
methylphenidate HCl (Novartis)   **CII**

OTHER BRAND NAMES: Ritalin LA (Novartis) - Ritalin SR (Novartis)

THERAPEUTIC CLASS: Sympathomimetic amine

INDICATIONS: (Cap; Extended-Release, Tab; Tab, Extended-Release) Treatment of
attention deficit disorders. (Tab; Tab, Extended-Release) Treatment of narcolepsy.

DOSAGE: *Adults:* (Tab) 10-60mg/day given bid-tid 30-45 min ac. Take last dose before 6
pm if insomnia occurs. (Tab, ER) May use in place of immediate release (IR) when the 8

hr dose corresponds to the titrated 8 hr IR dose. Swallow whole; do not chew or crush. (Cap, ER) Initial: 20mg qam. Titrate: Adjust weekly by 10mg. Max: 60mg qam. *Pediatrics:* ≥6 yrs: (Tab) Initial: 5mg bid before breakfast and lunch. Titrate: Increase gradually by 5-10mg weekly. Max: 60mg/day. (Tab, ER) May use in place of immediate release (IR) when the 8 hr dose corresponds to the titrated 8 hr IR dose. Swallow whole; do not chew or crush. (Cap, ER) Initial: 20mg qam. Titrate: Adjust weekly by 10mg. Max: 60mg qam. Previous Methylphenidate Use: May use as qd in place of IR dosed bid or daily dose of methylphenidate-SR. Swallow whole or sprinkle over spoonful of applesauce. Do not crush, chew, or divide. Reduce dose or d/c if paradoxical aggravation of symptoms occurs. D/C if no improvement after appropriate dose adjustment over 1 month.

HOW SUPPLIED: Cap, Extended-Release (Ritalin LA): 10mg, 20mg, 30mg, 40mg; Tab (Ritalin): 5mg, 10mg*, 20mg*; Tab, Extended-Release (Ritalin SR): 20mg *scored

CONTRAINDICATIONS: Marked anxiety, tension, and agitation; glaucoma; motor tics or family history or diagnosis of Tourette's syndrome; during or within 14 days of MAOI use.

WARNINGS/PRECAUTIONS: Monitor growth in children. Not for severe depression or fatigue. May exacerbate symptoms of behavior disturbance and thought disorder in psychotic children. Care should be taken in using stimulants to treat patients with comorbid bipolar disorder because of concern for possible induction of mixed/manic episode in such patients. Stimulants at usual doses can cause treatment emergent psychotic or manic symptoms (hallucinations, delusional thinking, mania) in children and adolescents without prior history of psychotic illness. Aggressive behavior or hostility reported in clinical trials and the postmarketing experience of some medications indicated for the treatment of ADHD. May lower seizure threshold, especially with prior history of seizures or with prior EEG abnormalities; d/c if seizures occur. Caution with HTN and other underlying conditions that may be compromised such as heart failure, recent MI, or hyperthyroidism. Visual disturbances may occur (rare). Monitor CBC, differential, and platelets with prolonged use. Caution with emotionally-unstable patients or prior history of drug dependence or alcoholism; chronic use may lead to tolerance and psychological dependence. Monitor during withdrawal. Periodically d/c to assess condition. Avoid with known structural cardiac abnormalities or other serious cardiac problems.

ADVERSE REACTIONS: Nervousness, insomnia, hypersensitivity reactions, anorexia, nausea, dizziness, palpitations, headache, dyskinesia, drowsiness, BP and pulse changes, tachycardia, angina, arrhythmia, abdominal pain.

INTERACTIONS: See Contraindications. May decrease hypotensive effect of guanethidine. Caution with <ALPHA/>β_2-agonist (eg, clonidine) and pressor agents. Potentiates anticoagulants, anticonvulsants (eg, phenobarbital, diphenylhydantoin, primidone), phenylbutazone, TCAs (eg, imipramine, clomipramine, desipramine); monitor plasma drug levels or PT/INR. (Cap, Extended-Release) Antacids or acid suppressants may alter release characteristics of cap.

PREGNANCY: Category C, caution in nursing.

MECHANISM OF ACTION: Sympathomimetic amine; CNS stimulant, blocks reuptake of norepinephrine and dopamine into presynaptic neuron and increases release of monoamines into extraneuronal space.

PHARMACOKINETICS: Absorption: Children: (Tab, ER) T_{max}=4.7 hrs; (Tab) 1.9 hrs. **Metabolism:** α-phenyl-2-piperidine acetic acid (major metabolite). **Elimination:** Urine (78-97%), feces (1-3%); $T_{1/2}$=3.5 hrs (adults), 2.5 hrs (children).

ROBAXIN
methocarbamol (Schwarz)

RX

OTHER BRAND NAMES: Robaxin Injection (Baxter) - Robaxin-750 (Schwarz)

THERAPEUTIC CLASS: Muscular analgesic (central-acting)

INDICATIONS: Adjunct for relief of acute, painful musculoskeletal conditions.

DOSAGE: *Adults:* (PO) Initial: (500mg tab) 1500mg qid for 2-3 days. Maint: 1000mg qid. Initial: (750mg tab) 1500mg qid for 2-3 days. Maint: 750mg q4h or 1500mg tid. Max: 6g/d for 2-3 days; 8g/d if severe. (Inj) Moderate Symptoms: 10mL IV/IM. IV Max Rate: 3mL undiluted drug/min. IM Max: 5mL into each gluteal region. Severe/Post-Op Condition: Max: 20-30mL/day up to 3 consecutive days. If feasible, continue with PO. Teta-

nus: 10-20mL up to 30mL. May repeat q6h until NG tube can be inserted. Continue with crushed tabs. Max: 24g/day PO.
Pediatrics: Tetanus: Initial: 15mg/kg or 500mg/m². Repeat q6h prn. Max: 1.8g/m² for 3 consecutive days. Administer by injection into tubing or IV infusion.

HOW SUPPLIED: Inj: 100mg/mL (10mL); Tab: 500mg, 750mg

CONTRAINDICATIONS: (Inj) Renal pathology with injection due to propylene glycol content.

WARNINGS/PRECAUTIONS: May impair mental/physical abilities required for operating machinery or driving a motor vehicle. May cause color interference in certain screening tests for 5-hydroxy-indoleacetic acid (5-HIAA) and vanillylmandelic acid (VMA). Caution in epilepsy with the injection. Injection rate should not exceed 3mL/min. Avoid extravasation with injection. Avoid use of injection particularly during early pregnancy.

ADVERSE REACTIONS: Lightheadedness, dizziness, drowsiness, nausea, urticaria, pruritus, rash, conjunctivitis, nasal congestion, blurred vision, headache, fever, seizures, syncope, flushing.

INTERACTIONS: Additive adverse effects with alcohol and other CNS depressants. May inhibit effect of pyridostigmine; caution in patients with myasthemia gravis receiving anticholinergics.

PREGNANCY: Category C, caution in nursing.

MECHANISM OF ACTION: Carbamate derivative of guaifenesin; not established, suspected to have CNS depressant with sedative and musculoskeletal relaxant properties.

PHARMACOKINETICS: Distribution: Plasma protein binding (46-50%). **Distribution:** Found in breast milk. **Metabolism:** Via dealkylation, hydroxylation, and conjugation pathways. **Elimination:** Urine; $T_{1/2}$=1-2 hrs.

ROBINUL   RX
glycopyrrolate (Sciele)

OTHER BRAND NAME: Robinul Forte (Sciele)

THERAPEUTIC CLASS: Anticholinergic

INDICATIONS: Adjunct treatment of peptic ulcer.

DOSAGE: *Adults:* Usual: (Tab) 1mg tid (am, pm and hs); may increase to 2mg qhs if needed. Maint: 1mg bid. (Forte) 2mg bid-tid. Max: 8mg/day.
Pediatrics: ≥12 yrs: Usual: (Tab) 1mg tid (am, pm & hs); may increase to 2mg qhs if needed. Maint: 1mg bid. (Forte) 2mg bid-tid. Max: 8mg/day.

HOW SUPPLIED: Tab: 1mg*, (Forte) 2mg* *scored

CONTRAINDICATIONS: Glaucoma, obstructive uropathy, GI tract obstruction, paralytic ileus, intestinal atony of elderly or debilitated, unstable cardiovascular status in acute hemorrhage, severe ulcerative colitis, toxic megacolon complicating ulcerative colitis, myasthenia gravis.

WARNINGS/PRECAUTIONS: May produce drowsiness and blurred vision; avoid operating machinery. Risk of heat prostration with high environmental temperature. Diarrhea may be early symptom of incomplete intestinal obstruction especially with ileostomy or colostomy. Caution in elderly, autonomic neuropathy, hepatic/renal disease, ulcerative colitis, hyperthyroidism, coronary heart disease, CHF, tachyarrhythmias, tachycardia, HTN, prostatic hypertrophy, hiatal hernia associated with reflux esophagitis.

ADVERSE REACTIONS: Blurred vision, dry mouth, urinary retention and hesitancy, increased ocular tension, tachycardia, decreased sweating, xerostomia, loss of taste, headache.

PREGNANCY: Safety in pregnancy is not known; not for use in nursing.

MECHANISM OF ACTION: Anticholinergic; inhibits action of acetylcholine on structures innervated by postganglionic cholinergic nerves and smooth muscles that respond to acetylcholine but lack cholinergic innervation. Diminishes volume and free acidity of gastric secretions and controls excessive pharyngeal, tracheal, and bronchial secretion.

ROBINUL INJECTION

RX

glycopyrrolate (Baxter)

THERAPEUTIC CLASS: Anticholinergic

INDICATIONS: Preoperative antimuscarinic to reduce salivary tracheobronchial, and pharyngeal secretions; decrease gastric sections; and block cardiac vagal inhibitory reflexes during anesthesia induction and intubation. Intra-operatively to counteract drug-induced or vagal traction reflexes associated with arrhythmias. To protect against peripheral muscarinic effects of cholinergic agents. Adjunct therapy for treatment of peptic ulcer when rapid anticholinergic effect is desired or when oral medication is not tolerated.

DOSAGE: *Adults:* Preanesthesia: 0.002mg/lb IM 30-60 min before anesthesia induction or at time of preanesthetic narcotic/sedative. Intraoperatively: 0.1mg IV, repeat prn every 2-3 min. Reverse Neuromuscular Blockade: 0.2mg IV for each 1mg neostigmine or 5mg pyridostigmine. Peptic Ulcer: 0.1mg IV/IM q4h, tid-qid. May use 0.2mg if needed. *Pediatrics:* Preanesthesia: 1 month-12 yrs: 0.002mg/lb IM 30-60 min before anesthesia induction or at time of preanesthetic narcotic/sedative. 1 month-2 yrs: May require up to 0.004mg/lb. Intraoperatively: 0.002mg/lb IV. Max: 0.1mg single dose. May repeat prn every 2-3 min. Reverse Neuromuscular Blockade: 0.2mg IV for each 1mg neostigmine or 5mg pyridostigmine. Peptic Ulcer: ≥12 yrs: 0.1mg IV/IM q4h, tid-qid. May use 0.2mg if needed.

HOW SUPPLIED: Inj: 0.2mg/mL

CONTRAINDICATIONS: Newborns (<1 month) due to benzyl alcohol content. For long treatment duration: Glaucoma, obstructive uropathy, obstructive disease of GI tract, paralytic ileus, intestinal atony of elderly or debilitated, unstable cardiovascular status in acute hemorrhage, severe ulcerative colitis, toxic megacolon complicating ulcerative colitis, myasthenia gravis.

WARNINGS/PRECAUTIONS: Caution with CAD, CHF, arrhythmias, HTN, hyperthyroidism, elderly, autonomic neuropathy, hepatic or renal disease, ulcerative colitis, or hiatal hernia. May produce drowsiness and blurred vision; caution when operating machinery. Risk of fever and heat stroke due to decreased sweating in high environmental temperature. Diarrhea may be early symptom of incomplete intestinal obstruction.

ADVERSE REACTIONS: Drowsiness, blurred vision, dry mouth, urinary retention and hesitancy, increased ocular tension, tachycardia, palpation, decreased sweating, loss of taste.

INTERACTIONS: Increased anticholinergic side effects with other anticholinergics, phenothiazines, antiparkinson drugs, TCAs. Increased severity of GI lesions with potassium chloride in a wax matrix.

PREGNANCY: Category B, caution in nursing.

MECHANISM OF ACTION: Anticholinergic; inhibits action of acethylcholine on structures innervated by postganglionic cholinergic nerves and on smooth muscles that respond to acethycholine but lack cholinergic innervation. Diminishes volume and free acidity of gastric secretions and controls excessive pharyngeal, tracheal, and bronchial secretions.

PHARMACOKINETICS: Absorption: (6mcg/kg, IV) AUC=8.64mcg/L•hr; (8mcg/kg, IM) C_{max}=3.47mcg/L, T_{max}=27.48 min, AUC=6.64mcg/L•hr. **Distribution:** V_d=0.42L/kg. **Elimination:** (IV) Urine (85%), bile; $T_{1/2}$=0.83 hrs. (IM) Urine, bile; $T_{1/2}$=0.55-1.25 hrs.

ROCALTROL

RX

calcitriol (Roche Labs)

THERAPEUTIC CLASS: Vitamin D analog

INDICATIONS: Predialysis: Management of secondary hyperparathyroidism and resultant metabolic bone disease with moderate to severe chronic renal failure (CrCl 15-55mL/min). Dialysis: Management of hypocalcemia and resultant metabolic bone disease. Hypoparathyroidism: Management of hypocalcemia and manifestations of postsurgical hypoparathyroidism, idiopathic hypoparathyroidism, and pseudohypoparathyroidism.

DOSAGE: *Adults:* Predialysis: Initial: 0.25mcg/day. Max: 0.5mcg/day. Hypoparathyroidism: Initial: 0.25mcg/day every am. Titrate: May increase at 2-4 week intervals to 0.5-

2mcg/day. Elderly: Start at low end of dosing range. Dialysis: Initial: 0.25mcg/day. Titrate: May increase by 0.25mcg/day every 4-8 weeks to 0.5-1mcg/day. Monitor serum calcium levels twice weekly during titration. Normal to slightly reduced serum calcium, give 0.25mcg every other day. Discontinue with hypercalcemia; when calcium levels return to normal continue therapy and decrease dose by 0.25 mcg.
Pediatrics: Predialysis: ≥3 yrs: Initial: 0.25mcg/day. Max: 0.5mcg/day. <3yrs: Initial: 10-15ng/kg/day. Hypoparathyroidism: ≥6 yrs: Initial: 0.25mcg/day every am. Titrate: May increase at 2-4 week intervals to 0.5-2mcg/day. 1-5yrs: Initial: 0.25mcg/day every am. Titrate: May increase at 2-4 week intervals up to 0.75mcg/day. Monitor serum calcium levels twice weekly during titration. Discontinue with hypercalcemia; when calcium levels return to normal continue therapy and decrease dose by 0.25 mcg.

HOW SUPPLIED: Cap: 0.25mcg, 0.5mcg; Sol: 1mcg/mL (15mL)

CONTRAINDICATIONS: Hypercalcemia or vitamin D toxicity.

WARNINGS/PRECAUTIONS: Use non-aluminum phosphate binders and low phosphate diet to control serum phosphate. Chronic hypercalcemia can cause calcification of soft tissues. Monitor calcium levels twice a week initially. Avoid dehydration. Monitor serum creatinine. Maintain adequate calcium intake of at least 600mg/day. Caution in elderly. If treatment switched from ergocalciferol, may take several months for ergocalciferol level to decrease to baseline. May increase inorganic phosphate levels; ectopic calcification reported with renal failure. Monitor phosphorus, magnesium, alkaline phosphatase, and 24-hour urine periodically.

ADVERSE REACTIONS: Weakness, nausea, vomiting, dry mouth, constipation, muscle and bone pain, metallic taste, polyuria, polydipsia, weight loss, pancreatitis, photophobia, pruritus, decreased libido.

INTERACTIONS: Avoid vitamin D products and derivatives during therapy. Hypermagnesemia may occur with magnesium-containing antacids, especially in chronic renal dialysis. Caution with digoxin; hypercalcemia may precipitate arrhythmias. Reduced intestinal absorption with cholestyramine. May need to increase dose if given with phenytoin or phenobarbital. Caution with thiazides; risk of hypercalcemia. Ketoconazole may effect metabolism. Corticosteroids antagonize activity. Changes in diet or uncontrolled intake of calcium preparations can cause hypercalcemia. Adjust dose phosphate-binding agents.

PREGNANCY: Category C, not for use in nursing.

MECHANISM OF ACTION: Synthetic vitamin D analog. Regulates absorption of calcium from the GI tract and its utilization in the body.

PHARMACOKINETICS: Absorption: Rapidly absorbed (intestine). $C_{max}=131\pm17pg/mL$; $T_{max}=3-6$ hrs. **Distribution:** Plasma protein binding (99.9%); crosses placenta; found in breast milk. **Metabolism:** Liver via hydroxylation. 1,25R(OH)$_2$-26, 23S-lactone D$_3$ lactone (major metabolite). **Elimination:** Urine (16%), feces (49%); $T_{1/2}=5-8$ hrs. Refer to prescribing guidelines for pediatric parameters.

ROCEPHIN   RX
ceftriaxone sodium (Roche Labs)

THERAPEUTIC CLASS: Cephalosporin (3rd generation)

INDICATIONS: Treatment of lower respiratory tract, skin and skin structure, bone and joint, intra-abdominal and urinary tract infections, acute otitis media, uncomplicated gonorrhea, pelvic inflammatory disease, bacterial septicemia, and meningitis caused by susceptible strains of microorganisms. Surgical prophylaxis during surgical procedures classified as contaminated or potentially contaminated.

DOSAGE: *Adults:* Usual: 1-2g/day IV/IM given qd-bid. Max: 4g/day. Gonorrhea: 250mg IM single dose. Surgical Prophylaxis: 1g IV 1/2-2 hrs before surgery. Avoid diluents containing calcium.
Pediatrics: Skin Infections: 50-75mg/kg/day IV/IM given qd-bid. Max: 2g/day. Otitis Media: 50mg/kg (up to 1g) IM single dose. Serious Infections: 50-75mg/kg/day IM/IV given q12h. Max: 2g/day. Meningitis: Initial: 100mg/kg (up to 4g), then 100mg/kg/day given qd-bid for 7-14 days. Max: 4g/day. Avoid diluents containing calcium.

HOW SUPPLIED: Inj: 250mg, 500mg, 1g, 2g, 10g

CONTRAINDICATIONS: Avoid use in hyperbilirubinemic neonates esp. prematures. Avoid concurrent use with calcium-containing solutions/products in newborns.

WARNINGS/PRECAUTIONS: Cross-sensitivity to PCNs and other cephalosporins may occur. *Clostridium difficile*-associated diarrhea reported. May result in overgrowth of nonsusceptible organisms. Altered PT, transient BUN, and serum creatinine elevations may occur. Do not exceed 2g/day and monitor blood levels with both hepatic dysfunction and significant renal disease. Caution with history of GI disease. D/C if gallbladder disease develops. May alter PT; monitor with impaired vitamin K synthesis or low vitamin K stores.

ADVERSE REACTIONS: Injection-site reactions, eosinophilia, thrombocytosis, diarrhea, SGOT and SGPT elevations.

INTERACTIONS: See Contraindications. Do not administer calcium containing products within 48 hrs of last administration of drug.

PREGNANCY: Category B, caution in nursing.

MECHANISM OF ACTION: Broad-spectrum cephalosporin; bactericidal activity results from inhibition of cell-wall synthesis.

PHARMACOKINETICS: Absorption: (Adults) Complete; T_{max}=2-3 hrs. (Pediatrics) Bacterial meningitis: C_{max}=216mcg/mL (50mg/kg), 275mcg/mL (75mg/kg). Middle ear fluid: C_{max}=35mcg/mL; T_{max}=24 hrs. **Distribution:** (Adults) V_d=5.78-13.5L. (Pediatrics) Bacterial meningitis: V_d=338mL/kg (50mg/kg), 373mL/kg (75mg/kg). **Elimination:** Urine (33-67%), feces. (Adults) $T_{1/2}$=5.8-8.7 hrs. (Pediatrics) Bacterial meningitis: $T_{1/2}$=4.6 hrs (50mg/kg), 4.3 hrs (75mg/kg); Middle ear fluid: $T_{1/2}$=25 hrs.

ROMAZICON
flumazenil (Roche Labs)

RX

THERAPEUTIC CLASS: Benzodiazepine antagonist

INDICATIONS: Complete or partial reversal of sedative effects of benzodiazepines (BZDs) given with general anesthesia, or diagnostic and therapeutic procedures, and for the management of BZD overdose in adults. For reversal of BZD-induced conscious sedation in pediatrics (1-17 yrs old).

DOSAGE: *Adults:* Reversal of Conscious Sedation/General Anesthesia: Give IV over 15 seconds. Initial: 0.2mg. May repeat dose after 45 seconds and again at 60 second intervals up to a max of 4 additional times until reach desired level of consciousness. Max Total Dose: 1mg. In event of resedation, repeated doses may be given at 20-min intervals. Max: 1mg/dose (0.2mg/min) and 3mg/hr. BZD Overdose: Give IV over 30 seconds. Initial: 0.2mg. May repeat with 0.3mg after 30 seconds and then 0.5mg at 1-min intervals until reach desired level of consciousness. Max Total Dose: 3mg. In event of resedation, repeated doses may be given at 20-min intervals. Max: 1mg/dose (0.5mg/min); 3mg/hr.
Pediatrics: >1yr: Give IV over 15 seconds. Initial: 0.01mg/kg (up to 0.2mg). May repeat dose after 45 seconds and again at 60-second intervals up to a max of 4 additional times until reach desired level of consciousness. Max Total Dose: 0.05mg/kg or 1mg, whichever is lower.

HOW SUPPLIED: Inj: 0.1mg/mL

CONTRAINDICATIONS: Patients given BZDs for life-threatening conditions (eg, control of ICP or status epilepticus), signs of serious cyclic antidepressant overdose.

WARNINGS/PRECAUTIONS: Caution in overdoses involving multiple drug combinations. Risk of seizures, especially with long-term BZD-induced sedation, cyclic antidepressant overdose, concurrent major sedative-hypnotic drug withdrawal, recent therapy with repeated doses of parenteral BZDs, myoclonic jerking or seizure prior to flumazenil administration. Monitor for resedation, respiratory depression, or other residual BZD effects (up to 2 hrs). Avoid use in the ICU; increased risk of unrecognized BZD dependence. Caution with head injury, alcoholism, and other drug dependencies. Does not reverse respiratory depression/hypoventilation or cardiac depression. May provoke panic attacks with history of panic disorder. Adjust subsequent doses in hepatic dysfunction. Not for use as treatment for BZD dependence or for management of protracted abstinence syndromes. May trigger dose-dependent withdrawal syndromes. Extravasation may occur; administer IV into a large vein.

ADVERSE REACTIONS: N/V, dizziness, injection-site pain, increased sweating, headache, abnormal or blurred vision, agitation.

INTERACTIONS: Avoid use until neuromuscular blockade effects are reversed. Toxic effects (eg, convulsions, cardiac dysrhythmias) may occur with mixed drug overdose (eg, cyclic antidepressants).

PREGNANCY: Category C, caution in nursing.

MECHANISM OF ACTION: Benzodiazepine receptor antagonist; inhibits activity at the benzodiazepine recognition site on the GABA/benzodiazepine receptor complex.

PHARMACOKINETICS: Absorption: C_{max}=24ng/mL; AUC=15ng•hr/mL. **Distribution:** V_d=1L/kg (steady state); plasma protein binding (50%). **Metabolism:** Complete (99%). **Elimination:** Urine (90-95%), feces (5-10%); $T_{1/2}$=54 min.

RONDEC RX
carbinoxamine maleate - pseudoephedrine HCl (Biovail)

OTHER BRAND NAMES: Rondec Oral Drops (Biovail) - Rondec-TR (Biovail)

THERAPEUTIC CLASS: Antihistamine/decongestant

INDICATIONS: (Drops) Seasonal/perennial allergic and vasomotor rhinitis. (Tab, Tab, Extended-Release) Relief of upper respiratory symptoms associated with allergic rhinitis and the common cold.

DOSAGE: *Adults:* (Tab) 1 tab qid; (Tab, Extended-Release) 1 tab bid. *Pediatrics:* (Sol) Give qid. 12-24 months: 1mL. 6-12 months: 3/4mL. 3-6 months: 1/2mL. 1-3 months: 1/4mL. (Tab) ≥6 yrs:1 tab qid. (Tab, Extended-Release) ≥12 yrs: 1 tab bid.

HOW SUPPLIED: (Carbinoxamine-Pseudoephedrine) Sol: 1mg-15mg/mL (30mL); Tab: 4mg-60mg; Tab, Extended-Release: (Rondec TR) 8mg-120mg

CONTRAINDICATIONS: Severe HTN or CAD, MAOIs, narrow-angle glaucoma, urinary retention, peptic ulcer, during asthma attack.

WARNINGS/PRECAUTIONS: Caution in asthma, DM, HTN, heart disease, hyperthyroidism, increased IOP, prostatic hypertrophy, elderly. May cause excitability, especially in children.

ADVERSE REACTIONS: Sedation, dizziness, diplopia, vomiting, diarrhea, dry mouth, headache, nervousness, nausea, convulsions, CNS stimulation, cardiac arrhythmias, respiratory difficulty, increased HR or BP.

INTERACTIONS: May enhance effects of TCAs, benzodiazepines, barbiturates, alcohol, other CNS depressants. Increased sympathomimetic effects with MAOIs, β-blockers. May reduce antihypertensive effects of reserpine, veratrum alkaloids, methyldopa, mecamylamine.

PREGNANCY: Category C, safety in nursing not known.

MECHANISM OF ACTION: Carbinoxamine: H_1 antihistaminic activity with mild anticholinergic and sedative effects. Pseudoephedrine: Sympathomimetic; acts as decongestant to respiratory tract mucous membranes.

PHARMACOKINETICS: Elimination: Carbinoxamine: Urine; $T_{1/2}$=10-20 hrs. Pseudoephedrine: Urine; $T_{1/2}$=6-8 hrs.

RONDEC SYRUP RX
brompheniramine maleate - pseudoephedrine HCl (Biovail)

THERAPEUTIC CLASS: Antihistamine/decongestant

INDICATIONS: Symptomatic relief of seasonal and perennial allergic rhinitis and vasomotor rhinitis.

DOSAGE: *Adults:* 5mL qid. *Pediatrics:* ≥6 yrs: 5mL qid. 2-6 yrs: 2.5mL qid.

HOW SUPPLIED: (Brompheniramine-Pseudoephedrine) Syrup: 4mg-45mg/5mL

CONTRAINDICATIONS: Severe HTN or CAD, MAOIs, narrow-angle glaucoma, urinary retention, peptic ulcer, during asthma attack.

WARNINGS/PRECAUTIONS: Caution in asthma, DM, HTN, heart disease, hyperthyroidism, increased IOP, prostatic hypertrophy, elderly. May cause excitability, especially in children.

ADVERSE REACTIONS: Sedation, dizziness, diplopia, vomiting, diarrhea, dry mouth, headache, nervousness, nausea, convulsions, CNS stimulation, cardiac arrhythmias, respiratory difficulty, increased HR or BP.

INTERACTIONS: May enhance effects of TCAs, benzodiazepines, barbiturates, alcohol, other CNS depressants. Increased sympathomimetic effects with MAOIs, β-blockers. May reduce antihypertensive effects of reserpine, veratrum alkaloids, methyldopa, mecamylamine.

PREGNANCY: Category C, safety in nursing not known.

MECHANISM OF ACTION: Brompheniramine: H_1 antihistaminic activity and mild anticholinergic and sedative effects. Pseudoephedrine: Sympathomimetic; acts as decongestant to respiratory tract mucous membranes.

PHARMACOKINETICS: Absorption: Brompheniramine: T_{max}=5 hrs. **Metabolism:** Brompheniramine: Liver. **Elimination:** Brompheniramine: Urine. Pseudoephedrine: Urine; $T_{1/2}$=6-8 hrs.

RONDEC-DM DROPS   RX
carbinoxamine maleate - dextromethorphan HBr - pseudoephedrine HCl
(Biovail)

THERAPEUTIC CLASS: Antihistamine/decongestant/antitussive

INDICATIONS: Relief of coughs and upper respiratory symptoms associated with allergy or the common cold.

DOSAGE: *Pediatrics:* Give qid. 12-24 months: 1mL. 6-12 months: 3/4mL. 3-6 months: 1/2mL. 1-3 months: 1/4mL.

HOW SUPPLIED: (Carbinoxamine-Dextromethorphan-Pseudoephedrine) Sol: 1mg-4mg-15mg/mL (30mL)

CONTRAINDICATIONS: Severe HTN or CAD, during or within 2 weeks of MAOIs, narrow-angle glaucoma, urinary retention, peptic ulcer, during asthma attack.

WARNINGS/PRECAUTIONS: Caution with HTN, DM, heart disease, asthma, hyperthyroidism, increased IOP, prostatic hypertrophy and in atopic children, elderly, sedated, debilitated, or confined to supine positions. May cause excitability especially in children.

ADVERSE REACTIONS: Sedation, drowsiness, dizziness, diplopia, nausea, vomiting, diarrhea, dry mouth, headache, nervousness, convulsions, CNS stimulation, arrhythmias, increased HR or BP, tremors.

INTERACTIONS: Avoid during or within 2 weeks of MAOIs. May enhance effects of TCAs, barbiturates, alcohol, other CNS depressants. May reduce antihypertensive effects of reserpine, veratrum alkaloids, methyldopa, mecamylamine. Increased sympathomimetic effect with MAOIs, β-blockers. Additive cough-suppressant effect with narcotic antitussives.

PREGNANCY: Category C, safety in nursing not known.

MECHANISM OF ACTION: Carbinoxamine: H_1 antihistamine activity with mild anticholinergic and sedative effects. Pseudoephedrine: Sympathomimetic amine; acts as decongestant to repiratory tract mucous membranes. Dextromethorphan: Nonnarcotic/antitussive; acts in the medulla oblongata to elevate the cough threshold.

PHARMACOKINETICS: Elimination: Carbinoxamine: Urine; $T_{1/2}$=10-20 hrs. Pseudoephedrine: Urine; $T_{1/2}$=6-8 hrs. Dextromethophran: Urine (conjugated metabolites).

RONDEC-DM SYRUP   RX
brompheniramine maleate - dextromethorphan HBr - pseudoephedrine HCl
(Biovail)

OTHER BRAND NAMES: Carbofed DM (Hi-Tech) - Cardec DM (Alpharma)

THERAPEUTIC CLASS: Antihistamine/decongestant/antitussive

INDICATIONS: Relief of coughs and upper respiratory symptoms, including nasal congestion, associated with allergy or the common cold.

DOSAGE: *Adults:* 5mL qid.
Pediatrics: >6 yrs: 5mL qid. 2-6 yrs: 2.5mL qid.

HOW SUPPLIED: Syrup: (Brompheniramine-Dextromethorphan-Pseudoephedrine) 4mg-15mg-45mg/5mL (120mL, 480mL)

CONTRAINDICATIONS: Severe HTN or CAD, narrow-angle glaucoma, urinary retention, peptic ulcer, acute asthma attack, with MAOI therapy.

WARNINGS/PRECAUTIONS: Caution with HTN, DM, ischemic heart disease, hyperthyroidism, BPH, asthma, and increased IOP. May produce CNS stimulation with convulsion, cardiovascular collapse and hypotension. Excitability reported especially in children. Do not exceed recommended doses. Caution in atopic children, elderly, sedated/debilitated, and patients confined to supine positions.

ADVERSE REACTIONS: Sedation, drowsiness, dizziness, diplopia, nausea, vomiting, diarrhea, dry mouth, headache, arrhythmias, increased heart rate, tremors, nervousness, insomnia, heartburn, dysuria, polyuria, increased BP.

INTERACTIONS: May enhance effects of TCAs, barbiturates, alcohol, other CNS depressants. May diminish antihypertensive effects of reserpine, veratrum alkaloids, methyldopa, mecamylamine. Increased sympathomimetic effect with β-blockers and MAOIs. Additive cough-suppressant effect with narcotic antitussives. Do not use within 14 days of MAOI therapy.

PREGNANCY: Category C, caution in nursing.

MECHANISM OF ACTION: Brompheniramine: H_1 antihistamine activity; mild anticholinergic and sedative effects. Pseudoephedrine: Oral sympathomimetic amine; acts as decongestant to respiratory tract mucous membranes. Dextromethorphan: Nonnarcotic antitussive with effectiveness equal to codeine; acts in medulla oblongata to elevate the cough threshold.

PHARMACOKINETICS: Absorption: Brompheniramine: T_{max}=5 hrs. **Metabolism:** Brompheniramine: Liver. **Elimination:** Brompheniramine: Urine. Pseudoephedrine: Urine; $T_{1/2}$=6-8 hrs. Dextromethorphan: Urine (conjugated metabolites).

Rosac RX
sulfacetamide sodium - sulfur (Stiefel)

THERAPEUTIC CLASS: Sulfonamide/sulfur combination

INDICATIONS: Topical control of acne vulgaris, acne rosacea, and seborrheic dermatitis.

DOSAGE: *Adults:* Apply a thin film qd-tid.
Pediatrics: ≥12 yrs: Apply a thin film qd-tid.

HOW SUPPLIED: Cre: (Sulfacetamide-Sulfur) 10%-5% (45g)

CONTRAINDICATIONS: Kidney disease.

WARNINGS/PRECAUTIONS: D/C if irritation or hypersensitivity reaction occurs. Avoid contact with eyes. Caution if denuded or abraded skin. May cause reddening and scaling of epidermis.

ADVERSE REACTIONS: Local irritation.

PREGNANCY: Category C, caution in nursing.

MECHANISM OF ACTION: Sulfonamide/sulfur combination. Sulfacetamide: Acts as a competitive antagonist to para-aminobenzoic acid (PABA), an essential component for bacterial growth. Sulfur: Not established. Inhibits the growth of *Propionibacterium acnes* and the formation of free fatty acids.

PHARMACOKINETICS: Absorption: Sulfacetamide: (PO) Readily absorbed. **Distribution:** Small amounts of orally administered sulfonamides have been found in breast milk. **Elimination:** Sulfacetamide: Urine (unchanged).

ROSULA
sulfacetamide sodium – sulfur (Doak)   RX

THERAPEUTIC CLASS: Sulfonamide/sulfur combination

INDICATIONS: Topical treatment of acne vulgaris, acne rosacea, and seborrheic dermatitis.

DOSAGE: *Adults:* (Gel) Apply thin film qd-tid. (Cleanser) Wash for 10-20 seconds qd-bid. *Pediatrics:* ≥12 yrs: (Gel) Apply thin film qd-tid. (Cleanser) Wash for 10-20 seconds qd-bid.

HOW SUPPLIED: (Sulfacetamide-Sulfur) Gel: 10%-5% (45mL); Cleanser: 10%-5% (355mL)

CONTRAINDICATIONS: Kidney disease.

WARNINGS/PRECAUTIONS: D/C if irritation or hypersensitivity reaction occurs. Avoid contact with eyes, lips, and mucous membranes. Caution with denuded or abraded skin. Can cause reddening and scaling of epidermis.

ADVERSE REACTIONS: Local irritation.

PREGNANCY: Category C, caution in nursing.

MECHANISM OF ACTION: Sulfonamide/sulfur combination. Sulfacetamide: Acts as a competitive antagonist to para-aminobenzoic acid (PABA), an essential component for bacterial growth. Sulfur: Not established. Inhibits the growth of *Propionibacterium acnes* and the formation of free fatty acids.

PHARMACOKINETICS: Absorption: (PO) Readily absorbed. **Elimination:** Urine (unchanged).

ROSULA NS
sulfacetamide sodium – urea (Doak)   RX

THERAPEUTIC CLASS: Sulfonamide

INDICATIONS: Topical treatment of bacterial infections of the skin including *P.acne* and seborrheic dermatitis.

DOSAGE: *Adults:* Apply to affected area qd-bid. *Pediatrics:* ≥12 yrs: Apply to affected area qd-bid.

HOW SUPPLIED: Swab: (Sulfacetamide-Urea) 10%-10% (30^s)

CONTRAINDICATIONS: Kidney disease

WARNINGS/PRECAUTIONS: D/C if irritation or hypersensitivity reaction occurs. Avoid contact with eyes, lips, and mucous membranes. Caution with denuded or abraded skin. Cases of Stevens-Johnson syndrome and drug-induced systemic lupus erythematosus reported.

ADVERSE REACTIONS: Local hypersensitivity, instances of Stevens-Johnson syndrome.

INTERACTIONS: Incompatible with silver preparations.

PREGNANCY: Category C, caution in nursing.

MECHANISM OF ACTION: Sulfonamide: Sulfacetamide; possesses bacteriostatic activity against susceptible gram-positive and gram-negative microorganisms, including *P. acne*. Acts as a competitive antagonist to para-aminobenzoic acid (PABA), an essential component for bacterial growth.

PHARMACOKINETICS: Absorption: Sulfacetamide: (PO) Readily absorbed. **Elimination:** Urine (unchanged).

ROTATEQ
rotavirus vaccine, live (Merck)   RX

THERAPEUTIC CLASS: Vaccine

INDICATIONS: Prevention of rotavirus gastroenteritis in infants and children caused by the serotypes G1, G2, G3, and G4 when administered as a 3-dose series to infants between the ages of 6-32 weeks. The first dose should be administered between 6-12 weeks of age.

DOSAGE: *Pediatrics:* Administer series of 3 doses orally starting at 6-12 weeks of age, with subsequent doses administered at 4-10 week intervals. Third dose should not be given after 32 weeks of age. Do not mix with any other vaccines or solutions. Do not reconstitute or dilute.

HOW SUPPLIED: Sus: 2mL

WARNINGS/PRECAUTIONS: Consider delaying use with febrile illness. Vaccination may not result in complete protection in all recipients. May increase risk of intussusception.

ADVERSE REACTIONS: Bronchiolitis, gastroenteritis, pneumonia, fever, UTI.

INTERACTIONS: Immunosuppressive therapies including irradiation, antimetabolites, alkylating agents, cytotoxic drugs, and corticosteroids (used in greater than physiologic doses) may reduce the immune response to vaccines.

PREGNANCY: Safety in pregnancy and nursing not known.

MECHANISM OF ACTION: Immunologic mechanism not established; may replicate in small intestine and induce immunity against rotavirus gastroenteritis.

RYNATAN PEDIATRIC   RX
chlorpheniramine tannate - phenylephrine tannate (MedPointe)

THERAPEUTIC CLASS: Antihistamine/sympathomimetic

INDICATIONS: Symptomatic relief of coryza and nasal congestion with the common cold, sinusitis, allergic rhinitis, and other upper respiratory tract conditions.

DOSAGE: *Pediatrics:* >6 yrs: 5-10mL q12h. 2 to 6 yrs: 2.5-5mL q12h. <2 yrs: Titrate individually.

HOW SUPPLIED: Sus: (Chlorpheniramine-Phenylephrine) 4.5mg-5mg/5mL

CONTRAINDICATIONS: Newborns and nursing mothers.

WARNINGS/PRECAUTIONS: Caution with HTN, cardiovascular disease, hyperthyroidism, DM, narrow-angle glaucoma, prostatic hypertrophy, and elderly. May impair mental alertness. Contains tartrazine.

ADVERSE REACTIONS: Drowsiness, sedation, dryness of mucous membranes, GI effects.

INTERACTIONS: Increased anticholinergic and sympathomimetic effects with MAOIs; avoid during or within 14 days of use. Additive CNS effects with alcohol or other CNS depressants (eg, sedative-hypnotics, tranquilizers).

PREGNANCY: Category C, not for use in nursing.

MECHANISM OF ACTION: Antihistamine/symphatomimetic nasal decongestant.

RYNATUSS   RX
carbetapentane tannate - chlorpheniramine tannate - ephedrine tannate - phenylephrine tannate (MedPointe)

OTHER BRAND NAME: Rynatuss Pediatric (MedPointe)

THERAPEUTIC CLASS: Antitussive/antihistamine/bronchodilator/sympathomimetic combination

INDICATIONS: Symptomatic relief of cough associated with respiratory tract conditions such as the common cold, bronchial asthma, acute and chronic bronchitis.

DOSAGE: *Adults:* 1-2 tabs q12h.
Pediatrics: >6 yrs: 5-10mL q12h. 2-6 yrs: 2.5-5mL q12h.

HOW SUPPLIED: (Carbetapentane-Chlorpheniramine-Ephedrine-Phenylephrine) Sus: (Rynatuss Pediatric) 30mg-4mg-5mg-5mg/5mL (240mL 480mL); Tab: (Rynatuss) 60mg-5mg-10mg-10mg* *scored

CONTRAINDICATIONS: Newborns, nursing mothers.

WARNINGS/PRECAUTIONS: Caution with HTN, cardiovascular disease, hyperthyroidism, DM, narrow angle glaucoma, elderly or prostatic hypertrophy. Suspension contains FD&C Yellow No. 5 which may cause allergic-type reactions.

ADVERSE REACTIONS: Drowsiness, sedation, dryness of mucous membranes, GI effects.

INTERACTIONS: Avoid MAOI use within 14 days. Additive CNS effects with alcohol or other CNS depressants.

PREGNANCY: Category C, not for use in nursing.

SAIZEN
somatropin (EMD Serono)

RX

THERAPEUTIC CLASS: Human growth hormone

INDICATIONS: Long-term treatment of children with growth failure due to inadequate secretion of endogenous growth hormone. For replacement of endogenous growth hormone in adults who have growth hormone deficiency either alone, or associated with multiple hormone deficiencies, as a result of pituitary disease, hypothalamic disease, surgery, radiation therapy or trauma; or in patients who were growth hormone deficient during childhood as a result of congenital, genetic, acquired or idiopathic causes.

DOSAGE: *Adults:* Initial: ≤0.005mg/kg/day SQ. Titrate: May increase after 4 weeks to ≤0.01mg/kg/day depending on patient tolerance. Without Consideration of Body Weight: Initial: 0.2mg/day (0.15-0.3mg/day) SQ. Titrate: May increase by increments of 0.1-0.2mg/day every 1-2 months. Consider dose reduction in elderly.
Pediatrics: Individualize dose. Usual: 0.06mg/kg IM/SQ 3x/week. If epiphyses are fused, d/c therapy.

HOW SUPPLIED: Inj: 4mg, 5mg, 8.8mg

CONTRAINDICATIONS: Acute critical illness due to complications following open heart or abdominal surgery, accidental trauma or acute respiratory failure. Active proliferative or severe non-proliferative diabetic retinopathy. Active malignancy, or evidence of progression or recurrence of intracranial tumor. Prader-Willi syndrome when severely obese or have severe respiratory impairment, and in pediatric patients with closed epiphyses. Avoid reconstitution with bacteriostatic water if sensitive to benzyl alcohol.

WARNINGS/PRECAUTIONS: Benzyl alcohol associated with toxicity in newborns; if sensitivity occurs, may reconstitute with SWFI. Insulin resistance reported; use caution with DM or family history of DM. Hypothyroidism may occur; bone maturation should be carefully followed. Increased incidence of slipped capital femoral epiphysis may develop with endocrine disorders; monitor for limping or hip/knee pain. Intracranial hypertension (IH) reported; d/c treatment if papilledema observed. Patients with Turner syndrome, chronic renal insufficiency or Prader-Willi syndrome may have increased risk for IH. If idiopathic IH confirmed, may restart therapy at lower dose after signs/symptoms resolve. Alternate injection sites to reduce development of tissue atrophy. Monitor for any malignant transformation of skin lesions.

ADVERSE REACTIONS: Arthalgia, headache, influenza-like symptoms, peripheral edema, back pain, myalgia, rhinitis, dizziness, upper respiratory tract infection, paraesthesia, hypoaesthesia, insomnia, nausea, generalized edema, depression.

INTERACTIONS: Diminished effects with concomitant glucocorticoid; adjust dose of accordingly. May alter clearance of CYP450 substrates (eg, corticosteroids, sex steroids, anticonvulsants, cyclosporine). May increase dose if taking oral estrogen replacement concomitantly. Adjust dose of insulin/oral antidiabetics when initiating therapy.

PREGNANCY: Category B, caution in nursing.

MECHANISM OF ACTION: Human growth hormone; stimulates skeletal growth, increases number and size of skeletal muscle cells, influences size and function of internal organs and increases red cell mass, stimulates protein synthesis, modulates carbohydrate metabolism, and mobilizes lipids.

PHARMACOKINETICS: Absorption: Absolute bioavailability (70-90%). **Distribution:** V_d=12.0L. **Metabolism:** Liver, kidneys. **Elimination:** $T_{1/2}$=1.75 hrs (SC), 3.4 hrs (IM), 0.6 hrs (IV).

SANDIMMUNE
cyclosporine (Novartis)

RX

> Give with adrenal corticosteroids but not with other immunosuppressives. Increased susceptibility to infection and development of lymphoma. Sandimmune and Neoral are not bioequivalent. Monitor blood levels to avoid toxicity.

THERAPEUTIC CLASS: Cyclic polypeptide immunosuppressant

INDICATIONS: Prophylaxis of organ rejection in kidney, liver, and heart allogeneic transplants with concomitant adrenal corticosteroids. Treatment of chronic rejection in patients previously treated with other immunosuppressives.

DOSAGE: *Adults:* Initial: PO: 15mg/kg single dose 4-12 hrs before transplant; continue same dose qd for 1-2 weeks. Usual: Taper by 5% per week until 5-10mg/kg/day. May mix oral solution with milk, chocolate milk, or orange juice. IV: 1/3 PO dose. Initial: 5-6mg/kg/day single dose; begin 4 to 12 hrs prior to transplantation. Maint: Continue single daily dose until PO forms are tolerated. Due to risk of anaphylaxis, only use injection if unable to take oral agents.
Pediatrics: Initial: PO: 15mg/kg single dose 4-12 hrs before transplant; continue same dose qd for 1-2 weeks. Usual: Taper by 5% per week until 5-10mg/kg/day. May mix oral solution with milk, chocolate milk, or orange juice. IV: 1/3 PO dose. Initial: 5-6mg/kg/day single dose; begin 4 to 12 hrs prior to transplantation. Maint: Continue single daily dose until PO forms are tolerated. Due to risk of anaphylaxis, only use injection if unable to take oral agents.

HOW SUPPLIED: Cap: 25mg, 100mg; Inj: 50mg/mL; Sol: 100mg/mL (50mL)

CONTRAINDICATIONS: Hypersensitivity to Cremophor EL (polyoxyethylated castor oil).

WARNINGS/PRECAUTIONS: May cause hepatotoxicity and nephrotoxicity. Convulsions, elevated serum creatinine, and BUN levels reported. Thrombocytopenia and microangiopathic hemolytic anemia may develop. Monitor for hyperkalemia. Increases risk for development of lymphomas and other malignancies. Observe for 30 minutes after the start of infusion and frequently thereafter. Caution with malabsorption.

ADVERSE REACTIONS: Renal dysfunction, tremor, hirsutism, HTN, gum hyperplasia, glomerular capillary thrombosis, cramps, acne, convulsions, headache, diarrhea, hepatotoxity, abdominal discomfort, paresthesia, flushing.

INTERACTIONS: Ciprofloxacin, gentamicin, tobramycin, vancomycin, SMZ/TMP, amphotericin B, ketoconazole, melphalan, diclofenac, azapropazon, sulindac, naproxen, colchicine, cimetidine, ranitidine, tacrolimus, bezafirate, fenofibrate may potentiate renal dysfunction. Diltiazem, nicardipine, colchicine, fluconazole, itraconazole, ketoconazole, verapamil, azithromycin, clarithromycin, erythromycin, quinupristin/dalfopristin, allopurinol, amiodarone, bromocriptine, danazol, imatinib, metoclopramide, oral contraceptives, HIV protease inhibitors may increase levels. St. John's wort, grapefruit juice, carbamazepine, phenobarbital, phenytoin, rifampin, sulfinpyrazone, octreotide, orlistat, terbinafine, ticlopidine, and naficillin may decrease levels. Avoid with potassium-sparing diuretics. Caution with ACEIs, angiotensin II blockers, NSAIDs. Digitalis toxicity reported. Myotoxicity with statins, frequent gingival hyperplasia with nifedipine, and convulsions with high dose methylprednisolone reported. Increased levels of sirolimus; give 4 hrs after cyclosporine. Avoid live vaccines during therapy.

PREGNANCY: Category C, not for use in nursing.

MECHANISM OF ACTION: Cyclic polypeptide immunosuppressant; not fully established. May cause specific and reversible inhibition of immunocompetent lymphocytes in the G_0- or G_1-phase of the cell cycle. T lymphocytes are preferentially inhibited with T-helper cell as main target while also possibly suppressing T-suppressor cells. Also inhibits lymphokine production and release (eg, interleukin-2, T-cell growth factor).

PHARMACOKINETICS: **Absorption:** Incomplete and variable. Absolute bioavailability (30%)(PO); $C_{max}=1ng/mL/mg$; $T_{max}=3.5$ hrs. **Distribution:** Plasma protein binding (90%). **Metabolism:** Extensively metabolized via hydroxylation, cyclic ether formation, and N-demethylation. **Elimination:** Urine (6%); $T_{1/2}=19$ hrs.

SECONAL SODIUM

secobarbital sodium (Ranbaxy)

CII

THERAPEUTIC CLASS: Barbiturate

INDICATIONS: Hypnotic, for the short-term treatment of insomnia (may lose effectiveness after 2 weeks); Preanesthetic.

DOSAGE: *Adults:* Hypnotic: 100mg hs; Preoperatively: 200-300mg, 1-2 hrs before surgery; Elderly/Debilitated/Renal or Hepatic Dysfunction: Reduce dose.
Pediatrics: Preoperatively: 2-6mg/kg. Max: 100mg.

HOW SUPPLIED: Cap: 100mg

CONTRAINDICATIONS: History of manifest or latent porphyria, marked impairment of liver function, or respiratory disease in which dyspnea or obstruction is evident.

WARNINGS/PRECAUTIONS: May be habit-forming; avoid abrupt cessation after prolonged use. Tolerance, psychological and physical dependence may occur with continued use. Use with caution, if at all, in patients who are mentally depressed, have suicidal tendencies, or have a history of drug abuse. In patients with hepatic damage, use with caution and initially reduce dose. Caution when administering to patients with acute or chronic pain. May impair mental and/or physical abilities. Avoid alcohol.

ADVERSE REACTIONS: Agitation, confusion, hyperkinesia, ataxia, CNS depression, somnolence, bradycardia, hypotension, nausea, vomiting, constipation, headache, hypersensitivity reactions, liver damage.

INTERACTIONS: May increase metabolism and decrease response to oral anticoagulants and enhance metabolism of exogenous corticosteroids. May interfere with absorption of griseofulvin, decreasing its blood level. May shorten half-life of doxycycline for up to 2 weeks after being discontinued. Variable effect on phenytoin and increased levels with sodium valproate and valproic acid; monitor blood levels and adjust dose appropriately. May cause additive depressant effects with other CNS depressants (eg, sedatives/hypnotics, antihistamines, tranquilizers, alcohol). Prolonged effects with MAOIs. May decrease effect of estradiol; alternative contraceptive methods should be suggested.

PREGNANCY: Category D, caution in nursing.

MECHANISM OF ACTION: Barbiturates, nonselective CNS depressants; depress sensory cortex, decrease motor activity, alter cerebellar function, and produce drowsiness, sedation, and hypnosis.

PHARMACOKINETICS: Absorption: Rapidly absorbed. **Distribution:** Crosses placenta, found in breast milk. **Metabolism:** Liver. **Elimination:** Urine and feces; $T_{1/2}$=28 hrs.

SEMPREX-D

acrivastine - pseudoephedrine HCl (Celltech)

RX

THERAPEUTIC CLASS: Antihistamine/decongestant

INDICATIONS: Relief of symptoms associated with seasonal allergic rhinitis.

DOSAGE: *Adults:* 1 cap q4-6h, qid.
Pediatrics: ≥12 yrs: 1 cap q4-6h, qid.

HOW SUPPLIED: Cap: (Acrivastine-Pseudoephedrine) 8mg-60mg

CONTRAINDICATIONS: Severe HTN, CAD, MAOIs during or within 14 days of use. Hypersensitivity to alkylamine antihistamines.

WARNINGS/PRECAUTIONS: Not for use >14 days. Caution with HTN, DM, increased IOP, ischemic heart disease, hyperthyroidism, BPH, renal impairment, peptic ulcer, pyloroduodenal obstruction, and elderly. Sedation reported. Avoid with CrCl ≤48mL/min.

ADVERSE REACTIONS: Somnolence, headache, dry mouth, insomnia, dizziness, nervousness, pharyngitis.

INTERACTIONS: See Contraindications. MAOIs and β-agonists increase effects of sympathomimetics; avoid use during or within 14 days of MAOIs. Increased sedation with CNS depressants, alcohol.

PREGNANCY: Category B, caution in nursing.

MECHANISM OF ACTION: Acrivastine: Alkylamine antihistamine; acts by exhibiting H1-antihistaminic activity and sedative effects. Pseudoephedrine: Indirect sympathomimetic agent; releases norepinephrine from adrenergic nerves.

PHARMACOKINETICS: Absorption: Acrivastine: Rapid; C_{max}=227ng/mL; T_{max}=1.14hr. Pseudoephedrine: Rapid; C_{max}=498ng/mL. **Distribution:** Acrivastine: V_d=0.46L/kg; plasma protein binding (50%). Pseudoephedrine: V_d=3.0L/kg; excreted in breast milk. **Metabolism:** Acrivastine: Propionic acid metabolite. **Elimination:** Acrivastine: Urine (67% unchanged), (11% as propionic acid) and (6% as unknown metabolite), feces (13%); $T_{1/2}$=1.9 hrs. Propionic acid: $T_{1/2}$=3.8 hrs. Pseudoephedrine: Urine (55-75% unchanged); $T_{1/2}$=6.2 hrs, increases in acidic urine.

SENOKOT OTC
senna (Purdue Products)

THERAPEUTIC CLASS: Stimulant laxative

INDICATIONS: To relieve functional constipation. Senokot-S also contains a stool softener.

DOSAGE: *Adults:* Take at bedtime. (Senokot/Senokot-S) 2 tabs qd. Max: 4 tabs bid. (SenokotXTRA) 1 tab qd. Max: 2 tabs bid. (Granules) 5mL qd. Max: 15mL bid. Granules may be eaten plain, mixed with liquids, or sprinkled on food.
Pediatrics: Take at bedtime. (Senokot/Senokot-S) ≥12 yrs: 2 tabs qd. Max: 4 tabs bid. 6-12 yrs: 1 tab qd. Max: 2 tabs bid. 2-6 yrs: 1/2 tab qd. Max: 1 tab bid. (SenokotXTRA) ≥12 yrs: 1 tab qd. Max: 2 tabs bid. 6-12 yrs: 1/2 tab qd. Max: 1 tab bid. (Granules) ≥12 yrs: 1 tsp qd. Max: 2 tsp bid. 6-12 yrs: 1/2 tsp qd. Max: 1 tsp bid. 2-6 yrs: 1/4 tsp qd. Max: 1/2 tsp bid. Granules may be eaten plain, mixed with liquids, or sprinkled on food.

HOW SUPPLIED: Granules: 15mg/dose; Tab (Sennoside A and B): (Senokot) 8.6mg, (SenokotXTRA) 17mg; (Docusate Sodium-Sennoside A and B) (Senokot-S) 50mg-8.6mg

WARNINGS/PRECAUTIONS: Do not use with abdominal pain, nausea, or vomiting. Should not be used for longer than 1 week. Rectal bleeding or failure to have a bowel movement after use may indicate serious condition.

INTERACTIONS: Avoid mineral oil with Senokot-S.

PREGNANCY: Safety in pregnancy and nursing not known.

SENSORCAINE WITH EPINEPHRINE RX
bupivacaine HCl - epinephrine (Abraxis)

OTHER BRAND NAME: Sensorcaine-MPF w/Epinephrine (Abraxis)

THERAPEUTIC CLASS: Local anesthetic

INDICATIONS: Production of local or regional anesthesia for surgery, oral surgery procedures, diagnostic and therapeutic procedures, and for obstetrical procedures. Only 0.25% and 0.5% are indicated for obstetrical anesthesia.

DOSAGE: *Adults:* Individualize dose. Dosage varies depending on procedure, area to be anesthetized, vascularity of tissues, number of neural segments to be blocked, depth and duration of anesthesia, degree of muscle relaxation required, and patient tolerance and physical condition. Single Dose Max: 225mg. May repeat once every 3 hrs. Total Daily Dose Max: 400mg. Epidural Anesthesia: 0.5% or 0.75% in 3-5mL increments. In obstetrics, use only 0.25% or 0.5%. Use 3-5mL increments of 0.5% solution not to exceed 50-100mg at any dosing interval. Repeat doses should be preceded by test dose containing epinephrine if not contraindicated. Young/Elderly/Debilitated/Cardiac or Liver Disease: Reduce dose.
Pediatrics: ≥12 yrs: Individualize dose. Dosage varies depending on procedure, area to be anesthetized, vascularity of tissues, number of neural segments to be blocked, depth and duration of anesthesia, degree of muscle relaxation required, and patient tolerance and physical condition. Single Dose Max: 225mg. May repeat once every 3 hrs. Total Daily Dose Max: 400mg. Epidural Anesthesia: 0.5% or 0.75% in 3-5mL increments. In obstetrics, use only 0.25% or 0.5%. Use 3-5mL increments of 0.5% solution not to exceed 50-100mg at any dosing interval. Repeat doses should be preceded by test dose containing epinephrine if not contraindicated.

HOW SUPPLIED: Inj: (Bupivacaine-Epinephrine) 0.25%/1:200,000, 0.5%/1:200,000; (MPF) 0.25%/1:200,000, 0.5%/1:200,000, 0.75%/1:200,000

CONTRAINDICATIONS: Obstetrical paracervical block anesthesia.

WARNINGS/PRECAUTIONS: The 0.75% strength is not recommended for obstetrical anesthesia. Acidosis, cardiac arrest, death reported from delay in toxicity management. Local anesthetic solutions containing antimicrobial preservatives should not be used for epidural or caudal anesthesia. Not recommended for IV regional anesthesia. Bupivacaine with epinephrine solutions contain sodium metabisulfite which may cause allergic-type reactions in susceptible people. Monitor cardiovascular and respiratory vital signs and state of consciousness after each injection. Caution when local anesthetic solutions containing a vasoconstrictor are used in areas of the body supplied by end arteries or having otherwise compromised blood supply; ischemic injury or necrosis may result with hypertensive vascular disease. Caution with hepatic disease and impaired cardiovascular function. Monitor circulation and respiration with injections into head and neck area. Respiratory arrest following local anesthetic injection during retrobulbar blocks has been reported.

ADVERSE REACTIONS: Restlessness, anxiety, dizziness, tinnitus, blurred vision, tremors, convulsions, NV, chills, hypotension, bradycardia, ventricular arrhythmias, urticaria, pruritus, erythema, edema.

INTERACTIONS: Avoid use with any other local anesthetics. Anesthetic solutions containing epinephrine or norepinephrine with MAOIs or TCAs may produce severe, prolonged HTN; avoid concurrent use or monitor closely if concurrent use is necessary. Concurrent administration of vasopressors and ergot-type oxytocic drugs may cause severe, persistent HTN or CVA. Phenothiazines and butyrophenones may reduce or reverse the pressor effect of epinephrine. Serious dose-related cardiac arrhythmias may occur with use during or following administration of potent inhalation anesthetics.

PREGNANCY: Category C, not for use in nursing.

MECHANISM OF ACTION: Long-acting amide-type local anaesthetic; causes a reversible blockade of impulse propagation along nerve fibres by preventing the inward movement of sodium ions through the cell membrane of the nerve fibres.

PHARMACOKINETICS: Absorption: Complete and biphasic. C_{max}=1-4mg/L; T_{max}=20-45 minutes. **Distribution:** V_d=73L; plasma protein binding (96%); crosses placenta; found in breast milk. **Metabolism:** Liver (extensive), through aromatic hydroxylation and N-dealkylation, via: CYP3A4 to PPX and 4-hydroxy-bupivacaine. **Elimination:** Urine (1%, unchanged); $T_{1/2}$=2.7 hrs (adults), $T_{1/2}$=8 hrs (neonates).

SENSORCAINE-MPF
bupivacaine HCl (Abraxis)

RX

THERAPEUTIC CLASS: Local anesthetic

INDICATIONS: Production of local or regional anesthesia for surgery, oral surgery procedures, diagnostic and therapeutic procedures, and for obstetrical procedures. Only 0.25% and 0.5% are indicated for obstetrical anesthesia.

DOSAGE: *Adults:* Individualize dose. Dosage varies depending on procedure, area to be anesthetized, vascularity of tissues, number of neural segments to be blocked, depth and duration of anesthesia, degree of muscle relaxation required, and patient tolerance and physical condition. Single Dose Max: 175mg. May repeat once every 3 hrs. Total Daily Dose Max: 400mg. Epidural Anesthesia: 0.5% or 0.75% in 3-5mL increments. In obstetrics, use only 0.25% or 0.5%. Use 3-5mL increments of 0.5% solution not to exceed 50-100mg at any dosing interval. Repeat doses should be preceded by test dose containing epinephrine if not contraindicated. Young/Elderly/Debilitated/Cardiac or Liver Disease: Reduce dose.
Pediatrics: ≥12 yrs: Individualize dose. Dosage varies depending on procedure, area to be anesthetized, vascularity of tissues, number of neural segments to be blocked, depth and duration of anesthesia, degree of muscle relaxation required, and patient tolerance and physical condition. Single Dose Max: 175mg. May repeat once every 3 hrs. Total Daily Dose Max: 400mg. Epidural Anesthesia: 0.5% in 3-5mL increments. In

obstetrics, use only 0.25% or 0.5%. Use 3-5mL increments of 0.5% solution not to exceed 50-100mg at any dosing interval. Repeat doses should be preceded by test dose containing epinephrine if not contraindicated.

HOW SUPPLIED: Inj: 0.25%, 0.5%; (MPF) 0.25%, 0.5%, 0.75%

CONTRAINDICATIONS: Obstetrical paracervical block anesthesia.

WARNINGS/PRECAUTIONS: The 0.75% strength is not recommended for obstetrical anesthesia. Acidosis, cardiac arrest, death reported from delay in toxicity management. Local anesthetic solutions containing antimicrobial preservatives should not be used for epidural or caudal anesthesia. Not recommended for IV regional anesthesia. Monitor cardiovascular and respiratory vital signs and state of consciousness after each injection. Caution with hepatic disease and impaired cardiovascular function. Monitor circulation and respiration with injections into head and neck area. Respiratory arrest following local anesthetic injection during retrobulbar blocks has been reported.

ADVERSE REACTIONS: Restlessness, anxiety, dizziness, tinnitus, blurred vision, tremors, convulsions, nausea, vomiting, chills, hypotension, bradycardia, ventricular arrhythmias, urticaria, pruritus, erythema, edema.

INTERACTIONS: Avoid use with any other local anesthetics.

PREGNANCY: Category C, not for use in nursing.

MECHANISM OF ACTION: A long-acting amide-type local anaesthetic; causes a reversible blockade of impulse propagation along nerve fibers by preventing the inward movement of sodium ions through the cell membrane of the nerve fibers.

PHARMACOKINETICS: Absorption: Complete and biphasic. C_{max}=1-4mg/L; T_{max}= 20-45 min. **Distribution:** V_d=73L; plasma protein binding (96%); crosses placenta, found in breast milk. **Metabolism:** Liver (extensive), through aromatic hydroxylation and N-dealkylation, via CYP3A4 to PPX and 4-hydroxy-bupivacaine. **Elimination:** Urine (1%, unchanged); $T_{1/2}$=2.7 hrs (adults), 8 hrs (neonates).

SEPTOCAINE WITH EPINEPHRINE RX
articaine HCl - epinephrine (Septodont)

THERAPEUTIC CLASS: Anesthetic agent

INDICATIONS: For local, infiltrative, or conductive anesthesia in both simple and complex dental and periodontal procedures.

DOSAGE: *Adults:* Submucosal Infiltration: 0.5-2.5mL. Nerve Block: 0.5-3.4mL. Oral Surgery: 1-5.1mL. Max: 7mg/kg (0.175mL/kg) or 3.2mg/lb (0.0795mL/lb).
Pediatrics: ≥4 yrs: Submucosal Infiltration/Nerve Block/Oral Surgery: up to 7mg/kg (0.175mL/kg) or 3.2mg/lb (0.0795mL/lb).

HOW SUPPLIED: Inj: (Articaine-Epinephrine) 4%-1:100,000/1.7mL, 4%-1:200,000/1.7ml.

CONTRAINDICATIONS: Hypersensitivity to sodium metabisulfite.

WARNINGS/PRECAUTIONS: Avoid intravascular injection; aspirate needle before use. Intravascular injection is associated with convulsions, followed by CNS or cardiorespiratory depression and coma progressing to respiratory arrest. Epinephrine can cause local tissue necrosis or systemic toxicity. Contains sodium metabisulfite which can cause allergic reactions. Exaggerated vasoconstrictive response may occur with peripheral vascular disease and hypertensive vascular disease. CNS or cardiovascular effects may occur with systemic absorption. Local anesthetics are capable of producing methemoglobinemia, with signs of cyanosis, fatigue, and weakness.

ADVERSE REACTIONS: Face edema, headache, infection, pain, gingivitis, swelling, paresthesia, trismus.

INTERACTIONS: MAOIs or TCAs may produce severe, prolonged HTN. Phenothiazines and butyrphenones may reduce or reverse pressor effect of epinephrine.

PREGNANCY: Category C, caution in nursing.

MECHANISM OF ACTION: Anaesthetic used in dental procedures.

SEPTRA

sulfamethoxazole - trimethoprim (King)

RX

OTHER BRAND NAMES: Septra DS (King) - Sulfatrim Pediatric (Alpharma)

THERAPEUTIC CLASS: Sulfonamide/tetrahydrofolic acid inhibitor

INDICATIONS: Treatment of urinary tract infections (UTI), acute otitis media, acute exacerbations of chronic bronchitis (AECB), *Pneumocystis carinii* pneumonia (PCP), traveler's diarrhea, and shigellosis caused by susceptible strains of microorganisms.

DOSAGE: *Adults:* UTI/Shigellosis: 800mg-160mg PO q12h for 10-14 days (UTI) or 5 days (shigellosis). AECB: 800mg-160mg PO q12h for 14 days. Traveler's Diarrhea: 800mg-160mg PO q12h for 5 days. PCP Treatment: 15-20mg/kg TMP and 75-100mg/kg SMX per 24 hrs given PO q6h for 14-21 days. PCP Prophylaxis: 800mg-160mg PO qd. Renal Impairment: CrCl 15-30mL/min: 50% usual dose. CrCl <15mL/min: Not recommended. *Pediatrics:* ≥2 months: UTI/Otitis Media/Shigellosis: 4mg/kg TMP and 20mg/kg SMX q12h for 10 days (UTI/otitis media) or 5 days (shigellosis). PCP Treatment: 15-20mg/kg TMP and 75-100mg/kg SMX per 24 hrs given q6h for 14-21 days. PCP Prophylaxis: 150mg/m^2/day TMP and 750mg/m^2/day SMX PO given bid, on 3 consecutive days per week. Max: 320mg TMP and 1600mg SMX per day. Renal Impairment: CrCl 15-30mL/min: 50% usual dose. CrCl <15mL/min: Not recommended.

HOW SUPPLIED: (Sulfamethoxazole (SMX)-Trimethoprim (TMP)) Sus: (Sulfatrim Pediatric, Septra) 200mg-40mg/5mL (100mL, 473mL); Tab: (Septra) *400mg-80mg**; Tab, DS: (Septra DS) *800mg-160mg** *scored*

CONTRAINDICATIONS: Megaloblastic anemia due to folate deficiency, pregnancy at term, nursing, infants <2 months old.

WARNINGS/PRECAUTIONS: Fatal hypersensitivity reactions (eg, Stevens-Johnson syndrome, toxic epidermal necrolysis, fulminant hepatic necrosis, agranulocytosis, aplastic anemia) may occur. Cough, SOB, and pulmonary infiltrates reported. Avoid with group A β-hemolytic streptococcal infections. *Clostridium difficile*-associated diarrhea reported. Caution with hepatic/renal impairment, elderly, folate deficiency (eg, chronic alcoholics, anticonvulsants, malabsorption, malnutrition), bronchial asthma, and other allergies. In G6PD deficiency, hemolysis may occur. Increased incidence of adverse events in AIDS patients. Maintain adequate fluid intake.

ADVERSE REACTIONS: Anorexia, NV, rash, urticaria, cough, SOB, cholestatic jaundice, agranulocytosis, anemia, hyperkalemia, renal failure, interstitial nephritis, hyponatremia, convulsions.

INTERACTIONS: Increase risk of thrombocytopenia with purpura with diuretics (especially thiazides) in the elderly. Caution with warfarin; may prolong PT. Increased effects of phenytoin, methotrexate. Concomitant ACE inhibitor therapy may cause hyperkalemia.

PREGNANCY: Category C, not for use in nursing.

MECHANISM OF ACTION: Sulfamethoxazole: Inhibits bacterial synthesis of dihydrofolic acid by competing with para-aminobenzoic acid (PABA). Trimetophrim: Blocks production of tetrahydrofolic acid from dihydrofolic acid by binding to and reversibly inhibiting required enzyme, dihydrofolate reductase; thus drug blocks 2 consecutive steps in biosynthesis of nucleic acids and proteins essential to many bacteria.

PHARMACOKINETICS: Absorption: Rapid; T_{max}=1-4 hrs. **Distribution:** Trimethoprim: Plasma protein binding (44%); Sulfamethoxazole: Plasma protein binding (70%). Crosses placenta, found in breast milk. **Metabolism:** Sulfamethoxazole: N_4 acetylation. Trimethoprim: 1-and 3-oxide, 3'-and 4'-hydroxy derivative (principal metabolites). **Elimination:** Urine, trimethoprim (66.8%), sulfamethoxazole (84.5%; 30% as free and remaining as N_4 acetylated metabolite); $T_{1/2}$=10 hr (sulfamethoxazole), 8-10 hr (trimethoprim).

SEREVENT

salmeterol xinafoate (GlaxoSmithKline)

RX

> Long-acting β$_2$-adrenergic agonists, such as salmeterol, may increase the risk of asthma-related deaths.

THERAPEUTIC CLASS: Beta$_2$ -agonist

SIMULECT

INDICATIONS: Long-term maintenance treatment of asthma and COPD. Prevention of bronchospasm with reversible obstructive airway disease (including nocturnal asthma) when regular treatment with inhaled short-acting β_2-agonists is required. Prevention of exercise-induced bronchospasm (EIB).

DOSAGE: *Adults:* Asthma/COPD: 1 inh bid, am and pm (12 hrs apart). EIB Prevention: 1 inh 30 min before exercise (do not give preventive doses if already on bid dose). *Pediatrics:* ≥4 yrs: Asthma: 1 inh bid, am and pm (12 hrs apart). EIB Prevention: 1 inh 30 min before exercise (do not give preventive doses if already on bid dose).

HOW SUPPLIED: Disk: 50mcg (28, 60 blisters)

WARNINGS/PRECAUTIONS: Avoid with significantly worsening or acutely deteriorating asthma. Not for acute treatment or substitute for oral/inhaled corticosteroids. Monitor for increasing use of inhaled β_2 agonists. QTc interval prolongation reported when exceeded recommended dose. D/C if paradoxical bronchospasm occurs. Immediate hypersensitivity and upper airway symptom reactions reported. Caution with cardiovascular disorder (eg, coronary insufficiency, arrhythmia, HTN), convulsive disorders, thyrotoxicosis, if usually unresponsive to sympathomimetic amines. May cause hypokalemia.

ADVERSE REACTIONS: Nasal/sinus congestion, pallor, rhinitis, headache, tracheitis/bronchitis, influenza, throat irritation.

INTERACTIONS: Caution with non-potassium-sparing diuretics. Extreme caution within 14 days of using MAOIs or TCAs. Avoid with β-blockers. Caution with >8 inhalations of short-acting β_2-agonists.

PREGNANCY: Category C, not for use in nursing.

MECHANISM OF ACTION: β_2-adrenergic agonist; increases cAMP levels causing relaxation of bronchial smooth muscles and inhibits the release of mediators of immediate hypersensitivity from mast cells.

PHARMACOKINETICS: Absorption: C_{max}=167pg/mL; T_{max}=20 min. **Distribution:** Plasma protein binding (96%). **Metabolism:** Liver (aliphatic oxidation) via CYP3A4. (Metabolite) α-hydroxysalmeterol. **Elimination:** $T_{1/2}$=5.5 hrs.

SIMULECT
basiliximab (Novartis)

RX

> **Manage patient in facility with adequate lab and supportive resources. Prescribing physician should be experienced with immunosuppressives and transplantation. Physician should have complete information requisite for patient follow-up.**

THERAPEUTIC CLASS: Monoclonal antibody/IL-2R alpha (CD25) blocker

INDICATIONS: Prophylaxis of acute organ rejection in renal transplantation.

DOSAGE: *Adults:* 20mg within 2 hrs prior to transplant, repeat 4 days after transplant. Withhold 2nd dose if graft loss or complications occur.
Pediatrics: ≥35kg: 20mg within 2 hrs prior to transplant, repeat 4 days after transplant. <35kg: 10mg within 2 hrs prior to transplant, repeat 4 days after transplant. Withhold 2nd dose if graft loss or complications occur.

HOW SUPPLIED: Inj: 10mg, 20mg

WARNINGS/PRECAUTIONS: Only administer under qualified medical supervision. Increased risk of developing lymphoproliferative disorder and opportunistic infections. Anaphylaxis and other severe hypersensitivity reactions (eg, hypotension, cardiac failure, bronchospasm, respiratory failure, etc) reported and may necessitate discontinuation. Anti-idiotype antibodies may develop.

ADVERSE REACTIONS: GI effects, peripheral edema, fever, viral infection, hyperkalemia, hypokalemia, hyperglycemia, hypercholesterolemia, hypophosphatemia, hyperuricemia, UTI, dyspnea, upper respiratory infection, acne, HTN, headache, tremor, insomnia, anemia.

PREGNANCY: Category B, not for use in nursing.

MECHANISM OF ACTION: Monoclonal antibody/IL-2Rα (CD25) blocker; acts as an IL-2 receptor antagonist by binding to the IL-2 receptor complex and inhibiting IL-2 binding. Specifically targeted against IL-2Rα, which is selectively expressed on the surface of activated T-lymphocytes. Binding to IL-2Rα causes competitive inhibition of IL-2-mediated activation of lymphocytes, a critical pathway in the cellular immune response involved in allograft rejection.

PHARMACOKINETICS: Absorption: C_{max}=7.1ng/mL (adult). **Distribution:** V_d=8.6L (adult); 4.8L (1-11 yrs); 7.8L (12-16 yrs). **Elimination:** $T_{1/2}$=7.2 days (adult); 9.5 days (1-11 yrs); 9.1 days (12-16 yrs).

SINGULAIR

montelukast sodium (Merck)

RX

THERAPEUTIC CLASS: Leukotriene receptor antagonist

INDICATIONS: Prophylaxis and chronic treatment of asthma (≥12 months). Relief of symptoms of seasonal allergic rhinitis (≥2 yrs) and perennial allergic rhinitis (≥6 months). Prevention of exercise-induced bronchoconstriction (EIB) (≥15 yrs).

DOSAGE: *Adults:* Asthma: 10mg qpm. Allergic Rhinitis: 10mg qd. EIB: 10mg 2 hrs before exercise. Do not take additional dose within 24 hrs of previous dose.
Pediatrics: Asthma:≥15 yrs: 10mg qpm. 6-14 yrs: 5mg qpm. 2-5 yrs: 4mg qpm. 6-23 months: 4mg qpm. Seasonal/Perennial Allergic Rhinitis: ≥15 yrs: 10mg qd. 6-14 yrs: 5mg qd. 2-5 yrs: 4mg qd. Perennial Allergic Rhinitis: 6-23 months: 4mg qd. EIB: ≥15 yrs: 10mg 2 hrs before exercise. Do not take additional dose within 24 hrs of previous dose. Granules may be mixed with applesauce, carrots, rice, or ice cream; give within 15 min of opening pkt.

HOW SUPPLIED: Granules: 4mg/pkt; Tab, Chewable: 4mg, 5mg; Tab: 10mg

WARNINGS/PRECAUTIONS: Not for treatment of acute asthma attacks. Do not abruptly substitute for inhaled or oral corticosteroids. Eosinophilic conditions reported (rare).

ADVERSE REACTIONS: (Adults, Pediatrics) Headache, abdominal pain, dyspepsia, cough, flu. (Pediatrics) Pharyngitis, flu, fever, sinusitis, nausea, diarrhea, dyspepsia, otitis, viral infection, laryngitis.

INTERACTIONS: Monitor with potent CYP450 inducers (eg, phenobarbital, rifampin).

PREGNANCY: Category B, caution in nursing.

MECHANISM OF ACTION: Leukotriene receptor antagonist; binds to cysteinyl leukotriene receptors found on airway smooth muscle cells and macrophages and other pro-inflammatory cells (eg, eosinophils); inhibits physiologic actions of leukotrienes.

PHARMACOKINETICS: Absorption: Rapid. (10mg) Bioavailability (64%) T_{max}=3-4 hrs. (5mg) T_{max}=2-2.5 hrs. Bioavailability (73%, fasted), (63%, fed). Fasted 2-5 yrs: (4mg Chewable) T_{max}=2 hrs. (4mg Granules) T_{max}=2.3 hrs (fasted), 6.4 hrs (fed). **Distribution:** V_d=8-11L; plasma protein binding (99%). **Metabolism:** Liver (extensive); CYP3A4, 2C9. **Elimination:** Biliary (major); $T_{1/2}$=2.7-5.5 hrs.

SKELAXIN

metaxalone (King)

RX

THERAPEUTIC CLASS: Muscular analgesic (central-acting)

INDICATIONS: Adjunct for acute, painful musculoskeletal conditions.

DOSAGE: *Adults:* 800mg tid-qid.
Pediatrics: >12 yrs: 800mg tid-qid.

HOW SUPPLIED: Tab: 800mg* *scored

CONTRAINDICATIONS: Tendency for drug-induced, hemolytic, and other anemias. Significant renal or hepatic impairment.

WARNINGS/PRECAUTIONS: Caution with pre-existing liver damage. Monitor hepatic function. False-positive Benedict's test reported.

ADVERSE REACTIONS: Nausea, vomiting, GI upset, drowsiness, dizziness, headache, nervousness, leukopenia, hemolytic anemia, jaundice.

INTERACTIONS: May enhance the effects of alcohol, barbiturates and other CNS depressants.

PREGNANCY: Not for use in pregnancy or nursing.

MECHANISM OF ACTION: Centrally acting muscular analgesic; not established; activity may be due to general depression of CNS.

PHARMACOKINETICS: Absorption: (400mg) C_{max}=983ng/mL, T_{max}= 3.3 hrs, AUC=7479ng•hr/mL; (800mg) C_{max}=1816ng/mL, T_{max}=3.0 hrs, AUC=15044ng•hr/mL. **Distribution:** Extensive in tissues; V_d=800L. **Metabolism:** Liver. **Elimination:** Urine (metabolites); $T_{1/2}$=9 hrs.

SOLAQUIN FORTE

RX

hydroquinone (Valeant)

THERAPEUTIC CLASS: Depigmenting agent

INDICATIONS: For the gradual bleaching of hyperpigmented skin conditions (eg, chloasma, melasma, freckles, senile lentigines).

DOSAGE: *Adults:* Apply bid.
Pediatrics: ≥12 yrs: Apply bid.

HOW SUPPLIED: Cre: 4% (28.4g); Gel: 4% (28.4g)

WARNINGS/PRECAUTIONS: Avoid sun exposure on bleached skin. Solaquin Forte contains sunscreen. May produce unwanted cosmetic effects if not used as directed. Test for skin sensitivity. D/C if no lightening effect after 2 months. Contains sodium metabisulfite, may cause serious allergic type reactions. Limit treatment to small areas of body at one time. Avoid contact with eyes.

ADVERSE REACTIONS: Cutaneous hypersensitivity (contact dermatitis).

PREGNANCY: Category C, caution in nursing.

MECHANISM OF ACTION: Reversible depigmentaion of the skin by inhibition of enzymatic oxidation of tyrosine to 3,4-dihydroxyphenylalanine (dopa) and suppression of other melanocyte metabolic processes.

SOLODYN

RX

minocycline HCl (Medicis)

THERAPEUTIC CLASS: Tetracycline derivative

INDICATIONS: Treatment of inflammatory lesions of non-nodular moderate to severe acne vulgaris in patients ≥12 yrs.

DOSAGE: *Adults:* 1mg/kg qd for 12 weeks. Reduce dose with renal impairment.
Pediatrics: ≥12 yrs: 1mg/kg qd for 12 weeks. Reduce dose with renal impairment.

HOW SUPPLIED: Tab, Extended-Release: 45mg, 90mg, 135mg.

WARNINGS/PRECAUTIONS: May cause fetal harm during pregnancy. Use during tooth development (last half of pregnancy, infancy, <8yrs) may cause permanent discoloration of the teeth or enamel hypoplasia; avoid use during this period. May decrease bone growth in premature infants. May cause pseudomembranous colitis. Renal toxicity, hepatotoxicity, photosensitivity, increased BUN, superinfection, pseudotumor cerebri may occur. Caution in renal impairment; may lead to azotemia, hyperphosphatemia, and acidosis. Long-term use has been associated with lupus-like syndrome, autoimmune hepatitis and vasculitis. May cause serum sickness. May induce hyperpigmentation.

ADVERSE REACTIONS: Headache, fatigue, dizziness, pruritus, malaise, mood alteration, Stevens-Johnson syndrome, photosensitivity.

INTERACTIONS: May require downward regulation of anticoagulant therapy. May interfere with bactericidal action of penicillin; avoid concurrent. May decrease efficacy of oral contraceptives. Impaired absorption with antacids containing aluminum, calcium or magnesium, and iron-containing preparations. Fatal renal toxicity with methoxyflurane reported.

PREGNANCY: Category D, not for use in nursing.

MECHANISM OF ACTION: Tetracycline derivative; inhibits bacterial protein synthesis.

PHARMACOKINETICS: Absorption: C_{max}=2.63mcg/mL; T_{max}=3.5-4 hrs; AUC=33.32mcg•hr/mL.

SOLU-CORTEF

RX

hydrocortisone sodium succinate (Pharmacia & Upjohn)

THERAPEUTIC CLASS: Corticosteroid

INDICATIONS: Steroid-responsive disorders.

DOSAGE: *Adults:* Initial: 100-500mg IV/IM, depending on condition severity. May repeat dose at 2, 4, or 6 hrs based on clinical response. High dose therapy usually not >48-72 hrs; may use antacids prophylactically.
Pediatrics: Use lower adult doses. Determine dose by severity of condition and response. Dose should not be <25mg/day.

HOW SUPPLIED: Inj: 100mg, 250mg, 500mg, 1g

CONTRAINDICATIONS: Premature infants, systemic fungal infections.

WARNINGS/PRECAUTIONS: May need to increase dose before, during, and after stressful situations. May mask signs of infection or cause new infections. Prolonged use may produce glaucoma, optic nerve damage, secondary ocular infections. Increases BP, salt/water retention, potassium and calcium excretion. More severe/fatal course of infections reported with chickenpox, measles. Enhanced effect with hypothyroidism or cirrhosis. Caution with Strongyloides, latent TB, ocular herpes simplex, HTN, diverticulitis, fresh intestinal anastomoses, ulcerative colitis, osteoporosis, myasthenia gravis, renal insufficiency, peptic ulcer disease. Kaposi's sarcoma reported. Monitor for psychic disturbances. Acute myopathy with high doses. Avoid abrupt withdrawal. Monitor growth and development of children on prolonged therapy. Hypernatremia may occur with high dose therapy >48-72 hrs.

ADVERSE REACTIONS: Fluid and electrolyte disturbances, HTN, osteoporosis, muscle weakness, cushingoid state, menstrual irregularities, vertigo, headache, impaired wound healing, DM, ulcerative esophagitis, peptic ulcer, pancreatitis, increased sweating, increases intracranial pressure, carbohydrate intolerance, glaucoma, cataracts.

INTERACTIONS: Reduced efficacy and increased clearance with hepatic enzyme inducers (eg, phenobarbital, phenytoin, and rifampin). Increases clearance of chronic high dose ASA. Caution with ASA in hypoprothrombinemia. Effects on oral anticoagulants are variable; monitor PT/INR. Increased insulin and oral hypoglycemic requirements in DM. Avoid live vaccines with immunosuppressive doses. Possible decreased vaccine response with killed or inactivated vaccines with immunosuppressive doses. Decreased clearance with ketoconazole and troleandomycin.

PREGNANCY: Safety in pregnancy and nursing not known.

MECHANISM OF ACTION: Anti-inflammatory glucocorticoid; causes profound and varied metabolic effects and modifies the body's immune responses to diverse stimuli.

PHARMACOKINETICS: Absorption: (IM) Rapidly absorbed. T_{max}=1 hr. **Distribution:** Found in breast milk. **Elimination:** $T_{1/2}$=12 hrs.

SOLU-MEDROL

RX

methylprednisolone sodium succinate (Pharmacia & Upjohn)

THERAPEUTIC CLASS: Glucocorticoid

INDICATIONS: Steroid-responsive disorders.

DOSAGE: *Adults:* Usual: Initial: 10-40mg IV over several min. May repeat IV/IM dose at intervals based on clinical response. High-Dose Therapy: 30mg/kg IV over at least 30 min, may repeat q4-6h for 48 hrs. High dose therapy usually not >48-72 hrs. Give antacids prophylactically. Multiple Sclerosis: (4mg methylprednisolone=5mg prednisolone): 200mg/day prednisolone for 1 week, then 80mg every other day for 1 month.
Pediatrics: Use lower adult doses. Determine dose by severity of condition and response. Dose should not be <0.5mg/kg q24h.

HOW SUPPLIED: Inj: 40mg, 125mg, 500mg, 1g, 2g

CONTRAINDICATIONS: Premature infants (due to benzyl alcohol diluent) and systemic fungal infections.

WARNINGS/PRECAUTIONS: May need to increase dose before, during, and after stressful situations. May mask signs of infection or cause new infections. Prolonged use may produce cataracts, glaucoma, secondary ocular infections. Increases BP, salt/water retention, calcium/potassium excretion. More severe/fatal course of infections reported with chickenpox, measles. Caution with latent TB, hypothyroidism, cirrhosis, ocular herpes simplex, HTN, diverticulitis, fresh intestinal anastomoses, ulcerative colitis, osteoporosis, myasthenia gravis, renal insufficiency, peptic ulcer disease. Kaposi's sarcoma reported. Growth and development of children on prolonged therapy should be monitored. Monitor for psychic disturbances. Avoid abrupt withdrawal. Reports of cardiac arrhythmias, circulatory collapse, cardiac arrest following rapid administration of large IV doses. Effectiveness not established for the treatment of sepsis syndrome and septic shock. Bradycardia reportedwith high doses.

ADVERSE REACTIONS: Fluid and electrolyte disturbances, HTN, osteoporosis, muscle weakness, cushingoid state, menstrual irregularities, insomnia, impaired wound healing, DM, ulcerative esophagitis, excessive sweating, increases intracranial pressure, carbohydrate intolerance, glaucoma, cataracts, nausea.

INTERACTIONS: Reduced efficacy with hepatic enzyme inducers (eg, phenobarbital, phenytoin, and rifampin). Increases clearance of chronic high dose ASA. Caution with ASA in hypoprothrombinemia. Effects on oral anticoagulants are variable; monitor PT/INR. Increased insulin and oral hypoglycemic requirements in DM. Avoid live vaccines with immunosuppressive doses. Possible decreased vaccine response with killed or inactivated vaccines with immunosuppressive doses. Mutual inhibition of metabolism with cyclosporine; convulsions reported. Decreased clearance with ketoconazole and troleandomycin.

PREGNANCY: Safety in pregnancy and nursing not known.

MECHANISM OF ACTION: Anti-inflammatory glucocorticoid; causes profound and varied metabolic effects and modifies the body's immune responses to diverse stimuli.

SOMA   RX
carisoprodol (MedPointe)

THERAPEUTIC CLASS: Skeletal muscle relaxant (central-acting)

INDICATIONS: Relief of discomfort associated with acute, painful musculoskeletal conditions.

DOSAGE: *Adults:* ≤65 yrs: 250-350mg tid and hs for 2-3 weeks.
Pediatrics: ≥16 yrs: 250-350mg tid and hs for 2-3 weeks.

HOW SUPPLIED: Tab: 250mg, 350mg

CONTRAINDICATIONS: Acute intermittent porphyria and hypersensitivity to a carbamate.

WARNINGS/PRECAUTIONS: May have sedative properties. Cases of drug abuse, dependence and withdrawal reported. Caution in addiction-prone patients. First-dose idiosyncratic reactions reported (rare). Occasionally within period of 1st-4th dose, allergic reactions have occured. Rare reports of seizures in postmarketing surveillance. Caution with liver or renal dysfunction. Seizures reported.

ADVERSE REACTIONS: Drowsiness, dizziness, headache, nausea, vomiting, tachycardia, postural hypotension, agitation, irritability, insomnia, seizures.

INTERACTIONS: Additive effects with alcohol, other CNS depressants, and psychotropic drugs. Concomitant use with meprobamate not recommended. Coadministration with CYP2C19 inhibitors (eg, omeprazole, fluvoxamine); may increase levels and CYP2C19 inducers (eg, St.Johns wort, rifampin); may decrease levels.

PREGNANCY: Category C, caution in nursing.

MECHANISM OF ACTION: Skeletal muscle relaxant; not clearly identified; suspected to relieve discomfort associated with acute painful musculoskeletal conditions.

PHARMACOKINETICS: Absorption: Carisoprodol: (250mg) C_{max}=1.2mcg/mL, T_{max}=1.5 hrs, AUC=4.5mcg•hr/mL; (350mg) C_{max}=1.8mcg/mL, T_{max}=1.7 hrs, AUC=7.0mcg•hr/mL. Meprobamate: (250mg) C_{max}=1.8mcg/mL, T_{max}= 3.6 hrs, AUC=32mcg•hr/mL; (350mg) C_{max}=2.5mcg/mL, T_{max}=4.5 hr, AUC=46mcg•hr/mL. **Distribution:** Found in breast milk. **Metabolism:** Liver via CYP2C19. Meprobamate (metabolite). **Elimination:** Urine, carisoprodol: $T_{1/2}$=1.7 hrs (250mg), 2.0 hrs (350mg). Meprobamate: $T_{1/2}$=9.7 hrs (250mg), 9.6 hrs (350mg).

SOMA CMPD/CODEINE `CIII`
aspirin - carisoprodol - codeine phosphate (MedPointe)

THERAPEUTIC CLASS: Central muscle relaxant/analgesic

INDICATIONS: Adjunct for relief of pain, muscle spasm, and limited mobility associated with acute, painful musculoskeletal conditions.

DOSAGE: *Adults:* 1-2 tabs qid.
Pediatrics: ≥12 yrs: 1-2 tabs qid.

HOW SUPPLIED: Tab: (Carisoprodol-Codeine-Aspirin) 200mg-16mg-325mg

CONTRAINDICATIONS: Acute intermittent porphyria, bleeding disorders.

WARNINGS/PRECAUTIONS: First-dose idiosyncratic reactions reported (rare). Contains sodium metabisulfate; may cause allergic type reactions. Caution with liver or renal dysfunction, elderly, peptic ulcer, gastritis, addiction-prone patients and anticoagulant therapy. Caution in individuals who are ultra rapid metabolizers of codeine.

ADVERSE REACTIONS: Drowsiness, dizziness, vertigo, ataxia, nausea, vomiting, gastritis, occult bleeding, constipation, diarrhea, miosis, allergic-skin rash, postural hypotension.

INTERACTIONS: Enhances methotrexate toxicity and hypoglycemia with oral antidiabetics. Corticosteroids and antacids decrease plasma levels. Increases GI bleeding risk with alcohol. Potentiated by urine acidifiers (eg, ammonium chloride). Antagonizes uricosuric effects of probenecid, sulfinpyrazone. Additive effects with alcohol, other CNS depressants, psychotropic drugs. Increases bleeding risk with anticoagulants.

PREGNANCY: Category C, not for use in nursing.

MECHANISM OF ACTION: Carisoprodol: Centrally acting muscle relaxant; does not directly relax tense skeletal muscle. Action in relieving acute muscle spasm not established; may be related to its sedative properties. ASA: Inhibits prostaglandin biosynthesis producing anti-inflammatory, analgesic, and antipyretic properties. Codeine: Centrally acting narcotic-analgesic.

PHARMACOKINETICS: Absorption: ASA: Rapid. **Distribution:** Carisoprodol, ASA, and Codeien: Found in breast milk. **Metabolism:** Carisoprodol: Liver. ASA: Hydrolyzed to salicylic acid. Codeine: Liver. **Elimination:** Carisoprodol: Urine; $T_{1/2}$=2.4 hr (parent), 10 hr (metabolite). ASA: Urine; $T_{1/2}$=15 min. Codeine: Urine (5-15% unchanged). $T_{1/2}$=2.5-4 hr.

SOMA COMPOUND RX
aspirin - carisoprodol (MedPointe)

THERAPEUTIC CLASS: Central muscle relaxant/analgesic

INDICATIONS: Adjunct for pain, muscle spasm and limited mobility associated with acute, painful musculoskeletal conditions.

DOSAGE: *Adults:* 1-2 tabs qid.
Pediatrics: ≥12 yrs: 1-2 tabs qid.

HOW SUPPLIED: Tab: (Carisoprodol-ASA) 200mg-325mg

CONTRAINDICATIONS: Acute intermittent porphyria, bleeding disorders.

WARNINGS/PRECAUTIONS: First-dose idiosyncratic reactions reported (rare). Caution with liver or renal dysfunction, elderly, peptic ulcer, gastritis, addiction-prone patients and anticoagulant therapy.

ADVERSE REACTIONS: Drowsiness, dizziness, vertigo, ataxia, nausea, vomiting, gastritis, occult bleeding, constipation, diarrhea.

INTERACTIONS: Enhances methotrexate toxicity and hypoglycemia with oral antidiabetics. Corticosteroids and antacids decrease plasma levels. Increases GI bleeding risk with alcohol. Potentiated by urine acidifiers (eg, ammonium chloride). Antagonizes uricosuric effects of probenecid, sulfinpyrazone. Additive effects with alcohol, other CNS depressants, psychotropic drugs. Increases bleeding risk with anticoagulants.

PREGNANCY: Category C, not for use in nursing.

MECHANISM OF ACTION: Carisoprodol: Centrally acting muscle relaxant; does not directly relax tense skeletal muscle. Action in relieving acute muscle spasm not established; may be related to its sedative properties. ASA: Inhibits prostaglandin biosynthesis producing anti-inflammatory, analgesic, and antipyretic properties.

PHARMACOKINETICS: Absorption: ASA: Rapid. **Distribution:** Carisoprodol, ASA: Found in breast milk. **Metabolism:** Carisoprodol: Liver. ASA: Hydrolyzed to salicylic acid. **Elimination:** Carisoprodol: Urine. ASA: Urine; $T_{1/2}$=15 min.

SPECTRACEF   RX
cefditoren pivoxil (Cornerstone)

THERAPEUTIC CLASS: Cephalosporin (3rd generation)

INDICATIONS: Treatment of acute bacterial exacerbations of chronic bronchitis (ABECB), pharyngitis/tonsillitis, community-acquired pneumonia (CAP), and uncomplicated skin and skin structure infections (SSSI) caused by susceptible strains of microorganisms.

DOSAGE: *Adults:* ABECB: 400mg bid for 10 days. Pharyngitis/Tonsillitis/SSSI: 200mg bid for 10 days. CAP: 400mg bid for 14 days. CrCl 30-49mL/min: 200mg bid. CrCl <30mL/min: 200mg qd. Take with meals.
Pediatrics: ≥12 yrs: ABECB: 400mg bid for 10 days. Pharyngitis/Tonsillitis/SSSI: 200mg bid for 10 days. CAP: 400mg bid for 14 days. CrCl 30-49mL/min: 200mg bid. CrCl <30mL/min: 200mg qd. Take with meals.

HOW SUPPLIED: Tab: 200mg

CONTRAINDICATIONS: Milk protein hypersensitivity, carnitine deficiency.

WARNINGS/PRECAUTIONS: Cross sensitivity to PCNs and other cephalosporins may occur. Pseudomembranous colitis reported. Not recommended for prolonged antibiotic therapy. Prolonged therapy may cause superinfection. May decrease PT.

ADVERSE REACTIONS: Diarrhea, nausea, vaginal moniliasis, headache.

INTERACTIONS: Avoid concomitant antacids and H_2 receptor antagonists. Increased plasma levels with probenecid.

PREGNANCY: Category B, caution in nursing.

MECHANISM OF ACTION: 3rd generation cephalosporin; inhibits cell-wall synthesis via affinity for penicillin-binding proteins (PBPs).

PHARMACOKINETICS: Absorption: C_{max}=1.8mcg/mL (200mg, fasting), 3.1mcg/mL (200mg, high-fat meal), 4.4mcg/mL (400mg, high-fat meal); T_{max}=1.5-3 hrs (fasting). Absolute bioavailability: 14% (fasting), 16.1 (low-fat meal). **Distribution:** V_d=9.3L; plasma protein binding: 88%; found in breast milk. **Metabolism:** Hydrolysis, via esterases to cefditoren (active component). **Elimination:** Urine; $T_{1/2}$=1.6 hrs.

STRATTERA   RX
atomoxetine HCl (Lilly)

> Increased risk of suicidal ideation in short-term studies in children or adolescents with ADHD. Closely monitor for suicidality, clinical worsening, or unusual changes in behavior. Close observation/communication with prescriber by families and caregivers is advised.

THERAPEUTIC CLASS: Selective norepinephrine reuptake inhibitor

INDICATIONS: Treatment of attention-deficit hyperactivity disorder (ADHD).

DOSAGE: *Adults:* Initial: 40mg/day given qam or evenly divided doses in the am and late afternoon/early evening. Titrate: Increase after minimum of 3 days to target dose of about 80mg/day. After 2-4 weeks, may increase to max of 100mg/day. Max: 100mg/day. Hepatic Insufficiency: Moderate (Child-Pugh Class B): Reduce initial and target doses to 50% of normal dose. Severe (Child-Pugh Class C): Reduce initial and target doses to 25% of normal dose. Concomitant CYP450 2D6 inhibitor (eg, paroxetine, fluoxetine, quinidine): Initial: 40mg/day. Titrate: Only increase to 80mg/day if symptoms fail to improve after 4 weeks.
Pediatrics: ≥6 yrs: ≤70kg: Initial: 0.5mg/kg/day given qam or evenly divided doses in the am and late afternoon or early evening. Titrate: Increase after minimum of 3 days to target dose of about 1.2mg/kg/day. Max: 1.4mg/kg/day or 100mg, whichever is less.

>70kg: Initial: 40mg/day given qam or evenly divided doses in the am and late afternoon/early evening. Titrate: Increase after minimum of 3 days to target dose of about 80mg/day. After 2-4 weeks, may increase to max of 100mg/day. Max: 100mg/day. Hepatic Insufficiency: Moderate (Child-Pugh Class B): Reduce initial and target doses to 50% of the normal dose. Severe (Child-Pugh Class C): Reduce initial and target doses to 25% of normal dose. Concomitant CYP450 2D6 inhibitor (eg, paroxetine, fluoxetine, quinidine): ≥6 yrs: ≤70kg: Initial: 0.5mg/kg/day. Titrate: Only increase to 1.2mg/kg/day if symptoms fail to improve after 4 weeks. >70kg: Initial: 40mg/day, Titrate: Only increase to 80mg/day if symptoms fail to improve after 4 weeks.

HOW SUPPLIED: Cap: 10mg, 18mg, 25mg, 40mg, 60mg, 80mg, 100mg

CONTRAINDICATIONS: During or within 14 days of MAOI use; narrow angle glaucoma.

WARNINGS/PRECAUTIONS: Monitor for clinical worsening and/or suicidality. Allergic reactions, orthostatic hypotension and syncope reported. Monitor growth. May increase BP and HR; caution with HTN, tachycardia, cardiovascular or cerebrovascular disease. May increase urinary retention and urinary hesitation. Rare cases of priapism reported. May cause severe liver injury in rare cases; monitor liver enzymes and d/c with jaundice or liver injury. Reports of MI, stroke and sudden death in adults. Avoid with known structural cardiac abnormalities or other serious cardiac problems. Physical exam and evaluation of patient history is necessary. Stimulants at usual doses can cause treatment-emergent psychotic or manic symptoms (eg, hallucinations, delusional thinking, mania) in children and adolescents without prior history of psychotic illness. Monitor for appearance or worsening of aggressive behavior or hostility.

ADVERSE REACTIONS: (Adults) Dry mouth, headache, insomnia, nausea, decreased appetite, constipation, dysmenorrhea, erectile disturbance, urinary retention. (Pediatrics) Upper abdominal pain, headache, vomiting, decreased appetite, irritability, dizziness, somnolence.

INTERACTIONS: See Contraindications. May potentiate the cardiovascular effects of albuterol or other β_2 agonists. Caution with pressor agents. Increased levels in extensive metabolizers with CYP2D6 inhibitors (eg, paroxetine, fluoxetine, quinidine); atomoxetine may need dose adjustment.

PREGNANCY: Category C, caution in nursing.

MECHANISM OF ACTION: Selective norepinephrine reuptake inhibitor; inhibits the presynaptic norepinephrine transporter, as determined in *ex vivo* uptake.

PHARMACOKINETICS: Absorption: (PO) rapid; T_{max}=1-2 hrs. **Distribution:** Plasma protein binding (98%). **Metabolism:** Via CYP2D6; 4-hydroxyatomoxetine (major metabolite). **Elimination:** Urine (>80%), feces (<17%); $T_{1/2}$=5 hrs;

STREPTOMYCIN

RX

streptomycin sulfate (Various)

> Risk of severe neurotoxic reactions (eg, vestibular and cochlear disturbances) increased significantly with renal dysfunction or pre-renal azotemia. Optic nerve dysfunction, peripheral neuritis, arachnoiditis, and encephalopathy may occur. Monitor renal function; reduce dose with renal impairment and/or nitrogen retention. Do not exceed peak serum level of 20-25mcg/mL with kidney damage. Avoid other neurotoxic and/or nephrotoxic drugs (eg, neomycin, kanamycin, gentamicin, cephaloridine, paromomycin, viomycin, polymyxin B, colistin, tobramycin, cyclosporine). Respiratory paralysis can occur, especially if given soon after anesthesia or muscle relaxants. Reserve parenteral form when adequate lab and audiometric testing is available.

THERAPEUTIC CLASS: Aminoglycoside

INDICATIONS: Treatment of moderate to severe infections such as mycobacterium tuberculosis (TB) and non-TB infections (eg, plague, tularemia, chancroid, granuloma inguinale, *H.influenzae* and *K.pneumoniae* infections, UTI, gram-negative bacillary bacteremia, endocardial infections).

DOSAGE: *Adults:* IM only. TB: 15mg/kg/day (Max: 1g), or 25-30mg/kg twice weekly (Max: 1.5g), or 25-30mg/kg three times weekly (Max: 1.5g). Do not exceed a total dose of 120g over the course of therapy unless no other therapeutic options exist. Elderly (>60 yrs): Reduce dose. Treat for minimum of 1 year if possible. Tularemia: 1-2g/day in divided doses for 7-14 days until afebrile for 5-7 days. Plague: 1g bid for minimum of 10 days. Streptococcal Endocarditis: With PCN, 1g bid for week 1, then 500mg bid for week 2. Elderly (>60 yrs): 500mg bid for 2 weeks. Enterococcal Endocarditis: With PCN,

1g bid for 2 weeks, then 500mg bid for 4 weeks. Renal Impairment: Reduce dose. Moderate/Severe Infections: 1-2g/day in divided doses q6-12h. Max: 2g/day. *Pediatrics:* IM only. TB: 20-40mg/kg/day (Max: 1g), or 25-30mg/kg twice weekly (Max: 1.5g), or 25-30mg/kg three times weekly (Max: 1.5g). Do not exceed a total dose of 120g over the course of therapy unless no other therapeutic options exist. Treat for minimum of 1 year if possible. Moderate/Severe Infections: 20-40mg/kg/day (8-20mg/lb/day) in divided doses q6-12h.

HOW SUPPLIED: Inj: 1g

WARNINGS/PRECAUTIONS: Vestibular and auditory dysfunction may occur. Contains sodium metabisulfite. Can cause fetal harm in pregnancy. Caution with dose selection in renal impairment. Alkalinize urine to minimize or prevent renal irritation with prolonged therapy. CNS depression (eg, stupor, flaccidity) reported in infants with higher than recommended doses. If syphilis is suspected when treating venereal infections, perform dark field exam before initiate treatment, and monthly serologic tests for at least 4 months. Overgrowth of nonsusceptible organisms may occur. Terminate therapy when toxic symptoms appear, when impending toxicity is feared, when organisms become resistant, or when full treatment effect has been obtained. Contains sodium metabisulfite, a sulfite that may cause allergic type reactions including anaphylaxis.

ADVERSE REACTIONS: Vestibular ototoxicity (NV, vertigo), paresthesia of face, rash, fever, urticaria, angioneurotic edema, eosinophilia, nephrotoxicity (rare).

INTERACTIONS: See Black Box Warning. Increased ototoxicity with ethacrynic acid, furosemide, mannitol and possibly other diuretics.

PREGNANCY: Category D, not for use in nursing.

MECHANISM OF ACTION: Aminoglycoside agent; interferes with normal protein synthesis.

PHARMACOKINETICS: Absorption: C_{max}=25-50mcg/mL; T_{max}=1 hr. **Distribution:** Passes through placenta; found in breast milk. **Elimination:** Urine (29-89%).

STROMECTOL
ivermectin (Merck)

RX

THERAPEUTIC CLASS: Avermectins derivative

INDICATIONS: Treatment of strongyloidiasis of the intestinal tract due to *Strongyloides stercoralis*, and onchocerciasis due to *Onchocerca volvulus*. Has no activity against adult *Onchocerca volvulus* parasites.

DOSAGE: *Adults:* Strongyloidiasis: 200mcg/kg single dose. Onchocerciasis: 150mcg/kg single dose. For mass distribution in international treatment programs, the usual dosing interval is 12 months. Usual dosing interval for retreatment for individual patients can be as short as 3 months. Take on empty stomach with water. To verify eradication of infection perform follow-up stool exams.
Pediatrics: ≥15kg: Strongyloidiasis: 200mcg/kg single dose. Onchocerciasis: 150mcg/kg single dose. For mass distribution in international treatment programs, the usual dosing interval is 12 months. Usual dosing interval for retreatment for individual patients can be as short as 3 months. Take on empty stomach with water. To verify eradication of infection perform follow-up stool exams.

HOW SUPPLIED: Tab: 3mg, 6mg* *scored

WARNINGS/PRECAUTIONS: May cause cutaneous and/or systemic reactions of varying severity (the Mazzotti reaction) and ophthalmological reactions. Patients with hyperreactive onchodermatitis (sowda) may be more likely to experience severe advisers reactions, especially edema and aggravation of onchodermatitis. Risk of serious or even fatal encephalopathy with onchocerciasis and *Loa loa* infection. Pretreatment assessment for loiasis and careful posttreatment follow-up should be performed in patients who were exposed to *Loa loa*-endemic areas of West or Central Africa.

ADVERSE REACTIONS: Diarrhea, nausea, dizziness, pruritis, decrease in leukocyte count, arthralgia/synovitis, axillary/cervical/inguinal lymph node enlargement, rash, fever, peripheral edema, tachycardia.

PREGNANCY: Category C, caution in nursing.

MECHANISM OF ACTION: Avermectin derivative; binds selectively and with high affinity to glutamate-gated chloride ion channels, which occur in invertebrate nerve and muscle cells. This leads to increase in permeability of cell membrane to chloride ions with hyperpolarization of nerve and muscle cell, resulting in paralysis and death of parasite.

PHARMACOKINETICS: Absorption: Administration of variable doses resulted in different parameters. **Metabolism:** Liver. **Elimination:** Feces, urine (≤1%); $T_{1/2}$=18 hrs.

SUBLIMAZE
fentanyl citrate (Akorn)

THERAPEUTIC CLASS: Opioid analgesic

INDICATIONS: For analgesic action of short duration during the anesthetic periods, pre-medication, induction and maintenance, and in the immediate postoperative period (recovery room) as the need arises. For use as a narcotic analgesic supplement in general or regional anesthesia. For administration with a neuroleptic as an anesthetic pre-medication, for the induction of anesthesia and as an adjunct in the maintenance of general and regional anesthesia. For use as an anesthetic agent with oxygen in selected high risk patients, such as those undergoing open heart surgery or certain complicated neurological or orthopedic procedures.

DOSAGE: *Adults:* ≥12 yrs: Individualize dose. Premedication: 50-100mcg IM 30-60 min prior to surgery. Adjunct to General Anesthesia: Low-Dose: Total Dose: 2mcg/kg for minor surgery. Maint: 2mcg/kg. Moderate Dose: Total Dose: 2-20mcg/kg for major surgery. Maint: 2-20mcg/kg or 25-100mcg IM or IV if surgical stress or lightening of analgesia. High-Dose: Total Dose: 20-50mcg/kg for open heart surgery, complicated neurosurgery, or orthopedic surgery. Maint: 20-50mcg/kg. Adjunct to Regional Anesthesia: 50-100mcg IM or slow IV over 1-2 min. Post-op: 50-100mcg IM, repeat q 1-2 hrs as needed. General Anesthetic: 50-100mcg/kg with oxygen and a muscle relaxant, up to 150mcg/kg may be used.
Pediatrics: 2-12 yrs: Individualize dose. Induction/Maint: 2-3mcg/kg.

HOW SUPPLIED: Inj: 50mcg/mL

WARNINGS/PRECAUTIONS: Should only be administered by persons specifically trained in the use of IV anesthetics and management of the respiratory effects of potent opioids. An opioid antagonist, resuscitative and intubation equipment and oxygen should be readily available. Fluids and other countermeasures to manage hypotension should be available with tranquilizers. Initial dose reduction recommended with narcotic analgesia for recovery. May cause muscle rigidity particularly with muscles used for respiration. Adequate facilities should be available for postoperative monitoring and ventilation. Caution in respiratory depression susceptible patients (eg, comatose patients with head injury or brain tumor). Reduce dose for elderly and debilitated patients. Caution with obstructive pulmonary disease, decreased respiratory reserve, liver and kidney dysfunction, cardiac bradyarrhythmias. Monitor vital signs routinely.

ADVERSE REACTIONS: Respiratory depression, apnea, rigidity, bradycardia, HTN, hypotension, dizziness, blurred vision, nausea, emesis, diaphoresis, pruritus, urticaria, laryngospasms, anaphylaxis, euphoria, miosis, bradycardia, and bronchoconstriction.

INTERACTIONS: Severe and unpredictable potentiation by MAOIs has been reported. Appropriate monitoring and availability of vasodilators and β-blockers for the treatment of hypertension is indicated. Additive or potentiating effects with other CNS depressants (eg, barbiturates, tranquilizers, narcotics, general anesthetics). Reduce dose of other CNS depressants. Reports of cardiovascular depression with nitrous oxide. Alteration of respiration with certain forms of conduction anesthesia (eg, spinal anesthesia, some peridural anesthesia). Decreased pulmonary arterial pressure and hypotension with tranquilizers. Elevated BP, with and without pre-existing hypertension, slower normalcy of EEG patterns with neuroleptics. Extreme caution with neuroleptics in presence of risk factors for development of prolonged QT syndrome and torsade de pointes; ECG monitoring indicated.

PREGNANCY: Category C, caution with nursing.

MECHANISM OF ACTION: Opioid analgesic; produces analgesic and sedative effects. Alters respiratory rate and aveolar ventilation, which may last longer than analgesic effects.

PHARMACOKINETICS: Distribution: V_d=4L/kg; found in skeletal muscle and fat. **Metabolism:** Liver. **Elimination:** Urine (75%, <10% unchanged), feces (10%); $T_{1/2}$=219 min.

SUBOXONE

CIII

buprenorphine - naloxone (Reckitt Benckiser)

OTHER BRAND NAME: Subutex (Reckitt Benckiser)

THERAPEUTIC CLASS: Partial opioid agonist/opioid antagonist

INDICATIONS: Opioid dependence.

DOSAGE: *Adults:* Give either agent SL as a single daily dose in the range of 12-16mg/day. Hold tabs under tongue until dissolved; swallowing tabs reduces bioavailability. Induction: Subutex: Give at least 4 hrs after last short-acting opioid (eg, heroin) use or preferably when early signs of opioid withdrawal appear. Maint: Suboxone: Range: 4mg-24mg/day. Target dose: 16mg/day. Titrate: Adjust by 2mg or 4mg to a level that maintains treatment and suppresses opioid withdrawal effects. Hepatic Impairment: Adjust dose and observe for precipitated opioid withdrawal. Concomant CNS Depressants: Consider dose reduction.
Pediatrics: ≥16 yrs: Give either agent SL as a single daily dose in the range of 12-16mg/day. Hold tabs under tongue until dissolved; swallowing tabs reduces bioavailability. Induction: Subutex: Give at least 4 hrs after last short-acting opioid (eg, heroin) use or preferably when early signs of opioid withdrawal appear. Maint: Suboxone: Range: 4mg-24mg/day. Target dose: 16mg/day. Titrate: Adjust by 2mg or 4mg to a level that maintains treatment and suppresses opioid withdrawal effects. Hepatic Impairment: Adjust dose and observe for precipitated opioid withdrawal. Concomant CNS Depressants: Consider dose reduction.

HOW SUPPLIED: Suboxone (Buprenorphine-Naloxone) Tab, SL: 2mg-0.5mg, 8mg-2mg. Subutex (Buprenorphine) Tab, SL: 2mg, 8mg

WARNINGS/PRECAUTIONS: Significant respiratory depression reported with buprenorphine; caution with compromised respiratory function. Naloxone may not be effective in reversing any respiratory depression produced by buprenorphine. Cytolytic hepatitis and hepatitis with jaundice reported. Obtain LFTs prior to initiation and periodically thereafter. Acute and chronic hypersensitivity reactions reported. May increase CSF pressure; caution with head injury, intracranial lesions. May cause miosis, changes in level of consciousness, and orthostatic hypotension. Caution with elderly, debilitated, myxedema, hypothyroidism, acute alcoholism, Addison's disease, CNS depression or coma, toxic psychoses, prostatic hypertrophy, urethral stricture, delirium tremens, kyphoscoliosis, biliary tract dysfunction or severe hepatic/renal/pulmonary impairment. Suboxone may cause opioid withdrawal symptoms. May obscure diagnosis of acute abdominal conditions. May produce dependence.

ADVERSE REACTIONS: Headache, infection, pain (general, abdomen, back), withdrawal syndrome, constipation, nausea, insomnia, sweating, asthenia, anxiety, depression, rhinitis.

INTERACTIONS: May need dose reduction with CYP3A4 inhibitors (eg, azole antifungals, macrolides and HIV protease inhibitors). General anesthetics, other narcotic analgesics, benzodiazepines, phenothiazines, other tranquilizers, sedative/hypnotics or other CNS depressants (including alcohol) may increase risk of CNS depression; consider dose reduction of one or both agents. Monitor closely with CYP3A4 inducers (eg, phenobarbital, carbamazepine, phenytoin, rifampicin).

PREGNANCY: Category C, not for use in nursing.

MECHANISM OF ACTION: Buprenorphine: Partial agonist at the mu-opioid receptor, antagonist at the kappa-opioid receptor. Naloxone: Inhibits mu-opioid receptor activity.

PHARMACOKINETICS: Absorption: (Suboxone 16mg) C_{max}=5.95ng/mL, AUC=34.89 hr•ng/mL. (Subtex 16mg) C_{max}=5.47ng/mL, AUC=32.63 hr•ng/mL. Refer to PI for more detailed information. **Distribution:** Plasma protein binding 96% (buprenorphine), 45% (naloxone). **Metabolism:** Buprenorphine: Through N-dealkylation and glucuronidation pathways; norbuprenorphine (active metabolite). Naloxone: Through glucuronidation, N-dealkylation, and reduction. **Elimination:** Urine (30%), feces (69%), $T_{1/2}$=37 hrs (Buprenorphine), 1.1 hrs (Naloxone).

SUDAFED
pseudoephedrine HCl (McNeil)

OTC

THERAPEUTIC CLASS: Decongestant

INDICATIONS: For the temporary relief of nasal congestion due to common cold, hay fever, or other upper respiratory allergies and nasal congestion associated with sinusitus.

DOSAGE: *Adults:* Tab, ER: 120mg q12h or 240mg q24h. Max: 240mg/24h.
Pediatrics: >12 yrs: Liquid/Tab/Tab, Chew: 60mg q4-6h. Max 240mg/24hrs. Tab, ER: 120mg q12h or 240mg q24h. Max: 240mg/24hrs. 6 to <12 yo: (Liquid/Tab/Tab, Chew) 30mg q4-6h. Max: 4 doses/24hrs. 2 to <6 yo: (Liquid/Tab/Tab, Chew) 15mg q4-6h. Max: 4 doses/24hrs.

HOW SUPPLIED: Liq: 15mg/5mL; Tab: 30mg, 60mg; Tab, Chewable: 15mg; Tab, Extended-Release: 120mg, 240mg

WARNINGS/PRECAUTIONS: Do not exceed recommended dosage. If nervousness, dizziness, or sleeplessness occurs, d/c use. Avoid with heart disease, high BP, thyroid disease, diabetes, or difficulty in urination due to prostate enlargement.

INTERACTIONS: Do not take with MAOI or 14 days after discontinuation.

PREGNANCY: Not rated in pregnancy or nursing.

MECHANISM OF ACTION: Relieves nasal congestion associated with sinusitis. Reduces swelling of nasal passages and relieves sinus pressure.

SUFENTA
sufentanil citrate (Akorn)

CII

THERAPEUTIC CLASS: Opioid analgesic

INDICATIONS: Analgesic adjunct in the maintenance of balanced general anesthesia in patients who are intubated and ventilated. Primary anesthetic agent of the induction and maintenance of anesthesia with 100% oxygen in patients undergoing major surgical procedures who are intubated or ventilated, such as cardiovascular surgery or neurosurgical procedures in the sitting position, to provide favorable myocardial and cerebral oxygen balance or when extended postoperative ventilation is anticipated. For epidural administrations an analgesic combined with low dose bupivacaine, usually 12.5mg per administration during labor and vaginal delivery.

DOSAGE: *Adults:* ≥12 yrs: Individualize dose. Premedication: Based on patients needs. Analgesic: Total Dose: 1-8mcg/kg. Maint: Incremental: 10-50mcg. Infusion: Based on induction dose not to exceed 1mcg/kg/hr. Anesthetic: Total Dose: 8-30mcg/kg. Maint: Incremental 0.5-10mcg/kg. Infusion: Based on induction dose not to exceed 30mcg/kg. Epidural: 10-15mcg with 10mL bupivacaine 0.125% with or without epinephrine. May repeat for a total of 3 doses in not less than 1 hour intervals.
Pediatrics: Individualize dose. 10-25mcg/kg with 100% oxygen. Maint: 25-50mcg supplemental doses.

HOW SUPPLIED: Inj: 50mcg/mL

WARNINGS/PRECAUTIONS: Should only be administered by persons specifically trained in the use of IV and epidural anesthetics and management of the respiratory effects of potent opioids. An opioid antagonist, resuscitative and intubation equipment and oxygen should be readily available. Prior to catheter insertion, the physician should be familiar with patient conditions (such as infection at the injection site, bleeding diathesis, anticoagulation therapy) which call for special evaluation of the benefit versus risk potential. May cause muscle rigidity of the neck and extremities. Adequate facilities should be available for postoperative monitoring and ventilation. Monitor vital signs routinely. Reduce dose for elderly and debilitated patients. Caution with pulmonary disease, decreased respiratory reserve, liver and kidney dysfunction, cardiac bradyarrhythmias. Reports of bradycardia responsive to atropine. May obscure clinical course of patients with head injuries.

ADVERSE REACTIONS: Respiratory depression, skeletal muscle rigidity, bradycardia, HTN, hypotension, chest wall rigidity, somnolence, pruritus, NV.

INTERACTIONS: Reports of cardiovascular depression with nitrous oxide. High doses of pancuronium may produce increase in heart rate. Reports of bradycardia and hypotension with other muscle relaxants. Greater incidence and degree of bradycardia and hypotension with chronic CCB and β-blocker therapy. Additive or potentiating effects with other CNS depressants (eg, barbiturates, tranquilizers, narcotics, general anesthetics). Reduce dose of either agent. Decrease in mean arterial pressure and systemic vascular resistance with benzodiazepines.

PREGNANCY: Category C, caution in nursing.

MECHANISM OF ACTION: An opioid analgesic.

PHARMACOKINETICS: Distribution: Plasma protein binding (healthy males: 93%, mothers: 91%, neonates: 79%). **Elimination:** $T_{1/2}$=164 min (adults), 97 min (neonates).

SULFACET-R RX
sulfacetamide sodium - sulfur (Dermik)

THERAPEUTIC CLASS: Sulfonamide/sulfur combination

INDICATIONS: Topical treatment of acne vulgaris, acne rosacea, and seborrheic dermatitis.

DOSAGE: *Adults:* Shake well before use. Apply qd-tid. Expires after 4 months.
Pediatrics: ≥12 yrs: Shake well before use. Apply qd-tid. Expires after 4 months.

HOW SUPPLIED: Lot: (Sulfacetamide-Sulfur) 10%-5% (25g)

CONTRAINDICATIONS: Kidney disease.

WARNINGS/PRECAUTIONS: D/C if irritation or hypersensitivity reaction occurs. Avoid eye contact. Contains sulfites. Caution with denuded or abraded skin. May cause reddening and scaling of epidermis.

ADVERSE REACTIONS: Local irritation.

PREGNANCY: Category C, caution in nursing.

MECHANISM OF ACTION: Sulfonamide/sufur combination. Sulfacetamide: Acts as a competitive antagonist to para-aminobenzoic acid (PABA), an essential component for bacterial growth. Sulfur: Not established. Inhibits the growth of *P. acnes* and the formation of free fatty acids.

PHARMACOKINETICS: Absorption: (PO) Readily absorbed. **Distribution:** Orally administered sulfonamides are found in breast milk. **Elimination:** Urine (unchanged).

SULFAMYLON RX
mafenide acetate (Mylan Bertek)

THERAPEUTIC CLASS: Sulfonamide

INDICATIONS: (Cre) Adjunctive therapy for 2nd- and 3rd-degree burns. (Sol) Adjunctive therapy for excised burn wounds.

DOSAGE: *Adults:* (Cre) Clean and debride wound, then apply qd-bid. Cre should cover wound at all times. Continue application until healing progressing well or site ready for grafting. (Sol) Cover grafted area with mesh gauze and wet with solution using irrigation syringe/tubing q4h or prn to keep wet. If irrigation tube is not used, moisten gauze q6-8h or prn to keep wet. May use solution up to 5 days with same dressing.
Pediatrics: (Cre) Clean and debride wound, then apply qd-bid. Cre should cover wound at all times. Continue application until healing progressing well or site ready for grafting. (Sol) 3 months-16 yrs: Cover grafted area with mesh gauze and wet with solution using irrigation syringe/tubing q4h or prn to keep wet. If irrigation tube is not used, moisten gauze q6-8h or prn to keep wet. May use solution up to 5 days with same dressing.

HOW SUPPLIED: Cre: 85mg/g (60g, 120g, 453.6g); Sol: 50g/pkt (1^s, 5^s)

WARNINGS/PRECAUTIONS: Fatal hemolytic anemia with DIC related to G6PD deficiency reported. Cream contains sodium metabisulfite. Monitor acid-base balance with pulmonary or renal dysfunction; risk of metabolic acidosis due to carbonic anhydrase inhibition. Fungal colonization may occur. D/C if hypersensitivity occurs, and for 24-48 hrs if acidosis occurs. Caution with acute renal failure.

ADVERSE REACTIONS: Facial edema, rash, burning sensation, pruritus, erythema, swelling, hyperventilation, tachypnea, acidosis.

INTERACTIONS: Possible cross sensitivity to other sulfonamides.

PREGNANCY: Category C, not for use in nursing.

MECHANISM OF ACTION: Sulfonamide; not established. Exerts broad bacteriostatic action against susceptible gram-negative and gram-positive organisms.

PHARMACOKINETICS: Absorption: T_{max}=2 hrs (cream), 4 hrs (solution). **Elimination:** Kidneys.

SUMYCIN
tetracycline HCl (Par)

RX

THERAPEUTIC CLASS: *Streptomyces* derived bacteriostatic agent

INDICATIONS: Treatment of respiratory tract, urinary tract, and skin and skin structure infections, lymphogranuloma, psittacosis, trachoma, uncomplicated urethral/endocervical/rectal infection caused by *Chlamydia*, nongonococcal urethritis, chancroid, plague, cholera, brucellosis, and others. When PCN is contraindicated, treatment of uncomplicated gonorrhea, syphilis, listeriosis, anthrax, *Clostridium* species, and others. Adjunct therapy for amebicides and severe acne.

DOSAGE: *Adults:* Mild-Moderate: 250mg qid or 500mg bid. Severe: 500mg qid. Continue for 24-48 hrs after symptoms subside (minimum 10 days with Group A β-hemolytic streptococci). Severe Acne: Initial: 1g/day in divided doses. Maint: After improvement, 125-500mg/day. Brucellosis: 500mg qid for 3 weeks plus streptomycin 1g IM bid for 1 week, then qd for 1 week. Syphilis: 30-40g equally divided over 10-15 days. Gonorrhea: 500mg q6h for 7 days. *Chlamydia:* 500mg qid for at least 7 days. Renal Dysfunction: Reduce dose or extend dose interval.
Pediatrics: >8 yrs: Usual: 25-50mg/kg divided bid-qid. Continue for 24-48 hrs after symptoms subside (minimum 10 days with Group A β-hemolytic streptococci). Severe Acne: Initial: 1g/day in divided doses. Maint: After improvement, 125-500mg/day. Renal Dysfunction: Reduce dose or extend dose interval.

HOW SUPPLIED: Sus: 125mg/5mL; Tab: 250mg, 500mg

WARNINGS/PRECAUTIONS: May cause fetal harm with pregnancy, permanent tooth discoloration during tooth development (last half of pregnancy and children <8 yrs). May increase BUN. Photosensitivity, enamel hypoplasia reported. Superinfection with prolonged use. Suspension contains sodium metabisulfite. Bulging fontanels in infants and benign intracranial HTN in adults reported. Monitor renal/hepatic and hematopoietic function with long-term use. Caution with history of asthma, hay fever, urticaria, and allergy.

ADVERSE REACTIONS: GI effects, photosensitivity, increased BUN, hypersensitivity reactions, blood dyscrasias, dizziness, headache.

INTERACTIONS: May decrease PT; adjust anticoagulants. May interfere with bactericidal agents (eg, penicillin). May decrease effects of oral contraceptives. Take 1 hr before or 2 hrs after dairy products. Aluminum-, calcium-, iron- and magnesium-containing products impair absorption. Fatal renal toxicity reported with concurrent methoxyflurane.

PREGNANCY: Category D, not for use in nursing.

MECHANISM OF ACTION: Tetracycline agent; inhibits bacterial protein synthesis.

PHARMACOKINETICS: Absorption: Adequate/incomplete. **Distribution:** Plasma protein binding (65%); excellent penetration into most bodily fluids and tissues; crosses placental barrier and enters fetal circulation and amniotic fluid; found in breast milk. **Elimination:** Urine, feces.

SUPPRELIN LA
histrelin acetate (Indevus)

RX

THERAPEUTIC CLASS: Gonadotropin-releasing hormone analog

INDICATIONS: Treatment of children with central precocious puberty.

DOSAGE: *Pediatrics:* ≥2 yrs: 50mg every 12 months. Inject SQ into inner aspect of upper arm. Remove after 12 months of therapy.

HOW SUPPLIED: Implant: 50mg

CONTRAINDICATIONS: Women who are or may become pregnant.

WARNINGS/PRECAUTIONS: Transient increase in estradiol in females and testosterone in both sexes with initial therapy. Proper surgical technique is critical during implant insertion and removal. Monitor LH, FSH, and estradiol or testosterone at 1 month post-implantation, then every 6 months. Assess height and bone age every 6-12 months.

ADVERSE REACTIONS: Implant site reactions, wound infection, dysmenorrhea, epistaxis, erythema, gynecomastia, headache, weight increase.

PREGNANCY: Category X, not for use in nursing.

MECHANISM OF ACTION: Gonadotropin secretion inhibitor; reversible down-regulation of GnRH receptor in pituitary gland and desensitization of pituitary gonadotropes, resulting in decreased levels of LH and FSH.

PHARMACOKINETICS: Absorption: C_{max}=0.43ng/mL.

SUPRANE
desflurane (Baxter)

RX

THERAPEUTIC CLASS: Inhalation anesthetic

INDICATIONS: Induction and/or maintenance of anesthesia for inpatient and outpatient surgery in adults. Maintenance of anesthesia in infants and children after induction of anesthesia with other agents and tracheal intubation.

DOSAGE: *Adults:* Individualize dose. MAC Values: 70 yrs: 5.2 with oxygen 100% or 1.7 with nitrous oxide 60%. 45 yrs: 6 with oxygen 100% or 2.8 with nitrous oxide 60%. 25 yrs: 7.3 with oxygen 100% or 4 with nitrous oxide 60%. With Fentanyl or Midazolam: 31-65 yrs: No Fentanyl: 6.3. With 3mcg/kg Fentanyl: 3.1. With 6mcg/kg Fentanyl: 2.3. No Midazolam: 5.9. With Midazolam 25mcg/kg: 4.9. With Midazolam 50mcg/kg: 4.9. 18-30 yrs: No Fentanyl: 6.4. With Fentanyl 3mcg/kg: 3.5. With Fentanyl 6mcg/kg: 3. No Midazolam: 6.9.
Pediatrics: Individualize dose. MAC Values: 7 yrs: 8.1 with oxygen 100%. 4 yrs: 8.6 with oxygen 100%. 3 yrs: 6.4 with nitrous oxide 60%. 2 yrs: 9.1 with oxygen 100%. 9 months: 10 with oxygen 100% or 7.5 with nitrous oxide 60%. 10 weeks: 9.4 with oxygen 100%. 2 weeks: 9.2 with oxygen 100%.

HOW SUPPLIED: Liq: (240mL)

CONTRAINDICATIONS: Known or suspected susceptibility to malignant hyperthermia.

WARNINGS/PRECAUTIONS: Not recommended for induction of general anesthesia via mask in infants or children. Produces dose-dependent decreases in BP. Concentrations >1 MAC may increase HR. Administer at 0.8 MAC or less, in conjunction with barbiturate induction and hyperventilation. Maintain normal hemodynamics with CAD. May cause sensitivity hepatitis in patients who have been sensitized by previous exposure to halogenated anesthetics. May trigger malignant hyperthermia. May produce a dose-dependent increase in CSF pressure when administered to patients with intracranial space occupying lesions. Not recommended for maintenance of anesthesia in non-intubated children.

ADVERSE REACTIONS: Coughing, breathholding, apnea, laryngospasm, oxyhemoglobin desaturation, increased secretions, bronchospasm, nausea, vomiting.

INTERACTIONS: Decreased MAC with benzodiazepines and opioids. May decrease the required dose of neuromuscular blocking agents.

PREGNANCY: Category B, caution in nursing.

MECHANISM OF ACTION: Inhalation anesthetic agent.

SUPRAX
cefixime (Lupin)

RX

THERAPEUTIC CLASS: Cephalosporin (3rd generation)

INDICATIONS: Otitis media, pharyngitis, tonsillitis, acute bronchitis, acute exacerbation of chronic bronchitis, uncomplicated UTIs, and cervical/urethral gonorrhea caused by susceptible strains.

DOSAGE: *Adults:* Usual: 400mg qd. Gonorrhea: 400mg single dose. CrCl 21-60mL/min/ Hemodialysis: Give 75% of standard dose. CrCl <20mL/min/CAPD: Give 50% of standard dose.
Pediatrics: >12 yrs or >50kg: (Tab/Sus) Usual: 400mg qd. ≥6 months: (Sus) 8mg/kg qd or 4mg/kg bid. Treat for at least 10 days with *S. pyogenes*. CrCl 21-60mL/min/ Hemodialysis: Give 75% of standard dose. CrCl <20mL/min/CAPD: Give 50% of standard dose.

HOW SUPPLIED: Tab: 400mg; Sus:100mg/5mL (50mL, 75mL, 100mL)

WARNINGS/PRECAUTIONS: Caution with PCN or other allergy, GI disease (eg, colitis). Anaphylactic/anaphylactoid reactions, pseudomembranous colitis reported. May cause false (+) direct Coombs test or false (+) reaction for urinary glucose using Benedict's/Fehling's solution or Clinitest.

ADVERSE REACTIONS: Diarrhea, abdominal pain, nausea, dyspepsia, flatulence, superinfection.

INTERACTIONS: May increase carbamazepine levels. Increased PT with anticoagulants (eg, warfarin).

PREGNANCY: Category B, not for use in nursing.

MECHANISM OF ACTION: 3rd-generation cephalosporin; inhibits cell-wall synthesis.

PHARMACOKINETICS: Absorption: 40-50% absorbed. C_{max}=2mcg/mL (200mg tab), 3.7mcg/mL (400mg tab), 3mcg/mL (200mg sus), 4.6mcg/mL (400mg sus); T_{max}=2-6 hrs (200mg tab, 400mg tab/sus), 2-5 hrs (200mg sus). **Distribution:** Serum protein binding (65%). **Elimination:** Urine (50% unchanged); $T_{1/2}$=3-4 up to 9 hrs.

SURMONTIL
trimipramine maleate (Odyssey)

RX

> **Antidepressants increased the risk of suicidal thinking and behavior (suicidality) in short-term studies in children, adolescents, and young adults with Major Depressive Disorder (MDD) and other psychiatric disorders. Trimipramine is not approved for use in pediatric patients.**

THERAPEUTIC CLASS: Tricyclic antidepressant

INDICATIONS: Relief of symptoms of depression.

DOSAGE: *Adults:* Outpatient: Initial: 75mg/day in divided doses. Titrate: Increase to 150mg/day. Maint: 50-150mg/day. Max: 200mg/day. Hospitalized Patients: Initial: 100mg/day in divided doses. Titrate: Increase gradually to 200mg/day. If no improvement after 2-3 weeks, may increase up to 250-300mg/day. Elderly: Initial: 50mg/day. Titrate: Increase gradually to 100mg/day. Take hs for at least 3 months.
Pediatrics: Adolescents: Initial: 50mg/day. Titrate: Increase gradually to 100mg/day. Take hs for at least 3 months.

HOW SUPPLIED: Cap: 25mg, 50mg, 100mg

CONTRAINDICATIONS: Acute recovery period post-MI, within 14 days of MAOI therapy.

WARNINGS/PRECAUTIONS: Caution with cardiovascular disease, increased IOP, urinary retention, narrow-angle glaucoma, hyperthyroidism, seizure disorder, liver dysfunction. May impair ability to operate machinery. May alter glucose levels. May activate psychosis in schizophrenia. Manic or hypomanic episodes may occur. May increase hazards with electroshock therapy.

ADVERSE REACTIONS: Hypotension, HTN, arrhythmia, confusion, insomnia, incoordination, GI complaints, allergic reactions, gynecomastia, blood dyscrasias, dry mouth, blurred vision, urinary retention.

INTERACTIONS: Cimetidine inhibits elimination. Alcohol may exaggerate effects. May potentiate catecholamine or anticholinergic effects. Potentiated by CYP2D6 inhibitors (eg, quinidine) and substrates (eg, other antidepressants, phenothiazines, propafenone, flecainide). Caution with SSRIs; wait 5 weeks after fluoxetine withdrawal before initiating therapy. Avoid MAOIs.

PREGNANCY: Category C, safety in nursing not known.

MECHANISM OF ACTION: Tricyclic antidepressant with anxiety-reducing sedative component to its action.

SUSTIVA
efavirenz (Bristol-Myers Squibb)

RX

THERAPEUTIC CLASS: Non-nucleoside reverse transcriptase inhibitor

INDICATIONS: Treatment of HIV-1 infection in combination with other antiretrovirals.

DOSAGE: *Adults:* Initial: 600mg qd. Take on an empty stomach, preferably at bedtime. *Pediatrics:* ≥3 yrs: 10 to <15kg: 200mg qd. 15 to <20kg: 250mg qd. 20 to <25kg: 300mg qd. 25 to <32.5kg: 350mg qd. 32.5 to <40kg: 400mg qd. ≥40kg: 600mg qd. Take on an empty stomach, preferably at bedtime.

HOW SUPPLIED: Cap: 50mg, 100mg, 200mg; Tab: 600mg

CONTRAINDICATIONS: Concomitant astemizole, bepridil, cisapride, midazolam, pimozide, triazolam, ergot derivatives, or standard doses of voriconazole.

WARNINGS/PRECAUTIONS: Not for monotherapy. Severe skin rash reported. Avoid pregnancy; use barrier contraception with other contraception methods and obtain (-) pregnancy test before therapy. Monitor LFTs with known or suspected hepatitis B or C. Monitor cholesterol and triglycerides. High fat meals may increase absorption. Possible redistribution or accumulation of body fat. Serious psychiatric and CNS adverse experiences (dizziness, insomnia, impaired concentration, somnolence, abnormal dreams, hallucinations) reported.

ADVERSE REACTIONS: CNS symptoms (eg, dizziness, insomnia, impaired concentration, somnolence, abnormal dreams), psychiatric symptoms (eg, severe depression), rash, GI effects.

INTERACTIONS: Avoid astemizole, cisapride, midazolam, triazolam, voriconazole, St. John's wort, or ergot derivatives. St. John's wort decreases efavirenz to suboptimal levels; increases risk of resistance. Significantly decreased levels of voriconazole. CYP3A4 inducers (eg, phenobarbital, rifampin, rifabutin) may decrease plasma levels. Increased levels of ethinyl estradiol. Decreased levels of clarithromycin; consider alternative. Decreased levels of indinavir and rifabutin; adjust doses. Increased levels of ritonavir and efavirenz with concomitant use; monitor LFTs. Decreased levels of saquinavir, sertraline. May decrease methadone levels; monitor for signs of withdrawal. May affect warfarin levels. May decrease itraconazole, ketoconazole, amprenavir levels. Decreased levels of anticonvulsants (eg, phenytoin, phenobarbital, carbamazepine) and efavirenz; monitor anticonvulsant levels.

PREGNANCY: Category D, not for use in nursing.

MECHANISM OF ACTION: Non-nucleoside reverse transcriptase inhibitor.

PHARMACOKINETICS: Absorption: C_{max}=12.9µM, T_{max}=3-5 hrs; AUC=184µM•h. **Distribution:** Plasma protein binding (99.5-99.75%). **Metabolism:** CYP3A4,2B6 (hydroxylation, glucuronidation). **Elimination:** Urine, feces; $T_{1/2}$=40-55 hrs.

SYMBICORT
budesonide fumarate dihydrate - formoterol (AstraZeneca)

RX

> Long-acting β_2-adrenergic agonists (formoterol) may increase the risk of asthma-related death.

THERAPEUTIC CLASS: Corticosteroid/beta$_2$ agonist

INDICATIONS: Long-term maintenance treatment of asthma in patients ≥12 yrs.

DOSAGE: *Adults:* Current Medium-High Dose Inhaled CS: 2 inh bid of 160/4.5. Current Low to Medium Doses Inhaled CS: 2 inh bid of 80/4.5. No Current Inhaled CS: 2 inh bid of 80/4.5 or 160/4.5 depending on asthma severity. Max: 640mcg/18mcg (2 inh bid of 160/4.5). Patients not responding to the starting dose after 1-2 weeks of therapy with 80/4.5, replace with 160/4.5 for better asthma control. Rinse mouth after use.

Pediatrics: ≥12 yrs: Current Medium-High Dose Inhaled CS: 2 inh bid of 160/4.5. Current Low to Medium Doses Inhaled CS: 2 inh bid of 80/4.5. No Current Inhaled CS: 2 inh bid of 80/4.5 or 160/4.5 depending on asthma severity. Max: 640mcg/18mcg (2 inh bid of 160/4.5). Patients not responding to the starting dose after 1-2 weeks of therapy with 80/4.5, replace with 160/4.5 for better asthma control. Rinse mouth after use.

HOW SUPPLIED: MDI: (Budesonide-Formoterol) 80mcg-4.5mcg/inh, 160mcg-4.5mcg/inh (10.2g)

CONTRAINDICATIONS: Primary treatment of status asthmaticus or other acute asthma attacks.

WARNINGS/PRECAUTIONS: Do not use in patients with significantly worsening or acutely deteriorating asthma. Not for acute treatment of symptoms. Monitor for increasing use of inhaled, short-acting β_2-agonists. Deaths due to adrenal insufficiency have occured with transfer from systemic corticosteroids to inhaled corticosteroids. Resume oral corticosteroids during stress or severe asthma attack. Transferring from oral to inhalation therapy may unmask allergic conditions (eg, rhinitis, conjunctivitis, eczema). Observe for adrenal insufficiency, systemic corticosteroid withdrawal effects, and growth suppression (children). More susceptible to infections. Not for acute bronchospasm. Do not use any additional inhaled long-acting β_2-agonist for prevention of exercise induced bronchospasm or the maintenance treatment of asthma. D/C if paradoxical bronchospasm occurs. Immediate hypersensitivity and upper airway symptom reactions reported. Caution with cardiovascular disorder (eg, coronary insufficiency, arrhythmia, HTN), seizures, thyroid and hepatic problems, diabetes, osteoporosis. QTc interval prolongation reported.

ADVERSE REACTIONS: Nasopharyngitis, headache, upper respiratory tract infections, sinusitis, back pain, nasal/sinus congestion, oral candidiasis, influenza, rhinitis, pharyngolaryngeal pain, vomiting.

INTERACTIONS: Oral ketoconazole increases plasma levels. CYP3A4 inhibitors (eg, itraconazole, clarithromycin, erythromycin) may inhibit metabolism and increase systemic exposure. Caution with non-K^+-sparing diuretics. Extreme caution within 14 days of using MAOIs or TCAs. Avoid with β-blockers.

PREGNANCY: Category C, not for use in nursing.

MECHANISM OF ACTION: Budesonide: Corticosteroid; shown to have inhibitory effects on multiple cell types (mast cells, eosinophils, neutrophils, macrophages and lymphocytes) and mediators (histamine, eicosanoids, leukotrienes and cytokines) involved in inflammatory and asthmatic response. Formoterol: β_2-adrenergic agonist; stimulates intracellular adenyl cyclase, which catalyzes conversion of ATP to cAMP, to produce relaxation of bronchial smooth muscle and inhibition of release of mediators of immediate hypersensitivity from cells (mast cells).

PHARMACOKINETICS: Absorption: Budesonide: Rapid (lungs). C_{max}=4.5nmol/L, T_{max}=20 min. Formoterol: Rapid (GI). C_{max}=136pmol, T_{max}=5-10 min. **Distribution:** Budesonide: V_d=3L/kg; plasma protein binding (85-90%). Formoterol: Plasma protein binding (RR enantiomer, 46%), (SS enantiomer, 58%). **Metabolism:** Budesonide: Liver (biotransformation) via CYP3A4. Formoterol: Liver (direct glucuronidation and O-demethylation) via CYP2D6, 2C. **Elimination:** Budesonide: $T_{1/2}$=2-3 hrs. Formoterol: Urine (8%).

SYMMETREL
amantadine HCl (Endo)

RX

THERAPEUTIC CLASS: Dopamine agonist

INDICATIONS: Prophylaxis and treatment of uncomplicated influenza A infections. Treatment of parkinsonism and drug-induced extrapyramidal reactions.

DOSAGE: *Adults:* Influenza A Virus Prophylaxis/Treatment: 200mg qd or 100mg bid. Elderly: ≥65 yrs: 100mg qd. Parkinsonism: Initial: 100mg bid. Serious Associated Illness/ Concomitant High Dose Antiparkinson Agent: Initial: 100mg qd. Titrate: May increase to 100mg bid after 1 to several weeks. Max: 400mg/day. Drug-Induced Extrapyramidal Reactions: 100mg bid. Titrate: May increase to 300mg/day in divided doses. CrCl 30-50mL/min: 200mg on Day 1, then 100mg qd. CrCl 15-29mL/min: 200mg on Day 1, then 100mg every other day. CrCl <15mL/min/Hemodialysis: 200mg every 7 days. *Pediatrics:* Influenza A Virus Prophylaxis/Treatment: 9-12 yrs: 100mg bid. 1-9 yrs: 4.4-8.8mg/kg/day. Max: 150mg/day.

HOW SUPPLIED: Syrup: 50mg/5mL; Tab: 100mg

WARNINGS/PRECAUTIONS: Deaths reported from overdose. Suicide attempts, NMS reported. Caution with CHF, peripheral edema, orthostatic hypotension, renal or hepatic dysfunction, recurrent eczematoid rash, uncontrolled psychosis or severe psychoneurosis. Avoid in untreated angle closure glaucoma. Do not d/c abruptly in Parkinson's disease. May increase seizure activity.

ADVERSE REACTIONS: Nausea, dizziness, insomnia, depression, anxiety, hallucinations, confusion, anorexia, dry mouth, constipation, ataxia, livedo reticularis, peripheral edema, orthostatic hypotension, agranulocytosis.

INTERACTIONS: Caution with CNS stimulants. Anticholinergic agents may potentiate the anticholinergic side effects. Increased tremor in elderly Parkinson's patients with thioridazine. Increased plasma levels with trimethoprim-sulfamethoxazole, quinine, or quinidine. Avoid use of Attenuated Influenza Vaccine within 2 weeks before or 48 hours after.

PREGNANCY: Category C, not for use in nursing.

MECHANISM OF ACTION: Antiviral; appears to prevent release of infectious viral nucleic acid into host cell by interfering with function of transmembrane domain of viral M2 protein, preventing virus assembly during replication.

PHARMACOKINETICS: Absorption: (Tab) C_{max}=0.51mcg/mL, T_{max}=2-4 hrs. (Syrup) C_{max}=0.24mcg/mL, T_{max}=2-4 hrs. **Distribution**: (IV) V_d=3-8L/Kg; plasma protein binding (67%).

SYNAGIS RX
palivizumab (MedImmune)

THERAPEUTIC CLASS: Monoclonal antibody/RSV F-protein blocker

INDICATIONS: Prevention of serious lower respiratory tract disease caused by respiratory syncytial virus (RSV) in pediatrics at high risk of RSV.

DOSAGE: *Pediatrics:* 15mg/kg IM; give 1st dose before start of RSV season (November-April), then monthly throughout season. Give monthly also if develop RSV infection. Safety and efficacy established in infants with bronchopulmonary dysplasia (BPD) and infants with history of prematurity (≤35 weeks gestational age).

HOW SUPPLIED: Inj: 50mg, 100mg

WARNINGS/PRECAUTIONS: Anaphylactoid reactions reported. Caution with thrombocytopenia or any coagulation disorder due to IM injection. Safety and efficacy not demonstrated for treatment of established RSV disease.

ADVERSE REACTIONS: Upper respiratory infection, otitis media, rash, cough, diarrhea, vomiting, liver function abnormality, fever, rhinitis, hernia, gastroenteritis, wheezing.

PREGNANCY: Category C, safety in nursing not known.

MECHANISM OF ACTION: Monoclonal antibody; exhibits neutralizing and fusion-inhibitory activity against RSV.

PHARMACOKINETICS: Elimination: $T_{1/2}$=20 days.

SYNALAR RX
fluocinolone acetonide (Medicis)

THERAPEUTIC CLASS: Corticosteroid

INDICATIONS: Corticosteroid responsive dermatoses.

DOSAGE: *Adults:* Apply bid-qid. May use occlusive dressings for psoriasis or recalcitrant conditions; d/c dressings if infection develops.
Pediatrics: Apply bid-qid. May use occlusive dressings for psoriasis or recalcitrant conditions; d/c dressings if infection develops.

HOW SUPPLIED: Cre, Oint: 0.025% (15g, 60g); Sol: 0.01% (20mL, 60mL)

WARNINGS/PRECAUTIONS: May produce reversible HPA axis suppression, manifestations of Cushing's syndrome, hyperglycemia, and glucosuria. Caution when applied to large surface areas or under occlusive dressings. Use appropriate antifungal or antibacterial agent with dermatological infections; d/c if infection does not clear. Peds may be more susceptible to systemic toxicity. Avoid eyes. D/C if irritation occurs.

ADVERSE REACTIONS: Burning, itching, irritation, dryness, folliculitis, hypertrichosis, acneiform eruptions, premolar dermatitis, hypopigmentation, allergic dermatitis, skin maceration, secondary infection, skin atrophy.

PREGNANCY: Category C, caution with nursing.

MECHANISM OF ACTION: Corticosteroid; possesses anti-inflammatory, antipruritic, and vasoconstrictive actions. Anti-inflammatory activity not established.

PHARMACOKINETICS: Absorption: Percutaneous; occlusion, inflammation, and other disease states may increase absorption. **Distribution:** Systemically administered corticosteroids are found in breast milk. **Metabolism:** Liver. **Excretion:** Kidneys, bile.

SYNAREL   RX
nafarelin acetate (G.D. Searle)

THERAPEUTIC CLASS: Gonadotropin-releasing hormone analog

INDICATIONS: Management of endometriosis, including pain relief and reduction of lesions. Treatment of central precocious puberty (CPP) (gonadotropin-dependent precocious puberty) in children of both sexes.

DOSAGE: (Endometriosis) *Adults:* ≥18 yrs: 1 spray (200mcg) into one nostril qam and 1 spray into other nostril qpm. Initiate therapy between days 2-4 of menstrual cycle. Increase to 1 spray per nostril qam and qpm after 2 months (800mcg/day) if amenorrhea has not occurred. Treat for 6 months.
(CPP) *Pediatrics:* Usual: 2 sprays (400mcg) per nostril qam and qpm. Total Daily Dose: 1600mcg. Increase to 3 sprays into alternating nostrils tid (1800mcg daily) if needed 30 seconds should elapse between sprays. Continue until resumption of puberty is desired.

HOW SUPPLIED: Spray: 200mcg/inh (8mL)

CONTRAINDICATIONS: Pregnancy, women who may become pregnant, nursing, undiagnosed abnormal vaginal bleeding.

WARNINGS/PRECAUTIONS: (Endometriosis) Ovarian cysts reported in adult women. Caution if risk factors for decreased bone mineral content present. Avoid sneezing during or after administration. Use nonhormonal methods of contraception. (CPP) Determine diagnosis before initiating therapy. Monitor regularly. Assess growth and bone age velocity within 3 to 6 months of initiation. Avoid sneezing during or after administration.

ADVERSE REACTIONS: (Endometriosis) Hot flashes, decreased libido, vaginal dryness, headache, emotional lability, myalgia, acne, nasal irritation, reduced breast size, insomnia, edema, seborrhea, weight gain, depression, hirsutism. (CPP) Acne, breast enlargement, vaginal bleeding, emotional lability, transient increase in pubic hair, rhinitis, body odor, seborrhea, white or brownish vaginal discharge.

INTERACTIONS: Avoid topical decongestants within 2 hrs after dosing.

PREGNANCY: Category X, not for use in nursing.

MECHANISM OF ACTION: Gonadotropin-releasing hormone analog. Initially, stimulates the release of the pituitary gonadotropins, LH and FSH, resulting in a temporary increase in gonadal steroidogenesis. Repeated dosing abolishes the stimulatory effects on the pituitary glands. Decreased secretions of gonadal steroids cause gonadal steroid-dependent tissues and functions to become quiescent.

PHARMACOKINETICS: Absorption: Rapidly absorbed. Children: C_{max}=2.2ng/mL (400µg), 6.6ng/mL (600µg); T_{max}=10-45 min. Adult women: C_{max}=0.6ng/mL (200µg), 1.8ng/mL (400µg); T_{max}=10-40 min. Bioavailability: 2.8% (400µg). **Distribution:** Plasma protein binding (80%); found in breast milk. **Metabolism:** Tyr-D(2)-Nal-Leu-Arg-Pro-Gly-NH₂(5-10) (major metabolite). **Elimination:** Urine (44-55%) (3% unchanged), feces (18.5-44.2%).

SYNERA
RX
lidocaine - tetracaine (Endo)

THERAPEUTIC CLASS: Acetamide local anesthetic

INDICATIONS: For use on intact skin to provide local dermal analgesia for superficial venous access and superficial dermatological procedures such as excision, electrodessication, and shave biopsy of skin lesions.

DOSAGE: *Adults:* Venipuncture or IV Cannulation: Apply to intact skin for 20-30 min prior to procedure. Superficial Dermatological Procedures: Apply to intact skin for 30 min prior to procedure.
Pediatrics: ≥3 yrs: Venipuncture or IV Cannulation: Apply to intact skin for 20-30 min prior to procedure. Superficial Dermatological Procedure: Apply to intact skin for 30 min prior to procedure.

HOW SUPPLIED: Patch: (Lidocaine-Tetracaine) 70mg-70mg

CONTRAINDICATIONS: PABA hypersensitivity.

WARNINGS/PRECAUTIONS: Serious adverse events may occur in children or pets if ingested. Caution in acutely ill or debilitated. Risk of allergic/anaphylactoid reactions (urticaria, angioedema, bronchospasm, shock). Increased risk of toxicity in severe hepatic disease. Avoid broken or inflamed skin, eye contact, larger area or longer duration than recommended.

ADVERSE REACTIONS: Erythema, blanching, edema, urticaria, angioedema, bronchospasm, shock.

INTERACTIONS: Additive toxic effect with concomitant Class I antiarrhythmics (eg, tocainide, mexiletine). Consider total amount absorbed from all formulations with other local anesthetics.

PREGNANCY: Category B, caution in nursing.

MECHANISM OF ACTION: Lidocaine: Amide-type local anesthetic; blocks Na^+ channels required for initiation and conduction of neuronal impulses. Tetracaine: Ester-type local anesthetic; blocks Na^+ channels required for initiation and conduction of neuronal impulses.

PHARMACOKINETICS: **Absorption:** C_{max}=1.7ng/mL (lidocaine), <0.9ng/mL (tetracaine); T_{max}=1.7 hrs. (lidocaine). **Distribution:** Lidocaine: V_d=0.8-1.3 L/kg; plasma protein binding (75%); crosses placenta. **Metabolism:** Lidocaine: CYP1A2, CYP3A4 (N-deethylation). Monoethylglycinexylidide, glycinexylidide (active metabolites). Tetracaine: Plasma esterases (hydrolysis). **Elimination:** Lidocaine: Urine; $T_{1/2}$=1.8 hrs.

SYNERCID
RX
dalfopristin - quinupristin (King)

THERAPEUTIC CLASS: Streptogramin

INDICATIONS: Treatment of serious or life-threatening infections associated with vancomycin-resistant *Enterococcus faecium* (VREF) bacteremia and complicated skin and skin structure infections (cSSSI) caused by *Staphylococcus aureus* (methicillin-susceptible) or *Streptococcus pyogenes*.

DOSAGE: *Adults:* ≥16 yrs: VREF: 7.5mg/kg IV q8h. Duration depends on site and severity of infection. cSSSI: 7.5mg/kg IV q12h for at least 7 days. Hepatic Cirrhosis (Child Pugh A or B): May need dose reduction.
Pediatrics: ≥16 yrs: VREF: 7.5mg/kg IV q8h. Duration depends on site and severity of infection. cSSSI: 7.5mg/kg IV q12h for at least 7 days. Hepatic Cirrhosis (Child Pugh A or B): May need dose reduction.

HOW SUPPLIED: Inj: (Dalfopristin-Quinupristin) 350mg-150mg per 500mg vial

WARNINGS/PRECAUTIONS: Pseudomembranous colitis reported. Flush vein with 5% dextrose after infusion to minimize venous irritation. Arthralgia, myalgia, and bilirubin elevation reported.

ADVERSE REACTIONS: Infusion site reactions (inflammation, pain, edema), nausea, diarrhea, rash.

INTERACTIONS: Significant inhibiton of CYP3A4; caution with drugs metabolized by this enzyme system (eg, cyclosporin A, tacrolimus, midazolam, nifedipine, verapamil, diltiazem, astemizole, terfenadine, delaviridine, nevirapine, indinavir, ritonavir, vinca alkaloids, docetaxel, paclitaxel, diazepam, HMG-CoA reductase inhibitors, methylpred-nisolone, carbamazepine, quinidine, lidocaine, disopyramide). Monitor cyclosporine levels. Avoid drugs metabolized by CYP3A4 that prolong QTc interval. May inhibit gut metabolism of digoxin.

PREGNANCY: Category B, caution in nursing.

MECHANISM OF ACTION: Bacteriostatic agent; acts on bacterial ribosome. Dalfopristin: Inhibits the early phase of protein synthesis. Quinipristin: Inhibits the late phase of pro-tein synthesis.

PHARMACOKINETICS: Absorption: Quinipristin: C_{max}=3.2mcg/mL, AUC=7.2mcg•hr/mL; Dalfopristin: C_{max}=7.96mcg/mL, AUC=10.57mcg•hr/mL. **Distribution:** Quinipristin: V_d=0.45L/kg, plasma protein binding (moderate); Dalfopristin: V_d=0.24L/kg, plasma pro-tein binding (moderate). **Metabolism:** Quinipristin: 2 conjugated metabolites (1 with glu-tathione; 1 with cysteine); Dalfopristin: 1 nonconjugated metabolite; active metabolites. **Elimination:** Urine: 15% (quinipristin), 19% (dalfopristin), feces (75-77%); $T_{1/2}$=0.85 hrs. (quinipristin), 0.7 hrs. (dalfopristin).

SYNTHROID
levothyroxine sodium (Abbott)

RX

THERAPEUTIC CLASS: Thyroid replacement hormone

INDICATIONS: Hypothyroidism. As a pituitary TSH suppressant in the treatment and pre-vention of euthyroid goiters, including thyroid nodules, lymphocytic thyroiditis, and mul-tinodular goiter. Adjunct to surgery and radioiodine therapy for thyrotropin-dependent well-differentiated thyroid cancer.

DOSAGE: *Adults:* Hypothyroidism: Usual: 1.7mcg/kg/day PO. Titrate: May increase by 12.5-25mcg every 6-8 weeks until euthyroid. >200mcg/day (seldom). Elderly/ Cardiovascular Disease: Initial: 12.5-50mcg qd PO. Titrate: Increase by 12.5-25mcg every 3-6 weeks until euthyroid. Give 1/2 of oral dose for IV/IM. Pregnancy: May require increased doses. Subclinical Hypothyroidism: Lower doses required.
Pediatrics: Hypothyroidism: 0-3 months: 10-15mcg/kg/day. 3-6 months: 8-10mcg/kg/ day. 6-12 months: 6-8mcg/kg/day. 1-5 yrs: 5-6mcg/kg/day. 6-12 yrs: 4-5mcg/kg/day. >12 yrs (growth/puberty complete): 2-3mcg/kg/day. Cardiac Risk: Lower starting dose. Infants with Serum T_4 <5mcg/dL: Initial: 50mcg/day. Chronic/Severe Hypothyroidism: Children: Initial: 25mcg/day. Titrate: Increase by 25mcg for 2 weeks then every 2-4 weeks until euthyroid. May crush tab and sprinkle over food (applesauce) or mix with 5-10mL water, formula (non-soy), or breast milk.

HOW SUPPLIED: Tab: 25mcg*, 50mcg*, 75mcg*, 88mcg*, 100mcg*, 112mcg*, 125mcg*, 137mcg*, 150mcg*, 175mcg*, 200mcg*, 300mcg* *scored

CONTRAINDICATIONS: Untreated thyrotoxicosis, uncorrected adrenal insufficiency.

WARNINGS/PRECAUTIONS: Do not use in the treatment of obesity; larger doses in euthy-roid patients can cause serious or even life threatening toxicity. Caution with cardio-vascular disorders, angina, CAD, HTN and the elderly. May aggravate DM, diabetes insipidus, or adrenal cortical insufficiency. Treatment of myxedema coma may require glucocorticoids. May lower seizure threshold.

ADVERSE REACTIONS: Craniosynostosis in infants, transient hair loss, pseudotumor cerebri in pediatrics (rare), hypersensitivity reactions, seizures (rare).

INTERACTIONS: Increased risk of coronary insufficiency with sympathomimetics and CAD. May potentiate oral anticoagulant effects; adjust dose and monitor PT/INR. Lith-ium blocks release of T_4 and T_3. Antidiabetic agents may need adjustment. Decreased absorption with cholestyramine resin, colestipol, ferrous sulfate, aluminum hydroxide, sodium polystyrene sulfonate, soybean flour (infant formula), sucralfate. Altered protein binding with clofibrate, estrogens, androgens/anabolic hormones, asparaginase, 5-FU, furosemide, glucocorticoids, meclofenamic acid, mefenamic acid, methadone, per-phenazine, phenytoin, phenylbutazone, tamoxifen, salicylates. Altered thyroid hormone or TSH levels with aminoglutethimide, p-aminosalicyclic acid, amiodarone, androgens/ anabolic hormones, complex anions (eg, thiocyanate, perchlorate, pertechnetate), antithyroid drugs, β-adrenergic blockers, carbamazepine, chloral hydrate, diazepam, dopamine/dopamine agonists, ethionamide, glucocorticoids, heparin, hepatic enzyme inducers, insulin, iodinated cholestographic agents, iodine-containing compounds, levodopa, lovastatin, lithium, 6-mercaptopurine, metoclopramide, mitotane, nitroprusside, phenobarbital, phenytoin, resorcinol, rifampin, somatostatin analogs, sulfonamides, sulfonylureas, thiazide diuretics. Adrenocorticoid clearance is decreased with hypothyroidism and increased with hyperthyroidism. May potentiate anticoagulants. Cytokines, amiodarone may induce hypo- or hyperthyroidism. Increased risk of arrhythmias with maprotiline. HTN and tachycardia reported with ketamine. Sympathomimetics may increase risk of coronary insufficiency with CAD. Adverse effects of both drugs with TCAs. Decreased clearance of theophylline with hypothyroidism. Impaired β-blocker effects. Decreased digitalis effects. Decreased uptake of iodine-containing radiolabeled ions. Altered levels of theophylline may occur. Use with somatrem/somatropin may accelerate epiphyseal closure. Additive effects of both agents with TCAs. Avoid mixing crushed tabs with foods/formula with large amounts of iron, soybean or fiber.

PREGNANCY: Category A, caution in nursing.

MECHANISM OF ACTION: Thyroid hormone; not understood, suspected to control DNA transcription and protein synthesis.

PHARMACOKINETICS: Distribution: Plasma protein binding (99%); found in breast milk. **Metabolism:** Deiodination and conjugation in the liver (mainly), kidneys, and other tissues. **Elimination:** Urine, feces; (approximately 20% unchanged). (T_4) $T_{1/2}$=6-7days, and (T_3) $T_{1/2}$≤2days.

TALWIN NX CIV
naloxone HCl - pentazocine HCl (Sanofi-Aventis)

> For oral use only. Severe, potentially lethal reactions may result from misuse by injection alone, or in combination with other agents.

THERAPEUTIC CLASS: Opioid agonist-antagonist analgesic

INDICATIONS: Relief of moderate to severe pain.

DOSAGE: *Adults:* Usual: 1 tab q3-4h. May increase to 2 tabs q3-4h. Max: 12 tabs/day. *Pediatrics:* ≥12 yrs: Usual: 1 tab q3-4h. May increase to 2 tabs q3-4h. Max: 12 tabs/day.

HOW SUPPLIED: Tab: (Pentazocine-Naloxone) 50mg-0.5mg* *scored

WARNINGS/PRECAUTIONS: Caution with elderly, drug dependence, head injury, increased ICP, certain respiratory conditions, acute CNS manifestations, renal or hepatic dysfunction, biliary surgery, and MI.

ADVERSE REACTIONS: Hypotension, tachycardia, hallucinations, dizziness, sedation, euphoria, sweating, NV, constipation, diarrhea, anorexia, facial edema, dermatitis, visual problems, chills, insomnia, urinary retention, paresthesia.

INTERACTIONS: Increased CNS depressant effects with alcohol. Withdrawal symptoms with narcotics.

PREGNANCY: Category C, caution in nursing.

MECHANISM OF ACTION: Pentazocine: Acts as analgesic and sedative. Naloxone: Acts as antagonist to pentazocine and pure antagonist to narcotic analgesics.

PHARMACOKINETICS: Absorption: Pentazocine: GI tract (well absorbed), T_{max}=1-3 hrs. **Distribution:** Pentazocine: Crosses placenta. **Metabolism:** Pentazocine: Liver. **Elimination:** Pentazocine: Urine; $T_{1/2}$=2-3 hrs.

TAMBOCOR RX
flecainide acetate (Graceway)

THERAPEUTIC CLASS: Class IC antiarrhythmic

INDICATIONS: Prevention of paroxysmal supraventricular tachycardias (PSVT), paroxysmal atrial fibrillation/flutter (PAF) associated with disabling symptoms in patients without structural heart disease. Prevention of life-threatening ventricular arrhythmias such as sustained ventricular tachycardia (VT).

DOSAGE: *Adults:* PSVT/PAF: Initial: 50mg q12h. Titrate: May increase by 50mg bid every 4 days. Max: 300mg/day. Sustained VT: Initial: 100mg q12h. Titrate: May increase by 50mg bid every 4 days. Max: 400mg/day. CrCl ≤35mL/min: Initial: 100mg qd or 50mg bid. Reduce dose by 50% with amiodarone.

Pediatrics: <6 months: Initial: 50mg/m^2/day given bid-tid. ≥6 months: Initial: 100mg/m^2/day given bid-tid. Max: 200mg/m^2/day. Reduce dose by 50% with amiodarone.

HOW SUPPLIED: Tab: 50mg, 100mg*, 150mg* *scored

CONTRAINDICATIONS: Right bundle branch block associated with left hemiblock (without a pacemaker), pre-existing 2nd- or 3rd-degree AV block, cardiogenic shock.

WARNINGS/PRECAUTIONS: Avoid with non-life-threatening ventricular arrhythmias. Increased mortality and non-cardiac arrests reported. Ventricular proarrhythmic effects may occur with atrial fibrillation/flutter. May cause or worsen CHF, arrhythmias. Slows cardiac conduction; dose related increases in PR, QRS, and QT intervals reported. Conduction changes may cause sinus pause, sinus arrest, bradycardia, 2nd- or 3rd-degree AV block. Extreme caution with sick sinus syndrome. May increase endocardial pacing thresholds and suppress ventricular escape with pacemakers. Correct hypokalemia or hyperkalemia before therapy. Monitor with significant hepatic impairment. Initiate treatment of sustained VT in the hospital.

ADVERSE REACTIONS: Arrhythmias, hepatic dysfunction, cardiac arrest, CHF, flushing, anxiety, vomiting, diarrhea, tinnitus.

INTERACTIONS: Additive negative inotropic effects with β-blockers (eg, propranolol). Potentiated by cimetidine, amiodarone, CYP2D6 inhibitors (eg, quinidine). Increases digoxin levels. Increased elimination with phenytoin, phenobarbital, carbamazepine. Diltiazem, nifedipine, verapamil, disopyramide not recommended.

PREGNANCY: Category C, safety in nursing unknown.

MECHANISM OF ACTION: Class 1C antiarrhythmic agent with local anesthetic activity; decreases intracardiac conduction in all parts of the heart with greatest effect on His-Purkinje system (H-V conduction).

PHARMACOKINETICS: Absorption: Complete. T_{max}=3 hrs. **Metabolism:** Extensive, via CYP2D6. Meta-O-dealkylated flecainide (active metabolite). **Elimination:** Urine (30% unchanged), feces (5%); $T_{1/2}$=20 hrs, 29 hrs (at birth), 11-12 hrs (3 months), 6 hrs (1 yr), 8 hrs (1-12 yrs), and 11-12 hrs (12-15 yrs).

TAMIFLU

RX

oseltamivir phosphate (Roche Labs)

THERAPEUTIC CLASS: Neuraminidase inhibitor

INDICATIONS: Treatment of uncomplicated acute illness due to influenza in adults and children ≥1 yr who have been symptomatic for no more than 2 days. Prophylaxis of influenza in adults and children ≥1 yr.

DOSAGE: *Adults:* Prophylaxis: Begin within 2 days of exposure to infection. 75mg qd for at least 10 days, up to 6 weeks with community outbreak. CrCl 10-30mL/min: 75mg every other day or 30mg qd. Treatment: Begin therapy within 2 days of symptom onset. 75mg bid for 5 days. CrCl 10-30mL/min: 75mg qd for 5 days.

Pediatrics: Prophylaxis: ≥13 yr: Begin within 2 days of exposure to infection. 75mg qd for at least 10 days, up to 6 weeks with community outbreak. ≥1 yr: (Sus) ≤15kg: 30mg qd. >15-23kg: 45mg qd. >23-40kg: 60mg qd. >40kg: 75mg qd. Duration: 10 days. Treatment: ≥13 yrs: Begin therapy within 2 days of symptom onset. 75mg bid for 5 days. ≥1 yr: (Sus) ≤15kg: 30mg bid. >15-23kg: 45mg bid. >23-40kg: 60mg bid. >40kg: 75mg bid. Duration: 5 days.

HOW SUPPLIED: Cap: 30mg, 45mg, 75mg; Sus: 12mg/mL (25mL)

WARNINGS/PRECAUTIONS: Efficacy not known with chronic cardiac disease, respiratory disease, and immunocompromised. Not a substitute for influenza vaccine. Adjust dose with renal dysfunction. Postmarketing neuropsychiatric events (self-injury and delirium) reported. Caution with kidney disease, heart disease, respiratory disease, or any serious health condition. Sorbitol in Tamiflu may cause upset stomach and diarrhea in patients with history of fructose intolerance.

ADVERSE REACTIONS: NV, diarrhea, cough, headache, fatigue, abdominal pain, bronchitis, dizziness.

INTERACTIONS: Avoid administration of attenuated influenza vaccine within 2 weeks before or 48 hours after; may inhibit replication of live vaccine virus.

PREGNANCY: Category C, caution in nursing.

MECHANISM OF ACTION: Neuraminidase inhibitor; inhibits influenza virus neuraminidase, affecting release of viral particles.

PHARMACOKINETICS: Absorption: (GI tract). Oseltamivir: C_{max}=65.2ng/mL; AUC_{0-12h}=112ng•hr/mL Oseltamivir carboxylate (metabolite). C_{max}=348ng/mL; AUC_{0-12h}=2719ng•hr/mL. **Distribution:** Oseltamivir carboxylate: (IV): V_d=23-26L; plasma protein binding (3%). Oseltamivir: Plasma protein binding (42%). **Metabolism:** Oseltamivir: Hepatic (esterases). Metabolite: (Oseltamivir carboxylate). **Elimination:** Oseltamivir carboxylate: Renal (>99%); feces (<20%).

TAPAZOLE
methimazole (King)

RX

THERAPEUTIC CLASS: Thyroid hormone synthesis inhibitor

INDICATIONS: Treatment of hyperthyroidism. To ameliorate hyperthyroidism prior to subtotal thyroidectomy or radioactive iodine therapy. Also indicated when thyroidectomy is contraindicated or not advisable.

DOSAGE: *Adults:* Initial: Mild Hyperthyroidism: 5mg q8h. Moderately Severe Hyperthyroidism: 30-40mg/day, in divided doses q8h. Severe Hyperthyroidism: 20mg q8h. Maint: 5-15mg/day.
Pediatrics: Initial: 0.4mg/kg/day, in divided doses q8h. Maint: 1/2 of initial dose.

HOW SUPPLIED: Tab: 5mg*, 10mg* *scored

CONTRAINDICATIONS: Nursing mothers.

WARNINGS/PRECAUTIONS: Can cause fetal harm. Agranulocytosis, leukopenia, thrombocytopenia, aplastic anemia may occur; monitor bone marrow function. D/C with agranulocytosis, aplastic anemia, or exfoliative dermatitis. D/C with liver abnormality (eg, hepatitis) including transaminases >3x ULN. Monitor thyroid function periodically. May cause hypoprothrombinemia and bleeding; monitor PT.

ADVERSE REACTIONS: Rash, urticaria, nausea, vomiting, arthralgia, paresthesia, myalgia, neuritis, vertigo, edema, altered taste, hair loss, lymphadenopathy, lupuslike syndrome, insulin autoimmune syndrome.

INTERACTIONS: May potentiate anticoagulants. β-blockers, digitalis, theophylline may need dose reduction when patient becomes euthyroid. Caution with other drugs that cause agranulocytosis.

PREGNANCY: Category D, contraindicated in nursing.

MECHANISM OF ACTION: Inhibits synthesis of thyroid hormones.

PHARMACOKINETICS: Absorption: Readily absorbed (GI tract). **Distribution:** Crosses placenta and found in breast milk. **Elimination:** Urine.

TAVIST ALLERGY
clemastine fumarate (Novartis Consumer)

OTC

THERAPEUTIC CLASS: Antihistamine

INDICATIONS: Temporarily reduces symptoms of common cold, hay fever, or other respiratory allergies.

DOSAGE: *Adults:* 1 tab q12h. Max: 2 tabs/24 hrs.
Pediatrics: ≥12 yrs: 1 tab q12h. Max: 2 tabs/24 hrs.

HOW SUPPLIED: Tab: 1.34mg* *scored

WARNINGS/PRECAUTIONS: May cause excitability in children. Caution with respiratory problems (eg, emphysema, chronic bronchitis), glaucoma, and enlarged prostate gland. May impair mental/physical abilities.

ADVERSE REACTIONS: Drowsiness, dizziness.

INTERACTIONS: Alcohol, sedatives, and tranquilizers may increase drowsiness.

PREGNANCY: Safety in pregnancy and nursing not known.

TAZICEF
ceftazidime (Hospira)

RX

THERAPEUTIC CLASS: Cephalosporin (3rd generation)

INDICATIONS: Treatment of lower respiratory tract (eg, pneumonia), skin and skin structure (SSSI), bone and joint, gynecologic, intra-abdominal, CNS (eg, meningitis), and urinary tract infections (UTI), bacterial septicemia, and sepsis caused by susceptible strains of microorganisms.

DOSAGE: *Adults:* Usual: 1g IV q8-12h. Uncomplicated UTI: 250mg IV q12h. Complicated UTI: 500mg IV q8-12h. Bone and Joint Infections: 2g IV q12h. Uncomplicated Pneumonia/SSSI: 500mg-1g IV q8h. Gynecological/Intra-Abdominal/Meningitis/Severe Life-Threatening Infection: 2g IV q8h. Lung Infection caused by *Pseudomonas* in Cystic Fibrosis (normal renal function): 30-50mg/kg IV q8h. Max: 6g/day. Renal Impairment: CrCl 31-50mL/min: 1g q12h. CrCl 16-30mL/min: 1g q24h. CrCl 6-15mL/min: 500mg q24h. CrCl <5mL/min: 500mg q48h. For severe infections (6g/day), increase renal impairment dose by 50% or increase dosing interval. Apply reduced dosage recommendations after initial 1g LD is given. Hemodialysis: Give 1g LD before and 1g after each hemodialysis period. Intra-Peritoneal Dialysis/Continuous Ambulatory Peritoneal Dialysis: Give 1g LD followed by 500mg q24h, or add to fluid at 250mg/2L.
Pediatrics: Neonates (0-4 weeks): 30mg/kg IV q12h. 1 month-12 yrs: 30-50mg/kg IV q8h. Max: 6g/day. Higher doses for patients with cystic fibrosis or when treating meningitis. Renal Impairment: CrCl 31-50mL/min: 1g q12h. CrCl 16-30mL/min: 1g q24h. CrCl 6-15mL/min: 500mg q24h. CrCl <5mL/min: 500mg q48h. Hemodialysis: Give 1 g before and 1 g after each hemodialysis. For severe infections (6g/day), increase renal impairment dose by 50% or increase dosing interval. Apply reduced dosage recommendations after initial 1g LD is given. Hemodialysis: Give 1g LD before and 1g after each hemodialysis period. Intra-Peritoneal Dialysis/Continuous Ambulatory Peritoneal Dialysis: Give 1g followed by 500mg q24h, or add to fluid at 250mg/2L.

HOW SUPPLIED: Inj: 1g, 2g, 6g

WARNINGS/PRECAUTIONS: Monitor renal function; potential for nephrotoxicity. May result in overgrowth of nonsusceptible organisms. Possible cross-sensitivity between PCNs, cephalosporins, and other β-lactams. Pseudomembranous colitis reported. Elevated levels with renal insufficiency can lead to seizures, encephalopathy, asterixis, and neuromuscular excitability. Possible decrease in PT; caution with renal or hepatic impairment, poor nutritional state; monitor PT and give vitamin K if needed. Caution with colitis and other GI diseases. Distal necrosis may occur after inadvertent intra-arterial administration. Continue for 2 days after signs/symptoms of infection resolve; may require longer therapy with complicated infections. Caution in elderly.

ADVERSE REACTIONS: Phlebitis and inflammation at injection site, pruritus, rash, fever, diarrhea, NV.

INTERACTIONS: Nephrotoxicity reported with aminoglycosides or potent diuretics (eg, furosemide). Avoid with chloramphenicol; may decrease effect of β-lactam antibiotics.

PREGNANCY: Category B, caution in nursing.

MECHANISM OF ACTION: 3rd-generation cephalosporin; inhibits enzymes responsible for cell-wall synthesis.

PHARMACOKINETICS: Absorption: C_{max}=90mcg/mL (1g IV), 39mcg/mL (1g IM); see PI for detailed info. **Distribution:** Plasma protein binding (<10%); found in breast milk. **Elimination:** Urine (80-90% unchanged); $T_{1/2}$=1.9 hrs (IV).

TAZORAC
tazarotene (Allergan)

RX

THERAPEUTIC CLASS: Retinoid

INDICATIONS: (Gel 0.05%, 0.1%) Stable plaque psoriasis of up to 20% body surface area involvement. (Gel 0.1%) Acne vulgaris of mild to moderate severity.

DOSAGE: *Adults:* Psoriasis: Start with 0.05% Gel, increase to 0.1% if tolerated. Apply thin film to psoriatic lesions qpm. Acne: Cleanse and dry skin. Apply thin film of 0.1% Gel to acne lesions qpm.

Pediatrics: ≥12 yrs: Psoriasis: Start with 0.05% Gel, increase to 0.1% if tolerated. Apply thin film to psoriatic lesions qpm. Acne: Cleanse and dry skin. Apply thin film of 0.1% Gel to acne lesions qpm.

HOW SUPPLIED: Gel: 0.05%, 0.1% (30g, 100g)

CONTRAINDICATIONS: Women who are or may become pregnant.

WARNINGS/PRECAUTIONS: Use adequate birth control measures. Avoid mouth, eyes, eyelids, exposure to sunlight or sunlamps, or eczematous skin. D/C if pruritus, burning, skin redness, or peeling. Weather extremes (eg, wind, cold) may be irritating.

ADVERSE REACTIONS: Pruritus, burning/stinging, erythema, worsening of psoriasis, irritation, skin pain, desquamation, dry skin, rash, fissuring, localized edema, skin discoloration.

INTERACTIONS: Avoid topical agents that have a strong drying effect. Caution with photosensitizers (eg, thiazides, tetracyclines, fluoroquinolones, phenothiazines, sulfonamides).

PREGNANCY: Category X, caution in nursing.

MECHANISM OF ACTION: Retinoic acid derivative; binds to all 3 members of the retinoic acid receptor RAR (RAR_α, RAR_β, and RAR_{gamma}). Treatment of psoriasis not established. Suppresses expression of MRP8, a marker of inflammation; induces expression of a gene which may be a growth suppressor in keratinocytes, and may inhibit epidermal hyperproliferation in treated plaques. Treatment of acne not established; may be due to anti-hyperproliferative, normalizing-of-differentiation, and anti-inflammatory actions.

PHARMACOKINETICS: Absorption: Percutaneous; C_{max}=18.9ng/mL; AUC_{0-24hr}=172ng•hr/mL. **Distribution:** Plasma protein binding (>99%). **Metabolism:** Esterase hydrolysis to form tazarotenic acid (active metabolite). **Excretion:** Urine, feces; $T_{1/2}$=18 hrs.

TEGRETOL   RX
carbamazepine (Novartis)

> Serious and fatal dermatologic reactions, including toxic epiderml necrolysis (TEN), Stevens-Johnson syndrome (SJS), and presence of HLA-B*1502 allele reported. Aplastic anemia and agranulocytosis reported. Obtain complete pretreatment hematological testing as a baseline. D/C if evidence of bone marrow depression develops.

OTHER BRAND NAME: Tegretol-XR (Novartis)

THERAPEUTIC CLASS: Carboxamide

INDICATIONS: Treatment of partial seizures with complex symptomatology, general tonic-clonic seizures, and mixed seizure patterns of these or other partial or generalized seizures. Treatment of trigeminal or glossopharyngeal neuralgia pain.

DOSAGE: *Adults:* Epilepsy: Initial: (Immediate- or Extended-Release Tabs) 200mg bid or (Sus) 100mg qid. Titrate: (Immediate-Release Tabs/Sus) Increase weekly by 200mg/day given tid-qid. (Extended-Release Tabs) Increase weekly by 200mg/day given bid. Maint: 800-1200mg/day. Max: 1200mg/day. Trigeminal Neuralgia: Initial (Day 1): (Immediate- or Extended-Release Tabs) 100mg bid or (Sus) 50mg qid. Titrate: May increase by 100mg q12h (Tabs) or 50mg qid (Sus). Maint: 400-800mg/day. Max: 1200mg/day. Re-evaluate every 3 months. Extended-Release tabs should be swallowed whole and not crushed or chewed.
Pediatrics: Epilepsy: >12 yrs: Initial: (Immediate- or Extended-Release Tabs) 200mg bid or (Sus) 100mg qid. Titrate: (Immediate-Release Tabs/Sus) Increase weekly by 200mg/day given tid-qid. (Extended-Release Tabs) Increase weekly by 200mg/day given bid. Max: 12-15 yrs: 1000mg/day. >15 yrs: 1200mg/day. 6-12 yrs: Initial: (Immediate- or Extended-Release Tabs) 100mg bid or (Sus) 50mg qid. Titrate: (Immediate-Release Tabs/Sus) Increase weekly by 100mg/day given tid-qid. (Extended-Release Tabs) Increase weekly by 100mg/day given bid. Maint: 400-800mg/day. Max: 1000mg/day. 6 months-6 yrs: Initial: (Immediate-Release Tabs) 10-20mg/kg/day given bid-tid or (Sus) 10-20mg/kg/day given qid. Titrate: (Immediate-Release Tabs/Sus) Increase weekly tid-qid. Max: 35mg/kg/day. Extended-Release tabs should be swallowed whole and not crushed or chewed.

HOW SUPPLIED: Sus: 100mg/5mL (450mL); Tab: (Tegretol) 200mg*; Tab, Chewable: 100mg*; Tab, Extended-Release: (Tegretol-XR) 100mg, 200mg, 400mg *scored*

CONTRAINDICATIONS: History of bone marrow depression, MAOI use within 14 days, hypersensitivity to TCAs. Co-administration with nefazodone.

WARNINGS/PRECAUTIONS: Lyell's syndrome, Stevens-Johnson syndrome, multi-organ hypersensitivity reactions, and presence of HLA-B*1502 reported. Caution with history of adverse hematologic reaction to any drug, increased IOP, the elderly, mixed seizure disorder with atypical absence seizure. Fetal harm with pregnancy. May activate latent psychosis. Caution with cardiac (eg, conduction disturbance including second and third degree AV block), hepatic, or renal damage. Perform eye exam and monitor LFTs and renal function at baseline and periodically. Suspension produces higher peak levels than the tablet. Avoid in hepatic porphyria (eg, acute intermittent porphyria, variegate porphyria, porphyria cutanea tarda). Withdraw gradually to minimize the potential of increased seizure frequency.

ADVERSE REACTIONS: Dizziness, drowsiness, unsteadiness, nausea, vomiting, bone marrow depression, rash, urticaria, photosensitivity reactions, CHF, edema, HTN, hypotension, Stevens-Johnson syndrome, toxic epidermal necrolysis.

INTERACTIONS: Do not give suspension with other medicinal liquids or diluents. Metabolism is inhibited by CYP3A4 inhibitors (eg, cimetidine, macrolides) and induced by CYP3A4 inducers (eg, rifampin, phenytoin). Decreases oral contraceptive effectiveness. Increases plasma levels of clomipramine, phenytoin and primidone. Decreases levels of APAP, alprazolam, clonazepam, clozapine, dicumarol, doxycycline, ethosuximide, haloperidol, lamotrigine, methsuximide, oral contraceptives, phensuximide, phenytoin, theophylline, tiagabine, topiramate, valproate, and warfarin. Increased risk of neurotoxic side effects with lithium. Avoid MAOIs.

PREGNANCY: Category D, not for use in nursing.

MECHANISM OF ACTION: Anticonvulsant; reduces polysynaptic response and blocks past-tetanic potentiation.

PHARMACOKINETICS: Absorption: T_{max}=1.5 hrs (oral); T_{max}=4-5 hrs(conventional tab); T_{max} = 3-12 hrs (XR tab). **Distribution:** Plasma protein binding (76%). Found in placenta and breast milk. **Metabolism:** Liver via cytochrome P450 3A4. Carbamazepine-10,11-epoxide (metabolite). **Elimination:** Urine (3% unchanged); $T_{1/2}$=25-65 hrs (single dose); $T_{1/2}$=12-17 hrs (multiple doses).

TEMOVATE

RX

clobetasol propionate (GlaxoSmithKline)

OTHER BRAND NAMES: Temovate Scalp (GlaxoSmithKline) - Temovate-E (GlaxoSmithKline)

THERAPEUTIC CLASS: Corticosteroid

INDICATIONS: Corticosteroid responsive dermatoses. Temovate-E is also used to treat moderate to severe plaque-type psoriasis.

DOSAGE: *Adults:* Apply bid. Max: 50g/week or 50mL/week. Moderate-Severe Psoriasis: (Temovate-E) Apply bid for up to 4 weeks. May use on 5-10% of BSA. Max: 50g/week. Limit treatment to 2 consecutive weeks. Avoid with occlusive dressings.
Pediatrics: ≥12 yrs: Apply bid. Max: 50g/week or 50mL/week. Moderate-Severe Psoriasis; ≥16 yrs: (Temovate-E) Apply bid for up to 4 weeks. May use on 5-10% of BSA. Max: 50g/week. Limit treatment to 2 consecutive weeks. Avoid with occlusive dressings.

HOW SUPPLIED: Cre, Oint: 0.05% (15g, 30g, 45g, 60g); Gel: 0.05% (15g, 30g, 60g); (Temovate-E) Cre: 0.05% (15g, 30g, 60g); (Temovate Scalp) Sol: 0.05% (25mL)

CONTRAINDICATIONS: (Scalp Sol) Primary scalp infections.

WARNINGS/PRECAUTIONS: Not for use on face, groin, or axillae, or for treatment of rosacea or perioral dermatitis. May produce reversible HPA axis suppression, manifestations of Cushing's syndrome, hyperglycemia, and glucosuria. Use appropriate antifungal or antibacterial agent with dermatological infections; d/c if infection does not clear. Peds may be more susceptible to systemic toxicity. Avoid eyes. D/C if irritation occurs.

ADVERSE REACTIONS: Burning, stinging, pruritus, skin atrophy, cracking/fissuring of the skin, erythema, folliculitis, numbness of fingers, telangiectasia, tingling (Sol), folliculitis (Sol).

PREGNANCY: Category C, caution in nursing.

MECHANISM OF ACTION: Corticosteroid; possesses anti-inflammatory, antipruritic, and vasoconstrictive properties. Anti-inflammatory effects not established. Suspected to act by induction of phospholipase A_2 inhibitory proteins, lipocortins. Lipocortins control biosynthesis of potent inflammation mediators (eg, prostaglandins, leukotrienes) by inhibiting release of their common precursor, arachidonic acid.

PHARMACOKINETICS: Absorption: Occlusion, inflammation, other disease states may increase absorption. Use of occlusive dressings ≤24 hrs does not increase penetration; use of occlusive dressings for 96 hrs markedly enhances penetration.

TERBUTALINE   RX
terbutaline sulfate (Various)

THERAPEUTIC CLASS: Beta$_2$ -agonist

INDICATIONS: Prevention and reversal of bronchospasm in asthma, and reversible bronchospasm in bronchitis and emphysema.

DOSAGE: *Adults:* (PO) Usual: 5mg tid. May reduce to 2.5mg tid. Max: 15mg/24hrs. (Inj) Usual: 0.25mg SQ into lateral deltoid area. May repeat within 15-30 min if no improvement. Max: 0.5mg/4hrs.
Pediatrics: (PO) 12-15 yrs: Usual: 2.5mg tid. Max: 7.5mg/24hrs. (Inj) ≥12 yrs: Usual: 0.25mg SQ into lateral deltoid area. May repeat within 15-30 min if no improvement. Max: 0.5mg/4hrs.

HOW SUPPLIED: Inj: 1mg/mL (1mL); Tab: 2.5mg*, 5mg* *scored

CONTRAINDICATIONS: Hypersensitivity to sympathomimetic amines.

WARNINGS/PRECAUTIONS: Caution with ischemic heart disease, HTN, arrhythmias, hyperthyroidism, DM, seizures. Not approved for tocolysis. Hypersensitivity and exacerbation of bronchospasm reported. Monitor for transient hypokalemia.

ADVERSE REACTIONS: Nervousness, tremor, headache, somnolence, palpitations, dizziness, tachycardia, nausea.

INTERACTIONS: Avoid other sympathomimetic agents (except aerosol bronchodilators). Extreme caution with MAOIs and TCAs during or within 14 days of treatment. Decreased effects with β-blockers. Possible ECG changes and hypokalemia with loop or thiazide diuretics.

PREGNANCY: Category B, caution in nursing.

MECHANISM OF ACTION: β$_2$-adrenergic agonist; stimulates intracellular adenyl cyclase, which catalyzes conversion of ATP to cAMP, to produce relaxation of bronchial smooth muscle and inhibition of release of mediators of immediate hypersensitivity from cells (mast cells).

PHARMACOKINETICS: Absorption: (SC) C_{max}=9.6ng/mL; T_{max}=0.5 hrs; AUC=29.4h•ng/mL. (Tab) C_{max}=8.3ng/mL; T_{max}=2 hrs; AUC=54.6h•ng/mL. (Sol) C_{max}=8.6ng/mL; T_{max}=1.5 hrs; AUC=53.1h•ng/mL. **Metabolism:** Sulfate conjugate (metabolite). **Elimination:** SC: Urine (60%); $T_{1/2}$=5.7 hrs. (PO) Urine (30-50%), feces; $T_{1/2}$=3.4 hrs (asthmatics).

TESSALON   RX
benzonatate (Forest)

THERAPEUTIC CLASS: Non-narcotic antitussive

INDICATIONS: Symptomatic relief of cough.

DOSAGE: *Adults:* Usual: 100-200mg tid as needed. Max: 600mg/day.
Pediatrics: >10 yrs: Usual: 100-200mg tid as needed. Max: 600mg/day.

HOW SUPPLIED: Cap: 100mg, 200mg

WARNINGS/PRECAUTIONS: Severe hypersensitivity reactions; confusion and hallucinations reported in combination with other prescribed drugs. Swallow capsules without sucking/chewing to avoid local anesthesia adverse effects.

ADVERSE REACTIONS: Sedation, headache, dizziness, confusion, hallucinations, constipation, nausea, GI upset, pruritus.

PREGNANCY: Category C, caution in nursing.

MECHANISM OF ACTION: Non-narcotic/antitussive agent; acts peripherally by anesthesizing stretch receptors located in respiratory passages, lungs, and pleura by dampening their activity, thereby reducing cough reflex at its source.

TESTRED
methylTESTOSTERONE (Valeant)

THERAPEUTIC CLASS: Androgen

INDICATIONS: Testosterone replacement therapy in males with primary hypogonadism or hypogonadotrophic hypogonadism. To stimulate puberty in males with delayed puberty. Secondary treatment of advancing inoperable metastatic (skeletal) breast cancer in females 1-5 yrs postmenopausal.

DOSAGE: *Adults:* Dose based on age, sex and diagnosis. Adjust dose according to clinical response and adverse events. Male Replacement Therapy: 10-50mg/day. Breast Carcinoma: 50-200mg/day.
Pediatrics: Dose based on age, sex and diagnosis. Adjust dose according to clinical response and adverse events. Delayed Puberty: Use lower range of 10-50mg/day for 4-6 months. Caution in children.

HOW SUPPLIED: Cap: 10mg

CONTRAINDICATIONS: Pregnancy. Males with breast or prostate carcinoma.

WARNINGS/PRECAUTIONS: D/C if hypercalcemia occurs in breast cancer; monitor calcium levels. Monitor for virilization in females. Risk of compromised stature in children; monitor bone growth every 6 months. Risk of hepatic damage with long-term use. D/C if jaundice, cholestatic hepatitis occurs. Risk of edema; caution with pre-existing cardiac, renal or hepatic disease. Caution in the elderly; increased risk of prostatic hypertrophy and prostatic carcinoma. Should not be used for enhancement of athletic performance. Monitor LFTs, Hct, and Hgb periodically.

ADVERSE REACTIONS: Amenorrhea, virilization, menstrual irregularities, gynecomastia, excessive frequency/duration of penile erections, male pattern baldness, increased/decreased libido, oligospermia, hirsutism, acne, fluid and electrolyte disturbances, nausea, hypercholesterolemia, clotting factor suppression, polycythemia, altered LFTs, priapism, anxiety, depression.

INTERACTIONS: Potentiates oral anticoagulants and oxyphenbutazone. May decrease blood glucose and insulin requirements in diabetics.

PREGNANCY: Category X, not for use in nursing.

MECHANISM OF ACTION: Endogenous androgen (derivative of testosterone); responsible for normal growth and development of male sex organs and maintenance of secondary sex characteristics.

PHARMACOKINETICS: Metabolism: Gut, liver. **Elimination:** Urine, feces; $T_{1/2}$=10-100 min.

TETANUS & DIPHTHERIA TOXOIDS ADSORBED RX
diphtheria toxoid - tetanus toxoid (Sanofi Pasteur)

THERAPEUTIC CLASS: Toxoid combination

INDICATIONS: Active immunization against tetanus and diphtheria (Td).

DOSAGE: *Adults:* 0.5mL IM in the vastus lateralis or deltoid. Repeat 4-8 weeks later. Give 3rd dose 6-12 months after 2nd dose. Booster: 0.5mL IM every 10 yrs.
Pediatrics: >7 yrs: 0.5mL IM in the vastus lateralis or deltoid. Repeat 4-8 weeks later. Give 3rd dose 6-12 months after 2nd dose. Booster: 0.5mL IM every 10 yrs.

HOW SUPPLIED: Inj: 5LFU-2LFU/0.5mL

CONTRAINDICATIONS: Neurological or systemic allergic reaction to previous dose. Defer during febrile illness, acute infection, or an outbreak of poliomyelitis. Thimerosal hypersensitivity.

WARNINGS/PRECAUTIONS: Suboptimal response may occur in immunocompromised patients. Avoid booster more frequently than every 10 yrs especially with Arthus-type hypersensitivity reactions or temperature >39.4°C after a previous dose of tetanus toxoid. Caution with IM injection in thrombocytopenia or any coagulation disorder. Increased risk of local/systemic reactions to boosters doses. Have epinephrine available.

ADVERSE REACTIONS: Injection site reaction, fever, malaise, hypotension, nausea, arthralgia.

INTERACTIONS: Immunosuppressive therapy may reduce response to active immunization. Caution with anticoagulants.

PREGNANCY: Category C, safety in nursing not known.

MECHANISM OF ACTION: Toxoid combination; activates neutralizing antibodies to diphtheria and tetanus toxins for protection against diphtheria and tetanus.

PHARMACOKINETICS: Absorption: Complete.

TETANUS TOXOID ADSORBED RX
tetanus toxoid (Sanofi Pasteur)

THERAPEUTIC CLASS: Toxoid

INDICATIONS: Active immunization against tetanus.

DOSAGE: *Adults:* Primary Immunization: 0.5mL IM. Repeat 4-8 weeks later. Give 3rd dose 6-12 months after 2nd dose. Booster: 0.5mL IM every 10 yrs.
Pediatrics: <1 yr: 3 doses of 0.5mL IM 4 to 8 weeks apart, then 4th dose (0.5mL) 6 to 12 months after the 3rd dose. Last dose before 4 yrs. Give booster of 0.5mL at 4-6 yrs. No booster needed if last primary dose was given after 4 yrs. ≥1 yrs: Primary Immunization: 0.5mL IM. Repeat 4-8 weeks later. Give 3rd dose 6-12 months after 2nd dose. Booster: 0.5mL IM every 10 yrs.

HOW SUPPLIED: Inj: 5 LFU/0.5mL

CONTRAINDICATIONS: Neurological or systemic allergic reaction to previous dose. Defer during febrile illness, acute infection, or an outbreak of poliomyelitis. Thimerosal hypersensitivity.

WARNINGS/PRECAUTIONS: Suboptimal response may occur in immunocompromised patients. Avoid booster more frequently than every 10 yrs especially with Arthus-type hypersensitivity reactions or temperature >103°F after a previous dose of tetanus toxoid. Caution with IM injections in thrombocytopenia or any coagulation disorders. Have epinephrine injection available. Increased incidence of local/systemic reaction to booster doses.

ADVERSE REACTIONS: Local erythema, malaise, transient fever, pain, hypotension, nausea, arthralgia.

INTERACTIONS: Caution with anticoagulants. Immunosuppresive therapy (eg, radiation, corticosteroids, chemotherapy) may reduce antibody response to vaccine; defer routine vaccination. Separate syringes and sites should be used when Tetanus Immune Globulin (human) and vaccine are given concurrently.

PREGNANCY: Category C, safety in nursing not known.

MECHANISM OF ACTION: Development of neutralizing antibodies against tetanus toxin.

TEV-TROPIN RX
somatropin (Gate)

THERAPEUTIC CLASS: Human growth hormone

INDICATIONS: Long-term treatment of children who have growth failure due to an inadequate secretion of normal endogenous growth hormone.

DOSAGE: *Pediatrics:* 0.1mg/kg (0.3 IU/kg) SQ 3x week.

HOW SUPPLIED: Inj: 5mg

CONTRAINDICATIONS: Prader-Willi syndrome (PWS) with severe obesity or severe respiratory impairment. Growth failure due to PWS. Acute critical illness due to complications following open heart or abdominal surgery, multiple accidental traumas, acute respiratory failure; closed epiphyses; progression of an underlying intracranial lesion; active neoplasia, benzyl alcohol sensitivity.

WARNINGS/PRECAUTIONS: Reports of fatalities in pediatric patients with PWS. In PWS, evaluate for upper airway obstruction prior to initiation; monitor weight, for sleep apnea, signs of upper airway obstruction (eg, suspend therapy with onset of or increased snoring), respiratory infections (treat early and aggressively if occur). Monitor GHD secondary to intracranial lesion for progression/recurrence; glucose intolerance; hypothyroidism; intracranial hypertension (perform fundoscopic exam at start and periodically). Slipped capital femoral epiphysis may occur. Monitor for malignant transformation of any skin lesion. When injected SQ in same site over long period of time, may cause tissue atrophy; rotate injection site.

ADVERSE REACTIONS: Headaches, injection site reactions (pain, bruise), leukemia.

INTERACTIONS: Decreased effects with glucocorticoids.

PREGNANCY: Category C, caution with nursing.

MECHANISM OF ACTION: Human growth hormone; stimulates linear growth synthesis, metabolizes lipids, reduces body fat stores by increasing cellular protein, and increases plasma fatty acids.

PHARMACOKINETICS: Absorption: C_{max}=80ng/mL. T_{max}=7 hrs. **Elimination:** (IV): $T_{1/2}$=0.42 hrs. (SQ) $T_{1/2}$=2.7 hrs.

THALOMID
thalidomide (Celgene)

RX

> Severe, life-threatening human birth defects if taken during pregnancy. Women of childbearing potential should have a pregnancy test before starting therapy, then weekly for 1st month, and monthly thereafter. Males must use latex condoms during sexual contact with females of childbearing potential. Effective contraception must be used 4 weeks before, during, and 4 weeks after therapy. Only prescribers and pharmacists registered with the *S.T.E.P.S.*® distribution program can prescribe and dispense. The use of thalidomide in multiple myeloma results in an increased risk of venous thromboembolic events (eg, DVT, PE).

THERAPEUTIC CLASS: Immunomodulatory agent

INDICATIONS: Acute treatment of the cutaneous manifestations of moderate to severe erythema nodosum leprosum (ENL). Maintenance therapy for prevention and suppression of the cutaneous manifestations of ENL recurrence. In combination with dexamethasone for the treatment of newly diagnosed multiple myeloma.

DOSAGE: *Adults:* Acute ENL: Initial: 100-300mg qhs with water at least 1 hr after evening meal. <50kg: Start therapy at lower end of dosing range. Severe Cutaneous ENL: Initial: 400mg qhs with water at least 1 hr after evening meal. Use with corticosteroids in moderate to severe neuritis with severe ENL. Taper steroid where neuritis is ameliorated. Duration of therapy is usually 2 weeks. Taper Dose: Decrease by 50mg every 2-4 weeks. Maintenance Therapy for Prevention/Suppression of ENL Recurrence: Use minimum dose to control reaction. Taper Dose: Every 3-6 months, attempt to decrease dose by 50mg every 2-4 weeks. Multiple Myeloma: 200mg qhs at least 1 hr after evening meal. Give with dexamethasone in 28 day treatment cycles.
Pediatrics: ≥12 yrs: Acute ENL: Initial: 100-300mg qhs with water at least 1 hr after evening meal. <50kg: Start therapy at lower end of dosing range. Severe Cutaneous ENL: Initial: 400mg qhs with water at least 1 hour after evening meal. Use with corticosteroids in moderate to severe neuritis with severe ENL. Taper steroid where neuritis is ameliorated. Duration of therapy is usually 2 weeks. Taper Dose: Decrease by 50mg every 2-4 weeks. Maintenance Therapy for Prevention/Suppression of ENL Recurrence: Use minimum dose to control reaction. Taper Dose: Every 3-6 months, attempt to decrease dose by 50mg every 2-4 weeks. Multiple Myeloma: 200mg qhs at least 1 hr after evening meal. Give with dexamethasone in 28-day treatment cycles.

HOW SUPPLIED: Cap: 50mg, 100mg, 200mg

CONTRAINDICATIONS: Women of childbearing potential unless alternative therapies are considered inappropriate and if precautions are taken to avoid pregnancy. Sexually mature males unless they comply with the *S.T.E.P.S.*® program and mandatory contraceptive measures.

WARNINGS/PRECAUTIONS: See Black Box Warning. If hypersensitivity reaction occurs such as rash, fever, or tachycardia, d/c drug. Stevens-Johnson syndrome and toxic epidermal necrolysis reported. May cause severe birth defects. Drowsiness and somnolence reported, caution when operating machinery. May cause neuropathy, monitor for symptoms. If symptoms of neuropathy arise, d/c immediately. Do not initiate if ANC <750/mm^3. Measure viral load of HIV patients after 1st and 3rd month of therapy and every 3 months thereafter.

ADVERSE REACTIONS: Drowsiness, somnolence, peripheral neuropathy, dizziness, orthostatic hypotension, neutropenia, increased HIV viral load, rash, constipation, hypocalcemia, thrombosis/embolism, dyspnea.

INTERACTIONS: Enhanced sedation with barbiturates, alcohol, chlorpromazine, and reserpine. Caution with drugs associated with peripheral neuropathy.

PREGNANCY: Category X, not for use in nursing.

MECHANISM OF ACTION: Immunomodulatory agent; not fully established. Possesses immunomodulatory, anti-inflammatory, and anti-angiogenic properties. Immunologic effects may be caused by suppression of excessive TNF-α production and down-modulation of selected cell surface adhesion molecules involved in leukocyte migration. Also causes suppression of macrophage involvement in prostaglandin synthesis and modulation of interleukin-10 and 12 production by peripheral blood mononuclear cells. In multiple myeloma, increased circulating natural killer cells and plasma levels of interleukin-2 and INF-gamma are also seen.

PHARMACOKINETICS: Absorption: Slow; T_{max}=2.9-5.7 hrs. **Distribution:** Plasma protein binding (55-66%); found in semen. **Metabolism:** Non-enzymatic hydrolysis. **Elimination:** Urine (<0.7% unchanged); $T_{1/2}$=5-7 hrs.

THEO-24   RX
theophylline (UCB Pharma)

THERAPEUTIC CLASS: Xanthine bronchodilator

INDICATIONS: Treatment of symptoms and reversible airflow obstruction associated with chronic asthma and other chronic lung diseases.

DOSAGE: *Adults:* Initial: 300-400mg/day. Titrate: After 3 days increase to 400-600mg/day if tolerated. May increase to >600mg/day if needed and tolerated after 3 more days. Renal/Liver Dysfunction/Elderly/CHF: Max: 400mg/day. May give in divided doses q12h in fast metabolizers. Swallow tab whole with full glass of water, do not crush. Dose should be titrated based on serum levels.
Pediatrics: 12-15 yrs: <45kg: Initial: 12-14mg/kg/day. Max: 300mg/day. Titrate: After 3 days increase to 16mg/kg/day. Max: 400mg/day. May increase to 20mg/kg/day if tolerated and needed after 3 more days. Max: 600mg/day. 12-15 yrs (>45kg): Follow adult dose schedule. Renal/Liver Dysfunction/CHF: Max: 16mg/kg/day or 400mg/day. May give in divided doses q12h in fast metabolizers. Swallow tab whole with full glass of water, do not crush. Dose should be titrated based on serum levels.

HOW SUPPLIED: Cap, Extended-Release: 100mg, 200mg, 300mg, 400mg

WARNINGS/PRECAUTIONS: Extreme caution in PUD, seizure disorders, and/or cardiac arrhythmias (except bradycardia). Caution in neonates, children <1 yr, and the elderly. Caution in pulmonary edema, CHF, fever ≥102°F for 24 hrs, cor-pulmonale, hypothyroidism, liver disease, reduced renal function, sepsis, shock, and HTN. If toxicity develops (eg, repetitive vomiting) monitor serum levels and adjust dosage.

ADVERSE REACTIONS: Diarrhea, nausea, vomiting, abdominal pain, nervousness, headache, insomnia, seizures, dizziness, tachycardia, arrhythmias, restlessness, tremor, transient diuresis.

INTERACTIONS: Potentiated by propranolol, allopurinol, erythromycin, cimetidine, interferon, ciprofloxacin, clarithromycin, disulfiram, enoxacin, methotrexate, β-adrenergic blockers, oral contraceptives, fluvoxamine, CCBs, corticosteroid, thyroid hormones, thiabendazole, ticlopidine, troleandomycin, carbamazepine, pentoxifylline, diuretics, tacrine, and isoniazid. Diminishes the effects of adenosine, diazepam, lithium, lorazepam, midazolam, and pancuronium. Synergistic CNS effects with ephedrine. Diminished effects with aminoglutethemide, phenytoin, phenobarbital, carbamazepine, rifampin, barbiturates, hydantoins, ketoconazole, diuretics sympathomimetics, and isoproterenol.

PREGNANCY: Category C, caution in nursing.

MECHANISM OF ACTION: Methylxanthine; not established, suspected to act by relaxation of smooth muscle and suppression of response of airways to stimuli.

PHARMACOKINETICS: Absorption: Rapid, complete; C_{max}=18.1mcg/mL. **Distribution**: V_d=0.45L/kg; plasma protein binding (40%); crosses placenta; excreted in breast milk. **Metabolism**: Liver (N-demethylation); metabolite: Caffeine. Liver (demethylation) via CYP1A2; metabolite: 3-methylxanthine. Liver (hydroxylation) via CYP2E1 and 3A3. **Elimination**: (Neonates) Urine (50%). (>3mo) Urine (10%).

THIOGUANINE
thioguanine (GlaxoSmithKline)

RX

THERAPEUTIC CLASS: Purine analog

INDICATIONS: For remission induction, remission consolidation, and maintenance therapy of acute nonlymphocytic leukemias.

DOSAGE: *Adults:* Monotherapy: 2mg/kg/day. After 4 weeks, may increase to 3mg/kg/day if no improvement and leukocyte or platelet depression. Usual therapy is with other agents in combination.
Pediatrics: Monotherapy: 2mg/kg/day. After 4 weeks, may increase to 3mg/kg/day if no improvement and leukocyte or platelet depression. Usual therapy is with other agents in combination.

HOW SUPPLIED: Tab: 40mg* *scored

CONTRAINDICATIONS: Prior resistance to this drug.

WARNINGS/PRECAUTIONS: Dose-related bone-marrow suppression. Increased sensitivity to myelosuppression with thioguanine methyltransferase (TPMT) deficiency. D/C temporarily at 1st sign of abnormally large fall in any formed elements of the blood. Withhold therapy with toxic hepatitis or biliary stasis. Monitor Hgb, Hct, platelets, WBCs, and differential frequently. Monitor LFTs weekly at start of therapy, monthly thereafter.

ADVERSE REACTIONS: Myelosuppression, hyperuricemia, hepatotoxicity, nausea, vomiting, anorexia, stomatitis.

INTERACTIONS: May be cross-resistant with mercaptopurine. Caution with TPMT inhibitors such as aminosalicylate derivatives (eg, olsalazine, mesalazine, sulfasalazine); increased sensitivity to myelosuppression. May need dose reduction with other drugs whose primary toxicity is myelosuppression. Esophageal varices reported with busulfan. Veno-occlusive liver disease reported with combination chemotherapy.

PREGNANCY: Category D, not for use in nursing.

MECHANISM OF ACTION: Purine analog; competes with hypoxanthine and guanine for the enzyme hypoxanthine-guanine phosphoribosyltransferase (HGPTase).

PHARMACOKINETICS: Absorption: (30%) Incomplete and variable. (2-amino-6-methylthiopurine (MTG)) T_{max}= 6-8 hrs. **Metabolism:** Rapid via methylation to MTG (active) and inactive compounds. **Elimination:** Urine, (MTG) $T_{1/2}$=12-22 hrs.

THIORIDAZINE
thioridazine HCl (Various)

RX

> Prolongation of QTc interval reported in a dose related manner. Associated with torsade de pointes and sudden death; reserve for patients who fail to respond to or cannot tolerate other antipsychotics.

THERAPEUTIC CLASS: Piperidine phenothiazine

INDICATIONS: Management of schizophrenia in patients not responsive to or intolerant to other antipsychotics.

DOSAGE: *Adults:* Initial: 50-100mg tid. Titrate: Increase gradually. Usual: 200-800mg/day given bid-qid. Max: 800mg/day.
Pediatrics: Initial: 0.6mg/kg/day given in divided doses. Titrate: Increase gradually. Max: 3mg/kg/day.

HOW SUPPLIED: Tab: 10mg, 15mg, 25mg, 50mg, 100mg, 150mg, 200mg

CONTRAINDICATIONS: Severe CNS depression, comatose states, severe hypo- or hypertensive heart disease. Drugs that prolong QTc interval, congenital long QT syndrome, cardiac arrhythmias, drugs that inhibit CYP450 2D6 (eg, fluoxetine, paroxetine), patients with reduced activity of CYP450 2D6.

435

WARNINGS/PRECAUTIONS: Perform baseline ECG and measure baseline potassium level; monitor periodically thereafter. May develop tardive dyskinesia. NMS, seizures, leukopenia, agranulocytosis reported. Caution with activities requiring alertness. May elevate prolactin levels.

ADVERSE REACTIONS: Tardive dyskinesia, ECG changes, drowsiness, dry mouth, blurred vision, peripheral edema, galactorrhea, nausea, vomiting, gynecomastia, impotence, constipation, diarrhea.

INTERACTIONS: See Contraindications. May potentiate CNS depressants, alcohol, atropine, and phosphorus insecticides. Propranolol, fluvoxamine, pindolol increases thioridazine plasma levels; avoid concomitant use. Avoid CYP2D6 inhibitors (eg, fluoxetine, paroxetine); increased risk of arrhythmias.

PREGNANCY: Safety in pregnancy and nursing not known.

MECHANISM OF ACTION: Phenothiazine; associated with minimal extrapyramidal stimulation.

THYROGEN   RX
thyrotropin alfa (Genzyme)

THERAPEUTIC CLASS: Recombinant human thyroid stimulating hormone

INDICATIONS: Adjunctive diagnostic tool for serum thyroglobulin testing with or without radioiodine imaging in thyroid cancer. Adjunctive treatment for radioiodine ablation of thyroid tissue remnants in patients who have undergone a near-total or total thyroidectomy for well-differentiated thyroid cancer and who do not have evidence of metastatic thyroid cancer.

DOSAGE: *Adults:* 0.9mg IM q24h for 2 doses into buttock. Radioiodine Imaging or Remnant Ablation: Administer radioiodine 24 hrs following final injection. Perform diagnostic scanning 48 hrs after radioiodine administration. Serum Thyroglobulin (Tg) Testing: Obtain serum sample 72 hrs after final injection.
Pediatrics: ≥16 yrs: 0.9mg IM q24h for 2 dose into buttock. Radioiodine Imaging or Remnant Ablation: Administer radioiodine 24 hrs following final injection. Perform diagnostic scanning 48 hrs after radioiodine administration. Serum Thyroglobulin (Tg) Testing: Obtain serum sample 72 hrs after final injection.

HOW SUPPLIED: Inj: 1.1mg

WARNINGS/PRECAUTIONS: Tg antibodies may confound the Tg assay and render Tg levels uninterpretable; may need to evaluate patients further with, eg, a confirmatory thyroid hormone withdrawal scan. Caution if previously treated with bovine TSH, particularly if hypersensitivity reactions occurred. Caution with history of heart disease and significant residual thyroid tissue. May prolong elevation of TSH levels in dialysis-dependent ESRD patients. IM use only. Caution in elderly.

ADVERSE REACTIONS: Headache, nausea, asthenia, hypercholesterolemia, paresthesia, influenza-like symptoms.

INTERACTIONS: Pretreatment with glucocorticoids may be considered in patients whom local tumor expansion may compromise vital anatomic structures.

PREGNANCY: Category C, caution in nursing.

MECHANISM OF ACTION: Recombinant human thyroid stimulating hormone; binds to TSH receptors on normal thyroid epithelial cells or thyroid cancer tissues and stimulates iodine reuptake and organification, and synthesis and secretion of thyroglobulin, T_3, T_4.

PHARMACOKINETICS: Absorption: (0.9mg IM) C_{max}=116mU/L, T_{max}=3-24 hrs. **Elimination:** $T_{1/2}$=25 hrs.

THYROLAR   RX
liotrix (Forest)

THERAPEUTIC CLASS: Thyroid replacement hormone

INDICATIONS: Hypothyroidism. As a pituitary TSH suppressant in the treatment or prevention of euthyroid goiters. Diagnostic agent in suppression tests to differentiate suspected hyperthyroidism or thyroid gland autonomy. Management of thyroid cancer.

DOSAGE: *Adults:* Hypothyroidism: Usual: 12.5mcg-50mcg to 25mcg-100mcg qd. Elderly/ Coronary Artery Disease: Initial: 6.25mcg-25mcg qd. Chronic Myxedema: 3.1mcg-12.5mcg qd. Titrate: Increase by 3.1mcg-12.5mcg/d q 2-3 weeks. Reduce dose if angina occurs. Myxedema Coma: 400mcg IV levothyroxine sodium (100mcg/mL rapidly) followed by 100-200mcg/day IV. Switch to PO when stable. Thyroid Suppression: 1.56mg/kg/d levothyroxine (T$_4$) for 7-10 days.
Pediatrics: Hypothyroidism: >12 yrs: 18.75mcg-75mcg qd. 6-12 yrs: 12.5mcg-50mcg to 18.75mcg-75mcg qd. 1-5 yrs: 9.35mcg-37.5mcg to 12.5mcg-50mcg qd. 6-12 months: 6.25mcg-25mcg to 9.35mcg-37.5mcg qd. 0-6 months: 3.1mcg-12.5mcg to 6.25mcg-25mcg qd.

HOW SUPPLIED: (T3-T4) Tab: (1/4) 3.1mcg-12.5mcg, (1/2) 6.25mcg-25mcg, (1) 12.5mcg-50mcg, (2) 25mcg-100mcg, (3) 37.5mcg-150mcg

CONTRAINDICATIONS: Untreated thyrotoxicosis, uncorrected adrenal cortical insufficiency.

WARNINGS/PRECAUTIONS: Do not use in the treatment of obesity; larger doses in euthyroid patients can cause serious or even life-threatening toxicity. Caution with angina pectoris and elderly; use lower doses. May aggravate diabetes mellitus or insipidus and adrenal cortical insufficiency. Excessive doses may cause craniosynostosis. Extreme caution with long-standing myxedema especially with cardiovascular impairment.

INTERACTIONS: May increase insulin or oral hypoglycemic requirements. Decreased absorption with cholestyramine and colestipol; space dosing by 4-5 hrs. Altered effect of oral anticoagulants; monitor PT/INR. Estrogens increase thyroxine-binding globulin; increase in thyroid dose may be needed. Serious or life-threatening side effects can occur with sympathomimetic amines. Androgens, corticosteroids, estrogens, iodine-containing preparations, and salicylates may interfere with thyroid lab tests.

PREGNANCY: Category A, caution in nursing.

MECHANISM OF ACTION: Thyroid hormone; not understood, suspected to enhance oxygen consumption by most tissues of the body, increase basal metabolic rate and metabolism of carbohydrates, lipids, and proteins.

TIMENTIN
RX

clavulanate potassium - ticarcillin disodium (GlaxoSmithKline)

THERAPEUTIC CLASS: Broad-spectrum penicillin/beta-lactamase inhibitor

INDICATIONS: Treatment of lower respiratory tract, bone and joint, skin and skin structure, urinary tract (UTI), gynecologic, and intra-abdominal infections, and septicemia caused by susceptible strains of microorganisms.

DOSAGE: *Adults:* ≥60kg: UTI/Systemic Infection: 3g-100mg (3.1g vial) IV q4-6h. Gynecologic Infections: Moderate: 200mg/kg/day ticarcillin IV given q6h. Severe: 300mg/kg/day ticarcillin IV given q4h. <60kg: Usual: 200-300mg/kg/day ticarcillin IV given q4-6h. Renal Impairment (based on ticarcillin): LD: 3.1g. Maint: CrCl >60mL/min: 3.1g q4h. CrCl 30-60mL/min: 2g IV q4h. CrCl 10-30mL/min: 2g IV q8h. CrCl <10mL/min: 2g IV q12h (2g IV q24h with hepatic dysfunction). Peritoneal Dialysis: 3.1g IV q12h. Hemodialysis: 2g IV q12h, and 3.1g after each dialysis.
Pediatrics: ≥3 months: ≥60kg: Mild to Moderate: 3g-100mg (3.1g vial) IV q6h. Severe: 3g-100mg (3.1g vial) IV q4h. <60 kg: Mild to Moderate: 50mg/kg ticarcillin IV q6h. Severe: 50mg/kg ticarcillin IV q4h. Renal Impairment (based on ticarcillin): LD: 3.1g vial. Maint: CrCl >60mL/min: 3.1g q4h. CrCl 30-60mL/min: 2g IV q4h. CrCl 10-30mL/min: 2g IV q8h. CrCl <10mL/min: 2g IV q12h (2g IV q24h with hepatic dysfunction). Peritoneal Dialysis: 3.1g IV q12h. Hemodialysis: 2g IV q12h, and 3.1g after each dialysis.

HOW SUPPLIED: Inj: (Ticarcillin-Clavulanate) 3g-100mg, 3g-100mg/100mL, 30g-1g

WARNINGS/PRECAUTIONS: Serious, sometimes fatal, hypersensitivity reactions reported with PCN therapy. *Clostridium difficile*-associated diarrhea reported. Prolonged use may result in overgrowth of nonsusceptible organisms. Risk of convulsions with high doses especially with renal impairment. Monitor renal, hepatic, hematopoietic functions, and serum K$^+$ with prolonged therapy. Caution with fluid and electrolyte imbalance; hypokalemia reported. Clotting time, platelet aggregation, and PT abnormalities may occur especially with renal impairment; d/c therapy. Continue therapy for at least 2 days after signs/symptoms disappear. Caution in elderly patients with impaired renal function.

ADVERSE REACTIONS: Hypersensitivity reactions, headache, giddiness, taste/smell disturbances, stomatitis, flatulence, NV, diarrhea, hematologic disturbances, hepatic/renal function tests abnormalities, local reactions.

INTERACTIONS: May inactivate aminoglycoside if mixed together in parenteral solution. Increased serum levels and prolonged half-life with probenecid. May reduce efficacy of combined oral estrogen/progesterone contraceptives.

PREGNANCY: Category B, caution in nursing.

MECHANISM OF ACTION: Ticarcillin: Broad-spectrum antibiotic with bactericidal activity against many gram-positive and gram-negative aerobic and anerobic bacteria. Clavulanic acid: β-lactam, which possesses ability to inactivate wide range of β-lactamase enzymes.

PHARMACOKINETICS: Absorption: Ticarcillin: C_{max}=330mcg/mL, AUC=485mcg•hr/mL. Clavulanic acid: C_{max}=8mcg/mL, AUC=8.2mcg•hr/mL. **Distribution:** Ticarcillin: Plasma protein binding (45%). Clavulanic acid: Plasma protein binding (25%). **Elimination:** Ticarcillin: Urine (unchanged 60-70%); $T_{1/2}$=1.1 hrs, 4.4 hrs (neonates), 1 hr (infants/children). Clavulanic acid: Urine (35-45% unchanged); $T_{1/2}$=1.1hrs, 1.9 hrs (neonates), 0.9 hr (infants/children).

Tᴍᴅᴀᴍᴀx RX
tinidazole (Mission)

> Avoid unnecessary use. Reserve only for indicated conditions. Although none reported, potential risk of carcinogenicity exists and has been observed in rats and mice treated chronically with metronidazole, a structurally related drug with similar biologic effects.

THERAPEUTIC CLASS: Antiprotozoal agent

INDICATIONS: Treatment of trichomoniasis caused by *Trichomonas vaginalis*, giardiasis caused by *Giardia duodenalis*, intestinal amebiasis and amebic liver abscess caused by *Entamoeba histolytica*, and bacterial vaginosis in non-pregnant women.

DOSAGE: *Adults:* Take with food. Trichomoniasis/Giardiasis: 2g single dose. Amebiasis: Intestinal: 2g qd for 3 days. Amebic Liver Abscess: 2g qd for 3-5 days. Hemodialysis: Give additional dose equivalent to one-half of recommended dose at the end of dialysis. For trichomoniasis, treat sexual partner with the same dose. Bacterial Vaginosis: 2g qd for 2 days or 1g qd for 5 days.
Pediatrics: >3 yrs: Take with food. Giardiasis: 50mg/kg single dose. Amebiasis: Intestinal: 50mg/kg qd for 3 days. Amebic Liver Abscess: 50mg/kg qd for 3-5 days. Max (for all): 2g/day. May crush tabs in cherry syrup.

HOW SUPPLIED: Tab: 250mg*, 500mg* *scored

CONTRAINDICATIONS: Treatment during 1st trimester of pregnancy, nursing mothers during therapy and 3 days following last dose.

WARNINGS/PRECAUTIONS: Seizures, peripheral neuropathy reported. D/C if abnormal neurological signs occur. Caution with hepatic impairment, blood dyscrasias, or CNS diseases. May develop vaginal candidiasis. May develop drug resistance if presribed in absence of proven or strongly suspected bacterial infection.

ADVERSE REACTIONS: Metallic/bitter taste, nausea, anorexia, flatulence, urinary tract infection, pelvic pain, vulvo-vaginal discomfort, vaginal odor, menorrhagia, upper respiratory infection, convulsions, peripheral neuropathy.

INTERACTIONS: Avoid alcohol during and for 3 days after use and within 2 weeks of disulfiram. May potentiate oral anticoagulants. May reduce clearance of phenytoin (IV), fluorouracil. May increase levels of lithium, cyclosporine, tacrolimus, fluorouracil. Separate dosing with cholestyramine. Phenobarbital, rifampin, phenytoin, other hepatic enzyme inducers may decrease levels. Cimetidine, ketoconazole, other hepatic enzyme inhibitors may increase levels. Antagonized by oxytetracycline.

PREGNANCY: Category C, not for use in nursing.

MECHANISM OF ACTION: Antiprotozoal; antibacterial agent; nitro group of tinidazole is reduced by cell extracts of *Trichomonas*. Free nitro radical generated as a result of this reduction may be responsible for antiprotozoal activity.

PHARMACOKINETICS: Absorption: Rapid, complete. (Fasted) C_{max}=47.7mcg/mL, T_{max}=1.6 hrs, AUC=901.6mcg/hr/mL. **Distribution:** V_d= 50L; plasma protein binding (12%);

crosses blood-brain and placental barrier; found in breast milk. **Metabolism:** Mainly via oxidation, hydroxylation, conjugation; CYP3A4 mainly involved. **Elimination:** Urine (20-25% unchanged), feces (12%); $T_{1/2}$=12-14 hrs.

TOBI RX

tobramycin (Chiron)

THERAPEUTIC CLASS: Aminoglycoside

INDICATIONS: Management of cystic fibrosis patients with *P.aeruginosa*.

DOSAGE: *Adults:* Inhale via nebulizer 300mg q12h for 28 days, then stop for 28 days. Resume therapy for next 28 day on/28 day off cycle.
Pediatrics: ≥6 yrs: Inhale via nebulizer 300mg q12h for 28 days, then stop for 28 days. Resume therapy for next 28 day on/28 day off cycle.

HOW SUPPLIED: Sol: 60mg/mL (300mg/amp)

WARNINGS/PRECAUTIONS: Caution with muscular disorders (eg, myasthenia gravis, Parkinson's disease), and renal, auditory, vestibular, or neuromuscular dysfunction. May cause hearing loss, bronchospasm. Can cause fetal harm in pregnancy. D/C if nephrotoxicity occurs until serum level <2mcg/mL.

ADVERSE REACTIONS: Voice alteration, taste perversion, tinnitus.

INTERACTIONS: Avoid neurotoxic or ototoxic drugs. Hearing loss reported with previous or concomitant systemic aminoglycosides. Avoid ethacrynic acid, furosemide, urea, and mannitol.

PREGNANCY: Category D, not for use in nursing.

MECHANISM OF ACTION: Aminoglycoside antibiotic; inhibits protein synthesis in bacterial cell.

PHARMACOKINETICS: Absorption: C_{max}=1237mcg/g (sputum), 0.95mcg/mL (serum). **Distribution:** Crosses placenta. **Elimination:** Glomerular filtration, sputum expectoration (unchanged); $T_{1/2}$=approximately 2 hrs (IV).

TOBRADEX RX
dexamethasone - tobramycin (Alcon)

THERAPEUTIC CLASS: Aminoglycoside/corticosteroid

INDICATIONS: Ocular inflammation associated with infection or risk of infection.

DOSAGE: *Adults:* (Sus) 1-2 drops q4-6h. May increase to 1-2 drops q2h for first 24-48 hrs. (Oint) Apply 1/2 inch in conjunctival sac up to tid-qid. Max: 20mL or 8g for initial RX.
Pediatrics: ≥2 yrs: (Sus) 1-2 drops q4-6h. May increase to 1-2 drops q2h for first 24-48 hrs. (Oint) Apply 1/2 inch in conjunctival sac up to tid-qid. Max: 20mL or 8g for initial RX.

HOW SUPPLIED: Oint: (Tobramycin-Dexamethasone) 0.3-0.1% (3.5g); Sus: 0.3-0.1% (2.5mL, 5mL, 10mL)

CONTRAINDICATIONS: Viral diseases of the cornea and conjunctiva including epithelial herpes simplex keratitis, vaccinia, and varicella. Mycobacterial infection and fungal diseases of the eye.

WARNINGS/PRECAUTIONS: Not for injection into the eye. Prolonged use may result in glaucoma, optic nerve damage, visual acuity and fields of vision defects, cataracts, secondary ocular infections (eg, fungal infections).

ADVERSE REACTIONS: Conjunctival erythema, hypersensitivity, lid itching and swelling, secondary infection.

PREGNANCY: Category C, caution in nursing.

MECHANISM OF ACTION: Tobramycin: Aminoglycoside antibiotic; inhibits synthesis of proteins in bacterial cells. Dexamethasone: Corticoid; suppresses inflammatory response and probably delays or slows healing.

TOBRAMYCIN RX
tobramycin sulfate (Various)

> Potential ototoxicity, nephrotoxicity, and neurotoxicity. Monitor peak and trough serum levels to avoid toxicity. Avoid prolonged serum levels >12mcg/mL. Rising trough levels (>2mcg/mL) may indicate tissue accumulation. Tissue accumulation, excessive peak levels, advanced age, and cumulative dose may contribute to ototoxicity and nephrotoxicity. Monitor urine, BUN, SrCr, and CrCl periodically. Obtain serial audiograms. D/C or adjust dose with renal, vestibular, or auditory dysfunction. Caution in premature and neonatal infants, advanced age, and dehydration. Avoid other neurotoxic or nephrotoxic agents, particularly other aminoglycosides, cephaloridine, viomycin, polymyxin B, colistin, cisplatin, and vancomycin. Avoid potent diuretics (eg, ethacrynic acid, furosemide). Risk of fetal harm during pregnancy.

THERAPEUTIC CLASS: Aminoglycoside

INDICATIONS: Treatment of serious lower respiratory tract, CNS (eg, meningitis), intra-abdominal, bone, skin and skin structure, and complicated/recurrent urinary tract infections, and septicemia.

DOSAGE: *Adults:* IM/IV: Serious Infections: 3mg/kg/day given q8h. Life-Threatening Infections: Up to 5mg/kg/day given tid-qid. Reduce to 3mg/kg/day as soon as clinically indicated. Max: 5mg/kg/day unless serum levels monitored. Treat for 7-10 days; may need longer course in difficult and complicated infections. Severe Cystic Fibrosis: Initial: 10mg/kg/day given qid. Measure levels to determine subsequent doses. Renal Impairment: LD: 1mg/kg, followed by reduced doses given q8h or normal doses given at prolonged intervals based on either CrCl or SrCr. Do not use either method during dialysis. Obese Patients: Calculate dose based on estimated LBW plus 40% of excess as basic weight on which to figure mg/kg. ADD-Vantage vials not for IM use.
Pediatrics: >1 week: IM/IV: 6-7.5mg/kg/day given tid-qid (eg, 2-2.5mg/kg q8h or 1.5-1.89mg/kg q6h). ≤1 week: Up to 2mg/kg q12h. Treat for 7-10 days; may need longer course in difficult and complicated infections. Severe Cystic Fibrosis: Initial: 10mg/kg/day given qid. Measure levels to determine subsequent doses. Renal Impairment: LD: 1mg/kg, followed by reduced doses given q8h or normal doses given at prolonged intervals based on either CrCl or SrCr. Do not use either method during dialysis. Obese Patients: Calculate dose based on estimated LBW plus 40% of excess as basic weight on which to figure mg/kg. ADD-Vantage vials not for IM use.

HOW SUPPLIED: Inj: 10mg/mL, 40mg/mL, 1.2g

CONTRAINDICATIONS: History of serious toxic reactions to aminoglycosides.

WARNINGS/PRECAUTIONS: Increased risk of ototoxicity, nephrotoxicity, and neurotoxicity if treatment >10 days. Contains sodium bisulfite. D/C if allergic reaction occurs. Monitor serum calcium, magnesium, and sodium. For peak levels, measure about 30 min after IV infusion or 1 hr after IM injection. For trough levels, measure at 8 hrs or just before next dose. Prolonged or secondary apnea may occur with massive transfusions of citrated blood. Caution with muscular disorders (eg, myasthenia gravis, parkinsonism). Increased risk of neurotoxicity and nephrotoxicity after absorption from body surfaces with local irrigation or application. Not for intraocular and/or subconjunctival use. Overgrowth of nonsusceptible organisms may occur.

ADVERSE REACTIONS: Neurotoxicity (eg, dizziness, tinnitus, hearing loss, numbness, skin tingling, muscle twitching, convulsions), nephrotoxicity (eg, rising BUN/nonprotein nitrogen/serum creatinine, oliguria, cylindruria, increased proteinuria), blood dyscrasias, fever, rash, exfoliative dermatitis, urticaria, NV, diarrhea, headache, lethargy, injection-site pain, confusion, disorientation, increased serum transaminases.

INTERACTIONS: See Black Box Warning. Increased nephrotoxicity with cephalosporins. Do not premix with other drugs; administer separately. Possibility of prolonged or secondary apnea in anesthetized patients receiving neuromuscular blockers (eg, succinylcholine, tubocurarine, decamethonium).

PREGNANCY: Category D, safety not known in nursing.

MECHANISM OF ACTION: Aminoglycoside antibiotic; inhibits synthesis of proteins in bacterial cells.

PHARMACOKINETICS: Absorption: (IM) Rapidly absorbed; C_{max}=4mcg/mL; T_{max}=30-90 min. **Distribution:** Crosses placenta, distributed in body fluids. **Elimination**: Renal, biliary; $T_{1/2}$=2 hrs.

TOFRANIL
imipramine HCl (Mallinckrodt)

RX

> Antidepressants increased the risk of suicidal thinking and behavior (suicidality) in short-term studies in children, adolescents, and young adults with Major Depressive Disorder (MDD) and other psychiatric disorders. Imipramine HCl is not approved for use in pediatric patients except for patients with nocturnal enuresis.

THERAPEUTIC CLASS: Tricyclic antidepressant

INDICATIONS: Treatment of depression. Temporary adjunct in childhood enuresis in ≥6 yrs.

DOSAGE: *Adults:* Depression: Initial: (Inpatient) 100mg/day in divided doses. Titrate: Increase to 200mg/day; up to 250-300mg/day after 2 weeks if needed. (Outpatient) 75mg/day. Titrate: Increase to 150mg/day. Maint: 50-150mg/day. Max: 200mg/day. Elderly/Adolescents: Initial: 30-40mg/day. Max: 100mg/day.
Pediatrics: Depression: Adolescents: Initial: 30-40mg/day. Max: 100mg/day. Enuresis: ≥6 yrs: Initial: 25mg/day 1 hour before bedtime. Titrate: 6-12 yrs: If inadequate response in 1 week, increase to 50mg before bedtime. ≥12 yrs: Increase to 75mg before bedtime after 1 week if needed. Max: 2.5mg/kg/day.

HOW SUPPLIED: Tab: 10mg, 25mg, 50mg

CONTRAINDICATIONS: Within 14 days of MAOI therapy, or during acute recovery period following MI.

WARNINGS/PRECAUTIONS: Caution with elderly, serious depression, cardiovascular disease, hyperthyroidism, urinary retention, narrow-angle glaucoma, increased IOP, seizure disorders, renal and hepatic impairment. May activate psychosis in schizophrenia; reduce dose. Limit electroshock therapy. May alter blood glucose levels. Photosensitivity reported. D/C prior to elective surgery, or with hypomanic or manic episodes. D/C with pathological neutrophil depression.

ADVERSE REACTIONS: Orthostatic hypotension, HTN, confusion, hallucinations, numbness, tremors, dry mouth, urticaria, nausea, vomiting, diarrhea, gynecomastia (male), breast enlargement (female), galactorrhea.

INTERACTIONS: See Contraindications. Increased levels with methylphenidate, CYP2D6 inhibitors (eg, quinidine, cimetidine, SSRIs) and enzyme substrates (eg, phenothiazines, other antidepressants, propafenone, flecainide). Wait 5 weeks after discontinuing SSRIs before initiating TCAs. Decreased levels with enzyme inducers (eg, barbiturates, phenytoin). May block effects of clonidine, guanethidine. Additive effects with anticholinergics, CNS depressants, alcohol. Caution with drugs that lower BP and thyroid drugs. Paralytic ileus with anticholinergics. Avoid preparations that contain a sympathomimetic amine (eg, epinephrine, norepinephrine); may potentiate catecholamine effect.

PREGNANCY: Safety in pregnancy not known; not for use in nursing.

MECHANISM OF ACTION: Tricyclic antidepressant; mechanism unknown. Suspected to potentiate adrenergic synapses by blocking uptake of norepinephrine at nerve endings.

TOFRANIL-PM
imipramine pamoate (Mallinckrodt)

RX

> Antidepressants increased the risk of suicidal thinking and behavior (suicidality) in short-term studies in children, adolescents, and young adults with Major Depressive Disorder (MDD) and other psychiatric disorders. Imipramine pamoate is not approved for use in pediatric patients.

THERAPEUTIC CLASS: Tricyclic antidepressant

INDICATIONS: Treatment of depression.

DOSAGE: *Adults:* (Inpatient) Initial: 100-150mg/day. Titrate: May increase to 200mg/day. After 2 weeks may increase up to 250-300mg/day if needed. (Outpatient) Initial: 75mg/day. Titrate: May increase to 150mg/day. Max: 200mg/day. (Inpatient/Outpatient) Maint: Following remission, maintain at lowest possible dose. Usual: 75-150mg/day. Elderly/Adolescents: Initiate with Tofranil 25-50mg/day. Switch to Tofranil-PM with doses

≥75mg. Max: 100mg/day.
Pediatrics: Adolescents: Initiate with Tofranil 25-50mg/day. Switch to Tofranil-PM with doses ≥75mg. Max: 100mg/day.

HOW SUPPLIED: Cap: 75mg, 100mg, 125mg, 150mg

CONTRAINDICATIONS: Within 14 days of MAOI therapy or during acute recovery period following MI.

WARNINGS/PRECAUTIONS: Caution with elderly, serious depression, cardiovascular disease, hyperthyroidism, urinary retention, narrow-angle glaucoma, increased IOP, seizure disorders, renal and hepatic impairment. May activate psychosis in schizophrenia; reduce dose. Limit electroshock therapy. May alter blood glucose levels. Photosensitivity reported. D/C prior to elective surgery, or with hypomanic or manic episodes. D/C with pathological neutrophil depression.

ADVERSE REACTIONS: Orthostatic hypotension, HTN, confusion, hallucinations, numbness, tremors, dry mouth, urticaria, nausea, vomiting, diarrhea, gynecomastia (male), breast enlargement (female), galactorrhea.

INTERACTIONS: See Contraindications. Increased levels with methylphenidate, CYP2D6 inhibitors (eg, quinidine, cimetidine, SSRIs) and enzyme substrates (eg, phenothiazines, other antidepressants, propafenone, flecainide). Wait 5 weeks after discontinuing SSRIs before initiating TCAs. Decreased levels with enzyme inducers (eg, barbiturates, phenytoin). Blocks effects of clonidine, guanethidine. Additive effects with anticholinergics, CNS depressants, alcohol. Caution with drugs that lower BP and thyroid drugs. Paralytic ileus with anticholinergics. Avoid preparations that contain a sympathomimetic amine (eg, epinephrine, norepinephrine); may potentiate catecholamine effect.

PREGNANCY: Safety in pregnancy not known; not for use in nursing.

MECHANISM OF ACTION: Tricyclic antidepressant; mechanism unknown. Suspected to potentiate adrenergic synapses by blocking uptake of norepinephrine at nerve endings.

TOLMETIN RX
tolmetin sodium (Various)

> NSAIDs may cause an increased risk of serious cardiovascular thrombotic events, MI, stroke, and serious GI adverse events including bleeding, ulceration and perforation of the stomach or intestines. Contraindicated for the treatment of perioperative pain in the setting of coronary artery bypass graft (CABG) surgery.

OTHER BRAND NAMES: Tolectin 600 (Ortho-McNeil) - Tolectin DS (Ortho-McNeil)

THERAPEUTIC CLASS: NSAID

INDICATIONS: Treatment of acute flares and the long-term management of rheumatoid arthritis (RA) and osteoarthritis (OA). Treatment of juvenile rheumatoid arthritis (JRA).

DOSAGE: *Adults:* OA/RA: Initial: 400mg tid. Usual: 200-600mg tid. Max: 1800mg/day. Take with antacids other than sodium bicarbonate if GI upset occurs.
Pediatrics: JRA: ≥2 yrs: Initial: 20mg/kg/day given tid-qid. Usual: 15-30mg/kg/day. Max: 30mg/kg/day. Take with antacids other than sodium bicarbonate if GI upset occurs.

HOW SUPPLIED: Cap: (DS) 400mg; Tab: 200mg*, 600mg *scored

CONTRAINDICATIONS: ASA or other NSAID allergy that precipitates asthma, rhinitis, urticaria, or allergic-type reactions. Treatment of perioperative pain in the setting of CABG surgery.

WARNINGS/PRECAUTIONS: May cause adverse ocular events. Prolongs bleeding time. Risk of renal toxicity with heart failure, liver dysfunction, and elderly. Caution with compromised cardiac function, HTN, or other conditions predisposing to fluid retention. Borderline LFT elevations may occur. Decreased bioavailability with milk or food. Can cause serious skin adverse reactions such as exfoliative dermatitis, SJS, and TEN, which can be fatal. Avoid with ASA-sensitive asthma and caution with preexisting asthma. Cannot be expected to substitute for corticosteroids or to treat corticosteroid insufficiency. Notable elevations of ALT or AST reported. Rare cases of severe hepatic reactions, including jaundice and fatal fulminant hepatitis, liver necrosis, and hepatic failure. Patients on long-term treatment should have Hgb or Hct checked if exhibit signs or symptoms of anemia.

ADVERSE REACTIONS: Dyspepsia, GI distress, diarrhea, flatulence, vomiting, headache, asthenia, elevated blood pressure, dizziness, edema, weight gain/loss.

INTERACTIONS: Increased PT and bleeding with warfarin. May enhance methotrexate toxicity. May diminish the antihypertensive effect of ACEIs. Concomitant administration with ASA not recommended; potential for increased adverse effects. Can reduce the natriuretic effect of furosemide and thiazides. Can produce elevation of plasma lithium levels and reduction in renal lithium clearance.

PREGNANCY: Category C, not for use in nursing.

MECHANISM OF ACTION: NSAID; not established, suspected to inhibit prostaglandin synthetase, lowers plasma level of PGE.

PHARMACOKINETICS: Absorption: Rapid; C_{max}=40mcg/mL (400 mg); T_{max}=30-60 min. **Elimination:** Urine; $T_{1/2}$=5 hrs.

TOPAMAX RX
topiramate (Ortho-McNeil)

OTHER BRAND NAME: Topamax Sprinkle Capsules (Ortho-McNeil)

THERAPEUTIC CLASS: Sulfamate-substituted monosaccharide antiepileptic

INDICATIONS: Monotherapy in patients 10 yrs of age and older with partial onset or primary generalized tonic-clonic seizures. Adjunct therapy in patients 2-16 yrs of age and older with partial onset seizures, primary generalized tonic-clonic seizures, and seizures associated with Lennox-Gastaut syndrome. Migraine prophylaxis in adults.

DOSAGE: *Adults:* Seizures: Monotherapy: Initial: 25mg qam for 1 week. Titrate: Increase am and pm dose by 25mg every week until 200mg/day, then increase by 50mg every week until 400mg/day. Adjunct Therapy: ≥17 yrs: Initial: 25-50mg/day. Titrate: Increase by 25-50mg/week. Usual: Partial: 100-200mg bid. Tonic-Clonic: 200mg bid. Max: 1600mg/day. Migraine Prophylaxis: Titrate: Week 1: 25mg qpm. Week 2: 25mg bid. Week 3: 25mg qam and 50mg qpm. Week 4: 50mg bid. Usual: 50mg bid. Renal Dysfunction: 50% of usual dose. Swallow caps whole or sprinkle over food.
Pediatrics: Seizures: Monotherapy: ≥10 yrs: Initial: 25mg qam and qpm for 1 week. Titrate: Increase am and pm dose by 25mg every week until 200mg/day, then increase by 50mg every week until 400mg/day. Adjunct Therapy: 2-16 yrs: Initial: 1-3mg/kg nightly for 1 week. Titrate: Increase by 1-3mg/kg/day every 1-2 weeks. Usual: 2.5-4.5mg/kg bid. Swallow caps whole or sprinkle over food.

HOW SUPPLIED: Cap, Sprinkle: 15mg, 25mg; Tab: 25mg, 50mg, 100mg, 200mg

WARNINGS/PRECAUTIONS: Hyperchloremic, nonanion gap, metabolic acidosis reported; obtain baseline and periodic serum bicarbonate levels. Withdraw gradually. Psychomotor slowing, difficulty with concentration, speech/language problems, paresthesia, acute myopia with secondary angle closure glaucoma, oligohidrosis, hyperthermia, and dose-related depression or mood problems reported. May cause hyperammonemia and encephalopathy if used concomitantly with valproic acid. Risk of kidney stones; maintain adequate fluid intake. Caution with renal or hepatic dysfunction.

ADVERSE REACTIONS: Somnolence, fatigue, dizziness, ataxia, speech disorders, psychomotor slowing, abnormal vision, memory difficulty, paresthesia, diplopia, depression, anorexia, anxiety, mood problems, pancreatitis, hepatic failure.

INTERACTIONS: Phenytoin, carbamazepine, valproic acid decrease levels. Increases phenytoin, decreases valproic acid levels. May decrease AUC of digoxin. May potentiate CNS depression with alcohol, other CNS depressants. Increased risk of kidney stones with carbonic anhydrase inhibitors. May increase metformin levels; monitor diabetics regularly.

PREGNANCY: Category C, caution in nursing.

MECHANISM OF ACTION: Sulfamate-substituted monosaccharide; unknown mechanism. Suspected to block voltage-dependent Na^+ channels, augment activity of the neurotransmitter gamma-aminobutyrate at some subtypes of the GABA-A receptor, antagonizes the AMPA/kainate subtype of the glutamate receptor, and inhibits the carbonic anhydrase enzyme, particularly isoenzymes II and IV.

PHARMACOKINETICS: Absorption: Rapid; T_{max}=2 hrs. **Distribution:** Plasma protein binding (15-41%); found in breast milk. **Metabolism:** Metabolized via hydroxylation, hydrolysis, and glucoronidation. **Elimination:** Urine: (70% unchanged); $T_{1/2}$=21 hrs. For pediatric parameters refer to PI.

TOPICORT
desoximetasone (Taro)

RX

OTHER BRAND NAME: Topicort LP (Taro)

THERAPEUTIC CLASS: Corticosteroid

INDICATIONS: Corticosteroid-responsive dermatoses.

DOSAGE: *Adults:* Apply bid.
Pediatrics: (Cre, Gel) Apply bid. ≥10 yrs: (Oint) Apply bid.

HOW SUPPLIED: Cre: (LP) 0.05% (15g, 60g), 0.25% (15g, 60g. 100g); Gel: 0.05% (15g, 60g); Oint: 0.25% (15g, 60g)

WARNINGS/PRECAUTIONS: May produce reversible HPA axis suppression, manifestations of Cushing's syndrome, hyperglycemia, and glucosuria. Caution when applied to large surface areas or under occlusive dressings. Use appropriate antifungal or antibacterial agent with dermatological infections; d/c if infection does not clear or if irritation occurs. Peds may be more susceptible to systemic toxicity. Avoid eyes.

ADVERSE REACTIONS: Burning, itching, irritation, dryness, folliculitis, hypertrichosis, acneiform eruptions, hypopigmentation, perioral dermatitis, allergic contact dermatitis, skin maceration, secondary infection, skin atrophy, striae, miliaria.

PREGNANCY: Category C, caution in nursing.

MECHANISM OF ACTION: Corticosteroid; possesses anti-inflammatory, anti-pruritic, and vasoconstrictive properties. Anti-inflammatory activity not established.

PHARMACOKINETICS: Absorption: Percutaneous; occlusion, inflammation, and other disease states may increase absorption. **Metabolism:** Liver. **Excretion:** Urine (major), bile.

TOPROL-XL
metoprolol succinate (AstraZeneca)

RX

THERAPEUTIC CLASS: Selective beta$_1$-blocker

INDICATIONS: Treatment of hypertension, angina pectoris, and stable symptomatic (NYHA Class II or III) heart failure of ischemic, hypertensive or cardiomyopathic origin.

DOSAGE: *Adults:* HTN: Initial: 25-100mg qd. Titrate: May increase weekly. Max: 400mg/day. Angina: Initial: 100mg qd. Titrate: May increase weekly. Max: 400mg/day. Heart Failure: Initial: (NYHA Class II) 25mg qd for 2 weeks. Severe Heart Failure: 12.5mg qd for 2 weeks. Titrate: Double dose every 2 weeks as tolerated. Max: 200mg/day. *Pediatrics:* ≥6 yrs: HTN: 1mg/kg qd. Max: 50mg/day. Dose adjust according to BP response. Doses above 2mg/kg have not been studied.

HOW SUPPLIED: Tab, Extended-Release: 25mg*, 50mg*, 100mg*, 200mg* *scored

CONTRAINDICATIONS: Severe bradycardia, >1st-degree heart block, cardiogenic shock, sick sinus syndrome (unless a pacemaker is present), decompensated cardiac failure.

WARNINGS/PRECAUTIONS: Exacerbation of angina pectoris and MI reported following abrupt withdrawal; taper over 1-2 weeks. Caution with heart failure, bronchospastic disease, DM, hepatic dysfunction, hyperthyroidism, or peripheral vascular disease. May mask symptoms of hyperthyroidism and hypoglycemia. Withdrawal prior to surgery is controversial.

ADVERSE REACTIONS: Bradycardia, shortness of breath, fatigue, dizziness, depression, diarrhea, pruritus, rash, hepatitis, arthralgia.

INTERACTIONS: Additive effects with catecholamine-depleting drugs (eg, reserpine, MAOIs). CYP2D6 inhibitors (eg, quinidine, fluoxetine, paroxetine, propafenone) may increase levels. May exacerbate rebound hypertension following clonidine withdrawal. Caution when used with CCBs of the verapamil and diltiazem type. Concomitant use of digitalis glycosides and β-blockers can increase the risk of bradycardia.

PREGNANCY: Category C, caution with nursing.

MECHANISM OF ACTION: β_1-selective (cardioselective) adrenergic receptor blocking agent; slows sinus rate and decreases AV nodal conduction.

PHARMACOKINETICS: Absorption: Rapid and complete. **Distribution:** Crosses blood-brain barrier. Plasma protein binding (12%). **Metabolism:** Metabolized via CYP2D6. **Elimination:** Liver. $T_{1/2}$=3-7 hrs. Urine.

TRACLEER

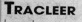
bosentan (Actelion)

RX

Potential liver injury; monitor LFTs before therapy, then monthly. Contraindicated in pregnancy; obtain monthly pregnancy tests. Prescribe through Tracleer Access Program.

THERAPEUTIC CLASS: Endothelin receptor antagonist

INDICATIONS: Treatment of pulmonary arterial hypertension in patients with WHO Class III or IV symptoms, to improve exercise ability and decrease rate of clinical worsening.

DOSAGE: *Adults:* Initial: 62.5mg bid. Titrate/Maint: Increase to 125mg bid after 4 weeks. Low Weight (<40kg): Initial/Maint: 62.5mg bid. Adjust if Develop LFT Abnormality: >3 to ≤5x ULN: Reconfirm LFTs. Reduce dose or interrupt therapy. Monitor LFTs every 2 weeks. If LFTs return to pre-treatment levels, reintroduce or continue therapy. >5 to ≤8x ULN: Reconfirm LFTs. Stop treatment and monitor LFTs every 2 weeks. If LFTs return to pre-treatment values, may reintroduce therapy. >8x ULN: Stop treatment, do not reintroduce.
Pediatrics: >12 yrs: <40kg: Initial/Maint: 62.5mg bid.

HOW SUPPLIED: Tab: 62.5mg, 125mg

CONTRAINDICATIONS: Pregnancy, cyclosporine A, glyburide.

WARNINGS/PRECAUTIONS: May decrease Hgb and Hct; monitor 1 and 3 months after initiation, then every 3 months. Caution in elderly or mild hepatic impairment. Avoid with moderate to severe hepatic impairment, or LFTs >3x ULN. D/C gradually. Patients with severe chronic heart failure had an increased incidence of hospitalization for CHF associated with weight gain and increased leg edema during the first 4-8 weeks of treatment. Consider intervention with diuretic, fluid management, or hospitalization for decompensating heart failure. If signs of pulmonary edema occur, possibility of associated Pulmonary Veno-Occlusive Disease should be considered. D/C therapy..

ADVERSE REACTIONS: Headache, nasopharyngitis, flushing, hepatic dysfunction, lower limb edema, hypotension, palpitations, dyspepsia, edema, fatigue, pruritus, thrombocytopenia.

INTERACTIONS: Do not rely on hormonal contraception alone. Cyclosporine A may increase levels. Glyburide may increase risk of elevated LFTs. May reduce statin efficacy; monitor cholesterol levels. May decrease levels of drugs metabolized by CYP450 3A4 (eg, statins) and 2C9. CYP450 3A4 inhibitors (eg, ketoconazole) increase levels.

PREGNANCY: Category X, not for use in nursing.

MECHANISM OF ACTION: Endothelin receptor antagonist; a neurohormone; binds to ET_A and ET_B receptors in the endothelium and vascular smooth muscle. Specific and competitive antagonist at endothelin receptors types with slightly higher affinity for ET_A receptors than ET_B receptors.

PHARMACOKINETICS: Absorption: Absolute bioavailabilty (50%). T_{max}=3-5 hrs. **Distribution:** V_d=18L; plasma protein binding (>98%). **Metabolism:** Liver via (CYP2C9, CYP3A4, and CYP2C19). **Elimination:** Biliary, and urine (<3%); $T_{1/2}$=5 hrs.

TRANXENE-SD

clorazepate dipotassium (Ovation)

CIV

OTHER BRAND NAMES: Tranxene T-Tab (Ovation) - Tranxene-SD Half Strength (Ovation)

THERAPEUTIC CLASS: Benzodiazepine

INDICATIONS: Management of anxiety disorders. Adjunct therapy for partial seizures. Symptomatic relief of acute alcohol withdrawal.

DOSAGE: *Adults:* Anxiety: Initial: (Tab) 15mg qhs. Usual: 30mg/day in divided doses. Max: 60mg/day. Elderly/Debilitated: Initial: 7.5-15mg/day. (Tab, Extended-Release)

22.5mg q24h, (may substitute for 7.5mg tid) or 11.25mg q24h (may substitute for 3.75mg tid). Do not use Extended-Release for initial therapy. Alcohol Withdrawal: Day 1: (Tab) 30mg, then 30-60mg/day. Day 2: 45-90mg/day. Day 3: 22.5-45mg/day. Day 4: 15-30mg. Give in divided doses. Reduce dose and continue with 7.5-15mg/day; discontinue when stable. Max: 90mg/day. Antiepileptic Adjunct: Initial: (Tab) 7.5mg tid. Titrate: Increase by no more than 7.5mg/week. Max: 90mg/day.

Pediatrics: >9 yrs: Anxiety: Initial: (Tab) 15mg qhs. Usual: 30mg/day in divided doses. Max: 60mg/day. (Tab, Extended-Release) 22.5mg q24h, (may substitute for 7.5mg tid) or 11.25mg q24h (may substitute for 3.75mg tid). Do not use Extended-Release for initial therapy. >12 yrs: Antiepileptic Adjunct: Initial: (Tab) 7.5mg tid. Titrate: Increase by no more than 7.5mg/week. Max: 90mg/day. 9-12 yrs: Initial: 7.5mg bid. Titrate: Increase by no more than 7.5mg/week. Max: 60mg/day.

HOW SUPPLIED: Tab: (Tranxene T-Tab) 3.75mg*, 7.5mg*, 15mg*; Tab, Extended-Release: (Tranxene-SD) 22.5mg, (Tranxene-SD Half Strength) 11.25mg *scored

CONTRAINDICATIONS: Acute narrow-angle glaucoma.

WARNINGS/PRECAUTIONS: Avoid with depressive neuroses or psychotic reactions. Withdrawal symptoms with abrupt withdrawal; taper gradually. Caution with known drug dependency, renal/hepatic impairment. Suicidal tendencies reported; give lowest effective dose. Monitor LFTs and blood counts periodically with long-term therapy. Use lowest effective dose in elderly.

ADVERSE REACTIONS: Drowsiness, dizziness, GI complaints, nervousness, blurred vision, dry mouth, headache, mental confusion.

INTERACTIONS: Additive CNS depression with CNS depressants, alcohol. Potentiated by barbiturates, narcotics, phenothiazines, MAOIs, other antidepressants. Increased sedation with hypnotics.

PREGNANCY: Safety in pregnancy not known, not for use in nursing.

MECHANISM OF ACTION: Benzodiazepine; antianxiety/hypnotic agent which has CNS depressant effect.

PHARMACOKINETICS: Absorption: Orally absorbed; completely decarboxylated to nordiazepam. **Distribution:** Plasma protein binding (97-98%) **Metabolism:** Hydroxylation. **Elimination:** Urine (62-67%), feces (15-19%); $T_{1/2}$=40-50 hrs.

TRAUMEEL INJECTION   RX
botanical/Mineral substances (Heel)

THERAPEUTIC CLASS: Homeopathic Complex

INDICATIONS: Treatment of symptoms associated with inflammatory, exudative, and degenerative processes due to acute trauma (eg, contusions, lacerations, fractures, sprains, post-op wounds), repetitive or overuse injuries (eg, tendonitis, bursitis, epicondylitis), and for minor aches and pains associated with such conditions. Treatment of minor aches and minor pain from rheumatoid arthritis, osteoarthritis, gouty arthritis, and ankylosing spondylitis.

DOSAGE: *Adults:* 1 amp qd for acute disorders or 1-2 amps 1-3 times weekly. May administer IV, IM, SQ, or intradermally.
Pediatrics: >6 yrs: 1 amp qd for acute disorders or 1-2 amps 1-3 times weekly. 2-6 yrs: Use 1/2 of the adult dosage. May administer IV, IM, SQ, or intradermally.

HOW SUPPLIED: Inj: 2.2mL amps (10^9)

WARNINGS/PRECAUTIONS: Carefully re-evaluate if pain persists or worsens, if new symptoms occur, or if redness or swelling is present.

ADVERSE REACTIONS: Allergic reactions, anaphylactic reactions.

PREGNANCY: Category C, caution in nursing.

TRAUMEEL TOPICAL
botanical/Mineral substances (Heel)

OTC

THERAPEUTIC CLASS: Homeopathic Complex

INDICATIONS: Temporary relief of symptoms associated with inflammatory, exudative, and degenerative processes due to acute trauma (eg, contusions, lacerations, fractures, sprains, post-op wounds), repetitive or overuse injuries (eg, tendonitis, bursitis, epicondylitis), and for temporary relief of minor aches and pains associated with such conditions. Temporary relief of minor aches and pains associated with backache, muscular aches, and minor pain from rheumatoid arthritis, osteoarthritis, gouty arthritis, and ankylosing spondylitis.

DOSAGE: *Adults:* Individualize dose. Apply to affected area(s) 2-3 times daily. Max: 5x/day. May apply using mild compression and/or occlusive bandaging. Avoid applying over large areas, over broken skin, or directly into open wounds.
Pediatrics: Individualize dose. Apply to affected area(s) 2-3 times daily. Max: 5x/day. May apply using mild compression and/or occlusive bandaging. Avoid applying over large areas, over broken skin, or directly into open wounds.

HOW SUPPLIED: Gel: (50g, 250g); Oint: (50g, 100g)

WARNINGS/PRECAUTIONS: Avoid administration for pain for >10 days for adults or 5 days for children. Persistent or worsening pain, occurrence of new symptoms, or presence of redness or swelling may signify a serious condition. Consult physician before use in children with arthritis pain.

ADVERSE REACTIONS: Allergic reactions, anaphylactic reactions.

PREGNANCY: Category C, caution in nursing.

MECHANISM OF ACTION: Acts to relieve pain, joint pain, sports injuries, and bruising.

TRECATOR
ethionamide (Wyeth)

RX

THERAPEUTIC CLASS: Peptide synthesis inhibitor

INDICATIONS: Treatment of active TB in patients with *M.tuberculosis* resistant to isoniazid or rifampin, or where there is intolerance to other drugs.

DOSAGE: *Adults:* 15-20mg/kg qd with food. May give in divided doses with poor GI tolerance. Max: 1g/day. Alternate Regimen: Initial: 250mg qd then titrate gradually to optimal doses as tolerated, or 250mg qd for 1-2 days, then 250mg bid for 1-2 days, then 1g/day in 3-4 divided doses. Continue therapy until bacteriological conversion has become permanent and maximal clinical improvement occurs.
Pediatrics: ≥12 yrs: 10-20 mg/kg/day in divided doses given bid or tid with food, or 15mg/kg/day as single dose. Continue therapy until bacteriological conversion has become permanent and maximal clinical improvement occurs.

HOW SUPPLIED: Tab: 250mg

CONTRAINDICATIONS: Severe hepatic impairment.

WARNINGS/PRECAUTIONS: Rapid development of resistance if used alone; should be used with at least 1 or 2 other drugs. Perform ophthalmologic exams before and periodically during therapy. Measure serum transaminases prior to initiation and monthly thereafter. Risk of hypoglycemia in diabetics; monitor blood glucose prior to initiation then periodically. Hypothyroidism reported; monitor TFTs.

ADVERSE REACTIONS: NV , diarrhea, abdominal pain, excessive salivation, metallic taste, stomatitis, anorexia, psychotic disturbances, drowsiness, dizziness, hypersensitivity reactions, increase in serum bilirubin, SGOT or SGPT.

INTERACTIONS: Discontinue all antituberculous medication with elevated serum transaminases until resolved; reintroduce sequentially to determine which drug is responsible. May raise isoniazid levels. May potentiate adverse effects of other antituberculous drugs. Convulsions reported with cycloserine. Risk of psychotic reactions with excessive ethanol ingestion. Give with pyridoxine.

PREGNANCY: Category C, not for use in nursing.

MECHANISM OF ACTION: Peptide synthesis inhibitor; may be bacteriostatic or bactericidal in action.

PHARMACOKINETICS: Absorption: Completely absorbed; C_{max}=2.16mcg/mL, T_{max}=1.02 hrs, AUC=7.67mcg•hr/mL. **Distribution:** V_d=93.5L; plasma protein binding (30%); widely distributed into body tissues. **Metabolism:** Liver (extensive). **Elimination:** Urine ≤1%; $T_{1/2}$=1.92 hrs.

TRILEPTAL RX
oxcarbazepine (Novartis)

THERAPEUTIC CLASS: Dibenzazepine

INDICATIONS: Monotherapy or adjunct therapy in adults and children 4-16 yrs with partial seizures.

DOSAGE: *Adults:* Monotherapy: Initial: 300mg bid. Titrate: Increase by 300mg/day every 3rd day. Maint: 1200mg/day. Adjunct Therapy: Initial: 300mg bid. Titrate: Increase weekly by a maximum of 600mg/day. Maint: 600mg bid. Conversion to Monotherapy: Initial: 300mg bid while reducing other AEDs. Titrate: Increase weekly by 600mg/day. Withdraw other AEDs over 3-6 weeks. Maint: 2400mg/day. Renal Impairment: CrCl <30mL/min: Initial: 300mg qd. Titrate: Increase gradually.
Pediatrics: 4-16yrs: Monotherapy: Initial: 4-5mg/kg bid. Titrate: Increase by 5mg/kg/day every 3rd day. Maint (mg/day): 20kg: Initial: 600mg. Max: 900mg. 25-30kg: Initial: 900mg. Max: 1200mg. 35-40kg: Initial: 900mg. Max: 1500mg. 45kg: Initial: 1200mg. Max: 1500mg. 50-55kg: Initial: 1200mg. Max: 1800mg. 60-65kg: Initial: 1200mg. Max: 2100mg. 70kg: Initial: 1500mg. Max: 2100mg. Adjunct Therapy: Initial: 4-5mg/kg bid. Max: 600mg/day. Titrate: Increase over 2 weeks. Maint (mg/day): 20-29kg: 900mg. 29.1-39kg: 1200mg. >39kg: 1800mg. Conversion to Monotherapy: Initial: 4-5mg/kg bid while reducing other AEDs. Titrate: Increase weekly by max of 10mg/kg/day to target dose. Withdraw other AEDs over 3-6 weeks. Renal Impairment: CrCl <30mL/min: Initial: 300mg qd. Titrate: Increase gradually.

HOW SUPPLIED: Sus: 300mg/5mL (250mL); Tab: 150mg*, 300mg*, 600mg* *scored

WARNINGS/PRECAUTIONS: Risk of hyponatremia. Cross sensitivity with carbamazepine. Avoid abrupt withdrawal. Adjust dose in renal impairment. Reports of serious dermatologic reactions (eg, Stevens-Johnson syndrome, toxic epidermal necrolysis). CNS effects reported (eg, psychomotor slowing, concentration difficulty, speech or language problems, somnolence or fatigue, coordination abnormalities). Reports of multi-organ hypersensitivity reactions in close temporal association to initiation of therapy. Rare cases of anaphylaxis and angioedema involving the larynx, glottis, lips and eyelids reported.

ADVERSE REACTIONS: Dizziness, somnolence, diplopia, nausea, vomiting, asthenia, nystagmus, ataxia, abnormal vision, tremor, abnormal gait, headache.

INTERACTIONS: Additive sedative effect with alcohol. Verapamil, carbamazepine, phenytoin, phenobarbital, valproic acid may decrease levels. Decreased plasma levels of felodipine and oral contraceptives. Increased plasma levels of phenytoin, phenobarbital.

PREGNANCY: Category C, not for use in nursing.

MECHANISM OF ACTION: Dibenzazepine; mechanism unknown. Oxcarbazepine and 10-monohydroxy metabolite (MHD) suspected to exert antiseizure effects through blockade of voltage-sensitive Na^+ channels, resulting in stabilization of hyperexcited neural membranes, inhibition of repetitive neuronal firing, and diminution of propagation of synaptic impulses. Also, increased K^+ conductance and modulation of high-voltage activated calcium channels may contribute to anticonvulsant activity.

PHARMACOKINETICS: Absorption: Completely absorbed; T_{max}=4.5 hrs (Tab), 6 hrs (Sus). **Distribution:** V_d=49L (MHD). Plasma protein binding (40%) (metabolite). Found in breast milk. **Metabolism:** Liver; reduced to MHD (active metabolite), then conjugated. **Elimination:** Urine (>95%), feces (<4%). $T_{1/2}$=2 hrs (parent drug), 9 hrs (MHD). In pediatrics, MHD clearance decreases as age/weight increase, approaching that of adults.

TRIPEDIA

RX

diphtheria toxoid - pertussis vaccine, acellular - tetanus toxoid (Sanofi Pasteur)

THERAPEUTIC CLASS: Vaccine/toxoid combination

INDICATIONS: Active immunization against diphtheria, tetanus, and pertussis in pediatrics 6 weeks to 7 yrs of age (prior to 7th birthday). Combined with ActHIB for active immunization in pediatrics 15-18 months previously immunized against diphtheria, tetanus, and pertussis with 3 doses of whole-cell pertussis DTP or acellular pertussis vaccine and 3 or fewer doses of ActHIB® within 1st year of life for prevention of *H. influenzae* type b, diphtheria, tetanus, and pertussis.

DOSAGE: *Pediatrics:* <7 yrs: Primary Series: 3 doses of 0.5mL IM at 4-8 week intervals. 1st dose usually at 2 months, but can give at 6 weeks up to 7th birthday. Booster: 4th dose (0.5mL IM) at 15-20 months, at least 6 months after 3rd dose, 5th dose at 4-6 yrs; prior to school entry. May give to complete 4th or 5th dose of primary series of 3 doses of whole-cell pertussis DTP (4th dose at 15-20 months and 5th dose before school if 4th dose not given on or before 4th birthday). May combine with ActHIB® for 4th dose at 15-18 months.

HOW SUPPLIED: Inj: 0.5mL

CONTRAINDICATIONS: Hypersensitivity to thimersal and gelatin, immediate anaphylactic reaction associated with previous dose, encephalopathy not due to an identifiable cause within 7 days of prior pertussis immunization. Defer during poliomyelitis outbreak or acute febrile illness.

WARNINGS/PRECAUTIONS: Caution if within 48 hrs of previous whole-cell DTP or acellular DTP vaccine, fever ≥105°F not due to another identifiable cause, collapse or shock-like state, or inconsolable crying lasting ≥3 hrs occurs, or if convulsions occur within 3 days. For high seizure risk, give APAP at time of vaccination and q4-6h for 24 hrs. Caution with neurologic or CNS disorders. Avoid with coagulation disorders. Have epinephrine available. Suboptimal response may occur in immunocompromised patients.

ADVERSE REACTIONS: Local erythema and swelling, irritability, drowsiness, anorexia, fever.

INTERACTIONS: Avoid with anticoagulants. Immunosuppressive therapy (eg, irradiation, antimetabolites, alkylating agents, cytotoxic drugs, corticosteroids) may decrease response. Do not combine through reconstitution with any vaccine for infants <15 months.

PREGNANCY: Category C, safety in nursing not known.

MECHANISM OF ACTION: Active immunization against diphtheria, tetanus, and pertussis (whooping cough).

TRISENOX

RX

arsenic trioxide (Cephalon)

> Administer under supervision of a physician experienced in the management of acute leukemia. Acute promyelocytic leukemia (APL) differentiation syndrome reported. Can cause QT interval prolongation and complete AV block. Monitor ECG, serum electrolytes, and creatinine before and during therapy.

THERAPEUTIC CLASS: DNA fragmentation agent

INDICATIONS: For induction of remission and consolidation of APL refractory to or relapsed from retinoid and anthracycline chemotherapy, and has t(15;17) translocation or PML/RAR-alpha gene expression.

DOSAGE: *Adults:* Induction: 0.15mg/kg IV qd until bone marrow remission. Max: 60 doses. Consolidation: 0.15mg/kg IV qd for 25 doses over 5 weeks. Begin 3-6 weeks after complete induction therapy. *Pediatrics:* ≥5 yrs: Induction: 0.15mg/kg IV qd until bone marrow remission. Max: 60 doses. Consolidation: 0.15mg/kg IV qd for 25 doses over 5 weeks. Begin 3-6 weeks after complete induction therapy.

HOW SUPPLIED: Inj: 1mg/mL

WARNINGS/PRECAUTIONS: Hyperleukocytosis, QT interval prolongation, torsade de pointes, and complete AV block reported. Caution with renal failure. Monitor electrolyte, hematologic, and coagulation profiles at least twice weekly, and more frequently in unstable patients during induction. Obtain ECG weekly, and more frequently for unstable patients. May cause fetal harm; avoid pregnancy.

ADVERSE REACTIONS: Fatigue, pyrexia, edema, chest pain, injection site pain, nausea, vomiting, abdominal pain, constipation, hypokalemia, hypomagnesemia, hyperglycemia, increased ALT, headache, insomnia, dyspnea.

INTERACTIONS: Caution with agents that prolong the QT interval (eg, certain antiarrhythmics, thioridazine) or lead to electrolyte abnormalities (eg, diuretics, amphotericin B).

PREGNANCY: Category D, not for use in nursing.

MECHANISM OF ACTION: DNA fragmentation agent; suspected to cause morphological changes in cells and DNA fragmentation characteristic of apoptosis, and damage or degradation of fushion protein PML/RAR-Alpha.

PHARMACOKINETICS: Metabolism: Liver via reduction and methylation. **Elimination:** Urine.

TRIZIVIR   RX
abacavir sulfate - lamivudine - zidovudine (GlaxoSmithKline)

> Fatal hypersensitivity reactions reported; discontinue if hypersensitivy reaction suspected and do not restart. Hematologic toxicities, lactic acidosis, and severe hepatomegaly with steatosis (including fatal cases) reported. Severe exacerbations of hepatitis B in patients co-infected with HIV upon discontinuation; monitor hepatic function.

THERAPEUTIC CLASS: Nucleoside analog combination

INDICATIONS: Treatment of HIV-1 infection alone or in combination with other antiretrovirals.

DOSAGE: *Adults:* >40kg and CrCl >50mL/min: 1 tab bid.
Pediatrics: Adolescents: >40kg and CrCl >50mL/min: 1 tab bid.

HOW SUPPLIED: Tab: (Abacavir-Lamivudine-Zidovudine) 300mg-150mg-300mg

WARNINGS/PRECAUTIONS: Hypersensitivity; d/c if suspected and register patients by calling 1-800-270-0425. Caution with bone marrow compromise. Prolonged use associated with myopathy and myositis with pathological changes. Avoid with mild to moderate hepatic impairment or liver cirrhosis. Recurrent hepatitis upon discontinuation of lamivudine reported in hepatitis B patients. Lamivudine-resistant hepatitis B virus reported.

ADVERSE REACTIONS: NV, diarrhea, loss of appetite, insomnia, fever, chills, fatigue.

INTERACTIONS: Ethanol decreases elimination. Ganciclovir, interferon-alpha, and other bone marrow suppressors or cytotoxic agents may increase hematologic toxicity. Antagonistic effects with stavudine. Increased lamivudine exposure with trimethoprim 160mg/sulfamethoxazole 800mg. Avoid zalcitabine. Hepatic decompensation reported in patients on combination antiretroviral therapy for HIV and interferon alfa with or without ribavarin; monitor closely for treatment-associated toxicities.

PREGNANCY: Category C, not for use in nursing.

MECHANISM OF ACTION: Abacavir: Carbocyclic nucleoside analogue; inhibits HIV-1 reverse transcriptase (RT) by competing with natural substrate dGTP and incorporating into viral DNA. Lamivudine/Zidovudine: Nucleoside analogue; inhibits RT via DNA chain termination.

PHARMACOKINETICS: Absorption: Abacavir: Rapid; bioavailability (86%). Lamivudine: Rapid; bioavailability (86%). Zidovudine: Rapid; bioavailability (64%). **Distribution:** Abacavir: V_d=0.86L/kg; plasma protein binding (50%). Lamivudine: V_d=1.3L/kg; plasma protein binding (low). Zidovudine: V_d=1.6L/kg; plasma protein binding (low). **Metabolism:** Abacavir: Hepatic, via alcohol dehydrogenase and glucuronyl transferase. Lamivudine: Metabolite (trans-sulfoxide). Zidovudine: Hepatic, via glucuronyl transferase. Major metabolite: (3'-azido-3'-deoxy-5'-O-β-D-glucopyranuronosylthymidine (GZDV). **Elimination:** Abacavir: $T_{1/2}$=1.45 hrs. Lamivudine: (IV): Urine (70%); $T_{1/2}$=5-7 hrs. Zidovudine: Urine (14%); (GZDV): Urine (74%); $T_{1/2}$=0.5-3 hrs.

TRUSOPT
dorzolamide HCl (Merck)

RX

THERAPEUTIC CLASS: Carbonic anhydrase inhibitor

INDICATIONS: Treatment of open-angle glaucoma and ocular hypertension.

DOSAGE: *Adults:* 1 drop tid. Space dosing other ophthalmic drugs by 10 min.
Pediatrics: 1 drop tid. Space dosing other ophthalmic drugs by 10 min.

HOW SUPPLIED: Sol: 2% (5mL, 10mL)

WARNINGS/PRECAUTIONS: Systemically absorbed. Avoid with sulfonamide allergy or severe renal impairment. Caution with hepatic impairment. Not studied in acute angle-closure glaucoma. Local ocular adverse effects (conjunctivitis, lid reactions) reported with chronic use. Bacterial keratitis reported with contaminated containers.

ADVERSE REACTIONS: Ocular burning, stinging, discomfort, superficial punctate keratitis, bitter taste, blurred vision, eye redness, tearing, dryness, photophobia, ocular allergic reactions, lid reactions, conjunctivitis.

INTERACTIONS: Caution with high-dose salicylates. Acid-base disturbances with oral carbonic anhydrase inhibitors. Avoid oral carbonic anhydrase inhibitors due to additive effects. Wait 10 minutes before using another ophthalmic drug.

PREGNANCY: Category C, not for use in nursing.

MECHANISM OF ACTION: Carbonic anhydrase inhibitor; catalyzes reversible reaction involving hydration of carbon dioxide and dehydration of carbonic acid; also decreases aqueous humor secretion in ciliary processes of the eye by slowing the formation of bicarbonate ions with subsequent reduction in Na^+ and fluid transport, which results in reduction in IOP.

PHARMACOKINETICS: Distribution: Plasma protein binding (33%). **Metabolism:** Metabolites: N-desethyl. **Elimination:** Urine (unchanged, metabolite).

TUCKS OINTMENT
mineral oil - pramoxine HCl - zinc oxide (McNeil)

OTC

THERAPEUTIC CLASS: Anesthetic agent

INDICATIONS: Temporary relief of pain, soreness, burning, and itching associated with hemorrhoids and anorectal disorders.

DOSAGE: *Adults:* Cleanse area with soap and water, then rinse and dry. Apply externally to affected area. Max: 5 times/day for 7 days. To use dispensing cap, attach it to tube, lubricate well, then gently insert part way into anal canal. Squeeze tube to deliver medication.
Pediatrics: ≥12 yrs: Cleanse area with soap and water, then rinse and dry. Apply externally to affected area. Max: 5 times/day for 7 days. To use dispensing cap, attach it to tube, lubricate well, then gently insert part way into anal canal. Squeeze tube to deliver medication.

HOW SUPPLIED: Oint: (Mineral Oil-Pramoxine-Zinc Oxide) 46.6%-1%-12.5% (30g)

WARNINGS/PRECAUTIONS: Allergic reactions may develop. D/C if redness, irritation, swelling, pain, other symptoms develop or increase, or if condition worsens within 7 days. Do not administer into rectum by using fingers or any mechanical device or applicator.

PREGNANCY: Safety in pregnancy and nursing not known.

TUCKS SUPPOSITORIES
starch (McNeil)

OTC

THERAPEUTIC CLASS: Anesthetic agent

INDICATIONS: To give temporary relief from itching, burning, and discomfort associated with hemorrhoids and other anorectal disorders.

DOSAGE: *Adults:* Cleanse area with soap and water, then rinse and dry. Insert 1 sup rectally. Max: 6 times/day for 7 days.
Pediatrics: ≥12 yrs: Cleanse area with soap and water, then rinse and dry. Insert 1 sup rectally. Max: 6 times/day for 7 days.

HOW SUPPLIED: Sup: 51% (12ˢ, 24ˢ)

WARNINGS/PRECAUTIONS: D/C if rectal bleeding occurs or if condition worsens or does not improve within 7 days.

PREGNANCY: Safety in pregnancy and nursing not known.

TUSSEND   **CIII**
chlorpheniramine maleate - hydrocodone bitartrate - pseudoephedrine HCl
(King)

THERAPEUTIC CLASS: Cough suppressant

INDICATIONS: Relief of cough and congestion of the respiratory tract. Relief of hay fever symptoms.

DOSAGE: *Adults:* 1 tab or 10mL q4-6h. Max: 4 doses/24 hrs.
Pediatrics: >12 yrs: 1 tab or 10mL q4-6h. Max: 4 doses/24 hrs. 6-12 yrs: 1/2 tab or 5mL q4-6h. Max: 4 doses/24 hrs.

HOW SUPPLIED: (Hydrocodone-Chlorpheniramine-Pseudophedrine) Syrup: 2.5mg-2mg-30mg/5mL; Tab: 5mg-4mg-60mg

CONTRAINDICATIONS: Severe CAD, MAOI therapy, narrow-angle glaucoma, urinary retention, peptic ulcer, during an asthma attack, nursing mothers and infants. Hypersensitivity to other sympathomimetic amines.

WARNINGS/PRECAUTIONS: Caution with HTN, ischemic heart disease, DM, asthma, increased IOP, elderly/debilitated, severe impairment of hepatic or renal function, hyperthyroidism, or prostatic hypertrophy. Caution with head injury, intracranial lesions or pre-existing increase in ICP. May obscure diagnosis/clinical course with acute abdominal conditions. May impair mental and physical abilities.

ADVERSE REACTIONS: Lightheadedness, dizziness, sedation, nausea, vomiting, constipation, urethral spasm, urinary retention.

INTERACTIONS: See Contraindications. Narcotics, antipsychotics, antianxiety agents, alcohol, and other CNS depressants may potentiate CNS depression. Increased effect of antidepressant or hydrocodone with MAOIs or TCAs. Anticholinergics may produce paralytic ileus. Digitalis glycosides may increase risk of cardiac arrhythmias. Decreased hypotensive effects of guanethidine, mecamylamine, methyldopa, reserpine, and veratrum alkaloids. TCAs may antagonize the effects of pseudoephedrine. Risk of hypertensive crises with pseudoephedrine and MAOIs, indomethacin, or with β-adrenergic blockers and methyldopa.

PREGNANCY: Category C, not for use in nursing.

TUSSEND EXPECTORANT   **CIII**
guaifenesin - hydrocodone bitartrate - pseudoephedrine HCl (King)

THERAPEUTIC CLASS: Cough suppressant/expectorant/decongestant

INDICATIONS: For exhausting, nonproductive cough accompanying respiratory tract congestion associated with the common cold, influenza, sinusitis and bronchitis.

DOSAGE: *Adults:* 10mL q4-6h. Max: 10mL qid prn. May take with meals.
Pediatrics: 6-12 yrs: 5mL q4-6h. Max: 5mL qid prn. May take with meals.

HOW SUPPLIED: Sol: (Hydrocodone-Guaifenesin-Pseudoephedrine) 2.5mg-100mg-30mg/5mL

CONTRAINDICATIONS: Severe HTN, severe CAD, MAOI therapy and nursing women. Hypersensitivity to sympathomimetics and phenanthrene derivatives.

WARNINGS/PRECAUTIONS: Caution with severe respiratory impairment , HTN, DM, ischemic heart disease, hyperthyroidism, increased IOP, prostatic hypertrophy, and in elderly or debilitated patients. May impair mental and physical abilities. May produce drug dependence of the morphine type.

ADVERSE REACTIONS: GI upset, nausea, drowsiness, constipation, tachycardia, palpitations, headache, dizziness.

INTERACTIONS: Hydrocodone may potentiate effects of narcotics, general anesthetics, tranquilizers, sedatives and hypnotics, alcohol, and other CNS depressants. Increased effect of antidepressant or hydrocodone with MAOIs or TCAs. Decreased hypotensive effects of mecamylamine, methyldopa, reserpine, and veratrum alkaloids. MAOIs and β-adrenergic blockers potentiate the sympathomimetic effect of pseudoephedrine.

PREGNANCY: Category C, not for use in nursing.

TUSSI-12

RX

carbetapentane tannate - chlorpheniramine tannate (Wallace)

THERAPEUTIC CLASS: Antitussive/antihistamine

INDICATIONS: Symptomatic relief of cough.

DOSAGE: *Adults:* 1-2 tabs q12h.
Pediatrics: >6 yrs: 5-10mL q12h. 2-6 yrs: 2.5-5mL q12h.

HOW SUPPLIED: (Carbetapentane-Chlorpheniramine) Sus: 30mg-4mg/5mL (118mL); Tab: 60mg-5mg* *scored

CONTRAINDICATIONS: Newborns, nursing mothers.

WARNINGS/PRECAUTIONS: Caution with HTN, CVD, hyperthyroidism, DM, elderly, narrow angle glaucoma, or prostatic hypertrophy. Excitation in children may occur. Suspension contains tartrazine.

ADVERSE REACTIONS: Drowsiness, sedation, dryness of mucous membranes, GI effects.

INTERACTIONS: Avoid with or within 14 days of discontinuation of MAOIs. Additive CNS effects with alcohol, CNS depressants.

PREGNANCY: Category C, not for use in nursing.

MECHANISM OF ACTION: Carbetapentane: Produces antitussive actions. Phenylephrine: Produces decongestant effect.

TUSSIONEX PENNKINETIC

CIII

chlorpheniramine polistirex - hydrocodone polistirex (UCB)

THERAPEUTIC CLASS: Opioid antitussive/antihistamine

INDICATIONS: Relief of cough and upper respiratory symptoms associated with allergy and cold.

DOSAGE: *Adults:* ≥12 yrs: 5mL q12h. Max: 10mL/24 hrs.
Pediatrics: 6-11 yrs: 2.5mL q12h. Max: 5mL/24 hrs.

HOW SUPPLIED: Sus: (Hydrocodone-Chlorpheniramine) 10mg-8mg/5mL

CONTRAINDICATIONS: Should not be used in children less than 6 years of age due to the risk of fatal respiratory depression.

WARNINGS/PRECAUTIONS: May produce dose-related respiratory depression. Caution with pulmonary disease, post-surgery, head injury, intracranial lesions or pre-existing increase in ICP, narrow angle glaucoma, asthma, BPH, elderly, debilitated, impaired hepatic/renal functions, hypothyroidosis, Addison's disease or urethral stricture. May mask acute abdominal conditions and the clinical course of head injuries. May cause obstructive bowel disease. Consider risk/benefit ratio in pediatrics, especially with croup. Impairment of mental and physical performance.

ADVERSE REACTIONS: Sedation, drowsiness, lethargy, anxiety, dysphoria, euphoria, dizziness, psychotic dependence, rash, pruritus, nausea, vomiting, ureteral spasm, urinary retention, respiratory depression, dryness of the pharynx, tightness of the chest.

INTERACTIONS: Additive CNS depression with narcotics, antipsychotics, antianxiety agents, and alcohol. Increased effect of antidepressant or hydrocodone with MAOIs or TCAs. Concurrent anticholinergics may cause paralytic ileus.

PREGNANCY: Category C, not for use in nursing.

MECHANISM OF ACTION: Hydrocodone: Opioid antitussive/antihistamine; not established. Suspected to act directly on cough center. Chlorpheniramine: H_1-receptor antagonist; possesses anticholinergic and sedative activity. Prevents released histamine from dilating capillaries and causing edema of the respiratory mucosa.

PHARMACOKINETICS: Absorption: Hydrocodone: C_{max}=22.8ng/mL, T_{max}=3.4 hrs. Chlorpheniramine: C_{max}=58.4ng/mL, T_{max}=6.3 hrs. **Elimination:** Hydrocodone: $T_{1/2}$=4 hrs. Chlorpheniramine: $T_{1/2}$=16 hrs.

TWINJECT   RX
epinephrine (Verus)

THERAPEUTIC CLASS: Sympathomimetic catecholamine

INDICATIONS: Emergency treatment of severe allergic reactions (type 1) including anaphylaxis to insect stings or bites, allergens, foods, drugs, diagnostic testing substances, as well as idiopathic or exercise-induced anaphylaxis.

DOSAGE: *Adults:* Administer SQ or IM into thigh. 15-30kg: (Twinject 0.15mg) 0.15mg. May repeat if needed. ≥30kg: (Twinject 0.3mg) 0.3mg. May repeat if needed.
Pediatrics: Administer SQ or IM into thigh. 15-30kg: (Twinject 0.15mg) 0.15mg. May repeat if needed. ≥30kg: (Twinject 0.3mg) 0.3mg. May repeat if needed.

HOW SUPPLIED: Inj: (Twinject 0.15mg, Twinject 0.3mg) 1mg/mL

WARNINGS/PRECAUTIONS: Inject into anterolateral aspect of thigh; avoid injecting into hands, feet, or buttock. Avoid IV use. Contains sodium bisulfite. Caution with cardiac arrhythmias, coronary artery or organic heart disease, or HTN. May precipitate/aggravate angina pectoris or produce ventricular arrhythmias with coronary insufficiency or ischemic heart disease. Light-sensitive; store in tube provided.

ADVERSE REACTIONS: Anxiety, apprehensiveness, restlessness, tremor, weakness, dizziness, sweating, palpitations, pallor, nausea, vomiting, headache, respiratory difficulties, HTN.

INTERACTIONS: Monitor for cardiac arrhythmias with cardiac glycosides or diuretics. Effects may be potentiated by TCAs, MAOIs, levothyroxine, and certain antihistamines (notably chlorpheniramine, tripelennamine, diphenhydramine). Cardiostimulating and bronchodilating effects antagonized by β-adrenergic blockers (eg, propranolol). Vasoconstricting and hypertensive effects antagonized by α-adrenergic blockers (eg, phentolamine). Ergot alkaloids and phenothiazines may reverse pressor effects.

PREGNANCY: Category C, safety in nursing not known.

MECHANISM OF ACTION: Acts on α- and β-adrenergic receptors.

TYLENOL   OTC
acetaminophen (McNeil Consumer)

OTHER BRAND NAMES: Tylenol 8 Hour (McNeil Consumer) - Tylenol Arthritis Pain (McNeil Consumer) - Tylenol Children's (McNeil Consumer) - Tylenol Extra Strength (McNeil Consumer) - Tylenol Infants' (McNeil Consumer) - Tylenol Junior (McNeil Consumer) - Tylenol Regular Strength (McNeil Consumer)

THERAPEUTIC CLASS: Analgesic

INDICATIONS: Temporary relief of minor aches and pains. Temporary reduction of fever.

DOSAGE: *Adults:* ≥12 yrs: (Regular Strength) 650mg q4-6h prn. Max: 3900mg/day. (Extra Strength GoTabs, EZ Tabs, Rapid Release Gels, Caplets, Cool Caplets) 1000mg q4-6h prn. Max: 4000mg/day. (Arthritis Pain, 8 Hour) 2 caplets or geltabs q8h with water. Max: 6 caplets or geltabs/day.
Pediatrics: Max: 5 doses/day. 0-3 months (6-11 lbs): 40mg q4h prn. 4-11 months (12-17 lbs): 80mg q4h prn. 12-23 months (18-23 lbs): 120mg q4h prn. 2-3 yrs (24-35 lbs): 160mg q4h prn. 4-5 yrs (36-47 lbs): 240mg q4h prn. 6-8 yrs (48-59 lbs): 320mg q4h prn. 9-10 yrs (60-71 lbs): 400mg q4h prn. 11 yrs (72-95 lbs): 480mg q4h prn. 12 yrs (≥96 lbs): 640mg q4h prn. Older Children: Regular Strength: 6-11 yrs: 325mg q4-6h prn. Max: 1625mg/day.

HOW SUPPLIED: Caplets: (Arthritis Pain, 8 Hour) 650mg; Drops: (Infants') 80mg/0.8mL (15mL, 30mL); Geltabs: (Arthritis Pain) 650mg; Sol: (Extra Strength) 500mg/15mL; Sus:

(Children's) 160mg/5mL; Tab: (Regular Strength) 325mg; (Extra Strength EZ Tabs, GoTabs, Caplets, Cool Caplets, Rapid Release Gels) 500mg; Tab, Chewable: (Children's) 80mg, (Junior) 160mg

WARNINGS/PRECAUTIONS: May cause liver damage.

INTERACTIONS: Increased risk of hepatotoxicity with excessive alcohol use (≥3 drinks/day).

PREGNANCY: Safety in pregnancy or nursing not known.

Tylenol with Codeine   CIII
acetaminophen - codeine phosphate (Ortho-McNeil)

OTHER BRAND NAME: Acetaminophen w/Codeine Elixir (Various)

THERAPEUTIC CLASS: Opioid analgesic

INDICATIONS: Relief of mild to moderately severe pain.

DOSAGE: *Adults:* (Tab) Usual: 15-60mg codeine/dose and 300-1000mg APAP/dose up to q4h prn. Max: 60mg codeine/dose, 360mg codeine/day, and 4g APAP/day. (Elixir): 15mL q4h prn.
Pediatrics: (Elixir): Usual: 7-12 yrs: 10mL tid-qid. 3-6 yrs: 5mL tid-qid.

HOW SUPPLIED: (Codeine-APAP) Elixir: (CV) 12-120mg/5mL; Tab: (#3, CIII) 30-300mg, (#4, CIII) 60-300mg

WARNINGS/PRECAUTIONS: Respiratory depressant effects may be exacerbated with head injury or increased ICP. May obscure head injuries, acute abdominal conditions. Caution in the elderly, debilitated, severe hepatic or renal dysfunction, hypothyroidism, Addison's disease, prostatic hypertrophy, or urethral stricture. Potential for physical dependence, tolerance. Tabs contain sulfites.

ADVERSE REACTIONS: Lightheadedness, dizziness, sedation, SOB, NV, allergic reactions, euphoria, dysphoria, constipation, abdominal pain, pruritus.

INTERACTIONS: Additive CNS depression with narcotic analgesics, antipsychotics, anti-anxiety agents, alcohol, other CNS depressants. Anticholinergics may produce para-lytic ileus.

PREGNANCY: Category C, caution in nursing.

MECHANISM OF ACTION: Codeine: Narcotic analgesic and antitussive; produces centrally-acting analgesic effects. APAP: Nonopiate, nonsalicyclate analgesic and anti-pyretic.

PHARMACOKINETICS: Absorption: Codeine: Rapidly absorbed. APAP: Rapidly absorbed. **Distribution:** Codeine: Found in liver, spleen, kidneys; crosses blood brain barrier; found in fetal tissue and breast milk. APAP: Found in breast milk. **Metabolism:** APAP: Liver (con-jugation). **Elimination:** Codeine: Urine (90%) (parent compound and metabolites); $T_{1/2}$=2.9 hrs. APAP: Urine (85%); $T_{1/2}$=1.25-3 hrs.

Tyzeka   RX
telbivudine (Idenix)

> **Lactic acidosis and severe hepatomegaly with steatosis reported. Discontinuation may result in severe acute exacerbations of hepatitis; monitor hepatic function closely for at least several months following discontinuation of therapy.**

THERAPEUTIC CLASS: Nucleoside analogue

INDICATIONS: Treatment of chronic hepatitis B.

DOSAGE: *Adults:* CrCl ≥50mL/min: 600mg qd. CrCl 30-49mL/min: 600mg every 48 hrs. CrCl <30mL/min (not requiring dialysis): 600mg every 72 hrs. ESRD: 600mg every 96 hrs.
Pediatrics: ≥16 yrs: CrCl ≥50mL/min: 600mg qd. CrCl 30-49mL/min: 600mg every 48 hrs. CrCl <30mL/min (not requiring dialysis): 600mg every 72 hrs. ESRD: 600mg every 96 hrs.

HOW SUPPLIED: Tab: 600mg

WARNINGS/PRECAUTIONS: Myopathy reported; interrupt therapy if myopathy suspected and d/c if myopathy diagnosed. Monitor renal function.

ADVERSE REACTIONS: Upper respiratory tract infection, fatigue, malaise, abdominal pain, nasopharyngitis, headache, elevated blood CPK, cough, nausea, vomiting, influenza, flu-like symptoms, diarrhea, loose stools, pharyngolaryngeal pain.

INTERACTIONS: Drugs that alter renal function may alter plasma concentrations of telbivudine.

PREGNANCY: Category B, not for use in nursing.

MECHANISM OF ACTION: Thymidine nucleoside analogue; inhibits HBV DNA polymerase by competing with thymidine 5'-triphosphate and inhibits viral replication by incorporating into viral DNA causing DNA chain termination.

PHARMACOKINETICS: Absorption: C_{max}=3.69mcg/mL, T_{max}=2 hrs, AUC=26.1mcg•h/mL. **Distribution:** Plasma protein binding (3.3%). **Elimination:** Urine; $T_{1/2}$=40-49 hrs.

ULTIVA
remifentanil HCl (Abbott)

THERAPEUTIC CLASS: Opioid analgesic

INDICATIONS: As an analgesic agent for use during the induction and maintenance of general anesthesia. For continuation as an analgesic into the immediate postoperative period in adults under the direct supervision of an anesthesia practitioner in a postoperative anesthesia care unit or intensive care setting. As an analgesic component of monitored anesthesia care in adults.

DOSAGE: *Adults:* Continuous IV Infusion: Induction: 0.5-1mcg/kg/min. Maint: 0.4mcg/kg with nitrous oxide 66%; 0.25mcg/kg with isoflurane (0.4-1.25 MAC); 0.25 with propofol (100-200mcg/kg/min). Post-Op Continuation: 0.1mcg/kg/min. CABG: Induction/Maint/Continuation: 1mcg/kg/min. Elderly (>65 yrs): Use 50% of adult dose. Titrate carefully. *Pediatrics:* Anesthesia Maint: Continuous IV Infusion: 1-12 yrs: 0.25mcg/kg/min with halothane (0.3-1.5 MAC), sevoflurane (0.3-1.5 MAC, or isoflurane (0.4-1.5 MAC). Range: 0.05-1.3mcg/kg/min. Birth-2 months: 0.4mcg/kg/min. Range: 0.4-1mcg/kg/min.

HOW SUPPLIED: Inj: 1mg, 2mg, 5mg

CONTRAINDICATIONS: Epidural or intrathecal administration, hypersensitivity to fentanyl analogs.

WARNINGS/PRECAUTIONS: Administer only with infusion device. IV bolus administration should be used only during the maintenance of general anesthesia. Interruption of infusion will result in rapid offset of effect. Use associated with apnea and respiratory depression. Not for use in diagnostic or therapeutic procedures outside the monitored anesthesia care setting. Resuscitative and intubation equipment, oxygen, and opioid antagonist must be readily available. May cause skeletal muscle rigidity and is related to the dose and speed of administration. Do not administer into the same IV tubing with blood due to potential inactivation by nonspecific esterases in blood products. Continuously monitor vital signs and oxygenation. Bradycardia, hypotension, intraoperative awareness reported. Not recommended as sole agent for induction of anesthesia.

ADVERSE REACTIONS: NV, hypotension, muscle rigidity, bradycardia, shivering, fever, dizziness, visual disturbances, respiratory depression, apnea.

INTERACTIONS: Synergism with thiopental, propofol, isoflurane, midazolam; reduce doses of these drugs by up to 75%.

PREGNANCY: Category C, caution in nursing.

MECHANISM OF ACTION: Opioid analgesic.

PHARMACOKINETICS: Distribution: V_d=100mL/kg, 350mL/kg (initial, steady-state), plasma protein binding (70%). **Metabolism:** Hydrolysis via nonspecific blood and tissue esterases to carboxylic acid metabolite. **Elimination:** $T_{1/2}$=10-20 min.

ULTRAVATE
halobetasol propionate (Ranbaxy)   RX

THERAPEUTIC CLASS: Corticosteroid

INDICATIONS: Corticosteroid-responsive dermatoses.

DOSAGE: *Adults:* Apply qd-bid. Rub in gently. Limit treatment to 2 weeks. Max: 50g/week.

Pediatrics: ≥12 yrs: Apply qd-bid. Rub in gently. Limit treatment to 2 weeks. Max: 50g/week.

HOW SUPPLIED: Cre, Oint: 0.05% (15g, 50g)

WARNINGS/PRECAUTIONS: Avoid face, groin, or axillae. Not for treatment of rosacea or perioral dermatitis. May produce reversible HPA axis suppression, manifestations of Cushing's syndrome, hyperglycemia, and glucosuria. Caution when applied to large surface areas or under occlusive dressings. Use appropriate antifungal or antibacterial agent with dermatological infections; d/c if infection does not clear. Pediatrics may be more susceptible to systemic toxicity. Avoid eyes. D/C if irritation occurs. Re-assess if no improvement after 2 weeks.

ADVERSE REACTIONS: Stinging, burning, itching, irritation, dryness, folliculitis, hypertrichosis, acneiform eruptions, hypopigmentation, perioral dermatitis, allergic contact dermatitis, skin maceration, secondary infection, skin atrophy, striae, miliaria.

PREGNANCY: Category C, caution in nursing.

MECHANISM OF ACTION: Corticosteroid; possesses anti-inflammatory, antipruritic, and vasoconstrictive properties. Anti-inflammatory activity not established; suspected to act by induction of phospholipase A_2 inhibitory proteins called lipocortins. Lipocortins control biosynthesis of potent inflammation mediators (eg, prostaglandins, leukotrienes) by inhibiting release of their common precursor, arachidonic acid.

PHARMACOKINETICS: Absorption: Percutaneous; occlusion, inflammation, and other disease states may increase absorption. **Distribution:** Systemically administered corticosteroids appear in breast milk.

UNASYN
RX

ampicillin sodium - sulbactam sodium (Pfizer)

THERAPEUTIC CLASS: Semisynthetic penicillin/beta-lactamase inhibitor

INDICATIONS: Treatment of skin and skin structure (SSSI), intra-abdominal, and gynecological infections caused by susceptible microorganisms.

DOSAGE: *Adults:* 1.5-3g (ampicillin+sulbactam) IM/IV q6h. Max: 4g sulbactam/day. Renal Impairment: CrCl ≥30mL/min: 1.5-3g q6-8h. CrCl 15-29mL/min: 1.5-3g q12h. CrCl 5-14mL/min: 1.5-3g q24h.

Pediatrics: ≥1 yr: 300mg/kg/day (ampicillin+sulbactam) IV in equally divided doses q6h. Max: 4g sulbactam/day. ≥40kg: Dose according to adult recommendations.

HOW SUPPLIED: Inj: (Ampicillin-Sulbactam) 1g-0.5g, 2g-1g, 10g-5g

WARNINGS/PRECAUTIONS: Serious, sometimes fatal, hypersensitivity reactions reported with PCN therapy. *Clostridium difficile*-associated diarrhea reported. Increased risk of skin rash with mononucleosis; use alternate agent.

ADVERSE REACTIONS: Injection site pain, thrombophlebitis, diarrhea.

INTERACTIONS: Probenecid increases and prolongs blood levels. Increased incidence of rash with allopurinol. Do not reconstitute with aminoglycosides; may inactivate aminoglycosides.

PREGNANCY: Category B, caution in nursing.

MECHANISM OF ACTION: Ampicillin: Broad-spectrum antibacterial agent; inhibits cell-wall mucopeptide biosynthesis. Sulbactam: Broad-spectrum antibacterial agent; good inhibitory activity against clinically important plasmid mediated β-lactamases most frequently responsible for transferred drug resistance.

PHARMACOKINETICS: Absorption: IV/IM administration of variable doses resulted in different parameters. **Distribution:** Plasma protein binding (28% ampicillin), (38% sulbactam). **Elimination:** Urine (75-80% unchanged); $T_{1/2}$=1 hr.

UNIPHYL

RX

theophylline (Purdue Pharmaceutical)

THERAPEUTIC CLASS: Xanthine bronchodilator

INDICATIONS: Treatment of the symptoms and reversible airflow obstruction associated with chronic asthma and other chronic lung disease (eg, emphysema, chronic bronchitis).

DOSAGE: *Adults:* Initial: 300-400mg qd for 3 days with meals. Titrate: Increase to 400-600mg qd. After 3 days and if needed/tolerated, increase dose according to blood levels. Tab may be split in half; do not chew or crush. Renal Dysfunction/Elderly (>60 yrs): Max: 400mg/day. Conversion from Immediate-Release Theophylline: Give same daily dose as once daily.
Pediatrics: 12-15 yrs: (<45kg): Initial: 12-14mg/kg/day up to 300mg qd for 3 days with meals. Titrate: Increase to 16mg/kg/day up to 400mg qd. After 3 days if needed/tolerated increase to 20mg/kg/day up to 600mg qd. (>45kg): Follow adult dose schedule. Tab may be split in half; do not chew or crush. Conversion from Immediate-Release Theophylline: ≥12 yrs: Give same daily dose as once daily. Renal Dysfunction: Max: 400mg qd.

HOW SUPPLIED: Tab, Extended-Release: 400mg*, 600mg* *scored

WARNINGS/PRECAUTIONS: Extreme caution in peptic ulcer disease, seizure disorders and/or cardiac arrhythmias (except bradycardia). Caution in neonates, children <1 yr, and the elderly. Caution in pulmonary edema, CHF, fever ≥102°F for 24 hrs, cor-pulmonale, hypothyroidism, liver disease, reduced renal function, sepsis, shock, and HTN. If toxicity develops (eg, repetitive vomiting) monitor serum levels and adjust dosage.

ADVERSE REACTIONS: Vomiting, headache, insomnia, diarrhea, restlessness, tremors, hematemesis, hypokalemia, hyperglycemia, tachycardia, hypotension/shock, nervousness, disorientation, arrhythmias, seizures.

INTERACTIONS: Diminished effects with charcoal broiled food, phenytoin, carbamazepine, phenobarbital, hydantoins, rifampin, ritonavir, aminoglutethimide, barbiturates, ketoconazole, sulfinpyrazone, INH, loop diuretics, sympathomimetics, high protein/low carbohydrate diet, St. John's wort. Potentiated by propranolol, allopurinol, erythromycin, troleandomycin, ciprofloxacin, quinolone antibiotics, oral contraceptives, CCBs, corticosteroids, disulfiram, ephedrine, influenza virus vaccine, interferon, macrolides, mexiletine, thiabendazole, thyroid hormones, carbamazepine, loop diuretics.

PREGNANCY: Category C, caution in nursing.

MECHANISM OF ACTION: Methylxanthine; acts via smooth muscle relaxation and suppression of airway response to stimuli. Bronchodilatation suggested to be mediated by inhibiting isozymes of phosphodiesterase. Also increases the force of contraction of diaphragmatic muscles due to enhancement of calcium uptake through adenosine-mediated channel.

PHARMACOKINETICS: **Absorption:** Rapid, complete; (800 qam, fed) C_{max}=12.1mcg/mL, C_{min}=4.5mcg/mL, T_{max}=8.8 hrs, AUC=203mcg•hr/mL. (600 qd, fed) C_{max}=12.91mcg/mL, C_{min}=5.52mcg/mL, T_{max}=8.62 hrs, AUC=209mcg•hr/mL. Bioavailability Ratio 600/400: 98.8%. **Distribution:** V_d=0.45L/kg; plasma protein binding (40%). **Metabolism:** Extensive; CYP1A2, 2E1, 3A3; Caffeine and 3-methylxanthine (active metabolites). **Elimination:** Urine (10% unchanged), $T_{1/2}$=8 hrs.

UNISOM

OTC

doxylamine succinate (Chattem)

THERAPEUTIC CLASS: Antihistamine

INDICATIONS: As a sleep aid 30 minutes before retiring.

DOSAGE: *Adult:* 1 tab 30 min prior to going to bed. Max: 1 tab qhs.
Pediatrics: >12 yrs: 1 tab 30 min prior to going to bed. Max: 1 tab qhs.

HOW SUPPLIED: Tab: 25mg

CONTRAINDICATIONS: Pregnancy, nursing, asthma, glaucoma, prostate enlargement.

WARNINGS/PRECAUTIONS: Caution in emphysema, chronic bronchitis, glaucoma, and difficulty in urination due to BPH. Caution with alcohol. Re-evaluate therapy if sleeplessness persists >2 weeks.

ADVERSE REACTIONS: Anticholinergic effects.

PREGNANCY: Not for use in pregnancy or nursing.

MECHANISM OF ACTION: Antihistamine; helps reduce difficulty falling asleep.

UNITHROID   RX
levothyroxine sodium (Lannett)

THERAPEUTIC CLASS: Thyroid replacement hormone

INDICATIONS: Hypothyroidism. As a pituitary TSH suppressant in the treatment and prevention of euthyroid goiters, including thyroid nodules, lymphocytic thyroiditis, and multinodular goiter. Adjunct to surgery and radioiodine therapy for thyrotropin-dependent well-differentiated thyroid cancer.

DOSAGE: *Adults:* Take in AM at least 1/2-1 hr before food. Hypothyroid: Usual: 1.7mcg/kg/day. >200mcg/day (seldom). >50 yrs/<50 yrs with Cardiac Disease: Initial: 25-50mcg/day. Titrate: Increase by 12.5-25mcg/day every 6-8 weeks until euthyroid. Elderly with Cardiac Disease: Initial: 12.5-25mcg/day. Titrate: Increase by 12.5-25mcg/day every 4-6 weeks until euthyroid. Severe Hypothyroidism: Initial: 12.5-25mcg/day. Titrate: Increase by 25mcg/day every 2-4 weeks until euthyroid. Pregnancy: May increase dose requirements. Subclinical Hypothyroidism: Lower doses required. *Pediatrics:* Take in AM at least 1/2-1 hr before food. Hypothyroidism: 0-3 months: 10-15mcg/kg/day. 3-6 months: 8-10mcg/kg/day. 6-12 months: 6-8mcg/kg/day. 1-5 yrs: 5-6mcg/kg/day. 6-12 yrs: 4-5mcg/kg/day. >12 yrs: 2-3mcg/kg/day. Growth/Puberty Complete: 1.7mcg/kg/day. Cardiac Risk: Initial: Use lower dose. Titrate: Increase dose every 4-6 weeks until euthyroid. Infants with Serum T_4 <5mcg/dL: Initial: 50mcg/day. Chronic/Severe Hypothyroidism: Children: Initial: 25mcg/day. Titrate: Increase by 25mcg/day every 2-4 weeks until desired effect. Minimize Hyperactivity in Older Children: Initial: Give 1/4 of full replacement dose. Titrate: Increase by same amount weekly until full dose achieved. May crush tab and mix with 5-10mL water.

HOW SUPPLIED: Tab: 25mcg*, 50mcg*, 75mcg*, 88mcg*, 100mcg*, 112mcg*, 125mcg*, 150mcg*, 175mcg*, 200mcg*, 300mcg* *scored

CONTRAINDICATIONS: Untreated thyrotoxicosis, acute MI, uncorrected adrenal insufficiency.

WARNINGS/PRECAUTIONS: Do not use in the treatment of obesity; larger doses in euthyroid patients can cause serious or even life threatening toxicity. Caution with cardiovascular disease, CAD, adrenal insufficiency, autonomous thyroid tissue, hypothalamic/pituitary hormone deficiencies, and the elderly with risk of occult cardiac disease. Carefully titrate dose to avoid over or under treatment. Decreased bone mineral density with long term use. With adrenal insufficiency supplement with glucocorticoids before therapy.

INTERACTIONS: Sympathomimetics may increase risk of coronary insufficiency with CAD. Upward dose adjustments needed for insulin and oral hypoglycemic agents. Decreased absorption with soybean flour (infant formula), cotton seed meal, walnuts, and fiber. May potentiate oral anticoagulant effects; adjust dose and monitor PT/INR. May decrease levels and effects of digitalis glycosides. Cholestyramine, colestipol, ferrous sulfate, aluminum hydroxide, sodium polystyrene, soybean flour, sucralfate may decrease absorption. Reduced TSH secretion with dopamine/dopamine agonists, glucocorticoids, octreotide. Decreased thyroid hormone secretion with aminoglutethimide, amiodarone, iodine (including iodine-containing radiographic contrast agents), lithium, methimazole, PTU, sulfonamides, tolbutamide. Increased thyroid hormone secretion with amiodarone, iodide (including iodine-containing radiographic contrast agents). Decreased T_4 absorption with antacids (aluminum & magnesium hydroxides), simethicone, bile acid sequestrants (cholestyramine, colestipol), calcium carbonate, cation exchange resins (eg, Kayexalate), ferrous sulfate, sucralfate. Increased serum TBG concentration with clofibrate, estrogens, heroin/methadone, 5-FU, mitotane, tamoxifen. Decreased serum TBG concentration with androgens/anabolic steroids, asparaginase, glucocorticoids, nicotinic acid (slow-release). Protein-binding site displacement with furosemide, heparin, hydantoins, NSAIDs, salicylates. Increased hepatic metabolism with carbamazepine, hydantoins, phenobarbital, rifampin. Decreased conversion of T_4 to T_3 levels with amiodarone, β-adrenergic antagonists (propranolol >160mg/day), glucocorticoids (dexamethasone >4mg/day), PTU. Additive effects of both agents with antidepressants. Interferon-(alpha) may cause development of antithyroid microsomal antibodies causing transient hypothyroidism, hyperthyroidism, or both. Interleukin-2 has been associated with transient painless thyroiditis. Excessive use with growth hormones may accelerate epiphyseal closure. Ketamine use may produce marked HTN and tachycardia. May reduce uptake of iodine-containing radiographic contrast agents. Altered levels of thyroid hormone and/or TSH level with choral hydrate, diazepam, ethionamide, lovastatin, metoclopramide, 6-mercaptopurine, nitroprusside, para-aminosalicylate sodium, perphenazine, resorcinol (excessive topical use), thiazide diuretics.

PREGNANCY: Category A, caution in nursing.

MECHANISM OF ACTION: Thyroid hormone; not understood, suspected to control DNA transcription and protein synthesis.

PHARMACOKINETICS: Distribution: Plasma protein binding (99%), found in breast milk. **Metabolism:** Liver via sequential deiodination (major pathway), conjugation in liver (mainly), kidneys, other tissues. **Elimination:** Urine, feces (20% unchanged), (T_4) $T_{1/2}$=6-7 days, (T_3) $T_{1/2}$≤2days.

URISED RX

atropine sulfate - benzoic acid - hyoscyamine sulfate - methenamine - methylene blue - phenyl salicylate (PolyMedica)

THERAPEUTIC CLASS: anticholinergic/antiseptic/antibacterial/analgesic

INDICATIONS: Relief of lower urinary tract discomfort due to hypermotility. Treatment of formaldehyde-susceptible cystitis, urethritis, trigonitis.

DOSAGE: *Adults:* Usual: 2 tabs qid with plenty of fluid.
Pediatrics: ≥6 yrs: Individualize dose. Take with plenty of fluid.

HOW SUPPLIED: Tab: Atropine 0.03mg-Benzoic Acid 4.5mg-Hyoscyamine 0.03mg-Methenamine 40.8mg-Methylene Blue 5.4mg-Phenyl Salicylate 18.1mg

CONTRAINDICATIONS: Glaucoma, pyloric or duodenal obstruction, urinary bladder neck obstruction, or cardiospasm.

WARNINGS/PRECAUTIONS: Caution with cardiovascular disorders. May precipitate acute urinary retention in prostatic hypertrophy.

ADVERSE REACTIONS: Rash, dry mouth, flushing, difficult micturition, rapid pulse, dizziness, blurred vision, urine/feces discoloration.

INTERACTIONS: Avoid alkalinizing agents/foods. Sulfonamides may precipitate in the urine; avoid concomitant use.

PREGNANCY: Category C, caution in nursing.

MECHANISM OF ACTION: Methenamine: Hydrolyses in acidic urine releasing formaldehyde, which provides mild antiseptic action. Methylene Blue/Benzoic acid: Has mild but effective antiseptic activity. Phenyl Salicylate: Has mild analgesic and antipyretic with weak antiseptic. Hyoscyamine/Atropine: Stimulates parasympatholytic action; leads to relaxing of smooth muscle spasm.

PHARMACOKINETICS: Absorption: Rapid (Methenamine, Phenyl Salicylate, Methylene Blue and Benzoic acid). **Metabolism:** Methenamine: Hydrolyses in acidic urine to formaldehyde. **Elimination:** Urine.

URISPAS RX

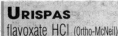

flavoxate HCl (Ortho-McNeil)

THERAPEUTIC CLASS: Smooth muscle antispasmodic

INDICATIONS: Relief of dysuria, urgency, nocturia, suprapubic pain, frequency and incontinence.

DOSAGE: *Adults:* 100-200mg tid-qid. Reduce dose with improvement.
Pediatrics: ≥12 yrs: 100-200mg tid-qid. Reduce dose with improvement.

HOW SUPPLIED: Tab: 100mg

CONTRAINDICATIONS: Pyloric or duodenal obstruction, obstructive intestinal lesions or ileus, achalasia, GI hemorrhage, and obstructive uropathies of the lower urinary tract.

WARNINGS/PRECAUTIONS: Caution with glaucoma and while operating machinery where alertness is required. Drowsiness, blurred vision may occur.

ADVERSE REACTIONS: Drowsiness, dry mouth, nausea, vomiting, tachycardia, palpitations, leukopenia, vertigo, nervousness, confusion, fatigue, headache, hyperpyrexia, urticaria, blurred vision.

PREGNANCY: Category B, caution in nursing.

MECHANISM OF ACTION: Urinary tract spasmolytic; counteracts smooth muscle spasm of urinary tract and exerts effect directly on muscle.

UROGESIC BLUE
RX

hyoscyamine sulfate - methenamine - methylene blue - phenyl salicylate - sodium biphosphate (Edwards)

THERAPEUTIC CLASS: anticholinergic/antibacterial/antiseptic/analgesic/Acidifier

INDICATIONS: Treatment of symptoms of irritative voiding. Relief of lower urinary tract discomfort.

DOSAGE: *Adults:* 1 tab qid with plenty of fluid.
Pediatrics: >6 yrs: Individualize dose. Take with plenty of fluid.

HOW SUPPLIED: Tab: Hyoscyamine 0.12mg-Methenamine, 81.6mg-Methylene Blue, 10.8mg-Phenyl Salicylate, 36.2mg-Sodium Biphosphate 40.8mg

CONTRAINDICATIONS: Consider risk-benefit with: cardiac disease, GI tract obstructive disease, glaucoma, myasthenia gravis, obstructive uropathy.

WARNINGS/PRECAUTIONS: D/C if rapid pulse, dizziness, or blurred vision occurs. Delay in gastric emptying may obscure gastric ulcer therapy. Caution in elderly.

ADVERSE REACTIONS: Rapid pulse, flushing, blurred vision, dizziness, shortness of breath, difficult micturition, acute urinary retention, dry mouth, NV, urine/feces discoloration.

INTERACTIONS: May decrease absorption of other oral agents (dose 2 hrs after ketoconazole). Reduced effectiveness with urinary alkaliners, thiazide diuretics, antacids/antidiarrheals (space dosing by 1 hr). Antimuscarinic effects potentiated with other antimuscarinics, MAOIs. Caution with antimyasthenics. Increased risk of constipation with opioids. Sulfonamides may precipitate in the urine.

PREGNANCY: Category C, safety in nursing not known.

MECHANISM OF ACTION: Hyoscyamine: Parasympatholytic; relaxes smooth muscle and produces antispasmodic effect. Methenamine: Hydrolyses in acidic urine releasing formaldehyde which provides bactericidal and bacteriostatic action. Methylene Blue: Has mild but effective antiseptic activity. Phenyl Salicylate: Mild analgesic. Sodium biphosphate: Helps to maintaine acidic pH in urine for methenamine degredation.

PHARMACOKINETICS: Absorption: Well absorbed (Hyoscyamine, Methenamine, and Methylene Blue). **Metabolism:** Hyoscyamine: Hepatic. Methenamine: Hydrolysis to formaldehyde. **Elimination:** Hyoscyamine: Urine (13-50% unchanged); $T_{1/2}$=12 hrs. Methenamine: Urine (70-90% unchanged); $T_{1/2}$=24 hrs.

VAGISTAT-1
OTC

tioconazole (Novartis)

THERAPEUTIC CLASS: Azole antifungal

INDICATIONS: Treatment of recurrent vaginal yeast infections.

DOSAGE: *Adults:* Insert applicatorful intravaginally hs single dose.
Pediatrics: ≥12 yrs: Insert applicatorful intravaginally hs single dose.

HOW SUPPLIED: Oint: 6.5% (4.6g)

WARNINGS/PRECAUTIONS: Do not use if abdominal pain, fever (>100°F), chills, nausea, vomiting, diarrhea, or foul smelling discharge. Do not use with tampons. Do not rely on condoms or diaphragm to prevent STDs or pregnancy until 3 days after last use.

PREGNANCY: Not for use in pregnancy, safety in nursing not known.

MECHANISM OF ACTION: Azole Antifungal.

VALIUM   CIV
diazepam (Roche Labs)

THERAPEUTIC CLASS: Benzodiazepine

INDICATIONS: Management of anxiety disorders and short-term relief of anxiety symptoms. Symptomatic relief of acute alcohol withdrawal. Adjunct therapy in skeletal muscle spasm and convulsive disorders.

DOSAGE: *Adults:* Anxiety: 2-10mg bid-qid. Alcohol Withdrawal: 10mg tid-qid for 24 hours. Maint: 5mg tid-qid prn. Skeletal Muscle Spasm: 2-10mg tid-qid: Seizure Disorders: 2-10mg bid-qid. Elderly/Debilitated: 2-2.5mg qd-bid initially; may increase gradually as needed and tolerated.
Pediatrics: ≥6 months: 1-2.5mg tid-qid initially; may increase gradually as needed and tolerated.

HOW SUPPLIED: Tab: 2mg*, 5mg*, 10mg* *scored

CONTRAINDICATIONS: Acute narrow angle glaucoma, untreated open angle glaucoma, patients <6 months.

WARNINGS/PRECAUTIONS: Monitor blood counts and LFTs in long-term use. Neutropenia and jaundice reported. Increase in grand mal seizures reported. Avoid abrupt withdrawal. Caution with kidney or hepatic dysfunction.

ADVERSE REACTIONS: Drowsiness, fatigue, ataxia, paradoxical reactions, minor EEG changes.

INTERACTIONS: Phenothiazines, narcotics, barbiturates, MAOIs, and other antidepressants may potentiate effects. Delayed clearance with cimetidine. Avoid alcohol and other CNS-depressants. Risk of seizure with flumazenil.

PREGNANCY: Not for use during pregnancy, safety in nursing not known.

MECHANISM OF ACTION: Benzodiazepine; exerts anxiolytic, sedative, muscle-relaxant, anticonvulsant and amnestic effect. Facilitates GABA, an inhibitory neurotransmitter in CNS.

PHARMACOKINETICS: Absorption: T_{max}=0.25-2.5 hrs. **Distribution:** V_d=0.8-1.0 L/kg, plasma protein binding (98%), crosses blood-brain and placental barrier, appears in breast milk. **Metabolism:** Via N-desmethylation, hydroxylation, glucuronidation to N-desmethyldiazepam, temazepam, oxazepam by CYP3A4, CYP2C19 enzymes. **Elimination:** Urine; $T_{1/2}$=48 hrs, $T_{1/2}$(N-desmethyldiazepam)=100 hrs.

VALTREX   RX
valacyclovir HCl (GlaxoSmithKline)

THERAPEUTIC CLASS: Nucleoside analogue

INDICATIONS: Treatment of herpes zoster (shingles) and herpes labialis (cold sores). Treatment or suppression of genital herpes in immunocompetent patients and for the suppression of recurrent genital herpes in HIV-infected patients.

DOSAGE: *Adults:* Herpes Zoster: 1g q8h for 7 days. Start within 48-72 hrs after onset of rash. CrCl 30-49mL/min: 1g q12h. CrCl 10-29mL/min: 1g q24h. CrCl <10mL/min: 500mg q24h. Genital Herpes: Initial: 1g q12h for 10 days. Start within 48-72 hrs after onset of symptoms. CrCl 10-29mL/min: 1g q24h. CrCl <10mL/min: 500mg q24h. Recurrent Episodes: Treatment: 500mg bid for 3 days. Start within 24 hrs after onset of symptoms. CrCl ≤29mL/min: 500mg q24h. Suppressive Therapy with Normal Immune Function:1g q24h. CrCl ≤29mL/min: 500mg q24h. Alternative: (≤9 episodes/yr) 500mg q24h. CrCl ≤29mL/min: 500mg q48h. Suppressive Therapy with HIV and CD4 ≥100cells/mm³: 500mg q12h. CrCl ≤29mL/min: 500mg q24h. Herpes Labialis: 2g q12h for 1 day. Start at earliest symptom of cold sore. CrCl 30-49mL/min: 1g q12h. CrCl 10-29mL/min: 500mg q12h. <10mL/min: 500mg single dose. Administer therapy for 1 day. Initiate at earliest symptoms of a cold sore.
Pediatrics: Post-Pubertal: Herpes Zoster: 1g q8h for 7 days. Start within 48-72 hrs after onset of rash. CrCl 30-49mL/min: 1g q12h. CrCl 10-29mL/min: 1g q24h. CrCl <10mL/min:

500mg q24h. Genital Herpes: Initial: 1g q12h for 10 days. Start within 48-72 hrs after onset of symptoms. CrCl 10-29mL/min: 1g q24h. CrCl <10mL/min: 500mg q24h. Recurrent Episodes: Treatment: 500mg bid for 3 days. Start within 24 hrs after onset of symptoms. CrCl ≤29mL/min: 500mg q24h. Suppressive Therapy with Normal Immune Function:1g q24h. CrCl ≤29mL/min: 500mg q24h. Alternative: (≤9 episodes/yr) 500mg q24h. CrCl ≤29mL/min: 500mg q48h. Suppressive Therapy with HIV and CD4 ≥100cells/mm^3: 500mg q12h. CrCl ≤29mL/min: 500mg q24h. Herpes Labialis: 2g q12h for 1 day. Start at earliest symptom of cold sore. CrCl 30-49mL/min: 1g q12h. CrCl 10-29mL/min: 500mg q12h. <10mL/min: 500mg single dose. Administer therapy for 1 day. Initiate at earliest symptoms of a cold sore.

HOW SUPPLIED: Tab: 500mg, 1g

CONTRAINDICATIONS: Acyclovir hypersensitivity.

WARNINGS/PRECAUTIONS: Thrombotic thrombocytopenic purpura/hemolytic uremic syndrome reported with advanced HIV disease, allogenic bone marrow or renal transplants. Reduce dose with renal dysfunction. Possible renal and CNS toxicity in elderly.

ADVERSE REACTIONS: NV, headache, dizziness, abdominal pain.

INTERACTIONS: Renal and CNS toxicity with nephrotoxic drugs.

PREGNANCY: Category B, caution in nursing.

MECHANISM OF ACTION: Nucleoside analogue; inhibits replication of herpes viral DNA by inhibiting viral DNA polymerase, incorporating and terminating growing viral DNA chain, and inactivating viral DNA polymerase.

PHARMACOKINETICS: Absorption: Rapid (GI tract). Oral administration of variable doses resulted in different parameters. **Distribution:** Plasma protein binding (13.5-17.9%). **Metabolism:** Hepatic/Intestinal (1st pass). **Elimination:** Urine (45.6%), feces (47.12%); $T_{1/2}$=2.5-3.3 hrs.

VALTROPIN RX
somatropin (LG Life)

THERAPEUTIC CLASS: Human growth hormone

INDICATIONS: Treatment of pediatric patients who have growth failure due to inadequate secretion of endogenous growth hormone. Treatment of growth failure associated with Turner syndrome in pediatric patients who have open epiphyses. Long-term replacement therapy in adults with growth hormone deficiency (GHD) of either adult or childhood onset etiology

DOSAGE: *Adults:* Individualize dose. Initial: 0.33mg/day SQ 6 days a week. Dosage may be increased to individual patient requirement to maximum of 0.66mg/day after 4 weeks. Alternative Dosing: 0.2mg/day (Range: 0.15-0.3mg/day). May increase gradually every 1-2 months by 0.1-0.2mg/day based on individual patient requirements. *Pediatrics:* Individualize dose. Divide weekly dose into equal amounts given either daily or 6 days a week by SQ injection. GHD: 0.17-0.3mg/kg of body weight/week. Turner Syndrome: Up to 0.375mg/kg of body weight/week.

HOW SUPPLIED: Inj: 5mg

CONTRAINDICATIONS: Pediatrics with closed epiphyses. Active proliferative and severe non-proliferative diabetic retinopathy. Presence of active malignancy. Acute critical illness due to complications following open heart surgery, abdominal surgery, or multiple accidental trauma, or those with acute respiratory failure. Patients with Prader-Willi syndrome who are severely obese or have severe respiratory impairment.

WARNINGS/PRECAUTIONS: Known sensitivity to supplied diluent (metacresol). Caution in pediatric pateints with Prader-Willi syndrome with 1 or more risk factors (severe obesity, history of upper airway destruction or sleep apnea, or unidentified respiratory infection). May decrease insulin sensitivity. Patients with GHD secondary to intracranial lesion should be monitered closely for progression or recurrence of underlying disease process. Intracranial HTN reported. Monitor closely with DM, glucose intolerance, hypopituitarism. Fundoscopic exam recommended at initiation and periodically during course of therapy. Monitor carefully for any malignant transformation of skin lesions.

ADVERSE REACTIONS: Headache, pyrexia, cough, respiratory tract infection, diarrhea, vomiting, pharyngitis.

INTERACTIONS: Growth-promoting effects may be inhibited by glucocorticoids. May alter clearance of compounds metabolized by CP450 liver enzymes (eg, corticosteroids, sex steroids, anticonvulsants, cyclosporine); monitor closely. May need insulin adjustment.

PREGNANCY: Category B, caution in nursing.

MECHANISM OF ACTION: Human growth hormone; stimulates linear growth synthesis, metabolizes lipids, reduces body fat stores by increasing cellular protein, and increases plasma fatty acids.

PHARMACOKINETICS: Absorption: C_{max}=43.97ng/mL, T_{max}=4 hrs, AUC=369.9ng•hr/mL. **Metabolism:** Liver, kidneys (protein catabolism). **Elimination:** $T_{1/2}$=3.03 hrs.

VANCOCIN ORAL   RX
vancomycin HCl (Viro Pharma)

THERAPEUTIC CLASS: Tricyclic glycopeptide antibiotic

INDICATIONS: Treatment of enterocolitis caused by *Staphylococcus aureus* and antibiotic-associated pseudomembranous colitis caused by *C.difficile.*

DOSAGE: *Adults:* 500mg-2g/day given tid-qid for 7-10 days.
Pediatrics: 40mg/kg/day given tid-qid for 7-10 days. Max: 2g/day.

HOW SUPPLIED: Cap: 125mg, 250mg

WARNINGS/PRECAUTIONS: Not effective for other types of infection. Caution with inflammatory disorders of intestinal mucosa, renal impairment; increased risk of systemic absorption. Ototoxicity reported. Monitor auditory function.

ADVERSE REACTIONS: Nephrotoxicity, ototoxicity, reversible neutropenia, anaphylactoid reactions (hypotension, wheezing, "Red Man Syndrome," pruritus), superinfection.

INTERACTIONS: Monitor renal function with aminoglycosides.

PREGNANCY: Category B, not for use in nursing.

MECHANISM OF ACTION: Tricyclic glycopeptide antibiotic; inhibits cell-wall biosynthesis, altering bacterial cell membrane permeabilty and RNA synthesis.

PHARMACOKINETICS: Absorption: Poor. **Elimination:** Urine, feces.

VANCOMYCIN INJECTION   RX
vancomycin HCl (Various)

THERAPEUTIC CLASS: Tricyclic glycopeptide antibiotic

INDICATIONS: Treatment of serious or severe infections caused by susceptible strains of methicillin-resistant (β-lactam resistant) staphylococci. Indicated for PCN-allergic patients, for patients who cannot receive or have failed to respond to other drugs, and for infections caused by vancomycin-susceptible organisms that are resistant to other antimicrobials. Indicated for initial therapy when methicillin-resistant staphylococci are suspected, but after susceptibility data are available, therapy should be adjusted accordingly. Effective in the treatment of staphylococcal endocarditis; effectiveness has been documented in other infections due to staphylococci, including septicemia, bone infections, lower respiratory tract infections, and skin and skin-structure infections. Reported to be effective alone or incombination with an aminoglycoside for endocarditis caused by *S.viridans* or *S.bovis.* Reported to be effective only in combination with an aminoglycoside for endocarditis caused by enterococci (eg, *E.faecalis*). Reported to be effective for treatment of diphtheroid endocarditis. Successfully used in combination with either rifampin, an aminoglycoside, or both in early-onset prosthetic valve endocarditis caused by *S.epidermidis* or diphtheroids. Parenteral form may be administered orally for treatment of antibiotic-associated pseudomembranous colitis produced by *C.difficile* and for staphylococcal enterocolitis.

DOSAGE: *Adults:* Inj: Usual: 500mg IV q6h or 1g IV q12h. Administer at not >10mg/min or over at least 60 min, whichever is longer. Max Conc: 5mg/mL. Max Rate: 10mg/min. Renal Impairment: Initial: Not <15mg/kg. Dosage per day in mg is about 15x the GFR in mL/min (refer to table in PI). Elderly: Require greater dose reductions than expected. Functionally Anephric: Initial: 15mg/kg, then 1.9mg/kg/24 hrs. Marked Renal Impairment: 250-1000mg every several days. Anuria: 1000mg every 7-10 days. PO: 500-

2000mg/day in 3-4 divided doses for 7-10 days. Max: 2000mg/day. May dilute in 1oz of water.

Pediatrics: Inj: Usual: 10mg/kg IV q6h. Infants/Neonates: Initial: 15mg/kg, then 10mg/kg q12h for neonates in 1st week of life and q8h thereafter until 1 month of age. Administer over at least 60 min. Renal Impairment: Initial: Not <15mg/kg. Dosage per day in mg is about 15x the GFR in mL/min (refer to table in PI). Premature Infants: Require greater dose reduction. ADD-Vantage vials should not be used in neonates, infants, and pediatrics who require doses <500mg. PO: 40mg/kg/day in 3-4 divided doses for 7-10 days. Max: 2000mg/day. May dilute in 1oz of water.

HOW SUPPLIED: Inj: 500mg, 1g, 5g, 500mg/100mL, 1g/200mL

WARNINGS/PRECAUTIONS: Rapid bolus administration may cause hypotension and cardiac arrest (rare); administer in diluted solution over ≥60 min. Frequency of infusion-related events may increase with concomitant use of anesthetic agents. Ototoxicity reported; monitor auditory function. Caution with renal insufficiency and adjust dose with renal dysfunction. Pseudomembranous colitis reported. Alters the normal flora of the colon and may permit overgrowth of clostridia. Prolonged use may result in overgrowth of nonsusceptible organisms. Reversible neutropenia reported; monitor leukocyte count. Administer via IV route; pain, avoid IM route. Thrombophlebitis may occur; rotate injection sites. Safety and efficacy of administration via the intraperitoneal and intrathecal (intralumbar and intraventricular) routes has not been established. Administration via intraperitoneal route during CAPD has resulted in a syndrome of chemical peritonitis. Adjust dosing schedules in elderly.

ADVERSE REACTIONS: Infusion-related events, hypotension, wheezing, pruritus, pain, chest and head muscle spasm, dyspnea, urticaria, "Red Man Syndrome," nephrotoxicity, pseudomembranous colitis, ototoxicity, neutropenia, phlebitis.

INTERACTIONS: Concomitant use of anesthetic agents has been associated with erythema, histamine-like flushing, and anaphylactoid reactions. Concurrent and/or sequential systemic or topical use of other potentially neurotoxic and/or nephrotoxic drugs (eg, amphotericin B, aminoglycosides, bacitracin, polymyxin B, colistin, viomycin, cisplatin) requires careful monitoring.

PREGNANCY: Category C, not for use in nursing.

MECHANISM OF ACTION: Tricyclic glycopeptide antibiotic; inhibits cell-wall biosynthesis, alters bacterial cell membrane permeability and RNA synthesis.

PHARMACOKINETICS: Absorption: (1g at 2 hrs) C_{max} =23mcg/mL; (500mg at 2 hrs) C_{max} = 19mcg/mL. **Distribution:** Serum protein binding (55%). **Elimination:** Urine (75% in 24 hrs); $T_{1/2}$=4-6 hrs.

VANIQA

eflornithine HCl (SkinMedica)

RX

THERAPEUTIC CLASS: Ornithine decarboxylase inhibitor

INDICATIONS: Reduction of unwanted facial hair in women. Usage is limited to the face and areas under the chin.

DOSAGE: *Adults:* Apply to affected areas bid, at least 8 hrs apart. Rub in thoroughly. May wash area after 4 hrs. May apply 5 min after other hair removal techniques. May apply sunscreen or cosmetics after cream dries.
Pediatrics: ≥12 yrs: Apply to affected areas bid, at least 8 hrs apart. Rub in thoroughly. May wash area after 4 hrs. May apply 5 min after other hair removal techniques. May apply sunscreen or cosmetics after cream dries.

HOW SUPPLIED: Cre: 13.9% (30g)

WARNINGS/PRECAUTIONS: D/C if hypersensitivity or continued irritation occurs. Transient stinging/burning with abraded/broken skin. Condition may return to pretreatment levels 8 weeks after discontinuation.

ADVERSE REACTIONS: Acne, stinging/tingling skin, burning/dry skin, pseudofolliculitis barbae, alopecia.

PREGNANCY: Category C, caution in nursing.

MECHANISM OF ACTION: Ornithine decarboxylase inhibitor; inhibits cell division and synthetic functions that effect the rate of hair growth (animal study).

PHARMACOKINETICS: Absorption: C_{max}=10ng/mL; AUC=92ng•hr/mL. **Elimination:** Urine (unchanged); $T_{1/2}$=8 hrs.

VANOS   RX
fluocinonide (Medicis)

THERAPEUTIC CLASS: Corticosteroid

INDICATIONS: Corticosteroid-responsive dermatoses.

DOSAGE: *Adults:* Apply thin layer to affected area qd-bid. Max: 60g/week. Do not exceed 2 weeks.
Pediatrics: ≥12 yrs: Appy thin layer to affected area qd-bid. Max: 60g/week. Do not exceed 2 weeks.

HOW SUPPLIED: Cre: 0.1% (30g, 60g)

WARNINGS/PRECAUTIONS: May produce reversible HPA axis suppression, manifestations of Cushing's syndrome, hyperglycemia, and glucosuria. Caution when applied to large surface areas or under occlusive dressings. Use appropriate antifungal or antibacterial agent with dermatological infections. D/C if infection does not clear or irritation develops. Do not use for more than 2 weeks at a time.

ADVERSE REACTIONS: Headache, application site burning, nasopharyngitis, nasal congestion, unspecified application site reaction.

PREGNANCY: Category C, not for use in nursing.

MECHANISM OF ACTION: Corticosteroid; possesses anti-inflammatory, antipruritic, and vasoconstrictive properties. Anti-inflammatory activity not established; suspected to act by induction of phospholipase A_2 inhibitory proteins, lipocortins. Lipocortins control biosynthesis of potent inflammation mediators (eg, prostaglandins, leukotrienes) by inhibiting release of their common precursor, arachidonic acid.

PHARMACOKINETICS: Absorption: Percutaneous; inflammation and/or other disease states may increase absorption. **Distribution:** Systemically administered corticosteroids appear in breast milk.

VANTIN   RX
cefpodoxime proxetil (Pharmacia & Upjohn)

THERAPEUTIC CLASS: Cephalosporin (3rd generation)

INDICATIONS: Treatment of acute otitis media, pharyngitis/tonsillitis, community-acquired pneumonia (CAP), acute bacterial exacerbation of chronic bronchitis (ABECB), acute uncomplicated urethral and cervical gonorrhea, acute uncomplicated anorectal infections in women, uncomplicated skin and skin structure infections (SSSI), acute maxillary sinusitis, and uncomplicated urinary tract infections (UTI) caused by susceptible strains of microorganisms.

DOSAGE: *Adults:* Take tabs with food. Pharyngitis/Tonsillitis: 100mg q12h for 5-10 days. CAP: 200mg q12h for 14 days. ABECB: 200mg q12h for 10 days. Uncomplicated Gonorrhea (Men/Women)/Rectal Gonococcal Infections (Women): 200mg single dose. SSSI: 400mg q12h for 7-14 days. Sinusitis: 200mg q12h for 10 days. UTI: 100mg q12h for 7 days. CrCl <30mL/min: Increase interval to q24h. Hemodialysis: Dose 3 times weekly after dialysis.
Pediatrics: ≥12 yrs: Take tabs with food. Pharyngitis/Tonsillitis: 100mg q12h for 5-10 days. CAP: 200mg q12h for 14 days. ABECB: 200mg q12h for 10 days. Uncomplicated Gonorrhea (Men/Women)/Rectal Gonococcal Infections (Women): 200mg single dose. SSSI: 400mg q12h for 7-14 days. Sinusitis: 200mg q12h for 10 days. UTI: 100mg q12h for 7 days. 2 months-12 yrs: Otitis Media: 5mg/kg q12h for 5 days. Max: 200mg/dose. Pharyngitis/Tonsillitis: 5mg/kg q12h for 5-10 days. Max: 100mg/dose. Sinusitis: 5mg/kg q12h for 10 days. Max: 200mg/dose. CrCl <30mL/min: Increase interval to q24h. Hemodialysis: Dose 3 times weekly after dialysis.

HOW SUPPLIED: Sus: 50mg/5mL (50mL, 75mL, 100mL), 100mg/5mL (50mL, 75mL, 100mL); Tab: 100mg, 200mg

WARNINGS/PRECAUTIONS: Cross-sensitivity to PCNs and other cephalosporins may occur. *Clostridium difficile*-associated diarrhea reported. Positive direct Coombs' tests reported. Caution with renal impairment; dose reduction may be needed. May result in overgrowth of nonsusceptible organisms.

ADVERSE REACTIONS: Diarrhea, nausea.

INTERACTIONS: Decreased plasma levels and absorption with antacids and H_2-blockers. Delayed peak plasma levels with anticholinergics. Probenecid inhibits renal excretion. Closely monitor renal function with nephrotoxic agents. Caution with potent diuretics.

PREGNANCY: Category B, not for use in nursing.

MECHANISM OF ACTION: Cephalosporin; inhibits cell-wall synthesis.

PHARMACOKINETICS: Absorption: C_{max}(100mg)=1.4mcg/mL, T_{max}=2-3 hrs. **Distribution:** Plasma protein binding (22-31%). **Metabolism:** Via desterification. **Elimination:** Urine; $T_{1/2}$= 2.09-2.84 hrs.

VAQTA   RX
hepatitis A Vaccine (Inactivated) (Merck)

THERAPEUTIC CLASS: Vaccine

INDICATIONS: Active immunization against hepatitis A virus in persons 12 months of age and older. Give primary immunization at least 2 weeks before expected exposure.

DOSAGE: *Adults:* ≥19 yrs: 1mL (50 U) IM followed by a booster of 1mL (50 U) 6-18 months later.
Pediatrics: 1-18 yrs: 0.5mL (25 U) IM followed by a booster of 0.5mL (25 U) 6-18 months later.

HOW SUPPLIED: Inj: 25 U/0.5mL, 50 U/mL

WARNINGS/PRECAUTIONS: Have epinephrine (1:1000) available. May not prevent hepatitis A with unrecognized infection. Caution with bleeding disorders. Defer use with acute infection or febrile illness. Suboptimal response may occur in immunocompromised patients.

ADVERSE REACTIONS: Injection-site pain, tenderness, erythema, swelling, warmth, fever.

INTERACTIONS: Immunosuppressive therapy may reduce response to active immunization.

PREGNANCY: Category C, caution in nursing.

MECHANISM OF ACTION: Vaccine; produces an antibody response against hepatitis A virus.

VARIVAX   RX
varicella virus vaccine live (Merck)

THERAPEUTIC CLASS: Vaccine

INDICATIONS: Vaccination against varicella.

DOSAGE: *Adults:* 0.5mL SQ at elected date, repeat 4-8 weeks later.
Pediatrics: 12 months-12 yrs: 0.5mL SQ. ≥13 yrs: 0.5mL SQ at elected date, repeat 4-8 weeks later.

HOW SUPPLIED: Inj: 1350PFU/0.5mL

CONTRAINDICATIONS: Pregnancy (avoid pregnancy for 3 months after vaccine); gelatin hypersensitivity; anaphylactoid reactions to neomycin, blood dyscrasias, leukemia, lymphomas, malignant neoplasms affecting bone marrow or lymphatic system, febrile infection, active untreated TB, immunosuppressive therapy, immunosuppressant doses of corticosteroids, immunodeficiency states.

WARNINGS/PRECAUTIONS: Children and adolescents with ALL in remission can receive the vaccine under an investigational protocol. Defer vaccine for at least 5 months after blood or plasma transfusions, or administration of immune globulin or varicella zoster immune globulin. Defer vaccine with family history of congenital, hereditary immunodeficiency until immune system evaluated. Rarely, vaccine virus transmission through varicella-like rash can occur; avoid close association with susceptible high-risk individuals for up to six weeks (eg, immunocompromised patients, pregnant women without history of chickenpox, newborns of mothers without documented history of chickenpox). Have epinephrine available.

ADVERSE REACTIONS: Fever, local reactions, pain, varicella-like rashes.

INTERACTIONS: Avoid immune globulins for 2 months after vaccination. Avoid salicylates for 6 weeks after vaccination. Contraindicated with immunosuppressive therapy or immunosuppressant doses of corticosteroids.

PREGNANCY: Category C, contraindicated in pregnancy and caution in nursing.

MECHANISM OF ACTION: Vaccine; cell-mediated immune response stimulation against varicella zoster virus (VZV) infection.

Vasocon-A OTC
antazoline phosphate - naphazoline HCl (Novartis Ophthalmics)

THERAPEUTIC CLASS: Antihistamine/decongestant

INDICATIONS: Temporary relief of minor allergic symptoms of the eye, including itching and redness due to pollen and animal hair.

DOSAGE: *Adults:* 1-2 drops prn. Max: 4 doses/day.
Pediatrics: >6 yrs: 1-2 drops prn. Max: 4 doses/day.

HOW SUPPLIED: Sol: (Antazoline-Naphazoline) 0.5%-0.05% (15mL)

WARNINGS/PRECAUTIONS: Do not use if solution changes color or becomes cloudy. D/C if develop eye pain, vision changes, redness or irritaton continues, or if condition worsens or persists >72hrs. Supervision required with heart disease, HTN, or narrow angle glaucoma.

PREGNANCY: Safety in pregnancy and nursing not known.

Vasotec RX
enalapril maleate (Merck)

> **ACE inhibitors can cause death/injury to developing fetus during 2nd and 3rd trimesters. Stop therapy if pregnancy detected.**

THERAPEUTIC CLASS: ACE inhibitor

INDICATIONS: Treatment of hypertension. Treatment of symptomatic CHF usually in combination with diuretics and digitalis. To decrease overt heart failure development and hospitalization in stable asymptomatic left ventricular dysfunction.

DOSAGE: *Adults:* HTN: If possible, d/c diuretic 2-3 days prior to therapy. Initial: 5mg qd, 2.5mg qd with concomitant diuretic. Usual: 10-40mg/day given qd or bid. Resume diuretic if BP not controlled. CrCl ≤30mL/min: Initial: 2.5mg/day. Dialysis: 2.5mg/day on dialysis days. Heart Failure: Initial: 2.5mg/day. Usual: 2.5-20mg given bid. Max: 40mg/day. Left Ventricular Dysfunction: Initial: 2.5mg bid. Titrate: Increase to 20mg/day. Hyponatremia or SrCr 1.6mg/dL with Heart Failure: Initial: 2.5mg qd. Titrate: Increase to 2.5mg bid, then 5mg bid. Max: 40mg/day.
Pediatrics: HTN: 1 month-16 yrs: Initial: 0.08mg/kg (up to 5mg) qd. Titrate: Adjust according to response. Max: 0.58mg/kg/dose (or 40mg/dose). Avoid if GFR <30mL/min/1.73m^2. (To prepare 200mL of 1mg/mL sus: Add 50mL of Bicitra® to polyethylene terephthalate bottle with ten 20mg tabs and shake for at least 2 min. Let stand for 60 min, then shake again for 1 min. Add 150mL of Ora-Sweet SF™ and shake, then refrigerate. Can store up to 30 days.)

HOW SUPPLIED: Tab: 2.5mg*, 5mg*, 10mg, 20mg *scored

CONTRAINDICATIONS: History of ACE inhibitor associated angioedema and hereditary or idiopathic angioedema.

WARNINGS/PRECAUTIONS: D/C if angioedema, jaundice, or if marked LFT elevation occurs. Risk of hyperkalemia with DM, renal dysfunction. Persistent nonproductive cough reported. Monitor WBCs in renal or collagen vascular disease. Anaphylactoid reactions reported. Fetal/neonatal morbidity and death reported. Monitor for hypotension in high-risk patients (heart failure, surgery/anesthesia, hyponatremia, high-dose diuretic therapy, severe volume and/or salt depletion, etc). Caution with CHF, obstruction to left ventricle outflow tract, renal dysfunction, and renal artery stenosis. Less effective on BP in blacks and more reports of angioedema than nonblacks. Intestinal angioedema reported.

ADVERSE REACTIONS: Fatigue, orthostatic effects, asthenia, diarrhea, NV, headache, dizziness, cough, rash, hypotension.

INTERACTIONS: May increase lithium levels. Hypotension risk with diuretics. May further decrease renal dysfunction with NSAIDs. Increase risk of hyperkalemia with K+-sparing diuretics, K+-containing salt substitutes or K+ supplements. Augmented effect by antihypertensives that cause renin release (eg, thiazides). NSAIDs may diminish antihypertensive effect.

PREGNANCY: Category C (1st trimester) and D (2nd and 3rd trimesters), not for use in nursing.

MECHANISM OF ACTION: ACE inhibitor; inhibition results in decreased plasma angiotensin II, which leads to decreased vasopressor activity and decreased aldosterone secretion.

PHARMACOKINETICS: Absorption: T_{max}=1, 3-4 hrs (enalapril, enalaprilat). **Metabolism:** Via hydrolysis, enalaprilat (metabolite). **Elimination:** Urine, feces; $T_{1/2}$=11 hrs (enalaprilat).

VECURONIUM RX
vecuronium bromide (Various)

> **Administer by adequately trained individuals familiar with actions, characteristics, and hazards.**

THERAPEUTIC CLASS: Skeletal muscle relaxant (nondepolarizing)

INDICATIONS: Adjunct to general anesthesia, to facilitate endotracheal intubation, and to provide skeletal muscle relaxation during surgery or mechanical ventilation.

DOSAGE: *Adults:* Individualize dose. Initial: 0.08-0.1mg/kg IV bolus. Maint: 0.01-0.015mg/kg IV within 25-40 min of initial dose. Administer subsequent doses at 12-15 min intervals under balanced anesthesia and slightly longer with inhalation agents. Max: 0.15-0.28mg/kg. Prior Succinylcholine: Reduce dose to 0.04-0.06mg/kg with inhalation anesthesia and 0.05-0.06mg/kg with balanced anesthesia. Continuous Infusion: Initial: 1mcg/kg/min administered 20-40 min after intubating dose of 80-100mcg/kg. Administer infusion after evidence of recovery from bolus. Adjust infusion rate to maintain 90% suppression of twitch response. Maint: 0.8-1.2mcg/kg/min. Concurrent Steady-State Enflurane/Isoflurane: Reduce rate 25-60%, 45-60 min after intubating dose.
Pediatrics: 10-17 yrs: Individualize dose. Initial: 0.08-0.1mg/kg IV bolus. Maint: 0.01-0.015mg/kg IV within 25-40 min of initial dose. Administer subsequent dose at 12-15 min intervals under balanced anesthesia and slightly longer with inhalation agents. Max: 0.15-0.28mg/kg. Prior Succinylcholine: Reduce dose to 0.04-0.06mg/kg with inhalation anesthesia and 0.05-0.06mg/kg with balanced anesthesia. Continuous Infusion: Initial: 1mcg/kg/min administered 20-40 min after intubating dose of 80-100mcg/kg. Administer infusion after evidence of recovery from bolus. Adjust infusion rate to maintain 90% suppression of twitch response. Maint: 0.8-1.2mcg/kg/min. Concurrent Steady-State Enflurane/Isoflurane: Reduce rate 25-60%, 45-60 min after intubating dose. 1-10 yrs: May require a slightly higher initial dose and may also require supplementation slightly more often than adults.

HOW SUPPLIED: Inj: 10mg, 20mg

WARNINGS/PRECAUTIONS: May have profound effect in myasthenia gravis or myasthenic (Eaton Lambert) syndrome; use small test dose and monitor closely. Prolongation of neuromuscular blockade may occur in anephric patients; consider lower initial dose. Conditions associated with slower circulation time in cardiovascular disease, old age, and edematous states may delay onset time; dosage should not be increased. Prolonged recovery time reported with cirrhosis or cholestasis. In ICU, long-term use may be associated with prolonged paralysis and/or skeletal muscle weakness. Monitor neuromuscular transmission of ICU patients continuously with a nerve stimulator. Severe obesity and neuromuscular disease may pose airway or ventilatory problems. Electrolyte imbalances may alter neuromuscular blockade.

ADVERSE REACTIONS: Skeletal muscle weakness and paralysis.

INTERACTIONS: Enhanced neuromuscular blocking action with pancuronium, d-tubocurarine, metocurine, gallamine, enflurane, isoflurane, halothane, aminoglycosides, tetracyclines, bacitracin, polymyxin B, colistin, sodium colistimethate, and magnesium salts. Possible synergistic or antagonistic effects with other muscle relaxants. Prior administration of succinylcholine may enhance neuromuscular blocking effect.

PREGNANCY: Category C, safety in nursing not known.

MECHANISM OF ACTION: Nondepolarizing neuromuscular blocking agent; acts by competing for cholinergic receptors at the motor end-plate.

PHARMACOKINETICS: Distribution: Vd=300-400mL/kg; plasma protein binding (60-80%). **Metabolism:** Liver. **Elimination:** Bile (25-50%); urine (3-35%); $T_{1/2}$=65-75 mins.

VENTOLIN HFA   RX
albuterol sulfate (GlaxoSmithKline)

THERAPEUTIC CLASS: Beta$_2$ -agonist

INDICATIONS: Prevention and treatment of bronchospasm with reversible obstructive airway disease. Prevention of Exercise-Induced Bronchospasm (EIB).

DOSAGE: *Adults:* Bronchospasm: 2 inh q4-6h or 1 inh q4h. EIB: 2 inh 15-30 min before activity.
Pediatrics: ≥4 yrs: Bronchospasm: 2 inh q4-6h or 1 inh q4h. EIB: 2 inh 15-30 min before activity.

HOW SUPPLIED: MDI: 90mcg/inh (18g)

WARNINGS/PRECAUTIONS: D/C if paradoxical bronchospasm or cardiovascular events occur. Avoid excessive use. Caution with coronary insufficiency, arrhythmias, HTN, DM, hyperthyroidism, seizures, sensitivity to sympathomimetics. Hypersensitivity reactions may occur. May cause transient hypokalemia.

ADVERSE REACTIONS: Throat irritation, viral respiratory infections, upper respiratory inflammation, cough, musculoskeletal pain.

INTERACTIONS: Avoid other short-acting sympathomimetic bronchodilators; caution with oral sympathomimetics. Extreme caution with MAOIs, TCAs during or within 2 weeks of discontinuation. May cause severe bronchospasm with β-blockers. Decreases digoxin levels. ECG changes and/or hypokalemia with nonpotassium-sparing diuretics.

PREGNANCY: Category C, not for use in nursing.

MECHANISM OF ACTION: β$_2$-adrenergic bronchodilator; stimulates adenyl cylase, the enzyme that catalyzes formation of cAMP from ATP. Increased cAMP levels associated with relaxation of bronchial smooth muscle and inhibition of release of mediators of immediate hypersensitivity.

PHARMACOKINETICS: Absorption: C_{max}=3ng/mL, T_{max}=0.42 hrs.

VERAMYST   RX
fluticasone furoate (GlaxoSmithKline)

THERAPEUTIC CLASS: Corticosteroid

INDICATIONS: Treatment of the symptoms of seasonal and perennial allergic rhinitis in patients ≥2 yrs.

DOSAGE: *Adults:* Initial: 2 sprays per nostril qd. Maint: 1 spray per nostril qd.
Pediatrics: ≥12 yrs: Initial: 2 sprays per nostril qd. Maint: 1 spray per nostril qd. 2-11 yrs: Initial: 1 spray per nostril qd. Titrate: If inadequate response, may increase to 2 sprays per nostril.

HOW SUPPLIED: Spray: 27.5mcg/spray (10g)

WARNINGS/PRECAUTIONS: Excessive use may cause hypercorticism and adrenal suppression. Risk of adrenal insufficiency and withdrawal symptoms when replacing systemic corticosteroids with topical corticosteroids. Caution with active or quiescent TB, ocular herpes simplex, or untreated bacterial, fungal, and systemic viral infections. Risk for more severe/fatal course of infections (eg, chickenpox, measles); avoid exposure in patients who have not had disease or have not been properly immunized. Epistaxis and nasal ulcerations may occur. Candida infection of nose reported. Avoid with recent nasal trauma, ulcers, or surgery. May result in glaucoma and cataracts. Potential for growth velocity reduction in pediatrics.

ADVERSE REACTIONS: Headache, epistaxis, nasopharyngitis, pyrexia, pharyngolaryngeal pain, cough, nasal ulceration, back pain.

INTERACTIONS: Ketoconazole or other potent CYP3A4 inhibitors may increase serum fluticasone levels; co-administer with caution. Increased levels with ritonavir; avoid use.

PREGNANCY: Category C, caution in nursing.

MECHANISM OF ACTION: Corticosteroid; unknown. Anti-inflammatory agent with wide range of effects on multiple cell types (eg, mast cells, eosinophils, neutrophils, macrophages, lymphocytes) and mediators (eg, histamine, eicosanoids, cytokines, leukotrienes) involved in inflammation.

PHARMACOKINETICS: Absorption: Incomplete absorption, absolute bioavailability (0.5%). **Distribution:** Plasma protein binding (99%). **Metabolism:** Hepatic (extensive) via CYP3A4. **Elimination:** Feces.

VERDESO
desonide (Stiefel)

RX

THERAPEUTIC CLASS: Corticosteroid

INDICATIONS: Mild to moderate atopic dermatitis.

DOSAGE: *Adults:* Apply thin layer to affected area(s) bid. Max Duration: 4 consecutive weeks. Not to dispense directly on face; use hands to gently massage. Avoid occlusive dressings.
Pediatrics: ≥3 months: Apply thin layer to affected area(s) bid. Max Duration: 4 consecutive weeks. Not to dispense directly on face; use hands to gently massage. Avoid occlusive dressings.

HOW SUPPLIED: Foam: 0.05% (50g, 100g)

WARNINGS/PRECAUTIONS: May produce reversible HPA axis suppression, manifestations of Cushing's syndrome, hyperglycemia, and glucosuria. D/C if irritation occurs. Caution when applied to large surface areas. Pediatrics may be more susceptible to systemic toxicity. Use appropriate antifungal or antibacterial with concomitant skin infections; d/c if infection does not clear.

ADVERSE REACTIONS: Application site burning, upper respiratory tract infection, cough.

PREGNANCY: Category C, caution in nursing.

MECHANISM OF ACTION: Corticosteroid; possesses anti-inflammatory, antipruritic, and vasoconstrictive properties. Anti-inflammatory activity not established. Suspected to act by induction of phospholipase A_2 inhibitory proteins, lipocortins. Lipocortins control biosynthesis of potent mediators of inflammation (eg, prostaglandins, leukotrienes) by inhibiting release of their common precursor, arachidonic acid.

PHARMACOKINETICS: Absorption: Percutaneous; occlusion, inflammation, and other disease states may increase absorption. **Distribution:** Systemically administered corticosteroids found in breast milk. **Metabolism:** Liver. **Elimination:** Kidneys (major), bile.

VESANOID
tretinoin (Roche Labs)

RX

> Administer under strict supervision of experienced physician and institution. Risk of retinoic acid-APL syndrome and leukocytosis. High risk of teratogenic effects.

THERAPEUTIC CLASS: Retinoid

INDICATIONS: Induction of remission in acute promyelocytic leukemia (APL) in those resistant to anthracycline therapy or those where anthracycline-based therapy is contraindicated.

DOSAGE: *Adults:* 45mg/m^2/day in 2 divided doses. D/C 30 days after achieving complete remission or after 90 days of therapy, whichever occurs 1st.
Pediatrics: ≥1 yrs: 45mg/m^2/day in 2 divided doses. D/C 30 days after achieving complete remission or after 90 days of therapy, whichever occurs 1st.

HOW SUPPLIED: Cap: 10mg

CONTRAINDICATIONS: Sensitivity to parabens.

WARNINGS/PRECAUTIONS: May cause abortion or fetal abnormalities. Females should use contraception during and 1 month after therapy. Confirm APL diagnosis. Pseudotumor cerebri reported, especially in pediatrics. Reversible hypercholesterolemia, hypertriglyceridemia reported. Elevated LFTs reported; d/c if >5x ULN. Monitor for signs of respiratory compromise or leukocytosis. Check hematologic profile, coagulation profile, LFTs, and cholesterol frequently.

ADVERSE REACTIONS: Malaise, shivering, hemorrhage, infections, peripheral edema, pain, chest discomfort, edema, disseminated intravascular coagulation, weight change, injection site reactions, dyspnea, pleural effusion, respiratory insufficiency, pneumonia.

INTERACTIONS: Possible interactions with drugs that affect CYP450 system. Aggravated symptoms of hypervitaminosis A with vitamin A. Cases of fatal thrombotic complications with antifibrinolytic agents (eg, tranexamic acid, aminocaproic acid). Increased risk of pseudotumor cerebri/intracranial HTN with tetracyclines.

PREGNANCY: Category D, not for use in nursing.

MECHANISM OF ACTION: Retinoid; not known. Induces cytodifferentiation and decreases proliferation of APL cells.

PHARMACOKINETICS: Absorption: C_{max}=394ng/mL, T_{max}=1-2 hrs; AUC=537ng•h/mL. **Distribution:** Plasma protein binding (>95%). **Metabolism:** Oxidation via CYP450. **Elimination:** $T_{1/2}$=0.5-2 hrs.

VIBRAMYCIN   RX
doxycycline hyclate (Pfizer)

OTHER BRAND NAME: Vibra-Tabs (Pfizer)

THERAPEUTIC CLASS: Tetracycline derivative

INDICATIONS: Treatment of the following infections caused by susceptible microorganisms: Rocky Mountain spotted fever; typhus fever and the typhus group; Q fever; rickettsialpox; tick fevers; respiratory tract infections; lymphogranuloma venereum; psittacosis (ornithosis); trachoma; inclusion conjunctivitis; uncomplicated urethral, endocervical, or rectal infections; nongonococcal urethritis; relapsing fever; chancroid; plague; tularemia; cholera; *Camphylobacter fetus* infections; brucellosis; bartonellosis; granuloma inguinale; respiratory tract and urinary tract infections; anthrax. Treatment of infections caused by *Escherichia coli, Enterobacter aerogenes, Shigella* species, *Acinetobacter* species. When penicillin is contraindicated, treatment of the following infections caused by susceptible microorganisms: uncomplicated gonorrhea, syphilis, yaws, listeriosis, Vincent's infection, actinomycosis, infections caused by *Clostridium* species. Adjunct in acute intestinal amebiasis and severe acne. Prophylaxis of malaria.

DOSAGE: *Adults:* Usual: 100mg q12h on Day 1, then 100mg qd or 50mg q12h. Severe Infection: 100mg q12h. Treat for 10 days with strep infection. Uncomplicated Gonococcal Infection (Except Anorectal in Men): 100mg bid for 7 days or 300mg followed by 300mg in 1 hr. Uncomplicated Urethral/Endocervical/Rectal Infection and Nongonococcal Urethritis: 100mg bid for 7 days. Syphilis: 100mg bid for 2 weeks. Syphilis for >1 yr: 100mg bid for 4 weeks. Acute Epididymo-orchitis: 100mg bid for at least 10 days. Inhalation Anthrax (Post-Exposure): 100mg bid for 60 days. Malaria Prophylaxis: 100mg qd. Begin 1-2 days before travel and continue for 4 weeks after leaving malarious area.
Pediatrics: >8 yrs: ≤100 lbs: 1mg/lb bid on Day 1, then 1mg/lb qd or 0.5mg/lb bid. Severe Infections: Maint: 2mg/lb. >100 lbs: Usual: 100mg q12h on Day 1, then 100mg qd or 50mg q12h. Severe Infection: 100mg q12h. Treat for 10 days with strep infection. Inhalation Anthrax (Post-Exposure): <100 lbs: 1mg/lb bid for 60 days. ≥100 lbs: 100mg bid for 60 days. Malaria Prophylaxis: >8 yrs: 2mg/kg qd. Max: 100mg/day. Begin 1-2 days before travel and continue for 4 weeks after leaving malarious area.

HOW SUPPLIED: Cap: (Doxycycline Hyclate) 50mg, 100mg; Syrup: (Doxycycline Calcium) 50mg/5mL; Sus: (Doxycycline Monohydrate) 25mg/5mL (60mL); Tab: (Vibra-Tabs) 100mg

WARNINGS/PRECAUTIONS: May cause fetal harm with pregnancy. Permanent tooth discoloration during tooth development (last half of pregnancy, infancy, and children <8 yrs) reported. *Clostridium difficile*-associated diarrhea reported. May increase BUN. Photosensitivity, enamel hypoplasia reported. Superinfection with prolonged use. Syrup contains sodium metabisulfite. Bulging fontanels in infants and benign intracranial HTN in adults reported. Monitor renal/hepatic and hematopoietic function with long-term use. Take adequate fluids with caps or tabs to reduce esophageal irritation. Take with food or milk if GI irritation occurs.

ADVERSE REACTIONS: GI effects (eg, anorexia, nausea, vomiting, diarrhea), photosensitivity, increased BUN, hypersensitivity reactions, hemolytic anemia, thrombocytopenia, neutropenia, eosinophilia.

INTERACTIONS: May decrease PT, adjust anticoagulants. May interfere with bactericidal agents (eg, penicillin). May decrease effects of oral contraceptives. Aluminum-, calcium-, iron-, and magnesium-containing products and bismuth subsalicylate impair absorption. Decreased half-life with barbiturates, carbamazepine, and phenytoin. Fatal renal toxicity with methoxyflurane.

PREGNANCY: Category D, not for use in nursing.

MECHANISM OF ACTION: Tetracycline derivative; thought to inhibit protein synthesis.

PHARMACOKINETICS: Absorption: (PO) completely absorbed, C_{max}=2.6 mcg/mL, T_{max}=2 hrs. **Distribution:** Crosses placenta. **Elimination:** Urine, feces.

VICOPROFEN

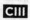

hydrocodone bitartrate - ibuprofen (Abbott)

OTHER BRAND NAME: Reprexain (Centrix)

THERAPEUTIC CLASS: Opioid analgesic

INDICATIONS: Short-term (generally <10 days) management of acute pain.

DOSAGE: *Adults:* Usual: 1 tab q4-6h prn. Max: 5 tabs/day. Elderly: Use lowest dose or longest interval.
Pediatrics: ≥16 yrs: Usual: 1 tab q4-6h prn. Max: 5 tabs/day.

HOW SUPPLIED: (Hydrocodone-Ibuprofen) Tab: (Vicoprofen) 7.5mg-200mg; (Reprexain) 5mg-200mg, 7.5mg-200mg *scored

CONTRAINDICATIONS: ASA or other NSAID allergy that precipitates asthma, urticaria, or other allergic reaction.

WARNINGS/PRECAUTIONS: May produce dose-related respiratory depression. May obscure acute abdominal conditions or head injuries. Avoid with ASA triad, late pregnancy, advanced renal disease, ASA-sensitive asthma. Caution in elderly, debilitated, dehydration, renal disease, intrinsic coagulation defects, severe hepatic dysfunction, asthma, hypothyroidism, Addison's disease, prostatic hypertrophy, urethral stricture, heart failure, HTN, ulcer disease, pulmonary disease, postoperative use. May be habit-forming. Suppresses cough reflex. Risk of GI ulceration, bleeding, perforation. Anemia, fluid retention, edema, severe hepatic reactions reported. Possible risk of aseptic meningitis, especially in SLE patients. Increased risk of serious cardiovascular thrombotic events, MI and stroke. Fluid retention and edema observed. Skin reactions (eg, exfoliative dermatitis, TEN, SJS) can occur.

ADVERSE REACTIONS: Headache, somnolence, dizziness, constipation, dyspepsia, NV, infection, edema, nervousness, anxiety, pruritus, diarrhea, asthenia, abdominal pain, insomnia, dry mouth, sweating.

INTERACTIONS: Additive CNS depression with other narcotics, antihistamines, antipsychotics, antianxiety agents, alcohol, CNS depressants. Increased effect of antidepressant or hydrocodone with MAOIs or TCAs. May produce paralytic ileus with anticholinergics. May decrease effects of furosemide and thiazide diuretics, ACE-inhibitors. Avoid ASA. Risk of serious GI bleeding with warfarin. May enhance methotrexate toxicity. Monitor for lithium toxicity.

PREGNANCY: Category C, not for use in nursing.

MECHANISM OF ACTION: Hydrocodone: Opioid analgesic and antitussive. Not known; suspected to be related to existence of opiate receptors in CNS. Produces actions similiar to codeine; most occur in CNS and smooth muscle. Ibuprofen: Non-steroidal anti-inflammatory agent. Not established; suspected to inhibit cyclooxygenase activity and prostaglandin synthesis. Peripherally acting analgesic; has no known effects on opiate receptors. Possesses antipyretic activity.

PHARMACOKINETICS: Absorption: Hydrocodone: C_{max}=27ng/mL; T_{max}=1.7 hrs. Ibuprofen: C_{max}=30mcg/mL; T_{max}=1.8 hrs. **Distribution:** Ibuprofen: Plasma protein binding (99%). **Metabolism:** Hydrocodone: CYP2D6, via O-demethylation to hydromorphone (active metabolite); CYP3A4 via N-demethylation; 6-keto reduction. Ibuprofen: Inter-conversion from R-isomer to S-isomer; (+)-2-4'-(2-hydroxy-2-methyl-propyl) phenyl propi-onic acid and (+)-2-4-(2-carboxypropyl) phenyl propionic acid (primary metabolites). **Elimination:** Hydrocodone: Urine (primary); $T_{1/2}$=4.5 hrs. Ibuprofen: Urine (50-60% metab-olites, 15% unchanged, conjugate), $T_{1/2}$=2.2 hrs.

VIDEX RX
didanosine (Bristol-Myers Squibb)

> **Fatal/nonfatal pancreatitis, lactic acidosis, and severe hepatomegaly with steatosis reported. Suspend therapy if suspect pancreatitis and discontinue if pancreatitis confirmed. Fatal lactic acidosis reported in pregnant women receiving concomitant stavudine.**

OTHER BRAND NAME: Videx EC (Bristol-Myers Squibb)

THERAPEUTIC CLASS: Nucleoside analogue

INDICATIONS: Treatment of HIV-1 infection in combination with other antiretrovirals (use Videx EC when management requires once daily dosing or alternative didanosine for-mulation).

DOSAGE: *Adults:* ≥60kg: (Cap) 400mg qd; (Sol) 200mg bid or 400mg qd. <60kg: (Cap) 250mg qd; (Sol) 125mg bid or 250mg qd. CrCl 30-59mL/min: ≥60kg: (Cap) 200mg qd; (Sol) 200mg qd or 100mg qd. <60kg: (Cap) 125mg qd; (Sol) 150mg qd or 75mg bid. CrCl 10-29mL/min: ≥60kg: (Cap) 125mg qd; (Sol) 150mg qd. <60kg: (Cap) 125mg qd; (Sol) 100mg qd. CrCl <10mL/min: ≥60kg: (Cap) 125mg qd; (Sol) 100mg qd. <60kg: (Sol) 75mg qd. Concomitant Viread: CrCl ≥60mL/min :≥60kg: 250mg qd; <60kg: 200mg qd. Take on empty stomach at least 30 min before or 2 hrs after meals. Swallow caps whole.
Pediatrics: 2 weeks-8 months: (Sol) 100mg/m² bid. >8 months: 120mg/m² bid.

HOW SUPPLIED: Sol: 2g, 4g (120mL, 240mL); Cap, Delayed-Release: (Videx EC) 125mg, 200mg, 250mg, 400mg

WARNINGS/PRECAUTIONS: Risk of toxicity with CrCl <60mL/min; reduce dose. Retinal changes and optic neuritis reported; perform periodic retinal exams. Peripheral neu-ropathy reported. Caution with hepatic dysfunction. May cause asymptomatic hyperu-ricemia. Twice daily dosing is preferred over once daily dosing. Chewable tabs contain phenylalanine. Caution with sodium restricted diets; buffered powder solution contains 1380mg sodium. Monitor for lactic acidosis in pregnancy if used with stavudine. Possible redistribution or accumulation of fat. Immune reconstitution syndrome has been reported in patients treated with combination antiretroviral therapy. Fatal and non-fatal pancreatitis reported; increased risk in combination with stavudine, with or without hydroxyurea.

ADVERSE REACTIONS: Pancreatitis, lactic acidosis, hepatomegaly, visual changes, diar-rhea, neuropathy, abdominal pain, headache, NV, rash, elevated LFTs.

INTERACTIONS: Extreme caution with drugs that may cause pancreatitis. Increase risk of peripheral neuropathy with neurotoxic agents (eg, stavudine). Aluminum- and magnesium-containing antacids may potentiate adverse events. Space dose by 2 hrs of drugs whose absorption can be affected by stomach acidity (eg, ketoconazole, itraconazole). Increased serum levels with oral ganciclovir. Space dose by 2 hrs after or 6 hrs before ciprofloxacin. Avoid allopurinol. Decreased serum levels with methadone. Caution with tenofovir or ribavirin; monitor closely for didanosine-related toxicities and suspend therapy if signs of pancreatitis, symptomatic hyperlactatemia, or lactic acido-sis develop.

PREGNANCY: Category B, not for use in nursing.

MECHANISM OF ACTION: Antiviral agent; inhibits activity of HIV-1 reverse transcriptase both by competing with natural substrate deoxyadenosine 5-triphosphate and by incorporation into viral DNA, causing termination of viral DNA chain elongation.

PHARMACOKINETICS: Absorption: Rapid. T_{max}=0.25-1.5 hrs. **Distribution:** V_d=1.08+/-0.22L/kg, <5% protein bound. **Elimination:** $T_{1/2}$=1.5+/-0.4 hrs. Refer to PI for pediatric guide-lines.

VIGAMOX
moxifloxacin HCl (Alcon)

RX

THERAPEUTIC CLASS: Fluoroquinolone

INDICATIONS: Treatment of bacterial conjunctivitis.

DOSAGE: *Adults:* 1 drop tid for 7 days.
Pediatrics: ≥1 yr: 1 drop tid for 7 days.

HOW SUPPLIED: Sol: 0.5% (3mL)

WARNINGS/PRECAUTIONS: Not for injection. Do not inject subconjunctivally or into the anterior chamber of the eye. Superinfection may result with prolonged use. Fatal hypersensitivity reactions reported after first dose of systemic quinolone therapy. Avoid contact lenses when symptoms are present.

ADVERSE REACTIONS: Conjunctivitis, decreased visual acuity, dry eye, keratitis, ocular discomfort/hyperemia, ocular pain/pruritus, subconjunctival hemorrhage, tearing.

PREGNANCY: Category C, caution in nursing.

MECHANISM OF ACTION: Fluoroquinolone antibiotic; inhibits topoisomerase II (DNA gyrase) and topoisomerase IV. DNA gyrase is essential enzyme involved in replication, transcription, and repair of bacterial DNA. Topoisomerase IV is enzyme known to play key role in partitioning of chromosomal DNA during bacterial cell division.

PHARMACOKINETICS: Absorption: C_{max}=2.7ng/mL; AUC=45ng•hr/mL. **Distribution:** Presumed to be excreted in breast milk.

VINBLASTINE
vinblastine sulfate (Various)

RX

> For IV use only; fatal if given intrathecally. Considerable irritation if leakage occurs into surrounding tissue. If this occurs, d/c and restart in another vein. Heat and hyaluronidase minimize discomfort and cellulitis.

THERAPEUTIC CLASS: Vinca alkaloid

INDICATIONS: Palliative treatment of generalized Hodgkin's disease (Stages III and IV), lymphocytic lymphoma, histiocytic lymphoma, advanced mycosis fungoides, advanced testis carcinoma, Kaposi's sarcoma, Letterer-Siwe disease, and resistant choriocarcinoma and unresponsive breast carcinoma.

DOSAGE: *Adults:* Dose at intervals of ≤7 days. 1st Dose: $3.7mg/m^2$. 2nd Dose: $5.5mg/m^2$. 3rd Dose: $7.4mg/m^2$. 4th Dose: $9.25mg/m^2$. 5th Dose: $11.1mg/m^2$. Max: $18.5mg/m^2$. Do not increase dose after that dose which reduces WBC to 3000 cells/mm^3. Maint: Use dose of 1 increment smaller than this dose at weekly intervals. Reduce to 50% dose if direct serum bilirubin >3mg/100mL. Only dose if WBC ≥4000 cells/mm^3.
Pediatrics: Letterer-Swine Disease as Single Agent: Initial: $6.5mg/m^2$. Hodgkin's Disease in Combination Therapy: Initial: $6mg/m^2$. Testicular Germ Cell Carcinoma in Combination Therapy: Initial: $3mg/m^2$.

HOW SUPPLIED: Inj: 1mg/mL (10mL)

CONTRAINDICATIONS: Significant granulocytopenia (unless result of disease being treated), bacterial infections.

WARNINGS/PRECAUTIONS: Avoid pregnancy. Acute shortness of breath, severe bronchospasm, aspermia, stomatitis, neurologic toxicity reported. Increased toxicity with hepatic insufficiency. Monitor for infection with WBC <2000 cells/mm^3. Avoid with malignant-cell infiltration of bone marrow, or in older persons with cachexia or ulcerated skin. Small daily amounts for long periods is not advised. Avoid eye contamination. Monitor WBCs. May cause fetal harm during pregnancy. Caution with ischemic cardiac disease.

ADVERSE REACTIONS: Leukopenia (granulocytopenia), anemia, thrombocytopenia, alopecia, constipation, anorexia, nausea, vomiting, abdominal pain, diarrhea, HTN, paresthesis.

INTERACTIONS: May increase phenytoin metabolism/elimination, or decrease phenytoin absorption. Caution with CYP3A inhibitors (eg, erythromycin, doxorubicin, etoposide), or with hepatic dysfunction; may cause earlier onset and/or an increased severity of side effects. Increased risk of acute shortness of breath and severe bronchospasm with mitomycin-C.

PREGNANCY: Category D, not for use in nursing.

MECHANISM OF ACTION: Vinca alkaloid; inhibits microtubule formation in mitotic spindle, resulting in cell division arrest.

PHARMACOKINETICS: Metabolism: CYP3A. **Elimination:** $T_{1/2}$=24.8 hrs.

VINCRISTINE RX
vincristine sulfate (Various)

> Properly position IV needle or catheter before injection; considerable irritation with extravasation. Use hyaluronidase and heat to minimize discomfort and cellulitis with extravasation. Fatal with intrathecal use. For IV use only.

THERAPEUTIC CLASS: Vinca alkaloid

INDICATIONS: For treatment of acute leukemia. As an adjunct in the treatment of Hodgkin's disease, non-Hodgkin's malignant lymphomas, rhabdomyosarcoma, neuroblastoma, and Wilms' tumor.

DOSAGE: *Adults;* Usual: 1.4mg/m^2 IV at weekly intervals. Bilirubin >3mg/dL: 50% dose reduction. If given together with L-asparaginase, give 12-24 hrs before the enzyme. *Pediatrics;* Usual: 2mg/m2 IV at weekly intervals. ≤10kg: Initial: 0.05mg/kg IV once weekly. Bilirubin >3mg/dL: 50% dose reduction. If given together with L-asparaginase, give 12-24 hrs before the enzyme.

HOW SUPPLIED: Inj: 1mg/mL

CONTRAINDICATIONS: Demyelinating form of Charcot-Marie-Tooth syndrome.

WARNINGS/PRECAUTIONS: Acute uric acid nephropathy may occur. May require additional agents with CNS leukemia. Neurotoxicity is dose-limiting toxicity. Perform CBC before each dose. Determine serum uric acid levels frequently during 1st 3-4 weeks. Acute shortness of breath, severe bronchospasm reported. Monitor with pre-existing neuromuscular disease. Avoid eye contamination. May cause fetal harm during pregnancy.

ADVERSE REACTIONS: Alopecia, abdominal cramps, weight loss, nausea, vomiting, diarrhea, constipation, paralytic ileus, HTN, hypotension, polyuria, dysuria, urinary retention, sensory impairment, paresthesia, neuritic pain, motor difficulties, rash, fever.

INTERACTIONS: Reduced levels of phenytoin and increased seizures reported. Increased risk of acute shortness of breath and severe bronchospasm with mitomycin-C. Monitor with other neurotoxic agents. Discontinue drugs known to cause urinary retention for 1st few days after administration. Give 12-24 hrs before L-asparaginase therapy to minimize toxicity. Do not give with radiation therapy through ports that include the liver. Do not dilute in solutions that raise or lower the pH outside the range of 3.5-5.5.

PREGNANCY: Category D, not for use in nursing.

MECHANISM OF ACTION: Antineoplastic agent; inhibits microtubule formation in mitotic spindle, resulting in arrest of dividing cells at metaphase stage.

PHARMACOKINETICS: Distribution: Crosses blood-brain barrier. **Metabolism:** Liver, via CYP450 isoenzyme 3A **Elimination:** Feces (80%), urine (10-20%); $T_{1/2}$=85 hrs.

VIOKASE RX
amylase - lipase - protease (Axcan Scandipharm)

THERAPEUTIC CLASS: Pancreatic enzyme supplement

INDICATIONS: Treatment of pancreatic exocrine insufficiency (eg, cystic fibrosis, chronic pancreatitis, pancreatectomy, and pancreatic ductal obstruction).

DOSAGE: *Adults;* (Powder) Cystic Fibrosis: 0.7g (1/4 tsp) with meals. (Tab) Cystic Fibrosis/Pancreatitis: 8,000-32,000 U Lipase with meals. Pancreatectomy/Pancreatic Duct Obstruction: 8,000-16,000 U Lipase q2h.

Pediatrics: (Powder) Cystic Fibrosis: 0.7g (1/4 tsp) with meals. (Tab) Cystic Fibrosis/Pancreatitis: 8,000-32,000 U Lipase with meals. Pancreatectomy/Pancreatic Duct Obstruction: 8,000-16,000 U Lipase q2h.

HOW SUPPLIED: (Amylase-Lipase-Protease) Powder: 70,000 U-16,800 U-70,000 U/0.7g (240g); Tab: (Viokase 8) 30,000 U-8,000 U-30,000 U; (Viokase 16) 60,000 U-16,000 U-60,000 U

CONTRAINDICATIONS: Pork protein hypersensitivity.

WARNINGS/PRECAUTIONS: May have allergic reactions if previously sensitized to trypsin, pancreatin or pancrelipase. Irritating to oral mucosa if held in mouth. Inhalation of powder can cause an asthma attack. High doses can cause hyperuricemia and hyperuricosuria.

ADVERSE REACTIONS: Irritation to nasal mucosa and respiratory tract with inhaled powder.

PREGNANCY: Category C, caution in nursing.

MECHANISM OF ACTION: Panrealipase; pancreatic enzyme concentrate of porcine origin. Natural digestive enzyme; acts to hydrolyze fats into fatty acid and glycerol, split protein into amino acids, and convert carbohydrates to dextrins and short chain sugars.

VIRACEPT   RX
nelfinavir mesylate (Pfizer)

THERAPEUTIC CLASS: Protease inhibitor

INDICATIONS: Treatment of HIV infection in combination with other antiretrovirals.

DOSAGE: *Adults:* 1250mg bid or 750mg tid. Concomitant rifabutin: Reduce rifabutin dose by one-half and nelfinavir 1250mg bid is preferred dose. Take with a meal or light snack. May crush or dissolve whole tab in water or mix in food and consume immediately. May store mixture under refrigeration up to 6 hrs.
Pediatrics: 2-13 yrs: 20-30mg/kg tid. Take with a meal or light snack. May mix powder with non-acidic liquid (eg, water, milk, formula, etc.); consume immediately. May store up to 6 hrs under refrigeration.

HOW SUPPLIED: Sus: (powder) 50mg/g (144g); Tab: 250mg, 625mg

CONTRAINDICATIONS: Concomitant pimozide, triazolam, midazolam, ergot derivatives, amiodarone or quinidine.

WARNINGS/PRECAUTIONS: Powder contains phenylalanine. New-onset DM, exacerbation of DM and hyperglycemia reported. Register pregnant patients (800-258-4263). Caution with hepatic dysfunction. Increased bleeding reported. Possible redistribution or accumulation of fat.

ADVERSE REACTIONS: Diarrhea, nausea, flatulence, rash, redistribution of body fat, jaundice, hypersensitivity reactions, bilirubinemia, hyperglycemia, metabolic acidosis.

INTERACTIONS: See Contraindications. Avoid pimozide, triazolam, midazolam, ergot derivatives, amiodarone or quinidine; potential for life-threatening adverse events. Avoid rifampin. Avoid lovastatin or simvastatin; caution with other HMG-CoA reductase inhibitors. May increase sildenafil or other PDE5 inhibitor levels and adverse effects. Avoid St. John's wort; may decrease levels of nelfinavir. May increase levels of drugs metabolized by CYP450 3A (eg, dihydropyridine CCBs, immunosuppressants, etc). Use alternative or additional contraception with oral contraceptives. May increase levels of cyclosporine, tacrolimus, sirolimus, atorvastatin, cerivastatin, fluticasone, azithromycin. Carbamazepine, phenobarbital may decrease levels of nelfinavir. May decrease levels of phenytoin, methadone. Give didanosine 1 hr before or 2 hrs after nelfinavir. Omeprazole decreases levels of nelfinavir; concomitant use with proton pump inhibitors may lead to loss of virologic response and development of resistance.

PREGNANCY: Category B, not for use in nursing.

MECHANISM OF ACTION: HIV-1 protease inhibitor; prevents cleavage of *gag* and *gag-pol* polyprotein resulting in production of immature, non-infectious virus.

PHARMACOKINETICS: Absorption: (1250mg bid) C_{max}=4mg/L; AUC=52.8mg•h/L. (750mg tid) C_{max}=3mg/L; AUC=43.6mg•h/L. **Distribution:** V_d=2-7L/kg; plasma protein binding (>98%). **Metabolism:** CYP3A, 2C19 (oxidation). **Elimination:** Feces (22%), urine (1-2%); $T_{1/2}$=3.5-5 hrs.

VIRAMUNE

RX

nevirapine (Boehringer Ingelheim)

> Severe, life-threatening, in some cases fatal, hepatotoxicity and skin reactions (eg, Stevens-Johnson syndrome, toxic epidermal necrolysis, hypersensitivity) reported. Women, including pregnant women, and/or patients with higher CD4 counts are at higher risk of hepatotoxicity. Permanently d/c following severe hepatitic, skin or hypersensitivity reactions. Monitoring during the first 18 weeks of therapy is essential; extra vigilance is warranted during the first 6 weeks of therapy.

THERAPEUTIC CLASS: Non-nucleoside reverse transcriptase inhibitor

INDICATIONS: Treatment of HIV-1 infection in combination with other antiretrovirals.

DOSAGE: *Adults:* 200mg qd for 14 days (lead-in period), then 200mg bid. If severe rash occurs, d/c therapy. If mild-to-moderate rash occurs during 14-day lead-in period, do not increase dose until rash resolves. If dosing interrupted for >7 days, restart 14-day lead-in dosing.
Pediatrics: ≥15 days:150mg/m² qd for 14 days, followed by 150mg/m² bid. Max: 400mg/day. If severe rash occurs, d/c therapy. If mild-to-moderate rash occurs during 14-day lead-in period, do not increase dose until rash resolves. If dosing interrupted for >7 days, restart lead-in dosing.

HOW SUPPLIED: Sus: 50mg/5mL (240mL); Tab: 200mg* *scored

CONTRAINDICATIONS: Moderate or severe (Child Pugh Class B or C) hepatic impairment.

WARNINGS/PRECAUTIONS: Avoid with severe hepatic impairment. Caution with moderate impairment and dialysis. Perform laboratory tests (eg, LFTs) at baseline and during first 18 weeks of therapy. Possible redistribution or accumulation of body fat.

ADVERSE REACTIONS: Headache, fever, severe rash, GI effects, fatigue, thrombocytopenia, fatigue, hepatotoxicity, granulocytopenia (pediatrics), rhabdomyolysis.

INTERACTIONS: Avoid use of prednisone for prevention of therapy-associated rash. Decreased levels of clarithromycin; consider alternative. Decreased levels of efavirenz, indinavir, nelfinavir, saquinavir. May decrease effectiveness of oral contraceptives and other hormonal contraceptives; use alternate or additional method of contraception. Increased levels with fluconazole. Avoid with ketoconazole, St. John's wort, rifampin. Decreased levels of lopinavir; adjust lopinavir/ritonavir doses. May decrease levels of methadone; monitor for signs of withdrawal. Increased levels of rifabutin. Possible decreased levels with antiarrhythmics (eg, amiodarone, disopyramide, lidocaine), anticonvulsants (eg, carbamazepine, clonazepam, ethosuximide), itraconazole, CCBs (eg, diltiazem, nifedipine, verapamil), cyclophosphamide, ergotamine, immunosuppressants (eg, cyclosporine, tacrolimus, sirolimus), cisapride, fentanyl. Monitor with warfarin.

PREGNANCY: Category B, not for use in nursing.

MECHANISM OF ACTION: Non-nucleoside reverse transcriptase inhibitor; binds directly to reverse transcriptase and blocks RNA-dependent DNA polymerase activities by causing disruption of the enzyme's catalytic site.

PHARMACOKINETICS: Absorption: Absolute bioavailability: 93+/- 9% (tab), 91+/-8% (sol); C_{max}=2+/-0.4 Mcg/mL; T_{max}=4 hrs. **Distribution:** V_d=1.21±0.09L/Kg; plasma protein binding (60%); readily crosses placenta; found in breast milk. **Metabolism:** Liver; oxidative metabolism, via CYP3A4 and CYP2B6 (extensively); glucoronide metabolites. **Elimination:** Urine (<3% excreted as parent drug); $T_{1/2}$=45 hrs.

VIRAZOLE

RX

ribavirin (Valeant)

> Sudden deterioration of respiratory function associated with initiation in infants. Monitor respiratory function carefully. Not for use in adults. Use with mechanical ventilator assistance with staff familiar with mode of administration and specific type of ventilator.

THERAPEUTIC CLASS: Nucleoside analogue

INDICATIONS: Treatment of hospitalized infants and young children with severe lower respiratory tract infections due to respiratory syncytial virus.

DOSAGE: *Pediatrics:* Continuous aerosol administration of 20mg/mL in the drug reservoir of the SPAG-2 unit for 12-18 hrs/day for 3-7 days.

HOW SUPPLIED: Sol, Inhalation: 6g

CONTRAINDICATIONS: Women who are or may become pregnant during exposure to drug.

WARNINGS/PRECAUTIONS: Monitor respiratory function and fluid status according to SPAG-2 manual. Accumulation of drug precipitate can result in mechanical ventilator dysfunction and associated increased pulmonary pressures.

ADVERSE REACTIONS: Worsening of respiratory status, bronchospasm, pulmonary edema, hypoventilation, cyanosis, dyspnea, bacterial pneumonia, pneumothorax, apnea, atelectasis, ventilator dependence, cardiac arrest, hypotension, bradycardia.

INTERACTIONS: Digoxin toxicity reported.

PREGNANCY: Category X, safety in nursing not known.

MECHANISM OF ACTION: Nucleoside analogue; mechanism unknown. Suspected to be analogue of guanosine or xanthosine.

PHARMACOKINETICS: Elimination: $T_{1/2}$=9.5 hrs.

VIROPTIC
trifluridine (King)

RX

THERAPEUTIC CLASS: Fluorinated pyrimidine nucleoside antiviral

INDICATIONS: Treatment of primary keratoconjunctivitis and recurrent epithelial keratitis due to herpes simplex virus, types 1 and 2.

DOSAGE: *Adults:* 1 drop q2h while awake until re-epithelialization. Max: 9 drops/day. Following Re-epithelialization: 1 drop q4h while awake for 7 days; minimum of 5 drops/day. If no improvement after 7 days or if complete re-epithelialization has not occurred after 14 days, consider other therapy. Avoid using >21 days.
Pediatrics: ≥6 yrs: 1 drop q2h while awake until re-epithelialization. Max: 9 drops/day. Following Re-epithelialization: 1 drop q4h while awake for 7 days; minimum of 5 drops/day. If no improvement after 7 days or if complete re-epithelialization has not occurred after 14 days, consider other therapy. Avoid using >21 days.

HOW SUPPLIED: Sol: 1% (7.5mL)

WARNINGS/PRECAUTIONS: Only use with a clinical diagnosis of herpetic keratitis. May cause transient, mild local irritation of the conjunctiva and cornea when instilled.

ADVERSE REACTIONS: Burning, stinging, palpebral edema, superficial punctate keratopathy, epithelial keratopathy, hypersensitivity reaction, stromal edema, irritation, keratitis sicca, hyperemia, increased IOP.

PREGNANCY: Category C, caution in nursing.

MECHANISM OF ACTION: Fluorinated pyrimidine nucleoside antiviral; unknown, suspected to interfere with DNA synthesis.

PHARMACOKINETICS: Absorption: Penetrates intact cornea. **Metabolism:** 5-carboxy-2'-deoxyuridine (major metabolite).

VISINE A.C.
tetrahydrozoline HCl - zinc sulfate (McNeil)

OTC

THERAPEUTIC CLASS: Decongestant/astringent

INDICATIONS: Temporary relief of discomfort and redness of the eyes due to minor eye irritations.

DOSAGE: *Adults:* 1-2 drops in affected eye up to qid.
Pediatrics: ≥6 yrs: 1-2 drops in affected eye up to qid.

HOW SUPPLIED: Sol: (Tetrahydrozoline-Zinc) 0.05%-0.25% (15mL, 30mL)

WARNINGS/PRECAUTIONS: May temporarily enlarge pupils. Overuse may cause more redness. Remove contact lenses before use. Do not touch container tip to any surface to avoid contamination. D/C if eye pain or vision changes occur, if redness or irritation continues, or if condition worsens or continues >72 hrs. Supervision required with glaucoma.

ADVERSE REACTIONS: Brief tingling sensation.

PREGNANCY: Safety in pregnancy and nursing not known.

VISINE ADVANCED RELIEF OTC
dextran 70 - polyethylene glycol 400 - povidone - tetrahydrozoline HCl
(McNeil)

THERAPEUTIC CLASS: Decongestant/lubricant

INDICATIONS: Relief of eye redness due to minor eye irritations. Use as a protectant against further irritation or to relieve eye dryness.

DOSAGE: *Adults:* 1-2 drops in affected eye up to qid.
Pediatrics: ≥6 yrs: 1-2 drops in affected eye up to qid.

HOW SUPPLIED: Sol: (Dextran 70-Polyethylene Glycol 400-Povidone, Tetrahydrozoline) 0.1%-1%-1%-0.05% (15mL, 30mL)

WARNINGS/PRECAUTIONS: May temporarily enlarge pupils. Overuse may cause more redness. Remove contact lenses before use. Do not touch container tip to any surface to avoid contamination. D/C if eye pain or vision changes occur, if redness or irritation continues, or if condition worsens or continues >72 hrs. Supervision required with glaucoma.

PREGNANCY: Safety in pregnancy and nursing not known.

VISINE FOR CONTACTS OTC
glycerin - hydroxypropyl methylcellulose (McNeil)

THERAPEUTIC CLASS: Lubricant

INDICATIONS: To moisten daily wear soft lenses while on the eyes during the day. To moisten extended wear soft lenses upon awakening, prior to retiring at night, and as needed during the day.

DOSAGE: *Adults:* Use prn throughout the day. Minor Irritation/Discomfort/Blurring With Lenses: Instill 1-2 drops on eye and blink 2-3 times. If discomfort continues; remove lenses.
Pediatrics: Use prn throughout the day. Minor Irritation/Discomfort/Blurring With Lenses: Instill 1-2 drops on eye and blink 2-3 times. If discomfort continues; remove lenses.

HOW SUPPLIED: Sol: (15mL, 30mL)

WARNINGS/PRECAUTIONS: Eye problems including corneal ulcers can occur; remove contacts if eye discomfort, excessive tearing, vision changes or eye redness occur. Do not touch container tip to any surface to avoid contamination.

ADVERSE REACTIONS: Eye irritation, excessive tearing, unusual eye secretions, eye redness, reduced visual acuity, blurred vision, photophobia, dry eyes.

PREGNANCY: Safety in pregnancy and nursing not known.

VISINE L.R. OTC
oxymetazoline HCl (McNeil)

THERAPEUTIC CLASS: Decongestant

INDICATIONS: Relief of eye redness due to minor eye irritations.

DOSAGE: *Adults:* 1-2 drops in affected eye q6h prn.
Pediatrics: ≥6 yrs: 1-2 drops in affected eye q6h prn.

HOW SUPPLIED: Sol: 0.025% (15mL, 30mL)

WARNINGS/PRECAUTIONS: Overuse may cause more redness. Remove contact lenses before use. Do not touch container tip to any surface to avoid contamination. D/C if eye pain or vision changes occur, if redness or irritation continues, or if condition worsens or continues >72 hrs. Supervision required with glaucoma.

PREGNANCY: Safety in pregnancy and nursing not known.

VISINE ORIGINAL
tetrahydrozoline HCl (McNeil)
OTC

THERAPEUTIC CLASS: Decongestant

INDICATIONS: Relief of eye redness due to minor eye irritations.

DOSAGE: *Adults:* 1-2 drops in affected eye up to qid.
Pediatrics: ≥6 yrs: 1-2 drops in affected eye up to qid.

HOW SUPPLIED: Sol: 0.05% (15mL, 30mL)

WARNINGS/PRECAUTIONS: May temporarily enlarge pupils. Overuse may cause more redness. Remove contact lenses before use. Do not touch container tip to any surface to avoid contamination. D/C if eye pain or vision changes occur, if redness or irritation continues, or if condition worsens or continues >72 hrs. Supervision required with glaucoma.

PREGNANCY: Safety in pregnancy and nursing not known.

VISINE PURE TEARS
glycerin - hydroxypropyl methylcellulose - polyethylene glycol 400 (McNeil)
OTC

THERAPEUTIC CLASS: Lubricant

INDICATIONS: Temporary relief of burning and irritation due to dryness of the eye and protection against further irritation.

DOSAGE: *Adults:* 1-2 drops prn.
Pediatrics: ≥6 yrs: 1-2 drops prn.

HOW SUPPLIED: Sol: (Glycerin-Hydroxypropyl Methylcellulose-Polyethylene Glycol 400) 0.2%-0.2%-1% (portables: 4^s, 28^s; single drop dispenser: 9mL)

WARNINGS/PRECAUTIONS: Remove contact lenses before use. Do not touch container tip to any surface to avoid contamination. Do not reuse, once opened; discard. D/C if eye pain, vision changes or redness/irritation worsens or lasts >72 hrs.

PREGNANCY: Safety in pregnancy and nursing not known.

VISINE TEARS
glycerin - hydroxypropyl methylcellulose - polyethylene glycol 400 (McNeil)
OTC

THERAPEUTIC CLASS: Lubricant

INDICATIONS: Temporary relief of burning and irritation due to dryness of the eye and protection against further irritation.

DOSAGE: *Adults:* 1-2 drops prn.
Pediatrics: ≥6 yrs: 1-2 drops prn.

HOW SUPPLIED: Sol: (Glycerin-Hydroxypropyl Methylcellulose-Polyethylene Glycol 400) 0.2%-0.2%-1% (15mL, 30mL)

WARNINGS/PRECAUTIONS: Remove contact lenses before use. Do not touch container tip to any surface to avoid contamination. D/C if eye pain or vision changes occur, if redness or irritation continues, or if condition worsens or continues >72 hrs.

PREGNANCY: Safety in pregnancy and nursing not known.

VISINE-A
naphazoline HCl - pheniramine maleate (McNeil)
OTC

THERAPEUTIC CLASS: Decongestant/antihistamine

INDICATIONS: Temporary relief of itchy, red eyes due to pollen, ragweed, grass, animal hair, and dander.

DOSAGE: *Adults:* 1-2 drops in affected eye up to qid.
Pediatrics: ≥6 yrs: 1-2 drops in affected eye up to qid.

HOW SUPPLIED: Sol: (Naphazoline-Pheniramine) 0.025%-0.3% (15mL)

WARNINGS/PRECAUTIONS: May temporarily enlarge pupils. Overuse may cause more redness. Remove contact lenses before use. Do not touch container tip to any surface to avoid contamination. D/C if eye pain or vision changes occur, if redness or irritation continues, or if condition worsens or continues >72 hrs. Supervision required with glaucoma, heart disease, HTN, and enlarged prostate gland.

ADVERSE REACTIONS: Brief tingling sensation.

PREGNANCY: Safety in pregnancy and nursing not known.

VITRASERT   RX
ganciclovir (Bausch & Lomb)

THERAPEUTIC CLASS: Nucleoside analogue

INDICATIONS: Treatment of cytomegalovirus (CMV) retinitis in AIDS patients.

DOSAGE: *Adults:* Each implant releases 4.5mg over 5-8 months. Remove and replace when there is evidence of progression of retinitis.
Pediatrics: ≥9 yrs: Each implant releases 4.5mg over 5-8 months. Remove and replace when there is evidence of progression of retinitis.

HOW SUPPLIED: Implant: 4.5mg

CONTRAINDICATIONS: Hypersensitivity to acyclovir, patients with contraindication for intraocular surgery (eg, external infection, severe thrombocytopenia).

WARNINGS/PRECAUTIONS: For intravitreal implantation only. Monitor for extraocular CMV disease. Implant does not treat systemic CMV. Complications from surgery include vitreous loss or hemorrhage, cataract formation, retinal detachment, uveitis, endophthalmitis, decrease in visual acuity. Immediate decrease in visual acuity will last 2-4 weeks postop. Maintain sterility of the surgical field, implant. Handle implant by suture tab to avoid damage to polymer coating. Handling and disposal of the implant should follow guidelines for antineoplastics.

ADVERSE REACTIONS: Visual acuity loss, vitreous hemorrhage, retinal detachments, cataract formation/lens opacities, macular abnormalities, IOP spikes, optic disk/nerve changes, uveitis, hyphemas.

PREGNANCY: Category C, not for use in nursing.

MECHANISM OF ACTION: Nucleoside analogue antiviral; inhibits replication of herpes viruses.

VIVACTIL   RX
protriptyline HCl (Various)

> Antidepressants increased the risk of suicidal thinking and behavior (suicidality) in short-term studies in children, adolescents, and young adults with Major Depressive Disorder (MDD) and other psychiatric disorders. Protriptyline is not approved for use in pediatric patients.

THERAPEUTIC CLASS: Tricyclic antidepressant

INDICATIONS: Treatment of symptoms of depression in those under close medical supervision.

DOSAGE: *Adults:* Usual: 15-40mg/day taken tid-qid. Titrate: May increase to 60mg/day. Max: 60mg/day. Elderly: Initial: 5mg tid. Titrate: Increase gradually if needed. Monitor cardiovascular system with doses >20mg/day.
Pediatrics: Adolescents: Initial: 5mg tid. Titrate: Increase gradually if needed.

HOW SUPPLIED: Tab: 5mg, 10mg

CONTRAINDICATIONS: Within 14 days of MAOI therapy, cisapride, acute recovery period following MI.

WARNINGS/PRECAUTIONS: Caution with history of seizures, urinary retention, increased IOP, cardiovascular disorders, hyperthyroidism, elderly. May aggravate psychotic symptoms in schizophrenia, manic symptoms in manic-depressive psychosis, and anxiety/agitation in overactive/agitated patients. D/C several days before elective surgery. Both elevation and lowering of blood sugar levels reported.

VISUAL IDENTIFICATION GUIDE*

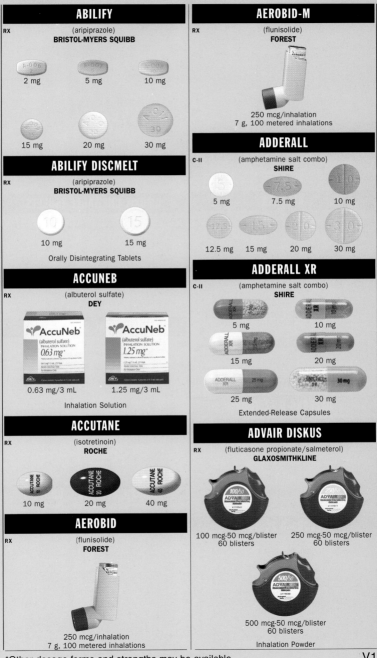

ABILIFY

RX

(aripiprazole)
BRISTOL-MYERS SQUIBB

2 mg   5 mg   10 mg

15 mg   20 mg   30 mg

ABILIFY DISCMELT

RX

(aripiprazole)
BRISTOL-MYERS SQUIBB

10 mg   15 mg

Orally Disintegrating Tablets

ACCUNEB

RX

(albuterol sulfate)
DEY

0.63 mg/3 mL   1.25 mg/3 mL

Inhalation Solution

ACCUTANE

RX

(isotretinoin)
ROCHE

10 mg   20 mg   40 mg

AEROBID

RX

(flunisolide)
FOREST

250 mcg/inhalation
7 g, 100 metered inhalations

AEROBID-M

RX

(flunisolide)
FOREST

250 mcg/inhalation
7 g, 100 metered inhalations

ADDERALL

C-II

(amphetamine salt combo)
SHIRE

5 mg   7.5 mg   10 mg

12.5 mg   15 mg   20 mg   30 mg

ADDERALL XR

C-II

(amphetamine salt combo)
SHIRE

5 mg   10 mg

15 mg   20 mg

25 mg   30 mg

Extended-Release Capsules

ADVAIR DISKUS

RX

(fluticasone propionate/salmeterol)
GLAXOSMITHKLINE

100 mcg-50 mcg/blister
60 blisters

250 mcg-50 mcg/blister
60 blisters

500 mcg-50 mcg/blister
60 blisters

Inhalation Powder

*Other dosage forms and strengths may be available

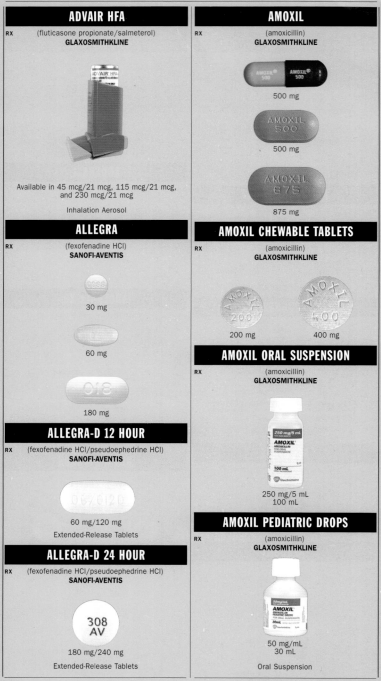

ADVAIR HFA

RX   (fluticasone propionate/salmeterol)
GLAXOSMITHKLINE

Available in 45 mcg/21 mcg, 115 mcg/21 mcg, and 230 mcg/21 mcg

Inhalation Aerosol

ALLEGRA

RX   (fexofenadine HCl)
SANOFI-AVENTIS

30 mg

60 mg

180 mg

ALLEGRA-D 12 HOUR

RX   (fexofenadine HCl/pseudoephedrine HCl)
SANOFI-AVENTIS

60 mg/120 mg

Extended-Release Tablets

ALLEGRA-D 24 HOUR

RX   (fexofenadine HCl/pseudoephedrine HCl)
SANOFI-AVENTIS

308
AV

180 mg/240 mg

Extended-Release Tablets

AMOXIL

RX   (amoxicillin)
GLAXOSMITHKLINE

500 mg

500 mg

875 mg

AMOXIL CHEWABLE TABLETS

RX   (amoxicillin)
GLAXOSMITHKLINE

200 mg   400 mg

AMOXIL ORAL SUSPENSION

RX   (amoxicillin)
GLAXOSMITHKLINE

250 mg/5 mL
100 mL

AMOXIL PEDIATRIC DROPS

RX   (amoxicillin)
GLAXOSMITHKLINE

50 mg/mL
30 mL

Oral Suspension

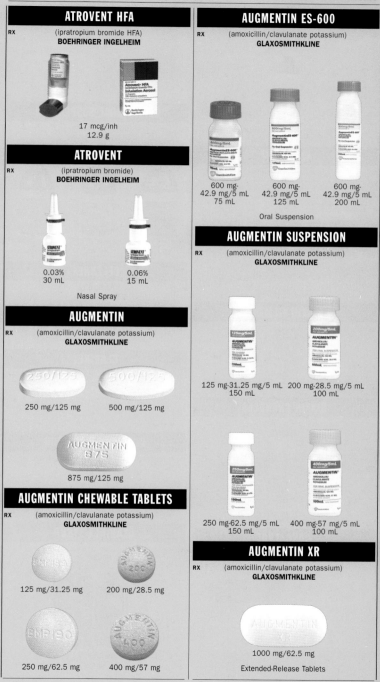

ATROVENT HFA

RX

(ipratropium bromide HFA)
BOEHRINGER INGELHEIM

17 mcg/inh
12.9 g

ATROVENT

RX

(ipratropium bromide)
BOEHRINGER INGELHEIM

0.03%
30 mL

0.06%
15 mL

Nasal Spray

AUGMENTIN

RX

(amoxicillin/clavulanate potassium)
GLAXOSMITHKLINE

250 mg/125 mg

500 mg/125 mg

875 mg/125 mg

AUGMENTIN CHEWABLE TABLETS

RX

(amoxicillin/clavulanate potassium)
GLAXOSMITHKLINE

125 mg/31.25 mg

200 mg/28.5 mg

250 mg/62.5 mg

400 mg/57 mg

AUGMENTIN ES-600

RX

(amoxicillin/clavulanate potassium)
GLAXOSMITHKLINE

600 mg-
42.9 mg/5 mL
75 mL

600 mg-
42.9 mg/5 mL
125 mL

600 mg-
42.9 mg/5 mL
200 mL

Oral Suspension

AUGMENTIN SUSPENSION

RX

(amoxicillin/clavulanate potassium)
GLAXOSMITHKLINE

125 mg-31.25 mg/5 mL
150 mL

200 mg-28.5 mg/5 mL
100 mL

250 mg-62.5 mg/5 mL
150 mL

400 mg-57 mg/5 mL
100 mL

AUGMENTIN XR

RX

(amoxicillin/clavulanate potassium)
GLAXOSMITHKLINE

1000 mg/62.5 mg

Extended-Release Tablets

V3

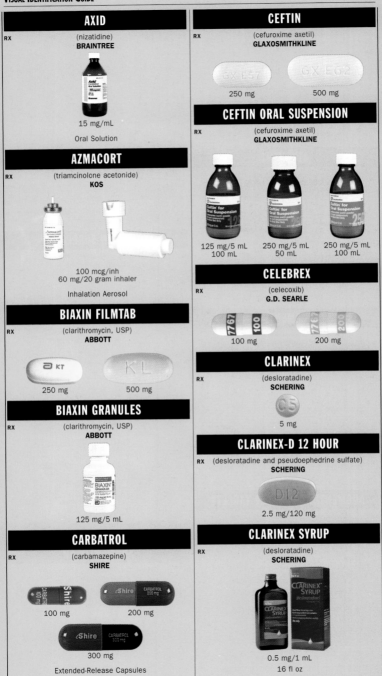

AXID

RX

(nizatidine)
BRAINTREE

15 mg/mL

Oral Solution

AZMACORT

RX

(triamcinolone acetonide)
KOS

100 mcg/inh
60 mg/20 gram inhaler

Inhalation Aerosol

BIAXIN FILMTAB

RX

(clarithromycin, USP)
ABBOTT

250 mg   500 mg

BIAXIN GRANULES

RX

(clarithromycin, USP)
ABBOTT

125 mg/5 mL

CARBATROL

RX

(carbamazepine)
SHIRE

100 mg   200 mg

300 mg

Extended-Release Capsules

CEFTIN

RX

(cefuroxime axetil)
GLAXOSMITHKLINE

250 mg   500 mg

CEFTIN ORAL SUSPENSION

RX

(cefuroxime axetil)
GLAXOSMITHKLINE

125 mg/5 mL   250 mg/5 mL   250 mg/5 mL
100 mL   50 mL   100 mL

CELEBREX

RX

(celecoxib)
G.D. SEARLE

100 mg   200 mg

CLARINEX

RX

(desloratadine)
SCHERING

5 mg

CLARINEX-D 12 HOUR

RX   (desloratadine and pseudoephedrine sulfate)
SCHERING

2.5 mg/120 mg

CLARINEX SYRUP

RX

(desloratadine)
SCHERING

0.5 mg/1 mL
16 fl oz

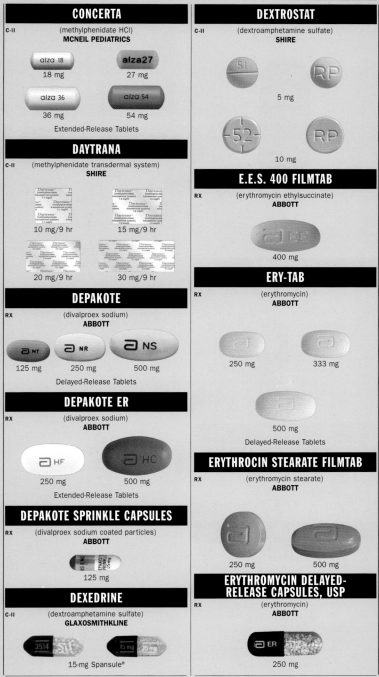

CONCERTA

C-II · (methylphenidate HCl)
MCNEIL PEDIATRICS

alza 18 — 18 mg
alza27 — 27 mg
alza 36 — 36 mg
alza 54 — 54 mg

Extended-Release Tablets

DAYTRANA

C-II · (methylphenidate transdermal system)
SHIRE

10 mg/9 hr
15 mg/9 hr
20 mg/9 hr
30 mg/9 hr

DEPAKOTE

RX · (divalproex sodium)
ABBOTT

NT — 125 mg
NR — 250 mg
NS — 500 mg

Delayed-Release Tablets

DEPAKOTE ER

RX · (divalproex sodium)
ABBOTT

HF — 250 mg
HC — 500 mg

Extended-Release Tablets

DEPAKOTE SPRINKLE CAPSULES

RX · (divalproex sodium coated particles)
ABBOTT

125 mg

DEXEDRINE

C-II · (dextroamphetamine sulfate)
GLAXOSMITHKLINE

3514 · 15 mg

15-mg Spansule®

DEXTROSTAT

C-II · (dextroamphetamine sulfate)
SHIRE

51 · RP — 5 mg
52 · RP — 10 mg

E.E.S. 400 FILMTAB

RX · (erythromycin ethylsuccinate)
ABBOTT

400 mg

ERY-TAB

RX · (erythromycin)
ABBOTT

250 mg
333 mg
500 mg

Delayed-Release Tablets

ERYTHROCIN STEARATE FILMTAB

RX · (erythromycin stearate)
ABBOTT

250 mg
500 mg

ERYTHROMYCIN DELAYED-RELEASE CAPSULES, USP

RX · (erythromycin)
ABBOTT

ER — 250 mg

V5

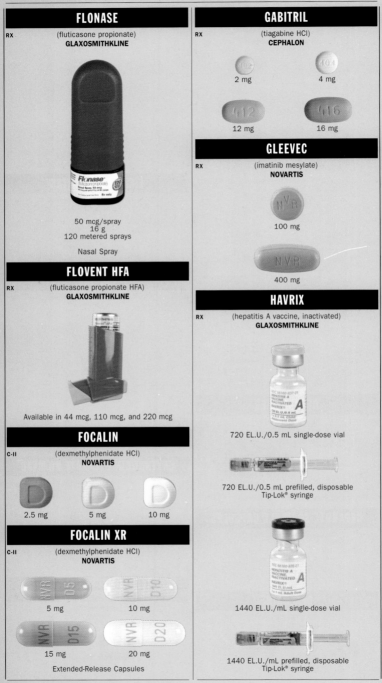

FLONASE

RX

(fluticasone propionate)
GLAXOSMITHKLINE

50 mcg/spray
16 g
120 metered sprays

Nasal Spray

FLOVENT HFA

RX

(fluticasone propionate HFA)
GLAXOSMITHKLINE

Available in 44 mcg, 110 mcg, and 220 mcg

FOCALIN

C-II

(dexmethylphenidate HCl)
NOVARTIS

2.5 mg   5 mg   10 mg

FOCALIN XR

C-II

(dexmethylphenidate HCl)
NOVARTIS

5 mg   10 mg

15 mg   20 mg

Extended-Release Capsules

GABITRIL

RX

(tiagabine HCl)
CEPHALON

2 mg   4 mg

12 mg   16 mg

GLEEVEC

RX

(imatinib mesylate)
NOVARTIS

100 mg

400 mg

HAVRIX

RX

(hepatitis A vaccine, inactivated)
GLAXOSMITHKLINE

720 EL.U./0.5 mL single-dose vial

720 EL.U./0.5 mL prefilled, disposable
Tip-Lok® syringe

1440 EL.U./mL single-dose vial

1440 EL.U./mL prefilled, disposable
Tip-Lok® syringe

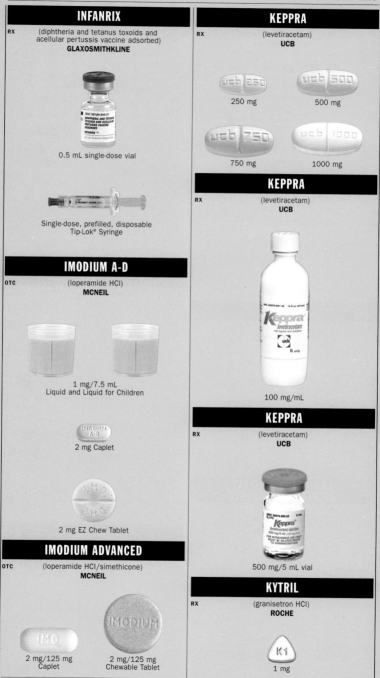

INFANRIX

RX

(diphtheria and tetanus toxoids and
acellular pertussis vaccine adsorbed)
GLAXOSMITHKLINE

0.5 mL single-dose vial

Single-dose, prefilled, disposable
Tip-Lok® Syringe

IMODIUM A-D

OTC

(loperamide HCl)
MCNEIL

1 mg/7.5 mL
Liquid and Liquid for Children

2 mg Caplet

2 mg EZ Chew Tablet

IMODIUM ADVANCED

OTC

(loperamide HCl/simethicone)
MCNEIL

2 mg/125 mg
Caplet

2 mg/125 mg
Chewable Tablet

KEPPRA

RX

(levetiracetam)
UCB

250 mg

500 mg

750 mg

1000 mg

KEPPRA

RX

(levetiracetam)
UCB

100 mg/mL

KEPPRA

RX

(levetiracetam)
UCB

500 mg/5 mL vial

KYTRIL

RX

(granisetron HCl)
ROCHE

1 mg

V7

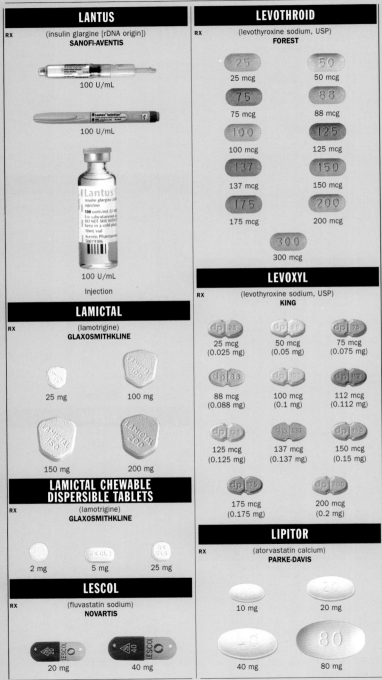

LANTUS

RX   (insulin glargine [rDNA origin])
SANOFI-AVENTIS

100 U/mL

100 U/mL

100 U/mL

Injection

LAMICTAL

RX   (lamotrigine)
GLAXOSMITHKLINE

25 mg   100 mg

150 mg   200 mg

LAMICTAL CHEWABLE DISPERSIBLE TABLETS

RX   (lamotrigine)
GLAXOSMITHKLINE

2 mg   5 mg   25 mg

LESCOL

RX   (fluvastatin sodium)
NOVARTIS

20 mg   40 mg

LEVOTHROID

RX   (levothyroxine sodium, USP)
FOREST

25 mcg   50 mcg

75 mcg   88 mcg

100 mcg   125 mcg

137 mcg   150 mcg

175 mcg   200 mcg

300 mcg

LEVOXYL

RX   (levothyroxine sodium, USP)
KING

25 mcg   50 mcg   75 mcg
(0.025 mg)   (0.05 mg)   (0.075 mg)

88 mcg   100 mcg   112 mcg
(0.088 mg)   (0.1 mg)   (0.112 mg)

125 mcg   137 mcg   150 mcg
(0.125 mg)   (0.137 mg)   (0.15 mg)

175 mcg   200 mcg
(0.175 mg)   (0.2 mg)

LIPITOR

RX   (atorvastatin calcium)
PARKE-DAVIS

10 mg   20 mg

40 mg   80 mg

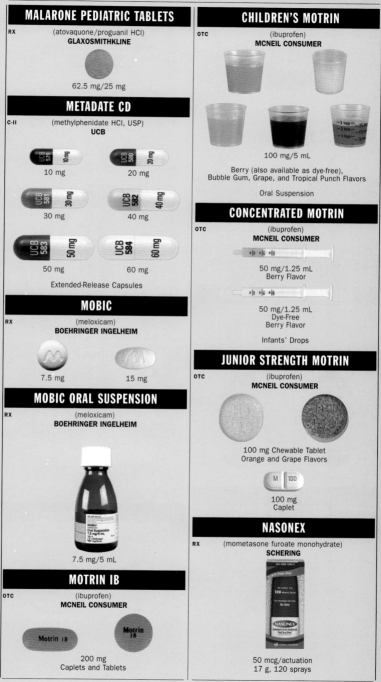

MALARONE PEDIATRIC TABLETS

RX

(atovaquone/proguanil HCl)
GLAXOSMITHKLINE

62.5 mg/25 mg

METADATE CD

C-II

(methylphenidate HCl, USP)
UCB

10 mg

20 mg

30 mg

40 mg

50 mg

60 mg

Extended-Release Capsules

MOBIC

RX

(meloxicam)
BOEHRINGER INGELHEIM

7.5 mg

15 mg

MOBIC ORAL SUSPENSION

RX

(meloxicam)
BOEHRINGER INGELHEIM

7.5 mg/5 mL

MOTRIN IB

OTC

(ibuprofen)
MCNEIL CONSUMER

200 mg
Caplets and Tablets

CHILDREN'S MOTRIN

OTC

(ibuprofen)
MCNEIL CONSUMER

100 mg/5 mL

Berry (also available as dye-free),
Bubble Gum, Grape, and Tropical Punch Flavors

Oral Suspension

CONCENTRATED MOTRIN

OTC

(ibuprofen)
MCNEIL CONSUMER

50 mg/1.25 mL
Berry Flavor

50 mg/1.25 mL
Dye-Free
Berry Flavor

Infants' Drops

JUNIOR STRENGTH MOTRIN

OTC

(ibuprofen)
MCNEIL CONSUMER

100 mg Chewable Tablet
Orange and Grape Flavors

100 mg
Caplet

NASONEX

RX

(mometasone furoate monohydrate)
SCHERING

50 mcg/actuation
17 g, 120 sprays

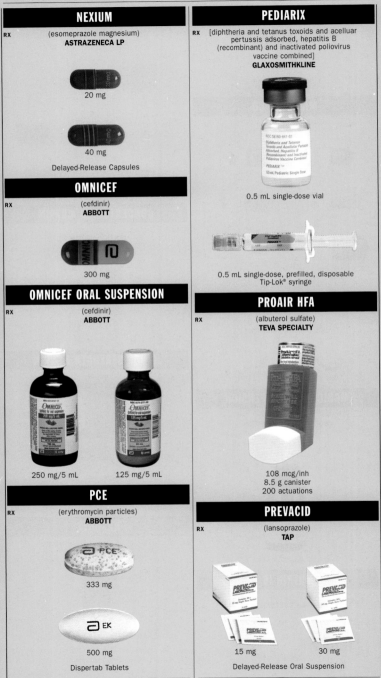

NEXIUM

RX

(esomeprazole magnesium)
ASTRAZENECA LP

20 mg

40 mg

Delayed-Release Capsules

OMNICEF

RX

(cefdinir)
ABBOTT

300 mg

OMNICEF ORAL SUSPENSION

RX

(cefdinir)
ABBOTT

250 mg/5 mL   125 mg/5 mL

PCE

RX

(erythromycin particles)
ABBOTT

333 mg

500 mg

Dispertab Tablets

PEDIARIX

RX

[diphtheria and tetanus toxoids and acelluar
pertussis adsorbed, hepatitis B
(recombinant) and inactivated poliovirus
vaccine combined]
GLAXOSMITHKLINE

0.5 mL single-dose vial

0.5 mL single-dose, prefilled, disposable
Tip-Lok® syringe

PROAIR HFA

RX

(albuterol sulfate)
TEVA SPECIALTY

108 mcg/inh
8.5 g canister
200 actuations

PREVACID

RX

(lansoprazole)
TAP

15 mg   30 mg

Delayed-Release Oral Suspension

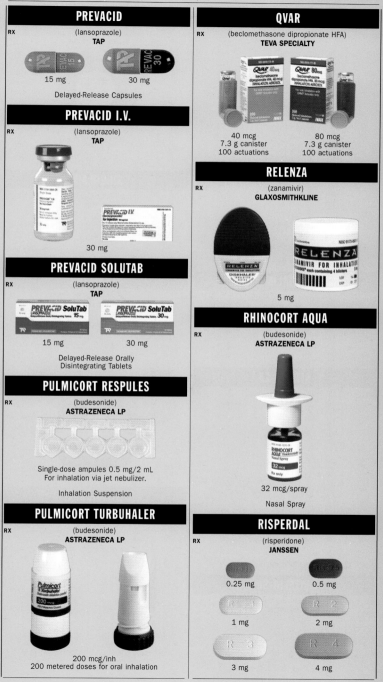

PREVACID

RX

(lansoprazole)
TAP

15 mg

30 mg

Delayed-Release Capsules

PREVACID I.V.

RX

(lansoprazole)
TAP

30 mg

PREVACID SOLUTAB

RX

(lansoprazole)
TAP

PREVACID SoluTab 15 mg

PREVACID SoluTab 30 mg

15 mg

30 mg

Delayed-Release Orally
Disintegrating Tablets

PULMICORT RESPULES

RX

(budesonide)
ASTRAZENECA LP

Single-dose ampules 0.5 mg/2 mL
For inhalation via jet nebulizer.

Inhalation Suspension

PULMICORT TURBUHALER

RX

(budesonide)
ASTRAZENECA LP

200 mcg/inh
200 metered doses for oral inhalation

QVAR

RX

(beclomethasone dipropionate HFA)
TEVA SPECIALTY

40 mcg
7.3 g canister
100 actuations

80 mcg
7.3 g canister
100 actuations

RELENZA

RX

(zanamivir)
GLAXOSMITHKLINE

5 mg

RHINOCORT AQUA

RX

(budesonide)
ASTRAZENECA LP

32 mcg/spray

Nasal Spray

RISPERDAL

RX

(risperidone)
JANSSEN

0.25 mg

0.5 mg

1 mg

2 mg

3 mg

4 mg

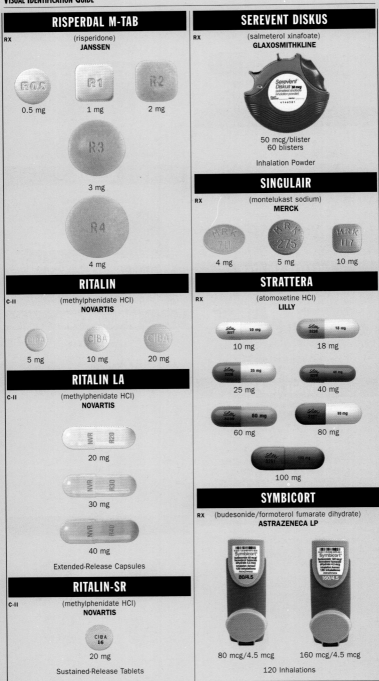

RISPERDAL M-TAB

RX

(risperidone)
JANSSEN

R 0.5 — 0.5 mg
R1 — 1 mg
R2 — 2 mg
R3 — 3 mg
R4 — 4 mg

RITALIN

C-II

(methylphenidate HCl)
NOVARTIS

CIBA — 5 mg
CIBA — 10 mg
CIBA — 20 mg

RITALIN LA

C-II

(methylphenidate HCl)
NOVARTIS

NVR R20 — 20 mg
NVR R30 — 30 mg
NVR R40 — 40 mg

Extended-Release Capsules

RITALIN-SR

C-II

(methylphenidate HCl)
NOVARTIS

CIBA 16 — 20 mg

Sustained-Release Tablets

SEREVENT DISKUS

RX

(salmeterol xinafoate)
GLAXOSMITHKLINE

Serevent Diskus 50 mcg
(salmeterol xinafoate inhalation powder)

50 mcg/blister
60 blisters

Inhalation Powder

SINGULAIR

RX

(montelukast sodium)
MERCK

MRK 711 — 4 mg
MRK 275 — 5 mg
MRK 117 — 10 mg

STRATTERA

RX

(atomoxetine HCl)
LILLY

Lilly 3227 — 10 mg
Lilly 3238 — 18 mg
Lilly 3228 — 25 mg
Lilly 3229 — 40 mg
Lilly 3239 — 60 mg
Lilly 3250 — 80 mg
Lilly 3251 — 100 mg

SYMBICORT

RX

(budesonide/formoterol fumarate dihydrate)
ASTRAZENECA LP

Symbicort 80/4.5 — 80 mcg/4.5 mcg
Symbicort 160/4.5 — 160 mcg/4.5 mcg

120 Inhalations

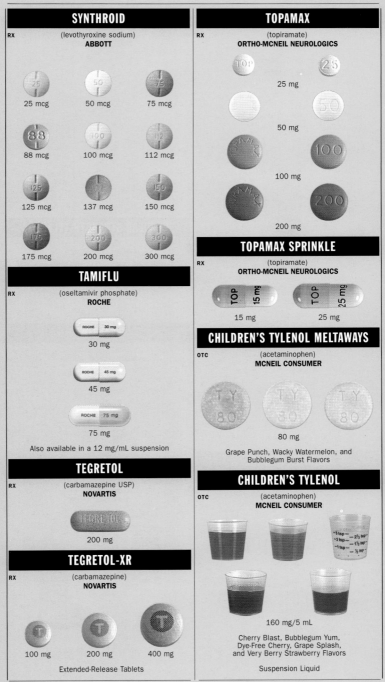

SYNTHROID

RX
(levothyroxine sodium)
ABBOTT

25 mcg 50 mcg 75 mcg
88 mcg 100 mcg 112 mcg
125 mcg 137 mcg 150 mcg
175 mcg 200 mcg 300 mcg

TAMIFLU

RX
(oseltamivir phosphate)
ROCHE

ROCHE 30 mg — 30 mg
ROCHE 45 mg — 45 mg
ROCHE 75 mg — 75 mg

Also available in a 12 mg/mL suspension

TEGRETOL

RX
(carbamazepine USP)
NOVARTIS

200 mg

TEGRETOL-XR

RX
(carbamazepine)
NOVARTIS

100 mg 200 mg 400 mg

Extended-Release Tablets

TOPAMAX

RX
(topiramate)
ORTHO-MCNEIL NEUROLOGICS

25 mg
50 mg
100 mg
200 mg

TOPAMAX SPRINKLE

RX
(topiramate)
ORTHO-MCNEIL NEUROLOGICS

TOP 15 mg — 15 mg
TOP 25 mg — 25 mg

CHILDREN'S TYLENOL MELTAWAYS

OTC
(acetaminophen)
MCNEIL CONSUMER

80 mg

Grape Punch, Wacky Watermelon, and
Bubblegum Burst Flavors

CHILDREN'S TYLENOL

OTC
(acetaminophen)
MCNEIL CONSUMER

160 mg/5 mL

Cherry Blast, Bubblegum Yum,
Dye-Free Cherry, Grape Splash,
and Very Berry Strawberry Flavors

Suspension Liquid

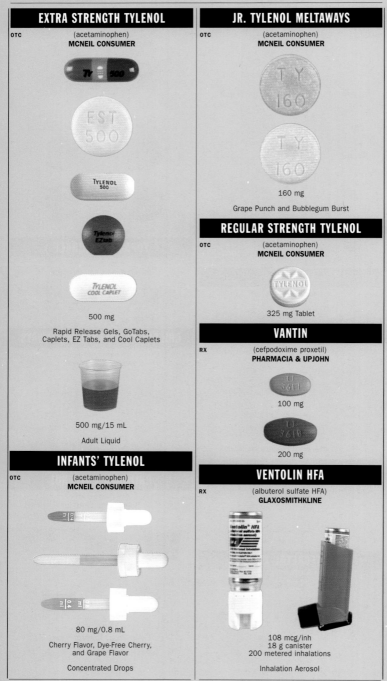

EXTRA STRENGTH TYLENOL

OTC

(acetaminophen)
MCNEIL CONSUMER

500 mg

Rapid Release Gels, GoTabs,
Caplets, EZ Tabs, and Cool Caplets

500 mg/15 mL

Adult Liquid

INFANTS' TYLENOL

OTC

(acetaminophen)
MCNEIL CONSUMER

80 mg/0.8 mL

Cherry Flavor, Dye-Free Cherry,
and Grape Flavor

Concentrated Drops

JR. TYLENOL MELTAWAYS

OTC

(acetaminophen)
MCNEIL CONSUMER

160 mg

Grape Punch and Bubblegum Burst

REGULAR STRENGTH TYLENOL

OTC

(acetaminophen)
MCNEIL CONSUMER

325 mg Tablet

VANTIN

RX

(cefpodoxime proxetil)
PHARMACIA & UPJOHN

100 mg

200 mg

VENTOLIN HFA

RX

(albuterol sulfate HFA)
GLAXOSMITHKLINE

108 mcg/inh
18 g canister
200 metered inhalations

Inhalation Aerosol

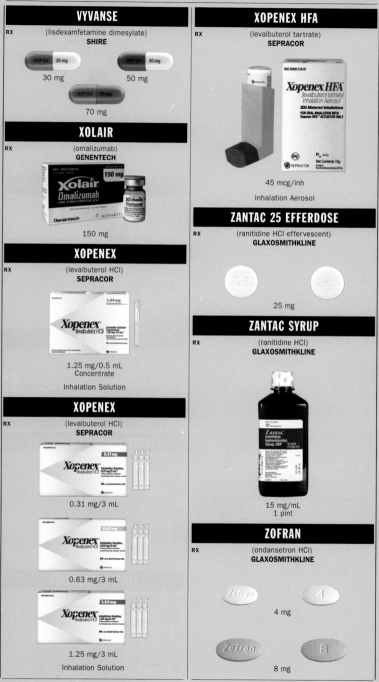

VYVANSE

RX (lisdexamfetamine dimesylate)
SHIRE

30 mg
50 mg
70 mg

XOLAIR

RX (omalizumab)
GENENTECH

150 mg

XOPENEX

RX (levalbuterol HCl)
SEPRACOR

1.25 mg/0.5 mL
Concentrate

Inhalation Solution

XOPENEX

RX (levalbuterol HCl)
SEPRACOR

0.31 mg/3 mL

0.63 mg/3 mL

1.25 mg/3 mL

Inhalation Solution

XOPENEX HFA

RX (levalbuterol tartrate)
SEPRACOR

45 mcg/inh

Inhalation Aerosol

ZANTAC 25 EFFERDOSE

RX (ranitidine HCl effervescent)
GLAXOSMITHKLINE

25 mg

ZANTAC SYRUP

RX (ranitidine HCl)
GLAXOSMITHKLINE

15 mg/mL
1 pint

ZOFRAN

RX (ondansetron HCl)
GLAXOSMITHKLINE

4 mg

8 mg

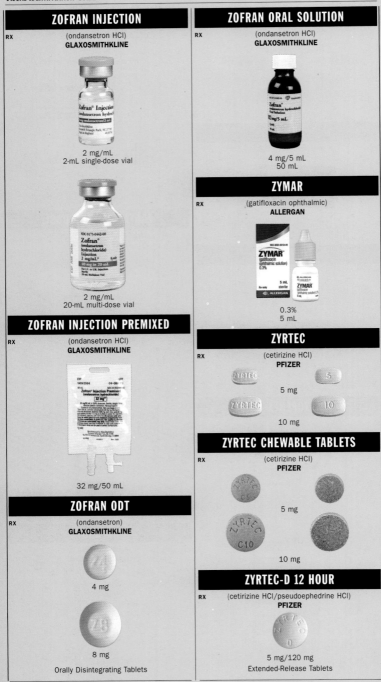

ZOFRAN INJECTION

RX

(ondansetron HCl)
GLAXOSMITHKLINE

2 mg/mL
2-mL single-dose vial

2 mg/mL
20-mL multi-dose vial

ZOFRAN INJECTION PREMIXED

RX

(ondansetron HCl)
GLAXOSMITHKLINE

32 mg/50 mL

ZOFRAN ODT

RX

(ondansetron)
GLAXOSMITHKLINE

4 mg

8 mg

Orally Disintegrating Tablets

ZOFRAN ORAL SOLUTION

RX

(ondansetron HCl)
GLAXOSMITHKLINE

4 mg/5 mL
50 mL

ZYMAR

RX

(gatifloxacin ophthalmic)
ALLERGAN

0.3%
5 mL

ZYRTEC

RX

(cetirizine HCl)
PFIZER

5 mg

10 mg

ZYRTEC CHEWABLE TABLETS

RX

(cetirizine HCl)
PFIZER

5 mg

10 mg

ZYRTEC-D 12 HOUR

RX

(cetirizine HCl/pseudoephedrine HCl)
PFIZER

5 mg/120 mg
Extended-Release Tablets

ADVERSE REACTIONS: Tachycardia, hypotension, confusion, anxiety, insomnia, nightmares, seizures, EPS, dizziness, headache, anticholinergic effects, rash, photosensitivity, blood dyscrasias, GI effects, impotence, decreased libido, flushing.

INTERACTIONS: See Contraindications. Risk of hyperpyrexia with anticholinergics and neuroleptics. Reduced hepatic metabolism with cimetidine. Enhanced seizure risk with tramadol. Enhanced response to alcohol, barbiturates, other CNS depressants. Use with CYP2D6 enzyme inhibitors (eg, quinidine, cimetidine, other antidepressants, phenothiazines, propafenone, flecainide, SSRIs) require lower doses for either TCA or other drug. Hyperpyretic crises, severe convulsions, and deaths reported with MAOIs. May block antihypertensive effect of guanethidine, or similarly acting compounds.

PREGNANCY: Safety in pregnancy and nursing not known.

MECHANISM OF ACTION: Unknown.

VoSoL HC
RX
acetic acid - hydrocortisone (Wallace)

OTHER BRAND NAME: Acetasol HC (Alpharma)

THERAPEUTIC CLASS: Antibacterial/corticosteroid combination

INDICATIONS: Treatment of superficial infections of the external auditory canal complicated by inflammation.

DOSAGE: *Adults:* Remove cerumen and debris. Insert cotton wick into ear canal; saturate cotton before or after insertion. Add 3-5 drops q4-6h to keep moist. Remove after 24 hrs; continue with 5 drops tid-qid as long as indicated.
Pediatrics: ≥3 yrs: Remove cerumen and debris. Insert cotton wick into ear canal; saturate cotton before or after insertion. Add 3-4 drops q4-6h to keep moist. Remove after 24 hrs; continue with 3-4 drops tid-qid as long as indicated.

HOW SUPPLIED: Sol: (Acetic Acid-Hydrocortisone) 2%-1% (10mL)

CONTRAINDICATIONS: Herpes simplex, vaccinia, varicella, perforated tympanic membrane.

WARNINGS/PRECAUTIONS: D/C promptly if sensitization occurs.

ADVERSE REACTIONS: Transient stinging, burning.

PREGNANCY: Safety in pregnancy and nursing not known.

VoSpire ER
RX
albuterol sulfate (Odyssey)

THERAPEUTIC CLASS: Beta$_2$ -agonist

INDICATIONS: Treatment of bronchospasm in reversible obstructive airway disease.

DOSAGE: *Adults:* Usual: 4-8mg q12h. Low Body Weight: Initial: 4mg q12h. Titrate: May increase to 8mg q12h. Max: 32mg/day in divided doses. Swallow whole with liquids; do not chew or crush.
Pediatrics: >12 yrs: Usual: 4-8mg q12h. Low Body Weight: Initial: 4mg q12h. Titrate: May increase to 8mg q12h. Max: 32mg/day in divided doses. 6-12 yrs: Usual: 4mg q12h. Max: 24mg/day in divided doses. Swallow whole with liquids; do not chew or crush.

HOW SUPPLIED: Tab, Extended-Release: 4mg, 8mg

WARNINGS/PRECAUTIONS: Hypersensitivity reactions reported. Caution with cardiovascular disorders, especially coronary insufficiency, arrhythmias and HTN. Increased doses may signify need for concomitant corticosteroids. Can produce paradoxical bronchospasm. Caution with DM, hyperthyroidism, seizures. May produce transient hypokalemia. Erythema multiforme and Stevens-Johnson (rare) reported in children.

ADVERSE REACTIONS: Tremor, headache, nervousness, tachycardia, palpitations, nausea, vomiting, muscle cramps.

INTERACTIONS: Avoid oral sympathomimetic agents. Extreme caution within 14 days of MAOI or TCA therapy. Monitor digoxin. May worsen ECG changes and/or hypokalemia with nonpotassium-sparing diuretics. Antagonized by β-blockers.

PREGNANCY: Category C, not for use in nursing.

MECHANISM OF ACTION: β_2-adrenergic bronchodilator; stimulates adenyl cylase, enzyme that catalyzes formation of cAMP from ATP. Increased cAMP levels associated with relaxation of bronchial smooth muscle and inhibition of release of mediators of immediate hypersensitivity.

PHARMACOKINETICS: Absorption: C_{max}=13.7ng/mL, T_{max}=6 hrs, AUC=134ng•hr/mL. **Elimination:** $T_{1/2}$=9.3 hrs.

VUMON   RX
teniposide (Bristol-Myers Squibb)

> **Cytotoxic. Severe myelosuppression, with resulting infection or bleeding, and/or hypersensitivity reactions may occur.**

THERAPEUTIC CLASS: Type II topoisomerase inhibitor

INDICATIONS: With other anticancer agents, for induction therapy of refractory childhood acute lymphoblastic leukemia.

DOSAGE: *Pediatrics:* 165mg/m^2 with cytarabine 300mg/m^2 IV twice weekly for 8-9 doses; or 250mg/m^2 with vincristine 1.5mg/m^2 IV weekly for 4-8 weeks and prednisone 40mg/m^2 PO for 28 days. Down Syndrome: Initial: Half usual dose. Maint: Increase based on degree of myelosuppression/mucositis.

HOW SUPPLIED: Inj: 10mg/mL (5mL)

CONTRAINDICATIONS: Hypersensitivity to Cremophor EL (polyoxyethylated castor oil).

WARNINGS/PRECAUTIONS: Monitor CBC, hepatic and renal function before and during therapy. Avoid rapid IV infusion. May cause fetal harm. Dose-limiting bone marrow suppression. D/C if significant hypotension occurs. Hypersensitivity (HS) reactions manifested by chills, fever, urticaria, tachycardia, bronchospasm, dyspnea, HTN, and hypotension may occur. If re-treating patient with earlier HS reaction, pretreat with corticosteroid and antihistamine. Continuously observe for at least 60 minutes after starting infusion and frequently thereafter. Use gloves when handling or preparing solution. Reduce dose or d/c if severe reactions occur.

ADVERSE REACTIONS: Myelosuppression, leukopenia, neutropenia, thrombocytopenia, anemia, mucositis, diarrhea, nausea, vomiting, infection, alopecia, bleeding, hypersensitivity reactions, rash, fever.

INTERACTIONS: Risk of CNS depression with antiemetics and high dose teniposide. Tolbutamide, sodium salicylate, and sulfamethizole displace protein-bound teniposide; may potentiate toxicity. Increased plasma clearance of methotrexate.

PREGNANCY: Category D, not for use in nursing.

MECHANISM OF ACTION: Podophyllotoxin derivative; acts in late S or early G_2 phase, preventing cells from entering mitosis; inhibits toposiomerase II, causing breaks in DNA and DNA-protein crosslinks.

PHARMACOKINETICS: Absorption: C_{max}≥40mcg/mL; T_{max}=1-2 hrs. **Distribution:** V_d=3.1L/m^2; plasma protein binding (>99%). **Elimination:** Urine (4-12%); $T_{1/2}$=5 hrs.

VYTONE   RX
hydrocortisone - iodoquinol (Dermik)

THERAPEUTIC CLASS: Corticosteroid/Anti-infective

INDICATIONS: "Possibly" Effective: Contact or atopic dermatitis, impetiginized eczema, nummular eczema, endogenous chronic infectious dermatitis, stasis dermatitis, pyoderma, nuchal eczema and chronic eczematoid otitis externa, acne urticata, localized or disseminated neurodermatitis, lichen simplex chronicus, anogenital pruritus (vulvae, scroti, ani), folliculitis, bacterial dermatoses, mycotic dermatoses such as tinea (capitis, cruris, corporis, pedis), monliasis, intertrigo.

DOSAGE: *Adults:* Apply to affected area(s) tid-qid.
Pediatrics: ≥12 yrs: Apply tid-qid.

HOW SUPPLIED: Cre: (Hydrocortisone-Iodoquinol) 1%-1% (30g)

WARNINGS/PRECAUTIONS: For external use only. Avoid eyes. D/C if irritation develops. May stain skin, hair, or fabrics. Risk of systemic absorption with treatment of extensive areas or use of occlusive dressings. Increased risk of systemic absorption in children. Iodoquinol may interfere with thyroid tests. False-positive phenylketonuria test reported.

ADVERSE REACTIONS: Burning, itching, irritation, dryness, folliculitis, hypertrichosis, acneiform eruptions, hypopigmentation, perioral dermatitis, allergic dermatitis, skin maceration, secondary infection, skin atrophy, striae, miliaria.

PREGNANCY: Category C, caution in nursing.

MECHANISM OF ACTION: Hydrocortisone: Corticosteroid; possesses anti-inflammatory, antipruritic, and vasoconstrictive properties; anti-inflammatory activity not established. Iodoquinol: Antifungal and antibacterial agent.

PHARMACOKINETICS: Absorption: Hydrocortisone: Percutaneous absorption; inflammation, other disease states, and use of occlusive dressings may increase absorption. **Metabolism:** Hydrocortisone: Liver. **Elimination:** Hydrocortisone: Urine (metabolites and parent compound).

VYVANSE CII
lisdexamfetamine dimesylate (Shire)

> High abuse potential; prolonged periods of administration may lead to dependence. Misuse of amphetamine may cause sudden death and serious cardiovascular events.

THERAPEUTIC CLASS: Sympathomimetic amine

INDICATIONS: Treatment of ADHD.

DOSAGE: *Adults:* Individualize dose. Usual: 30mg qam. Titrate: If needed, may increase in increments of 10mg or 20mg at weekly intervals. Max: 70mg/day. Swallow caps or dissolve contents in glass of water; do not store once dissolved. Re-evaluate periodically.
Pediatrics: 6-12 yrs: Individualize dose. Usual: 30mg qam. Titrate: If needed, may increase in increments of 10mg or 20mg at weekly intervals. Max: 70mg/day. Swallow caps or dissolve contents in glass of water; do not store once dissolved. Re-evaluate periodically.

HOW SUPPLIED: Cap: 20mg, 30mg, 40mg, 50mg, 60mg, 70mg

CONTRAINDICATIONS: Advanced arteriosclerosis, symptomatic CVD, moderate to severe HTN, hyperthyroidism, glaucoma, agitated states, history of drug abuse, during or within 14 days of MAOI use.

WARNINGS/PRECAUTIONS: Avoid use with structural cardiac abnormalities, cardiomyopathy, serious heart rhythm abnormalities, or other serious cardiac problems; sudden death reported. Assess presence of cardiac disease through cardiac evaluation. Caution with HTN, heart failure, recent MI, or ventricular arrhythmia; monitor BP and HR. May exacerbate symptoms of behavior disturbance and thought disorder in psychotic patients. Caution with comorbid bipolar disorder; concern for possible induction of mixed/manic episode. Treatment emergent psychotic or manic symptoms (eg, hallucinations, delusional thinking, or mania, without prior history of psychotic illness) may occur; d/c treatment if needed. Aggressive behavior or hostility reported; monitor condition as it worsens. Monitor growth in children. Stimulants may lower the convulsive threshold; d/c in the presence of seizures. Difficulties with accommodation and blurring of vision reported. May exacerbate motor or phonic tics and Tourette's syndrome.

ADVERSE REACTIONS: Ventricular hypertrophy, tic, vomiting, psychomotor hyperactivity, insomnia, rash, upper abdominal pain, decreased appetite, dizziness, dry mouth, irritability, weight loss, nausea, headache, affect lability.

INTERACTIONS: Urinary acidifying agents (eg, ammonium chloride, sodium acid phosphate) and methenamine decrease efficacy. Inhibits adrenergic blockers, antihistamines, and antihypertensives (veratrum alkaloids). Potentiated effects of both agents with TCAs. MAOIs and furazolidone metabolite may cause hypertensive crisis. Antagonized by chlorpromazine, haloperidol, and lithium carbonate. May delay absorption of ethosuximide, phenobarbital, and phenytoin. Potentiates meperidine, norepinephrine, phenobarbital, and phenytoin. Potentiated by propoxyphene overdose; fatal convulsions may occur.

PREGNANCY: Category C, not for use in nursing.

485

MECHANISM OF ACTION: Dextroamphetamine; blocks reuptake of norepinephrine and dopamine into presynaptic neuron and increases release of these monoamines into extraneuronal space.

PHARMACOKINETICS: Absorption: Rapidly absorbed; T_{max}=1 hr. **Metabolism:** 1st-pass intestinal and/or hepatic metabolism to dextroamphetamine and L-lysine. **Elimination:** Urine, feces; $T_{1/2} \leq$ 1hr.

WESTCORT   RX
hydrocortisone valerate (Ranbaxy)

THERAPEUTIC CLASS: Corticosteroid

INDICATIONS: Corticosteroid-responsive dermatoses.

DOSAGE: *Adults:* Apply bid-tid. May use occlusive dressings for psoriasis or recalcitrant conditions; d/c dressings if infection develops.
Pediatrics: Apply bid-tid. May use occlusive dressings for psoriasis or recalcitrant conditions; d/c dressings if infection develops.

HOW SUPPLIED: Cre, Oint: 0.2% (15g, 45g, 60g)

WARNINGS/PRECAUTIONS: May produce reversible HPA axis suppression, manifestations of Cushing's syndrome, hyperglycemia, and glucosuria. Caution when applied to large surface areas or under occlusive dressings. Use appropriate antifungal or antibacterial agent with dermatological infections; d/c if infection does not clear. Pediatrics may be more susceptible to systemic toxicity. Avoid eyes. D/C if irritation occurs.

ADVERSE REACTIONS: Burning, itching, dryness, irritation, folliculitis, hypertrichosis, acneiform eruptions, hypopigmentation, allergic contact dermatitis, skin maceration, secondary infection, skin atrophy, striae, miliaria.

PREGNANCY: Category C, caution in nursing.

MECHANISM OF ACTION: Corticosteroid; possesses anti-inflammatory, antipruritic, and vasoconstrictive properties. Anti-inflammatory effects not established; suspected to act by induction of phospholipase A_2 inhibitory proteins, lipocortins. Lipocortins control biosynthesis of potent inflammation mediators (eg, prostaglandins, leukotrienes) by inhibiting release of their common precursor, arachidonic acid.

PHARMACOKINETICS: Absorption: Percutaneous; inflammation and other disease states may increase absorption. Use of occlusive dressings for ≤24 hrs not shown to increase penetration; use for ≥96 hrs markedly enhances penetration. **Distribution:** Systemically administered corticosteroids found in breast milk.

WINRHO SDF   RX
rho (D) immune globulin (Baxter)

INDICATIONS: Treatment of non-splenectomized, Rh_o(D) positive children with chronic or acute immune thrombocytopenic purpura (ITP), adults with chronic ITP, or children and adults with ITP secondary to HIV infection. To prevent Rh isoimmunization in Rh_o (D) negative mothers who had not been previously sensitized to Rh_o (D) factor. To suppress Rh isoimmunization in non-sensitized, Rh_o(D) negative women within 72 hours after spontaneous or induced abortions, amniocentesis, chorionic villus sampling, ruptured tubal pregnancy, abdominal trauma or transplacental hemorrhage or in the normal course of pregnancy, unless fetus or father is known to be Rh_o(D) negative. To suppress Rh isoimmunization in Rh_o(D) negative female children and adults transfused with Rh_o(D) positive blood products.

DOSAGE: *Adults:* ITP: Initial: 50mcg/kg IV as a single dose or in 2 divided doses on separate days. Hgb <10g/dL: 25-40mcg/kg. Subsequent/Maint: 25-60mcg/kg. Hgb 8-10g/dL: 25-40mcg/kg. Hgb >10g/dL: 50-60mcg/kg. Hgb <8g/dL: Use caution. Rh Suppression: Pregnancy: Give as IM or IV. 28 Weeks Gestation: 300mcg. If early in pregnancy, give at 12 week intervals. Postpartum: With Rh Positive Baby: 120mcg at birth, but no later than 72 hours after. Rh Status of Baby Unknown at 72 Hours: Administer to mother at 72 hours after birth. May give up to 28 days after birth. Abortion/Amniocentesis or Other Manipulation After 34 Weeks Gestation: 120mcg dose within 72 hours. Amniocentesis Before 34 Weeks Gestation/Post Chorionic Villus Sampling: 300mcg dose immediately after procedure. Repeat every 12 weeks. Threatened Abortion: 300mcg as soon as possible. Transfusion: Exposure to Rh$_o$(D) Positive Blood: 9mcg/mL blood given as 600mcg q8h IV or 12mcg/mL blood given as 1200mcg q12h IM. Exposure to Rh$_o$(D) Positive RBCs: 18mcg/mL cells given as 600mcg q8h IV or 24mcg/mL cells given as 1200mcg q12h IM.

Pediatrics: ITP: Initial: 50mcg/kg IV as a single dose or in 2 divided doses on separate days. Hgb <10g/dL: 25-40mcg/kg. Subsequent/Maint: 25-60mcg/kg. Hgb 8-10g/dL: 25-40mcg/kg. Hgb >10g/dL: 50-60mcg/kg. Hgb <8g/dL: Use caution. Transfusion: Exposure to Rh$_o$(D) Positive Blood: 9mcg/mL blood given as 600mcg q8h IV or 12mcg/mL blood given as 1200mcg q12h IM. Exposure to Rh$_o$(D) Positive RBCs: 18mcg/mL cells given as 600mcg q8h IV or 24mcg/mL cells given as 1200mcg q12h IM.

HOW SUPPLIED: Inj: 120mcg (600 IU), 300mcg (1500 IU), 1000mcg (5000 IU)

CONTRAINDICATIONS: When used to prevent Rh alloimmunization, should not be adminstered to Rh$_o$(D) positive individuals including babies; Rh$_o$(D) negative women who are Rh immunized as evidenced by standard manual Rh antibody screening test; individuals with a history of anaphylactic or other severe systemic reaction to immune globulins. When used to treat patients with ITP, should not be administered to Rh$_o$(D) negative individuals; splenectomized individuals; individuals with known hypersensitivity to plasma products.

WARNINGS/PRECAUTIONS: May transmit disease. Avoid use in Rh$_o$(D) negative, Rh$_o$(D) negative who are Rh immunized, or spelenectomized patients. Not for replacement therapy for immuneglobulin deficiency syndromes. Caution with IgA deficiency; anaphylactic reactions may occur. (ITP): Monitor for intravascular hemolysis, clinically compromising anemia, renal insufficiency. If transfused, use Rh$_o$(D) negative RBCs. Caution if platelets from Rh$_o$(D) positive donors are transfused.

ADVERSE REACTIONS: Headache, chills, fever, decreased Hgb, back pain, intravascular hemolysis.

INTERACTIONS: May interfere with response to live vaccines; delay immunization for 3 months.

PREGNANCY: Category C, safety in nursing not known.

MECHANISM OF ACTION: Gamma globulin; not established. For ITP, thought to aid in formation of anti-Rh$_o$(D) (anti-D)-coated RBC complexes resulting in Fc receptor blockade, sparing antibody-coated platelets.

PHARMACOKINETICS: Absorption: (IV, IM) C_{max}=36-48ng/mL, 18-19ng/mL. (IV, IM) T_{max}=2 hrs, 5-10 days. **Elimination:** (IV, IM) $T_{1/2}$=24 days; 30 days.

XENICAL
orlistat (Roche Labs)

RX

THERAPEUTIC CLASS: Lipase inhibitor

INDICATIONS: For weight loss and weight maintenance and to reduce risk of weight regain after weight loss in obese patients with initial BMI ≥30kg/m^2 or ≥27kg/m^2 in presence of other risk factors.

DOSAGE: *Adults:* 120mg tid with each main meal containing fat. Take during or up to 1 hr after meals. Use with reduced-calorie diet with about 30% of calories from fat. Omit dose if meal is missed or contains no fat. Separate multivitamin (containing fat-soluble vitamins) by at least 2 hrs.

Pediatrics: ≥12 yrs: 120mg tid with each main meal containing fat. Take during or up to 1 hr after meals. Use with reduced-calorie diet with about 30% of calories from fat. Omit dose if meal is missed or contains no fat. Separate multivitamin (containing fat-soluble vitamins) by at least 2 hrs.

HOW SUPPLIED: Cap: 120mg

CONTRAINDICATIONS: Chronic malabsorption syndrome, cholestasis.

WARNINGS/PRECAUTIONS: Exclude organic causes of obesity. Caution with history of hyperoxaluria or calcium oxalate nephrolithiasis. GI effects may increase with a high-fat diet (>30%). Weight loss may improve metabolic control; monitor dosage of antidiabetic agents. Increased risk of cholelithiasis due to substantial weight loss.

ADVERSE REACTIONS: Oily spotting, flatus with discharge, fecal urgency, fatty/oily stool, oily evacuation, increased defecation, fecal incontinence.

INTERACTIONS: Monitor warfarin and cyclosporine (separate cyclosporine dose by 2 hrs). May decrease absorption of fat-soluble vitamins and β-carotene; supplement with fat-soluble multivitamin.

PREGNANCY: Category B, not for use in nursing.

MECHANISM OF ACTION: Lipase inhibitor; inhibits absorption of dietary fats. Acts in lumen of stomach and small intestine by forming covalent bond with active serine residue site of gastric and pancreatic lipases, inactivating enzymes making them unavailable to hydrolyze dietary fats.

PHARMACOKINETICS: Distribution: Plasma protein binding (>99%). **Metabolism:** GI wall. **Elimination:** Feces (83%); $T_{1/2}$=1-2 hrs.

XIFAXAN
rifaximin (Salix)

RX

THERAPEUTIC CLASS: Semisynthetic rifampin analog

INDICATIONS: Traveler's diarrhea caused by noninvasive strains of *E.coli*

DOSAGE: *Adults:* 1 tab tid for 3 days.
Pediatrics: ≥12 yrs: 1 tab tid for 3 days.

HOW SUPPLIED: Tab: 200mg

WARNINGS/PRECAUTIONS: Avoid in diarrhea complicated by fever or blood in the stool or diarrhea due to pathogens other than *E.coli*. D/C if diarrhea symptoms worsen or persist >24-48 hrs; consider alternative antibiotic therapy. Pseudomembranous colitis reported.

ADVERSE REACTIONS: Flatulence, headache, abdominal pain, rectal tenesmus, defecation urgency, nausea, constipation, pyrexia.

PREGNANCY: Category C; not for use in nursing.

MECHANISM OF ACTION: Antibacterial agent; binds to β-subunit of bacterial DNA-dependent RNA polymerase, resulting in inhibition of bacterial RNA synthesis.

PHARMACOKINETICS: Absorption: C_{max}=4.3ng/mL; T_{max}=1.25 hrs. **Metabolism:** CYP3A4. **Elimination:** Feces (97%), urine (0.32%).

XOLAIR
omalizumab (Genentech)

RX

> **Anaphylaxis, presenting as bronchospasm, hypotension, syncope, urticaria, and/or angioedema of the throat or tongue has been reported. Monitor patients closely for an appropriate time period after administration.**

THERAPEUTIC CLASS: Monoclonal antibody/IgE-blocker

INDICATIONS: Moderate-severe persistent asthma in those who have a positive skin test or *in vitro* reactivity to a perennial aeroallergen and whose symptoms are inadequately controlled with inhaled corticosteroids.

DOSAGE: *Adults:* 150-375mg SQ every 2 or 4 weeks based on body weight and pre-treatment serum total IgE level. Max: 150mg/site. 30-90kg & IgE ≥30-100 IU/mL: 150mg every 4 weeks. >90-150kg & IgE ≥30-100 IU/mL OR 30-90kg & IgE >100-200 IU/mL OR 30-60kg & IgE >200-300 IU/mL: 300mg every 4 weeks. >90-150kg & IgE >100-200 IU/mL OR >60-90kg & IgE >200-300 IU/mL OR 30-70kg & IgE >300-400 IU/mL: 225mg every 2 weeks. >90-150kg & IgE >200-300 IU/mL OR >70-90kg & IgE >300-400 IU/mL OR 30-70kg & IgE >400-500 IU/mL OR 30-60kg & IgE >500-600 IU/mL: 300mg every 2 weeks. >70-90kg & IgE >400-500 IU/mL OR >60-70kg & IgE >500-600 IU/mL OR 30-60kg & IgE >600-700 IU/mL: 375mg every 2 weeks.
Pediatrics: ≥12 yrs: 150-375mg SQ every 2 or 4 weeks based on body weight and pre-treatment serum total IgE level. Max: 150mg/site. 30-90kg & IgE ≥30-100 IU/mL: 150mg every 4 weeks. >90-150kg & IgE ≥30-100 IU/mL OR 30-90kg & IgE >100-200 IU/mL OR 30-60kg & IgE >200-300 IU/mL: 300mg every 4 weeks. >90-150kg & IgE >100-200 IU/mL OR >60-90kg & IgE >200-300 IU/mL OR 30-70kg & IgE >300-400 IU/mL: 225mg every 2 weeks. >90-150kg and IgE >200-300 IU/mL OR >70-90kg & IgE >300-400 IU/mL OR

30-70kg & IgE >400-500 IU/mL OR 30-60kg & IgE >500-600 IU/mL: 300mg every 2 weeks. >70-90kg & IgE >400-500 IU/mL OR >60-70kg & IgE >500-600 IU/mL OR 30-60kg & IgE >600-700 IU/mL: 375mg q2 weeks.

HOW SUPPLIED: Inj: 150mg (5mL)

WARNINGS/PRECAUTIONS: Malignant neoplasms reported. Not for use in treatment of acute bronchospasm or status asthmaticus. Systemic or inhaled corticosteroids should not be abruptly discontinued when initiating therapy.

ADVERSE REACTIONS: Anaphylaxis, malignancies, injection site reactions, viral infections, upper respiratory infection, sinusitis, headache, pharyngitis, pain, arthralgia.

PREGNANCY: Category B, caution in nursing.

MECHANISM OF ACTION: Monoclonal antibody/IgE blocker; inhibits binding of IgE to high-affinity IgE receptor on surface of mast cells and basophils and limits degree of release of mediators of allergic response.

PHARMACOKINETICS: Absorption:(SQ) Absolute bioavailability (62%); T_{max}=7-8 days. **Distribution:** V_d=78mL/kg; crosses placental barrier. **Elimination:** $T_{1/2}$=26 days.

XOPENEX
levalbuterol HCl (Sepracor)

RX

THERAPEUTIC CLASS: Beta$_2$ -agonist

INDICATIONS: Prevention and treatment of bronchospasm with reversible obstructive airway disease.

DOSAGE: *Adults:* Initial: 0.63mg tid, q6-8h. Severe Asthma: 1.25mg tid, q6-8h. Administer by nebulizer.
Pediatrics: ≥12 yrs: Initial: 0.63mg tid, q6-8h. Severe Asthma: 1.25mg tid, q6-8h. 6-11 yrs: 0.31mg tid. Max: 0.63mg tid. Administer by nebulizer.

HOW SUPPLIED: Sol: 0.31mg/3mL, 0.63mg/3mL, 1.25mg/3mL (3mL, 24^5)

WARNINGS/PRECAUTIONS: Hypersensitivity reactions reported. D/C immediately if paradoxical bronchospasm occurs. May produce ECG changes; caution with cardiovascular disorders, coronary insufficiency, arrhythmias, and HTN. Caution with convulsive disorders, hyperthyroidism, and diabetes. May produce transient hypokalemia.

ADVERSE REACTIONS: Tachycardia, migraine, dyspepsia, leg cramps, nervousness, dizziness, tremor, rhinitis, increased cough, chest pain, HTN, hypotention, diarrhea, dry mouth, anxiety, insomnia, paresthesia, wheezing.

INTERACTIONS: Avoid other sympathomimetic agents. Extreme caution with MAOIs and TCAs. Monitor digoxin. ECG changes and/or hypokalemia with nonpotassium-sparing diuretics. Antagonized by β-blockers.

PREGNANCY: Category C, not for use in nursing.

MECHANISM OF ACTION: β$_2$-adrenergic bronchodilator; stimulates adenyl cylase, the enzyme that catalyzes formation of cAMP from ATP. Increased cAMP levels associated with relaxation of bronchial smooth muscle and inhibition of release of mediators of immediate hypersensitivity.

PHARMACOKINETICS: Absorption: C_{max}(1.25, 5mg)=1.1, 4.5ng/ml; T_{max}(1.25, 5mg)=0.2, 0.2 hrs. **Metabolism:** GI tract by SULT1A3. **Elimination:** Renal (80-100%), urine (25-46% unchanged), feces (≤20%); $T_{1/2}$(1.25, 5mg)=3.3, 4 hrs.

XOPENEX HFA
levalbuterol tartrate (Sepracor)

RX

THERAPEUTIC CLASS: Beta$_2$ -agonist

INDICATIONS: Prevention and treatment of bronchospasm with reversible obstructive airway disease.

DOSAGE: *Adults:* 2 inh (90mcg) q4-6h or 1 inh (45mcg) q4h may be sufficient.
Pediatrics: ≥4 yrs: 2 inh (90mcg) q4-6h or 1 inh (45mcg) q4h may be sufficient.

HOW SUPPLIED: MDI: 45mcg/inh (15g)

WARNINGS/PRECAUTIONS: D/C immediately if paradoxical bronchospasm occurs. May produce ECG changes; caution with cardiovascular disorders, coronary insufficiency, arrhythmias, and HTN. Caution with convulsive disorders, hyperthyroidism, and diabetes. May produce transient hypokalemia.

ADVERSE REACTIONS: Asthma, pharyngitis, rhinitis, pain, vomiting.

INTERACTIONS: Avoid other sympathomimetic agents. Extreme caution with MAOIs and TCAs. Monitor digoxin. ECG changes and/or hypokalemia with nonpotassium-sparing diuretics. Antagonized by β-blockers.

PREGNANCY: Category C, not for use in nursing.

MECHANISM OF ACTION: β_2-adrenergic bronchodilator; stimulates adenyl cylase, the enzyme that catalyzes formation of cAMP from ATP. Increased cAMP levels associated with relaxation of bronchial smooth muscle and inhibition of release of mediators of immediate hypersensitivity.

PHARMACOKINETICS: Absorption: C_{max}=0.199ng/mL (≥12 yrs), 0.163ng/mL (4-11 yrs); T_{max}=0.54 hrs (≥12 yrs), 0.76 hrs (4-11 yrs); AUC=0.695ng•hr/mL (≥12 yrs), 0.579ng•hr/mL (4-11 yrs). **Metabolism:** GI tract by SULT1A3. **Elimination:** Renal (80-100%), urine (25-46% unchanged), feces (≤20%).

XYLOCAINE INJECTION   RX
lidocaine HCl (Abraxis)

OTHER BRAND NAME: Xylocaine-MPF (Abraxis)

THERAPEUTIC CLASS: Local anesthetic

INDICATIONS: For production of local or regional anesthesia by infiltration techniques such as percutaneous injection and IV regional anesthesia by peripheral nerve block techniques such as brachial plexus and intercostal and by central neural techniques such as lumbar and caudal epidural blocks.

DOSAGE: *Adults:* Dosage varies depending on procedure, depth, and duration of anesthesia, degree of muscular relaxation, and patient physical condition. Max: 4.5mg/kg or total dose of 300mg. Epidural/Caudal Anesthesia: Max: Intervals not less than 90 min. Paracervical Block: Max: 200mg/90 min. Regional Anesthesia: IV: Max: 4mg/kg. Children/Elderly/Debilitated/Cardiac or Liver Disease: Reduce dose. *Pediatrics:* >3 yrs: Max: 1.5-2mg/lb. Regional Anesthesia: IV: Max: 3mg/kg.

HOW SUPPLIED: Inj: 0.5%, 1%, 2%; (MPF) 0.5%, 1%, 1.5%, 2%

WARNINGS/PRECAUTIONS: Acidosis, cardiac arrest, death reported from delay in toxicity management. Local anesthetic solutions containing antimicrobial preservatives should not be used for epidural or spinal anesthesia. Use lowest effective dose. During epidural anesthesia, administer initial test dose and monitor for CNS and cardiovascular toxicity as well as for signs of unintended intrathecal administration. Reduce dose with debilitated, elderly, acutely ill, and children. Extreme caution when using lumbar and caudal epidural anesthesia with existing neurological disease, spinal deformities, septicemia, and severe HTN. Monitor cardiovascular and respiratory vital signs and state of consciousness after each injection. Caution with hepatic disease, cardiovascular disorders. Monitor circulation and respiration with injections to head and neck area.

ADVERSE REACTIONS: Lightheadedness, nervousness, euphoria, confusion, dizziness, drowsiness, tinnitus, blurred vision, vomiting, heat/cold sensations, twitching, tremors, convulsions, respiratory depression, bradycardia, hypotension, urticaria, edema, anaphylactoid reactions.

PREGNANCY: Category B, caution in nursing.

MECHANISM OF ACTION: Anesthetic; stabilizes neuronal membrane by inhibiting ionic fluxes required for initiation and conduction of impulses, thereby effecting local anesthetic action.

PHARMACOKINETICS: Absorption: Complete. **Distribution:** Crosses blood-brain and placental barriers. **Metabolism:** Liver (rapid), oxidative N-alkylation (major pathway), yields monoethylglycinexylidide and glycinexylidide (metabolites). **Elimination:** Urine, 90% (metabolites) and ≤10% (unchanged); $T_{1/2}$=1.5-2.0 hrs.

XYLOCAINE JELLY

RX

lidocaine HCl (AstraZeneca)

THERAPEUTIC CLASS: Acetamide local anesthetic

INDICATIONS: Prevention and control of pain in procedures involving the male and female urethra. Topical treatment of painful urethritis. Anesthetic lubricant for endotracheal intubation.

DOSAGE: *Adults:* Max: 600mg/12 hrs. Surface Anesthesia of Male Urethra: Instill about 15mL (300mg). Instill an additional dose of not more than 15mL if needed. Prior to Sounding or Cystoscopy: A total dose of 30mL (600mg) is usually required. Prior to Catheterization: 5-10mL usually adequate. Surface Anesthesia of Female Urethra: Instill 3-5mL. Elderly/Debilitated: Reduce dose.
Pediatrics: Determine dose by age and weight. Max: 4.5mg/kg.

HOW SUPPLIED: Jelly: 2% (Tube: 5mL, 30mL; Syringe: 10mL, 20mL)

WARNINGS/PRECAUTIONS: Avoid excessive dosage or frequent administration; may result in serious adverse effects requiring resuscitative measures. Caution with heart block and severe shock. Extreme caution if mucosa traumatized or sepsis is present in the area of application; risk of rapid systemic absorption.

ADVERSE REACTIONS: Lightheadedness, nervousness, confusion, euphoria, dizziness, drowsiness, blurred vision, tremors, convulsions, respiratory depression, bradycardia, hypotension, urticaria, edema, anaphylactoid reactions.

PREGNANCY: Category B, caution in nursing.

MECHANISM OF ACTION: Local anesthetic; stabilizes neuronal membrane by initiating ionic fluxes required for initiation and conduction of impulses.

PHARMACOKINETICS: Absorption: Rapid. **Metabolism:** Biotransformation. **Distribution:** Plasma protein binding (60-80%); crosses placenta. **Elimination:** Urine; $T_{1/2}$=1.5-2 hrs.

XYLOCAINE VISCOUS

RX

lidocaine HCl (AstraZeneca)

THERAPEUTIC CLASS: Acetamide local anesthetic

INDICATIONS: Topical anesthesia of irritated or inflamed mucous membranes of the mouth and pharynx. To reduce gagging during X-ray or dental procedures.

DOSAGE: *Adults:* Irritated/Inflamed Mucous Membranes: Usual: 15mL undiluted. (Mouth) Swish and spit out. (Pharynx) Gargle and may swallow. Do not administer in <3 hr intervals. Max: 8 doses/24hr; (Single Dose) 4.5mg/kg or total of 300mg.
Pediatrics: >3 yrs: Max: Determine by age and weight. Infants <3 yrs: Apply 1.25mL with cotton-tipped applicator to immediate area. Do not administer in <3 hour intervals. Max: 8 doses/24hr.

HOW SUPPLIED: Sol: 2% (100mL, 450mL)

WARNINGS/PRECAUTIONS: Reduce dose in elderly, debilitated, acutely ill and children. Caution with heart block, severe shock, and known drug sensitivities. Excessive dosage or too frequent administration may result in high plasma levels and serious adverse effects requiring resuscitative measures. Extreme caution if mucosa traumatized; risk of rapid systemic absorption. Overdose reported in pediatrics due to inappropriate dosing.

ADVERSE REACTIONS: Lightheadedness, nervousness, confusion, euphoria, dizziness, drowsiness, blurred vision, tremors, convulsions, respiratory depression, bradycardia, hypotension, urticaria, edema, anaphylactoid reactions.

PREGNANCY: Category B, caution in nursing.

MECHANISM OF ACTION: Local anesthetic; stabilizes neuronal membrane by inhibiting ionic fluxes required for initiation and conduction of nerve impulses.

PHARMACOKINETICS: Absorption: Well-absorbed. **Distribution:** Crosses blood-brain and placental barriers; plasma protein binding (60-80%). **Metabolism:** Liver (rapid), oxidative N-alkylation, ring hydoxylation, cleavage of amide linkage, conjugation; monoethylglycinexylidide and glyciexylidide (metabolites). **Elimination:** Urine (90% metabolites, <10% unchanged); $T_{1/2}$=1.5-2 hrs.

XYLOCAINE WITH EPINEPHRINE   RX
epinephrine - lidocaine HCl (AstraZeneca)

OTHER BRAND NAME: Xylocaine-MPF with Epinephrine (AstraZeneca)

THERAPEUTIC CLASS: Local anesthetic

INDICATIONS: For production of local or regional anesthesia by infiltration techniques such as percutaneous injection and IV regional anesthesia by peripheral nerve block techniques such as brachial plexus and intercostal and by central neural techniques such as lumbar and caudal epidural blocks.

DOSAGE: *Adults:* Dosage varies depending on procedure, depth and duration of anesthesia, degree of muscular relaxation, and patient physical condition. Max: 7mg/kg or total dose of 500mg. Epidural/Caudal Anesthesia: Max: Intervals not less than 90 min. Paracervical Block: Max: 200mg/90 min. Regional Anesthesia: IV: Max: 4mg/kg. Children/Elderly/Debilitated/Cardiac or Liver Disease: Reduce dose.
Pediatrics: >3 yrs: Max: 1.5-2mg/lb. Regional Anesthesia: IV: Max: 3mg/kg.

HOW SUPPLIED: Inj: (Lidocaine-Epinephrine) 0.5%/1:200000, 1%/1:100000, 2%/1:100000; (MPF) 1%/1:200000, 1.5%/1:200000, 2%/1:200000; (Dental) 2%/1:50000, 2%/1:100000.

WARNINGS/PRECAUTIONS: Acidosis, cardiac arrest, death reported from delay in toxicity management. Local anesthetic solutions containing antimicrobial preservatives should not be used for epidural or spinal anesthesia. Xylocaine with epinephrine solutions contain sodium metabisulfite which may cause allergic-type reactions in susceptible people. Use lowest effective dose. During epidural anesthesia, administer initial test dose and monitor for CNS and cardiovascular toxicity as well as for signs of unintended intrathecal administration. Reduce dose with debilitated, elderly, acutely ill, and children. Extreme caution when using lumbar and caudal epidural anesthesia with existing neurological disease, spinal deformities, septicemia, and severe HTN. Caution when local anesthetic injections containing a vasoconstrictor are used in areas of the body supplied by end arteries or having otherwise compromised blood supply; ischemic injury or necrosis may result with peripheral or hypertensive vascular disease due to exaggerated vasoconstrictor response. Monitor cardiovascular and respiratory vital signs and state of consciousness after each injection. Caution with hepatic disease, cardiovascular disorders. Monitor circulation and respiration with injections into head and neck area.

ADVERSE REACTIONS: Lightheadedness, nervousness, euphoria, confusion, dizziness, drowsiness, tinnitus, blurred vision, vomiting, heat/cold sensations, twitching, tremors, convulsions, respiratory depression, bradycardia, hypotension, urticaria, edema, anaphylactoid reactions.

INTERACTIONS: Anesthetic solutions containing epinephrine or norepinephrine with MAOIs or TCAs may produce severe, prolonged HTN; avoid concurrent use or monitor closely if concurrent use is essential. Phenothiazines and butyrophenones may reduce or reverse pressor effect of epinephrine; avoid concurrent use or monitor closely if concurrent use is essential. Vasopressors, ergot-type oxytocic drugs may cause severe, persistent HTN or CVA.

PREGNANCY: Category B, caution in nursing.

MECHANISM OF ACTION: Anesthetic; stabilizes neuronal membrane by inhibiting ionic fluxes required for initiation and conduction of impulses, thereby effecting local anesthetic action.

PHARMACOKINETICS: Absorption: Complete. **Distribution:** Crosses blood-brain and placental barriers. **Metabolism:** Liver (rapid). Oxidative N-alkylation yields monoethylglycinexylidide and glycinexylidide (metabolites). **Elimination:** Urine 90% (metabolites) and <10% (unchanged); $T_{1/2}$=1.5-2.0 hrs.

XYREM

CIII

sodium oxybate (Orphan Medical)

> Sodium oxybate is GHB (gamma hydroxybutyrate), a known drug of abuse. Do not use with alcohol or other CNS depressants. Associated with confusion, depression, and other neuropsychiatric events. Available only through the Xyrem Success Program, call 1-866-XYREM88.

THERAPEUTIC CLASS: CNS Depressant

INDICATIONS: Treatment of excessive daytime sleepiness and cataplexy in patients with narcolepsy.

DOSAGE: *Adults:* Initial: 2.25g qhs, then take 2.25g 2.5-4 hrs later. Titrate: Increase by 0.75g/dose every 1-2 weeks. Range: 6-9g/night. Max: 9g/night. Hepatic Insufficiency: Initial: Decrease by 50%. Titrate dose increments to effect. Take 1st dose at bedtime while in bed and the 2nd dose while sitting in bed. Dilute each dose with 2 ounces of water.
Pediatrics: ≥16 yrs: Initial: 2.25g qhs, then take 2.25g 2.5-4 hrs later. Titrate: Increase by 0.75g/dose every 1-2 weeks. Range: 6-9g/night. Max: 9g/night. Hepatic Insufficiency: Initial: Decrease by 50%. Titrate dose increments to effect. Take 1st dose at bedtime while in bed and the 2nd dose while sitting in bed. Dilute each dose with 2 ounces of water.

HOW SUPPLIED: Sol: 500mg/mL (180mL)

CONTRAINDICATIONS: Sedative hypnotic agents, succinic semialdehyde dehydrogenase deficiency.

WARNINGS/PRECAUTIONS: Rapid onset of CNS depressant effects; ingest only at bedtime and while in bed. Avoid engaging in activities requiring mental alertness for 6 hrs after ingestion. Daily sodium intake ranges from 0.5g (with 3g dose) to 1.6g (with 9g dose); caution in heart failure, HTN, or renal impairment. Caution with compromised respiratory function, hepatic insufficiency, history of depressive illness or suicide attempts, elderly. Evaluate patients who develop through disorders or behavior abnormalities. Sleepwalking reported. Rule out worsening sleep apnea or nocturnal seizures if incontinence develops.

ADVERSE REACTIONS: Headache, nausea, dizziness, pain, somnolence, pharyngitis, infection, flu syndrome, diarrhea, urinary incontinence, vomiting, rhinitis, asthenia, sinusitis, nervousness, back pain, confusion, sleepwalking, depression, dyspepsia, abdominal pain, abnormal dreams, insomnia.

INTERACTIONS: Avoid alcohol, sedative hypnotics, or other CNS depressants. Food decreases bioavailability.

PREGNANCY: Category B, caution in nursing.

MECHANISM OF ACTION: CNS depressant agent; effect on cataplexy not established, causes CNS depression.

PHARMACOKINETICS: Absorption: Rapid (incomplete); absolute bioavailabiltiy (25%). C_{max}=78mcg/mL (1st peak), 142mcg/mL (2nd peak); T_{max}=0.5-1.25 hr. **Distribution:** V_d=190-384mL/kg; plasma protein binding (<1%). **Metabolism:** Liver via CYP450. **Elimination:** By transformation to CO_2 eliminated by expiration. Urine (<5%), feces; $T_{1/2}$=0.5-1 hr.

XYZAL

RX

levocetirizine dihydrochloride (UCB)

THERAPEUTIC CLASS: H_1-antagonist

INDICATIONS: Relief of symptoms associated with seasonal and perennial allergic rhinitis. Treatment of uncomplicated skin manifestations of chronic idiopathic urticaria.

DOSAGE: *Adults:* 5mg qd in evening. Adjust dose with decreased renal function.
Pediatrics: ≥12 yrs: 5mg qd in evening. Adjust dose with decreased renal function. 6-11 yrs: 2.5mg (1/2 tab) qd in evening.

HOW SUPPLIED: Sol: 2.5mg/5mL; Tab: 5mg* *scored

CONTRAINDICATIONS: End stage renal disease (CrCl <10mL/min) or hemodialysis. Pediatrics 6-11 yrs with renal impairment.

YAZ

WARNINGS/PRECAUTIONS: May impair mental/physical abilities.

ADVERSE REACTIONS: Somnolence, fatigue, dry mouth, headache, nasopharyngitis, abdominal pain, cough, epistaxis, asthenia, pharyngitis.

INTERACTIONS: Avoid alcohol and CNS depressants. Possible decreased clearance with large doses of theophylline.

PREGNANCY: Category B, not for use in nursing.

MECHANISM OF ACTION: Antihistamine; inhibits H_1-receptor.

PHARMACOKINETICS: Absorption: Rapid, extensive; C_{max}=270ng/mL (single dose), 308ng/mL (multiple doses); T_{max}=0.9 hrs. **Distribution:** V_d=0.4L/kg; plasma protein binding (91-92%). Found in breast milk. **Metabolism:** Through aromatic oxidation, N and O-dealkylation and taurine conjugation pathways, via CYP3A4. **Elimination:** Urine (58.4%), feces (12.9%); $T_{1/2}$=8 hrs.

YAZ   RX
drospirenone - ethinyl estradiol (Berlex)

THERAPEUTIC CLASS: Estrogen/progestogen combination

INDICATIONS: Prevention of pregnancy. Treatment of symptoms of premenstrual dysphoric disorder (PMDD). Treatment of moderate acne vulgaris in women ≥14 yrs.

DOSAGE: *Adults:* 1 tab qd for 28 days (24 active plus 4 inert pills), then repeat. Start 1st Sunday after menses begin or 1st day of menses.
Pediatrics: ≥14 yrs: Acne: 1 tab qd for 28 days (24 active plus 4 inert pills), then repeat. Start 1st Sunday after menses begin or 1st day of menses.

HOW SUPPLIED: Tab: (Ethinyl Estradiol-Drospirenone) 0.02mg-3mg

CONTRAINDICATIONS: Renal or adrenal insufficiency, hepatic dysfunction, thrombophlebitis, thromboembolic disorders, history of deep vein thrombophlebitis, valvular heart disease with thrombogenic complications, severe HTN, DM with vascular involvement, HA with focal neurological symptoms, major surgery with prolonged immobilization, cerebrovascular or CAD, breast carcinoma, endometrial carcinoma, estrogen-dependent neoplasia, undiagnosed abnormal genital bleeding, cholestatic jaundice of pregnancy or jaundice with prior pill use, liver tumor, active liver disease, pregnancy, heavy smoking (>15 cigarettes daily) and >35 yrs.

WARNINGS/PRECAUTIONS: Cigarette smoking increases risk of serious CV side effects. Risk increases with age (especially >35 yrs) and with heavy smoking. Increased risk of MI, thromboembolism, thrombotic disease, cerebrovascular events, and gallbladder disease. Monitor K^+ levels during first cycle with conditions predisposing to hyperkalemia. Retinal thrombosis, hepatic neoplasia, carcinoma of breast and reproductive organs reported. May cause glucose intolerance. May increase BP, elevate LDL levels or cause other lipid changes, fluid retention, breakthrough bleeding and spotting. May cause or exacerbate migraine. May develop visual changes with contact lens. Increased risk of MI with HTN, hyperlipidemia, obesity and DM. D/C if jaundice, significant depression or ophthalmic irregularities develop. Use before menarche is not indicated.

ADVERSE REACTIONS: Nausea, vomiting, breakthrough bleeding, spotting, amenorrhea, migraine, mental depression, vaginal candidiasis, edema, weight changes, depression decrease in serum folate levels, aggravation of varicose veins, uritcaria, angioedema, severe reactions with respiratory and circulatory symptoms, dysmenorrhea.

INTERACTIONS: Reduced effects, increased breakthrough bleeding, and menstrual irregularities with rifampin, phenobarbital, phenytoin, carbamazepine, possibly with griseofulvin, ampicillin, tetracycline, St. John's wort, and phenylbutazone. Increased levels with atorvastatin, ascorbic acid and APAP. Risk of hyperkalemia with ACE inhibitors, angiotensin-II receptor antagonists, potassium-sparing diuretics, heparin, aldosterone antagonists, and NSAIDs; monitor K^+ levels during 1st cycle. Increased levels of cyclosporine, prednisolone, and theophylline. May decrease APAP levels and increase clearance of temazepam, salicylic acid, morphine, and clofibric acid.

PREGNANCY: Category X, not for use in nursing.

MECHANISM OF ACTION: Estrogen/progestogen oral contraceptive; acts by suppressing gonadotropins, inhibiting ovulation, and causing other alterations, including changes in the cervical mucus (which increases difficulty of sperm entry into uterus) and the endometrium (which reduces likelihood of implantation).

PHARMACOKINETICS: Absorption: Drospirenone (DRSP): Absolute bioavailability (76%); (Cycle 1/Day 21) C_{max}=70.3ng/mL; T_{max}=1.5 hrs; AUC=763ng•h/mL. Ethinyl estradiol (EE): Absolute bioavailability (40%); (Cycle 1/Day 21) C_{max}=45.1pg/mL; T_{max}=1.5 hrs; AUC=220pg•h/mL. **Distribution:** DRSP: V_d=4L/kg; serum protein binding (97%). EE: V_d=4-5L/kg; serum albumin binding (98.5%). **Metabolism:** DRSP: Liver, via CYP3A4 (minor). EE: Hydroxylation (via CYP3A4), conjugation (glucuronidation and sulfation). **Elimination:** DRSP: Urine, feces; $T_{1/2}$=30 hrs. EE: Urine, feces; $T_{1/2}$=24 hrs.

YF-VAX
RX
yellow fever vaccine (Sanofi Pasteur)

THERAPEUTIC CLASS: Vaccine

INDICATIONS: Active immunization of persons ≥9 months living or traveling to endemic areas or for international travel when required or laboratory personnel who might be exposed to virulent yellow fever virus.

DOSAGE: *Adults:* Primary Vaccination: 0.5mL (4.74 $\log_{10}$ PFU) SQ. Booster: 0.5mL (4.74 $\log_{10}$ PFU) every 10 yrs. Desensitization: 0.05mL of 1:10 dilution, then 0.05mL of full strength, then 0.10mL of full strength, then 0.15mL of full strength, then 0.20mL of full strength SQ at 15-20 min intervals.
Pediatrics: ≥9 months: Primary Vaccination: 0.5mL (4.74 $\log_{10}$ PFU) SQ. Booster: 0.5mL (4.74 $\log_{10}$ PFU) every 10 yrs. Desensitization: 0.05mL of 1:10 dilution, then 0.05mL of full strength, then 0.10mL of full strength, then 0.15mL of full strength, then 0.20mL of full strength SQ at 15-20 min intervals.

HOW SUPPLIED: Inj: 4.74 $\log_{10}$ PFU/0.5mL

CONTRAINDICATIONS: Hypersensitivity to eggs or egg products. Immunosuppressed patients due to illness (eg, HIV infection, leukemia, lymphoma, thymoma, generalized malignancy) or drug therapy (eg, corticosteroids, alkylating drugs, or antimetabolites) or radiation.

WARNINGS/PRECAUTIONS: Epinephrine (1:1000) should be immediately available. Vaccine-associated viscerotropic disease (rare) and vaccine-associated neurotropic disease (rare).

ADVERSE REACTIONS: Systemic: Headache, myalgia, low-grade fevers. Local: Edema, hypersensitivity, pain or mass at injection site.

INTERACTIONS: Prednisone and other corticosteroids may decrease immunogenicity and increase risk of adverse events.

PREGNANCY: Category C, not for use in nursing.

MECHANISM OF ACTION: Stimulates immune system to produce antibodies that may protect against yellow fever.

ZADITOR
OTC
ketotifen fumarate (Novartis Ophthalmics)

THERAPEUTIC CLASS: H_1-antagonist and mast cell stabilizer

INDICATIONS: Temporary prevention of itching of the eye due to allergic conjunctivitis.

DOSAGE: *Adults:* 1 drop q8-12h.
Pediatrics: ≥3 yrs: 1 drop q8-12h.

HOW SUPPLIED: Sol: 0.025% (5mL)

WARNINGS/PRECAUTIONS: Not for contact lens irritation. Do not wear a contact lens if eye is red. If eyes are not red, wait 10 minutes after instillation before inserting contacts. Soft contact lens can absorb benzalkonium chloride.

ADVERSE REACTIONS: Rhinitis, allergic reactions, burning, stinging, conjunctivitis, dry eye, eye pain, eyelid disorder, itching, keratitis, lacrimation disorder, mydriasis, photophobia, headache, rash.

PREGNANCY: Category C, caution in nursing.

ZANTAC
ranitidine HCl (GlaxoSmithKline)

RX

THERAPEUTIC CLASS: H_2-blocker

INDICATIONS: (PO) Short-term treatment of active duodenal (DU) and benign gastric ulcers (GU). Maintenance therapy for duodenal and gastric ulcers. Treatment of pathological hypersecretory conditions (eg, Zollinger-Ellison) and GERD. Treatment and maintenance of erosive esophagitis. (Inj) Hospitalized patients with pathological hypersecretory conditions or intractable duodenal ulcer. Short-term alternate to oral therapy.

DOSAGE: *Adults:* (PO) DU/GU: 150mg bid or (DU) 300mg after evening meal or qhs. Maint: 150mg qhs. GERD: 150mg bid. Erosive Esophagitis: 150mg qid. Maint: 150mg bid. Hypersecretory Conditions: 150mg bid. May give up to 6g/day with severe disease. (Inj) Usual: 50mg IV/IM q6-8 hrs or 6.25mg/hr continuous IV. Max: 400mg/day. Zollinger-Ellison: Initial: 1mg/kg/hr. Titrate: May increase after 4 hrs by 0.5mg/kg/hr increments. Max: 2.5mg/kg/hr or 220mg/hr. CrCl <50mL/min: 50mg IV q18-24 hrs or 150mg PO q24h. Give more frequent (q12h) if necessary. Hemodialysis: Give dose at end of treatment. Dissolve each 150mg effervescent tab in 6-8oz of water before administration.
Pediatrics: 1 month-16 yrs: (PO) DU/GU: 2-4mg/kg bid. Max: 300mg/day. Maint: 2-4mg/kg qd. Max: 150mg/day. GERD/Erosive Esophagitis: 2.5-5mg/kg bid. (Inj) DU: 2-4mg/kg/day IV given q6-8 hrs. Max: 50mg q6-8 hrs. CrCl <50mL/min: 50mg IV q18-24 hrs or 150mg PO q24h. Give more frequent (q12h) if necessary. Hemodialysis: Give dose at end of treatment. Dissolve each 25mg effervescent tab in 5mL of water before administration.

HOW SUPPLIED: Inj: 1mg/mL, 25mg/mL; Syrup: 15mg/mL; Tab: 150mg, 300mg; Tab, Effervescent: 25mg

WARNINGS/PRECAUTIONS: Do not exceed recommended infusion rates; bradycardia reported with rapid infusion. Caution with liver and renal dysfunction. Monitor SGPT if on IV therapy for ≥5 days at dose >100mg qid. Avoid use with history of acute porphyria. Symptomatic response does not preclude the presence of gastric malignancy. May cause false (+) urine protein test. Granules and effervescent tablets contain phenylalanine.

ADVERSE REACTIONS: Headache, constipation, diarrhea, nausea, abdominal discomfort, vomiting, hepatitis, blood dyscrasias, rash, injection site reactions (IV/IM).

INTERACTIONS: Increases plasma levels of triazolam. Monitor anticoagulants.

PREGNANCY: Category B, caution with nursing.

MECHANISM OF ACTION: H_2-blocker; competitive, reversible inhibitor of histamine action at histamine H_2-receptors, including those found on gastric cells.

PHARMACOKINETICS: Absorption: (PO, 150mg) C_{max}=440-545ng/mL, T_{max}=2-3 hrs; (IM) Rapid; C_{max}= 576ng/mL, T_{max}=15 min. **Distribution:** V_d = 1.4L/kg; plasma protein binding (15%); found in breast milk. **Metabolism:** Liver, N-oxide (principal metabolite). **Elimination:** Urine, (PO 30% unchanged); (IV 70% unchanged); (PO) $T_{1/2}$=2.5-3 hrs, (IV) $T_{1/2}$=2-2.5 hrs. Refer to PI for pediatric parameters.

ZANTAC OTC
ranitidine HCl (Boehringer Ingelheim)

OTC

OTHER BRAND NAMES: Zantac 150 (Boehringer Ingelheim) - Zantac 75 (Boehringer Ingelheim)

THERAPEUTIC CLASS: H_2-blocker

INDICATIONS: For prevention and relief of heartburn associated with acid indigestion and sour stomach brought on by certain foods and beverages.

DOSAGE: *Adults:* Treatment/Relief of Heartburn: 75-150mg with water. Heartburn Prevention: 75-150mg 30-60 min before eating food or drinking beverages that cause heartburn. Max: 300mg/24 hrs.
Pediatrics: ≥12 yrs: Treatment/Relief of Heartburn: 75-150mg with water. Heartburn Prevention: 75-150mg 30-60 min before eating food or drinking beverages that cause heartburn. Max: 300mg/24 hrs.

HOW SUPPLIED: Tab: 75mg, 150mg

WARNINGS/PRECAUTIONS: Do not use if trouble or pain swallowing food, vomiting with blood, or bloody or black stools; with other acid reducers; or in patients with kidney disease. D/C if heartburn continues/worsens or use for >14 days.

INTERACTIONS: Avoid other acid reducers.

PREGNANCY: Safety in pregnancy and nursing not known.

MECHANISM OF ACTION: H_2-blocker; competitive, reversible inhibitor of histamine action at histamine H_2-receptors, including those found on gastric cells.

PHARMACOKINETICS: Apsorption: C_{max}=440-545ng/mL, T_{max}=2-3 hrs (IV). **Distribution:** V_d=1.4L/kg; serum protein binding (15%). **Metabolism:** Liver. **Elimination:** Urine 80% (unchanged); $T_{1/2}$=2.5-3 hrs (PO).

ZARONTIN
ethosuximide (Parke-Davis)

RX

THERAPEUTIC CLASS: Succinimide

INDICATIONS: Control of absence (petit mal) epilepsy.

DOSAGE: *Adults:* 500mg qd. Titrate: May increase daily dose by 250mg every 4-7 days. Max: 1.5g/day.
Pediatrics: Initial: 3-6 yrs: 250mg qd. ≥6 yrs: 500mg qd. Titrate: May increase daily dose by 250mg every 4-7 days. Usual: 20mg/kg/day. Max: 1.5g/day.

HOW SUPPLIED: Cap: 250mg; Syrup: 250mg/5mL

WARNINGS/PRECAUTIONS: Extreme caution in liver and renal dysfunction. Monitor blood counts, liver and renal function periodically. SLE, blood dyscrasias reported. Adjust dose slowly and avoid abrupt withdrawal. May increase grand mal seizures in mixed types of epilepsy when used alone. Caution with mental/physical activities.

ADVERSE REACTIONS: Anorexia, nausea, vomiting, abdominal pain, blood dyscrasias, drowsiness, headache, urticaria, SLE, myopia.

INTERACTIONS: May increase phenytoin levels. Valproic acid may alter levels.

PREGNANCY: Safety in pregnancy and nursing not known.

MECHANISM OF ACTION: Succinimide anticonvulsant; suppresses paroxysmal 3 cycles/second spike and wave activity associated with lapses of consciousness, which is common in absence (petit mal) seizures. Frequency of attacks is reduced through depression of motor cortex and elevation of the CNS threshold to convulsive stimuli.

PHARMACOKINETICS: Distribution: Crosses placenta, found in breast milk.

ZEMPLAR IV
paricalcitol (Abbott)

RX

THERAPEUTIC CLASS: Vitamin D analog

INDICATIONS: Prevention and treatment of secondary hyperparathyroidism associated with chronic kidney disease Stage 5.

DOSAGE: *Adults:* Initial: 0.04-0.1mcg/kg bolus no more frequently than every other day during dialysis. Max: 0.24mcg/kg (16.8mcg). Titrate: May increase by 2-4mcg at 2-4 week intervals. Monitor serum Ca and phosphorus more frequently during dose adjustments. Reduce or interrupt dose if elevated Ca level or Ca x P product >75, may reinitiate at lower dose once normalized. May need dose decrease as PTH levels decrease (see PI).
Pediatrics: ≥5 yrs: (Inj) Initial: 0.04-0.1mcg/kg bolus no more frequently than every other day during dialysis. Max: 0.24mcg/kg (16.8mcg). Titrate: May increase by 2-4mcg at 2-4 week intervals. Monitor serum Ca and phosphorus more frequently during dose adjustments. Reduce or interrupt dose if elevated Ca level or Ca x P product >75, may reinitiate at lower dose once normalized. May need dose decrease as PTH levels decrease (see PI).

HOW SUPPLIED: Inj: 2mcg/mL, 5mcg/mL

CONTRAINDICATIONS: Vitamin D toxicity, hypercalcemia.

WARNINGS/PRECAUTIONS: Overdose may cause progressive hypercalcemia. Should supplement with calcium and restrict phosphorus. May need phosphate-binding compounds to control serum phosphorus levels. Avoid concomitant phosphate or vitamin D-related compounds.

ADVERSE REACTIONS: Nausea, vomiting, edema, chills, flu, GI bleeding, lightheadedness, pneumonia, pain, allergic reaction, headache, HTN, diarrhea, arthritis, rash.

INTERACTIONS: Digitalis toxicity potentiated by hypercalcemia. Avoid excessive use of aluminum containing compounds.

PREGNANCY: Category C, caution in nursing.

MECHANISM OF ACTION: Synthetic vitamin D analog; binds to vitamin D receptor, which results in selective activation of vitamin D pathways. Shown to reduce parathyroid hormone levels by inhibiting PTH synthesis and secretion.

PHARMACOKINETICS: Absorption: C_{max}=1.680ng/mL (hemodialysis), 1.832ng/mL (peritoneal dialysis); AUC= 14.51ng•h/mL (hemodialysis), 16.01ng•h/mL (peritoneal dialysis). **Distribution:** V_d=23.8L (healthy), 31L (hemodialysis), and 35L (peritoneal dialysis); plasma protein binding (≥99.8%). **Metabolism:** Hepatic, via hydroxylation and glucuronidation; CYP24, CYP3A4, UGT1A4. **Elimination:** Hepatobiliary excretion (primary), urine (19%), feces (63%); $T_{1/2}$=13.9 hrs (hemodialysis), 15.4 hrs (peritoneal dialysis).

ZEMURON   RX
rocuronium bromide (Organon USA)

THERAPEUTIC CLASS: Skeletal muscle relaxant (nondepolarizing)

INDICATIONS: Adjunct to general anesthesia to facilitate both rapid sequence and routine tracheal intubation, and to provide skeletal muscle relaxation during surgery or mechanical ventilation

DOSAGE: *Adults:* Individualize dose. Rapid Sequence Intubation: 0.6-1.2mg/kg; Tracheal Intubation: Initial: 0.6mg/kg. Maint: 0.1, 0.15, or 0.2mg/kg. Continous Infusion: Initial: 10-12mcg/kg/min. Range: 4-16mcg/kg/min.
Pediatrics: 3 months-14 yrs: Individualize dose. Initial: 0.6mg/kg.

HOW SUPPLIED: Inj: 10mg/mL

WARNINGS/PRECAUTIONS: Employ peripheral nerve stimulator to monitor drug response. May have profound effects with myasthenia gravis or myasthenic (Eaton-Lambert) syndrome; use small test dose and monitor closely. Do not mix with alkaline solutions (eg, barbiturate solutions) in the same syringe or administer simultaneously during IV infusion through the same needle. Anaphylactic reactions reported. Tolerance may develop during chronic administration. Not recommended for rapid sequence induction in Cesarean section. Caution with clinically significant hepatic disease. Conditions associated with slower circulation time (eg, cardiovascular disease or advanced age) may delay onset time. Electrolyte imbalances may enhance neuromuscular blockade.

ADVERSE REACTIONS: Arrhythmia, abnormal ECG, tachycardia, nausea, vomiting, asthma, hiccup, rash, injection site edema, pruritus.

INTERACTIONS: Use of inhalation anesthetics has been shown to enhance the activity of other neuromuscular blocking agents. Resistance observed with chronic anticonvulsant therapy. Certain antibiotics (eg, aminoglycosides, vancomycin; tetracyclines, bacitracin, polymyxins, colistin, and sodium colistimethate) may cause prolongation of neuromuscular block. Quinidine injection during recovery from use of other muscle relaxants suggests that recurrent paralysis may occur. Magnesium salts may enhance neuromuscular blockade.

PREGNANCY: Category C, safety in nursing not known.

MECHANISM OF ACTION: Non-depolarizing neuromuscular blocking agent; acts by competing for cholinergic receptors at the motor end-plate.

PHARMACOKINETICS: Distribution: V_d=0.25L/Kg; plasma protein binding (30%). **Metabolism:** Liver via CYP450. **Elimination:** $T_{1/2}$=1.4 hrs.

ZENAPAX
daclizumab (Roche Labs)

RX

THERAPEUTIC CLASS: Immunosuppressive agent

INDICATIONS: For prophylaxis of acute organ rejection in renal transplants, in combination with cyclosporine and corticosteroids.

DOSAGE: *Adults:* 1mg/kg IV over 15 min for 5 doses. Administer 1st dose no more than 24 hrs prior to transplant and remaining 4 doses at 14-day intervals.
Pediatrics: ≥11 months: 1mg/kg IV over 15 min for 5 doses. Administer 1st dose no more than 24 hrs prior to transplant and remaining 4 doses at 14-day intervals.

HOW SUPPLIED: Inj: 25mg/5mL

WARNINGS/PRECAUTIONS: Increased risk of lymphoproliferative disorder and opportunistic infections. Anaphylactic reactions reported. Caution in elderly. Re-administration after initial course of therapy has not been studied in humans.

ADVERSE REACTIONS: Constipation, nausea, vomiting, diarrhea, abdominal pain, pyrosis, dyspepsia, abdominal distention, epigastric pain.

PREGNANCY: Category C, not for use in nursing.

MECHANISM OF ACTION: IL-2 receptor antagonist; binds with high affinity to the Tac subunit of the high affinity IL-2 receptor complex and inhibits IL-2 binding.

PHARMACOKINETICS: Absorption: C_{max}=7.6µg/mL (adult); 5.0µg/mL (pediatric). **Elimination:** $T_{1/2}$=20 days (adult), 13 days (pediatric).

ZERIT
stavudine (Bristol-Myers Squibb)

RX

> Lactic acidosis and severe, fatal hepatomegaly reported. Fatal and non-fatal pancreatitis reported with didanosine.

THERAPEUTIC CLASS: Synthetic thymidine nucleoside analogue

INDICATIONS: Treatment of HIV-1 infection in combination with other antiretrovirals.

DOSAGE: *Adults:* ≥60kg: 40mg q12h. <60kg: 30mg q12h. Interrupt therapy if develop peripheral neuropathy, resume at 1/2 dose when neuropathy resolves. D/C permanently if neuropathy recurs after resumption. Suspend therapy if lactic acidosis or hepatotoxicity occurs. CrCl 26-50mL/min: ≥60kg: 20mg q12h. <60kg: 15mg q12h. CrCl 10-25mL/min: ≥60kg: 20mg q24h. <60kg: 15mg q24h.
Pediatrics: ≥60kg: 40mg q12h. 30-59 kg: 30mg q12h. ≥14 days and <30kg: 1mg/kg q12h. Birth-13 days: 0.5mg/kg q12h. Interrupt therapy if develop peripheral neuropathy, resume with 1/2 dose when neuropathy resolves. D/C permanently if neuropathy recurs after resumption. Suspend therapy if lactic acidosis or hepatotoxicity occurs. Renal Impairment: Reduce dose and/or increase interval.

HOW SUPPLIED: Cap: 15mg, 20mg, 30mg, 40mg; Sus: 1mg/mL (200mL)

WARNINGS/PRECAUTIONS: Obesity and prolonged nucleoside exposure may increase risk to lactic acidosis and hepatomegaly. Caution with risk factors for hepatic disease. Peripheral neuropathy reported. Monitor for lactic acidosis in pregnancy if used with didanosine. D/C if motor weakness develops.

ADVERSE REACTIONS: Peripheral neuropathy, rash, elevated LFTs and amylase, headache, diarrhea, NV.

INTERACTIONS: Avoid zidovudine. Increased risk of neuropathy with neurotoxic drugs (eg, didanosine). Increased risk of hepatotoxicity with didanosine and hydroxyurea. Motor weakness reported with other antiretrovirals.

PREGNANCY: Category C, not for use in nursing.

MECHANISM OF ACTION: Thymidine nucleoside analogue; inhibits activity of HIV-1 reverse transcriptase by competing with natural substrate thymidine triphosphate and by DNA chain termination following incorporation into viral DNA. Inhibits cellular DNA polymerases β and gamma and markedly reduces synthesis of mitochondrial DNA.

PHARMACOKINETICS: Absorption: Rapidly absorbed; C_{max}=536±146ng/mL; T_{max}=1 hr; AUC=2568±454ng.h/mL. **Distribution:** V_d=46±21L (adults); V_d=0.73+/-0.32L/kg (age 5

weeks to 15 yrs). **Elimination**: Renal (40%); $T_{1/2}$=1.15±0.35 hrs (IV, adult), 1.6±0.23 hrs (PO, adult); $T_{1/2}$=1.11+/-0.28 hrs (IV, age 5 weeks to 15 yrs); $T_{1/2}$= 0.96+/-0.26 hrs (PO, age 5 weeks to 15 yrs).

ZESTRIL
lisinopril (AstraZeneca)

RX

> ACE inhibitors can cause death/injury to developing fetus during 2nd and 3rd trimesters. D/C if pregnancy is detected.

THERAPEUTIC CLASS: ACE inhibitor

INDICATIONS: Treatment of HTN. Adjunct therapy in heart failure if inadequately controlled by diuretics and digitalis. Adjunct therapy in stable patients within 24 hrs of AMI to improve survival.

DOSAGE: *Adults:* HTN: If possible, d/c diuretic 2-3 days prior to therapy. Initial: 10mg qd, 5mg qd with diuretic. Usual: 20-40mg qd. Resume diuretic if BP not controlled. Max: 80mg/day. CrCl 10-30mL/min: Initial: 5mg/day. Max: 40mg/day. CrCl <10mL/min: Initial: 2.5mg/day. Max: 40mg/day. Heart Failure: Initial: 5mg qd. Usual: 5-40mg qd. May increase by 10mg every 2 weeks. Max: 40mg/day. Hyponatremia or CrCl ≤30mL/min: Initial: 2.5mg qd. AMI: Initial: 5mg within 24 hrs, then 5mg after 24 hrs, then 10mg after 48 hrs, then 10mg qd. Use 2.5mg during first 3 days with low SBP. Maint: 10mg qd for 6 weeks, 2.5-5mg with hypotension. D/C with prolonged hypotension. Elderly: Caution with dose adjustment.
Pediatrics: ≥6 yrs: HTN: Initial: 0.07mg/kg qd up to 5mg total. Dose adjust according to response. Max: 0.61mg/kg or 40mg.

HOW SUPPLIED: Tab: 2.5mg, 5mg, 10mg, 20mg, 30mg, 40mg

CONTRAINDICATIONS: History of ACE inhibitor-associated angioedema, hereditary or idiopathic angioedema.

WARNINGS/PRECAUTIONS: D/C if angioedema, jaundice, or marked LFT elevation occur. Risk of hyperkalemia, hypoglycemia with DM, renal dysfunction. Persistent nonproductive cough reported. Monitor WBCs in renal and collagen vascular disease. Anaphylactoid reactions during membrane exposure reported. Fetal/neonatal morbidity and death reported. Monitor for hypotension in high-risk patients (heart failure with SBP <100mmHg, surgery/anesthesia, hyponatremia, high-dose diuretic therapy, severe volume and/or salt depletion, etc). Caution with CHF, aortic stenosis/hypertrophic cardiomyopathy, renal dysfunction, and renal artery stenosis. Less effective on BP in blacks and more reports of angioedema than nonblacks.

ADVERSE REACTIONS: Hypotension, diarrhea, headache, dizziness, hyperkalemia, chest pain, cough, cutaneous pseudolymphoma.

INTERACTIONS: May increase lithium levels. Hypotension risk with diuretics. Concomitant use with antidiabetic medications may increase risk of hypoglycemia. Increase risk of hyperkalemia with K⁺-sparing diuretics, K⁺-containing salt substitutes, or K⁺ supplements. Indomethacin may reduce effects. Nitritoid reactions with gold.

PREGNANCY: Category C (1st trimester) and D (2nd and 3rd trimesters), not for use in nursing.

MECHANISM OF ACTION: ACE inhibitor; inhibition results in decreased plasma angiotensin II, which leads to decreased vasopressor activity and aldosterone secretion.

PHARMACOKINETICS: Absorption: T_{max}=7 hrs. **Elimination:** Urine (unchanged); $T_{1/2}$=12 hrs.

ZETACET
sulfacetamide sodium - sulfur (Various)

RX

OTHER BRAND NAME: Sufacetamide Sodium/Sulfur (Various)

THERAPEUTIC CLASS: Sulfonamide/sulfur combination

INDICATIONS: Topical treatment of acne vulgaris, acne rosacea, and seborrheic dermatitis.

DOSAGE: *Adults:* Apply a thin layer qd-tid. Shake well before use.
Pediatrics: ≥12 yrs: Apply a thin layer qd-tid. Shake well before use.

HOW SUPPLIED: Lot: (Sulfacetamide-Sulfur) 10%-5% (25g)

CONTRAINDICATIONS: Kidney disease.

WARNINGS/PRECAUTIONS: Caution with denuded or abraded skin. Caution in patients prone to hypersensitivity to topical sulfonamides. D/C if irritation occurs. For external use only; avoid eye contact. Can cause reddening and scaling of epidermis.

ADVERSE REACTIONS: Local irritation.

PREGNANCY: Category C, caution in nursing.

ZIAGEN
abacavir sulfate (GlaxoSmithKline)

RX

> Fatal hypersensitivity reactions, lactic acidosis, severe hepatomegaly with steatosis, including fatal cases reported. D/C if hypersensitivity reaction is suspected and do not restart.

THERAPEUTIC CLASS: Synthetic carbocyclic nucleoside analogue

INDICATIONS: Treatment of HIV-1 infection in combination with other antiretrovirals.

DOSAGE: *Adults:* >16 yrs: 300mg bid or 600mg qd.
Pediatrics: 3 months-16 yrs: 8mg/kg bid. Max: 300mg bid.

HOW SUPPLIED: Sol: 20mg/mL (240mL); Tab: 300mg

WARNINGS/PRECAUTIONS: Register abacavir hypersensitive patients at 800-270-0425. Caution with liver disease; lactic acidosis and severe hepatomegaly with steatosis, including fatal cases, reported. Not for monotherapy when antiretroviral regimens are changed. Immune reconstitution syndrome reported. Should not be coadministered with Epzicom or Trizivir.

ADVERSE REACTIONS: Hypersensitivity reactions (eg, fever, rash, fatigue, GI symptoms), NV, diarrhea, loss of appetite, insomnia, chills, headache, fatigue.

INTERACTIONS: Decreased elimination with ethanol.

PREGNANCY: Category C, not for use in nursing.

MECHANISM OF ACTION: Carbocyclic nucleoside analogue; inhibits HIV-1 reverse transcriptase (RT) by competing with natural substrate dGTP and incorporating into viral DNA.

PHARMACOKINETICS: **Absorption:** Rapid; absolute bioavailability (83%). (BID dosing) C_{max}= 3mcg/mL, AUC_{0-12h}=6.02mcg•hr/mL. (QD dosing) C_{max}= 4.26mcg/mL, AUC=11.95mcg•hr/mL. **Distribution:** (IV) V_d=0.86L/kg; plasma protein binding (50%). **Metabolism:** Hepatic, via alcohol dehydrogenase and glucuronyl transferase. **Elimination:** Urine (1.2%); (QD dosing) $T_{1/2}$=1.54 hrs.

ZIANA
clindamycin phosphate - tretinoin (Medicis)

RX

THERAPEUTIC CLASS: Lincosamide derivative/retinoid

INDICATIONS: Topical treatment of acne vulgaris.

DOSAGE: *Adults:* Apply pea-sized amount to entire face qd at bedtime. Avoid eyes, mouth, angles of nose, or mucous membranes. Not for oral, ophthalmic, or intravaginal use.
Pediatrics: ≥12 yrs: Apply pea-sized amount to entire face qd at bedtime. Avoid eyes, mouth, angles of nose, or mucous membranes. Not for oral, ophthalmic, or intravaginal use.

HOW SUPPLIED: Gel: (Clindamycin-Tretinoin) 1.2%-0.025% (2g, 30g, 60g)

CONTRAINDICATIONS: Regional enteritis, ulcerative colitis, or history of antibiotic-associated colitis.

WARNINGS/PRECAUTIONS: May cause severe colitis; d/c if significant diarrhea occurs. Avoid exposure to sunlight and sunlamps; wear sunscreen daily.

ADVERSE REACTIONS: Nasopharyngitis, erythema, scaling, itching, burning.

INTERACTIONS: Caution with concomitant topical medications, medicated/abrasive soaps and cleansers, soaps/cosmetics with strong drying effect, products with high concentrations of alcohol, astringents, spices, or lime. Avoid with erythromycin-containing products. Caution with neuromuscular blocking agents.

PREGNANCY: Category C, not for use in nursing.

MECHANISM OF ACTION: Clindamycin: Lincosamide antibiotic; binds to 50S ribosomal subunits of susceptible bacteria and prevents elongation of peptide chains by interfering with peptidyl transfer, thereby suppressing bacterial protein synthesis. Found to have activity against *P.acnes*. Tretinoin: Retinoid; mechanism not established. Suspected to decrease cohesiveness of follicular epithelial cells with decreased micromedo formation. Also responsible for stimulating miotic activity and increasing turnover of follicular epithelial cells, causing extrusion of comedones.

PHARMACOKINETICS: Absorption: Tretinoin: Percutaneous (minimal). **Distribution:** Orally and parenterally administered clindamycin found in breast milk. **Metabolism:** Tretinoin: 13-cis-retinoic acid and 4-oxo-13-cis-retinoic acid (metabolites).

ZINACEF   RX
cefuroxime (GlaxoSmithKline)

THERAPEUTIC CLASS: Cephalosporin (2nd generation)

INDICATIONS: Treatment of septicemia; meningitis; gonorrhea; lower respiratory tract, urinary tract, skin and skin structure (SSSI), and bone and joint infections caused by susceptible strains of microorganisms. For preoperative and perioperative surgical prophylaxis.

DOSAGE: *Adults:* Usual: 750mg-1.5g q8h for 5-10 days. Uncomplicated Pneumonia and UTI/SSSI/Disseminated Gonococcal Infections: 750mg q8h. Severe/Complicated Infections: 1.5g q8h. Bone and Joint Infections: 1.5g q8h. Life-Threatening Infections/ Infections With Susceptible Organisms: 1.5g q6h. Meningitis: Max: 3g q8h. Uncomplicated Gonococcal Infection: 1.5g IM single dose at 2 different sites with 1g PO probenecid. Surgical Prophylaxis: 1.5g IV 0.5-1 hr before incision, then 750mg IM/IV q8h with prolonged procedure. Open Heart Surgery (Perioperative): 1.5g IV at induction of anesthesia and q12h thereafter, for total of 6g. Renal Impairment: CrCl 10-20mL/min: 750mg q12h. CrCl <10mL/min: 750mg q24h. Hemodialysis: Give further dose at end of dialysis.
Pediatrics: >3 months: Usual: 50-100mg/kg/day in divided doses q6-8h. Severe Infections: 100mg/kg/day (not to exceed max adult dose). Bone and Joint Infections: 150mg/kg/day in divided doses q8h (not to exceed max adult dose). Meningitis: 200-240mg/kg/day IV in divided doses q6-8h. Renal Dysfunction: Modify dosing frequency consistent with adult recommendations.

HOW SUPPLIED: Inj: 750mg, 1.5g, 7.5g, 750mg/50mL, 1.5g/50mL

WARNINGS/PRECAUTIONS: Cross-sensitivity to PCNs and other cephalosporins may occur. *Clostridium difficile*-associated diarrhea reported, ranging in severity from mild diarrhea to fatal colitis. Monitor renal function. May result in overgrowth of nonsusceptible organisms. Caution with history of GI disease, particularly colitis. Hearing loss in peds being treated for meningitis. Risk of decreased prothrombin activity with renal or hepatic impairment, poor nutritional state, or protracted course of therapy. False (+) urine glucose with copper reduction tests and false (-) with ferricyanide test.

ADVERSE REACTIONS: Thrombophlebitis, GI symptoms, decreased Hgb and Hct, eosinophilia. Transient rise in SGOT, SGPT, alkaline phosphatase, bilirubin, and LDH.

INTERACTIONS: Possible nephrotoxicity with concomitant aminoglycosides. Caution with potent diuretics; may adversely affect renal function. May decrease prothrombin activity; caution with anticoagulants. May reduce efficacy of combined estrogen/ progesterone oral contraceptives.

PREGNANCY: Category B, caution in nursing.

MECHANISM OF ACTION: 2nd-generation cephalosporin; inhibits cell-wall synthesis.

PHARMACOKINETICS: Absorption: C_{max}(750mg IM, IV)=27mcg/mL, 50mcg/mL; T_{max}(750mg IM, IV)=45 min, 15 min. **Distribution:** Plasma protein binding (50%). **Elimination:** Urine; $T_{1/2}$=80 min.

ZITHROMAX
azithromycin (Pfizer)

RX

THERAPEUTIC CLASS: Macrolide

INDICATIONS: Treatment of the following infections caused by susceptible microorganisms: (PO) Acute bacterial exacerbations of COPD, acute bacterial sinusitis (ABS), community-acquired pneumonia (CAP), pharyngitis/tonsillitis, uncomplicated skin and skin structure, urethritis/cervicitis, genital ulcer disease (men), acute otitis media. Prevention (alone) or treatment (with ethambutol) of disseminated *Mycobacterium avium* complex (MAC) disease in advanced HIV infection. (IV) CAP and pelvic inflammatory disease (PID).

DOSAGE: *Adults:* PO: CAP/Pharyngitis/Tonsillitis (2nd-line therapy)/SSSI: 500mg on Day 1, then 250mg qd on Days 2-5. COPD: 500mg qd for 3 days or 500 mg on Day 1, then 250ng qd on Days 2-5. ABS: 500mg qd for 3 days. Genital Ulcer Disease and Nongonococcal Urethritis/Cervicitis: 1g single dose. Gonococcal Urethritis/Cervicitis: 2g single dose. MAC Prophylaxis: 1200mg once weekly. MAC Treatment: 600mg qd with ethambutol 15mg/kg/day. IV: CAP: 500mg qd for at least 2 days, then 500mg PO qd to complete 7-10 day course. PID: 500mg qd for 1-2 days, then 250mg PO qd to complete 7 day course.
Pediatrics: Sus: Otitis Media: ≥6 months: 30mg/kg single dose; 10mg/kg qd for 3 days; or 10mg/kg qd on Day 1, then 5mg/kg qd on Days 2-5. ABS: ≥6 months: 10mg/kg qd for 3 days. CAP: ≥6 months: 10mg/kg qd on Day 1, then 5mg/kg qd on Days 2-5. Sus/Tab: Pharyngitis/Tonsillitis: ≥2 yrs: 12mg/kg qd for 5 days. 1g sus not for pediatric use.

HOW SUPPLIED: Inj: 500mg; Sus: 100mg/5mL (15mL), 200mg/5mL (15mL, 22.5mL, 30mL), 1g/pkt (3^s, 10^9); Tab: 250mg (Z-PAK, 6 tabs), 500mg (TRI-PAK, 3 tabs), 600mg

WARNINGS/PRECAUTIONS: D/C if allergic reaction occurs. Oral therapy only for CAP of mild severity. Hypersensitivity reactions may recur after initial successful symptomatic treatment. *Clostridium difficile*-associated diarrhea reported. Caution with renal/hepatic dysfunction. 1g sus not for pediatric use.

ADVERSE REACTIONS: Diarrhea/loose stools, nausea, abdominal pain, taste/smell perversion.

INTERACTIONS: Monitor theophylline, terfenadine, cyclosporine, hexobarbital, phenytoin, warfarin. May increase digoxin, carbamazepine levels. Potentiates triazolam. Aluminum- and magnesium-containing antacids may reduce PO levels. Acute ergot toxicity may occur with ergotamine or dihydroergotamine. Monitor for side effects (eg, liver enzyme abnormalities, hearing impairment) with nelfinavir.

PREGNANCY: Category B, caution in nursing.

MECHANISM OF ACTION: Macrolide; inhibits protein synthesis by binding 50S ribosomal subunits of susceptible organisms.

PHARMACOKINETICS: Absorption: Administration of variable doses resulted in different parameters. **Distribution:** Plasma protein binding (7-51%). **Elimination:** Biliary (major), urine; $T_{1/2}$=68 hrs.

ZOCOR
simvastatin (Merck)

RX

THERAPEUTIC CLASS: HMG-CoA reductase inhibitor

INDICATIONS: May initiate with diet in patients with, or at high risk for, coronary heart disease (CHD). In high risk patients with CHD, diabetes, peripheral vessel disease, history of stroke or other cerebrovascular disease to reduce risk of total mortality by reducing CHD deaths, risk of non-fatal MI and stroke, need for revascularization procedures. To reduce elevated total-C, LDL-C, Apo B, TG, and increase HDL-C in primary hypercholesterolemia (heterozygous familial and nonfamilial) and mixed dyslipidemia (Types IIa and IIb). To treat hypertriglyceridemia (Type IV) and primary dysbetalipoproteinemia (Type III). To reduce total-C, LDL-C in homozygous familial hypercholesterolemia as adjunct to other lipid-lowering agents or if such treatments are unavailable. To reduce total-C, LDL-C, Apo B in adolescents 10-17 yrs old, at least 1 yr postmenarche, with heterozygous familial hypercholesterolemia. To reduce elevated LDL-C, TG in Type IIb hyperlipidemia.

DOSAGE: *Adults:* Initial: 20-40mg qpm. Usual: 5-80mg/day. Titrate: Adjust at ≥4-week intervals. High Risk for CHD Events: Initial: 40mg/day. Homozygous Familial Hypercholesterolemia: 40mg qpm or 80mg/day given as 20mg bid plus 40mg qpm. Concomitant Cyclosporine: Initial: 5mg/day. Max: 10mg/day. Concomitant Gemfibrozil (try to avoid): Max: 10mg/day. Concomitant Amiodarone/Verapamil: Max: 20mg/day. Severe Renal Insufficiency: 5mg/day; monitor closely.
Pediatrics: Heterozygous Familial Hypercholesterolemia: 10-17 yrs (at least 1 yr postmenarchal): Initial: 10mg qpm. Usual: 10-40mg/day. Titrate: Adjust at ≥4-week intervals. Max: 40mg/day.

HOW SUPPLIED: Tab: 5mg, 10mg, 20mg, 40mg, 80mg

CONTRAINDICATIONS: Active liver disease, unexplained persistent elevations of serum transaminases, pregnancy, nursing mothers.

WARNINGS/PRECAUTIONS: Caution with heavy alcohol use, severe renal insufficiency or history of hepatic disease. Monitor LFT's prior to therapy, periodically thereafter for 1st yr, or until 1 yr after last dose elevation (additional test at 3 months for 80mg dose). D/C if AST or ALT ≥3x ULN persist, if myopathy is suspected or diagnosed, a few days prior to major surgery. Rhabomyolysis (rare), myopathy reported.

ADVERSE REACTIONS: Abdominal pain, headache, CK and transaminase elevations, constipation, upper respiratory infection, hepatic failure.

INTERACTIONS: Avoid use with concomitant itraconazole, ketoconazole, erythromycin, clarithromycin, telithromycin, HIV protease inhibitors, nefazodone, grapefruit juice (>1 quart/day); increased risk of myopathy/rhabdomyolysis. Max 10mg/day with gemfibrozil, cyclosporine, danazol. Max 20mg/day with amiodarone, verapamil. Caution with other fibrates, ≥1g/day of niacin. Monitor digoxin, warfarin.

PREGNANCY: Category X, not for use in nursing.

MECHANISM OF ACTION: HMG-CoA reductase inhibitor; lipid-lowering agent.

PHARMACOKINETICS: Absorption: T_{max}=1.3-2.4 hrs. **Distribution:** Plasma protein binding (95%); crosses blood-brain barrier. **Metabolism:** Liver (1st pass); β-hydroxyacid; 6'hydroxy, 6'-hydroxymethyl, 6'-exomethylene (active metabolites). **Elimination:** Feces (60%), urine (13%).

ZOFRAN   RX
ondansetron (GlaxoSmithKline)

THERAPEUTIC CLASS: 5-HT$_3$-antagonist

INDICATIONS: (Inj) Prevention of nausea and vomiting associated with initial and repeat courses of emetogenic cancer chemotherapy, including high-dose cisplatin. Prevention of postoperative nausea and/or vomiting. (Sol/Tab) Prevention of nausea and vomiting associated with: highly emetogenic cancer chemotherapy, including cisplatin ≥50mg/m^2; initial and repeat courses of moderately emetogenic cancer chemotherapy; and radiotherapy in patients receiving either total body irradiation, single high-dose fraction to the abdomen, or daily fractions to the abdomen. Prevention of postoperative nausea and/or vomiting.

DOSAGE: *Adults:* Prevention of Chemotherapy-Induced Nausea/Vomiting: (Inj) 32mg single dose or three 0.15mg/kg doses, 1st dose 30 min before chemotherapy, then 4 and 8 hrs after 1st dose. Prevention of Nausea/Vomiting Associated With Highly Emetogenic Cancer Chemotherapy: (Tab) 24mg single dose tab 30 min before chemotherapy. Prevention of Nausea/Vomiting Associated With Moderately Emetogenic Cancer Chemotherapy: (Sol/Tab) 8mg bid, 1st dose 30 min before chemotherapy, then 8 hrs later, then bid for 1-2 days after chemotherapy. Prevention of Post-Op Nausea/Vomiting: (Inj) 4mg IM/IV immediately before anesthesia or post-op after surgery if nausea or vomiting occurs. (Sol/Tab) 16mg 1 hr before anesthesia. Prevention of Nausea/Vomiting Associated with Radiation Therapy: (Sol/Tab) Usual: 8mg tid. Total Body Irradiation: 8mg 1-2 hrs before therapy daily. Single High-Dose Therapy To Abdomen: 8mg 1-2 hrs before therapy then q8h after 1st dose for 1-2 days after completion of therapy. Daily Fractionated Therapy To Abdomen: 8mg 1-2 hrs before therapy then q8h after 1st dose. Severe Hepatic Dysfunction (Child-Pugh ≥10): Max: 8mg/day IV single dose infused over 15 min, start 30 min before chemotherapy or 8mg/day PO.
Pediatrics: Prevention of Chemotherapy-Induced Nausea/Vomiting: (Inj) 6 months-18 yrs: Three 0.15mg/kg doses, 1st dose 30 min before chemotherapy, then 4 and 8 hrs

after the 1st dose. (Sol/Tab) Prevention of Nausea/Vomiting Associated With Moderately Emetogenic Cancer Chemotherapy: ≥12 yrs: 8mg bid, 1st dose 30 min before chemotherapy, then 8mg 8 hrs later, then bid for 1-2 days. 4-11 yrs: 4mg tid, 1st dose 30 min before chemotherapy, then 4 and 8 hrs after 1st dose, then tid for 1-2 days. Prevention of Post-Op Nausea/Vomiting: (Inj) >12 yrs: 4mg IM/IV immediately before anesthesia or post-op after surgery if nausea or vomiting occurs. 1 month-12 yrs: ≤40kg: 0.1mg/kg single dose. >40kg: 4mg single dose. Severe Hepatic Dysfunction: Max: 8mg/day IV single dose infused over 15 min, start 30 min before chemotherapy or 8mg/day PO.

HOW SUPPLIED: Inj: 2mg/mL, 32mg/50mL; Sol: 4mg/5mL (50mL); Tab: 4mg, 8mg, 24mg; Tab, Disintegrating: 4mg, 8mg

WARNINGS/PRECAUTIONS: Hypersensitivity reactions reported in those hypersensitive to other 5-HT$_3$ receptor antagonists. Transient ECG changes including QT interval prolongation reported with IV administration. May mask progressive ileus or gastric distension. Orally disintegrating tabs contain phenylalanine; caution in phenylketonurics.

ADVERSE REACTIONS: Headache, diarrhea, dizziness, drowsiness, malaise/fatigue, constipation, LFT abnormalities.

INTERACTIONS: Ondansetron is metabolized by CYP450 enzymes; inducers or inhibitors of these enzymes may change the clearance and half-life of ondansetron.

PREGNANCY: Category B, caution in nursing.

MECHANISM OF ACTION: Serotonin 5-HT$_3$ receptor blocker; not established. Blocks 5-HT$_3$ receptors from serotonin which may stimulate vagal afferents through 5-HT$_3$ receptors which initiate vomiting reflex.

PHARMACOKINETICS: **Absorption:** IV and oral administration of variable ages resulted in different parameters. **Distribution:** Plasma protein binding (70-76%). **Metabolism:** Hydroxylation, conjugation. **Elimination:** Urine.

ZOLOFT
sertraline HCl (Pfizer)

RX

> Antidepressants increased the risk of suicidal thinking and behavior (suicidality) in short-term studies in children, adolescents, and young adults with Major Depressive Disorder (MDD) and other psychiatric disorders. Sertraline HCl is not approved for use in pediatric patients except for patients with obsessive compulsive disorder (OCD).

THERAPEUTIC CLASS: Selective serotonin reuptake inhibitor

INDICATIONS: Treatment of MDD, social anxiety disorder (SAD), OCD, panic disorder with or without agoraphobia, premenstrual dysphoric disorder (PMDD) and posttraumatic stress disorder (PTSD).

DOSAGE: *Adults:* MDD/OCD: 50mg qd. Titrate: Adjust dose at 1 week intervals. Max: 200mg/day. Panic Disorder/PTSD/SAD: Initial: 25mg qd. Titrate: Increase to 50mg qd after 1 week. Adjust dose at 1 week intervals. Max: 200mg/day. PMDD: Initial: 50mg qd continuous or limited to luteal phase of cycle. Titrate: Increase 50mg/cycle if needed up to 150mg/day for continuous or 100mg/day for luteal phase dosing. If 100mg/day is established for luteal phase dosing, a 50mg/day titration step for 3 days should take place at the beginning of each luteal phase dosing period. Hepatic Impairment: Use lower or less frequent doses. Dilute sol with 4oz water, ginger ale, lemon/lime soda, lemonade or orange juice. Take immediately after mixing.
Pediatrics: OCD: Initial: 6-12 yrs: 25mg qd. 13-17 yrs: 50mg qd. Titrate: Adjust dose at 1 week intervals. Max: 200mg/day. Hepatic Impairment: Use lower or less frequent doses. Dilute sol with 4oz water, ginger ale, lemon/lime soda, lemonade or orange juice. Take immediately after mixing.

HOW SUPPLIED: Sol: 20mg/mL (60mL); Tab: 25mg*, 50mg*, 100mg* *scored

CONTRAINDICATIONS: Concomitant use with MAOIs or pimozide. Concomitant disulfiram with solution.

WARNINGS/PRECAUTIONS: Activation of mania/hypomania reported. Monitor weight loss. Caution with conditions that could affect metabolism or hemodynamic responses, seizure disorder. Dose adjust with liver dysfunction. Altered platelet function and hyponatremia reported. Weak uricosuric effects reported. Caution with latex sensitivity; solution dropper dispenser contains rubber. Monitor for clinical worsening and/or suicidality, especially at initiation of therapy or dose changes. Avoid abrupt withdrawal. Monitor for discontinuation symptoms.

ADVERSE REACTIONS: Ejaculation failure, dry mouth, increased sweating, somnolence, tremor, anorexia, dizziness, headache, vomiting, diarrhea, dyspepsia, nausea, agitation, insomnia, nervousness, abnormal vision.

INTERACTIONS: See Contraindications. Increased levels with cimetidine. Avoid with alcohol, pimozide or MAOIs. Decreases clearance of tolbutamide. Rare reports of weakness, hyperreflexia, incoordination with an SSRI and sumatriptan. May potentiate drugs metabolized by CYP2D6 (eg, TCAs, Type 1C antiarrhythmics). Caution with CNS drugs (eg, diazepam). Monitor lithium. Caution with TCAs; may need dose adjustment. May shift concentrations with plasma protein-bound drugs (eg, warfarin, digitoxin). Monitor PT with warfarin. Caution with OTC products. May induce metabolism of cisapride. Caution with drugs that interfere with hemostasis (eg, non-selective NSAIDs, ASA, warfarin) due to increased risk of bleeding.

PREGNANCY: Category C, caution in nursing.

MECHANISM OF ACTION: SSRI; inhibits CNS neuronal uptake of serotonin.

PHARMACOKINETICS: Absorption: T_{max}=4.5-8.4 hrs. **Distribution:** Plasma protein binding (98%). **Metabolism:** Liver (extensive). **Elimination:** Feces 12-14% (unchanged), urine (minor); $T_{1/2}$=26 hrs.

ZONEGRAN   RX

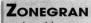
zonisamide (Eisai)

THERAPEUTIC CLASS: Sulfonamide anticonvulsant

INDICATIONS: Adjunctive therapy in the treatment of partial seizures.

DOSAGE: *Adults:* Initial: 100mg qd for 2 weeks. Titrate: May increase to 200mg/day for at least 2 weeks. May then increase to 300mg/day, then to 400mg/day for at least 2-week intervals. Max: 400mg/day.
Pediatrics: ≥16 yrs: Initial: 100mg qd for 2 weeks. Titrate: May increase to 200mg/day for at least 2 weeks. May then increase to 300mg/day, then to 400mg/day for at least 2-week intervals. Max: 400mg/day.

HOW SUPPLIED: Cap: 25mg, 100mg

CONTRAINDICATIONS: Sulfonamide hypersensitivity.

WARNINGS/PRECAUTIONS: Sulfonamide hypersensitivity reactions (eg, Stevens-Johnson syndrome, toxic epidermal necrolysis, fulminant hepatic necrosis, blood dyscrasias), cognitive/neuropsychiatric effects, kidney stones, sudden death reported. D/C with unexplained rash. Increased risk of oligohidrosis and hyperthermia in pediatrics; monitor for decreased sweating and increased body temperature. Advise females to use contraceptives to prevent pregnancy. Caution with renal/hepatic impairment. Avoid abrupt withdrawal. May cause cognitive/neuropsychiatric adverse events. Caution while driving, operating machinery, or performing hazardous tasks. Taper and d/c if CPK levels elevated or if patient manifests clinical signs and symptoms of pancreatitis.

ADVERSE REACTIONS: Headache, abdominal pain, anorexia, nausea, dizziness, ataxia, confusion, difficulty concentrating, memory difficulties, agitation/irritability, depression, insomnia, somnolence, fatigue, tiredness.

INTERACTIONS: Liver enzyme inducers increase metabolism and clearance and decrease half-life. Caution with drugs that predispose patients to heat-related disorders (eg, carbonic anhydrase inhibitors, anticholinergic drugs).

PREGNANCY: Category C, not for use in nursing.

MECHANISM OF ACTION: Sulfonamide; mechanism unknown. Found to block Na^+ channels and reduce voltage-dependent, transient inward currents (T-type Ca^{2+} currents), which then stabilize neuronal membranes and suppress neuronal hypersynchronization. Facilitates both dopaminergic and serotonergic neurotransmission.

PHARMACOKINETICS: Absorption: C_{max}=2-5mcg/mL; T_{max} =2 to 6 hrs. **Distribution:** V_d=1.45L/kg; plasma protein binding (40%). **Metabolism:** Liver, via acetylation and reduction by CYP3A4; N-acetyl zonisamide, 2-sulfamoylacetyl phenol (metabolites). **Elimination:** Urine (62%), feces (3%); $T_{1/2}$=63 hrs.

ZOSYN

piperacillin sodium - tazobactam (Wyeth)

THERAPEUTIC CLASS: Broad-spectrum penicillin/beta-lactamase inhibitor

INDICATIONS: Treatment of appendicitis, peritonitis, uncomplicated/complicated skin and skin structure infections, postpartum endometritis, pelvic inflammatory disease, moderate severity of community acquired pneumonia (CAP), and moderate to severe nosocomial pneumonia caused by susceptible strains of microorganisms.

DOSAGE: *Adults:* Usual: 3.375g q6h for 7-10 days. CrCl 20-40mL: 2.25g q6h. CrCl <20mL/min: 2.25g q8h. Hemodialysis/CAPD: 2.25g q12h. Give 1 additional 0.75g dose after each dialysis period. Nosocomial Pneumonia: 4.5g q6h for 7-14 days plus aminoglycoside. CrCl 20-40mL/min: 3.375g q6h. CrCl <20mL/min: 2.25g q6h. Hemodialysis/CAPD: Max: 2.25g q8h. Give 1 additional 0.75g dose after each dialysis period.
Pediatrics: Appendicitis/Peritonitis: ≤40kg: ≥9 months: 100mg piperacillin-12.5mg tazobactam/kg q8h. 2-9 months: 80mg piperacillin-10mg tazobactam/kg q8h. ≥40kg: Use adult dose.

HOW SUPPLIED: Inj: (Piperacillin-Tazobactam) 40mg-5mg/mL, 60mg-7.5mg/mL, 2g-0.25g, 3g-0.375g, 4g-0.5g, 2g-0.25g/50mL, 3g-0.375g/50mL, 4g-0.5g/100mL, 36g-4.5g

CONTRAINDICATIONS: History of allergic reactions to cephalosporins.

WARNINGS/PRECAUTIONS: Serious, fatal hypersensitivity reactions may occur with PCN allergy. *Clostridium difficile*-associated diarrhea reported. D/C if bleeding manifestations occur. May experience neuromuscular excitability or convulsions with higher doses. Contains 2.79mEq/g Na; caution with restricted salt intake. Increased incidence of rash and fever in cystic fibrosis. Monitor electrolyte periodically with low K$^+$ reserves. Therapy may lead to emergence of resistant organisms that can cause superinfections. Caution with renal impairment (CrCl <40mL/min).

ADVERSE REACTIONS: Diarrhea, headache, constipation, NV, insomnia, rash, dyspepsia, pruritus.

INTERACTIONS: May inactivate aminoglycosides. Probenecid prolongs half-life. Monitor coagulation parameters with heparin, oral anticoagulants, or drugs that affect blood coagulation system or thrombocyte function. May prolong neuromuscular blockade of vecuronium.

PREGNANCY: Category B, caution in nursing.

MECHANISM OF ACTION: Piperacillin: Broad-spectrum penicillin; exerts bactericidal activity by inhibiting septum formation and cell-wall synthesis of susceptible bacteria. Tazobactam: β-lactamase enzyme inhibitor.

PHARMACOKINETICS: Absorption: (2.25g, 3.375g, 4.5g of piperacillin): C_{max}=134mcg/mL, 242mcg/mL, 298mcg/mL. (2.25g, 3.375g, 4.5g of tazobactam): C_{max}= 15mcg/mL, 24mcg/mL, 34mcg/mL. **Distribution:** V_d=0.243L/kg; plasma protein binding (30%); wide distribution into tissues and bodily fluids; crosses placental barrier; found in breast milk. **Elimination:** Kidneys; Piperacillin: Urine (68% unchanged); Tazobactam: Urine (80% unchanged, 20% as single metabolite); $T_{1/2}$=0.7-1.2 hrs.

ZOVIRAX CREAM

acyclovir (Biovail)

THERAPEUTIC CLASS: Nucleoside analogue

INDICATIONS: Treatment of recurrent herpes labialis (cold sores).

DOSAGE: *Adults:* Apply 5x/day for 4 days. Initiate with 1st sign/symptom.
Pediatrics: ≥12 yrs: Apply 5x/day for 4 days. Initiate with 1st sign/symptom.

HOW SUPPLIED: Cre: 5% (2g, 5g)

WARNINGS/PRECAUTIONS: Cutaneous use only; not for use in the eye, mouth or nose.

ADVERSE REACTIONS: Dry lips, desquamation, dryness of skin, cracked lips, burning skin, pruritus, flakiness of skin, stinging on skin.

PREGNANCY: Category B, caution in nursing.

MECHANISM OF ACTION: Synthetic purine nucleoside analogue; possesses inhibitory activity against herpes simplex virus types 1 and 2, and varicella-zoster virus. Stops replication of herpes viral DNA by competitive inhibition of viral DNA polymerase, incorporation into and termination of growing viral DNA chain, and inactivation of viral DNA polymerase.

PHARMACOKINETICS: Absorption: Minimal systemic absorption.

ZOVIRAX INJECTION

RX

acyclovir sodium (GlaxoSmithKline)

THERAPEUTIC CLASS: Nucleoside analogue

INDICATIONS: Treatment of neonatal herpes simplex infections and herpes simplex encephalitis. Treatment of varicella-zoster (shingles), initial and recurrent mucosal and cutaneous herpes simplex in immunocompromised patients. Treatment of severe initial clinical episodes of herpes genitalis in immunocompetent patients.

DOSAGE: *Adults:* Initiate with 1st sign/symptom. Max: 20mg/kg q8h for any patient. Mucosal/Cutaneous Herpes Simplex Infections: 5mg/kg q8h for 7 days. Herpes Genitalis: 5mg/kg q8h for 5 days. Herpes Simplex Encephalitis: 10mg/kg q8h for 10 days. Varicella Zoster: 10mg/kg q8h for 7 days. Obese Patients: Dose according to IBW. CrCl 25-50mL/min: Give 100% of recommended dose q12h. CrCl 10-25: Give 100% of recommended dose q24h. CrCl 0-10mL/min: Give 50% of recommended dose q24h. Elderly: Reduce dose and monitor renal function.
Pediatrics: Initiate with 1st sign/symptom. Max: 20mg/kg q8h for any patient. Mucosal/Cutaneous Herpes Simplex: ≥12 yrs: 5mg/kg q8h for 7 days. <12 yrs: 10mg/kg q8h for 7 days. Herpes Genitalis: ≥12 yrs: 5mg/kg q8h for 5 days. Herpes Simplex Encephalitis: ≥12 yrs: 10mg/kg q8h for 10 days. 3 months-12 yrs: 20mg/kg q8h for 10 days. Neonatal Herpes Simplex: Birth-3 months: 10mg/kg q8h for 10 days. Varicella Zoster: ≥12 yrs: 10mg/kg q8h for 7 days. <12 yrs: 20mg/kg q8h for 7 days. Obese Patients: Dose according to IBW. CrCl 25-50mL/min: Give 100% of recommended dose q12h. CrCl 10-25: Give 100% of recommended dose q24h. CrCl 0-10mL/min: Give 50% of recommended dose q24h.

HOW SUPPLIED: Inj: 500mg, 1000mg

CONTRAINDICATIONS: Hypersensitivity to valacyclovir.

WARNINGS/PRECAUTIONS: Do not administer topically, IM, PO, SQ, or in the eye. Adjust dose in renal impairment and the elderly. Renal failure and death reported. Thrombotic thrombocytopenic purpura/hemolytic uremic syndrome in immunocompromised patients reported. Patient must be adequately hydrated. Caution with underlying neurologic abnormalities, electrolyte abnormalities, significant hypoxia, and serious renal or hepatic abnormalities. Infusion must not be given over <1 hr.

ADVERSE REACTIONS: Injection site inflammation, phlebitis, transient serum creatinine and BUN elevations, NV.

INTERACTIONS: Increased serum levels with probenecid. Avoid with nephrotoxic drugs.

PREGNANCY: Category B, caution in nursing.

MECHANISM OF ACTION: Synthetic purine nucleoside analogue; possesses inhibitory activity against herpes simplex virus types 1 and 2, and varicella-zoster virus. Stops replication of herpes viral DNA by competitive inhibition of viral DNA polymerase, incorporation into and termination of growing viral DNA chain, and inactivation of viral DNA polymerase.

PHARMACOKINETICS: Absorption: C_{max}=9.8mcg/mL (5mg/kg), 22.9mcg/mL (10mg/kg). **Distribution:** Plasma protein binding (9-33%); found in breast milk. **Metabolism:** 9-carboxymethoxymethylguanine (major metabolite). **Elimination:** Urine (62-91% unchanged) (14.1% metabolite). Refer to PI for detailed info regarding renal function and pediatrics.

ZOVIRAX ORAL RX
acyclovir (GlaxoSmithKline)

THERAPEUTIC CLASS: Nucleoside analogue

INDICATIONS: Acute treatment of herpes zoster (shingles). Treatment of initial and recurrent episodes of genital herpes. Treatment of chickenpox (varicella).

DOSAGE: *Adults:* Herpes Zoster: 800mg q4h, 5x/day for 7-10 days. Start within 72 hrs after onset of rash. Genital Herpes: Initial: 200mg q4h, 5x/day for 10 days. Chronic Therapy: 400mg bid or 200mg 3-5x/day up to 12 months, then re-evaluate. Intermittent Therapy: 200mg q4h, 5x/day for 5 days. Start with 1st sign/symptom of recurrence. Chickenpox: 800mg qid for 5 days. CrCl 10-25mL/min: For a dose of 800mg q4h, give 800mg q8h. CrCl 0-10mL/min: For a dose of 200mg q4h, give 200mg q12h. For a dose of 400mg q12h, give 200mg q12h. For a dose of 800mg q4h, give 800mg q12h. Elderly: Reduce dose.
Pediatrics: ≥2 yrs: ≤40kg: Chickenpox: 20mg/kg qid for 5 days. >40kg: 800mg qid for 5 days.

HOW SUPPLIED: Cap: 200mg; Sus: 200mg/5mL; Tab: 400mg, 800mg

CONTRAINDICATIONS: Hypersensitivity to valacyclovir.

WARNINGS/PRECAUTIONS: Adust dose in renal impairment, elderly. Renal failure and death reported. Thrombotic thrombocytopenic purpura/hemolytic uremic syndrome in immunocompromised patients reported.

ADVERSE REACTIONS: NV, diarrhea, headache, malaise, renal dysfunction.

INTERACTIONS: Probenecid increased levels of IV formulation. Caution with potentially nephrotoxic agents.

PREGNANCY: Category B, caution in nursing.

MECHANISM OF ACTION: Synthetic purine nucleoside analogue; possesses inhibitory activity against herpes simplex virus types 1 and 2, and varicella-zoster virus. Stops replication of herpes viral DNA by competitive inhibition of viral DNA polymerase, incorporation into and termination of growing viral DNA chain, and inactivation of viral DNA polymerase.

PHARMACOKINETICS: Absorption: Absolute bioavailability (10-20%). Oral administration of variable doses resulted in different parameters. **Distribution:** Plasma protein binding (9-33%). **Elimination:** $T_{1/2}$=2.5-3.3 hrs.

ZYFLO CR RX
zileuton (Critical Therapeutics)

THERAPEUTIC CLASS: Leukotriene inhibitor

INDICATIONS: Prophylaxis and chronic treatment of asthma.

DOSAGE: *Adults:* 1200mg bid within 1 hr after am and pm meals. Max: 2400mg/day.
Pediatrics: ≥12 yrs: 1200mg bid within 1 hr after am and pm meals. Max: 2400mg/day.

HOW SUPPLIED: Tab: Extended-Release: 600mg *scored

CONTRAINDICATIONS: Active liver disease or transaminase elevations (≥3x ULN).

WARNINGS/PRECAUTIONS: Not for treatment of acute attacks. Evaluate liver function prior to therapy and periodically thereafter. D/C if signs of liver disease occur.

ADVERSE REACTIONS: Headache, ALT elevation, dyspepsia, pain, nausea, asthenia, myalgia, sinusitis, pharyngolaryngeal pain.

INTERACTIONS: Monitor drugs metabolized by CYP450 3A4. Increases theophylline levels; reduce theophylline by 50% and monitor levels. Potentiates warfarin, propranolol.

PREGNANCY: Category C, not for use in nursing.

MECHANISM OF ACTION: Leukotriene inhibitor; anti-asthmatic agent, inhibits leukotriene (LTB_4, LTC_4, LTD_4, and LTE_4) formation by inhibiting the enzyme 5-lipoxygenase.

PHARMACOKINETICS: Absorption: T_{max}=4.3 hrs. **Distribution:** V_d=1.2L/kg; plasma protein binding (93%). **Metabolism:** Liver, via oxidation by CYP1A2, CYP2C9, CYP3A4; glucoronidation. **Elimination:** Urine, feces; $T_{1/2}$=3.2 hrs.

ZYLOPRIM

RX

allopurinol (Prometheus)

THERAPEUTIC CLASS: Xanthine oxidase inhibitor

INDICATIONS: Management of symptoms of primary and secondary gout. Management of hyperuricosuria and hyperuricemia due to chemotherapy. Management of recurrent calcium oxalate calculi in those with hyperuricosuria (uric acid excretion >800mg/day in males and >750mg/day in females).

DOSAGE: *Adults:* Gout: Initial: 100mg/day. Titrate: Increase by 100mg/week until serum uric acid level is ≤6mg/dL. Mild Gout: Usual: 200-300mg/day. Moderately Severe Gout: Usual: 400-600mg/day. Max: 800mg/day. Recurrent Calcium Oxalate Stones: Usual: 200-300mg/day. Prevention of Uric Acid Nephropathy with Chemotherapy: Usual: 600-800mg/day for 2-3 days with high fluid intake. CrCl 10-20mL/min: 200mg/day. CrCl <10mL/min: Max: 100mg/day. CrCl <3mL/min: Also increase dosing intervals. Take after meals. Divide dose if >300mg.
Pediatrics: Hyperuricemia with Malignancies: 6-10 yrs: 300mg/day. <6 yrs: 150mg/day. Evaluate response after 48 hrs. Take after meals.

HOW SUPPLIED: Tab: 100mg*, 300mg* *scored

WARNINGS/PRECAUTIONS: D/C if skin rash occurs. Severe hypersensitivity reactions, hepatotoxicity, and bone marrow depression reported. Monitor LFTs during early stages of therapy with liver disease. Caution with activities that require alertness. Caution with renal impairment. Renal failure reported with hyperuricemia secondary to neoplastic diseases. Fluid intake should yield ≥2L of urinary output/day. Maintain neutral or slightly alkaline urine. Acute gout attacks increase during early stages of therapy; give colchicine.

ADVERSE REACTIONS: Acute gout attacks, rash, diarrhea, SGOT/SGPT increase, alkaline phosphatase increase, nausea.

INTERACTIONS: Increased toxicity with thiazide diuretics or renal impairment; monitor renal function. Reduce mercaptopurine or azathioprine to 1/3 or 1/4 of usual dose. Potentiates dicumarol, chlorpropamide and cyclosporine. Decreased effects with uricosurics. Increased skin rash with ampicillin, amoxicillin. Enhanced bone marrow suppression with cytotoxic agents (eg, cyclophosphamide). Caution with sulfinpyrazone.

PREGNANCY: Category C, caution in nursing.

MECHANISM OF ACTION: Xanthine oxidase inhibitor; acts on purine catabolism; reduces production of uric acid by inhibiting biochemical reactions immediately preceding its formation.

PHARMACOKINETICS: Absorption: C_{max}=3mcg/mL, T_{max}=1.5 hrs; Oxipurinol: C_{max}=6.5mcg/mL, T_{max}=4.5 hrs. **Metabolism:** Oxidation, oxipurinol (metabolite). **Elimination:** Kidneys, feces (20%); $T_{1/2}$=1-2 hrs. Oxipurinol: $T_{1/2}$=15 hrs.

ZYMAR

RX

gatifloxacin (Allergan)

THERAPEUTIC CLASS: Fluoroquinolone

INDICATIONS: Treatment of bacterial conjunctivitis.

DOSAGE: *Adults:* 1 drop q2h while awake, up to 8x/day for 2 days; then 1 drop up to qid while awake for 5 days.
Pediatrics: ≥1 yr: 1 drop q2h while awake, up to 8x/day for 2 days; then 1 drop up to qid while awake for 5 days.

HOW SUPPLIED: Sol: 0.3% (5mL)

WARNINGS/PRECAUTIONS: Not for injection. Do not inject subconjunctivally or into the anterior chamber of the eye. Superinfection may result with prolonged use. Fatal hypersensitivity reactions reported after 1st dose of systemic quinolone therapy. Avoid contact lenses when symptoms are present.

ADVERSE REACTIONS: Conjunctival irritation, increased lacrimation, keratitis, papillary conjunctivitis, chemosis, conjunctival hemorrhage, dry eye, eye discharge/irritation/pain, red eye, eyelid edema, headache, reduced visual acuity, taste disturbance.

INTERACTIONS: Systemic quinolone therapy may increase theophylline levels, interfere with caffeine metabolism, enhance warfarin effects, and elevate serum creatinine with cyclosporine.

PREGNANCY: Category C, caution in nursing.

MECHANISM OF ACTION: Fluoroquinolone antibiotic; inhibits topoisomerase II (DNA gyrase) and topoisomerase IV. DNA gyrase is essential enzyme involved in replication, transcription, and repair of bacterial DNA. Topoisomerase IV is enzyme known to play key role in partitioning of chromosomal DNA during bacterial cell division.

ZYMASE
amylase - lipase - protease (Organon)

RX

THERAPEUTIC CLASS: Pancreatic enzyme supplement

INDICATIONS: Treatment of conditions with pancreatic enzyme deficiency with resultant inadequate fat digestion (eg, chronic pancreatitis, pancreatectomy, cystic fibrosis, steatorrhea).

DOSAGE: *Adults:* 1-2 caps with each meal or snack. Contents of cap may be mixed with liquids or soft foods that do not require chewing.
Pediatrics: 1-2 caps with each meal or snack. Contents of cap may be mixed with liquids or soft foods that do not require chewing.

HOW SUPPLIED: Cap, Delayed-Release: (Amylase-Lipase-Protease) 24,000 U-12,000 U-24,000 U

CONTRAINDICATIONS: Pork protein hypersensitivity.

WARNINGS/PRECAUTIONS: Do not chew or crush contents of capsules. High doses can cause hyperuricemia and hyperuricosuria.

PREGNANCY: Safety in pregnancy and nursing not known.

ZYRTEC
cetirizine HCl (Pfizer)

RX

THERAPEUTIC CLASS: H₁-antagonist

INDICATIONS: Seasonal or perennial allergic rhinitis. Chronic idiopathic urticaria.

DOSAGE: *Adults:* 5-10mg qd. Hepatic Impairment/Hemodialysis/CrCl <31mL/min: 5mg qd.
Pediatrics: ≥12 yrs: 5-10mg qd. 6-11 yrs: 5-10mg qd. 2-5 yrs: 2.5mg qd. Max: 5mg qd or 2.5mg q12h. Perennial Allergic Rhinitis/Urticaria: 6 months-23 months: 2.5mg qd. 12 months-23 months: May increase to max 5mg/day given as 2.5mL q12h. Hepatic Impairment/Hemodialysis/CrCl <31mL/min: ≥12 yrs: 5mg qd. 6-11 yrs: Use lower the recommended dose. <6 yrs: Not recommended.

HOW SUPPLIED: Syrup: 1mg/mL (120mL, 480mL); Tab: 5mg, 10mg; Tab, Chewable: 5mg, 10mg

CONTRAINDICATIONS: Hydroxyzine hypersensitivity.

WARNINGS/PRECAUTIONS: Adjust dose with hepatic or renal impairment. May impair mental/physical abilities.

ADVERSE REACTIONS: Somnolence, fatigue, dry mouth, headache, pharyngitis, abdominal pain, cough, epistaxis, diarrhea, bronchospasm.

INTERACTIONS: Avoid alcohol and CNS depressants. Possible decreased clearance with large doses of theophylline.

PREGNANCY: Category B, not for use in nursing.

ZYRTEC-D
cetirizine HCl - pseudoephedrine HCl (Pfizer)

OTC

THERAPEUTIC CLASS: Antihistamine/decongestant

INDICATIONS: Relief of nasal and non-nasal symptoms associated with seasonal or perennial allergic rhinitis.

DOSAGE: *Adults:* 1 tab bid. Hepatic Impairment/Renal Dysfunction (CrCl <31mL/min): 1 tab qd. Swallow tabs whole.

Pediatrics: ≥12 yrs: 1 tab bid. Hepatic Impairment/Renal Dysfunction (CrCl <31mL/min): 1 tab qd. Swallow tabs whole.

HOW SUPPLIED: Tab, Extended-Release: (Cetirizine-Pseudoephedrine) 5mg-120mg

CONTRAINDICATIONS: Narrow angle glaucoma, urinary retention, MAOIs during or within 14 days of use, severe HTN, severe CAD, hypersensitivity to adrenergics.

WARNINGS/PRECAUTIONS: Caution with HTN, DM, ischemic heart disease, increased IOP, hyperthyroidism, renal impairment, or prostatic hypertrophy. May produce CNS stimulation with convulsions or cardiovascular collapse. May impair mental/physical abilities.

ADVERSE REACTIONS: Insomnia, dry mouth, fatigue, somnolence.

INTERACTIONS: Avoid MAOIs during or within 14 days of use.

PREGNANCY: Category C, not for use in nursing.

MECHANISM OF ACTION: Cetirizine: Antihistamine/decongestant; selectively inhibits H1-receptors. Pseudoephedrine: orally active sympathomimetic amine; exerts a decongestant effect on the nasal mucosa.

PHARMACOKINETICS: Absorption: Cetirizine: C_{max}=114 ng/mL (single dose), 178ng/mL (multiple doses); T_{max}=2.2 hrs. Pseudoephedrine: C_{max}=309 ng/mL, 526ng/mL (multiple doses); T_{max}=4.4 hrs. **Distribution:** Found in breast milk. Cetirizine: Plasma protein binding (93%). Pseudoephedrine: V_d=2.6-3.3 L/kg. **Metabolism:** Cetirizine: Oxidative-O-dealkylation. Pseudoephedrine: N-demethylation; (1%-7%) metabolized to norpseudoephedrine. **Elimination:** Cetirizine: $T_{1/2mean}$=7.9 hrs; urine (70%), feces (10%). Pseudoephedrine: $T_{1/2}$=6hrs.

ZYVOX   RX
linezolid (Pharmacia & Upjohn)

THERAPEUTIC CLASS: Oxazolidinone class antibacterial

INDICATIONS: Treatment of vancomycin-resistant *Enterococcus faecium* (VRE) infections, nosocomial pneumonia caused by *Staphylococcus aureus* (methicillin-susceptible and -resistant strains) or *Streptococcus pneumoniae* (including multi drug-resistant strains (MDRSP)), complicated skin and skin structure infections (SSSI) including diabetic foot infections without concomitant osteomyelitis caused by *Staphylococcus aureus* (methicillin-susceptible and -resistant strains), *Streptococcus pyogenes*, or *Streptococcus agalactiae*, uncomplicated SSSI caused by *Staphylococcus aureus* (methicillin-susceptible only) or *Streptococcus pyogenes*, community-acquired pneumonia (CAP) caused by *Streptococcus pneumoniae* (MDRSP), including concurrent bacteremia, or *Staphylococcus aureus* (methicillin-susceptible strains only).

DOSAGE: *Adults:* Complicated SSSI/CAP/Nosocomial Pneumonia: 600mg IV/PO q12h for 10-14 days. VRE: 600mg IV/PO q12h for 14-28 days. Uncomplicated SSSI: 400mg PO q12h for 10-14 days.

Pediatrics: Complicated SSSI/CAP/Nosocomial Pneumonia: Treat for 10-14 days. ≥12 yrs: 600mg IV/PO q12h. Birth-11 yrs: 10mg/kg IV/PO q12h. VRE: Treat for 14-28 days: ≥12 yrs: 600mg IV/PO q12h; Birth-11 yrs: 10mg/kg IV/PO q8h. Uncomplicated SSSI: Treat for 10-14 days: ≥12 yrs: 600mg PO q12h; 5-11 yrs: 10mg/kg PO q12h; <5 yrs: 10mg/kg PO q8h. Neonates <7 days: Initiate with dosing regimen of 10mg/kg q12h; may increase to 10mg/kg q8h if suboptimal response. All neonatal patients should receive 10mg/kg q8h by 7 days of life.

HOW SUPPLIED: Inj: 2mg/mL (100mL, 200mL, 300mL); Sus: 100mg/5mL (150mL); Tab: 400mg, 600mg

WARNINGS/PRECAUTIONS: Myelosuppression including anemia, thrombocytopenia, pancytopenia, and leukopenia reported; monitor CBC weekly. *Clostridium difficile*-associated diarrhea reported. Oral sus contains phenylalanine. Peripheral and optic neuropathy reported; monitor visual function if on for extended periods (≥3 months). Lactic acidosis and convulsions reported. May promote overgrowth of nonsusceptible organisms.

ADVERSE REACTIONS: Diarrhea, headache, NV.

INTERACTIONS: Potential interaction with adrenergic and serotonergic agents. May enhance pressor response to sympathomimetics, vasopressors, and dopaminergic agents; caution with dopamine, epinephrine, pseudoephedrine, and phenylpropanolamine. Serotonin syndrome may occur with concomitant serotonergic agents, including antidepressants such as SSRIs. Avoid large quantities of tyramine-containing foods or beverages.

PREGNANCY: Category C, caution in nursing.

MECHANISM OF ACTION: Oxazolidinone antibacterial; inhibits bacterial protein synthesis; binds to a site on the bacterial 23S ribosomal RNA of the 50S subunit and prevents formation of functional 70S initiation complex, which is an essential component of the bacterial translation process.

PHARMACOKINETICS: Absorption: Rapid/extensive; absolute bioavailability (100%); T_{max}=1-2 hrs. **Distribution:** V_d=40-50L; plasma protein binding (31%); distributes to well-perfused tissues. **Metabolism:** Via oxidation; aminoethoxyacteic acid (A), hydroxyethyl glycine (B) (inactive metabolites). **Elimination:** Urine (30% as parent drug, 40% as B, 10% as A), feces (6% as B, 3% as A).

NeoFax® Drug Monographs

ACETAMINOPHEN

DOSE & ADMINISTRATION: Oral Loading dose: 20 to 25 mg/kg. Maintenance: 12 to 15 mg/kg per dose. **Rectal Loading dose:** 30 mg/kg. Maintenance: 12 to 18 mg/kg per dose. **Maintenance intervals:** Term infants: Q6 hours Preterm infants ≥ 32 weeks Postmenstrual Age: Q8 hours; Preterm infants < 32 weeks Postmenstrual Age: Q12 hours;

USES: Fever reduction and treatment of mild to moderate pain.

MONITORING: Assess for signs of pain. Monitor temperature. Assess liver function. Serum acetaminophen concentration is obtained only to assess toxicity.

ADVERSE EFFECTS/PRECAUTIONS: Liver toxicity occurs with excessive doses or after prolonged administration (>48 hours) of therapeutic doses. Rash, fever, thrombocytopenia, leukopenia, and neutropenia have been reported in children.

PHARMACOLOGY: Nonnarcotic analgesic and antipyretic. Peak serum concentration occurs approximately 60 minutes after an oral dose. Absorption after rectal administration is variable and prolonged. Extensively metabolized in the liver, primarily by sulfation with a small amount by glucuronidation. Metabolites and unchanged drug are excreted by the kidney. Elimination half-life is approximately 3 hours in term neonates, 5 hours in preterm neonates > 32 weeks gestation, and up to 11 hours in more immature neonates. Elimination is prolonged in patients with liver dysfunction.

SPECIAL CONSIDERATIONS/PREPARATION: Dosage forms: Drops: 100 mg/mL, 48 mg/mL (alcohol-free). Elixir: 16 mg/mL, 24 mg/mL, 32 mg/mL. Liquid: 32 mg/mL (alcohol-free). Liquid: 33.33 mg/mL (7% alcohol). Suppositories: 80,120, 325, and 650 mg. Inaccurate dosing may occur with rectal administration because of unequal distribution of acetaminophen in the suppositories. **Treatment of Serious Acetaminophen Toxicity:** N-acetylcysteine (NAC), 150 mg/kg in 5% dextrose or 1/2 NS given IV over 60 minutes (loading dose), followed by 50 mg/kg in 5% dextrose or 1/2 NS over 4 hours, then 100 mg/kg in 5% dextrose or 1/2 NS over 16 hours. NAC should be continued until clinical and biochemical markers of hepatic injury improve, and acetaminophen concentration is below the limits of detection. NAC solution concentrations of 40 mg/mL have been used to avoid fluid overload and hyponatremia in the neonate.

SELECTED REFERENCES
- Walls L, Baker CF, Sarkar S: Acetaminophen-induced hepatic failure with encephalopathy in a newborn. *J Perinatol* 2007;27:133-135.
- Anderson BJ, van Lingen RA, Hansen TG, et al: Acetaminophen developmental pharmacokinetics in premature neonates and infants. *Anesthesiology* 2002;96:1336-45.
- Isbister GK, Bucens IK, Whyte IM: Paracetamol overdose in a preterm neonate. *Arch Dis Child Fetal Neonatal Ed* 2001;85:F70-F72.
- Arana A, Morton NS, Hansen TG: Treatment with paracetamol in infants. *Acta Anaesthesiol Scand* 2001;45:20-29.
- Levy G, Khanna NN, Soda DM, et al: Pharmacokinetics of acetaminophen in the human neonate: Formation of acetaminophen glucuronide and sulfate in relation to plasma bilirubin concentration and D-glucaric acid excretion. *Pediatrics* 1975;55:818.
- Product Information, Cumberland (acetylcysteine), 2006

ACYCLOVIR

DOSE & ADMINISTRATION: 20 mg/kg per dose Q8 hours IV infusion by syringe pump over 1 hour. Prolong the dosing interval in premature infants <34 weeks PMA, or in patients with significant renal impairment or hepatic failure. Treat localized herpes simplex infections for 14 days, disseminated or CNS infections for 21 days. **Chronic suppression:** 75 mg/kg per dose PO Q12 hours.

USES: Treatment of neonatal herpes simplex infections, varicella zoster infections with CNS and pulmonary involvement, and herpes simplex encephalitis.

MONITORING: Periodic CBC. Serum concentrations two hours after a dose should be approximately 2 mcg/mL. Follow renal and hepatic function. Monitor IV site for phlebitis—if noted, make infusion solution more dilute.

ADVERSE EFFECTS/PRECAUTIONS: Neutropenia occurs in approximately 20% of patients - decrease dose or treat with GCSF if ANC remains less than 500/mm³. Phlebitis may occur at IV site due to alkaline pH of 10. Risk of transient renal dysfunction and crystalluria is minimized by slow infusion rates and adequate patient hydration. Resistant viral strains may emerge during long-term therapy; these patients are at high risk for progressive life-threatening disease.

PHARMACOLOGY: Antiviral drug that is preferentially taken up by infected cells; inhibits viral DNA synthesis. CSF concentrations are 30 to 50% of serum concentrations. Oral absorption is 15 to 30%. Most of administered dose is excreted unchanged in urine, primarily via glomerular filtration. Protein binding and metabolism are minimal. Serum half-life is 3 to 4 hours in patients with normal renal and hepatic function.

SPECIAL CONSIDERATIONS/PREPARATION: Intravenous formulations available as solution (50 mg/mL) or as powder for solution in 500-mg and 1-g vials. Prepare powder for solution by dissolving contents of 500-mg vial in 10 mL sterile water for injection. Reconstituted solution is stable at room temperature for 12 hours. **Do not refrigerate. Infusion solution concentration should be no greater than 7 mg/mL.** A 5-mg/mL dilution may be made by adding 1 mL of 50 mg/mL concentration to 9 mL of preservative-free normal saline. Dilution should be used within 24 hours. Oral suspension available in 200 mg/5 mL concentration. Store at room temperature. Shake well before administration.

Solution Compatibility: D_5W, $D_{10}W$, and NS.

Solution Incompatibility: Dex/AA.

Terminal Injection Site Compatibility: Amikacin, ampicillin, aminophylline, cefazolin, cefotaxime, cefoxitin, ceftazidime, ceftriaxone, chloramphenicol, cimetidine, clindamycin, dexamethasone, erythromycin lactobionate, famotidine, fluconazole, gentamicin, heparin, hydrocortisone succinate, imipenem/cilastatin, linezolid, lorazepam, meropenem, metoclopramide, metronidazole, milrinone, morphine, nafcillin, oxacillin, penicillin G, pentobarbital, piperacillin, potassium chloride, propofol, ranitidine, remifentanil, sodium bicarbonate, theophylline, ticarcillin/clavulanate, tobramycin, trimethoprim-sulfamethoxazole, vancomycin, and zidovudine.

Incompatibility: Fat emulsion. Aztreonam, caffeine citrate, cefepime, dobutamine,dopamine, and piperacillin-tazobactam.

SELECTED REFERENCES

- Tiffany KF, Benjamin DK Jr, Palasanthiran P, et al: Improved neurodevelopmental outcomes following long-term high-dose acyclovir therapy in infants with central nervous system and disseminated herpes simplex disease. *J Perinatol* 2005;25:156-161.
- Kimberlin DW, Lin C-Y, Jacobs RF, et al: Safety and efficacy of high-dose intravenous acyclovir in the management of neonatal herpes simplex infections. *Pediatrics* 2001;108:230-238.
- American Academy of Pediatrics. Herpes simplex. In: Pickering LK, ed. *2003 Red Book: Report of the Committee on Infectious Diseases.* 26th ed. Elk Grove Village, IL: American Academy of Pediatrics;2003: p 347.
- Rudd C, Rivadeneira ED, Gutman LT: Dosing considerations for oral acyclovir following neonatal herpes disease. *Acta Paediatr* 1994;83:1237-43.
- Whitley R, Arvin A, Prober C, et al: A controlled trial comparing vidarabine with acyclovir in neonatal herpes simplex virus infection. *N Engl J Med* 1991;324:444.
- Englund JA, Zimmerman BS, Swierkosz EM, et al: Herpes simplex virus resistant to acyclovir: A study in a tertiary care center. *Ann Intern Med* 1990;112:416.
- McDonald L, Tartaglione TA, Mendelman PM, et al: Lack of toxicity in two cases of neonatal acyclovir overdose. *Pediatr Infect Dis J* 1989;8:529.
- Sullender WM, Arvin AM, Diaz PS, et al: Pharmacokinetics of acyclovir suspension in infants and children. *Antimicrob Agents Chemother* 1987;31:1722.
- Hintz M, Connor JD, Spector SA, et al: Neonatal acyclovir pharmacokinetics in patients with herpes virus infections. *Am J Med* 1982;73(suppl):210.
- Product Information, Abraxis Pharmaceutical Products, 2006
- Product Information, GlaxoSmithKline, 2005

ADENOSINE

DOSE & ADMINISTRATION: Starting dose: 50 mcg/kg rapid IV push (1 to 2 seconds). Increase dose in 50 mcg/kg increments Q2 minutes until return of sinus rhythm. Usual maximum dose: 250 mcg/kg. Infuse as close to IV site as possible. Flush IV with saline immediately. Intraosseous administration has also been reported to be successful.

USES: Acute treatment of sustained paroxysmal supraventricular tachycardia. It may also be useful in establishing the cause of the SVT.

MONITORING: Continuous EKG and blood pressure monitoring.

ADVERSE EFFECTS/PRECAUTIONS: Flushing, dyspnea, and irritability occur frequently, but usually resolve within 1 minute. Transient (duration <1 minute) arrhythmias may occur between termination of SVT and onset of normal sinus rhythm. Apnea has been reported in one preterm infant. Recurrence of SVT occurs in approximately 30% of treated patients. Aminophylline/Theophylline and caffeine diminish adenosine's effect by competitive antagonism.

PHARMACOLOGY: Adenosine is the pharmacologically active metabolite of ATP. It acts by depressing sinus node automaticity and A-V node conduction. It does **not** have negative inotropic effects. Response should occur within 2 minutes of the dose. Estimated serum half-life is 10 seconds.

SPECIAL CONSIDERATIONS/PREPARATION: Supplied in 2 mL vials containing 6 mg adenosine in NS. Contains no preservative. Store at room temperature. **Do not refrigerate;** crystallization will occur. Solution must be clear at the time of use. Dilutions can be made with NS for doses <0.2 mL (600 mcg). Use 1 mL (3000 mcg) with 9 mL NS to make a solution with a final concentration of 300 mcg/mL.

Solution Compatibility: D_5W and NS

SELECTED REFERENCES

- Paret G, Steinmetz D, Kuint J et al: Adenosine for the treatment of paroxysmal supraventricular tachycardia in fullterm and preterm newborn infants. *Am J Perinatol* 1996;13:343-46.
- Friedman FD: Intraosseous adenosine for the termination of supraventricular tachycardia in an infant. *Ann Emerg Med* 1996;28:356-58.
- Crosson JE, Etheridge SP, Milstein S et al: Therapeutic and diagnostic utility of adenosine during tachycardia evaluation in children. *Am J Cardiol* 1994;74:155-60.
- Till J, Shinebourne EA, Rigby ML, et al: Efficacy and safety of adenosine in the treatment of supraventricular tachycardia in infants and children. *Br Heart J* 1989;62:204.
- Overholt ED, Rhuban KS, Gutgesell HP, et al: Usefulness of adenosine for arrhythmias in infants and children. *Am J Cardiol* 1988;61:336.
- Product Information, Astellas, 2005

ALBUTEROL

DOSE & ADMINISTRATION: Bronchodilation: 0.1 to 0.5 mg/kg per dose Q2 to 6 hours via nebulizer. 1 MDI actuation per dose (approx. 0.1 mg or 100 mcg) Q2 to 6 hours. **Oral:** 0.1 to 0.3 mg/kg per dose Q6 to 8 hours PO. **Treatment of hyperkalemia:** 0.4 mg/kg per dose Q2 hours via nebulizer.

USES: Bronchodilator. Treatment of hyperkalemia.

MONITORING: Assess degree of bronchospasm. Continuous EKG monitoring. **Consider not administering when heart rate is greater than 180 beats per minute.** Serum potassium.

ADVERSE EFFECTS/PRECAUTIONS: Tachycardia, arrhythmias, tremor, hypokalemia, and irritable behavior.

PHARMACOLOGY: Specific β_2-adrenergic agonist. Minimal cardiovascular effects unless used concurrently with aminophylline. Stimulates production of intracellular cyclic AMP, enhancing the binding of intracellular calcium to the cell membrane and endoplasmic reticulum, resulting in bronchodilation. Enhances mucociliary clearance. Drives potassium intracellular. Studies in vitro indicate that approximately 5% of a MDI dose administered using an in-line holding chamber/spacer device, versus less than 1% of a nebulizer dose, is delivered to the lung. Optimal aerosol dose in neonates is uncertain due to differences in aerosol drug delivery techniques. The therapeutic margin appears to be wide. Well absorbed when administered PO. Onset of action is 30 minutes; duration is 4 to 8 hours. Serum half-life is approximately 6 hours (adults). Time to peak serum concentration is 3 to 4 hours. Tolerance may develop.

SPECIAL CONSIDERATIONS/PREPARATION: Oral dosage form: Syrup, 2 mg/5 mL. **Inhalation solution:** Available as either 5 mg/mL, 0.83 mg/mL, 0.42 mg/mL, or 0.21 mg/mL. A 0.1 mg/mL dilution for inhalation may be made by adding 3 mL of 0.83 mg/mL albuterol concentration to 22 mL of preservative-free normal saline. Label for inhalation use only. Stable for 7 days refrigerated. **MDI:** Available in a pressurized hydrofluoroalkane metered dose inhaler (contains no chlorofluorocarbons (CFC)). Proventil ® HFA 100 mcg albuterol per actuation.

SELECTED REFERENCES

- Singh BS, Sadiq HF, Noguchi A, Keenan WJ: Efficacy of albuterol inhalation in treatment of hyperkalemia in premature neonates. *J Pediatr* 2002;141:16-20.
- Lugo RA, Kenney JK, Keenan J: Albuterol delivery in a neonatal ventilated lung model: nebulization versus chlorofluorocarbon- and, hydrofluoroalkane- pressurized metered dose inhalers. *Pediatr Pulmonol* 2001;31:247-254.

- Stefano JL, Bhutani VK, Fox WW: A randomized placebo-controlled study to evaluate the effects of oral albuterol on pulmonary mechanics in ventilator-dependent infants at risk of developing BPD. *Pediatr Pulmonol* 1991;10:183-90.
- Wong CS, Pavord ID, Williams J, et al: Bronchodilator, cardiovascular, and hypokalemic effects of fenoterol, salbutamol, and terbutaline in asthma. *Lancet* 1990;336:1396.
- Morgan DJ, Paull JD, Richmond BH, et al: Pharmacokinetics of intravenous and oral salbutamol and its sulphate conjugate. *Br J Clin Pharmacol* 1986;22:587.
- Beck R, Robertson C, Galdes-Sebaldt M, Levison H: Combined salbutamol and ipratropium bromide by inhalation in the treatment of severe acute asthma. *J Pediatr* 1985;107:605.
- Product information, Dey, 2007

ALPROSTADIL (PROSTAGLANDIN E₁)

DOSE & ADMINISTRATION: Initial dose: 0.05 to 0.1 mcg/kg per minute by continuous IV infusion. Titrate to infant's response—oxygenation *versus* adverse effects. **Maintenance dose:** May be as low as 0.01 mcg/kg per minute. Higher initial doses are usually no more effective and have a high incidence of adverse effects. May also be given via UAC positioned near ductus arteriosus.

Sample Dilution and Infusion Rate: Mix 1 ampule (500 mcg) in 49 mL of compatible solution (e.g., D₅W) yielding a concentration of 10 mcg/mL. Infuse at a rate of 0.6 mL/kg per hour to provide a dose of 0.1 mcg/kg per minute.

USES: To promote dilation of ductus arteriosus in infants with congenital heart disease dependent on ductal shunting for oxygenation/perfusion.

MONITORING: Closely monitor respiratory and cardiovascular status. Assess for improvement in oxygenation. Closely monitor infant's temperature. Ensure reliable IV access; duration of effect is short.

ADVERSE EFFECTS/PRECAUTIONS: Be prepared to intubate/resuscitate. Common (6% to 15%): Apnea (consider treating with aminophylline), fever, leukocytosis, cutaneous flushing, and bradycardia. Gastric outlet obstruction and reversible cortical proliferation of the long bones after prolonged treatment (>120 hours). **Uncommon (1% to 5%):** Seizures, hypoventilation, hypotension, tachycardia, cardiac arrest, edema, sepsis, diarrhea, and disseminated intravascular coagulation. **Rare (<1%):** Urticaria, bronchospasm, hemorrhage, hypoglycemia, and hypocalcemia. **Musculoskeletal changes:** Widened fontanels, pretibial and soft tissue swelling, and swelling of the extremities may occur after 9 days of therapy. Cortical hyperostosis and periostitis may occur with long-term (>3 months) therapy. These changes resolve over weeks after discontinuation of therapy.

PHARMACOLOGY: Alprostadil causes vasodilation of **all** arterioles. Inhibition of platelet aggregation. Stimulation of uterine and intestinal smooth muscle. Maximal drug effect usually seen within 30 minutes in cyanotic lesion; may take several hours in acyanotic lesions.

SPECIAL CONSIDERATIONS/PREPARATION: Supplied in 1 mL (500 mcg) ampules that must be refrigerated. **Dilute before administration to a concentration ≤ 20 mcg/mL.** Prepare fresh infusion solutions every 24 hours. Osmolality of undiluted (500 mcg/mL) solution is 23,250 mOsm/kg. Extravasation may cause tissue sloughing and necrosis. **Sample Dilution and Infusion Rate:** Mix 1 ampule (500 mcg) in 49 mL of compatible solution (e.g., D₅W) yielding a concentration of 10 mcg/mL. Infuse at a rate of 0.6 mL/kg per hour to provide a dose of 0.1 mcg/kg per minute.

Solution Compatibility: D₅W and NS. No data are currently available on Dex/AA.

Terminal Injection Site Compatibility: Aminophylline, atropine, caffeine citrate, calcium chloride, cefazolin, cimetidine, clindamycin, dexamethasone, digoxin, dopamine, epinephrine, furosemide, gentamicin, glycopyrrolate, heparin, hydralazine, hydrocortisone succinate, isoproterenol, lidocaine, metoclopramide, metronidazole, midazolam, morphine, nitroglycerin, nitroprusside, pancuronium, phenobarbital, potassium chloride, penicillin G, and ranitidine.

SELECTED REFERENCES

- Lim DS, Kulik TJ, Kim DW: Aminophylline for the prevention of apnea during prostaglandin E₁ infusion. *Pediatrics* 2003;112:e27-e29.
- Arav-Boger R, Baggett HC, Spevak PJ, Willoughby RE: Leukocytosis caused by prostaglandin E₁ in neonates. *J Pediatr* 2001;138:263-265.
- Kaufman MB, El-Chaar GM: Bone and tissue changes following prostaglandin therapy in neonates. *Ann Pharmacother* 1996;30:269.

- Peled N, Dagan O, Babyn P, et al: Gastric-outlet obstruction induced by prostaglandin therapy in neonates. *N Engl J Med* 1992;327:505.
- Gannaway WI, et al; Chemical stability of alprostadil (PGE-1) in combination with common injectable medications (abstract #P-152E). *American Society of Hospital Pharmacists Midyear Clinical Meeting Abstracts* 1989;24:75A.
- Roberts RJ: *Drug Therapy in Infants.* Philadelphia: WB Saunders Co, 1984, p 250.
- Lewis AB, Freed MD, Heymann MA, et al: Side effects of therapy with prostaglandin E₁ in infants with congenital heart disease. *Circulation* 1981;64:893.
- Heymann MA: Pharmacologic use of prostaglandin E₁ in infants with congenital heart disease. *Am Heart J* 1981;101:837.
- Product Information, Pfizer, 2002

ALTEPLASE

(TISSUE PLASMINOGEN ACTIVATOR (T-PA))

DOSE & ADMINISTRATION: Restoration of function to central venous catheter: Instill into dysfunctional catheter at a concentration of 1 mg/mL. Use 110% of the internal lumen volume of the catheter, not to exceed 2 mg in 2 mL. If catheter function is not restored in 120 minutes after 1 dose, a second dose may be instilled. **Dissolution of intravascular thrombi:** 200 mcg/kg per hour (0.2 mg/kg per hour). Duration of therapy is 6 to 48 hours. If administering directly into the thrombus, dose may be increased after 6 hours to a maximum of 500 mcg/kg per hour. If localized bleeding occurs, stop infusion for 1 hour and restart using 100 mcg/kg per hour. Discontinue heparin several hours prior to initiation of therapy. **Note:** Reports in the literature are a collection of cases gathered over several years. Some authors used loading doses, others did not. Infused doses ranged from 20 to 500 mcg/kg per hour. Complications were most often linked with higher doses and longer duration of therapy. Call 1-800-NOCLOTS for case reporting and treatment guidance.

USES: Dissolution of intravascular thrombi of recent onset that are either intraarterial or life-threatening. Adjuvant treatment of infective endocarditis vegetations.

MONITORING: Follow coagulation studies (PT, aPTT, fibrinogen, fibrin split products) prior to therapy and at least daily during treatment. Maintain fibrinogen levels greater than 100 mg/dL and platelets > 50,000/mm³. Echocardiography to assess clot lysis at least every 12 hours (Q6 hours optimal). Cranial ultrasound to assess for hemorrhage prior to therapy.

ADVERSE EFFECTS/PRECAUTIONS: Intracranial hemorrhage may occur, especially in premature infants treated for prolonged periods. Bleeding from venipuncture sites occurs in approximately half of treated patients. The risk of complications increases at doses above 450 mcg/kg per hour.

PHARMACOLOGY: Alteplase binds strongly and specifically to fibrin in a thrombus and converts the entrapped plasminogen to plasmin. This initiates local fibrinolysis with limited systemic proteolysis. Alteplase has a shorter half-life than streptokinase and does not cause anaphylactic reactions. It is cleared rapidly from the plasma, primarily via the liver.

SPECIAL CONSIDERATIONS/PREPARATION: Activase® is supplied as lyophilized powder in 50 mg and 100 mg vials. Reconstitute 50 mg vial by adding 50 mL sterile water for injection (do not use bacteriostatic water for injection) for a concentration of 1 mg/mL. Can be further diluted with NS or D₅W to a concentration of 0.5 mg/mL if necessary. Use reconstituted solution within 8 hours of mixing when stored refrigerated or at room temperature. Cathflo® Activase® is supplied as lyophilized powder in 2 mg vials. Reconstitute by adding 2.2 mL sterile water for injection to a final concentration of 1 mg/mL. Do not use bacteriostatic water for injection. Mix by gently swirling until the contents are completely dissolved. DO NOT SHAKE. Use reconstituted solution within 8 hours of mixing. Reconstituted solution may be stored refrigerated or at room temperature.

Solution Compatibility: NS, and D₅W

Terminal Injection Site Compatibility: Lidocaine, morphine, nitroglycerin, and propranolol.

Incompatibility: Dobutamine, dopamine, and heparin.

SELECTED REFERENCES

- Manco-Johnson M, Nuss R: Neonatal thrombotic disorders. *NeoReviews* 2000;1:e201.

- Hartmann J, Hussein A, Trowitzsch E, et al: Treatment of neonatal thrombus formation with recombinant tissue plasminogen activator: six years experience and review of the literature. *Arch Dis Child Fetal Neonatal Ed* 2001;85:F18-F22.
- Marks KA, Zucker N, Kapelushnik J, et al: Infective endocarditis successfully treated in extremely low birth weight infants with recombinant tissue plasminogen activator. *Pediatrics* 2002;109:153-158.
- Weiner GM, Castle VP, DiPietro MA, Faix RG: Successful treatment of neonatal arterial thromboses with recombinant tissue plasminogen activator. *J Pediatr* 1998;133:133-136.
- Product Information, Genentech, Inc., 2005.

AMIKACIN

DOSE & ADMINISTRATION: IV infusion by syringe pump over 30 minutes. Administer as a separate infusion from penicillin-containing compounds. IM injection is associated with variable absorption, especially in the very small infant. To use dosing chart, please refer to explanatory note in "How to Use This Book."

DOSING CHART

PMA (weeks)	Postnatal (days)	Dose (mg/kg)	Interval (hours)
≤29*	0 to 7	18	48
	8 to 28	15	36
	≥29	15	24
30 to 34	0 to 7	18	36
	≥8	15	24
≥35	ALL	15	24
* or significant asphyxia, PDA, or treatment with indomethacin			

USES: Restricted to treatment of infections caused by gram-negative bacilli that are resistant to other aminoglycosides. Usually used in combination with a β-lactam antibiotic.

MONITORING: Measure serum concentrations when treating for more than 48 hours. Obtain peak concentration 30 minutes after end of infusion, and trough concentration just prior to the next dose. When treating patients with serious infections or significantly changing fluid or renal status consider measuring the serum concentration 24 hours after a dose, and use the chart below for the suggested dosing interval. Blood samples obtained to monitor serum drug concentrations should be spun and refrigerated or frozen as soon as possible. Therapeutic serum concentrations: **Peak:** 20 to 30 mcg/mL (or C_{max}/MIC ratio greater than 8:1) (Draw 30 minutes after end of infusion, 1 hour after IM injection.) **Trough:** 2 to 5 mcg/mL

SUGGESTED DOSING INTERVALS

Level at 24 hrs (mcg/mL)	Half-life (hours)	Suggested Dosing Interval (hours)
≤5	≈9	24
5.1 to 8.0	≈12	36
8.1 to 10.5	≈16	48
≥10.6		Measure level in 24 hours

ADVERSE EFFECTS/PRECAUTIONS: Transient and reversible renal tubular dysfunction may occur, resulting in increased urinary losses of sodium, calcium, and magnesium. Vestibular and auditory ototoxicity. The addition of other nephrotoxic and/or ototoxic medications (e.g. furosemide, vancomycin) may increase these adverse effects. Increased neuromuscular blockade (i.e. neuromuscular weakness and respiratory failure) may occur when used with pancuronium or other neuromuscular blocking agents and in patients with hypermagnesemia.

PHARMACOLOGY: Dosing recommendations are based on: (1) Higher peak concentrations increase concentration-dependent bacterial killing; (2) There is a post-antibiotic effect on bacterial killing, especially when treating concurrently with a β-lactam antibiotic; (3) There may be less toxicity with less frequent dosing, due to less renal drug accumulation. Volume of distribution is increased and clearance is decreased in patients with PDA. Serum half-life is prolonged in premature and asphyxiated newborns. Inactivation of amikacin by penicillin-containing compounds appears to be a time-, temperature-, and concentration-dependent process. This is probably clinically significant only when penicillin-containing compounds are mixed in IV solutions or when the blood is at room temperature for several hours before the assay is performed.

SPECIAL CONSIDERATIONS/PREPARATION: Available in concentrations of 50 mg/mL and 250 mg/mL. For IV use, dilute with a compatible solution to a concentration of 5 mg/mL.

Solution Compatibility: D_5W, $D_{10}W$, $D_{20}W$, and NS.

Terminal Injection Site Compatibility: Dex/AA solutions. Acyclovir, aminophylline, amiodarone, aztreonam, caffeine citrate, calcium chloride, calcium gluconate, cefazolin, cefepime, cefotaxime, cefoxitin, ceftazidime, ceftriaxone, chloramphenicol, cimetidine, clindamycin, dexamethasone, enalaprilat, epinephrine, esmolol, fluconazole, furosemide, heparin (concentrations ≤1 unit/mL), hydrocortisone succinate, hyaluronidase, linezolid, lorazepam, metronidazole, midazolam, milrinone, morphine, nicardipine, pentobarbital, phenobarbital, potassium chloride, ranitidine, remifentanil, sodium bicarbonate, vancomycin, vitamin K_1, and zidovudine.

Incompatibility: Fat emulsion. Amphotericin B, ampicillin, azithromycin, carbenicillin, heparin (concentrations >1 unit/mL), imipenem/cilastatin, methicillin, mezlocillin, nafcillin, oxacillin, penicillin G, phenytoin, propofol, thiopental, and ticarcillin/clavulanate.

SELECTED REFERENCES

• Contopoulos-Ioannidis DG, Giotis ND, Baliatsa DV, Ioannidis JPA: Extended-interval aminoglycoside administration for children: a meta-analysis. *Pediatrics* 2004;114:e111-e118.
• Langhendries JP, Battisti O, Bertrand JM, et al: Adaptation in neonatology of the once-daily concept of aminoglycoside administration: Evaluation of a dosing chart for amikacin in an intensive care unit. *Biol Neonate* 1998;74:351-362.
• Product Information, Bedford Laboratories, 2004

AMINOPHYLLINE

DOSE & ADMINISTRATION: Loading dose: 8 mg/kg IV infusion over 30 minutes, or PO. **Maintenance:** 1.5 to 3 mg/kg per dose PO, or IV slow push Q8 to 12 hours (start maintenance dose 8 to 12 hours after the loading dose). In older infants (greater than 55 weeks PMA), dosage may need to be increased to 25 to 30 mg/kg per day in divided doses Q4 to 8 hours. If changing from IV to PO aminophylline: increase dose 20%. If changing from IV aminophylline to PO theophylline: no adjustment.

USES: Treatment of neonatal apnea, including post-extubation, post-anesthesia, and prostaglandin E_1-induced. Bronchodilator. May improve respiratory function.

MONITORING: Monitor heart rate and check blood glucose periodically with reagent strips. Assess for agitation and feeding intolerance. **Consider withholding next dose if heart rate is greater than 180 beats per minute.** When indicated by lack of efficacy or clinical signs of toxicity, serum trough concentration should be obtained. Therapeutic ranges are:

1) Apnea of prematurity: 7 to 12 mcg/mL.
2) Bronchospasm: 10 to 20 mcg/mL (older infants with bronchospasm may need these higher levels because of increased protein binding).

ADVERSE EFFECTS/PRECAUTIONS: GI irritation. Hyperglycemia. CNS irritability and sleeplessness. May be associated with renal calcifications when used concurrently with furosemide and/or dexamethasone. **Signs of toxicity:** Sinus tachycardia, failure to gain weight, vomiting, jitteriness, hyperreflexia, and seizures.

Treatment of Serious Theophylline Toxicity: Activated charcoal, 1 g/kg as a slurry by gavage tube Q2 to 4 hours. Avoid sorbitol-containing preparations: They may cause osmotic diarrhea.

PHARMACOLOGY: Stimulates central respiratory drive and peripheral chemoreceptor activity. May increase diaphragmatic contractility. Cerebral blood flow is acutely decreased following IV bolus dose. Renal effects include diuresis and increased urinary calcium excretion. Stimulates gastric acid secretion and may cause GE reflux. Cardiac output is increased due to higher sensitivity to catecholamines. Elimination in preterm infants is primarily as unchanged drug, although significant interconversion to caffeine occurs. In the very immature neonate, the serum half-life of theophylline is prolonged (20 to 30 hours). Theophylline metabolism and clearance mature to adult values by 55 weeks postmenstrual age. Aminophylline salt is 78.9% theophylline. Theophylline administered orally is approximately 80% bioavailable; therefore, no dosage adjustment is necessary when changing from IV aminophylline to PO theophylline.

SPECIAL CONSIDERATIONS/PREPARATION: Available as aminophylline for IV use (25 mg/mL) in 10- and 20-mL vials. Dilute 1 mL (25 mg) with 4 mL NS or D_5W to yield a final concentration of 5 mg/mL. Stable for 4 days refrigerated. Aminophylline oral solution is available in a concentration of 21 mg/mL. Dilute with sterile water to a final concentration of 2 to 4 mg/mL for oral use. Theophylline oral solution is available as an alcohol- and dye-free preparation in a concentration of 5.33 mg/mL.

Solution Compatibility: D_5W, $D_{10}W$, and NS.

Terminal Injection Site Compatibility: Dex/AA (white precipitate forms within 2 hours) solutions, fat emulsion. Acyclovir, ampicillin, amikacin, aztreonam, caffeine citrate, calcium gluconate, cefazolin, ceftazidime, chloramphenicol, cimetidine, dexamethasone, dopamine, enalaprilat, erythromycin lactobionate, esmolol, famotidine, fluconazole, flumazenil, furosemide, heparin, hydrocortisone succinate, isoproterenol, lidocaine, linezolid, meropenem, methicillin, metoclopramide, metronidazole, midazolam, morphine, nafcillin, netilmicin, nicardipine, nitroglycerin, nitroprusside, pancuronium bromide, pentobarbital, phenobarbital, piperacillin, piperacillin-tazobactam, potassium chloride, propofol, prostaglandin E_1, ranitidine, remifentanil, sodium bicarbonate, ticarcillin/clavulanate, tobramycin, vancomycin, and vecuronium.

Incompatibility: Amiodarone, cefepime, cefotaxime, ceftriaxone, ciprofloxacin, clindamycin, dobutamine, epinephrine, hydralazine, insulin, methadone, methylprednisolone, penicillin G, and phenytoin.

SELECTED REFERENCES
- Lim DS, Kulik TJ, Kim DW: Aminophylline for the prevention of apnea during prostaglandin E_1 infusion. Pediatrics 2003;112:e27-e29.
- Hochwald C, Kennedy K, Chang J, Moya F: A randomized, controlled, double-blind trial comparing two loading doses of aminophylline. J Perinatol 2002;22:275-278.
- Carnielli VP, Verlato G, Benini F, et al: Metabolic and respiratory effects of theophylline in the preterm infant. Arch Dis Child Fetal Neonatal Ed 2000;83:F39-F43.
- Zanardo V, Dani C, Trevisanuto D: Methylxanthines increase renal calcium excretion in preterm infants. Biol Neonate 1995;68:169-74.
- Reese J, Prentice G, Yu VYH: Dose conversion from aminophylline to theophylline in preterm infants. Arch Dis Child 1994;71:F51-F52.
- Kraus DM, Fischer JH, Reitz SJ, et al: Alterations in theophylline metabolism during the first year of life. Clin Pharmacol Ther 1993;54:351-59.
- Shannon M, Amitai Y, Lovejoy FH: Multiple dose activated charcoal for theophylline poisoning in young infants. Pediatrics 1987;80:368.
- Gal P, Boer HR, Toback J, et al: Effect of asphyxia on theophylline clearance in newborns. South Med J 1982;75:836.
- Srinivasan G, Pildes RS, Jaspan JB, et al: Metabolic effects of theophylline in preterm infants. J Pediatr 1981;98:815.
- Aranda JV, Sitar DS, Parsons WD, et al: Pharmacokinetic aspects of theophylline in premature newborns. N Engl J Med 1976;295:413.
- Product Information, Hospira, 2004

AMIODARONE

DOSE & ADMINISTRATION: IV Loading dose: 5 mg/kg IV infusion given over 30 to 60 minutes, preferably in a central vein. **Maintenance infusion:** 7 to 15 mcg/kg per minute (10 to 20 mg/kg per 24 hours). Begin at 7 mcg/kg per minute and titrate by monitoring effects. **Prepare fresh drug Q24 hours due to degradation of amiodarone in solution. Consider switching to oral therapy within 24 to 48 hours. PO:** 5 to 10 mg/kg per dose Q12 hours.

USES: Treatment of life-threatening or drug-resistant refractory supraventricular (SVT), ventricular tachyarrhythmias (VT), and postoperative junctional ectopic tachycardia (JET) - see Adverse Effects.

MONITORING: Continuous EKG and blood pressure (for IV). Follow AST and ALT. Monitor T_3, T_4, and TSH. Observe IV site for extravasation.

ADVERSE EFFECTS/PRECAUTIONS: Short term toxicity: Bradycardia and hypotension (possibly associated with rapid rates of infusion). Polymorphic ventricular tachycardia. Irritating to the peripheral vessels (concentrations > 2 mg/mL). Administer through central vein preferred. **Long term toxicity:** Hyperthyroidism (due to inhibition of T_4 to T_3) and hypothyroidism (due to high concentration of inorganic iodine). Contains 2% benzyl alcohol (20mg/mL). Hepatitis and cholestatic hepatitis (rare). Photosensitivity (10%), nausea and vomiting (10%), optic neuritis (4 to 9%), and pulmonary fibrosis (4 to 9%) have been reported with prolonged oral use in adults.

PHARMACOLOGY: Class III antiarrhythmic agent that is an iodinated benzofuran compound. Electrophysiologic activity is accomplished by prolonging the duration of the action potential and increasing the effective refractory period. Increases cardiac blood flow and decreases cardiac work and myocardial oxygen consumption. Highly protein bound (95%) in adults. Extensively metabolized to an active metabolite by the cytochrome CYP3A4 isoenzyme system (limited in preterm infants). Drug-drug interaction potentially occur when given in combination with drugs that inhibit cytochrome CYP3A4: phenytoin, fosphenytoin, clarithromycin, erythromycin, azole antifungals (e.g. fluconazole, ketoconazole, itraconazole), protease inhibitors (e.g. indinavir, ritonavir), class IA and class III antiarrhythmics (e.g. quinidine, procainamide, sotalol) and cimetidine (amiodarone levels increase). Amiodarone prevents the elimination of digoxin resulting in high digoxin levels. Half-life reported to be 26 to 107 days in adults. No data in preterm infants. Accumulates in tissues; serum levels can be detected for months. Contains 37.3% iodine by weight. Adheres to PVC tubing: low infusion rates in neonates may lead to reduced drug delivery during continuous infusions. Oral absorption is variable with approximately 50% bioavailability.

SPECIAL CONSIDERATIONS/PREPARATION: IV: Available as 50 mg/mL concentration in 3 mL ampules. Contains 2% (20 mg/mL) of benzyl alcohol and 10% (100 mg/mL) polysorbate (Tween) 80 as a preservative. Store at room temperature and protect from light. **Infusions greater than 1 hour, amiodarone IV concentrations should not exceed 2 mg/mL unless using a central line. PO:** Supplied in 200 mg tablets. An oral suspension with a final concentration of 5 mg/mL may be made as follows: crush a 200 mg tablet, slowly mix in 20 mL of 1% methylcellulose, then add in 20 mL of simple syrup to make a total volume of 40 mL. Stable for six weeks at room temperature and three months refrigerated when stored in glass or plastic.

Solution Compatibility: D_5W, and NS.

Solution Incompatibility: No data available for Dex/AA solutions.

Terminal Injection Site Compatibility: Amikacin, amphotericin B, atropine, calcium chloride, calcium gluconate, ciprofloxacin, ceftizoxime, ceftriaxone, cefuroxime, clindamycin, dobutamine, dopamine, epinephrine, famotidine, fentanyl, fluconazole, furosemide, esmolol, erythromycin, gentamicin, insulin, isoproterenol, lidocaine, lorazepam, metronidazole, midazolam, milrinone, morphine, nitroglycerin, norepinephrine, penicillin G, phentolamine, potassium chloride, procainamide, tobramycin, vancomycin, and vecuronium.

Incompatibility: Aminophylline, ampicillin, ceftazidime, cefazolin, digoxin, heparin, imipenem-cilastatin, mezlocillin, piperacillin, piperacillin-tazobactam, sodium bicarbonate, and sodium nitroprusside. No data available for Dex/AA solutions.

SELECTED REFERENCES

- Etheridge SP, Craig JE, Compton SJ. Amiodarone is safe and highly effective therapy for supraventricular tachycardia in infants. *Am Heart J* 2001;141:105-110.
- Yap SC, Hoomtje T, Sreeram N: Polymorphic ventricular tachycardia after use of intravenous amiodarone for postoperative junctional ectopic tachycardia. *Internat J Cardiol* 2000;76:245-247.
- Drago F, Mazza A, Guccione P, et al: Amiodarone used alone or in combination with propranolol: A very effective therapy for tachyarrhythmias in infants and children. *Pediatr Cardiol* 1998;19:445-449.
- Gandy J, Wonko N, Kantoch MJ, et al: Risks of intravenous amiodarone in neonates. *Can J Cardiol* 1998;14:855-858.
- Bowers PN, Fields J, Schwartz D, et al: Amiodarone induced pulmonary fibrosis in infancy. *PACE* 1998;21:1665-1667.
- Nahata MC, Morosco RS, Hipple TF: Stability of amiodarone in extemporaneously oral suspension prepared from commonly available vehicles. *J Pediatr Pharm Pract* 1999;4:186-189.
- Pramar YV: Chemical stability of amiodarone hydrocortisone in intravenous fluids. *Int J Pharm Comp* 1997;1:347-348.

- Perry JC, Fenrich AL, Hulse JE, et al: Pediatric use of intravenous amiodarone: Efficacy and safety in critically ill patients from a multicenter protocol. *J Am Coll Cardiol* 1996;27:1246-1250.
- Soult JA, Munoz M, Lopez JD, et al: Efficacy and safety of intravenous amiodarone for short-term treatment of paroxysmal supraventricular tachycardia in children. *Pediatr Cardiol* 1995;16:16-19.
- Figa FH, Gow RW, Hamilton RM, et al: Clinical efficacy and safety of intravenous amiodarone in infants and children. *Am J Cardiol* 1994;74:573-577.
- Product Information, Wyeth, 2006

AMPHOTERICIN B

DOSE & ADMINISTRATION: 0.5 to 1 mg/kg Q24 hours IV infusion over 2 to 6 hours. Dosage modification for renal dysfunction is only necessary if serum creatinine increases >0.4 mg/dL during therapy - hold dose for 2 to 5 days.

USES: Treatment of systemic fungal infections and severe superficial mycoses.

MONITORING: Monitor CBC, electrolytes, urine output, BUN, and serum creatinine at least every other day. Observe IV site for irritation—phlebitis is common. Serum amphotericin concentrations are not routinely followed.

ADVERSE EFFECTS/PRECAUTIONS: Decreases renal blood flow and GFR by 20% to 60%. Injures tubular epithelium with resultant urinary loss of potassium and magnesium, decreased reabsorption of sodium, and renal tubular acidosis. Sodium intake > 4 mEq/kg per day may prevent or decrease nephrotoxicity. Anemia, thrombocytopenia, hypokalemia, nausea/vomiting, and fever/chills. Consider analgesia before beginning infusion. Cardiac arrest has occurred in patients who received 10 times the recommended dose.

PHARMACOLOGY: Amphotericin B binds to ergosterol in the membrane of sensitive fungi and may be fungicidal or fungistatic. The therapeutic concentration range is not well-defined. Highly protein-bound (greater than 90%). Elimination half-life is approximately 15 days. Drug may accumulate in tissues to a significant concentration and be excreted renally for months.

SPECIAL CONSIDERATIONS/PREPARATION: Available as powder for injection in 50-mg vials. Reconstitute using D_5W or Preservative free SW to a concentration of 5 mg/mL, then dilute further using D_5W to a concentration no greater than 0.1 mg/mL for infusion. Reconstituted solution stable for 24 hours at room temperature or 7 days in refrigerator. **Do not flush IV or mix amphotericin with saline solution**— precipitation will occur. May filter if necessary; mean pore diameter should not be less than 1 micron. **Protect from light.**

Solution Compatibility: D_5W, $D_{10}W$, $D_{15}W$, and $D_{20}W$.

Solution Incompatibility: Dex/AA solutions and NS.

Terminal Injection Site Compatibility: Amiodarone, heparin, hydrocortisone, sodium bicarbonate, and zidovudine.

Incompatibility: Fat emulsion. Amikacin, aztreonam, calcium chloride, calcium gluconate, cefepime, cimetidine, ciprofloxacin, dopamine, enalaprilat, fluconazole, gentamicin, linezolid, magnesium sulfate, meropenem, netilmicin, penicillin G, piperacillin-tazobactam, potassium chloride, propofol, ranitidine, remifentanil, and tobramycin.

SELECTED REFERENCES

- Holler B, Omar SA, Farid MD, Patterson MJ: Effects of fluid and electrolyte management on amphotericin B-induced nephrotoxicity among extremely low birth weight infants. *Pediatrics* 2004;113:e608-e616.
- Chapman RL: *Candida* infections in the neonate. *Curr Opin Pediatr* 2003;15:97-102.
- Bliss JM, Wellington M, Gigliotti F: Antifungal pharmacotherapy for neonatal candidiasis. *Semin Perinatol* 2003;27:365-374.
- Lyman CA, Walsh TJ: Systemically administered antifungal agents: A review of their clinical pharmacology and therapeutic applications. *Drugs* 1992;44:9.
- Baley JE, Meyers C, Kliegman RM, et al: Pharmacokinetics, outcome of treatment, and toxic effects of amphotericin B and 5-fluorocytosine in neonates. *J Pediatr* 1990;116:791.
- Starke JR, Mason EL, Kramer WG, Kaplan SL: Pharmacokinetics of amphotericin B in infants and children. *J Infect Dis* 1987;155:766.
- Dodds Ashley ES, Lewis R, Lewis JS, et al. Pharmacology of systemic antifungal agents. *Clin Infect Dis* 2006;43:S29-39.
- Product Information, Bristol-Myers Squibb, 2006.

AMPHOTERICIN B LIPID COMPLEX

DOSE & ADMINISTRATION: 5 mg/kg per dose Q24 hours IV infusion by syringe pump over 2 hours.

USES: Treatment of systemic fungal infections resistant to conventional amphotericin B therapy or in patients with renal or hepatic dysfunction.

MONITORING: Serum amphotericin B concentrations are not routinely followed. Monitor urine output. Periodic CBC for thrombocytopenia, electrolytes for hypokalemia, BUN, serum creatinine, and hepatic transaminases.

ADVERSE EFFECTS/PRECAUTIONS: Anemia, thrombocytopenia, hypokalemia, nausea/vomiting, and fever/chills.

PHARMACOLOGY: ABELCET® consists of amphotericin B complexed with two phospholipids in a 1:1 drug-to-lipid ratio. Acts by binding to the sterol component of a cell membrane leading to alterations in the cell wall permeability and death. Penetrates the cell wall of susceptible fungi. Concentrates in the liver and spleen. Less nephrotoxic than conventional amphotericin B. Mean serum half-life in adults 24 to 38 hours. The pharmacokinetics of amphotericin B lipid complex is nonlinear.

SPECIAL CONSIDERATIONS/PREPARATION: Available as a ready-to-use admixture containing 100-mg ABELCET® in 20-mL suspension (5 mg/mL). Shake the vial gently until there is no evidence of any yellow sediment on the bottom. Withdraw the appropriate dose into a syringe using an 18 gauge needle. Remove the needle and replace with the supplied 5 micron filter needle. Inject the drug into a different syringe containing a measured amount of D_5W so that the **final infusion concentration is 1 to 2 mg/mL.** Shake until thoroughly mixed. Check for complete dispersion. The diluted admixture is stable for 48 hours refrigerated and an additional 6 hours at room temperature. **Do not freeze. Protect from light. Do not flush IV or mix ABELCET® with saline solutions - precipitation will occur.**

Solution Compatibility: D_5W at 1 to 2 mg/mL, $D_{10}W$ and $D_{15}W$ at 1 mg/mL dilution.

Solution Incompatibility: Dex/AA and NS.

Terminal Injection Site Compatibility: No available data.

SELECTED REFERENCES

- Adler-Shohet F, Waskin H, Lieberman J M: Amphotericin B lipid complex for neonatal invasive candidiasis. *Arch Dis Child Fetal Neonatal Ed* 2001;84:F131-F133.
- Walsh TJ, Seibel NL, Arndt C, et al: Amphotericin B lipid complex in pediatric patients with invasive fungal infections. *Pediatr Infect Dis J* 1999;18:702-708.
- Wong-Beringer A, Jacobs RA, Guglielmo BJ: Lipid formulations of amphotericin B: Clinical efficacy and toxicities. *Clin Infect Dis* 1998;27:603-618.
- Dodds Ashley ES, Lewis R, Lewis JS, et al. Pharmacology of systemic antifungal agents. *Clin Infect Dis* 2006;43:S29-39.
- Product Information, Enzon, 2002

AMPHOTERICIN B LIPOSOME

DOSE & ADMINISTRATION: 5 to 7 mg/kg per dose Q24 hours IV infusion by syringe pump over 2 hours.

USES: Treatment of systemic fungal infections resistant to conventional amphotericin B therapy or in patients with renal or hepatic dysfunction.

MONITORING: Serum amphotericin B concentrations are not routinely followed. Monitor urine output. Periodic CBC for thrombocytopenia, electrolytes for hypokalemia, BUN, serum creatinine, and hepatic transaminases.

ADVERSE EFFECTS/PRECAUTIONS: Anemia, thrombocytopenia, hypokalemia, nausea/vomiting, and fever/chills.

PHARMACOLOGY: AmBisome® consists of amphotericin B intercalated within a single bilayer liposomal drug delivery system. Acts by binding to the sterol component of a cell membrane leading to alterations in the cell wall permeability and death. Penetrates the cell wall of susceptible fungi. Concentrates in the liver and spleen but penetrates the CNS less than conventional amphotericin B. Less nephrotoxic than conventional amphotericin B. Mean serum half-life in adults 24 to 38 hours. The pharmacokinetics of amphotericin B liposome is nonlinear.

SPECIAL CONSIDERATIONS/PREPARATION: Available as powder for injection in 50 mg vials. Reconstitute by adding 12 mL of sterile water for injection to a yield a concentration of 4 mg/mL. Immediately shake vial vigorously for 30 seconds. Check for complete dispersion. Reconstituted suspension stable for 24 hours refrigerated. **Do not freeze. Protect from light**. Before administration, AmBisome® must be diluted with D_5W to a final concentration less than 2 mg/mL. A 1 mg/mL dilution may be made by filtering (using 5 micron filter) 1 mL of reconstituted solution into 3 mL of D_5W. Use one filter per vial of AmBisome®. Use dilution immediately. **Do not flush IV or mix Ambisome® with saline solutions**-precipitation will occur.

Solution Compatibility: D_5W.

Solution Incompatibility: Dex/AA and NS.

Terminal Injection Site Compatibility: No available data.

SELECTED REFERENCES

- Juster-Reicher A, Flidel-Rimon O, Amitay M, et al: High dose liposomal amphotericin B in the therapy of systemic candidiasis in neonates. *Eur J Clin Microbiol Infect Dis* 2003;22:603-07.
- Scarcella A, Pasquariello MB, Giugliano B, et al: Liposomal amphotericin B treatment for neonatal fungal infections. *Pediatr Infect Dis J* 1998;17:146-148.
- Evdoridou J, Roilides E, Bibashi E, Kremenopoulos G: Multifocal osteoarthritis due to Candida albicans in a neonate: Serum level monitoring of liposomal amphotericin B and literature review. *Infection* 1997;25:112.
- Weitkamp JH, Poets CF, Sievers R, et al: Candida infection in very low birthweight infants: Outcome and nephrotoxicity of treatment with liposomal amphotericin B (AmBisome®). *Infection* 1998;26:11-15.
- Dodds Ashley ES, Lewis R, Lewis JS, et al. Pharmacology of systemic antifungal agents. *Clin Infect Dis* 2006;43:S29-39.
- Product Information, Gilead Sciences, 2005

AMPICILLIN

DOSE & ADMINISTRATION: 25 to 50 mg/kg per dose by IV slow push, or IM. Some experts recommend 100 mg/kg/dose when treating meningitis and severe group B streptococcal sepsis. To use dosing chart, please refer to explanatory note in "How to Use This Book."

DOSING INTERVAL CHART

PMA (weeks)	PostNatal (days)	Interval (hours)
≤29	0 to 28 >28	12 8
30 to 36	0 to 14 >14	12 8
37 to 44	0 to 7 >7	12 8
≥45	ALL	6

USES: Broad-spectrum antibiotic useful against group B *streptococcus, Listeria monocytogenes,* and susceptible *E coli* species.

MONITORING: Serum concentration can be measured but is not usually necessary.

ADVERSE EFFECTS/PRECAUTIONS: Very large doses may result in CNS excitation or seizure activity. Hypersensitivity reactions (maculopapular rash, urticarial rash, or fever) are rare in neonates.

PHARMACOLOGY: Ampicillin is a semisynthetic penicillin that is bactericidal. Clearance is primarily by the renal route and is inversely related to postnatal age. Serum half-life in term infants younger than 7 days is approximately 4 hours.

SPECIAL CONSIDERATIONS/PREPARATION: Available as powder for injection in 125-, 250-, 500-mg, 1-g, and 2-g vials. Reconstitute using sterile water for injection. Maximum concentration for IV infusion is 100 mg/mL. Mix to a final concentration of 250 mg/mL for IM administration. Reconstituted solution must be used within 1 hour of mixing because of loss of potency.

Solution Compatibility: D_5W, and NS.

Solution Incompatibility: Dex/AA.

Terminal Injection Site Compatibility: Fat emulsion. Acyclovir, aminophylline, aztreonam, calcium gluconate, cefepime, chloramphenicol, cimetidine, clindamycin, dopamine, enalaprilat, epinephrine, famotidine, furosemide, heparin, hydrocortisone succinate, insulin, lidocaine, linezolid, metronidazole, milrinone, morphine, phytonadione, potassium chloride, propofol, ranitidine, remifentanil, sodium bicarbonate, and vancomycin.

Incompatibility: Amikacin, amiodarone, erythromycin lactobionate, fluconazole, gentamicin, hydralazine, metoclopramide, midazolam, nicardipine, and tobramycin.

SELECTED REFERENCES

- Shaffer CL, Davey AM, Ransom JL, et al: Ampicillin-induced neurotoxicity in very-low-birth-weight neonates. *Ann Pharmacother* 1998;32:482-484.
- Prober CG, Stevenson DK, Benitz WE: The use of antibiotics in neonates weighing less than 1200 grams. *Pediatr Infect Dis J* 1990;9:111.
- Kaplan JM, McCracken GH, Horton LJ, et al: Pharmacologic studies in neonates given large dosages of ampicillin. *J Pediatr* 1974;84:571.
- Boe RW, Williams CPS, Bennett JV, Oliver TK Jr: Serum levels of methicillin and ampicillin in newborn and premature infants in relation to postnatal age. *Pediatrics* 1967;39:194.
- Axline SG, Yaffe SJ, Simon HJ: Clinical pharmacology of antimicrobials in premature infants: II. Ampicillin, methicillin, oxacillin, neomycin, and colistin. *Pediatrics* 1967;39:97.
- Product Information, Sandoz 2004

ATROPINE

DOSE & ADMINISTRATION: IV: 0.01 to 0.03 mg/kg per dose IV over 1 minute, or IM. Dose can be repeated Q10 to 15 minutes to achieve desired effect, with a maximum total dose of 0.04 mg/kg. **ET:** 0.01 to 0.03 mg/kg per dose immediately followed by 1 mL NS. **PO:** Begin with 0.02 mg/kg per dose given Q4 to 6 hours. May increase gradually to 0.09 mg/kg per dose.

USES: Reversal of severe sinus bradycardia, particularly when parasympathetic influences on the heart (digoxin, beta-blocker drugs, hyperactive carotid sinus reflex) predominate. Also used to reduce the muscarinic effects of neostigmine when reversing neuromuscular blockade.

MONITORING: Heart rate.

ADVERSE EFFECTS/PRECAUTIONS: Cardiac arrhythmias can occur, particularly during the first 2 minutes following IV administration; usually a simple A-V dissociation, more often caused by smaller rather than larger doses. Fever, especially in brain-damaged infants. Abdominal distention with decreased bowel activity. Esophageal reflux. Mydriasis and cycloplegia.

PHARMACOLOGY: Anticholinergic. Increases heart rate by decreasing the effects of the parasympathetic system while increasing the effects of the sympathetic system. Peak tachycardia is 12 to 16 minutes after dose is given. Relaxes bronchial smooth muscle, thus reducing airway resistance and increasing dead space by 30%. Motor activity in the stomach and small and large intestines is reduced. Esophageal sphincter tone is reduced. Salivary secretion is inhibited. Duration of action is 6 hours. Primarily excreted renally unchanged.

SPECIAL CONSIDERATIONS/PREPARATION: Supplied in multiple concentrations (0.05-, 0.1-, 0.4-, and 1-mg/mL) for injection. Give IV dosage form PO. Prepare IV or PO dilution by mixing 1 mL of injectable atropine (0.4 mg/mL) in 7 mL of sterile water for injection to yield final concentration of 0.05 mg/mL. Stable for 28 days refrigerated.

Solution Compatibility: D_5W, $D_{10}W$, and NS.

Terminal Injection Site Compatibility: Dex/AA. Amiodarone, cimetidine, dobutamine, famotidine, fentanyl, furosemide, glycopyrrolate, heparin, hydrocortisone succinate, meropenem, metoclopramide, midazolam, milrinone, morphine, nafcillin, netilmicin, pentobarbital, potassium chloride, propofol, prostaglandin E_1, ranitidine, and sodium bicarbonate.

Incompatibility: Phenytoin, trimethoprim sulfamethoxazole.

SELECTED REFERENCES

- Miller BR, Friesen RH: Oral atropine premedication in infants attenuates cardiovascular depression during Halothane anesthesia. *Anesth Analg* 1988;67:180.
- Roberts RJ: *Drug Therapy in Infants.* Philadelphia: WB Saunders Co, 1984, p 284.
- Adams RG, Verma P, Jackson AJ, Miller RL: Plasma pharmacokinetics of intravenously administered atropine in normal human subjects. *J Clin Pharmacol* 1982;22:477.

- Kattwinkel J, Fanaroff AA, Klaus M: Bradycardia in preterm infants: Indications and hazards of atropine therapy. *Pediatrics* 1976;58:494.
- Unna KR, Glaser K, Lipton E, Patterson PR: Dosage of drugs in infants and children: I. Atropine. *Pediatrics* 1950;6:197.
- Product Information, Hospira, 2004

Azithromycin

DOSE & ADMINISTRATION: Treatment of Pertussis infections: 10 mg/kg per dose orally, once daily for 5 days. **Treatment of Chlamydia trachomatis conjunctivitis and pneumonitis:** 20 mg/kg per dose orally, once daily for 3 days. Intravenous treatment is limited to those who cannot be treated orally. To date no clinical studies have been conducted to evaluate the safety or efficacy of IV azithromycin in the pediatric population. Suggested IV dose: 5 mg/kg per dose once daily.

USES: Treatment and postexposure prophylaxis against *Bordetella pertussis*. As a substitute for penicillin in situations of significant allergic intolerance.

MONITORING: Assess gastrointestinal tolerance.

ADVERSE EFFECTS/PRECAUTIONS: Limited data in neonates. Diarrhea and/or vomiting occur in 5 to 12% of patients. Irritability, rash, and blood in stool have also been reported. There is one new case report of pyloric stenosis in 2 of 3 triplets treated with azithromycin for pertussis.

PHARMACOLOGY: Azithromycin is classified as an azalide, a subclass of macrolide antibiotics. In vitro activity has been demonstrated against *Bordetella pertussis*, as well as Streptococci (Groups C, F, G and Viridans), *Ureaplasma urealyticum*, and Peptostreptococcus species. Eradication of *B. pertussis* in unimmunized individuals (e.g., neonates) takes longer and requires higher doses than immunized individuals. Oral bioavailability is 38% in adults and children and is not affected by food. Primarily excreted unchanged in the bile, with some hepatic metabolism to inactive metabolites. The prolonged terminal half-life (approximately 80 hours) is thought to be due to extensive uptake and subsequent release of drug from tissues.

SPECIAL CONSIDERATIONS/PREPARATION: Oral suspension is available in 300, 600, 900, and 1,200 mg bottles. Reconstitute 300 mg bottle with 9 mL of water to provide a final concentration of 100 mg per 5 mL (20 mg/mL). Shake well before administration. Do not refrigerate. Use within 10 days once bottle has been opened. Azithromycin for intravenous injection is supplied in single use vials containing 500 mg lyophilized powder. Reconstitute by adding 4.8 mL Sterile Water for Injection, then shake the vial until all the drug is dissolved. The concentration of the reconstituted solution is 100 mg/mL. It is stable at room temperature for 24 hours. **Dilute prior to administration** using a compatible solution to a final concentration of 1 to 2 mg/mL. Diluted solution stable for 24 hours at room temperature or 7 days in refrigerator. Do not use higher concentrations due to local IV site reactions. **Infuse over at least 60 minutes.**

Solution Compatibility: D$_5$W, NS, 5% Dextrose in 0.45% NaCl with 20 mEq/L KCl, and Lactated Ringer's.

Terminal Injection Site Compatibility: Do not infuse other drugs through the same IV line.

Incompatibility: Amikacin, aztreonam, cefotaxime, ceftazidime, ceftriaxone, cefuroxime, clindamycin, famotidine, fentanyl, furosemide, gentamicin, imipenem-cilastatin, morphine, piperacillin-tazobactam, potassium chloride, ticarcillin-clavulanate, and tobramycin.

SELECTED REFERENCES

- American Academy of Pediatrics. Chlamydia trachomatis, and Pertussis. In: Pickering LK, Baker CJ, Long SS, McMillan JA, eds. *Red Book: 2006 Report of the Committee on Infectious Diseases*. 27th ed. Elk Grove Village, IL: American Academy of Pediatrics; 2006: pp 255, and 500-502.
- Centers for Disease Control and Prevention. Recommended antimicrobial agents for the treatment and postexposure prophylaxis of pertussis. 2005 CDC guidelines. *MMWR* 2005;54(No. RR-14):pp. 4, 10.
- Friedman DS, Curtis CR, Schauer SL, et al. Surveillance for transmission and antibiotic adverse events among neonates and adults exposed to a healthcare worker with pertussis. *Infect Control Hosp Epidemiol* 2004;25:967-73.
- Langley JM, Halperin SA, Boucher FD, et al. Azithromycin is as effective and better tolerated than erythromycin estolate for the treatment of pertussis. *Pediatrics* 2004;114:96-101.
- Jacobs RF, Maples HD, Aranda JV, et al. Pharmacokinetics of intravenously administered azithromycin in pediatric patients. *Pediatr Infect Dis J* 2005;24:34-39.

- Morrison W. Infantile hypertrophic pyloric stenosis in infants treated with azithromycin. *Pediatr Infect Dis J* 2007;26:186-188.
- Product Information, Pfizer, Inc., 2007.

AZTREONAM

DOSE & ADMINISTRATION: 30 mg/kg per dose IV slow push over 5 to 10 minutes, or IM. To use dosing chart, please refer to explanatory note in "How to Use This Book."

DOSING INTERVAL CHART

PMA (weeks)	PostNatal (days)	Interval (hours)
≤29	0 to 28 >28	12 8
30 to 36	0 to 14 >14	12 8
37 to 44	0 to 7 >7	12 8
≥ 45	ALL	6

USES: Treatment of neonatal sepsis caused by susceptible gram-negative organisms (e.g. *E coli, H influenzae, Klebsiella, Pseudomonas,* and *Serratia*). Generally used in combination with ampicillin (empirical treatment of sepsis) or an aminoglycoside (for synergism against *Pseudomonas* and *Enterobacteriaceae*).

MONITORING: Check serum glucose one hour after administration. Measuring serum concentration is not usually necessary. Periodic CBC, AST, ALT.

ADVERSE EFFECTS/PRECAUTIONS: Aztreonam contains 780 mg L-arginine per gram of drug (23.4 mg/kg body weight per dose). Adequate amounts of glucose must be provided to prevent hypoglycemia. Side effects are rare but include eosinophilia, elevation of serum transaminases, and phlebitis at the injection site.

PHARMACOLOGY: Aztreonam is a synthetically-produced monocyclic β-lactam antibiotic. Although bactericidal against aerobic gram-negative bacteria, it has virtually no activity against aerobic gram-positive and anaerobic bacteria, thereby producing little alteration of bowel flora. Good tissue and fluid penetration has been demonstrated in adults, along with protein-binding of 50 to 65%. Eliminated renally, primarily as unchanged drug. Serum half-life in neonates is 3 to 9 hours. Aztreonam does not interfere with bilirubin-albumin binding.

SPECIAL CONSIDERATIONS/PREPARATION: Available as powder for injection in 1-g, and 2-g vials. Reconstitute 1-g vial with 10 mL of either sterile water for injection or NS (100 mg/mL). **Shake immediately and vigorously.** Reconstituted solution stable for 48 hours at room temperature, 7 days refrigerated.

Solution Compatibility: D5W, D10W, and NS.

Terminal Injection Site Compatibility: Dex/AA and fat emulsion. Amikacin, aminophylline, ampicillin, bumetanide, calcium gluconate, cefazolin, cefepime, cefotaxime, cefoxitin, ceftazidime, ceftriaxone, cimetidine, clindamycin, dexamethasone, dobutamine, dopamine, enalaprilat, famotidine, fluconazole, furosemide, gentamicin, heparin, hydrocortisone succinate, imipenem, insulin, linezolid, metoclopramide, mezlocillin, morphine, netilmicin, nicardipine, piperacillin, piperacillin/tazobactam, potassium chloride, propofol, quinupristin/dalfopristin, ranitidine, remifentanil, sodium bicarbonate, ticarcillin/clavulanate, tobramycin, vancomycin, and zidovudine.

Incompatibility: Acyclovir, amphotericin B, azithromycin, ganciclovir, lorazepam, metronidazole, and nafcillin.

SELECTED REFERENCES

- Uauy R, Mize C, Argyle C, McCracken GH: Metabolic tolerance to arginine: Implications for the safe use of arginine salt-aztreonam combination in the neonatal period. *J Pediatr* 1991;118:965.
- Cuzzolin L, Fanos V, Zambreri D, et al: Pharmacokinetics and renal tolerance of aztreonam in premature infants. *Antimicrob Agents Chemother* 1991;35:1726.
- Prober CG, Stevenson DK, Benitz WE: The use of antibiotics in neonates weighing less than 1200 grams. *Pediatr Infect Dis J* 1990;9:111.

- Likitnukul S, McCracken GH, Threlkeld N, et al: Pharmacokinetics and plasma bactericidal activity of aztreonam in low-birth-weight infants. *Antimicrob Agents Chemother* 1987;31:81.
- Product Information, Bristol-Myers Squibb, 2007

BUMETANIDE

DOSE & ADMINISTRATION: 0.005 to 0.05 mg/kg per dose Q6 hours IV slow push, IM, or PO.

USES: Diuretic used in patients with renal insufficiency, congestive heart failure, or significant edema that is refractory to furosemide.

MONITORING: Serum electrolytes and urine output. Assess patients receiving digoxin concurrently for potassium depletion. Follow weight changes.

ADVERSE EFFECTS/PRECAUTIONS: Water and electrolyte imbalances occur frequently, especially hyponatremia, hypokalemia, and hypochloremic alkalosis. Potentially ototoxic, but less so than furosemide. May displace bilirubin from albumin binding sites when given in high doses or for prolonged periods.

PHARMACOLOGY: Bumetanide is 40 times more potent than furosemide with a similar mechanism of action. Inhibits chloride reabsorption in the ascending limb of Henle's loop and inhibits tubular sodium transport, causing major loss of sodium and chloride. Increases urinary losses of potassium, calcium, and bicarbonate. Urine sodium losses are lower with bumetanide than furosemide, but urine calcium losses are higher. Decreases CSF production by weak carbonic anhydrase inhibition. Decreases pulmonary transvascular fluid filtration. Increases renal blood flow and prostaglandin secretion. Highly protein bound (>97%). Data from adults indicate excellent oral bioavailability and significant hepatic metabolism (40%) via the cytochrome CYP pathway. Serum half-life is 2 to 6 hours in neonates.

SPECIAL CONSIDERATIONS/PREPARATION: Supplied as 2-, 4-, and 10-mL vials (0.25-mg/mL solution). Contains 1% (10 mg/mL) benzyl alcohol; pH adjusted to 7. A 0.125 mg/mL dilution may be made by adding 3 mL of 0.25 mg/mL injectable solution to 3 mL preservative-free normal saline for injection. Refrigerated dilution is stable for 24 hours. Discolors when exposed to light.

Solution Compatibility: D_5W and NS. No data are available on Dex/AA.

Terminal Injection Site Compatibility: Fat emulsion. Aztreonam, cefepime, furosemide, lorazepam, milrinone, morphine, piperacillin-tazobactam, and propofol.

Incompatibility: Dobutamine and midazolam.

SELECTED REFERENCES

- Sullivan JE, Witte MK, Yamashita TS, Myers CM, Blumer JL: Dose-ranging evaluation of bumetanide pharmacodynamics in critically ill infants. *Clin Pharmacol Ther* 1996;60:424. (2 other related articles by same authors in same issue).
- Shankaran S, Liang K-C, Ilagan N, Fleischmann L: Mineral excretion following furosemide compared with bumetanide therapy in premature infants. *Pediatr Nephrol* 1995;9:159-62.
- Wittner M, Stefano AD, Wangemann P, Greger R: How do loop diuretics act? *Drugs* 1991;41(suppl 3):1.
- Brater DC: Clinical pharmacology of loop diuretics. *Drugs* 1991;41(suppl 3):14.
- Product Information, Bedford, 2005

CAFFEINE CITRATE

DOSE & ADMINISTRATION: Loading dose: 20 to 25 mg/kg of caffeine citrate IV over 30 minutes or PO. (Equivalent to 10 to 12.5 mg/kg caffeine base). **Maintenance dose:** 5 to 10 mg/kg per dose of caffeine citrate IV slow push or PO Q24 hours. (Equivalent to 2.5 to 5 mg/kg caffeine base). Maintenance dose should be started 24 hours after the loading dose. May consider an additional loading dose and higher maintenance doses if able to monitor serum concentrations. (Please note that emphasis has changed to caffeine citrate due to commercially available product. This product (Cafcit®) may be administered both intravenously and orally).

USES: Treatment of neonatal apnea, including post-extubation and post-anesthesia. (More favorable therapeutic index than aminophylline).

MONITORING: If using the suggested doses above, measuring serum concentrations is probably not necessary. Monitoring of serum drug concentration should be based on a trough level determined on approximately day 5 of therapy. Therapeutic trough serum concentration is 5 to 25 mcg/mL. Concentrations greater than 40 to 50 mcg/mL are toxic. Assess for agitation. Monitor heart rate; **consider withholding dose if greater than 180 beats per minute.**

ADVERSE EFFECTS/PRECAUTIONS: Adverse effects are usually mild, and include restlessness, vomiting, and functional cardiac symptoms. There has been a suggested association with NEC, but causality has never been proven. Loading doses of 25 mg/kg caffeine (50 mg/kg caffeine citrate) have been reported to decrease cerebral and intestinal blood flow velocity.

PHARMACOLOGY: The pharmacological effects of caffeine are mediated by its antagonism of the actions of adenosine at cell surface receptors. It is rapidly distributed in the brain, with CNS levels approximating plasma levels. Caffeine increases the respiratory center output, chemoreceptor sensitivity to CO_2, smooth muscle relaxation, and cardiac output. Oxygen consumption may be increased and weight gain may be reduced. Renal effects include diuresis and increased urinary calcium excretion. Orally administered caffeine citrate is rapidly and completely absorbed. There is almost no first-pass metabolism. In neonates, approximately 86% is excreted unchanged in the urine, with the remainder metabolized via the CYP1A2 enzyme system. The serum half-life of caffeine ranges from 40 to 230 hours, decreasing with advancing postmenstrual age until 60 weeks PMA. Half-life is prolonged in infants with cholestatic hepatitis.

SPECIAL CONSIDERATIONS/PREPARATION: Both Cafcit® Oral Solution and Cafcit® Injection for intravenous administration are preservative free and available in 3-mL single use vials. Each mL of Cafcit® contains 20 mg of caffeine citrate (equivalent to 10 mg caffeine base). The osmolality is 160 mOsm/kg. Store at room temperature. Alternatively, an oral solution may be prepared by dissolving 2.5 g of caffeine anhydrous powder in 250 mL of water, yielding a final concentration of 10 mg/mL. Solution is stable for 4 weeks refrigerated. Crystals form when stored at low temperature but dissolve at room temperature without loss of potency. **Do not freeze.**

Solution Compatibility: D_5W, $D_{50}W$, and NS.

Terminal Injection Site Compatibility: Dex/AA solutions, fat emulsion. Amikacin, aminophylline, calcium gluconate, cefotaxime, cimetidine, clindamycin, fentanyl, dexamethasone, dobutamine, dopamine, doxapram, epinephrine, fentanyl, gentamicin, heparin (concentration < 1 Unit/mL), isoproterenol, lidocaine, metoclopramide, morphine, nitroprusside, pancuronium, penicillin G, phenobarbital, sodium bicarbonate, and vancomycin.

Incompatibility: Acyclovir, furosemide, lorazepam, oxacillin, and nitroglycerin.

SELECTED REFERENCES

- Schmidt B, Roberts RS, Davis P, et al: Long-term effects of caffeine therapy for apnea of prematurity. *N Engl J Med* 2007;357:1893-1902.
- Schmidt B, Roberts RS, Davis P, et al: Caffeine therapy for apnea of prematurity. *N Engl J Med* 2006;354:2112-2121.
- Steer P, Flenady V, Shearman A, et al: High dose caffeine citrate for extubation of preterm infants: a randomized controlled trial. *Arch Dis Child Fetal Neonatal Ed* 2004;89:F499-F503.
- Comer AM, Perry CM, Figgitt DP: Caffeine citrate: A review of its use in apnoea of prematurity. *Paediatr Drugs* 2001;3:61-70.
- Bauer J, Maier K, Linderkamp O, Hentschel R: Effect of caffeine on oxygen consumption and metabolic rate in very low birth weight infants with idiopathic apnea. *Pediatrics* 2001;107:660-663.
- Erenberg A, Leff RD, Haack DG, et al: Caffeine citrate for the treatment of apnea of prematurity: A double-blind, placebo-controlled study. *Pharmacotherapy* 2000;20:644-652.
- Anderson BJ, Gunn TR, Holford NHG, et al: Caffeine overdose in a premature infant: Clinical course and pharmacokinetics. *Anaesth Intensive Care* 1999;27:307-311.
- Lane AJP, Coombs RC, Evans DH, et al: Effect of caffeine on neonatal splanchnic blood flow. *Arch Dis Child Fetal Neonatal Ed* 1999;80:F-128-F129.
- Lee TC, Charles B, Steer P: Population pharmacokinetics of intravenous caffeine in neonates with apnea of prematurity. *Clin Pharmacol Ther* 1997;61:628-640.
- Falcao AC, Fernandez de Gatta MM, Delgado Iribarnegaray MF, et al: Population pharmacokinetics of caffeine in premature neonates. *Eur J Clin Pharmacol* 1997;52:211-217.
- Zanardo V, Dani C, Trevisanuto D: Methylxanthines increase renal calcium excretion in preterm infants. *Biol Neonate* 1995;68:169-74.
- Product Information, Watson, 2006

CALCIUM CHLORIDE 10%

DOSE & ADMINISTRATION: Symptomatic hypocalcemia - acute treatment: 35 to 70 mg/kg per dose (0.35 to 0.7 mL/kg per dose, equivalent to 10 to 20 mg/kg elemental calcium). Dilute in appropriate fluid, then infuse in IV over 10 to 30 minutes while monitoring for bradycardia. Stop infusion if heart rate is less than 100 beats per minute. **Do not give intra-arterially. Maintenance treatment:** 75 to 300 mg/kg per day (0.75 to 3 mL/kg per day, equivalent to 20 to 80 mg/kg elemental calcium). Administer by continuous IV infusion. Treat for 3 to 5 days, and follow serum concentrations periodically. **Exchange transfusion:** 33 mg per 100 mL citrated blood exchanged (equals 0.33 mL per 100 mL blood exchanged). Infuse IV over 10 to 30 minutes.

USES: Treatment and prevention of hypocalcemia, usually defined as a serum ionized calcium concentration less than approximately 4 mg/dL (or total serum calcium less than approximately 8 mg/dL).

MONITORING: If possible, measure ionized calcium directly. Avoid hypercalcemia during treatment. Correct hypomagnesemia if present. Observe IV infusion site closely for extravasation. Observe IV tubing for precipitates. Monitor continuously for bradycardia when giving bolus doses.

ADVERSE EFFECTS/PRECAUTIONS: Rapid administration is associated with bradycardia or cardiac standstill. Cutaneous necrosis or calcium deposition occurs with extravasation. Bolus infusions by UAC have been associated with intestinal bleeding and lower-extremity tissue necrosis.

PHARMACOLOGY: Calcium chloride may be more bioavailable than calcium gluconate, but it also is more likely to cause metabolic acidosis. Administration by continuous infusion is more efficacious than intermittent bolus dosing due to less renal calcium loss. Ionized calcium is the physiologically active fraction, accounting for approximately 50% of total blood calcium. The remainder is bound to albumin (40%) or complexed (10%) with citrate, phosphate, and bicarbonate. Early hypocalcemia is common in asphyxiated infants, premature infants, and infants of diabetic mothers. Significant decreases in ionized calcium may occur during acute alkalosis and following exchange transfusions with citrated blood. Clinical signs suggestive of hypocalcemia in neonates include muscle twitching, jitteriness, generalized seizures, and QTc above 0.4 second.

SPECIAL CONSIDERATIONS/PREPARATION: Calcium chloride 10% injection yields 27 mg/mL elemental calcium (1.36 mEq/mL). Osmolarity is 2040 mOsm/L. Injectable calcium salts should be stored at room temperature and are stable indefinitely.

Solution Compatibility: D_5W, $D_{10}W$, and NS.

Terminal Injection Site Compatibility: Dex/AA solutions, fat emulsion. Amikacin, amiodarone, chloramphenicol, dobutamine, dopamine, epinephrine, esmolol, hydrocortisone, isoproterenol, lidocaine, methicillin, milrinone, morphine, penicillin G, pentobarbital, phenobarbital, potassium chloride, prostaglandin E_1, and sodium nitroprusside.

Incompatibility: Amphotericin B, ceftriaxone, methylprednisolone, metoclopramide, sodium bicarbonate, and phosphate and magnesium salts when mixed directly.

SELECTED REFERENCES

- Rigo J, DeCurtis M: Disorders of calcium, phosphorus, and magnesium metabolism. In: Martin RJ, Fanaroff AA, Walsh MC (eds): *Neonatal-Perinatal Medicine: Diseases of the Fetus and Newborn*, ed 8. St. Louis: Mosby, 2005, pp 1508-1514.
- Mimouni F, Tsang RC: Neonatal hypocalcemia: to treat or not to treat? (A review). *J Am Coll Nutr* 1994;13:408-15.
- Broner CW, Stidham GL, Westernkirchner DF, Watson DC: A prospective, randomized, double-blind comparison of calcium chloride and calcium gluconate therapies for hypocalcemia in critically ill children. *J Pediatr* 1990;117:986.
- Scott SM, Ladenson JH, Aguanna JJ, et al: Effect of calcium therapy in sick premature infats with early neonatal hypocalcemia. *J Pediatr* 1984;104:747.
- Roberts RJ: *Drug Therapy in Infants*. Philadelphia: WB Saunders Co, 1984, p 294.
- Product Information, Abbott, 2002

CALCIUM GLUCONATE 10%

DOSE & ADMINISTRATION: Symptomatic hypocalcemia - acute treatment: 100 to 200 mg/kg per dose (1 to 2 mL/kg per dose, equivalent to 10 to 20 mg/kg elemental calcium). Dilute in appropriate fluid, then infuse in IV over 10 to 30 minutes while monitoring for bradycardia. Stop infusion if heart rate is less than 100 beats per minute. **Do not give intra-arterially. Maintenance treatment:** 200 to 800 mg/kg per day (2 to 8 mL/kg per day, equivalent to 20 to 80 mg/kg elemental calcium). Administer by continuous IV infusion. Treat for 3 to 5 days, and follow serum concentrations periodically. **May also be give orally in the same dose. Exchange transfusion:** 100 mg per 100 mL citrated blood exchanged (equals 1 mL per 100 mL blood exhanged). Infuse IV over 10 minutes.

USES: Treatment and prevention of hypocalcemia, usually defined as a serum ionized calcium concentration less than approximately 4 mg/dL (or total serum calcium less than approximately 8 mg/dL). Treatment of asymptomatic infants is controversial.

MONITORING: If possible, measure ionized calcium directly. Avoid hypercalcemia during treatment. Correct hypomagnesemia if present. Observe IV infusion site closely for extravasation. Observe IV tubing for precipitates. Monitor continuously for bradycardia when giving bolus doses. Assess for GI intolerance when treating PO.

PHARMACOLOGY: Ionized calcium is the physiologically active fraction, accounting for approximately 50% of total blood calcium. The remainder is bound to albumin (40%) or complexed (10%) with citrate, phosphate, and bicarbonate. Early hypocalcemia is common in asphyxiated infants, premature infants, and infants of diabetic mothers. Significant decreases in ionized calcium may occur during acute alkalosis and following exchange transfusions with citrated blood. Clinical signs suggestive of hypocalcemia in neonates include muscle twitching, jitteriness, generalized seizures, and QT_c above 0.4 second. Calcium chloride may be more bioavailable than calcium gluconate, but it also is more likely to cause metabolic acidosis. Administration by continuous infusion is more efficacious than intermittent bolus dosing due to less renal calcium loss.

SPECIAL CONSIDERATIONS/PREPARATION: Calcium gluconate 10% injection yields 9.3 mg/mL elemental calcium (0.46 mEq/mL). Osmolarity is 700 mOsm/L. Injectable calcium salts should be stored at room temperature and are stable indefinitely.

Solution Compatibility: D_5W, $D_{10}W$, and NS.

Terminal Injection Site Compatibility: Dex/AA solutions, fat emulsion. Amikacin, aminophylline, amiodarone, ampicillin, aztreonam, caffeine citrate, cefazolin, cefepime, chloramphenicol, dobutamine, enalaprilat, epinephrine, famotidine, furosemide, heparin, hydrocortisone, isoproterenol, lidocaine, linezolid, meropenem, methicillin, midazolam, milrinone, netilmicin, nicardipine, penicillin G, phenobarbital, piperacillin-tazobactam, potassium chloride, propofol, remifentanil, tobramycin, and vancomycin.

Incompatibility: Amphotericin B, ceftriaxone, clindamycin, esmolol, fluconazole, indomethacin, methylprednisolone, metoclopramide, sodium bicarbonate, and phosphate and magnesium salts when mixed directly.

SELECTED REFERENCES

- Rigo J, DeCurtis M: Disorders of calcium, phosphorus, and magnesium metabolism. In: Martin RJ, Fanaroff AA, Walsh MC (eds): *Neonatal-Perinatal Medicine: Diseases of the Fetus and Newborn*, ed 8. St. Louis: Mosby, 2005, pp 1508-1514.
- Porcelli PJ, Oh W: Effects of single dose calcium gluconate infusion in hypocalcemic preterm infants. *Am J Perinatol* 1995;12:18-21.
- Mimouni F, Tsang RC: Neonatal hypocalcemia: to treat or not to treat? (A review). *J Am Coll Nutr* 1994;13:408-15.
- Broner CW, Stidham GL, Westernkirchner DF, Watson DC: A prospective, randomized, double-blind comparison of calcium chloride and calcium gluconate therapies for hypocalcemia in critically ill children. *J Pediatr* 1990;117:986.
- Scott SM, Ladenson JH, Aguanna JJ, et al: Effect of calcium therapy in sick premature infats with early neonatal hypocalcemia. *J Pediatr* 1984;104:747.
- Roberts RJ: *Drug Therapy in Infants*. Philadelphia: WB Saunders Co, 1984, p 294.
- Product Information, APP, 2002

CALCIUM - ORAL

DOSE & ADMINISTRATION: 20 to 80 mg/kg elemental calcium per day PO in divided doses. **Calcium gluconate** 10% IV formulation (9.3 mg/mL elemental calcium): 2 to 8 mL/kg per day. **Calcium carbonate** 250 mg/mL suspension (100 mg/mL elemental calcium): 0.2 to 0.8 mL/kg per day **Calcium glubionate** 6.5% syrup (23 mg/mL elemental calcium): 1 to 3.5 mL/kg per day.

USES: Treatment of non-acute hypocalcemia in babies able to tolerate oral medications.

MONITORING: Periodically measure serum calcium concentrations. Assess GI tolerance. Assess serum phosphorus and vitamin D levels when indicated.

ADVERSE EFFECTS/PRECAUTIONS: Oral calcium preparations are hypertonic, especially calcium glubionate syrup. Gastric irritation and diarrhea occur often. Use with caution in infants who are at risk for necrotising enterocolitis.

PHARMACOLOGY: Absorption of calcium administered orally is approximately 50%. Absorption takes place throughout the small intestine, and is primarily regulated by 1,25-dihydroxy Vitamin D. Calcium carbonate significantly interferes with the absorption of levothyroxine. The osmolarity of calcium glubionate syrup is 2500 mOsm/L, and of calcium gluconate is 700 mOsm/L.

SPECIAL CONSIDERATIONS/PREPARATION: Calcium carbonate (Roxane) is available as a 250 mg/mL suspension (equivalent to 100 mg/mL elemental calcium) in 5-mL unit dose cups. Calcium glubionate 6.5% syrup (Rugby/Watson) yields 23 mg/mL elemental calcium (1.16 mEq/mL) and is available in 473 mL bottles. Osmolarity is 2500 mOsm/L.

SELECTED REFERENCES

- Hsu SC, Levine MA: Perinatal calcium metabolism: physiology and pathophysiology. *Semin Neonat* 2004;9:23-36.
- Singh N, Weisler SL, Hershman JM: The acute effect of calcium carbonate on the intestinal absorption of levothyroxine. *Thyroid* 2001;11:967-71.
- Product information, Roxane, 1996.

CAPTOPRIL

DOSE & ADMINISTRATION: Initial dose: 0.01 to 0.05 mg/kg per dose PO Q8 to 12 hours. Adjust dose and interval based on response. Administer 1 hour before feeding.

USES: Treatment of moderate to severe hypertension. Afterload reduction in patients with congestive heart failure.

MONITORING: Frequent assessment of blood pressure, particularly after the first dose. Periodic assessment of renal function and serum potassium.

ADVERSE EFFECTS/PRECAUTIONS: Neonates are more sensitive to the effects of captopril than are older infants and children. Significant decreases in cerebral and renal blood flow have occurred in premature infants with chronic hypertension who received higher doses (0.15 to 0.30 mg/kg per dose) than those recommended above. These episodes occurred unpredictably during chronic therapy, and some were associated with neurologic (seizures, apnea, lethargy) and renal (oliguria) complications. **The use of captopril is contraindicated in** patients with bilateral renovascular disease or with unilateral renal artery stenosis in a solitary kidney, as the loss of adequate renal perfusion could precipitate acute renal failure. Hyperkalemia occurs primarily in patients receiving potassium-sparing diuretics or potassium supplements.

PHARMACOLOGY: Captopril is an angiotensin-converting enzyme (ACE) inhibitor that blocks the conversion of angiotensin I to angiotensin II, a potent vasoconstrictor. It thereby decreases plasma and tissue concentrations of angiotensin II and aldosterone, and increases plasma and tissue renin activity. Captopril also prevents the breakdown of bradykinin, a potent vasodilator. Vascular resistance is reduced without reflex tachycardia. Beneficial effects are thought to be caused by a combination of afterload reduction and long-term inhibition of salt and water retention. Bioavailability is good in neonates, although food will decrease absorption. Onset of action is 15 minutes after a dose, with peak effects seen in 30 to 90 minutes. Duration of action is usually 2 to 6 hours, but may be significantly longer (>24 hours).

SPECIAL CONSIDERATIONS/PREPARATION: Captopril oral suspension can be made by dissolving 6.25 mg (one-half of a scored 12.5 mg tablet) in 10 mL of sterile water, adding 1000 mg of sodium ascorbate for injection (4 mL of 250 mg/mL solution) to decrease oxidation, then adding sufficient water to make a final volume of 200 mL. The final concentration is 0.03 mg/mL captopril and 5 mg/mL sodium ascorbate. Solution is stable for 14 days at room temperature, 56 days refrigerated. Some undissolved excipients will remain visible.

SELECTED REFERENCES

• Nahata MC, Morosco RS, Hipple TF: Stability of captopril in liquid containing ascorbic acid or sodium ascorbate. *Am J Hosp Pharm* 1994;1707-1708.
• Perlman JM, Volpe JJ: Neurologic complications of captopril treatment of neonatal hypertension. *Pediatrics* 1989;83:47.
• O'Dea RF, Mirkin BL, Alward CT: Treatment of neonatal hypertension with captopril. *J Pediatr* 1988;113:403.

CASPOFUNGIN

DOSE & ADMINISTRATION: 1 to 2 mg/kg per dose Q24h IV infusion via syringe pump over at least 1 hour. The above dosage is based on a small number of case reports in neonates, as there are no pharmacokinetic data in neonates available at this time. Pharmacokinetic studies in children suggest that a larger dose (50 mg/m^2) may be required to obtain serum concentrations similar to adults. Adults with moderate hepatic insufficiency require dosage reductions.

USES: Treatment of patients with refractory Candidemia, intra-abdominal abscesses, peritonitis and pleural space infections, and those patients intolerant of amphotericin B. Treatment of invasive Aspergillosis in patients who are refractory to or intolerant of other therapies. There are case reports, but not controlled clinical trials, treating endocarditis, osteomyelitis, and meningitis due to *Candida.*

MONITORING: Assess IV site for signs of irritation. Periodic measurement of serum potassium, calcium, and hepatic transaminases.

ADVERSE EFFECTS/PRECAUTIONS: Adverse effects reported in neonates (small number of patients): thrombophlebitis, hypercalcemia, hypokalemia, elevated liver enzymes, and isolated direct hyperbilirubinemia. In adult studies the primary adverse effects are fever, headache, vomiting, diarrhea, signs of histamine release and irritation at the injection site. These occurred less frequently than with amphotericin B or with AmBisome®.

PHARMACOLOGY: Caspofungin is the first of a new class of antifungal agents (echinocandins) that inhibit the synthesis of β-(1,3)-D-glucan, an integral component of the fungal cell wall. It is fungicidal against *Candida* species, but fungistatic against *Aspergillus.* The echinocandins are excreted primarily by the liver, presumably metabolized through an O-methyltransferase. They are not metabolized through the CYP enzyme system and therefore have significantly fewer drug-drug interactions than the azoles. Dexamethasone, phenytoin, carbamazepine, nevirapine, and rifampin all induce caspofungin drug clearance, lowering serum concentrations.

SPECIAL CONSIDERATIONS/PREPARATION: Cancidas® is supplied as a white to off-white powder cake in single use vials, containing either 50- or 70 mg. To prepare the 50 mg Cancidas® infusion: 1) Equilibrate the refrigerated vial to room temperature. 2) Aseptically add 10.5 mL Normal Saline or Sterile Water for Injection to the vial. The powder cake will dissolve completely with gentle mixing. This reconstituted solution can be stored at room temperature for up to one hour. Visually inspect the reconstituted solution for particulate matter or discoloration. Do not use if the solution is cloudy or has precipitated. 3) Aseptically transfer 10 mL of the reconstituted solution to 250 mL bag or bottle of 0.9%, 0.45%, or 0.225% Sodium Chloride Injection, or Lactated Ringer's Injection. This final patient infusion solution has a concentration of 0.2 mg/mL caspofungin, and can be stored for up to 24 hours at room temperature or up to 48 hours refrigerated. May also be diluted in 100 mL of compatible diluent for fluid restricted patients. **Do not use diluents containing dextrose.**

 Solution Compatibility: Normal Saline, Lactated Ringer's.

 Solution Incompatibility: All solutions containing dextrose.

 Terminal Injection Site Compatibility: Do not co-infuse with any other medications. (No data).

SELECTED REFERENCES

• Smith PB, Steinbach WJ, Cotton CM, et al. Caspofungin for the treatment of azole resistant candidemia in a premature infant. *J Perinatol* 2007;27:127-129.

- Manzar S, Kamat M, Pyati S. Caspofungin for refractory candidemia in neonates. *Pediatr Infect Dis J* 2006;25:282-283.
- Odio CM, Araya R, Pinto Le, et al. Caspofungin therapy of neonates with invasive candidiasis. *Pediatr Infect Dis J* 2004;23:1093-1097.
- Steinbach WJ, Benjamin DK. New agents under development in children and neonates. *Curr Opin Infect Dis* 2005;18:484-489.
- Pannaraj PS, Walsh TJ, Baker CJ. Advances in antifungal therapy. *Pediatr Infect Dis J* 2005;10:921-923.
- Walsh TJ, Adamson PC, Seibel NL, et al. Pharmacokinetics, safety, and tolerability of caspofungin in children and adolescents. *Antimicrob Agents Chemother* 2005;49:4536-4545.
- Dodds Ashley ES, Lewis R, Lewis JS, et al. Pharmacology of systemic antifungal agents. *Clin Infect Dis* 2006;43:S29-39.
- Product Information, Merck & Co., 2005.

Cefazolin

DOSE & ADMINISTRATION: 25 mg/kg per dose IV slow push, or IM. To use dosing chart, please refer to explanatory note in "How to Use This Book."

Dosing Interval Chart

PMA (weeks)	PostNatal (days)	Interval (hours)
≤29	0 to 28	12
	>28	8
30 to 36	0 to 14	12
	>14	8
37 to 44	0 to 7	12
	>7	8
≥ 45	ALL	6

USES: Use in neonates is generally limited to perioperative infection prophylaxis and treatment of urinary tract and soft tissue infections caused by susceptible organisms, e.g. penicillin-resistant *Staph. aureus*, *Klebsiella*, and *Proteus*.

MONITORING: Serum concentrations are not routinely monitored.

ADVERSE EFFECTS/PRECAUTIONS: Adverse effects are rare, but include phlebitis and eosinophilia.

PHARMACOLOGY: First generation cephalosporin that is bactericidal against many gram-positive and a few gram-negative organisms. Inactivated by β-lactamase producing organisms. Poor CNS penetration. Renally excreted as unchanged drug. Half-life in neonates is 3 to 5 hours.

SPECIAL CONSIDERATIONS/PREPARATION: Available as powder for injection in 500-mg, and 1000-mg vials. Reconstitute 500-mg vial using 2 mL of NS or sterile water for injection to a concentration of 225 mg/mL. Reconstituted solution stable for 24 hours at room temperature or 10 days in refrigerator. A 20 mg/mL dilution may be made by adding 1-mL of reconstituted solution to 10 mL sterile water for injection, or D_5W.

Solution Compatibility: D_5W, $D_{10}W$, and NS.

Terminal Injection Site Compatibility: Dex/AA and fat emulsion. Acyclovir, amikacin, aminophylline, aztreonam, calcium gluconate, clindamycin, enalaprilat, esmolol, famotidine, fluconazole, heparin, insulin, lidocaine, linezolid, midazolam, milrinone, morphine, metronidazole, multivitamins, nicardipine, pancuronium bromide, propofol, prostaglandin E_1, ranitidine, remifentanil, and vecuronium.

Incompatibility: Amiodarone, cimetidine, pentobarbital, and vancomycin. No data are currently available for potassium chloride.

SELECTED REFERENCES

- Saez-Llorens X, McCracken GH: Clinical pharmacology of antibacterial agents. In: Remington JS, Klein JO (eds): *Infectious Diseases of the Fetus and Newborn Infant*, ed 5. Philadelphia: WB Saunders Co, 2001.
- Pickering LK, O'Connor DM, Anderson D, et al: Clinical and pharmacologic evaluation of cefazolin in children. *J Infect Dis* 1973;128:S407.
- Product Information, Orchid Healthcare, 2006

CEFEPIME

DOSE & ADMINISTRATION: Term and preterm infants >14 days of age: 50 mg/kg per dose Q12 hr. **Term and preterm infants ≤14 days of age:** 30 mg/kg per dose Q12 hr. **Meningitis and severe infections** due to *Pseudomonas aeruginosa* or *Enterobacter* spp.: Doses above administered Q8 hours. Administer via IV infusion by syringe pump over 30 minutes, or IM. To reduce pain at IM injection site, cefepime may be mixed with 1% lidocaine without epinephrine.

USES: Treatment of serious infections caused by susceptible gram-negative organisms (e.g. *E coli, H influenzae, Enterobacter, Klebsiella, Morganella, Neisseria, Serratia,* and *Proteus* species), especially *Pseudomonas aeruginosa* that are resistant to 3rd generation cephalosporins. Treatment of serious infections caused by susceptible Gram-positive organisms (e.g. *Strep pneumoniae, Strep. pyogenes, Strep. agalactiae, and Staph. aureus*).

MONITORING: Measuring serum concentration is not usually necessary.

ADVERSE EFFECTS/PRECAUTIONS: Safety has been documented to be the same as commonly used second- and third-generation cephalosporins. Reported adverse effects are uncommon but include rash, diarrhea, elevated hepatic transaminases, eosinophilia, and positive Coombs' test.

PHARMACOLOGY: Cefepime is a fourth-generation cephalosporin with treatment efficacy equivalent to third-generation cephalosporins. Potential advantages include: more rapid penetration through the cell wall of Gram-negative pathogens; enhanced stability to hydrolysis by β-lactamases; and enhanced affinity for penicillin-binding proteins. The drug distributes widely in body tissues and fluids (i.e. CSF, bile, bronchial secretions, lung tissue, ascitic fluid, middle ear). Protein binding is low (≈ 20%), and it is primarily excreted unchanged in the urine. Serum half-life in infants older than 2 months of age is approximately 2 hours.

SPECIAL CONSIDERATIONS/PREPARATION: Available as powder for injection in 500-mg and 1-g, and 2-g vials. Reconstitute 500-mg vial with 5 mL of sterile water for injection to a concentration of 100 mg/mL. Maximum concentration for IV administration is 160 mg/mL, and for IM administration 280 mg/mL. Reconstituted solution stable for 24 hours at room temperature, 7 days refrigerated.

Solution Compatibility: D_5W, $D_{10}W$, D_5LR, and NS.

Terminal Injection Site Compatibility: Dex/AA solutions. Amikacin, ampicillin, aztreonam, bumetanide, calcium gluconate, clindamycin, dexamethasone, fluconazole, furosemide, heparin, hydrocortisone succinate, imipenem/cilastatin, lorazepam, methylprednisolone, metronidazole, milrinone, piperacillin-tazobactam, potassium chloride, ranitidine, sodium bicarbonate, ticarcillin/clavulanate, trimethoprim/sulfamethoxazole, and zidovudine.

Incompatibility: Acyclovir, aminophylline, amphotericin B, cimetidine, diazepam, dobutamine, dopamine, enalaprilat, famotidine, ganciclovir, gentamicin, magnesium sulfate, metoclopramide, morphine, netilmicin, tobramycin, and vancomycin.

SELECTED REFERENCES

- Capparelli E, Hochwald C, Rasmussen M, et al: Population pharmacokinetics of cefepime in the neonate. *Antimicrob Agents Chemother* 2005;49:2760-2766.
- Gutierrez K: Newer antibiotics: cefepime. *NeoReviews* 2004;5:e382-386.
- Blumer JL, Reed MD, Knupp C: Review of the pharmacokinetics of cefepime in children. *Pediatr Infect Dis J* 2001;20:337-342.
- Bradley JS, Arrieta A: Empiric use of cefepime in the treatment of lower respiratory tract infections in children. *Pediatr Infect Dis J* 2001;20:343-349.
- Saez-Llorens XO, O'Ryan M: Cefepime in the empiric treatment of meningitis in children. *Pediatr Infect Dis J* 2001;20:356-361.
- Kessler RE: Cefepime microbiologic profile and update. *Pediatr Infect Dis J* 2001; 20:331-336.
- Product Information, Bristol-Myers Squibb, 2007

CEFOTAXIME

DOSE & ADMINISTRATION: 50 mg/kg per dose IV infusion by syringe pump over 30 minutes, or IM. **Gonococcal infections:** 25 mg/kg per dose IV over 30 minutes, or IM. **Gonococcal ophthalmia prophylaxis in newborns whose mothers have gonorrhea at the time of delivery:** 100 mg/kg IV over 30 minutes or IM, single dose. (Note: topical antibiotic therapy alone is inadequate and is unnecessary if systemic treatment is administered.) To use dosing chart, please refer to explanatory note in "How to Use This Book."

DOSING INTERVAL CHART

PMA (weeks)	PostNatal (days)	Interval (hours)
≤29	0 to 28	12
	>28	8
30 to 36	0 to 14	12
	>14	8
37 to 44	0 to 7	12
	>7	8
≥45	ALL	6

USES: Treatment of neonatal meningitis and sepsis caused by susceptible gram-negative organisms (e.g. *E coli*, *H influenzae*, *Klebsiella*, and *Pseudomonas*). Treatment of disseminated gonococcal infections.

MONITORING: Measuring serum concentration is not usually necessary. Periodic CBC.

ADVERSE EFFECTS/PRECAUTIONS: Side effects are rare but include rash, phlebitis, diarrhea, leukopenia, granulocytopenia, and eosinophilia.

PHARMACOLOGY: Cefotaxime is one of many third-generation cephalosporin antibiotics. The mechanism of action appears to be by bacterial cell wall disruption. Metabolized in the liver to an active compound, desacetylcefotaxime. The drug distributes widely (i.e. CSF, bile, bronchial secretions, lung tissue, ascitic fluid, middle ear). Excreted renally. Serum half-life in the premature infant is approximately 3 to 6 hours.

SPECIAL CONSIDERATIONS/PREPARATION: Available as powder for injection in 500-mg, 1-g, and 2-g vials. The 500-mg vial is reconstituted with 10 mL sterile water for injection to yield a concentration of 50 mg/mL. Reconstituted solution stable for 24 hours at room temperature, 7 days refrigerated.

Solution Compatibility: D_5W, $D_{10}W$, and NS.

Terminal Injection Site Compatibility: Dex/AA solutions, fat emulsion. Acyclovir, amikacin, aztreonam, caffeine citrate, clindamycin, famotidine, heparin, lorazepam, metronidazole, midazolam, milrinone, morphine, potassium chloride, propofol, and remifentanil.

Incompatibility: Aminophylline, azithromycin, fluconazole, sodium bicarbonate, and vancomycin.

SELECTED REFERENCES

- Centers for Disease Control and Prevention: Sexually transmitted diseases treatment guidelines 2006. *MMWR* 2006;55(No. RR-11):47-48.
- Prober CG, Stevenson DK, Benitz WE: The use of antibiotics in neonates weighing less than 1200 grams. *Pediatr Infect Dis J* 1990;9:111.
- Kearns GL, Jacobs RF, Thomas BR, et al: Cefotaxime and desacetylcefotaxime pharmacokinetics in very low birth weight neonates. *J Pediatr* 1989;114:461.
- de Louvois J, Mulhall A, Hurley R: The safety and pharmacokinetics of cefotaxime in the treatment of neonates. *Pediatr Pharmacol* 1982;2:275.
- Kafetzis DA, Brater DC, Kapiki AN: Treatment of severe neonatal infections with cefotaxime: Efficacy and pharmacokinetics. *J Pediatr* 1982;100:483.
- Product Information, Abraxis Pharmaceutical Products, 2006

CEFOXITIN

DOSE & ADMINISTRATION: 25 to 33 mg/kg per dose IV infusion by syringe pump over 30 minutes. To use dosing chart, please refer to explanatory note in "How to Use This Book."

DOSING INTERVAL CHART

PMA (weeks)	PostNatal (days)	Interval (hours)
≤29	0 to 28	12
	>28	8
30 to 36	0 to 14	12
	>14	8
37 to 44	0 to 7	12
	>7	8
≥45	ALL	6

USES: Use in neonates is generally limited to treatment of skin, intra-abdominal and urinary tract infections caused by susceptible bacteria - anaerobes (e.g. *Bacteroides fragilis*), gram positives (e.g. *Staphylococcus aureus, Streptococcus pneumoniae,* and other streptococci except enterococcus) and gram negatives (e.g. *Haemophilus influenzae, Klebsiella* sp., *E. coli, Proteus vulgaris,* and *Neisseria gonorrhoeae*).

MONITORING: Serum concentrations are not routinely monitored.

ADVERSE EFFECTS/PRECAUTIONS: Adverse effects are rare. Transient eosinophilia and elevation of hepatic transaminases have been reported in < 3% of treated patients. Severe overdose can cause tachypnea, pallor, hypotonia, and metabolic acidosis.

PHARMACOLOGY: Broad spectrum bactericidal second generation cephalosporin that has enhanced activity against anaerobic bacteria. Inhibits bacterial cell wall synthesis by binding to one or more penicillin-binding proteins. Not inactivated by β-lactamase. Poor CNS penetration. Highly protein bound. Renally excreted as unchanged drug (85 to 90%). Half-life in term neonates is approximately 1.4 hours, and 2.3 hours in preterm neonates—considerably longer than children (0.6 hours) and adults (0.8 hours).

SPECIAL CONSIDERATIONS/PREPARATION: Available as powder for injection in 1-g, and 2-g vials. **IV administration:** Reconstitute 1-g vial with 9.5 mL sterile water for injection to a concentration of 100 mg/mL. A 40 mg/mL dilution may be made by adding 4 mL of reconstituted solution to 6 mL sterile water for injection, or D5W. Stable for 18 hours at room temperature or 7 days refrigerated.

Solution Compatibility: D5W, D10W, and NS.

Terminal Injection Site Compatibility: Dex/AA and fat emulsion. Acyclovir, amikacin, aztreonam, cimetidine, clindamycin, famotidine, fluconazole, gentamicin, heparin, insulin, lidocaine, linezolid, magnesium sulfate, metronidazole, morphine, multivitamins, potassium chloride, propofol, ranitidine, remifentanil, sodium bicarbonate, tobramycin and vecuronium.

Incompatibility: Vancomycin

SELECTED REFERENCES

- Regazzi MB, Chirico G, Cristiani D, et al: Cefoxitin in newborn infants. *Eur J Clin Pharmacol* 1983;25:507-509.
- Yogev R, Delaplane D, Wiringa K: Cefoxitin in a neonate. *Ped Infect Dis J* 1983;2:342-343.
- Farmer K: Use of cefoxitin in the newborn. *New Zealand Med J* 1982;95:398.
- Marget W: Tenfold overdose of cefoxitin in a newborn. *Infection* 1982;10:243.
- Brogden RN, Heel RC, Speight TM, et al: Cefoxitin: A review of its antibacterial activity, pharmacological properties and therapeutic use. *Drugs* 1979;17:1-37.
- Feldman WE, Moffitt S, Sprow N: Clinical and pharmacokinetic evaluation of parenteral cefoxitin in infants and children. *Antimicrob Agents Chemother* 1980;17:669-674.
- Product Information, Abraxis Pharmaceutical Produts, 2006

CEFTAZIDIME

DOSE & ADMINISTRATION: 30 mg/kg per dose IV infusion by syringe pump over 30 minutes, or IM. To reduce pain at IM injection site, ceftazidime may be mixed with 1% lidocaine without epinephrine. To use dosing chart, please refer to explanatory note in "How to Use This Book."

DOSING INTERVAL CHART

PMA (weeks)	PostNatal (days)	Interval (hours)
≤29	0 to 28	12
	>28	8
30 to 36	0 to 14	12
	>14	8
37 to 44	0 to 7	12
	>7	8
≥45	ALL	8

USES: Treatment of neonatal meningitis and sepsis caused by susceptible gram-negative organisms (e.g. *E coli, H influenzae, Neisseria, Klebsiella,* and *Proteus* species), especially *Pseudomonas aeruginosa.* Resistance among strains of *Serratia* and *Enterobacteriaceae* is increasing.

MONITORING: Measuring serum concentration is not usually necessary.

ADVERSE EFFECTS/PRECAUTIONS: Reported adverse effects are uncommon but include rash, diarrhea, elevated hepatic transaminases, eosinophilia, and positive Coombs' test.

PHARMACOLOGY: Ceftazidime is one of many third-generation cephalosporins. The drug distributes widely in body tissues and fluids (i.e. CSF, bile, bronchial secretions, lung tissue, ascitic fluid, middle ear). Protein binding is low, and it is excreted unchanged in the urine. Ceftazidime is synergistic with aminoglycosides. Serum half-life in neonates is 3 to 12 hours.

SPECIAL CONSIDERATIONS/PREPARATION: Available as powder for injection in 500-mg and 1-g, 2-g, and 6-g vials. **Intravenous solution:** Reconstitute 500-mg vial with 10 mL of sterile water for injection to make a concentration of 50 mg/mL. Reconstituted solution stable for 12 hours at room temperature, 3 days refrigerated. **Intramuscular solution:** Prepared by reconstituting 500-mg vial with 2.2 mL of 1% lidocaine without epinephrine or Sterile Water to a concentration of 200 mg/mL. Solution is stable for 12 hours at room temperature, 3 days refrigerated. All dosage forms approved for pediatric use contain sodium carbonate; when reconstituted, carbon dioxide bubbles will form. Using a vented needle may help reduce spraying and leaking.

Solution Compatibility: D_5W, $D_{10}W$, and NS.

Terminal Injection Site Compatibility: Dex/AA solutions, fat emulsion. Acyclovir, amikacin, aminophylline, aztreonam, cimetidine, ciprofloxacin, clindamycin, enalaprilat, esmolol, famotidine, furosemide, gentamicin, heparin, linezolid, metronidazole, milrinone, morphine, potassium chloride, propofol, ranitidine, remifentanil, sodium bicarbonate, tobramycin, and zidovudine.

Incompatibility: Amiodarone, azithromycin, erythromycin lactobionate, fluconazole, midazolam, nicardipine, and vancomycin.

SELECTED REFERENCES

- Prober CG, Stevenson DK, Benitz WE: The use of antibiotics in neonates weighing less than 1200 grams. *Pediatr Infect Dis J* 1990;9:111.
- Tessin I, Thiringer K, Trollfors B, Brorson JE: Comparison of serum concentrations of ceftazidime and tobramycin in newborn infants. *Eur J Pediatr* 1988;147:405.
- Odio CM, Umana MA, Saenz A, et al: Comparative efficacy of ceftazidime vs. carbenicillin and amikacin for treatment of neonatal septicemia. *Pediatr Infect Dis* 1987;6:371.
- McCracken GH, Threlkeld N, Thomas ML: Pharmacokinetics of ceftazidime in newborn infants. *Antimicrob Agents Chemother* 1984;26:583.
- Product Information, GlaxoSmithKline, 2007

CEFTRIAXONE

DOSE & ADMINISTRATION: Sepsis and disseminated gonococcal infection: 50 mg/kg Q24 hours. **Meningitis:** 100 mg/kg loading dose, then 80 mg/kg Q24 hours. **Uncomplicated gonococcal ophthalmia:** 50 mg/kg (maximum 125 mg) single dose. (Note: topical antibiotic therapy alone is inadequate and is unnecessary if systemic treatment is administered.) **IV administration:** Infusion by syringe pump over 30 minutes. Avoid administration of calcium-containing solutions or products within 48 hours of the last administration of ceftriaxone. **IM administration:** To reduce pain at the injection site, reconstitute with 1% lidocaine without epinephrine.

USES: Treatment of neonatal sepsis and meningitis caused by susceptible gram-negative organisms (e.g. *E coli, Pseudomonas, Klebsiella, H influenzae*). Treatment of gonococcal infections.

MONITORING: CBC for eosinophilia, thrombocytosis, leukopenia. Serum electrolytes, BUN, creatinine. AST, ALT, bilirubin. Consider abdominal ultrasonography.

ADVERSE EFFECTS/PRECAUTIONS: Not recommended for use in neonates with hyperbilirubinemia. Displaces bilirubin from albumin binding sites, resulting in higher free bilirubin serum concentrations. **Concurrent administration of ceftriaxone and calcium-containing solutions or products in newborns is not recommended.** Fatal reactions with calcium-ceftriaxone precipitates have been reported in neonates (lung and kidney). Administration of calcium-containing solutions or products within 48 hours of the last administration of ceftriaxone is not recommended. Eosinophilia, thrombocytosis, leukopenia. Increase in bleeding time. Diarrhea. Increase in BUN and serum creatinine. Increase in AST and ALT. Skin rash. Transient gallbladder precipitations occasionally associated with colicky abdominal pain, nausea, and vomiting.

PHARMACOLOGY: Ceftriaxone is one of many third-generation cephalosporin antibiotics. The drug distributes widely (i.e. CSF, bile, bronchial secretions, lung tissue, ascitic fluid, middle ear). It is eliminated unchanged by both biliary (40%) and renal mechanisms. Serum half-life in premature infants is 5 to 16 hours. Dosage adjustment is necessary only for patients with combined hepatic and renal failure.

SPECIAL CONSIDERATIONS/PREPARATION: Intravenous solution: Available as a powder for injection in 250-mg, 500-mg, 1-g, and 2-g vials. Prepared by reconstituting powder with compatible solution (sterile water for injection, D_5W, or $D_{10}W$) to a concentration of 100 mg/mL. Reconstituted solution is stable for 2 days at room temperature, 10 days refrigerated. A dark color may appear after reconstitution; however, potency is retained. To make 40-mg/mL solution add 6.2 mL to the 250-mg vial. **Intramuscular solution:** Prepared by reconstituting 250-mg vial with 0.9 mL of 1% lidocaine without epinephrine to a concentration of 250 mg/mL. Solution is stable for 24 hours at room temperature, 3 days refrigerated.

Solution Compatibility: D_5W, $D_{10}W$, and NS.

Solution Incompatibility: Any calcium-containing solution.

Terminal Injection Site Compatibility: Dex/AA solutions, fat emulsion. Acyclovir, amikacin, amiodarone, aztreonam, clindamycin, famotidine, gentamicin, heparin, lidocaine, linezolid, metronidazole, morphine, potassium chloride, propofol, remifentanil, sodium bicarbonate, and zidovudine.

Incompatibility: Aminophylline, azithromycin, calcium chloride, calcium gluconate, fluconazole and vancomycin.

SELECTED REFERENCES

- Centers for Disease Control and Prevention: Sexually transmitted diseases treatment guidelines 2006. *MMWR* 2006;55(No. RR-11):47-48.
- Prober CG, Stevenson DK, Benitz WE: The use of antibiotics in neonates weighing less than 1200 grams. *Pediatr Infect Dis J* 1990;9:111.
- Schaad UB, Suter S, Gianella-Borradori A, et al: A comparison of ceftriaxone and cefuroxime for the treatment of bacterial meningitis in children. *N Engl J Med* 1990;332:141.
- Fink S, Karp W, Robertson A: Ceftriaxone effect on bilirubin-albumin binding. *Pediatrics* 1987;80:873.
- Laga M, Naamara W, Brunham RC, et al: Single-dose therapy of gonococcal ophthalmia neonatorum with ceftriaxone. *N Engl J Med* 1986;315:1382.
- Yogev R, Shulman ST, Chadwick E, et al: Once daily ceftriaxone for central nervous system infections and other serious pediatric infections. *Pediatr Infect Dis J* 1986;5:298.
- Martin E, Koup JR, Paravicini U, Stoeckel K: Pharmacokinetics of ceftriaxone in neonates and infants with meningitis. *J Pediatr* 1984;105:475.
- Schaad UB, Stoeckel K: Single-dose pharmacokinetics of ceftriaxone in infants and young children. *Antimicrob Agents Chemother* 1982;21:248.
- Product Information, Roche, 2007.

CHLORAL HYDRATE

DOSE & ADMINISTRATION: 25 to 75 mg/kg per dose PO or PR. Oral preparation should be diluted or administered after a feeding to reduce gastric irritation.

USES: Sedative/hypnotic for short-term use only. Chloral hydrate has no analgesic properties; excitement may occur in patients with pain.

MONITORING: Assess level of sedation.

ADVERSE EFFECTS/PRECAUTIONS: Episodes of bradycardia are more frequent for up to 24 hours after a single dose in former premature infants. Gastric irritation and paradoxical excitement may also occur after a single dose. Other toxic effects have generally been reported in patients who received either repeated doses at regular intervals or acute overdoses. These effects may persist for days and include CNS, respiratory, and myocardial depression; cardiac arrhythmias; and ileus and bladder atony. Indirect hyperbilirubinemia may occur because TCE and bilirubin compete for hepatic conjugation. **Do not use in patients with significant hepatic and/or renal disease.**

PHARMACOLOGY: Well absorbed from the oral route, with the onset of action in 10 to 15 minutes. Chloral hydrate is rapidly converted by alcohol dehydrogenase to the active and potentially toxic metabolite trichloroethanol (TCEt), which is excreted renally after glucuronidation in the liver. It is also metabolized to trichloroacetic acid (TCA), which is carcinogenic in mice when given in very high doses. Both TCEt (8 to 64 hours) and TCA (days) have long serum half-lives in neonates and accumulate with repeated doses.

SPECIAL CONSIDERATIONS/PREPARATION: Chloral hydrate is available in syrup as 100-mg/mL concentration. Osmolality is 3285 mOsm/kg of water. **The preparations are light-sensitive: Store in a dark container.** Also available as 500 mg suppository. Inaccurate dosing may occur with rectal administration because of unequal distribution of chloral hydrate in the suppositories.

SELECTED REFERENCES

- Allegaert K, Daniels H, Naulaers G, et al: Pharmacodynamics of chloral hydrate in former premature infants. *Eur J Pediatr* 2005;164:403-407.
- American Academy of Pediatrics, Committee on Drugs and Committee on Environmental Health: Use of chloral hydrate for sedation in children. *Pediatrics* 1993;92:471.
- Mayers DJ, Hindmarsh KW, Gorecki DKJ, Sankaran K: Sedative/hypnotic effects of chloral hydrate in the neonate: Trichloroethanol or parent drug? *Dev Pharmacol Ther* 1992;19:141.
- Anyebuno MA, Rosenfeld CR: Chloral hydrate toxicity in a term infant. *Dev Pharmacol Ther* 1991;17:116.
- Mayers DJ, Hindmarsh KW, Sankaran K, et al: Chloral hydrate disposition following single-dose administration to critically ill neonates and children. *Dev Pharmacol Ther* 1991;16:71.
- Reimche LD, Sankaran K, Hindmarsh KW, et al: Chloral hydrate sedation in neonates and infants: Clinical and pharmacologic considerations. *Dev Pharmacol Ther* 1989;12:57.

CHLORAMPHENICOL

DOSE & ADMINISTRATION: Loading dose: 20 mg/kg IV infusion by syringe pump over 30 minutes. **Maintenance dose:** (Begin 12 hours after loading dose.) Premature infants under 1 month of age: 2.5 mg/kg per dose Q6 hours. Fullterm infants under 1 week of age and premature infants over 1 month of age: 5 mg/kg per dose Q6 hours. Fullterm infants over 1 week of age: 12.5 mg/kg per dose Q6 hours. (Absorption of oral chloramphenicol palmitate is erratic in newborns.)

USES: A wide-spectrum antimicrobial bacteriostatic agent. May be bactericidal to species such as *H influenzae* and *Neisseria meningitidis.*

MONITORING: Close monitoring of serum concentration is mandatory. Small changes in dose and interval can lead to disproportionately large changes in serum concentration. Therapeutic peak serum concentration: 10 to 25 mcg/mL. Monitor CBC and reticulocyte counts. Assess hepatic and renal function.

ADVERSE EFFECTS/PRECAUTIONS: Reversible bone marrow suppression, irreversible aplastic anemia. Serum concentration greater than 50 mcg/mL has been associated with the "gray baby" syndrome (i.e. abdominal distention, pallid cyanosis, vasomotor collapse; may lead to death within hours of onset). Fungal overgrowth.

PHARMACOLOGY: Both esters (succinate and palmitate) are biologically inactive prodrugs. Hydrolysis to the active compound is erratic in newborns. Metabolized by hepatic glucuronyl transferase. Hepatically and renally eliminated. Inhibits metabolism of phenobarbital, phenytoin, and other agents.

SPECIAL CONSIDERATIONS/PREPARATION: Chloramphenicol succinate is available as powder for injection in a 1-g vial. Reconstitute with 10 mL sterile water for injection, or D_5W to a concentration of 100 mg/mL.

Solution Compatibility: D$_5$W, D$_{10}$W, and NS.

Terminal Injection Site Compatibility: Dex/AA solutions, fat emulsion. Acyclovir, amikacin, aminophylline, ampicillin, calcium chloride, calcium gluconate, dopamine, enalaprilat, erythromycin lactobionate, esmolol, heparin, hydrocortisone succinate, lidocaine, magnesium sulfate, methicillin, metronidazole, morphine, nafcillin, nicardipine, oxacillin, penicillin G, pentobarbital, potassium chloride, ranitidine, sodium bicarbonate, and vitamin K$_1$.

Incompatibility: Fluconazole, metoclopramide, phenytoin, and vancomycin.

SELECTED REFERENCES

- Roberts RJ: *Drug Therapy in Infants.* Philadelphia: WB Saunders Co, 1984, p 70.
- Rajchgot P, Prober CG, Soldin S: Initiation of chloramphenicol therapy in the newborn infant. *J Pediatr* 1982;101:1018.
- Glazer JP, Danish MA, Plotkin SA, Yaffe SJ: Disposition of chloramphenicol in low birth weight infants. *Pediatrics* 1980;66:573.
- Product Information, Abraxis, 2006

CHLOROTHIAZIDE

DOSE & ADMINISTRATION: Diuresis: 10 to 20 mg/kg per dose Q12 hours PO. **Adjuvant treatment of central diabetes insipidus:** 5 mg/kg per dose Q12 hours PO. Administer with food (improves absorption). IV administration not recommended because of a lack of data. **Note: Do not confuse with hydrochlorothiazide.**

USES: Diuretic used in treating both mild to moderate edema and mild to moderate hypertension. Effects increased when used in combination with furosemide or spirono-lactone. May improve pulmonary function in patients with BPD. Adjuvant treatment of central diabetes insipidus.

MONITORING: Serum electrolytes, calcium, phosphorus, and glucose; urine output and blood pressure.

ADVERSE EFFECTS/PRECAUTIONS: Hypokalemia and other electrolyte abnormalities. Hyperglycemia. Hyperuricemia. **Do not use in patients with significant impairment of renal or hepatic function.**

PHARMACOLOGY: Limited data in neonates. Variable absorption from GI tract. Onset of action within 1 hour. Elimination half-life depends on GFR, and is approximately 5 hours. Major diuretic effect results from inhibition of sodium reabsorption in the distal nephron. Increases urinary losses of sodium, potassium, magnesium, chloride, bicarbonate, and phosphorus. Decreases renal excretion of calcium. Inhibits pancreatic release of insulin. Displaces bilirubin from albumin binding sites.

SPECIAL CONSIDERATIONS/PREPARATION: Available as a 250 mg/5mL suspension for oral use.

SELECTED REFERENCES

- Pogacar PR, Mahnke S, Rivkees SA: Management of central diabetes insipidus in infancy with low renal solute load formula and chlorothiazide. *Curr Opin Pediatr* 2000;12:405-411.
- Wells TG: The pharmacology and therapeutics of diuretics in the pediatric patient. *Pediatr Clin North Am* 1990;37:463.
- Albersheim SG, Solimano AJ, Sharma AK, et al: Randomized, double-blind, controlled trial of long-term diuretic therapy for bronchopulmonary dysplasia. *J Pediatr* 1989;115:615.
- Roberts RJ: *Drug Therapy in Infants.* Philadelphia: WB Saunders Co; 1984, p 244.
- Kao LC, Warburton D, Cheng MH, et al: Effect of oral diuretics on pulmonary mechanics in infants with chronic bronchopulmonary dysplasia: Results of a double-blind crossover sequential trial. *Pediatrics* 1984;74:37.
- Product Information, Merck, 2007

CIMETIDINE

DOSE & ADMINISTRATION: 2.5 to 5 mg/kg per dose Q6 to 12 hours PO or IV infusion over 15 to 30 minutes.

USES: Prevention and treatment of stress ulcers and GI hemorrhage aggravated by gastric acid secretion.

MONITORING: Gastric pH may be measured to assess efficacy. Observe for impaired consciousness and reduced spontaneous movements.

ADVERSE EFFECTS/PRECAUTIONS: Known adverse effects of cimetidine in adults include mental confusion, seizures, renal dysfunction, hepatic dysfunction, flushing and transpiration, neutropenia, diarrhea, hypothalamic-pituitary-gonadal dysfunction, and muscular pain. Cimetidine has been reported to increase the serum level and potentiate toxicity of other drugs such as aminophylline, carbamazepine, diazepam, lidocaine, morphine, phenytoin, procainamide, propranolol, quinidine, theophylline, and warfarin. **Contraindicated** in patients receiving cisapride due to precipitation of life-threatening arrhythmias.

PHARMACOLOGY: Inhibits gastric acid secretion by histamine H_2-receptor antagonism. Peak inhibition occurs in 15 to 60 minutes after both oral and IV administration. Metabolized in the liver via sulfation and hydroxylation to inactive compounds that are 90% renally eliminated. Half-life in neonates is 1.1 to 3.4 hours, and is prolonged in patients with renal or hepatic insufficiency. The sulfoxide metabolite may accumulate in the CNS and cause toxicity. Antacids interfere with absorption; therefore concomitant administration is not recommended.

SPECIAL CONSIDERATIONS/PREPARATION: Available as a 150-mg/mL injectable solution in 2-mL single-use vials and 8-mL multidose vials. A 15-mg/mL dilution may be made by adding 1 mL of 150 mg/mL concentration to 9 mL of preservative-free normal saline. Dilution stable for 48 hours. Manufacturer's oral solution (60 mg/mL) contains 2.8% alcohol. A 2.4 mg/mL oral dilution may be prepared by adding 1 mL (60 mg) of manufacturer's oral solution to 24 mL of sterile water. Stable for 14 days refrigerated. Also available in 200-, 300-, 400-, and 800-mg tablets.

Solution Compatibility: D_5W, $D_{10}W$, and NS.

Terminal Injection Site Compatibility: Dex/AA solutions, fat emulsion. Acetazolamide, acyclovir, amikacin, aminophylline, ampicillin, atropine, aztreonam, caffeine citrate, cefoxitin, ceftazidime, clindamycin, dexamethasone, diazepam, digoxin, enalaprilat, epinephrine, erythromycin lactobionate, esmolol, fentanyl, fluconazole, flumazenil, furosemide, gentamicin, glycopyrrolate, heparin, insulin, isoproterenol, lidocaine, linezolid, lorazepam, meperidine, meropenem, metoclopramide, midazolam, milrinone, morphine, nafcillin, nicardipine, nitroprusside, pancuronium, penicillin G, piperacillin-tazobactam, potassium chloride, propofol, prostaglandin E_1, protamine, remifentanil, sodium bicarbonate, vancomycin, vecuronium, vitamin K_1, and zidovudine.

Incompatibility: Amphotericin B (Immediate precipitation occurs), cefazolin, cefepime, indomethacin, pentobarbital, phenobarbital, and secobarbital.

SELECTED REFERENCES

- Vandenplas Y, Sacre L: The use of cimetidine in newborns. *Am J Perinatol* 1987;4:131.
- Lloyd CW, Martin WJ, Taylor BD: The pharmacokinetics of cimetidine and metabolites in a neonate. *Drug Intell Clin Pharm* 1985;19:203.
- Ziemniak JA, Wynn RJ, Aranda JV, et al: The pharmacokinetics and metabolism of cimetidine in neonates. *Dev Pharmacol Ther* 1984;7:30.
- Aranda JV, Outerbridge EW, Shentag JJ: Pharmacodynamics and kinetics of cimetidine in a premature newborn. *Am J Dis Child* 1983;137:1207.
- Product Information, Hospira, 2004

CLINDAMYCIN

DOSE & ADMINISTRATION: 5 to 7.5 mg/kg per dose IV infusion by syringe pump over 30 minutes, or PO. Increase dosing interval in patients with significant liver dysfunction. To use dosing chart, please refer to explanatory note in "How to Use This Book."

DOSING INTERVAL CHART

PMA (weeks)	PostNatal (days)	Interval (hours)
≤29	0 to 28	12
	>28	8
30 to 36	0 to 14	12
	>14	8
37 to 44	0 to 7	12
	>7	8
≥ 45	ALL	6

USES: Bacteriostatic antibiotic used for the treatment of bacteremia and pulmonary and deep tissue infections caused by anaerobic bacteria and some gram-positive cocci. Clindamycin should not be used in the treatment of meningitis.

MONITORING: Assess liver function. Monitor GI status closely. Therapeutic serum concentration ranges from 2 to 10 mcg/mL (bioassay yields variable results).

ADVERSE EFFECTS/PRECAUTIONS: The most serious adverse effect is pseudomembranous colitis, characterized by bloody diarrhea, abdominal pain, and fever. Discontinue clindamycin if any of these signs or symptoms occur, begin bowel rest and TPN, and consider treatment with oral metronidazole.

PHARMACOLOGY: Clindamycin inhibits bacterial protein synthesis and is primarily bacteriostatic at therapeutically attainable concentrations. Widely distributed into most tissues, especially the lung. Poor CSF penetration. Oral clindamycin is completely absorbed from the GI tract. Highly protein bound. Almost complete metabolism in the liver, with excretion via bile and feces. Available data in neonates suggest extremely variable clearance, especially in premature infants. No data are available regarding conversion of ester to active drug.

SPECIAL CONSIDERATIONS/PREPARATION: Oral preparation (clindamycin palmitate) is reconstituted with sterile water for injection, yielding a 75 mg per 5 mL solution. **Do not refrigerate.** Stable at room temperature for 2 weeks. IV preparation (clindamycin phosphate) is available as a 150 mg/mL solution in 2-mL, 4-mL, and 6-mL vials containing 9.45 mg/mL benzyl alcohol. It should be diluted using D_5W, NS, or LR to a maximum concentration of 18 mg/mL, and infused at a rate no greater than 30 mg/min. Also available in premixed bags (50 mL) without benzyl alcohol containing 300 mg, 600 mg or 900 mg of clindamycin.

Solution Compatibility: D_5W, $D_{10}W$, and NS.

Terminal Injection Site Compatibility: Dex/AA solutions, fat emulsion. Acyclovir, amikacin, amiodarone, ampicillin, aztreonam, caffeine citrate, cefazolin, cefepime, cefotaxime, cefoxitin, ceftazidime, ceftriaxone, cimetidine, enalaprilat, esmolol, gentamicin, heparin, hydrocortisone succinate, linezolid, magnesium sulfate, metoclopramide, metronidazole, midazolam, milrinone, morphine, netilmicin, nicardipine, penicillin G, piperacillin, piperacillin/tazobactam, potassium chloride, propofol, prostaglandin E_1, ranitidine, remifentanil, sodium bicarbonate, tobramycin, and zidovudine.

Incompatibility: Aminophylline, azithromycin, barbiturates, calcium gluconate, ciprofloxacin, fluconazole, and phenytoin.

SELECTED REFERENCES

- Koren G, Zarfin Y, Maresky D, et al: Pharmacokinetics of intravenous clindamycin in newborn infants. *Pediatr Pharmacol* 1986;5:287.
- Bell MJ, Shackelford P, Smith R, Schroeder K: Pharmacokinetics of clindamycin phosphate in the first year of life. *J Pediatr* 1984;105:482.
- Feigin RD, Pickering LK, Anderson D, et al: Clindamycin treatment of osteomyelitis and septic arthritis in children. *Pediatrics* 1975;55:213.
- Lwin N, Collipp PJ: Absorption and tolerance of clindamycin 2-palmitate in infants below 6 months of age. *Curr Ther Res Clin Exp* 1970;12:648.
- Product Information, Pfizer, 2003

CUROSURF®

(PORACTANT ALFA) INTRATRACHEAL SUSPENSION

DOSE & ADMINISTRATION: Initial dose is 2.5 mL/kg per dose intratracheally, divided into 2 aliquots followed by up to two subsequent doses of 1.25 mL/kg per dose administered at 12-hour intervals if needed.

Clear the trachea of secretions. Shorten a 5F end-hole catheter so the tip of the catheter will protrude just beyond end of ET tube above infant's carina. Slowly withdraw entire contents of vial into a plastic syringe through a large (greater than 20 gauge) needle. **Do not filter or shake.** Attach shortened catheter to syringe. Fill catheter with surfactant. Discard excess through catheter so only total dose to be given remains in syringe. Administer in two to four aliquots with the infant in different positions to enhance distribution in the lungs. The catheter can be inserted into the infant's endotracheal tube without interrupting ventilation by passing the catheter through a neonatal suction valve attached to the endotracheal tube. Alternatively, surfactant can be instilled through the catheter by briefly disconnecting the endotracheal tube from the ventilator. After administration of each aliquot, the dosing catheter is removed from the ET tube and the infant is ventilated for at least 30 seconds until stable.

PHARMACOLOGY: Pulmonary lung surfactants are essential for effective ventilation by modifying alveolar surface tension thereby stabilizing the alveoli. Curosurf® is a modified porcine-derived minced lung extract containing phospholipids, neutral lipids, fatty acids, and surfactant-associated proteins B and C. Each mL of surfactant contains 80 mg of total phospholipids (54 mg of phosphatidylcholine of which 30.5 mg dipalmitoyl phosphatidylcholine) and 1 mg of protein including 0.3 mg of SP-B.

SPECIAL CONSIDERATIONS/PREPARATION: Available in 1.5 mL (120 mg phospholipid) and 3 mL (240 mg phospholipid) vials. Refrigerate (2 °C to 8 °C (36 °F to 46 °F)) and protect from light. Inspect Curosurf for discoloration; normal color is creamy white. If settling occurs during storage, gently turn vial upside-down in order to uniformly suspend. **Do not shake.** Used vials with residual drug should be discarded. Unopened vials that have been warmed to room temperature one time may be refrigerated within 24 hours and stored for future use. Should not be warmed and returned to the refrigerator more than once.

SELECTED REFERENCES

- Collaborative European Multicenter Study Group: Surfactant replacement therapy for severe neonatal respiratory distress syndrome: A international randomized clinical trial. *Pediatrics* 1988;82:683-691.
- Bevilacqua G, Parmigiani S, Robertson B: Prophylaxis of respiratory distress syndrome by treatment with modified porcine surfactant at birth: a multicentre prospective prospective trial. *J Perinat Med* 1996;24:609-620.
- Egberts J, de Winter JP, Sedin G, et al: Comparison of prophylaxis and rescue treatment with Curosurf® in neonates less than 30 weeks' gestation: A randomized trial. *Pediatrics* 1993;92:768-774.
- Halliday HL, Tarnow-Mordi WO, Corcoran JD, et al: Multicentre randomised trial comparing high and low dose surfactant regimens for the treatment of respiratory distress syndrome (the Curosurf® 4 trials). *Arch Dis Child* 1993;69:276-280.
- Product Information, Dey, 2002

CYCLOPENTOLATE (OPHTHALMIC)

DOSE & ADMINISTRATION: 1 or 2 drops instilled in the eye 10 to 30 minutes prior to funduscopy. Use solutions containing concentrations of 0.5% or less in neonates. May be used in conjunction with 1 drop of phenylephrine 2.5% ophthalmic solution. Apply pressure to the lacrimal sac during and for 2 minutes after instillation to minimize systemic absorption.

USES: Induction of mydriasis and cycloplegia for diagnostic and therapeutic ophthalmic procedures.

MONITORING: Monitor heart rate and assess for signs of ileus prior to feeding.

ADVERSE EFFECTS/PRECAUTIONS: Feedings should be withheld for 4 hours following procedure. Systemic effects are those of anticholinergic drugs: Fever, tachycardia, vasodilatation, dry mouth, restlessness, delayed gastric emptying and decreased gastrointestinal motility, and urinary retention. The use of solutions with concentrations of 1% or greater have caused systemic toxicity in infants.

PHARMACOLOGY: Anticholinergic drug that produces pupillary dilation by inhibiting the sphincter pupillae muscle, and paralysis of accommodation. Maximal mydriasis occurs 30 to 60 minutes following administration. Recovery of accommodation occurs in 6 to 24 hours. Without lacrimal sac occlusion, approximately 80% of each drop may pass through the nasolacrimal system and be available for rapid systemic absorption by the nasal mucosa.

SPECIAL CONSIDERATIONS/PREPARATION: Supplied as ophthalmic solution in 0.5%, 1% and 2% concentrations in 2- to 15-mL bottles. Store away from heat. **Do not refrigerate.** A preparation containing cyclopentolate 0.2% and phenylephrine 1% (Cyclomydril®) is commercially available in 2- and 8-mL Drop-tainers. A combination eye drop solution ("Caputo drops") may be prepared in a 15-mL bottle with 3.75 mL of cyclopentolate 2%, 7.5 mL of tropicamide 1%, and 3.75 mL of phenylephrine 10%. The final solution contains cyclopentolate 0.5%, tropicamide 0.5%, and phenylephrine 2.5%.

SELECTED REFERENCES

- Bonthala S, Sparks JW, Musgrove KH, Berseth CL: Mydriatics slow gastric emptying in preterm infants. *J Pediatr* 2000;137:327-30.
- Wallace DK, Steinkuller PG: Ocular medications in children. *Clin Pediatr* 1998;37:645.

- Laws DE, Morton C, Weindling M, Clark D: Systemic effects of screening for retinopathy of prematurity. *Br J Ophthalmol* 1996;80:425-428.
- McGregor MLK: Anticholinergic agents, in Mauger TF, Craig EL (eds): *Havener's Ocular Pharmacology*, ed 6. St. Louis: Mosby-YearBook, 1994, pp 148-155.
- Caputo AR, Schnitzer RE, Lindquist TD, Sun S: Dilation in neonates: a protocol. *Pediatrics* 1982;69:77-80.
- Isenberg S, Everett S: Cardiovascular effects of mydriatics in low-birth-weight infants. *J Pediatr* 1984;105:111-112.
- Product Information, Falcon, 2004

DEXAMETHASONE

DOSE & ADMINISTRATION: DART trial protocol: 0.075 mg/kg per dose Q12 hours for 3 days, 0.05 mg/kg per dose Q12 hours for 3 days, 0.025 mg/kg per dose Q12 hours for 2 days, and 0.01 mg/kg per dose Q12 hours for 2 days. Doses may be administered IV slow push or PO.

USES: Anti-inflammatory glucocorticoid used to facilitate extubation and improve lung function in infants at high risk for developing chronic lung disease.

MONITORING: Assess for hyperglycemia and hyperlipidemia. Monitor blood pressure. Guaiac gastric aspirates. Echocardiogram if treating longer than 7 days.

ADVERSE EFFECTS/PRECAUTIONS: The February 2002 AAP and CPS statement strongly discourages routine use of dexamethasone. If dexamethasone is used for CLD risk reduction, 1) Treat only those infants at highest risk; 2) Use lower than traditional pharmacologic doses; 3) Begin treatment after Day 7 but before Day 14 of life; 4) Do not give concurrently with indomethacin; 5) Use preservative-free drug wherever possible. The DART trial found no association with long-term morbidity, but other studies have reported an increased risk of cerebral palsy. Most evidence suggests no increase in the incidence of ROP or the need for cryotherapy. Gastrointestinal perforation and GI hemorrhage occur more frequently in patients treated beginning on Day 1 and in those also being treated concurrently with indomethacin. Hyperglycemia and glycosuria occur frequently after the first few doses, and one case of diabetic ketoacidosis has been reported. Blood pressure increases are common, and hypertension occurs occasionally. Cardiac effects noted by Day 14 of therapy include increased left ventricular wall thickness with outflow tract obstruction and transient impairment of left ventricular filling, systolic anterior motion of the mitral valve, and ST-segment depression. Other potential short-term adverse effects include sodium and water retention, hypokalemia, hypocalcemia, hypertriglyceridemia, increased risk of sepsis, renal stones (in patients receiving furosemide), osteopenia, and inhibition of growth. Adrenal insufficiency may occur secondary to pituitary suppression.

PHARMACOLOGY: Stabilizes lysosomal and cell membranes, inhibits complement-induced granulocyte aggregation, improves integrity of alveolar-capillary barrier, inhibits prostaglandin and leukotriene production, rightward shifts oxygen-hemoglobin dissociation curve, increases surfactant production, decreases pulmonary edema, relaxes bronchospasm. Hyperglycemia is caused by inhibition of glucose uptake into cells and decreased glucokinase activity. Increased triglyceride synthesis is due to hyperinsulinemia and increased acetyl-CoA carboxylase activity. Blood pressure is increased due to increased responsiveness to endogenous catecholamines. Increases protein catabolism with potential loss of muscle tissue, increases urinary calcium excretion because of bone resorption, and suppresses pituitary ACTH secretion. Biologic half-life is 36 to 54 hours.

SPECIAL CONSIDERATIONS/PREPARATION: Dexamethasone sodium phosphate for injection is available in concentrations of 4 mg/mL (benzyl alcohol preservative 10 mg/mL) and 10 mg/mL (preservative free or benzyl alcohol preservative 10 mg/mL). A 0.2 mg/mL dilution may be made by adding 1 mL of the 4 mg/mL concentration to 19 mL preservative-free sterile water for injection. Dilution is stable for 24 hours refrigerated and may be used for PO administration.

Solution Compatibility: D_5W, $D_{10}W$, and NS.

Terminal Injection Site Compatibility: Dex/AA solutions, fat emulsion. Acyclovir, amikacin, aminophylline, aztreonam, caffeine citrate, cefepime, cimetidine, famotidine, fentanyl, fluconazole, furosemide, heparin, hydrocortisone succinate, lidocaine, linezolid, lorazepam, meropenem, metoclopramide, milrinone, morphine, nafcillin, netilmicin, piperacillin-tazobactam, potassium chloride, propofol, prostaglandin E_1, ranitidine, remifentanil, sodium bicarbonate, and zidovudine.

Incompatibility: Ciprofloxacin, glycopyrrolate, midazolam and vancomycin.

SELECTED REFERENCES

- Doyle LW, Davis PG, Morley CJ, et al. DART Study Investigators: Low-dose dexamethasone facilitates extubation among chronically ventilator-dependent infants: a multicenter, international, randomized, controlled trial. *Pediatrics* 2006;117:75-83.

REVIEWS

- Eichenwald EC, Stark AR: Are postnatal steroids ever justified to treat severe bronchopulmonary dysplasia? *Arch Dis Child Fetal Neonatal Ed* 2007;92:334-337.
- American Academy of Pediatrics, Canadian Paediatric Society: Postnatal corticosteroids to treat or prevent chronic lung disease in preterm infants. *Pediatrics* 2002;109:330.
- Kennedy KA: Controversies in the use of postnatal steroids. *Semin Perinatol* 2001;25:397-405.
- Halliday HL, Ehrenkranz RA, Doyle LW: Moderately early (7-14 days) postnatal corticosteroids for preventing chronic lung disease in preterm infants. (Cochrane Review). In: *The Cochrane Library*, Issue 1, 2003. Oxford: Update Software.

ADVERSE EFFECTS

- Stark AR, Carlo W, Tyson JE, et al: Adverse effects of early dexamethasone treatment extremely low birth weight infants. *N Engl J Med* 2001;344:95-101.
- Stoll BJ, Temprosa MS, Tyson JE, et al: Dexamethasone therapy increases infection in very low birth weight infants. *Pediatrics* 1999;104(5). URL: http://www.pediatrics.org/cgi/content/full/104(5)/e63.
- Amin SB Sinkin RA, McDermott MP, Kendig JW: Lipid intolerance in neonates receiving dexamethasone for bronchopulmonary dysplasia. *Arch Pediatr Adolesc Med* 1999;153:795-800.
- Bensky AS, Kothadia JM, Covitz, W: Cardiac effects of dexamethasone In very low birth weight infants. *Pediatrics* 1996;97:818.
- Wright K, Wright SP: Lack of association of glucocorticoid therapy and retinopathy of prematurity. *Arch Pediatr Adolesc Med* 1994;148:848.
- Ng PC: The effectiveness and side effects of dexamethasone in preterm infants with bronchopulmonary dysplasia. *Arch Dis Child* 1993;68:330.

DEVELOPMENTAL FOLLOW-UP

- Doyle LW, Davis PG, Morley CJ, et al. DART Study Investigators: Outcome at 2 years of age of infants from the DART study: a multicenter, international, randomized, controlled trial of low-dose dexamethasone. *Pediatrics* 2007;119:716-21.
- O'Shea TM, Kothadia JM, Klinepeter KL, et al: Randomized placebo-controlled trial of a 42-day tapering course of dexamethasone to reduce the duration of ventilator dependency in very low birth weight infants: Outcome of study participants at 1 year adjusted age. *Pediatrics* 1999;104:15-21.
- Shinwell ES, Karplus M, Reich D, et al: Early postnatal dexamethasone therapy and increased incidence of cerebral palsy. *Arch Dis Child Fetal Neonatal Ed* 2000; 83:F177-181.
- Product Information, Abraxis, 2006

DIAZOXIDE

DOSE & ADMINISTRATION: 2 to 5 mg/kg per dose PO given Q8 hours. Begin therapy at the higher dosage and taper by response.

USES: Treatment of persistent (more than a few days) or severe hypoglycemia due to hyperinsulinism. Positive responses are usually seen within 48 to 72 hours, and occur in less than 50% of neonates.

MONITORING: Periodic CBC and serum uric acid concentrations if treating long term.

ADVERSE EFFECTS/PRECAUTIONS: Sodium and fluid retention is common—consider concurrent treatment with chlorothiazide (which may also potentiate the hyperglycemic action of diazoxide). There are a few case reports of pulmonary hypertension and cardiac failure, perhaps due to a direct toxic vascular injury. Hyperuricemia, leukopenia, and neutropenia are rare complications. Excessive hair growth and coarse facial features develop with long term use. Ketoacidosis may occur during times of intercurrent illness.

PHARMACOLOGY: Diazoxide inhibits insulin release by opening ATP-sensitive potassium channels in normal pancreatic beta cells. The opening of these channels also occurs in cardiac and vascular smooth muscle, leading to decreases in blood pressure and the potential for other rare toxic cardiovascular effects. Diazoxide also reduces insulin release and counters the peripheral actions of insulin via catecholamine stimulation. The serum half-life is 10 to 24 hours in infants. Protein binding is more than 90% in adults, and it is primarily excreted unchanged by the kidneys.

SPECIAL CONSIDERATIONS/PREPARATION: Proglycem® is available as an oral suspension, 50 mg/mL concentration. Alcohol content is 7.25%. Shake well before use. Protect from light. Store at room temperature.

SELECTED REFERENCES

- Nebesio TD, Hoover WC, Caldwell RL, et al: Development of pulmonary hypertension in an infant treated with diazoxide. *J Pediatr Endocrinol Metab* 2007;20:939-44.
- Hoe FM, Thornton PS, Wanner LA, et al. Clinical features and insulin regulation in infants with a syndrome of prolonged neonatal hyperinsulinism. *J Pediatr* 2006;148:207-212.
- Schwitzgebel VM, Gitelman SE: Neonatal hyperinsulinism. *Clin Perinatol* 1998;25:1015-1038.
- Kane C, Lindley KJ, Johnson PRV, et al: Therapy for persistent hyperinsulinemic hypoglycemia of infancy: understanding the responsiveness of beta cells to diazoxide and somatostatin. *J Clin Investig* 1997;100:1888-1893.
- Stanley CA: Hyperinsulinism in infants and children. *Pediatr Clin North Am* 1997;44:363-374.
- Product Information, Ivax, 2003.

DIGOXIN

DOSE & ADMINISTRATION: Loading doses: ("Digitalization") are generally used only when treating arrhythmias and acute congestive heart failure. Give over 24 hours as 3 divided doses. Administer IV slow push over 5 to 10 minutes. Oral doses should be 25% greater than IV doses. Do not administer IM.

Note: These beginning doses are based primarily on studies that measured echocardiographic changes and EKG signs of toxicity and take into account renal maturation. We recommend titrating dosage based on clinical response. Decrease dose proportional to the reduction in creatinine clearance.

TOTAL LOADING DOSE

PMA weeks	IV mcg/kg	PO <mcg/kg
≤29	15	20
30 to 36	20	25
37 to 48	30	40
≥49	40	50
Divide into 3 doses over 24 hours		

MAINTENANCE DOSES

PMA weeks	IV mcg/kg	PO mcg/kg	Interval hours
≤29	4	5	24
30 to 36	5	6	24
37 to 48	4	5	12
≥49	5	6	12
Titrate based on clinical response			

USES: Treatment of heart failure caused by diminished myocardial contractility. Treatment of SVT, atrial flutter, and atrial fibrillation.

MONITORING: Follow heart rate and rhythm closely. Periodic EKGs to assess both desired effects and signs of toxicity. Follow closely (especially in patients receiving diuretics or amphotericin B) for decreased serum potassium and magnesium, or increased calcium and magnesium, all of which predispose to digoxin toxicity. Assess renal function. Be aware of drug interactions. May follow serum drug concentrations if assay is available that excludes endogenous digoxin-like substances. Therapeutic serum concentration is 1 to 2 ng/mL.

ADVERSE EFFECTS/PRECAUTIONS:

Toxic Cardiac Effects:
- PR interval prolongation
- Sinus bradycardia or SA block
- Atrial or nodal ectopic beats
- Ventricular arrhythmias

Nontoxic Cardiac Effects:
- QTc interval shortening
- ST segment sagging
- T-wave amplitude dampening
- Heart rate slowing

Other Effects: Feeding intolerance, vomiting, diarrhea, and lethargy.

Treatment of Life-Threatening Digoxin Toxicity: Digibind® Digoxin Immune Fab, IV over 30 minutes through 0.22 micron filter.

$$\text{Dose (\# of vials)} = \frac{\text{(weight [kg])} \times \text{(serum digoxin concentration)}}{100}$$

Each vial of digibind contains 38 mg (enough to bind 0.5 mg Digoxin).

PHARMACOLOGY: Digitalis glycoside with positive inotropic and negative chronotropic actions. Increases myocardial catecholamine levels (low doses) and inhibits sarcolemmal sodium-potassium-ATPase (higher doses) to enhance contractility by increasing systolic intracellular calcium-ion concentrations. Indirectly increases vagal activity, thereby slowing S-A node firing and A-V node conduction. Other effects include peripheral, splanchnic, and perhaps, pulmonary vasoconstriction, and reduced CSF production. Serum concentration peaks 30 to 90 minutes after an oral dose, with myocardial peak occurring in 4 to 6 hours. Large volume of distribution that increases with age during infancy. Rapid absorption of oral dose from small intestine; reduced by antacids and rapid transit times. 20% protein bound. Probably not significantly metabolized. Glomerular filtration and tubular secretion account for most of the total body clearance of digoxin, although significant nonrenal elimination has been proposed.

SPECIAL CONSIDERATIONS/PREPARATION: Pediatric dosage forms: Injectable (100 mcg/mL) and elixir (50 mcg/mL). Store at room temperature and protect from light. Dilute injectable as follows:

1) Draw up digoxin into syringe.
2) Inject desired amount of drug into second syringe containing a fourfold or greater volume of solution-compatible diluent. Use diluted product immediately.

Drug Interactions: Amiodarone, indomethacin, spironolactone, quinidine, and verapamil decrease digoxin clearance. Cisapride and metoclopramide decrease digoxin absorption. Spironolactone interferes with radioimmunoassay. Erythromycin may increase digoxin absorption.

Solution Compatibility: (only when diluted fourfold or greater): D_5W, $D_{10}W$, NS, and sterile water for injection.

Terminal Injection Site Compatibility: Dex/AA solutions, fat emulsion. Cimetidine, ciprofloxacin, famotidine, furosemide, heparin, hydrocortisone succinate, insulin, lidocaine, linezolid, meropenem, midazolam, milrinone, morphine, potassium chloride, propofol, prostaglandin E_1, ranitidine, and remifentanil.

Incompatibility: Amiodarone, dobutamine and fluconazole.

SELECTED REFERENCES

- Smith TW: Digitalis: Mechanisms of action and clinical use. *N Engl J Med* 1988;318:358.
- Roberts RJ: *Drug Therapy in Infants*. Philadelphia: WB Saunders Co, 1984, p 138.
- Johnson GL, Desai NS, Pauly TH, Cunningham MD: Complications associated with digoxin in low-birth-weight infants. *Pediatrics* 1982;69:463.
- Nyberg L, Wettrell G: Pharmacokinetics and dosage of digoxin in neonates and infants. *Eur J Clin Pharmacol* 1980;18:69.
- Pinsky WW, Jacobsen JR, Gillette PC, et al: Dosage of digoxin in premature infants. *J Pediatr* 1979;96:639.
- Product Information, GlaxoSmithKline, 2002

DOBUTAMINE

DOSE & ADMINISTRATION: 2 to 25 mcg/kg per minute continuous IV infusion. Begin at a low dose and titrate by monitoring effects. Use a large vein for IV.

Solution Preparation Calculations To calculate the AMOUNT of drug needed per defined final fluid volume:

Desired final concentration (mg/mL) × defined final fluid volume (mL) = **AMOUNT of drug to add to final infusion solution (mg).**

To calculate the AMOUNT of drug needed per defined final fluid volume:

$$\frac{\text{*AMOUNT of drug to add (mg)}}{\text{drug (vial) concentration (mg/mL)}} = \text{VOLUME of drug to add (mL)}$$

Example (for Dobutamine): Mix 30 mL of 800 mcg/mL solution using dobutamine concentration of 12.5 mg/mL. 800 mcg/mL = 0.8 mg/mL 0.8 mg/mL x 30 mL = 24 mg dobutamine

$$\frac{^*24 \text{ mg}}{12.5 \text{ mg/mL}} = 1.9 \text{ mL of dobutamine}$$

Add 1.9 mL of dobutamine (12.5 mg/mL) to 28.1 mL of compatible solution (eg, D₅W) to yield 30 mL of infusion solution with a concentration of 800 mcg/mL.

DOBUTAMINE TITRATION CHART

Concentration (mcg/mL)	Dose (mcg/kg/min)	IV Rate (mL/kg/hour)
500	2.5 5 7.5 10	0.3 0.6 0.9 1.2
800	2.5 5 7.5 10	0.19 0.38 0.56 0.75
1000	2.5 5 7.5 10	0.15 0.3 0.45 0.6
1600	2.5 5 7.5 10	0.094 0.19 0.28 0.38
2000	2.5 5 7.5 10	0.075 0.15 0.23 0.3
3200	2.5 5 7.5 10	0.047 0.094 0.14 0.19
4000	2.5 5 7.5 10	0.038 0.075 0.11 0.15

USES: Treatment of hypoperfusion and hypotension, especially if related to myocardial dysfunction.

MONITORING: Continuous heart rate and intra-arterial blood pressure monitoring preferable. Observe IV site for signs of extravasation.

ADVERSE EFFECTS/PRECAUTIONS: May cause hypotension if patient is hypovolemic. Volume loading is recommended before starting dobutamine therapy. Tachycardia occurs at high dosage. Arrhythmias, hypertension, and cutaneous vasodilation. Increases myocardial oxygen consumption. Tissue ischemia occurs with infiltration.

PHARMACOLOGY: Synthetic catecholamine with primarily β_1-adrenergic activity. Inotropic vasopressor. Increases myocardial contractility, cardiac index, oxygen delivery, and oxygen consumption. Decreases systemic and pulmonary vascular resistance (adults). Dobutamine has a more prominent effect on cardiac output than dopamine but less of an effect on blood pressure. Onset of action is 1 to 2 minutes after IV administration, with peak effect in 10 minutes. Must be administered by continuous IV infusion because of rapid metabolism of drug. Serum half-life is several minutes. Metabolized in the liver by sulfoconjugation to an inactive compound. There is wide interpatient variability in plasma clearance due to differences in metabolism and renal excretion.

SPECIAL CONSIDERATIONS/PREPARATION: Supplied as 250 mg per 20 mL vial (12.5 mg/mL). Diluted solutions for infusion should be used within 24 hours. There are no specific data regarding the compatibility of dobutamine and fat emulsions. Dobutamine is most stable in solutions with a pH at or below 5. In alkaline solutions, the catechol moieties are oxidized, cyclized, and polymerized to colored materials. All fat emulsions have pH ranges from 6 to 9. Caution is urged when co-infusing dobutamine and fat emulsion together; dobutamine may degrade over time in this alkaline pH resulting in lower than expected clinical effects.

Solution Compatibility: D_5W, D_5NS, $D_{10}W$, LR, and NS.

Terminal Injection Site Compatibility: Dex/AA solutions. Amiodarone, atropine, aztreonam, caffeine citrate, calcium chloride, calcium gluconate, ciprofloxacin, dopamine, enalaprilat, epinephrine, famotidine, fentanyl, fluconazole, flumazenil, heparin, hydralazine, insulin, isoproterenol, lidocaine, linezolid, lorazepam, magnesium sulfate, meropenem, midazolam, milrinone, morphine, nicardipine, nitroglycerin, nitroprusside, pancuronium bromide, phentolamine, potassium chloride, procainamide, propofol, propranolol, phytonadione, ranitidine, remifentanil, vecuronium, and zidovudine.

Incompatibility: Acyclovir, alteplase, aminophylline, cefepime, bumetanide, diazepam, digoxin, furosemide, indomethacin, phenytoin, piperacillin-tazobactam, and sodium bicarbonate.

SELECTED REFERENCES

- Noori S, Friedlich P, Seri I: The use of dobutamine in the treatment of neonatal cardiovascular compromise. *NeoReviews* 2004;5:e22-e26.

- Berg RA, Donnerstein RL, Padbury JF: Dobutamine infusion in stable, critically ill children: pharmacokinetics and hemodynamic actions. *Crit Care Med* 1993;21:678-86.

- Martinez AM, Padbury JF, Thio S: Dobutamine pharmacokinetics and cardiovascular responses in critically ill neonates. *Pediatrics* 1992;89:47.

- Leier CV, Unverferth DV: Dobutamine. *Ann Intern Med* 1983;99:490.

- Perkin RM, Levin DL, Webb R, et al: Dobutamine: A hemodynamic evaluation in children with shock. *J Pediatr* 1982;100:977.

- Product Information, Bedford, 2005

DOPAMINE

DOSE & ADMINISTRATION: 2 to 20 mcg/kg per minute continuous IV infusion. Begin at a low dose and titrate by monitoring effects. Use a large vein for IV.

Solution Preparation Calculations To calculate the AMOUNT of drug needed per defined final fluid volume:

Desired final concentration (mg/mL) × defined final fluid volume (mL) = AMOUNT of drug to add to final infusion solution (mg).

To calculate the VOLUME of drug needed per defined final fluid volume:

$$\frac{\text{*AMOUNT of drug to add (mg)}}{\text{drug (vial) concentration (mg/mL)}} = \text{VOLUME of drug to add (mL)}$$

Example (for Dopamine): Mix 30 mL of 800 mcg/mL solution using dopamine concentration of 40 mg/mL.
800 mcg/mL = 0.8 mg/mL
0.8 mg/mL x 30 mL = 24 mg dopamine

$$\frac{\text{*24 mg}}{\text{40 mg/mL}} = 0.6 \text{ mL of dopamine}$$

Add 0.6 mL of dopamine (40 mg/mL) to 29.4 mL of compatible solution (eg, D_5W) to yield 30 mL of infusion solution with a concentration of 800 mcg/mL.

DOPAMINE TITRATION CHART

Concentration (mcg/mL)	Dose (mcg/kg/min)	IV Rate (mL/kg/hour)
500	2.5	0.3
	5	0.6
	7.5	0.9
	10	1.2
800	2.5	0.19
	5	0.38
	7.5	0.56
	10	0.75
1000	2.5	0.15
	5	0.3
	7.5	0.45
	10	0.6
1600	2.5	0.094
	5	0.19
	7.5	0.28
	10	0.38
2000	2.5	0.075
	5	0.15
	7.5	0.23
	10	0.3
3200	2.5	0.047
	5	0.094
	7.5	0.14
	10	0.19

USES: Treatment of hypotension.

MONITORING: Continuous heart rate and intra-arterial blood pressure monitoring is preferable. Assess urine output and peripheral perfusion frequently. Observe IV site closely for blanching and infiltration.

ADVERSE EFFECTS/PRECAUTIONS: Tachycardia and arrhythmias. May increase pulmonary artery pressure. Reversible suppression of prolactin and thyrotropin secretion. Tissue sloughing may occur with IV infiltration. **Suggested treatment:** Inject a 1 mg/mL solution of phentolamine into the affected area. The usual amount needed is 1 to 5 mL, depending on the size of the infiltrate.

PHARMACOLOGY: Catecholamine. Metabolized rapidly. Serum half-life is 2 to 5 minutes, but clearance is quite variable. Dopamine increases blood pressure primarily by increasing systemic vascular resistance via α-adrenergic effects. Effects on cardiac output vary with gestational age and baseline stroke volume. Selective renal vasodilation associated with increases in urine output has been noted in preterm neonates at doses of 2 to 5 mcg/kg/minute. No changes in mesenteric or cerebral blood flow were observed. Mechanism of action in neonates is controversial. Relative effects of dopamine at different doses are uncertain because of developmental differences in 1) endogenous norepinephrine stores, 2) α-adrenergic, β-adrenergic, and dopaminergic receptor functions, and 3) the ability of the neonatal heart to increase stroke volume. Responses tend to be individualized. Use higher doses with caution in patients with persistent pulmonary hypertension of the newborn.

SPECIAL CONSIDERATIONS/PREPARATION: Available in 40-mg/mL, 80-mg/mL, and 160-mg/mL vials for injection and premixed bags in concentrations of 800-, 1600-, and 3200-mcg/mL. Diluted solutions stable for 24 hours. **Admixtures exhibiting a color change should not be used.** There are no specific data regarding the compatibility of dopamine and fat emulsions. Dopamine is most stable in solutions with a pH at or below 5. In alkaline solutions, the catechol moieties are oxidized, cyclized, and polymerized to colored materials. All fat emulsions have pH ranges from 6 to 9. Caution is urged when co-infusing dopamine and fat emulsion together; dopamine may degrade over time in this alkaline pH resulting in lower than expected clinical effects.

Solution Compatibility: D_5W, D_5NS, $D_{10}W$, LR, and NS.

Terminal Injection Site Compatibility: Dex/AA solutions. Aminophylline, amiodarone, ampicillin, aztreonam, caffeine citrate, calcium chloride, chloramphenicol, dobutamine, enalaprilat, epinephrine, esmolol, famotidine, fentanyl, fluconazole, flumazenil, gentamicin, heparin, hydrocortisone succinate, lidocaine, linezolid, lorazepam, meropenem, metronidazole, midazolam, milrinone, morphine, nicardipine, nitroglycerin, nitroprusside, oxacillin, pancuronium bromide, penicillin G, piperacillin-tazobactam, potassium chloride, propofol, prostaglandin E$_1$, ranitidine, tobramycin, vecuronium, and zidovudine.

Incompatibility: Acyclovir, alteplase, amphotericin B, cefepime, furosemide, indomethacin, insulin, and sodium bicarbonate.

SELECTED REFERENCES

- Valverde E, Pellicer A, Madero R, et al: Dopamine versus epinephrine for cardiovascular support in low birth weight infants: analysis of systemic effects and neonatal clinical outcomes. *Pediatrics* 2006;117:e1213-e1222.
- Lynch SK, Lemley KV, Polak MJ: The effect of dopamine on glomerular filtration rate in normotensive, oliguric premature neonates. *Pediatr Nephrol* 2003;18:649-652.
- Seri I, Abbasi S, Wood DC, Gerdes JS: Regional hemodynamic effects of dopamine in the sick preterm neonate. *J Pediatr* 1998;133:728-734.
- Seri I: Cardiovascular, renal, and endocrine actions of dopamine in neonates and children. *J Pediatr* 1995;126:333.
- Filippi L, Pezzati M, Cecchi A, et al: Dopamine infusion and anterior pituitary gland function in very low birth weight infants. *Biol Neonate* 2006;89:274-280.
- Van den Berghe G, de Zegher F, Lauwers P: Dopamine suppresses pituitary function in infants and children. *Crit Care Med* 1994;22:1747.
- Roze JC, Tohier C, Maingueneau C, et al : Response to dobutamine and dopamine in the hypotensive very preterm infant. *Arch Dis Child* 1993;69:59-63.
- Padbury JF, Agata Y, Baylen BG, et al: Dopamine pharmacokinetics in critically ill newborn infants. *J Pediatr* 1987;110:293.
- DiSessa TG, Leitner M, Ti CC, et al: The cardiovascular effects of dopamine in the severely asphyxiated neonate. *J Pediatr* 1981;99:772.
- Product Information, American Regent, 2001

DORNASE ALFA

DOSE & ADMINISTRATION: 1.25 mL to 2.5 mL via nebulizer, or 0.2 mL/kg instilled directly into the endotracheal tube. Administer once or twice per day.

USES: Treatment of atelectasis, secondary to mucus plugging, that is unresponsive to conventional therapies.

MONITORING: Monitor airway patency. Suction the airway as needed.

ADVERSE EFFECTS/PRECAUTIONS: Desaturation and/or airway obstruction may occur due to rapid mobilization of secretions.

PHARMACOLOGY: Pulmozyme® is a highly purified solution of recombinant human deoxyribonuclease (rhDNase, an enzyme that selectively cleaves DNA). The protein is produced by genetically engineered Chinese hamster ovary cells. Purulent pulmonary secretions contain very high concentrations of extracellular DNA released by degenerating leukocytes. rhDNase hydolyzes this DNA to decrease the viscoelasticity of the secretions. Clinical improvements in the thickness of secretions and ventilation usually occur within 3 hours of administration.

SPECIAL CONSIDERATIONS/PREPARATION: Pulmozyme® is supplied in single-use ampules. Each ampule contains 2.5 mL of a sterile, clear, colorless, aqueous solution containing 1 mg/mL dornase alfa (2.5 mg per ampule), 0.15 mg/mL calcium chloride dihydrate, and 8.77 mg/mL sodium chloride (22 mg per ampule) with no preservative. The nominal pH of the solution is 6.3. The ampules should be stored in their protective foil pouch under refrigeration (2-8° C, 36-46° F) and protected from strong light. Do not use beyond the expiration date on the ampule.

SELECTED REFERENCES

- Erdeve O, Uras N, Atasay B, Arsan S: Efficacy and safety of nebulized recombinant human DNase as rescue treatment for persistent atelectasis in newborns: case-series. *Croat Med J* 2007;48:234-239.
- Riethmueller J, Borth-Bruhns T, Kumpf M, et al: Recombinant human deoxyribonuclease shortens ventilation time in young, mechanically ventilated children. *Pediatr Pulmonol* 2006;41:61-66.
- Hendricks T, de Hoog M, Lequin MH, et al: DNase and atelectasis in non-cystic fibrosis patients. *Crit Care* 2005;9:R351-R356.
- Ratjen F: Dornase in non-CF. *Pediatr Pulmonol* 2004;26:S154-155.

- Kupeli S, Teksam O, Dogru D, Yurdakok M: Use of recombinant human DNase in a premature infant with recurrent atelectasis. *Pediatrics International* 2003;45:584-586.
- El Hassan NO, Chess PR, Huysman MWA, et al: Rescue use of DNase in critical lung atelectasis and mucus retention in premature neonates. *Pediatrics* 2001;108:468-471.
- Reiter PD, Townsend SF, Velasquez R: Dornase alfa in premature infants with severe respiratory distress and early bronchopulmonary dysplasia. *J Perinatol* 2000;20:530-534.
- Product information, Genentech, 2005.

DTAP-HEPB-IPV COMBINATION VACCINE

(Diptheria and tetanus toxoids and acellular pertussis adsorbed, Hepatitis B (recombinant) and inactivated poliovirus vaccine combined)

DOSE & ADMINISTRATION: 0.5 mL IM in the anterolateral thigh. Shake vial vigorously before withdrawing dose. PEDIARIX® should not be administered to any infant before the age of 6 weeks. Only monovalent hepatitis B vaccine can be used for the birth dose. Please refer to the most recent AAP/ACIP immunization schedule. It is recommended that premature infants should be immunized according to their postnatal age; however, inadequate seroconversion against hepatitis B may occur in chronically ill premature infants.

USES: Immunoprophylaxis against diphtheria, tetanus, pertussis, hepatitis B, and polio. Using PEDIARIX® to complete the hepatitis B vaccination series in infants who were born of HBsAg-positive mothers and who received monovalent Hepatitis B vaccine (Recombinant) has not been studied.

MONITORING: Cardiorespiratory monitoring and pulse oximetry are recommended for premature infants who remain hospitalized at the time of vaccination.

ADVERSE EFFECTS/PRECAUTIONS: Fever is more common (≈20%) after PEDIARIX® than with the individual component vaccines administered separately. Other local and systemic adverse events occur at similar rates. Apnea, bradycardia, and desaturation events are common in premature infants for 48 hours after vaccination.

PHARMACOLOGY: Each dose of PEDIARIX® contains the type and amount of diphtheria and tetanus toxoids and pertussis antigens as INFANRIX®, and hepatitis B virus antigens as Engerix-B®. The poliovirus component of DTaP-HepB-IPV contains the same strains and quantity of inactivated poliovirus Types 1, 2, and 3 as IPV from a different manufacturer (IPOL®, Aventis Pasteur, South Africa). The immunologic responses following 3 doses of DTaP-HepB-IPV are generally similar to those following 3 doses of the individual vaccines administered separately.

SPECIAL CONSIDERATIONS/PREPARATION: PEDIARIX® is supplied as a turbid white suspension in single dose (0.5 mL) vials, and in disposable prefilled Tip-Lock® syringes. Shake well prior to administration. Do not use if resuspension does not occur after vigorous shaking. Store refrigerated at 2° to 8°C (36°F to 46°F). **Do not freeze.** Discard if the vaccine has been frozen.

SELECTED REFERENCES

- Advisory Committee on Immunization Practices: Recommendations of the ACIP. Most recent updates available on the National Immunization Program website: http://www.cdc.gov/nip/publications/acip-list.htm
- Centers for Disease Control and Prevention: FDA licensure of diphtheria and tetanus toxoids and acellular pertussis adsorbed, hepatitis B (recombinant), and poliovirus vaccine combined, (PEDIARIX™) for use in infants. *MMWR* 2003;52(RR-10):202-203.
- Pfister RE, Aeschbach V, Niksic-Stuber V, et al: Safety of DTaP-based combined immunization in very-low-birth-weight premature infants: frequent but mostly benign cardiorespiratory events. *J Pediatr* 2004;145:58-66.
- Product information, GlaxoSmithKline Biologicals, 2007.

DTAP VACCINE

(DIPHTHERIA AND TETANUS TOXOIDS AND ACELLULAR PERTUSSIS VACCINE ADSORBED)

DOSE & ADMINISTRATION: 0.5 mL IM in the anterolateral thigh. Shake vial vigorously before withdrawing each dose. Immunize premature infants according to their postnatal age. Please refer to the most recent AAP/ACIP immunization schedule. **When giving multiple vaccines, use a separate syringe for each and give at different sites.** Care should be taken to draw back on the plunger of the syringe before injection to be certain the needle is not in a blood vessel.

DTaP Vaccine

USES: Preferred immunoprophylaxis against diphtheria, tetanus, and pertussis.

MONITORING: Minor reactions, such as drowsiness, irritability, fever, anorexia, and pain/erythema/induration at the injection site are similar to those observed with DTwP vaccine, but are significantly less frequent. Moderate to severe reactions are also less frequent. Refer to Precautions section for more information.

ADVERSE EFFECTS/PRECAUTIONS: It is prudent to delay the initial dose of DTaP vaccine in infants with neurologic disorders until further observation and study have clarified their neurologic status and the effect of treatment. Those infants with stable neurologic conditions, including well-controlled seizures, may be vaccinated. Infants who have had prior seizures are at increased risk for seizures following DTP vaccination; acetaminophen should be used to prevent postvaccination fever. **Precautions to further DTaP vaccination** (the benefits of administering DTaP may exceed risks in areas with a high incidence of pertussis; otherwise administer DT vaccine):

1) Temperature of $\geq$ 40.5 °C (105 °F) within 48 hours with no other cause. (Frequency approximately 1 per 3000 doses)
2) Hypotonic-hyporesponsive collapse or shock-like state within 48 hours. (Frequency approximately 1 per 10,000 doses)
3) Inconsolable crying ($\geq$ 3 hours) occurring within 48 hours. (Frequency approximately 1 per 2000 doses)
4) Convulsions with or without fever occurring within 3 days. (Frequency approximately 1 per 14,000 doses)

Contraindications to further DTaP vaccination: In children who develop encephalopathy within 7 days following any DTP vaccination, DT vaccine should be substituted for the remaining doses. In children who develop an immediate anaphylactic reaction, further immunization with any of the three antigens should be deferred.

PHARMACOLOGY: DTaP vaccines are aluminum-salt-adsorbed preparations. All acellular pertussis vaccines contain inactivated pertussis toxoid, but vary in the inclusion and concentration of four other pertussis antigens. Diphtheria and tetanus toxoids are prepared by formaldehyde treatment of the respective toxins. Daptacel®, Infanrix® and Tripedia® are thimerosal-free. Each dose of Daptacel® contains 15 Lf diphtheria toxoid, 5 Lf tetanus toxoid, 5 mcg fimbriae types 2 and 3, 5 mcg FHA, and 3 mcg pertactin, with 3.3 mg 2-phenoxyethanol as a preservative. Each dose of Infanrix® contains 25 Lf diphtheria toxoid, 10 Lf tetanus toxoid, 25 mcg inactivated toxin, 25 mcg FHA, and 8 mcg pertactin, with 2.5 mg 2-phenoxyethanol as a preservative. Each dose of Tripedia® contains 6.7 Lf diphtheria toxoid, 5 Lf tetanus toxoid, 23.4 mcg inactivated toxin, and 23.4 mcg FHA.

SPECIAL CONSIDERATIONS/PREPARATION: FDA-licensed DTaP vaccines as of March 2008: Infanrix® (GlaxoSmithKline), available in single-dose vials and single-dose prefilled syringes, Daptacel® (Sanofi Pasteur), available in single-dose vials and multi-dose vials, and Tripedia® (Sanofi Pasteur), available in single-dose vials.Store refrigerated at 2 °C to 8 °C (36 °F to 46 °F). **Do not freeze.** SHAKE VIAL WELL before withdrawing dose. Do not use if product contains clumps that cannot be resuspended with vigorous shaking. Normal appearance is a homogeneous (Tripedia® and Daptacel®) or turbid (Infanrix®) white suspension.

SELECTED REFERENCES

- American Academy of Pediatrics. Pertussis. In: Pickering LK, Baker CJ, Long SS, McMillan JA, eds. *Red Book: 2006 Report of the Committee on Infectious Diseases.* 27th ed. Elk Grove Village, IL: American Academy of Pediatrics; 2006: pp 505-513.
- American Academy of Pediatrics, Committee on Infectious Diseases: Acellular pertussis vaccine: recommendations for use as the initial series in infants and children. *Pediatrics* 1997;99:282.
- Advisory Committee on Immunization Practices: Recommendations of the ACIP. Most recent updates available on the National Immunization Program website: http://www.cdc.gov/nip/publications/acip-list.htm
- Product information, GlaxoSmithKline, 2007.
- Product information, Sanofi Pasteur, 2005, 2008.

DT Vaccine

(DIPHTHERIA AND TETANUS TOXOIDS FOR PEDIATRIC USE)

DOSE & ADMINISTRATION: 0.5 mL IM in the anterolateral thigh. Immunize premature infants according to their postnatal age. Please refer to most recent AAP/ACIP immunization schedule. **When giving multiple vaccines, use a separate syringe for each and give at different sites.** Care should be taken to draw back on the plunger of the syringe before injection to be certain the needle is not in a blood vessel.

USES: Immunoprophylaxis against diphtheria and tetanus for infants who have a contraindication for pertussis vaccine.

MONITORING: Observe injection site for erythema, induration (common), palpable nodule (uncommon), or sterile abscess (rare). Fever (common) may be treated with acetaminophen. Other common, self-limited, systemic effects are drowsiness, fretfulness, and anorexia. Rare anaphylactic reactions (i.e. hives, swelling of the mouth, hypotension, breathing difficulty, and shock) have been reported.

ADVERSE EFFECTS/PRECAUTIONS: Infants with stable neurologic conditions, including well-controlled seizures, may be vaccinated. Infants who have had prior seizures are at increased risk for seizures following DT vaccination; acetaminophen should be used to prevent postvaccination fever.

PHARMACOLOGY: Diphtheria and tetanus toxoids are prepared by formaldehyde treatment of the respective toxins. DT vaccine is an aluminum-salt-adsorbed preparation.

SPECIAL CONSIDERATIONS/PREPARATION: DT vaccine (for pediatric use) is available as 0.5-mL single-dose vials. Store refrigerated. Do not freeze. Shake vial well before withdrawing each dose. Do not use if product contains clumps that cannot be resuspended with vigorous shaking. Normal appearance is a turbid whitish suspension.

SELECTED REFERENCES

- American Academy of Pediatrics. Tetanus. In: Pickering LK, ed. *2006 Red Book: Report of the Committee on Infectious Diseases.* 27th ed. Elk Grove Village, IL: American Academy of Pediatrics; 2006: pp 67-71.
- Advisory Committee on Immunization Practices: Recommendations of the ACIP. Most recent updates available on the National Immunization Program website: http://www.cdc.gov/nip/publications/acip-list.htm.
- Product Information, Sanofi Pasteur, 2005

EMLA®

(EUTECTIC MIXTURE OF LOCAL ANESTHETICS)

DOSE & ADMINISTRATION: Apply 1 to 2 gm to distal half of the penis, then wrap with occlusive dressing. Allow dressing to remain intact for 60 to 90 minutes, remove and clean treated area completely prior to circumcision to avoid systemic absorption.

USES: Topical analgesia for circumcision. Not effective for heel lancing.

MONITORING: Blood methemoglobin concentration if concerned about toxicity.

ADVERSE EFFECTS/PRECAUTIONS: Blanching and redness resolve without treatment. When measured, blood levels of methemoglobin in neonates after the application of 1 g of EMLA cream have been well below toxic levels. Two cases of methemoglobinemia in infants occurred after >3 g of EMLA cream was applied; in 1 of these cases, the infant also was receiving sulfamethoxazole. EMLA cream should not be used in neonates who are receiving other drugs known to induce methemoglobinemia: sulfonamides, acetaminophen, nitrates, nitroglycerin, nitroprusside, phenobarbital, and phenytoin.

PHARMACOLOGY: EMLA cream, containing 2.5% lidocaine and 2.5% prilocaine, attenuates the pain response to circumcision when applied 60 to 90 minutes before the procedure. The analgesic effect is limited during the phases associated with extensive tissue trauma such as during lysis of adhesions and tightening of the clamp. Stabilizes the neuronal membranes by inhibiting the ionic fluxes required for conduction and initiation of nerve impulses. There is a theoretic concern about the potential for neonates to develop methemoglobinemia after the application of EMLA cream, because a metabolite of prilocaine can oxidize hemoglobin to methemoglobin. Neonates are deficient in methemoglobin NADH cytochrome b_5 reductase. Lidocaine is metabolized rapidly by the liver to a number of active metabolites and then excreted renally.

SPECIAL CONSIDERATIONS/PREPARATION: Available in 5-gm and 30-gm tubes with Tegaderm dressing. Each gram of EMLA contains lidocaine 25 mg and prilocaine 25 mg in a eutectic mixture. pH of the product is 9. Contains no preservatives.

SELECTED REFERENCES

- American Academy of Pediatrics, Task Force on Circumcision. Circumcision policy statement. *Pediatrics* 1999;103:686-693.
- Taddio A, Ohlsson A, Einarson TR, et al: A systematic review of lidocaine-prilocaine cream (EMLA) in the treatment of acute pain in neonates. *Pediatrics* 1998;101:1-9.
- Lander J, Brady-Fryer B, Metcalfe JB, et al: Comparison of ringblock, dorsal penile nerve block, and topical anesthesia for neonatal circumcision: A randomized controlled trial. *JAMA* 1997;278:2157-2162.
- Taddio A, Stevens B, Craig K, et al: Efficacy and safety of lidocaine-prilocaine cream for pain during circumcision. *N Engl J Med* 1997;336:1197-1201.
- Product Information, AstraZeneca, 2005.

ENALAPRILAT

DOSE & ADMINISTRATION: Begin with 10 mcg/kg per dose (0.01 mg/kg per dose) IV over 5 minutes Q24 hours. Titrate subsequent doses and interval based on amount and duration of response. Dosage may need to be increased every few days.

USES: Treatment of moderate to severe hypertension. Afterload reduction in patients with congestive heart failure.

MONITORING: Frequent assessment of blood pressure, particularly after the first dose. Periodic assessment of renal function and serum potassium.

ADVERSE EFFECTS/PRECAUTIONS: Use with extreme caution in patients with impaired renal function: oliguria and increased serum creatinine occur frequently. Hypotension occurs primarily in patients who are volume-depleted. Hyperkalemia occurs primarily in patients receiving potassium-sparing diuretics or potassium supplements. Cough has been reported frequently in adults.

PHARMACOLOGY: Enalaprilat is an ACE inhibitor which blocks the production of the potent vasoconstrictor angiotensin II. It thereby decreases plasma and tissue concentrations of angiotensin II and aldosterone, and increases plasma and tissue renin activity. Enalaprilat also prevents the breakdown of bradykinin, a potent vasodilator. Vascular resistance is reduced without reflex tachycardia. Beneficial effects are thought to be caused by a combination of afterload reduction and long-term inhibition of salt and water retention. Duration of action is quite variable in neonates, ranging from 8 to 24 hours.

SPECIAL CONSIDERATIONS/PREPARATION: Enalaprilat is supplied as a 1.25 mg/mL solution for injection in 1 mL and 2 mL vials. Benzyl alcohol content is 9 mg/mL. To make a dilution for IV use, take 1 mL (1.25 mg) of solution and add 49 mL NS to make a final concentration of 25 mcg/mL (0.025 mg/mL). Dilution stable for 24 hours.

Solution Compatibility: D_5W, D_5NS, and NS.

Terminal Injection Site Compatibility: Fat emulsion. Amikacin, aminophylline, ampicillin, aztreonam, calcium gluconate, cefazolin, ceftazidime, chloramphenicol, cimetidine, clindamycin, dobutamine, dopamine, erythromycin lactobionate, esmolol, famotidine, fentanyl, gentamicin, heparin, hydrocortisone succinate, lidocaine, linezolid, magnesium sulfate, meropenem, metronidazole, morphine, nafcillin, nicardipine, nitroprusside, penicillin G, phenobarbital, piperacillin, piperacillin-tazobactam, potassium chloride, propofol, ranitidine, remifentanil, tobramycin, trimethoprim-sulfamethoxazole, and vancomycin.

Incompatibility: Amphotericin B, cefepime, and phenytoin.

SELECTED REFERENCES

- Schilder JLAM, Van den Anker JN: Use of enalapril in neonatal hypertension. *Acta Paediatr* 1995;84:1426.
- Mason T, Polak MJ, Pyles L, et al: Treatment of neonatal renovascular hypertension with intravenous enalapril. *Am J Perinatol* 1992;9:254.
- Rasoulpour M, Marinelli KA: Systemic hypertension. *Clin Perinatol* 1992;19:121.
- Wells TG, Bunchman TE, Kearns GL: Treatment of neonatal hypertension with enalaprilat. *J Pediatr* 1990;117:665.
- Frenneaux M, Stewart RAH, Newman CMH, Hallidie-Smith KA: Enalapril for severe heart failure in infancy. *Arch Dis Child* 1989;64:219.
- Product Information, Hospira, 2006

ENALAPRIL MALEATE

DOSE & ADMINISTRATION: Begin with 40 mcg/kg per dose (0.04 mg/kg per dose) given PO Q24 hours. Usual maximum dose 150 mcg/kg per dose (0.15 mg/kg per dose), as frequently as Q6 hours. Titrate subsequent doses and interval based on amount and duration of response. Dosage may need to be increased every few days.

USES: Treatment of moderate to severe hypertension. Afterload reduction in patients with congestive heart failure.

MONITORING: Frequent assessment of blood pressure, particularly after the first dose. Periodic assessment of renal function and serum potassium.

ADVERSE EFFECTS/PRECAUTIONS: Use with extreme caution in patients with impaired renal function: oliguria and increased serum creatinine occur frequently. Hypotension occurs primarily in patients who are volume-depleted. Hyperkalemia occurs primarily in patients receiving potassium-sparing diuretics or potassium supplements. Cough has been reported frequently in adults.

PHARMACOLOGY: Enalapril is a prodrug that is hydrolyzed in the liver to form the active angiotensin-converting enzyme (ACE) inhibitor enalaprilat, which blocks the conversion of angiotensin I to angiotensin II, a potent vasoconstrictor. It thereby decreases plasma and tissue concentrations of angiotensin II and aldosterone, and increases plasma and tissue renin activity. Enalaprilat also prevents the breakdown of bradykinin, a potent vasodilator. Vascular resistance is reduced without reflex tachycardia. Beneficial effects are thought to be caused by a combination of afterload reduction and long-term inhibition of salt and water retention. Bioavailability of oral dosage form is uncertain in neonates, but is significantly less than the 60% reported in adults. Onset of action after oral dose is 1 to 2 hours. Duration of action is quite variable in neonates, ranging from 8 to 24 hours.

SPECIAL CONSIDERATIONS/PREPARATION: Supplied in 2.5-mg, 5-mg, 10-mg, and 20-mg tablets. Enalapril maleate oral suspension can be prepared by crushing a 2.5 mg tablet and adding to 25 mL of isotonic citrate buffer, yielding a final concentration of 100 mcg/mL (0.1 mg/mL). Suspension is stable for 30 days refrigerated.

SELECTED REFERENCES

- Schilder JLAM, Van den Anker JN: Use of enalapril in neonatal hypertension. *Acta Paediatr* 1995;84:1426.
- Nahata MC, Morosco RS, Hipple TF: Stability of enalapril maleate in three extemporaneously prepared oral liquids. *Am J Health Syst Pharm* 1998;55:1155-1157.
- Mason T, Polak MJ, Pyles L et al: Treatment of neonatal renovascular hypertension with intravenous enalapril. *Am J Perinatol* 1992;9:254.
- Rasoulpour M, Marinelli KA: Systemic hypertension. *Clin Perinatol* 1992;19:121.
- Wells TG, Bunchman TE, Kearns GL: Treatment of neonatal hypertension with enalaprilat. *J Pediatr* 1990;117:665.
- Frenneaux M, Stewart RAH, Newman CMH, Hallidie-Smith KA: Enalapril for severe heart failure in infancy. *Arch Dis Child* 1989;64:219.
- Product Information, Ivax Pharmaceuticals, Inc., 2003

ENOXAPARIN

(LOW MOLECULAR WEIGHT HEPARIN)

DOSE & ADMINISTRATION: Initial treatment of thrombosis: Term infants: 1.7 mg/kg per dose subQ every 12 hours. Preterm infants: 2 mg/kg per dose subQ every 12 hours. Adjust dosage to maintain anti-factor X_a level between 0.5 and 1.0 units/mL. It will usually take several days to attain levels in the target range. Dosage requirements to maintain target anti-factor X_a levels in preterm infants are quite variable, ranging from 0.8 to 3 mg/kg every 12 hours. Infants older than 3 months of age: 1 mg/kg per dose subQ every 12 hours. Call 1-800-NOCLOTS for case reporting and treatment guidance. **Low-risk prophylaxis:** 0.75 mg/kg per dose subQ every 12 hours. Infants older than 3 months of age: 0.5 mg/kg per dose subQ every 12 hours. Adjust dosage to maintain anti-factor X_a level between 0.1 and 0.4 units/mL. Administration may be aided by using a small plastic indwelling subcutaneous catheter (Insuflon®, Hypoguard USA). Adverse events related to these catheters are much more frequent in ELBW infants.

USES: Anticoagulation. Advantages over standard unfractionated heparin: (1) may be given subcutaneously, (2) more predictable pharmacokinetics, (3) dosing every 8 to 12 hours, (4) less frequent bleeding complications.

Epinephrine (Adrenaline)

MONITORING: Measure anti-factor X_a concentrations 4 hours after a dose (See above for desired range). Preterm infants are likely to require several dosage adjustments to achieve the target levels. After attaining target levels, dosage adjustments will be necessary once or twice a month, perhaps more often in preterm infants and infants with hepatic or renal dysfunction. Assess for signs of bleeding and thrombosis.

ADVERSE EFFECTS/PRECAUTIONS: Major bleeding may occur even with anti-factor X_a levels in the therapeutic range. The overall incidence is approximately 4%. Reported complications include major bleeding or hematoma at the administration site, compartment syndrome, intracranial hemorrhage, and gastrointestinal hemorrhage.

PHARMACOLOGY: Enoxaparin is a low-molecular weight heparin that has considerably less activity against thrombin than does standard heparin. Efficacy in neonates is decreased due to low antithrombin plasma concentrations. It is also much less likely to interfere with platelet function or cause osteoporosis. It activates antithrombin III, which progressively inactivates both thrombin and factor X_a, key proteolytic enzymes in the formation of fibrinogen and activation of prothrombin. Bioavailability is almost 100% after subcutaneous administration, with peak activity 2.5 to 4 hours later. The apparent half-life of anti-X_a activity is 4 to 5 hours. Clearance in neonates is more rapid than in older infants, children or adults.

SPECIAL CONSIDERATIONS/PREPARATION: Available as 100 mg/mL concentration as 30 mg/0.3 mL, 40 mg/0.4 mL, 60 mg/0.6 mL, 80 mg/0.8 mL, 100 mg/mL in preservative-free prefilled syringes. Multidose vial available in 100 mg/mL concentration with 15 mg benzyl alcohol per 1 mL as a preservative.

Solution Compatibility: NS and sterile water.

SELECTED REFERENCES

- Malowany JI, Monagle P, Knoppert DC, et al: Enoxaparin for neonatal thrombosis: a call for a higher dose in neonates. *Thrombosis Research* 2008; in press.
- Malowany JI, Knoppert DC, Chan AKC, et al: Enoxaparin use in the neonatal intensive care unit: experience over 8 years. *Pharmacotherapy* 2007;27:1263-1271.
- Streif W, Goebel G, Chan AKC, Massicotte MP: Use of low molecular mass heparin (enoxaparin) in newborn infants: a prospective cohort study of 62 newborn infants. *Arch Dis Child Fetal Neonatal Ed* 2003;88:F365-F370.
- Fareed J, Hoppensteadt D, Walenga J, et al: Pharmacodynamic and pharmacokinetic properties of enoxaparin. *Clin Pharmacokinet* 2003;42:1043-57.
- Edstrom CS, Christensen RD: Evaluation and treatment of thrombosis in the neonatal intensive care unit. *Clin Perinatol* 2000;27:623-41.
- Dunaway KK, Gal P, Ransom JL: Use of enoxaparin in a preterm infant. *Ann Pharmacother* 2000;34:1410-3.
- Klinger G, Hellmann J, Daneman A: Severe aortic thrombosis in the neonate - successful treatment with low-molecular-weight heparin: Two case reports and review of the literature. *Am J Perinatol* 2000;17:151-8.
- Product Information, Sanofi-Aventis, 2007

Epinephrine (Adrenaline)

DOSE & ADMINISTRATION: Resuscitation and severe bradycardia: 0.1 to 0.3 mL/kg 1:10,000 concentration; equal to 0.01 to 0.03 mg/kg (10 to 30 mcg/kg). IV push, or IC. May be given ET using higher doses, up to 0.1 mg/kg (100 mcg/kg), immediately followed by 1 mL NS. Do **not** administer these higher doses of epinephrine intravenously.
IV continuous infusion: Start at 0.1 mcg/kg per minute and adjust to desired response, to a maximum of 1 mcg/kg per minute. If possible, correct acidosis before administration of epinephrine to enhance the effectiveness of the drug.

Solution Preparation Calculations To calculate the AMOUNT of drug needed per defined final fluid volume:

Desired final concentration (mg/mL) × defined final fluid volume (mL) = AMOUNT of drug to add to final infusion solution (mg).

To calculate the VOLUME of drug needed per defined final fluid volume:

$$\frac{\text{*AMOUNT of drug to add (mg)}}{\text{drug (vial) concentration (mg/mL)}} = \text{VOLUME of drug to add (mL)}$$

Example (for Epinephrine): Mix 50 mL of 20 mcg/mL solution using epinephrine concentration of 1 mg/mL.
20 mcg/mL = 0.02 mg/mL
0.02 mg/mL x 50 mL = 1 mg epinephrine

$$\frac{^*1\ mg}{1\ mg/mL} = mL\ of\ epinephrine$$

Add 1 mL of epinephrine (1:1000) to 49 mL of compatible solution (eg, D_5W) to yield 50 mL of infusion solution with a concentration of 20 mcg/mL. Maximum concentration 64 mcg/mL.

EPINEPHRINE TITRATION CHART

Concentration (mcg/mL)	Dose (mcg/kg/min)	IV Rate (mL/kg/hour)
10	0.05 0.1 0.5 1	0.3 0.6 3 6
20	0.05 0.1 0.5 1	0.15 0.3 1.5 3
30	0.05 0.1 0.5 1	0.1 0.2 1 2
40	0.05 0.1 0.5 1	0.075 0.15 0.75 1.5
50	0.05 0.1 0.5 1	0.06 0.12 0.6 1.2
60	0.05 0.1 0.5 1	0.05 0.1 0.5 1

USES: Acute cardiovascular collapse. Short-term use for treatment of systemic hypotension. Despite the widespread use of epinephrine/adrenaline during resuscitation, no placebo-controlled studies have evaluated either the tracheal or intravenous administration of epinephrine at any stage during cardiac arrest in human neonates. Nonetheless, it is reasonable to continue to use epinephrine when adequate ventilation and chest compressions have failed to increase the heart rate to >60 beats per minute.

MONITORING: Monitor heart rate and blood pressure continuously. Observe IV site for signs of infiltration.

ADVERSE EFFECTS/PRECAUTIONS: Compared to dopamine, continuous infusions at doses yielding similar changes in blood pressure are more likely to cause hyperglycemia, tachycardia, and elevations in serum lactate. Cardiac arrhythmias (PVCs and ventricular tachycardia)are also more likely. Renal vascular ischemia may occur at higher doses. Bolus doses are associated with severe hypertension and intracranial hemorrhage. Increased myocardial oxygen requirements. IV infiltration may cause tissue ischemia and necrosis. Suggested treatment: Inject a 1 mg/mL solution of phentolamine into the affected area. The usual amount needed is 1 to 5 mL, depending on the size of the infiltrate.

PHARMACOLOGY: Epinephrine (adrenaline) is the major hormone secreted by the adrenal medulla. It is a potent stimulatator of both alpha and beta adrenergic receptors, with complex effects on body organ systems. Low doses are associated with systemic and pulmonary vasodilation. Higher doses increase blood pressure by direct myocardial stimulation, increases in heart rate, and vasoconstriction. Myocardial oxygen consumption is increased. Blood flow to skeletal muscle, brain, liver, and myocardium is increased. However, blood flow to the kidney is decreased due to increased vascular resistance.

SPECIAL CONSIDERATIONS/PREPARATION: Always use as a 1:10,000 concentration (0.1 mg/mL) for individual doses. Use 1:1000 (1 mg/mL) concentration to prepare continuous infusion solution. Protect from light.

Solution Compatibility: D_5W, $D_{10}W$, and NS.

Terminal Injection Site Compatibility: Dex/AA. Amikacin, amiodarone, ampicillin, caffeine citrate, calcium chloride, calcium gluconate, cimetidine, dobutamine, dopamine, famotidine, fentanyl, furosemide, heparin, hydrocortisone succinate, lorazepam, midazolam, milrinone, morphine, nicardipine, nitroglycerin, nitroprusside, pancuronium bromide, potassium chloride, propofol, prostaglandin E_1, ranitidine, remifentanil, vecuronium, and vitamin K_1.

Incompatibility: Aminophylline, hyaluronidase, and sodium bicarbonate.

SELECTED REFERENCES

- International Liaison Committee on Resuscitation: The International Liaison Committee on Resuscitation (ILCOR) consensus on science with treatment recommendations for pediatric and neonatal patients: neonatal resuscitation. *Pediatrics* 2006;117:e978-e988. URL: http://www.pediatrics.org/cgi/content/full/117/5/e978.
- Barber CA, Wyckoff MH: Use and efficacy of endotracheal versus intravenous epinephrine during neonatal cardiopulmonary resuscitation in the delivery room. *Pediatrics* 2006;118:1028-1034.
- Valverde E, Pellicer A, Madero R, et al: Dopamine versus epinephrine for cardiovascular support in low birth weight infants: analysis of systemic effects and neonatal clinical outcomes. *Pediatrics* 2006;117(6):e1213-22. URL: http://www.pediatrics.org/cgi/content/full/117/6/e1213.
- Pellicer A, Valverde E, Elorza MD, et al: Cardiovascular support for low birth weight infants and cerebral hemodynamics: a randomized, blinded clinical trial. *Pediatrics* 2005; 115: 15011512.
- Burchfield DJ: Medication use in neonatal resuscitation. *Clin Perinatol* 1999;26:683-691.

EPOETIN ALFA

DOSE & ADMINISTRATION: 200 to 400 units/kg/dose, 3 to 5 times per week, for 2 to 6 weeks. Total dose **per week** is 600 to 1400 units per kg. **Short course:** 300 units/kg per dose daily for 10 days. Administer subQ, or IV over at least 4 hours (even continuously in TPN). Supplemental iron therapy should be initiated concurrently

USES: To stimulate erythropoiesis and decrease the need for erythrocyte transfusions in high-risk preterm infants. Those most likely to benefit are infants with birth weights < 800 g and phlebotomy losses > 30 mL/kg.

MONITORING: Weekly CBC to check for neutropenia and monitor RBC response.

ADVERSE EFFECTS/PRECAUTIONS: The only adverse effect in premature neonates is neutropenia, which occurs rarely and resolves with discontinuation of the drug.

PHARMACOLOGY: Epoetin alfa is a 165-amino acid glycoprotein manufactured by recombinant DNA technology that has the same biological effects as endogenous erythropoietin. It acts on mature erythroid progenitors, CFU-E, by binding to cell surface receptors and stimulating differentiation and cell division. Noticeable effects on hematocrit and reticulocyte counts occur within 2 weeks. Adequate iron and protein intake is necessary for epoetin to be effective (additional Vitamin E intake may be necessary as well). Subcutaneously administered drug appears to be pharmacodynamically as effective as IV, despite only 40% bioavailability. Half- life of r-HuEPO in preterm infants is approximately 12 hours. Doses reported in the literature are all stated as Units/kg **per week**. Efficacy may be dose dependent in the range of 500 to 1500 Units/kg per week (see meta-analysis by Garcia et al), but no differences were observed in the randomized trial by Maier et al.

SPECIAL CONSIDERATIONS/PREPARATION: Available in preservative-free, single-use, 1-mL vials containing 2000, 3000, 4000, 10,000, or 40,000 Units formulated in an isotonic, sodium chloride/sodium citrate buffered solution with 2.5 mg human albumin. **Do not shake.** Undiluted epoetin is stable in plastic syringes for 2 weeks. For IV infusion, dilute epoetin in 2 mL of solutions containing at least 0.05% protein and infuse over 4 hours. These dilutions are stable for 24 hours. Product adapted for use in neonates is handled by Ortho Biotech, Inc. (Procrit®). A multidose 2-mL vial is also available from both Ortho Biotech (Procrit®) and Amgen (Epogen®) containing 20,000 Units in a 1% (10 mg/mL) benzyl alcohol solution with 2.5-mg albumin per mL.

SELECTED REFERENCES

- Reiter PD, Rosenberg AA, Valuck R, Novak K: Effect of short-term erythropoietin therapy in anemic premature infants. *J Perinatol* 2005;25:125-129.
- Ohls R: Human recombinant erythropoietin in the prevention and treatment of anemia of prematurity. *Paediatr Drugs* 2002;4:111-121.
- Garcia MG, Hutson AD, Christensen RD: Effect of recombinant erythropoietin on "late" transfusions in the neonatal intensive care unit: A meta-analysis. *J Perinatol* 2002;22:108-111.
- Donato H, Vain N, Rendo P, et al: Effect of early versus late administration of human recombinant human erythropoietin on transfusion requirements in premature infants: Results of a randomized, placebo-controlled, multicenter trial. *Pediatrics* 2000;105:1066.
- Maier RF, Obladen M, Kattner E, et al: High- versus low-dose erythropoietin in extremely low birth weight infants. *J Pediatr* 1998;132:866-870.
- Ohls RK, Christensen RD: Stability of recombinant human epoetin alfa in commonly used neonatal intravenous solutions. *Ann Pharmacother* 1996;30:466.
- Shannon KM, Keith JF, Mentzer WC, et al: Recombinant human erythropoietin stimulates erythropoiesis and reduces erythrocyte transfusions in very low birth weight preterm infants. *Pediatrics* 1995;95:1.
- Ohls RK, Osborne KA, Christensen RD: Efficacy and cost analysis of treating very low birth weight infants with erythropoietin during their first two weeks of life: A randomized placebo controlled trial. *J Pediatr* 1995;126:421.
- Meyer MP, Meyer JH, Commerford A, et al: Recombinant erythropoietin in the treatment of the anemia of prematurity: Results of a double-blind, placebo-controlled study. *Pediatrics* 1994;93:918.
- Product Information, Amgen, 2008

ERYTHROMYCIN

DOSE & ADMINISTRATION: Treatment of pneumonitis and conjunctivitis due to *Chlamydia trachomatis:* 12.5 mg/kg per dose PO Q6 hours for 14 **Other infections and prophylaxis:** 10 mg/kg per dose PO Q6 hours. Oral treatment with E. ethylsuccinate (e.g., E. E. S.®, EryPed®). **Treatment and prophylaxis of pertussis:** 12.5 mg/kg per dose PO Q6 hours for 14 days. The drug of choice in infants younger than 1 month of age is azithromycin. Administer with infant formula to enhance absorption of the ethylsuccinate and reduce possible GI side effects. **Severe infections when PO route unavailable:** 5 to 10 mg/kg per dose IV infusion by syringe pump over at least 60 minutes Q6 hours. **Do not administer IM. Prophylaxis of ophthalmia neonatorum:** Ribbon of 0.5% ointment instilled in each conjunctival sac. **Treatment of feeding intolerance due to dysmotility:** 10 mg/kg per dose PO every 6 hours for 2 days, followed by 4 mg/kg per dose PO every 6 hours for 5 days.

USES: Treatment of infections caused by *Chlamydia, Mycoplasma,* and *Ureaplasma.* Treatment for and prophylaxis against *Bordetella pertussis.* As a substitute for penicillin in situations of significant allergic intolerance. As a prokinetic agent in cases of feeding intolerance.

MONITORING: Watch for diarrhea and signs of abdominal discomfort. CBC for eosinophilia. **Monitor heart rate and blood pressure closely during IV administration.** Observe IV site for signs of infiltration.

ADVERSE EFFECTS/PRECAUTIONS: The risk of hypertrophic pyloric stenosis is increased 10-fold in neonates under 2 weeks of age who receive oral erythromycin for pertussis prophylaxis (1 additional case per every 42 infants treated). No studies of premature infants with feeding intolerance have been large enough to assess safety. Two reported cases of severe bradycardia and hypotension occurring during IV administration of erythromycin lactobionate. Intrahepatic cholestasis. Loose stools occur infrequently. Bilateral sensorineural hearing loss has been reported rarely in adults, usually associated with intravenous administration and renal or hepatic dysfunction. The hearing loss occurred after the first few doses and was reversible after discontinuing the drug. Venous irritation is common when using the IV dosage form.

PHARMACOLOGY: Erythromycin may be bacteriostatic or bactericidal depending on the tissue concentration of drug and the microorganism involved. IV administration of E. lactobionate to preterm infants, using doses of 6.25 to 10 mg/kg, yielded peak serum concentrations of 1.9 to 3.7 mcg/mL and a half-life of 2 hours. The drug penetrates poorly into the CNS, is concentrated in the liver and bile, and is excreted via the bowel. It is a motilin receptor agonist and induces stomach and small intestine motor activity. Plasma clearance of midazolam is reduced by 50%. Digoxin, midazolam, theophylline and carbamazepine serum concentrations may be significantly increased because of prolongation of their half-life.

SPECIAL CONSIDERATIONS/PREPARATION: E. ethylsuccinate oral suspension is available in concentrations of 200 mg- and 400 mg per 5 mL. Refrigeration not required except to preserve taste. Shake suspension well before administering. Available as powder for injection in 500-mg and 1-g vials. Reconstitute 500-mg vial with 10 mL of sterile water for injection to concentration of 50 mg/mL. Reconstituted solution stable for 24 hours at room temperature or 2 weeks in refrigerator. After reconstitution, dilute to a concentration of 1 to 5 mg/mL for infusion. To make a 5-mg/mL dilution, add 1 mL of reconstituted solution to 9 mL sterile water for injection. Use diluted drug within 8 hours.

Solution Compatibility: NS and sterile water for injection.

Solution Incompatibility: D_5W and $D_{10}W$ (unless buffered with 4% sodium bicarbonate to maintain stability).

Terminal Injection Site Compatibility: Dex/AA solutions, fat emulsion. Acyclovir, aminophylline, amiodarone, chloramphenicol, cimetidine, enalaprilat, esmolol, famotidine, heparin, hydrocortisone succinate, lidocaine, lorazepam, magnesium sulfate, methicillin, midazolam, morphine, nicardipine, penicillin G, pentobarbital, potassium chloride, ranitidine, sodium bicarbonate, and zidovudine.

Incompatibility: Ampicillin, ceftazidime, fluconazole, furosemide, linezolid, and metoclopramide.

SELECTED REFERENCES

- American Academy of Pediatrics. Chlamydia trachomatis. In: Pickering LK, Baker CJ, Long SS, McMillan JA, eds. *Red Book: 2006 Report of the Committee on Infectious Diseases.* 27th ed. Elk Grove Village, IL: American Academy of Pediatrics; 2006: p255.
- Centers for Disease Control and Prevention: Sexually transmitted diseases treatment guidelines 2006. *MMWR* 2006;55(No. RR-11).
- Nuntnarumit P, Kiatchoosakun P, Tantiprapa W, Boonkasidecha S: Efficacy of oral erythromycin for treatment of feeding intolerance in preterm infants. *J Pediatr* 2006;148:600605.
- Patole S, Rao S, Doherty D: Erythromycin as a prokinetic agent in preterm neonates: a systematic review. *Arch Dis Child Fetal Neonatal Ed* 2005;90:F301-F306.
- Oei J, Lui K: A placebo-controlled trial of low-dose erythromycin to promote feed tolerance in preterm infants. *Acta Paediatr* 2001;90:904-908.
- Pai MP, Graci DM, Amsden GW: Macrolide drug interactions: an update. *Ann Pharmacother* 2000;34:495-513.
- Honein MA, Paulozzi LJ, Himelright IM, et al: Infantile hypertrophic pyloric stenosis after pertussis prophylaxis with erythromycin: a case review and cohort study. *Lancet* 1999;354:2101-2105.
- Waites KB, Sims PJ, Crouse DT, et al: Serum concentrations of erythromycin after intravenous infusion in preterm neonates treated for *Ureaplasma* urealyticum infection. *Pediatr Infect Dis J* 1994;13:287.
- Farrar HC, Walsh-Sukys MC, Kyllonen K, Blumer JL: Cardiac toxicity associated with intravenous erythromycin lactobionate: Two case reports and a review of the literature. *Pediatr Infect Dis J* 1993;12:688.
- Ginsburg CM: Pharmacology of erythromycin in infants and children. *Pediatr Infect Dis* 1986;5:124.
- Gouyon JB, Benoit A, Betremieux P, et al: Cardiac toxicity of intravenous erythromycin lactobionate in preterm infants. *Pediatr Infect Dis J* 1994;13:840-841.
- Eichenwald H: Adverse reactions to erythromycin. *Pediatr Infect Dis* 1986;5:147.
- Product Information, Abbott, 2003

ESMOLOL

DOSE & ADMINISTRATION: Starting IV doses: Supraventricular tachycardia (SVT): 100 mcg/kg per minute continuous infusion. Increase in increments of 50 to 100 mcg/kg per minute every 5 minutes until control of the ventricular rate is achieved. **Acute managment of postoperative hypertension:** 50 mcg/kg per minute continuous infusion. Increase in increments of 25 to 50 mcg/kg per minute every 5 minutes until desired blood pressure is achieved. **Usual maximum dosage:** 200 mcg/kg per minute. Doses greater than 300 mcg/kg per minute are likely to cause hypotension.

USES: Short term treatment of postoperative hypertension, supraventricular tachycardia (SVT), and ventricular tachycardia (VT).

MONITORING: Continuous EKG monitoring during acute treatment of arrhythmias. Measure systemic blood pressure and heart rate frequently.

ADVERSE EFFECTS/PRECAUTIONS: May cause hypotension in high doses. Adverse effects reversable with discontinuation of drug. Monitor IV site closely for vein irriatation and phlebitis, especially at high concentrations (> 10 mg/mL).

PHARMACOLOGY: Esmolol is a potent cardio-selective beta-blocking agent with a uniquely short half-life (2.8 to 4.5 minutes) and a brief (10 to 15 minute) duration of action. There appears to be no correlation between age and pharmacodynamic response or pharmacokinetic profile. Esmolol is cleared primarily by red blood cell esterases. Renal or hepatic failure does not effect elimination.

SPECIAL CONSIDERATIONS/PREPARATION: Esmolol is supplied in preservative-free 10 mL (10 mg/mL) and a 5-mL (20 mg/mL) ready-to-use vials and 2500 mg/250 mL and 2000 mg/100 mL ready to use premixed bags. The pH is approximately 3.5-5.5. Osmolarity is 312 mOsm/L. Store at room temperature.

Solution Compatibility: D₅W, LR, and NS.

Terminal Injection Site Compatibility: Amikacin, aminophylline, atracurium, calcium chloride, cefazolin, ceftazidime, chloramphenicol, cimetidine, clindamycin, digoxin, dopamine, enalaprilat, erythromycin lactobionate, famoditine, fentanyl, gentamicin, heparin, hydrocortisone, insulin, lidocaine, linezolid, magnesium sulfate, metronidazole, midazolam, morphine, nafcillin, nicardipine, nitroglycerin, norepinephrine, pancuronium, penicillin G, phenytoin, piperacillin, potassium chloride, propofol, ranitidine, remifentanil, sodium nitroprusside, tobramycin, trimethoprim-sulfamethoxazole, vancomycin, and vecuronium.

Incompatibility: Amphotericin B, diazepam, furosemide, and procainamide.

SELECTED REFERENCES

- Wiest DB, Garner SS, Uber WE, et al: Esmolol for the management of pediatric hypertension after cardiac operations. *J Thoracic Cardiov Surg* 1998;115:890-897.
- Cuneo B, Zales VR, Blahunka PC, et al: Pharmacodynamics and pharmacokinetics of esmolol, a short-acting β-blocking agent, in children. *Pediatr Cardiol* 1994;15:296-301.
- Trippel MD, Wiest DB, Gillette PC: Cardiovascular and antiarrhythmic effects of esmolol in children. *J Pediatr* 1991;119:142-147.
- Wiest DB, Trippel MD, Gillette PC, et al: Pharmacokinetics of esmolol in children. *Clin Pharmacol Ther* 1991;49:618-623.
- Product Information, Baxter, 2007.

EXOSURF®

(SYNTHETIC SURFACTANT)

DOSE & ADMINISTRATION: 5 mL/kg per dose ET. **Prophylaxis** (for neonates less than 29 weeks gestation): The first dose is given as soon as possible after birth. Two additional doses are given at 12 and 24 hours if indicated. **Rescue treatment of RDS:** Two doses 12 hours apart; the first dose given as soon as possible after intubation for respiratory deterioration.

After ET suctioning, administer in two 2.5-mL/kg aliquots using the sideport on the supplied ET tube adapter without interrupting mechanical ventilation. Each half-dose is instilled over 1 to 2 minutes in small bursts timed with inspiration, with the infant's head in the midline position. After each half dose, the head and torso are turned 45° to the side for 30 seconds to improve distribution. After dosing, frequent assessments of oxygenation and ventilation should be performed to prevent postdose hyperoxia and hypocarbia. Suctioning should not be performed for 2 hours following administration, except when dictated by clinical necessity.

ADVERSE EFFECTS/PRECAUTIONS: Reflux of Exosurf® up the ET tube and falls in oxygenation occur frequently. If the infant becomes dusky or agitated, heart rate slows, oxygen saturation falls more than 15%, or Exosurf® backs up in the ET tube, dosing should be slowed or halted. If necessary, ventilator settings and/or FiO₂ should be turned up. Pulmonary hemorrhage occurs in 2% to 4% of treated infants, primarily the smallest patients with untreated PDA possibly the result of hemorrhagic pulmonary edema caused by the rapid fall in pulmonary vascular resistance and resulting increased pulmonary blood flow.

PHARMACOLOGY: Synthetic, protein-free surfactant, supplied as a sterile lyophilized powder. After reconstitution, each mL of Exosurf® suspension contains 13.5 mg colfosceril palmitate (DPPC, the major lipid component of natural surfactant), 1.5 mg cetyl alcohol (a spreading agent), and 1 mg tyloxapol (a nonionic surfactant that disperses the DPPC and cetyl alcohol).

SPECIAL CONSIDERATIONS/PREPARATION: Reconstitute immediately before administration using only preservative-free sterile water for injection (supplied). 1) Fill a 10-mL or 12-mL syringe with 8 mL of sterile water. 2) Allow vacuum in the Exosurf® vial to draw sterile water into vial. 3) Aspirate as much as possible out of vial back into syringe (while maintaining vacuum), then suddenly release syringe plunger. 4) Step 3 should be repeated 3 or 4 times to assure adequate mixing. 5) Draw appropriate dosage volume into syringe **from below froth** in vial. Each vial yields 7.5 to 8 mL of Exosurf® suspension (enough to treat an infant weighing up to ≈1600 g). The suspension appears milky white, has a pH of 5 to 7, and an osmolality of 185 mOsm/L. The reconstituted suspension is stable for 12 hours when stored at 2 °C to 30 °C (36 °F to 86 °F) .Exosurf® is no longer available in the United States.

SELECTED REFERENCES

• Corbet A: Clinical trials of synthetic surfactant in the respiratory distress syndrome of premature infants. *Clin Perinatol* 1993;20:737.
• The OSIRIS Collaborative Group: Early versus delayed neonatal administration of a synthetic surfactant: The judgment of OSIRIS. *Lancet* 1992;2(340):1363.

FAMOTIDINE

DOSE & ADMINISTRATION: IV: 0.25 to 0.5 mg/kg per dose Q24 hours, IV slow push; Continuous infusion of the daily dose in adults provides better gastric acid suppression than intermittent dosing. **PO:** 0.5 to 1 mg/kg per dose Q24 hours orally.

USES: Prevention and treatment of stress ulcers and GI hemorrhage aggravated by gastric acid secretion.

MONITORING: Gastric pH may be measured to assess efficacy (>4.0).

ADVERSE EFFECTS/PRECAUTIONS: No adverse events have been reported in infants and children, although data are limited to a few small studies. The most common (<5% of patients) adverse effects noted in adults were headache, dizziness, constipation, and diarrhea.

PHARMACOLOGY: Inhibits gastric acid secretion by histamine H_2-receptor antagonism. Elimination half-life is dependent on renal function, and decreases with age from 11 hours (range 5 to 22) in neonates to 8 hours (range 4 to 12) by 3 months of age. Oral bioavailability is 42 to 50%.

SPECIAL CONSIDERATIONS/PREPARATION: Available as 10-mg/mL solution for intravenous use in 2-mL preservative-free single-dose vials, and 4-mL multidose vials containing 0.9% (9 mg/mL) benzyl alcohol as a preservative. A 1-mg/mL dilution may be made by adding 1 mL of the 10 mg/mL concentrated solution to 9 mL of sterile water for injection. Dilution stable for 7 days at room temperature. Although diluted Pepcid® Injection has been shown to be physically and chemically stable for 7 days at room temperature, there are no data on the maintenance of sterility after dilution. Therefore, it is recommended that if not used immediately after preparation, diluted solutions of Pepcid® Injection should be refrigerated and used within 48 hours. Pepcid® for oral suspension is supplied as a powder containing 400 mg famotidine. Constitute by slowly adding 46 mL Purified Water and shaking vigorously for 5-10 seconds. Final concentration 40 mg/5 mL (8 mg/mL). Stable at room temperature for 30 days. Shake bottle before each use.

Solution Compatibility: D_5W, $D_{10}W$, NS. Dex/AA solutions, fat emulsion.

Terminal Injection Site Compatibility: Acyclovir, aminophylline, amiodarone, ampicillin, atropine, aztreonam, calcium gluconate, cefazolin, cefotaxime, cefoxitin, ceftazidime, ceftriaxone, dexamethasone, digoxin, dobutamine, dopamine, enalaprilat, epinephrine, erythromycin lactobionate, esmolol, fluconazole, flumazenil, furosemide, gentamicin, heparin, hydrocortisone succinate, imipenem/cilastatin, insulin, isoproterenol, lidocaine, linezolid, lorazepam, magnesium sulfate, metoclopramide, mezlocillin, midazolam, morphine, nafcillin, nicardipine, nitroglycerin, oxacillin, phenytoin, piperacillin, potassium chloride, procainamide, propofol, remifentanil, sodium bicarbonate, sodium nitroprusside, ticarcillin/clavulanate, vancomycin, and vitamin K_1.

Incompatibility: Azithromycin, cefepime and piperacillin-tazobactam.

SELECTED REFERENCES

• Wenning LA, Murphy MG, James LP, et al: Pharmacokinetics of famotidine in infants. *Clin Pharmacokinet* 2005;44:395-406.
• James LP, Marotti T, Stowe CD, et al: Pharmacokinetics and pharmacodynamics of famotidine in infants. *J Clin Pharmacol* 1998;38:1089-1095.
• James LP, Marshall JD, Heulitt MJ, et al: Pharmacokinetics and pharmacodynamics of famotidine in children. *J Clin Pharmacol* 1996;21:48-54.
• Bullock L, Fitzgerald JF, Glick MR: Stability of famotidine 20 and 50 mg/L in total nutrient admixtures. *Am J Hosp Pharm* 1989;46:2326-29.

- Product information, Merck Inc., 2006.
- Product information, Salix, 2007

FENTANYL

DOSE & ADMINISTRATION: Sedation and analgesia: 0.5 to 4 mcg/kg per dose IV slow push. Repeat as required (usually Q2 to 4 hours). **Infusion rate:** 1 to 5 mcg/kg per hour. Tolerance may develop rapidly following constant infusion. **Anesthesia:** 5 to 50 mcg/kg per dose.

USES: Analgesia. Sedation. Anesthesia.

MONITORING: Monitor respiratory and cardiovascular status closely. Observe for abdominal distention, loss of bowel sounds, and muscle rigidity.

ADVERSE EFFECTS/PRECAUTIONS: Respiratory depression occurs when anesthetic doses (>5 mcg/kg) are used and may also occur unexpectedly because of redistribution. Chest wall rigidity has occurred in 4% of neonates who received 2.2 to 6.5 mcg/kg per dose, occasionally associated with laryngospasm. This was reversible with administration of naloxone. Urinary retention may occur when using continuous infusions. Tolerance may develop to analgesic doses with prolonged use. Significant withdrawal symptoms have been reported in patients treated with continuous infusion for 5 days or longer.

PHARMACOLOGY: Synthetic opioid narcotic analgesic that is 50 to 100 times more potent than morphine on a weight basis. Extremely lipid soluble. Penetrates the CNS rapidly. Transient rebound in fentanyl serum concentration may reflect sequestration and subsequent release of fentanyl from body fat. Metabolized extensively in the liver by CYP 3A4 enzyme system and then excreted by the kidney. Serum half-life is prolonged in patients with liver failure. Highly protein bound. Wide variability in apparent volume of distribution (10 to 30 L/kg) and serum half-life (1 to 15 hours).

SPECIAL CONSIDERATIONS/PREPARATION: Naloxone should be readily available to reverse adverse effects. Available in 2-, 5-, 10-, and 20-mL ampules in a concentration of 50 mcg/mL. A 10 mcg/mL dilution may be made by adding 1 mL of the 50 mcg/mL concentration to 4 mL preservative-free normal saline. Stable for 24 hours refrigerated.

Solution Compatibility: D_5W, $D_{10}W$, and NS.

Terminal Injection Site Compatibility: Dex/AA solutions, fat emulsion. Amiodarone, atropine, caffeine citrate, cimetidine, dexamethasone, dobutamine, dopamine, enalaprilat, epinephrine, esmolol, furosemide, heparin, hydrocortisone succinate, lidocaine, linezolid, lorazepam, metoclopramide, midazolam, milrinone, mivacurium, morphine, nafcillin, nicardipine, pancuronium bromide, potassium chloride, propofol, ranitidine, remifentanil, sodium bicarbonate, and vecuronium.

Incompatibility: Azithromycin, pentobarbital and phenytoin.

SELECTED REFERENCES

- Anand KJS and the International Evidence-Based Group for Neonatal Pain: Consensus statement for the prevention and management of pain in the newborn. *Arch Pediatr Adolesc Med* 2001;155:173-180.
- Fahnenstich H, Steffan J, Kau N, Bartmann P: Fentanyl-induced chest wall rigidity and laryngospasm in preterm and term infants. *Crit Care Med* 2000;28:836-839.
- Saarenmaa E, Neuvonen PJ, Fellman V: Gestational age and birth weight effects on plasma clearance of fentanyl in newborn infants. *J Pediatr* 2000;136:767-770.
- Muller P and Vogtmann C: Three cases with different presentation of fentanyl-induced muscle rigidity-A rare problem in intensive care of neonates. *Am J Perinatol* 2000;17:23-26.
- Santeiro ML, Christie J, Stromquist C, et al: Pharmacokinetics of continuous infusion fentanyl in newborns. *J Perinatol* 1997;17:135-139.
- Arnold JH, Truog RD, Orav EJ, et al: Tolerance and dependence in neonates sedated with fentanyl during extracorporeal membrane oxygenation. *Anesthesiology* 1990;73:1136.
- Koehntop DE, Rodman JH, Brundage DM, et al: Pharmacokinetics of fentanyl in neonates. *Anesth Analg* 1986;65:227.
- Johnson KL, Erickson JP, Holley FO, Scott JC: Fentanyl pharmacokinetics in the pediatric population. *Anesthesiology* 1984;61:A441.
- Reilly CS, Wood AJ, Wood M: Variability of fentanyl pharmacokinetics in man. *Anaesthesia* 1984;40:837.
- Mather LE: Clinical pharmacokinetics of fentanyl and its newer derivatives. *Clin Pharmacokinet* 1983;8:422.
- Product Information, Hospira, 2005

FERROUS SULFATE

DOSE & ADMINISTRATION: 2 mg/kg per day of elemental iron for growing premature infants. (Maximum of 15 mg/day). Begin therapy after 2 weeks of age. Infants with birthweights less than 1000 grams may need 4 mg/kg per day. 6 mg/kg per day of elemental iron for patients receiving erythropoietin. Administer PO in 1 or 2 divided doses, preferably diluted in formula.

USES: Iron supplementation for prevention and treatment of anemia.

MONITORING: Monitor hemoglobin and reticulocyte counts during therapy. Observe stools, check for constipation.

ADVERSE EFFECTS/PRECAUTIONS: In growing premature infants, iron supplementation should not be started until adequate vitamin E is supplied in the diet; otherwise, iron may increase hemolysis. Nausea, constipation, black stools, lethargy, hypotension, and erosion of gastric mucosa.

PHARMACOLOGY: Well absorbed from stomach.

SPECIAL CONSIDERATIONS/PREPARATION: Drops: Contain 15 mg elemental iron per 0.6 mL (0.2% alcohol). **Elixir:** Contains 44 mg elemental iron per 5 mL (some with 5% alcohol).

SELECTED REFERENCES

- Rao R, Georgieff M: Microminerals. In: Tsang R, Uauy R, Koletzko B, Zlotkin S. *Nutrition of the Preterm Infant. Scientific Basis and Practical Guidelines.* Cincinnati, Ohio: Digital Publishing Inc; 2005: pp 277-288.
- Rao R, Georgieff MK: Neonatal iron nutrition. *Semin Neonatol* 2001;6:425-35.
- Siimes MA, Järvenpää A-L: Prevention of anemia and iron deficiency in very-low-birth-weight infants. J Pediatr 1982;101:277-280.
- Oski FA: Iron requirements of the premature infant, in Tsang R (ed): *Vitamin and Mineral Requirements in Preterm Infants.* New York: Marcel Dekker, 1985, p 18.
- Product Information, Mead Johnson, 2006

FLECAINIDE

DOSE & ADMINISTRATION: Begin at 2 mg/kg per dose Q12 hours PO. Adjust dose based on response and serum concentrations to a maximum of 4 mg/kg per dose Q12 hours. Correct preexisting hypokalemia or hyperkalemia before administration. Optimal effect may take 2 to 3 days of therapy to achieve, and steady-state plasma levels may not be reached until 3 to 5 days at a given dosage in patients with normal renal and hepatic function. Therefore, do not increase dosage more frequently than approximately once every 4 days.

USES: Treatment of supraventricular arrhythmias not responsive to conventional therapies. Contraindicated in patients with structurally abnormal hearts.

MONITORING: Continuous EKG during initiation of therapy, as this is the most common time to see drug-induced arrhythmias. Follow trough serum concentrations closely at initiation, 3 to 5 days after any dose change, and with any significant change in clinical status or diet. Therapeutic trough levels are 200 to 800 nanograms/mL.

ADVERSE EFFECTS/PRECAUTIONS: Flecainide can cause new or worsened arrhythmias, including AV block, bradycardia, ventricular tachycardia, torsades de pointes. There is also a negative inotropic effect. Dizziness, blurred vision, and headache have been reported in children.

PHARMACOLOGY: Flecainide is a Class I-C antiarrhythmic that produces a dose-related decrease in intracardiac conduction in all parts of the heart, thereby increasing PR, QRS and QT intervals. Effects upon atrioventricular (AV) nodal conduction time and intra-atrial conduction times are less pronounced than those on the ventricle. Peak serum concentrations occur 2 to 3 hours after an oral dose. Infant formula and milk products interfere with drug absorption. Plasma protein binding is about 40% in adults and is independent of plasma drug level. Children under 1 year of age have elimination half-life values of 11 to 12 hours. Elimination half-life in newborns after maternal administration is as long as 29 hours.

SPECIAL CONSIDERATIONS/PREPARATION: Supplied in 50-mg, 100-mg, and 150-mg tablets. An oral suspension with a final concentration of 5 mg/mL can be made as follows: crush 6 (six) 100-mg tablets, slowly mix in 20 mL of a 1:1 mixture of Ora-Sweet® and Ora-Plus®, or cherry syrup (cherry syrup concentrate diluted 1:4 with simple syrup) to form a uniform paste, then add to this mixture enough vehicle to make a final volume of 120 mL. Shake well and protect from light. Stable for 45 days refrigerated and at room temperature when stored in amber glass or plastic.

SELECTED REFERENCES

- O'Sullivan JJ, Gardiner HM, Wren C: Digoxin or flecainide for prophylaxis of supraventricular tachycardia in infants? *J Am Coll Cardiol* 1995;26:991-994.
- Luedtke SA, Kuhn RJ, McCaffrey FM: Pharmacologic management of supraventricular tachycardia in children. *Ann Pharmacother* 1997;31:1227-43.
- Perry JC, Garson A: Flecainide acetate for treatment of tachyarrhythmias in children: Review of world literature on efficacy, safety, and dosing. *Am Heart J* 1992;124:1614-21.
- Wiest DB, Garner SS, Pagacz LR, et al: Stability of flecainide acetate in an extemporaneously compounded oral suspension. *Am J Hosp Pharm* 1992;49:1467-70.

FLUCONAZOLE

DOSE & ADMINISTRATION: Systemic infections, including meningitis: 12 mg/kg loading dose, then 6 mg/kg per dose IV infusion by syringe pump over 30 minutes, or PO. **Prophylaxis:** 3 mg/kg per dose via IV infusion twice weekly. (Consider only in VLBW infants cared for in NICUs with high rates of invasive fungal disease). **Thrush:** 6 mg/kg on Day 1, then 3 mg/kg per dose Q24 hours PO. To use dosing chart, please refer to explanatory note in "How to Use This Book."

SYSTEMIC INFECTIONS DOSING INTERVAL CHART

PMA (weeks)	PostNatal (days)	Interval (hours)
≤29	0 to 14	72
	>14	48
30 to 36	0 to 14	48
	>14	24
37 to 44	0 to 7	48
	>7	24
≥45	ALL	24

USES: Treatment of systemic infections, meningitis, and severe superficial mycoses caused by *Candida* species. Resistance has been reported with *C glabrata* and *C krusei* and in patients receiving long-term suppressive therapy.

MONITORING: Serum fluconazole concentrations are not routinely followed. Assess renal function. Follow AST, ALT, and CBC for eosinophilia.

ADVERSE EFFECTS/PRECAUTIONS: Data in neonates are limited. Reversible elevations of transaminases have occurred in 12% of children. A retrospective study using historical controls reports direct hyperbilirubinemia in the absence of elevated transaminases in some infants treated prophylactically for 6 weeks. Interferes with metabolism of barbiturates and phenytoin. May also interfere with metabolism of aminophylline, caffeine, theophylline, and midazolam. **Contraindicated** in patients receiving **cisapride** due to precipitation of life-threatening arrhythmias.

PHARMACOLOGY: Water-soluble triazole antifungal agent. Inhibits cytochrome P-450-dependent ergosterol synthesis. Well absorbed after oral administration, with peak serum concentrations reached within 1 to 2 hours. Less than 12% protein binding. Good penetration into CSF after both oral and IV administration. Serum half-life is 30 to 180 hours in severely ill VLBW infants in the first 2 weeks of life and approximately 17 hours in children. Primarily excreted unchanged in the urine.

SPECIAL CONSIDERATIONS/PREPARATION: Available as a premixed solution for IV injection in concentrations of 200 mg/100 mL and 400 mg/200 mL in Viaflex® bags (2 mg/mL). Oral dosage form is available as powder for suspension in concentrations of 10mg/mL and 40 mg/mL. Prepare both concentrations by adding 24 mL distilled water to bottle of powder and shaking vigorously. Suspension is stable at room temperature for 2 weeks. Do not freeze.

Solution Compatibility: D_5W and $D_{10}W$.

Terminal Injection Site Compatibility: Dex/AA solutions, fat emulsion. Acyclovir, amikacin, aminophylline, amiodarone, aztreonam, cefazolin, cefepime, cefoxitin,

FLUCYTOSINE

cimetidine, dexamethasone, dobutamine, dopamine, famotidine, gentamicin, heparin, hydrocortisone succinate, intravenous immune globulin (human), linezolid, lorazepam, meropenem, metoclopramide, metronidazole, midazolam, morphine, nafcillin, nitroglycerin, oxacillin, pancuronium bromide, penicillin G, phenytoin, piperacillin/tazobactam, potassium chloride, propofol, quinupristin/dalfopristin, ranitidine, remifentanil, ticarcillin/clavulanate, tobramycin, vancomycin, vecuronium, and zidovudine.

Incompatibility: Amphotericin B, ampicillin, calcium gluconate, cefotaxime, ceftazidime, ceftriaxone, chloramphenicol, clindamycin, digoxin, erythromycin lactobionate, furosemide, imipenem, piperacillin, ticarcillin, and trimethoprim-sulfamethoxazole.

SELECTED REFERENCES

- Manzoni P, Stolfi I, Pugni L, et al: A multicenter, randomized trial of prophylactic fluconazole in preterm neonates. N Eng J Med 2007;356:2483-95.
- Kaufman D, Boyle R, Hazen KC, et al: Twice weekly fluconazole prophylaxis for prevention of invasive Candida infection in high-risk infants of <1000 grams birth weight. J Pediatr 2005;147:172-179.
- Aghai ZH, Mudduluru M, Nakhla TA, et al. Fluconazole prophylaxis in extremely low birth weight infants: association with cholestasis. J Perinatol 2006;26:550-555.
- Huttova M, Hartmanova I, Kralinsky K, et al: Candida fungemia in neonates treated with fluconazole: report of forty cases, including eight with meningitis. Pediatr Infect Dis J 1998;17:1012-1015.
- Driessen M, Ellis JB, Cooper PA, et al: Fluconazole vs. amphotericin B for the treatment of neonatal fungal septicemia: a prospective randomized trial. Pediatr Infect Dis J 1996;15;1107.
- Flynn PM, Cunningham CK, Kerkering T, et al: Oropharyngeal candidiasis in immuno-compromised children: a randomized, multicenter study of orally administered fluconazole suspension versus nystatin. The Multicenter Fluconazole Study Group. J Pediatr 1995;127:322.
- Fasano C, O'Keefe J, Gibbs D: Fluconazole treatment of neonates and infants with severe fungal infections not treatable with conventional agents. Eur J Clin Microbiol Infect Dis 1994;13:351.
- Saxen H, Hoppu K, Pohjavuori M: Pharmacokinetics of fluconazole in very low birth weight infants during the first two weeks of life. Clin Pharmacol Ther 1993;54:269.
- Dodds Ashley ES, Lewis R, Lewis JS, et al. Pharmacology of systemic antifungal agents. Clin Infect Dis 2006;43:S29-39.
- Product information, Pfizer, 2004

FLUCYTOSINE

DOSE & ADMINISTRATION: 12.5 to 37.5 mg/kg per dose Q6 hours PO. Increase dosing interval if renal dysfunction is present.

USES: Antifungal agent used in combination with amphotericin B or fluconazole for treatment of infections caused by Candida, Cryptococcus, and other sensitive fungi.

MONITORING: Desired peak serum concentration ranges from 50 to 80 mcg/mL. Assess renal function. Follow GI status closely. Twice-weekly CBC and platelet counts. Periodic AST, ALT.

ADVERSE EFFECTS/PRECAUTIONS: Toxicities are related to serum concentration above 100 mcg/mL, and are usually reversible if the drug is stopped or the dose is reduced. Fatal bone marrow depression (related to fluorouracil production), hepatitis, severe diarrhea, rash. Amphotericin B may increase toxicity by decreasing renal excretion.

PHARMACOLOGY: Well absorbed orally. Transformed within cell to fluorouracil, which interferes with RNA synthesis. Excellent penetration into CSF and body tissues. 90% renal elimination of unchanged drug, proportional to GFR. Serum half-life in adults is 3 to 5 hours if renal function is normal, but 30 to 250 hours if renal impairment is present. Limited pharmacokinetic data in premature infants. Resistance develops frequently if used alone. Synergistic with amphotericin even if treating resistant strain.

SPECIAL CONSIDERATIONS/PREPARATION: Flucytosine is available only in 250 and 500-mg capsules. A pediatric suspension (10 mg/mL) may be prepared using distilled water; adjust pH from 5 to 7 with dilute sodium hydroxide. The capsule contains talc, which forms large-particle precipitates of inactive compound. The remaining suspension, containing the active drug, may be decanted. Shake well before use. The suspension is stable for 7 days at room temperature.

SELECTED REFERENCES

- Marr B, Gross S, Cunningham C, et al: Candidal sepsis and meningitis in a very-low-birth-weight infant successfully treated with fluconazole and flucytosine. Clin Infect Dis 1994;19;795.
- Smego RA, Perfect JR, Durack DT: Combined therapy with amphotericin B and 5-fluorocytosine for Candida meningitis. Rev Infect Dis 1984;6:791.

- Johnson DE, Thompson TR, Green TP, Ferrieri P: Systemic candidiasis in very low-birth-weight infants (<1500 grams). *Pediatrics* 1984;73:138.
- Koldin MH, Medoff G: Antifungal chemotherapy. *Pediatr Clin North Am* 1983;30:49.
- Product Information, Valeant Pharmaceuticals, 2005

FLUMAZENIL

DOSE & ADMINISTRATION: IV: 5 to 10 mcg/kg per dose IV over 15 seconds. May repeat every 45 seconds until the patient is awake. Maximum reported dose should not exceed 50 mcg/kg (0.05 mg/kg) or 1 mg in infants, whichever is smaller. No reported maximum dose in neonates has been tested. Administer intravenously through a freely running large vein to minimize pain upon injection. **Intranasal:** 40 mcg/kg per dose divided equally between both nostrils. Administer via TB syringe for accurate equal dosing. **Rectal:** 15 to 30 mcg/kg per dose, may repeat if sedation not reversed within 15 to 20 minutes.

USES: Reversal of sedative effect from benzodiazepines, in cases of suspected benzodiazepines overdose, and in neonatal apnea secondary to prenatal benzodiazepine exposure.

MONITORING: Monitor for the return of sedation and respiratory depression. Continuous EKG and blood pressure.

ADVERSE EFFECTS/PRECAUTIONS: The reported experience in neonates is very limited. Use with caution in neonates with pre-existing seizure disorders. Hypotension has been reported in adults following rapid administration. Resedation has been reported in 10% of treated pediatric patients, occurring 19 to 50 minutes after initial dosing. May cause pain on injection. Observe IV site for extravasation.

PHARMACOLOGY: Imidazobenzodiazepine that is a benzodiazepine receptor antagonist. Competitively inhibits the activity at the benzodiazepine recognition site on the GABA/benzodiazepine receptor. Eliminated rapidly by hepatic metabolism to three inactive metabolites. Highly lipid soluble and penetrates the brain rapidly. Elimination half-life in children 20 to 75 minutes. Peak concentration reached in 3 minutes when delivered intravenously (children). Limited pharmacokinetic data in neonates.

SPECIAL CONSIDERATIONS/PREPARATION: Available in an injectable form as a 0.1 mg/mL concentration in 5- and 10-mL multi-dose vials. If drawn into a syringe or mixed with D_5W, LR, or NS, discard solution after 24 hours. Discard opened vials within 24 hours. Store at room temperature.

Solution Compatibility: D_5W, LR, and NS.

Terminal Injection Site Compatibility: Aminophylline, cimetidine, dobutamine, dopamine, famotidine, heparin, lidocaine, procainamide, and ranitidine.

SELECTED REFERENCES

- Phelps SJ, Hak EB: *Pediatric Injectable Drugs.* Maryland: American Society of Health System Pharmacists, 2004, p176.
- Zaw W, Knoppert DC, da Silva O: Flumazenil's reversal of myoclonic-like movements associated with midazolam in term newborns. *Pharmacotherapy* 2001;21:642-6.
- Carbajal R, Simon N, Blanc P, et al: Rectal flumazenil to reverse midazolam sedation in children. *Anest Analog* 1996;82:895.
- Richard P, Autret E, Bardol J, et al: The use of flumazenil in a neonate. *Clin Toxicol* 1991;29:137-40.
- Brogden RN, Goa KL: Flumazenil. A review of its benzodiazepine antagonist properties, intrinsic activity and therapeutic use. *Drugs* 1988;35:448-67.
- Product Information, Roche, 2007.

FOSPHENYTOIN

DOSE & ADMINISTRATION: Note: Fosphenytoin dosing is expressed in phenytoin equivalents (PE). (Fosphenytoin 1 mg PE = phenytoin 1 mg) **Loading dose:** 15 to 20 mg PE/kg IM or IV infusion over at least 10 minutes. **Maintenance dose:** 4 to 8 mg PE/kg Q24 hours IM or IV slow push. Begin maintenance 24 hours after loading dose. Maximum rate of infusion 1.5 mg PE/kg per minute. May be administered more rapidly than phenytoin due to less infusion-related toxicity. Flush IV with saline before and after administration. Term infants older than 1 week of age may require up to 8 mg PE/kg per dose Q8 to 12 hours.

USES: Anticonvulsant. Generally used to treat seizures that are refractory to phenobarbital. Can be administered with lorazepam for rapid onset of seizure control.

MONITORING: Monitor blood pressure closely during infusion. Measure trough serum phenytoin (**not** fosphenytoin) concentration; obtain 48 hours after IV loading dose. Therapeutic serum phenytoin concentration: Probably 6 to 15 mcg/mL (up to 10 to 20 mcg/mL). Collect blood samples in EDTA tubes to minimize fosphenytoin to phenytoin conversion in the tube.

ADVERSE EFFECTS/PRECAUTIONS: Clinical signs of toxicity, such as drowsiness, are difficult to identify in infants, but are dose and infusion rate dependent. Minor venous irritation upon IV administration. Fosphenytoin drug interactions are similar to phenytoin (i.e. carbamazepine, cimetidine, corticosteroids, digoxin, furosemide, phenobarbital, and valproate). **Use with caution in neonates with hyperbilirubinemia:** both fosphenytoin and bilirubin displace phenytoin from protein-binding sites, resulting in increased serum free phenytoin concentration.

PHARMACOLOGY: Fosphenytoin is a water-soluble prodrug of phenytoin rapidly converted by phosphatases in blood and tissue. It has no known intrinsic pharmacologic activity before conversion to phenytoin. Each 1.5 mg of fosphenytoin is metabolically converted to 1 mg phenytoin. Conversion half-life of fosphenytoin administered intravenously to young pediatric patients is approximately 7 minutes. Data obtained using spiked blood samples from term and preterm neonates demonstrated similar conversion rates. No drugs have been identified to interfere with the conversion of fosphenytoin to phenytoin. Fosphenytoin is highly protein bound (adults 95% to 99%) and does not penetrate the blood-brain barrier. Serum half-life reflects that of phenytoin (18 to 60 hours) due to rapid conversion. The conversion of fosphenytoin to phenytoin yields very small amounts of formaldehyde and phosphate. This is only significant in cases of large overdosage. Phenytoin serum concentrations measured up to two hours after IV and four hours after IM dose may be falsely elevated due to fosphenytoin interaction with immunoanalytic methods (e.g. TDx fluorescence polarization).

SPECIAL CONSIDERATIONS/PREPARATION: Available as an injectable solution in a concentration equivalent to 50 mg PE/mL, in 2- and 10-mL vials. Administer IM undiluted. Administer IV after diluting in NS or D_5W to a concentration of 1.5 to 25 mg PE/mL. The pH is 8.6 to 9.0. **Store refrigerated.** Stable for 48 hours at room temperature. Do not use vials containing particulate matter.

Solution Compatibility: D_5W, $D_{10}W$ and NS.

Terminal Injection Site Compatibility: Lorazepam, phenobarbital, and potassium chloride.

Incompatibility: Midazolam.

SELECTED REFERENCES

• Fischer JH, Patel TV, Fischer PA: Fosphenytoin: Clinical pharmacokinetics and comparative advantages in the acute treatment of seizures. *Clin Pharmacokinet* 2003;42:33-58.
• Takeoka M, Krishnamoorthy KS, Soman TB, et al: Fosphenytoin in infants. *J Child Neurol* 1998;13:537-540.
• Morton LD: Clinical experience with fosphenytoin in children. *J Child Neurol* 1998;13(Suppl 1): S19-S22.
• Hatzopoulus FK, Carlos MA, Fischer JH: Safety and pharmacokinetics of intramuscular fosphenytoin in neonates. *Pediatr Res* 1998;43:60A.
• Fischer JH, Cwik MJ, Luer MS, et al: Stability of fosphenytoin sodium with intravenous solutions in glass bottles, polyvinyl chloride bags, and polypropylene syringes. *Ann Pharmacother* 1997;31:553-559.
• English BA, Riggs RM, Webster KW: Y-site stability of fosphenytoin and sodium phenobarbital. *Int J Pharm Compound* 1999;3:64-66.
• Riggs RM, English BA, Webster AA, et al: Fosphenytoin Y-site stability studies with lorazepam and midazolam hydrochloride. *Int J Pharm Compound* 1999;3:235-238.
• Product Information, Teva, 2007

FUROSEMIDE

DOSE & ADMINISTRATION: Initial dose: 1 mg/kg IV slow push, IM, or PO. May increase to a maximum of 2 mg/kg per dose IV or 6 mg/kg per dose PO. **Initial intervals:** Premature infant: Q24 hours. Fullterm infant: Q12 hours. Fullterm infant older than 1 month: Q6 to 8 hours. Consider alternate-day therapy for long-term use.

USES: Diuretic that may also improve pulmonary function.

MONITORING: Follow urine output and serum electrolytes and phosphorus. Assess closely for potassium depletion in patients receiving digoxin concurrently. Follow weight changes.

ADVERSE EFFECTS/PRECAUTIONS: Water and electrolyte imbalances occur frequently, especially hyponatremia, hypokalemia, and hypochloremic alkalosis. Hypercalciuria and development of renal calculi occur with long-term therapy. Potentially ototoxic, especially in patients also receiving aminoglycosides. Cholelithiasis has been reported in patients with BPD or congenital heart disease who received long-term TPN and furosemide therapy.

PHARMACOLOGY: The diuretic actions of furosemide are primarily at the ascending limb of Henle's loop, and are directly related to renal tubular drug concentration. Furosemide causes major urinary losses of sodium, potassium, and chloride. Urinary calcium and magnesium excretion, and urine pH are also increased. Prostaglandin production is stimulated, with increases in renal blood flow and renin secretion. Free water clearance is increased and CSF production is decreased by weak carbonic anhydrase inhibition. Nondiuretic effects include decreased pulmonary transvascular fluid filtration and improved pulmonary function. Protein binding is extensive, but bilirubin displacement is negligible when using normal doses. Oral bioavailability is good. Time to peak effect when given IV is 1 to 3 hours; duration of effect is approximately 6 hours, although half-life may be as long as 67 hours in the most immature neonates.

SPECIAL CONSIDERATIONS/PREPARATION: Furosemide oral solution is available in 8-mg/mL and 10-mg/mL concentrations. Protect from light and discard open bottle after 90 days. The injectable solution may also be used for oral administration. Furosemide for injection is available as a 10-mg/mL concentration in 2-, 4-, and 10-mL single use vials. A 2-mg/mL dilution may be made by adding 2 mL of the 10 mg/mL injectable solution to 8 mL preservative-free normal saline for injection. Dilution should be used within 24 hours. Protect from light and do not refrigerate.

Solution Compatibility: NS and sterile water for injection. Acidic solutions (pH <5.5) such as D_5W, $D_{10}W$, and Dex/AA cause furosemide to degrade when they are mixed together for several hours.

Terminal Injection Site Compatibility: Fat emulsion. Amikacin, aminophylline, amiodarone, ampicillin, atropine, aztreonam, bumetanide, calcium gluconate, cefepime, ceftazidime, cimetidine, dexamethasone, digoxin, epinephrine, famotidine, fentanyl, heparin, hydrocortisone succinate, indomethacin, lidocaine, lorazepam, linezolid, meropenem, morphine, nitroglycerin, penicillin G, piperacillin-tazobactam, potassium chloride, propofol, prostaglandin E_1, ranitidine, remifentanil, sodium bicarbonate, sodium nitroprusside, and tobramycin.

Incompatibility: Azithromycin, ciprofloxacin, dobutamine, dopamine, erythromycin lactobionate, esmolol, fluconazole, gentamicin, hydralazine, isoproterenol, metoclopramide, midazolam, milrinone, netilmicin, nicardipine, and vecuronium.

SELECTED REFERENCES

- Stefano JL, Bhutani VK: Role of furosemide after booster-packed erythrocyte transfusions in infants with bronchopulmonary dysplasia. *J Pediatr* 1990;117:965.
- Rush MG, Engelhardt B, Parker RA, Hazinski TA: Double-blind, placebo-controlled trial of alternate-day furosemide therapy in infants with chronic bronchopulmonary dysplasia. *J Pediatr* 1990;117:112.
- Mirochnick MH, Miceli JJ, Kramer PA, et al: Furosemide pharmacokinetics in very low birth weight infants. *J Pediatr* 1988;112:653.
- Green TP: The pharmacologic basis of diuretic therapy in the newborn. *Clin Perinatol* 1987;14:951.
- Hufnagle KG, Khan SN, Penn D: Renal calcifications: A complication of long-term furosemide therapy in preterm infants. *Pediatrics* 1982;70:360.
- Ross BS, Pollak A, Oh W: The pharmacological effects of furosemide therapy in the low-birth-weight infant. *J Pediatr* 1978;92:149.
- Ghanekar AG, Das Gupta V, Gibbs CW Jr: Stability of furosemide in aqueous systems. *J Pharm Sci* 1978;67:808.
- Product Information, Roxane, 2007
- Product Information, Abraxis, 2006

GANCICLOVIR

DOSE & ADMINISTRATION: 6mg/kg per dose Q12 hours IV infusion by syringe pump over 1 hour. Treat for a minimum of 6 weeks if possible. Reduce the dose by half for significant neutropenia (<500 cells/mm^3). **Chronic oral suppression:** 30 to 40 mg/kg per dose Q8 hours PO.

USES: Prevention of progressive hearing loss in babies with symptomatic congenital CMV infection.

MONITORING: CBC every 2 to 3 days during first 3 weeks of therapy, weekly thereafter if stable.

ADVERSE EFFECTS/PRECAUTIONS: Significant neutropenia will occur in the majority of treated patients. Discontinue treatment if the neutropenia does not resolve after reducing the dosage by half. Anemia and thrombocytopenia may also occur.

PHARMACOLOGY: Ganciclovir is an acyclic nucleoside analog of guanine that inhibits replication of herpes viruses in vivo. There is large interpatient variability in pharmacokinetic parameters. Mean half-life in infants less than 49 days postnatal age is 2.4 hours. Metabolism is minimal; almost all drug is excreted unchanged in the urine via glomerular filtration and active tubular secretion.

SPECIAL CONSIDERATIONS/PREPARATION: Cytovene® is supplied as lyophilized powder for injection, 500 mg per vial. Reconstitute by injecting 10 mL of Sterile Water for Injection into the vial. Do not use bacteriostatic water for injection containing parabens; it is incompatible with ganciclovir and may cause precipitation. Shake the vial to dissolve the drug. Visually inspect the reconstituted solution for particulate matter and discoloration prior to proceeding with infusion solution. Discard the vial if particulate matter or discoloration is observed. Reconstituted solution in the vial is stable at room temperature for 12 hours. Do not refrigerate, may cause precipitation. The pH is approximately 11; use caution when handling. Osmolarity is 320 mOsm/kg. Based on patient weight, remove the appropriate volume of the reconstituted solution (ganciclovir concentration 50 mg/mL) from the vial and add to a compatible diluent fluid to make a final infusion concentration less than 10 mg/mL. Although stable for 14 days, the infusion solution must be used within 24 hours of dilution to reduce the risk of bacterial contamination. Refrigerate the infusion solution. Do not freeze. Available as 250-mg and 500-mg capsules. Do not open or crush ganciclovir capsules. Prepare oral suspension in a vertical-flow laminar hood. Oral suspension (100 mg/mL) may be prepared by emptying eighty (80) 250-mg capsules into a glass mortar wetted and triturated with Oral-Sweet® to a smooth paste. Add 50-mL of Oral-Sweet® to the paste, mix, and transfer contents to an amber polyethylene terephthalate bottle. Rinse the mortar with another 50 mL of Oral-Sweet® and transfer contents to the bottle. Add enough Oral-Sweet® to make a final volume of 200 mL. Stable for 123 days when stored at 23° to 25° C. Protect from light.

Solution Compatibility: NS, D5W, and LR.

Solution Incompatibility: Dex/AA.

Terminal Injection Site Compatibility: Enalaprilat, fluconazole, linezolid, propofol, and remifentanil.

Incompatibility: Aztreonam, cefepime, and piperacillin-tazobactam.

SELECTED REFERENCES

- Kimberlin DW, Lin C-Y, Sanchez PJ, et al: Effect of ganciclovir therapy on hearing in symptomatic congenital cytomegalovirus disease involving the central nervous system: a randomized, controlled trial. *J Pediatr* 2003;143:16-25.
- Michaels MG, Greenberg DP, Sabo DL, Wald ER: Treatment of children with cytomegalovirus infection with ganciclovir. *Pediatr Infect Dis J* 2003;22:504-08.
- Frenkel LM, Capparelli EV, Dankner WM, et al: Oral ganciclovir in children: pharmacokinetics, safety, tolerance, and antiviral effects. *J Infect Dis* 2000;182:1616-24.
- Anaizi NH, Swenson CF, and Dentinger PJ: Stability of ganciclovir in extemporaneously compounded oral liquids. *Am J Health Syst Pharm* 1999;56:1738-41.
- Product Information, Roche, 2006

GENTAMICIN

DOSE & ADMINISTRATION: IV infusion by syringe pump over 30 minutes. Administer as a separate infusion from penicillin-containing compounds. IM injection is associated with variable absorption, especially in the very small infant. To use dosing chart, please refer to explanatory note in "How to Use This Book."

DOSING CHART

PMA (weeks)	Postnatal (days)	Dose (mg/kg)	Interval (hours)
≤29*	0 to 7	5	48
	8 to 28	4	36
	≥29	4	24
30 to 34	0 to 7	4.5	36
	≥8	4	24
≥35	ALL	4	24
* or significant asphyxia, PDA, or treatment with indomethacin			

USES: Treatment of infections caused by aerobic gram-negative bacilli (e.g. *Pseudomonas, Klebsiella, E coli*). Usually used in combination with a β-lactam antibiotic.

MONITORING: Measure serum concentrations when treating for more than 48 hours. Obtain peak concentration 30 minutes after end of infusion, and trough concentration just prior to the next dose. When treating patients with serious infections or significantly changing fluid or renal status consider measuring the serum concentration 24 hours after a dose, and use the chart below for the suggested dosing interval. Blood samples obtained to monitor serum drug concentrations should be spun and refrigerated or frozen as soon as possible. Therapeutic serum concentrations: **Peak:** 5 to 12 mcg/mL (or C_{max}/MIC ratio greater than 8:1) **Trough:** 0.5 to 1 mcg/mL

SUGGESTED DOSING INTERVALS

Level at 24 hours (mcg/mL)	Half-life (hours)	Suggested Dosing Interval (hours)
≤1	≈8	24
1.1 to 2.3	≈12	36
2.4 to 3.2	≈15	48
≥3.3		Measure level in 24 hours

ADVERSE EFFECTS/PRECAUTIONS: Transient and reversible renal tubular dysfunction may occur, resulting in increased urinary losses of sodium, calcium, and magnesium. Vestibular and auditory ototoxicity. The addition of other nephrotoxic and/or ototoxic medications (e.g. furosemide, vancomycin) may increase these adverse effects. Increased neuromuscular blockade (i.e. neuromuscular weakness and respiratory failure) may occur when used with pancuronium or other neuromuscular blocking agents and in patients with hypermagnesemia.

PHARMACOLOGY: Dosing recommendations are based on: (1) Higher peak concentrations increase concentration-dependent bacterial killing; (2) There is a post-antibiotic effect on bacterial killing, especially when treating concurrently with a β-lactam antibiotic; (3) There may be less toxicity with less frequent dosing, due to less renal drug accumulation. Volume of distribution is increased and clearance is decreased in patients with PDA. Serum half-life is prolonged in premature and asphyxiated newborns. Inactivation of gentamicin by penicillin-containing compounds appears to be a time-, temperature-, and concentration-dependent process. This is probably clinically significant only when penicillin-containing compounds are mixed in IV solutions or when the blood is at room temperature for several hours before the assay is performed.

SPECIAL CONSIDERATIONS/PREPARATION: Pediatric injectable solution available in a concentration of 10 mg/mL.

Solution Compatibility: D_5W, $D_{10}W$, and NS.

Terminal Injection Site Compatibility: Dex/AA solutions, fat emulsion. Acyclovir, amiodarone, aztreonam, caffeine citrate, cefoxitin, ceftazidime, ceftriaxone, cimetidine, clindamycin, dopamine, enalaprilat, esmolol, famotidine, fluconazole, insulin, lorazepam, heparin (concentrations ≤1 unit/mL), linezolid, magnesium sulfate, meropenem, metronidazole, midazolam, milrinone, morphine, nicardipine, pancuronium bromide, prostaglandin E_1, ranitidine, remifentanil, vecuronium, and zidovudine.

Incompatibility: Amphotericin B, ampicillin, azithromycin, cefepime, furosemide, imipenem/cilastatin, heparin (concentrations >1 unit/mL), indomethacin, methicillin, mezlocillin, nafcillin, oxacillin, penicillin G, propofol, and ticarcillin/clavulanate.

SELECTED REFERENCES

- Contopoulos-Ioannidis DG, Giotis ND, Baliatsa DV, Ioannidis JPA: Extended-interval aminoglycoside administration for children: a meta-analysis. *Pediatrics* 2004;114:e111-e118.
- Stolk LML, Degraeuwe PLJ, Nieman FHM, et al: Population pharmacokinetics and relationship between demographic and clinical variables and pharmacokinetics of gentamicin in neonates. *Ther Drug Monit* 2002;24:527-31.
- Avent ML, Kinney JS, Istre GR, Whitfield JM: Gentamicin and tobramycin in neonates: comparison of a new extended dosing regimen with a traditional multiple daily dosing regimen. *Am J Perinatol* 2002;8:413-19.
- Giapros VI, Andronikou S, Cholevas VI, Papadopoulou ZL: Renal function in premature infants during aminoglycoside therapy. *Pediatr Nephrol* 1995;9:163.
- Daly JS, Dodge RA, Glew RH, et al: Effect of time and temperature on inactivation of aminoglycosides by ampicillin at neonatal dosages. *J Perinatol* 1997;17:42-45.
- Williams BS, Ransom JL, Gal P, et al: Gentamicin pharmacokinetics in neonates with patent ductus arteriosus. *Crit Care Med* 1997;25:273-75.
- Product Information, Hospira, 2004

GLUCAGON

DOSE & ADMINISTRATION: 200 mcg/kg per dose (0.2 mg/kg per dose) IV push, IM, or SC. **Maximum dose:** 1 mg. **Continuous infusion:** Begin with 10 to 20 mcg/kg per hour (0.5 to 1 mg per day). Rise in blood glucose should occur with one hour of starting infusion.

USES: Treatment of hypoglycemia refractory to intravenous dextrose infusions, or when dextrose infusion is unavailable, or in cases of documented glucagon deficiency.

MONITORING: Follow blood glucose concentration closely. Watch for rebound hypoglycemia. Rise in blood glucose will last approximately 2 hours.

ADVERSE EFFECTS/PRECAUTIONS: Nausea and vomiting, tachycardia, and ileus. Hyponatremia and thrombocytopenia have also been reported.

PHARMACOLOGY: Glucagon stimulates synthesis of cyclic AMP, especially in liver and adipose tissue. Stimulates gluconeogenesis. In high doses, glucagon has a cardiac inotropic effect. Inhibits small-bowel motility and gastric-acid secretion.

SPECIAL CONSIDERATIONS/PREPARATION: Supplied in 1-mg single-dose vials. Dissolve the lyophilized product in the supplied diluent. Precipitates in chloride solutions. One unit of glucagon and 1 mg of glucagon are equivalent. Use immediately after reconstitution.

Solution Compatibility: No data are currently available on Dex/AA and other intravenous solutions.

Terminal Injection Site Compatibility: No data are currently available.

SELECTED REFERENCES

- Charsha DS, McKinley PS, Whitfield JM: Glucagon infusion for treatment of hypoglycemia: efficacy and safety in sick, preterm neonates. *Pediatrics* 2003;111:220-1.
- Miralles RE, Lodha A, Perlman M, Moore AM: Experience with intravenous glucagon infusions as a treatment for resistant neonatal hypoglycemia. *Arch Pediatr Adolesc Med* 2002;156:99-1004.
- Hawdon JM, Aynsley-Green A, Ward Platt MP: Neonatal blood glucose concentrations: metabolic effect of intravenous glucagon and intragastric medium chain triglyceride. *Arch Dis Child* 1993;68:255.
- Mehta A, Wootton R, Cheng KN, et al: Effect of diazoxide or glucagon on hepatic production rate during extreme neonatal hypoglycemia. *Arch Dis Child* 1987;62:924.
- Davis SN, Granner DK: Insulin and oral hypoglycemic agents and the pharmacology of the endocrine pancreas, in Hardman JG, Limbird LE, Gilman AG (eds): *The Pharmacological Basis of Therapeutics*, ed 10. New York: Macmillan Co, 2001, pp 1707-08.
- Product Information, Eli Lilly, 2005

HAEMOPHILUS B (HIB) CONJUGATE VACCINE

DOSE & ADMINISTRATION: 0.5 mL IM in the anterolateral thigh. Please refer to the most recent AAP/ACIP immunization schedule. It is recommended that premature infants should be immunized according to their postnatal age; however, inadequate seroconversion may occur in chronically ill premature infants. For HbOC and PRP-T, second and third doses are given at 2-month intervals, followed by a fourth dose given at age 15 months. For PRP-OMP, only the second dose is given after a 2-month interval; the third dose is given at age 15 months. **When giving multiple vaccines, use a separate syringe for each and give at different sites.** Care should be taken to draw back on the plunger of the syringe before injection to be certain the needle is not in a blood vessel.

USES: Immunoprophylaxis against invasive disease caused by *Haemophilus influenzae* type b.

MONITORING: Observe injection site for local reactions.

ADVERSE EFFECTS/PRECAUTIONS: Soreness at the injection site with local erythema, swelling, tenderness, and fever.

PHARMACOLOGY: Three conjugate vaccines are currently approved for use in infants older than 2 months of age. These vaccines are derived from *H influenzae* type b capsular polysaccharide, polyribosylribitol phosphate (PRP), which is linked to a T-cell-dependent protein antigen to enhance immunogenicity.

SPECIAL CONSIDERATIONS/PREPARATION: HibTITER® is a clear, colorless solution supplied in single-dose (preservative-free) vials. Discard if discolored or turbid. Store refrigerated at 2 °C to 8 °C (36 °F to 46 °F). **Do not freeze.** ActHIB® is supplied as lyophilized powder. Store the lyophilized vaccine and diluent refrigerated at 2 °C to 8 °C (36 °F to 46 °F). **Do not freeze.** Reconstitute using only the 0.4% saline diluent provided in single-dose 0.6-mL vials and use immediately. Reconstituted vaccine is a clear, colorless solution. Liquid PedvaxHIB® is supplied in single-dose vials. It is a slightly opaque white suspension. Shake well before withdrawal and use. Store refrigerated at 2 °C to 8 °C (36 °F to 46 °F). **Do not freeze.**

PRODUCTS

Manufacturer	Abbreviation	Trade Name	Carrier Protein
Wyeth-Lederle Pharmaceuticals	HbOC	HibTITER®	CRM$_{197}$ (a nontoxic mutant diphtheria toxin)
Sanofi Pasteur	PRP-T	ActHIB®	Tetanus toxoid
Merck & Co, Inc	PRP-OMP Liquid	PedvaxHIB®	OMP (an outer membrane protein complex of N meningitidis)

SELECTED REFERENCES

- American Academy of Pediatrics. *Haemophilus Influenzae* Infections. In: Pickering LK, Baker CJ, Long SS, McMillan JA, eds. Red Book: 2006 Report of the Committee on Infectious Diseases. 27th ed. Elk Grove Village, IL: American Academy of Pediatrics; 2006: pp 315-317.
- Advisory Committee on Immunization Practices: Recommendations of the ACIP. Most recent updates available on the National Immunization Program website: http://www.cdc.gov/nip/publications/acip-list.htm
- Washburn LK, O'Shea TM, Gillis DC, et al: Response to *Haemophilus influenzae* type b conjugate vaccine in chronically ill premature infants. *J Pediatr* 1993;123:791.
- Product information, Wyeth-Lederle Pharmaceuticals, 2007.
- Product information, Sanofi Pasteur, 2005.
- Product information, Merck & Co, 2004.

HEPARIN

DOSE & ADMINISTRATION: Maintaining patency of peripheral and central vascular catheters: 0.5 to 1 unit/mL of IV fluid. **Treatment of thrombosis:** 75 units/kg bolus, followed by 28 units/kg per hour continuous infusion. Four hours after initiating therapy, measure aPTT, then adjust dose to achieve an aPTT that corresponds to an anti-factor X_a level of 0.3 to 0.7 (this is usually equivalent to an aPTT of 60 to 85 seconds). Treatment should be limited to 10 to 14 days. **Make certain correct concentration is used.**

USES: See above. Only continuous infusions (rather than intermittent flushes) have been demonstrated to maintain catheter patency. Treatment of renal vein thromboses is limited to those that are bilateral or extend into the IVC. Although data are limited, enoxaparin may be preferable to heparin for treatment of thromboses. Call 1-800-NOCLOTS for case reporting and treatment guidance.

MONITORING: Follow platelet counts every 2 to 3 days. When treating thromboses, maintain a prolonged aPTT in a range corresponding to an anti-factor X_a level of 0.3 to 0.7 units/mL. Assess for signs of bleeding and thrombosis.

ADVERSE EFFECTS/PRECAUTIONS: Data are insufficient to make specific recommendations regarding anticoagulation therapy. Heparin-induced thrombocytopenia (HIT) has been reported to occur in approximately 1% of newborns exposed to heparin. Heparin-associated antiplatelet antibodies were found in half of the newborns who were both thrombocytopenic and heparin-exposed. Although the thrombocytopenia resolved spontaneously in most patients upon stopping the heparin, a high incidence of ultrasonographic-documented aortic thrombosis was seen. Contraindicated in infants with evidence of intracranial or GI bleeding or thrombocytopenia (below 50,000/mm³). Long term use of therapeutic doses of heparin can lead to osteoporosis.

PHARMACOLOGY: Activates antithrombin III, which progressively inactivates both thrombin and factor X_a, key proteolytic enzymes in the formation of fibrinogen and activation of prothrombin. Efficacy in neonates is decreased due to low antithrombin plasma concentrations. Metabolized by liver. Renal excretion should occur within 6 hours, but may be delayed. Clearance in neonates is more rapid than in children or adults. Half-life is dose-dependent, but averages 1 to 3 hours.

SPECIAL CONSIDERATIONS/PREPARATION: Keep protamine sulfate on hand to manage hemorrhage (see Protamine monograph for appropriate dosing). Heparin available in 10 units/mL (for IV reservoirs); 100 units/mL; 1000 units/mL (for central catheters); 5000 units/mL, and 10,000 units/mL.

Solution Compatibility: D_5W, $D_{10}W$, and NS.

Terminal Injection Site Compatibility: Dex/AA solutions, fat emulsion. Acyclovir, aminophylline, amphotericin B, ampicillin, atropine, aztreonam, caffeine citrate, calcium gluconate, cefazolin, cefepime, cefotaxime, cefoxitin, ceftazidime, ceftriaxone, chloramphenicol, cimetidine, clindamycin, dexamethasone, digoxin, dobutamine, dopamine, enalaprilat, epinephrine, erythromycin lactobionate, esmolol, famotidine, fentanyl, fluconazole, flumazenil, furosemide, hydralazine, hydrocortisone succinate, insulin, isoproterenol, lidocaine, linezolid, lorazepam, meropenem, methicillin, metoclopramide, metronidazole, mezlocillin, midazolam, milrinone, morphine, nafcillin, naloxone, netilmicin, neostigmine, nitroglycerin, oxacillin, pancuronium bromide, penicillin G, phenobarbital, phytonadione, piperacillin, piperacillin-tazobactam, potassium chloride, procainamide, propofol, propranolol, prostaglandin E₁, ranitidine, remifentanil, sodium bicarbonate, sodium nitroprusside, ticarcillin/clavulanate, trimethoprim-sulfamethoxazole, vecuronium, and zidovudine.

Incompatibility: Alteplase, amikacin, amiodarone, ciprofloxacin, diazepam, gentamicin, hyaluronidase, methadone, phenytoin, tobramycin, and vancomycin.

SELECTED REFERENCES

- Monagle P, Chan A, Massicotte P, et al: Antithrombotic therapy in children: the seventh ACCP conference on antithrombotic and thrombolytic therapy. *Chest* 2004;126:645-687.
- Schmugge M, Risch L, Huber AR, et al: Heparin-induced thrombocytopenia-associated thrombosis in pediatric intensive care patients. *Pediatrics* 2002;109(1). URL:http://www.pediatrics.org/cgi/content/full/109/1/e10.
- Edstrom CS, Christensen RD: Evaluation and treatment of thrombosis in the neonatal intensive care unit. *Clin Perinatol* 2000;27:623-41.
- Chang GY, Leuder FL, DiMichele DM, et al: Heparin and the risk of intraventricular hemorrhage in premature infants. *J Pediatr* 1997;131:362-66.
- Paisley MK, Stamper M, Brown J, et al: The use of heparin and normal saline flushes in neonatal intravenous catheters. *Pediatr Nurs* 1997;23:521-27.
- Kotter RW: Heparin vs saline for intermittent intravenous device maintenance in neonates. *Neonat Network* 1996;15:43-47.
- Moclair A, Bates I: The efficacy of heparin in maintaining peripheral infusions in neonates. *Eur J Pediatr* 1995;154:567-70.
- Spadone D, Clark F, James E, et al: Heparin-induced thrombocytopenia in the newborn. *J Vasc Surg* 1992;15:306.
- Product Information, Baxter, 2006

HEPATITIS B IMMUNE GLOBULIN (HUMAN)

DOSE & ADMINISTRATION: 0.5 mL IM in the anterolateral thigh. Term and preterm newborns born to HBsAg-positive mother: Give within 12 hours of birth. Term and preterm newborns born to HBsAg status unknown mother with BW ≥ 2000 g: Give as soon as it is determined that the mother is HBsAg-positive, within 7 days of birth. Preterm newborns born to HBsAg status unknown mother with BW < 2000 g: If mothers status unavailable, give within 12 hours of birth. **When given at the same time as the first dose of hepatitis B vaccine, use a separate syringe and a different site.** Care should be taken to draw back on the plunger of the syringe before injection to be certain the needle is not in a blood vessel.

USES: Passive immunization of newborns whose mothers have acute hepatitis B infection at the time of delivery, or who are HBsAg-positive. Infants born to mothers who are HBeAg-positive have the highest risk.

MONITORING: No specific monitoring required.

ADVERSE EFFECTS/PRECAUTIONS: Local pain and tenderness may occur at the injection site. **Do not administer IV** because of the risk of serious systemic reactions. Serious complications of IM injections are rare. Universal precautions should be used with neonates born to HBsAg-positive mothers until they have been bathed carefully to remove maternal blood and secretions.

PHARMACOLOGY: Hepatitis B Immune Globulin (human) is a hyperimmune globulin solution prepared from pooled plasma of individuals with high titers of antibody to hepatitis B surface antigen (anti-HBsAg). All donors are HBsAg-negative and HIV-antibody negative. Nabi-HB™ (Nabi) and BayHep B™ (Bayer) are solvent detergent treated and thimerosal free hepatitis B immune globulin preparations.

SPECIAL CONSIDERATIONS/PREPARATION: Refrigerate. Supplied in 1-mL and 5-mL single-dose vials and 0.5-mL unit-dose syringes.

SELECTED REFERENCES

- American Academy of Pediatrics. Hepatitis B. In: Pickering LK, Baker CJ, Long SS, McMillan JA, eds. *Red Book: 2006 Report of the Committee on Infectious Diseases.* 27th ed. Elk Grove Village, IL: American Academy of Pediatrics; 2006: pp 341-347.
- Crumpacker CS: Hepatitis, in Remington JS, Klein JO (eds): *Infectious Diseases of the Fetus and Newborn Infant,* ed 5. Philadelphia: WB Saunders Co, 2001, pp 932-33.
- Product Information, Cangene, 2006

HEPATITIS B VACCINE (RECOMBINANT)

DOSE & ADMINISTRATION: Engerix-B® 10 mcg (0.5 mL) or Recombivax HB® 5 mcg (0.5 mL) IM. **Maternal HBsAg-Positive:** Administer first dose before 12 hours of age regardless of birth weight (administer HBIG also). Infants with BW < 2000 g should receive 3 additional vaccine doses, beginning at 1 to 2 months of age. **Maternal HBsAg Unknown:** Administer first dose before 12 hours of age regardless of birth weight. If BW < 2000 g, administer HBIG if mother tests HBsAg positive or if mother's HBsAg result is not available within 12 hours of age. Administer HBIG to newborns with BW ≥ 2000 g within 7 days of birth if the mother tests HBsAg positive. **Maternal HBsAg Negative:** Administer first dose shortly after birth, before hospital discharge. If BW < 2000 g and medically stable, administer first dose 1 to 30 days of chronologic age or at time of hospital discharge if before 30 days of chronologic age. Please refer to the most recent AAP/ACIP immunization schedule for subsequent doses. Engerix-B® also has an alternative four-dose schedule: Birth, 1, 2, and 12 to 18 months of age.

USES: Immunoprophylaxis against hepatitis B. Safe for use in infants born to HIV-positive mothers, although it may be less effective.

MONITORING: Testing for immunity 3 months after completion of the vaccination series is recommended for infants born to HBsAg-positive mothers and, perhaps, for premature infants who received an early first dose.

ADVERSE EFFECTS/PRECAUTIONS: The only common side effect is soreness at the injection site. Fever greater than 37.7 °C occurs in 1 to 6%.

PHARMACOLOGY: Recombinant hepatitis B vaccines are produced by *Saccharomyces cerevisiae* (common baker's yeast) that has been genetically modified to synthesize

HBsAg. Both vaccines are inactivated (noninfective) products that contain HBsAg protein adsorbed to aluminum hydroxide, and may be interchanged with comparable efficacy.

SPECIAL CONSIDERATIONS/PREPARATION: Recombivax HB® for infant use is supplied in 0.5 mL single-dose vials and single-dose prefilled syringes containing 5 mcg. Engerix-B® is supplied in 0.5 mL single-dose vials and 0.5 mL single-dose prefilled disposable syringes containing 10 mcg per 0.5 mL. Preservative free. The vaccine should be used as supplied; do not dilute. **Shake well before withdrawal and use.** Store refrigerated at **2 °C to 8 °C (36 °F to 46 °F). Do not freeze**-destroys potency.

SELECTED REFERENCES

- American Academy of Pediatrics. Hepatitis B. In: Pickering LK, Baker CJ, Long SS, McMillan JA, eds. *Red Book: 2006 Report of the Committee on Infectious Diseases.* 27th ed. Elk Grove Village, IL: American Academy of Pediatrics; 2006: pp 341-347.
- Centers for Disease Control and Prevention: A comprehensive immunization strategy to eliminate transmission of hepatitis B virus in the United States. Recommendations of the Advisory Committee on Immunization Practices (ACIP) part 1: immunization of infants, children and adolescents. *MMWR Recomm Rep* 2005;54 (RR-16):1-23.
- Saari TN, Committee on Infectious Diseases: Immunization of preterm and low birth weight infants. *Pediatrics* 2003;112:193-98.
- Product Information, Merck and Company, 2007
- Product Information, GlaxoSmithKline, 2006

HIB CONJUGATE/HEPATITIS B COMBINATION VACCINE

DOSE & ADMINISTRATION: 0.5 mL IM in the anterolateral thigh. Please refer to the most recent AAP/ACIP immunization schedule. It is recommended that premature infants should be immunized according to their postnatal age; some data, however, suggest delaying the first dose in chronically ill premature infants due to inadequate seroconversion against *H influenzae*. **When giving multiple vaccines, use a separate syringe for each and give at different sites.** Care should be taken to draw back on the plunger of the syringe before injection to be certain the needle is not in a blood vessel.

USES: COMVAX® is indicated for vaccination against invasive disease caused by Haemophilus influenzae type b and against infection caused by all known subtypes of hepatitis B virus in infants 6 weeks to 15 months of age born to HBsAg-negative mothers. COMVAX® should not be used in infants younger than 6 weeks of age.

MONITORING: Observe injection site for local reactions.

ADVERSE EFFECTS/PRECAUTIONS: Local pain and tenderness may occur at the injection site.

PHARMACOLOGY: COMVAX® (preservative-free) combines the antigenic components of Recombivax HB® and PedvaxHIB®. Each 0.5 mL dose contains 5 mcg HBsAg and 7.5 mcg *Haemophilus b* -PRP.

SPECIAL CONSIDERATIONS/PREPARATION: Supplied in 0.5-mL single-dose vial. Store refrigerated. **Do not freeze.**

SELECTED REFERENCES

- American Academy of Pediatrics. Hepatitis B. In: Pickering LK, Baker CJ, Long SS, McMillan JA, eds. Red Book: 2006 Report of the Committee on Infectious Diseases. 27th ed. Elk Grove Village, IL: American Academy of Pediatrics; 2006: pp 341-343.
- Product information, Merck & Co, 2004.

HYALURONIDASE

DOSE & ADMINISTRATION: Inject 1 mL (150 units) as 5 separate 0.2-mL subcutaneous injections around the periphery of the extravasation site. Use 25- or 26-gauge needle and change after each injection. The chances of therapeutic success may be increased by:

1) Initiating treatment within 1 hour of extravasation;
2) Subcutaneously flushing the affected area with up to 500 mL of normal saline after the hyaluronidase treatment;
3) Covering with a hydrogel dressing for 48 hours.

USES: Prevention of tissue injury caused by IV extravasation. Suggested indications (some anecdotal) are for extravasations involving drugs that are irritating to veins because of hyperosmolarity or extreme pH (e.g. aminophylline, amphotericin B, calcium, diazepam, erythromycin, gentamicin, methicillin, nafcillin, oxacillin, phenytoin, potassium chloride, rifampin, sodium bicarbonate, tromethamine, vancomycin, and TPN, and concentrated IV solutions). Hyaluronidase is **not** indicated for treatment of extravasations of vasoconstrictive agents (e.g. dopamine, epinephrine, and norepinephrine).

MONITORING: No specific monitoring required.

ADVERSE EFFECTS/PRECAUTIONS: Not recommended for IV use.

PHARMACOLOGY: Hyaluronidase is a mucolytic enzyme that disrupts the normal intercellular barrier and allows rapid dispersion of extravasated fluids through tissues.

SPECIAL CONSIDERATIONS/PREPARATION: Amphadase™ and Hydase™ are supplied as 150 USP units/mL in 2 mL glass vials. Store refrigerated. Do not freeze.

Solution Compatibility: D_5W, $D_{10}W$, and NS.

Terminal Injection Site Compatibility: Amikacin, pentobarbital, and sodium bicarbonate.

Incompatibility: Epinephrine, heparin, and phenytoin.

SELECTED REFERENCES

• Ramasethu J: Prevention and management of extravasation injuries in neonates. *NeoReviews* 2004;5:e491-e497.
• Casanova D, Bardot J, Magalon G: Emergency treatment of accidental infusion leakage in the newborn: report of 14 cases. *Br J Plast Surg* 2001;545:396-399.
• Davies J, Gault D, Buchdahl: Preventing the scars of neonatal intensive care. *Arch Dis Child* 1994;70:F50-F51.
• Raszka WV, Kueser TK, Smith FR, Bass JW: The use of hyaluronidase in the treatment of intravenous extravasation injuries. *J Perinatol* 1990;10:146.
• Lehr VT, Lulic-Botica M, Lindblad WJ, et al: Management of infiltration injury in neonates using duoderm hydroactive gel. *Am J Perinatol* 2004;21:409-414.
• Product information, Amphastar Pharmaceuticals, Inc., 2005
• Product information, Akorn, 2007

HYDRALAZINE

DOSE & ADMINISTRATION: IV: Begin with 0.1 to 0.5 mg/kg per dose Q6 to 8 hours. Dose may be gradually increased as required for blood pressure control to a maximum of 2 mg/kg per dose Q6 hours. **PO:** 0.25 to 1 mg/kg per dose Q6 to 8 hours, or approximately twice the required IV dose. Administer with food to enhance absorption. **Note:** Use with a beta-blocking agent is often recommended to enhance the antihypertensive effect and decrease the magnitude of the reflex tachycardia. This is expected to reduce hydralazine IV dosage requirements to less than 0.15 mg/kg per dose.

USES: Treatment of mild to moderate neonatal hypertension by vasodilation. Afterload reduction in patients with congestive heart failure.

MONITORING: Frequent assessment of blood pressure and heart rate. Guaiac stools. Periodic CBC during long-term use.

ADVERSE EFFECTS/PRECAUTIONS: Diarrhea, emesis, and temporary agranulocytosis have been reported in neonates. Tachycardia, postural hypotension, headache, nausea, and a lupus-like syndrome occur in 10% to 20% of adults. Uncommon reactions in adults include GI irritation and bleeding, drug fever, rash, conjunctivitis, and bone marrow suppression.

PHARMACOLOGY: Causes direct relaxation of smooth muscle in the arteriolar resistance vessels. Major hemodynamic effects: Decrease in systemic vascular resistance and a resultant increase in cardiac output. Increases renal, coronary, cerebral, and splanchnic blood flow. When administered orally, hydralazine has low bioavailability because of extensive first-pass metabolism by the liver and intestines. The rate of enzymatic metabolism is genetically determined by the acetylator phenotype—slow acetylators have higher plasma concentrations and a higher incidence of adverse effects.

SPECIAL CONSIDERATIONS/PREPARATION: Hydralazine hydrochloride injection for IV use (20 mg/mL) is available in 1 mL vial. A 1 mg/mL dilution may be made by diluting 0.5

mL of the 20 mg/mL concentrate with 9.5 mL of preservative-free normal saline for injection. Dilution is stable for 24 hours. Oral tablet strengths include 10-, 25-, 50-, and 100-mg. Oral formulations using simple syrups containing dextrose, fructose, or sucrose are unstable. To prepare an oral suspension, crush a 50 mg tablet and dissolve in 4 mL of 5% mannitol, then add 46 mL of sterile water to make a final concentration of 1 mg/mL. Protect from light. Stable for 7 days refrigerated.

Solution Compatibility: NS.

Terminal Injection Site Compatibility: Dex/AA. Dobutamine, heparin, hydrocortisone succinate, potassium chloride, and prostaglandin E_1.

Incompatibility: Aminophylline, ampicillin, diazoxide, furosemide, and phenobarbital.

SELECTED REFERENCES

- Artman M, Graham TP Jr: Guidelines for vasodilator therapy of congestive heart failure in infants and children. Am Heart J 1987;113:995.
- Gupta VD, Stewart KR, Bethea C: Stability of hydralazine hydrochloride in aqueous vehicles. J Clin Hosp Pharm 1986;11:215.
- Beekman RH, Rocchini AP, Rosenthal A: Hemodynamic effects of hydralazine in infants with a large ventricular septal defect. Circulation 1982;65:523.
- Fried R, Steinherz LJ, Levin AR, et al: Use of hydralazine for intractable cardiac failure in childhood. J Pediatr 1980;97:1009.
- Product Information, American Regent, 2003

HYDROCHLOROTHIAZIDE

DOSE & ADMINISTRATION: 1 to 2 mg/kg per dose Q12 hours PO. Administer with food (improves absorption) . **Note: Do not confuse with chlorothiazide.**

USES: Diuretic used in treating both mild to moderate edema and mild to moderate hypertension. Effects increased when used in combination with furosemide or spironolactone. May improve pulmonary function in patients with BPD.

MONITORING: Serum electrolytes, calcium, phosphorus, and glucose; urine output and blood pressure.

ADVERSE EFFECTS/PRECAUTIONS: Hypokalemia and other electrolyte abnormalities. Hyperglycemia. Hyperuricemia. **Do not use in patients with significant impairment of renal or hepatic function.**

PHARMACOLOGY: Limited data in neonates. Rapidly absorbed from GI tract. Onset of action is within 1 hour. Elimination half-life depends on GFR and is longer than that of chlorothiazide. Major diuretic effect results from inhibition of sodium reabsorption in the distal nephron. Increases urinary losses of sodium, potassium, magnesium, chloride, phosphorus, and bicarbonate. Decreases renal excretion of calcium. Inhibits pancreatic release of insulin. Displaces bilirubin from albumin.

SPECIAL CONSIDERATIONS/PREPARATION: Supplied as a 50-mg/5mL oral solution.

SELECTED REFERENCES

- Albersheim SG, Solimano AJ, Sharma AK, et al: Randomized, double-blind, controlled trial of long-term diuretic therapy for bronchopulmonary dysplasia. J Pediatr 1989;115:615.
- Roberts RJ: Drug Therapy in Infants. Philadelphia: WB Saunders Co, 1984, p 244.

HYDROCORTISONE

DOSE & ADMINISTRATION: Physiologic replacement: 7 to 9 mg/m^2 per day IV or PO, in 2 or 3 doses. **Treatment of pressor- and volume-resistant hypotension (Stress doses):** 20 to 30 mg/m^2 per day IV, in 2 or 3 doses, or approximately 1 mg/kg per dose every 8 hours. **Treatment of chorioamnionitis-exposed ELBW infants to decrease risk of CLD:** Initial dose: 0.5 mg/kg/dose IV Q12 hours for 12 days, followed by 0.25 mg/kg IV Q 12 hours for 3 days.

BODY SURFACE AREA

Weight (kg)	Surface Area (sq meters)
0.6	0.08
1	0.1
1.4	0.12
2	0.15
3	0.2
4	0.25

BSA (m²) = (0.05 x kg) + 0.05

USES: Treatment of cortisol deficiency. Treatment of pressor-resistant hypotension. Adjunctive therapy for persistent hypoglycemia. May improve survival and decrease CLD in ELBW infants exposed to chorioamnionitis.

MONITORING: Measure blood pressure and blood glucose frequently during acute illness.

ADVERSE EFFECTS/PRECAUTIONS: Hyperglycemia, hypertension, salt and water retention. There is an increased risk of GI perforations when treating concurrently with indomethacin. There is also an increased risk of disseminated *Candida* infections. Early, low-dose hydrocortisone treatment was not associated with increased cerebral palsy. Treated infants had indicators of improved developmental outcome.

PHARMACOLOGY: Hydrocortisone is the main adrenal corticosteroid, with primarily glucocorticoid effects. It increases the expression of adrenergic receptors in the vascular wall, thereby enhancing vascular reactivity to other vasoactive substances, such as norepinephrine and angiotensin II. Hypotensive babies who are cortisol deficient (< 15 mcg/dL) are most likely to respond, and blood pressure will increase within 2 hours of the first dose. Hydrocortisone also stimulates the liver to form glucose from amino acids and glycerol, and stimulates the deposition of glucose as glycogen. Peripheral glucose utilization is diminished, protein breakdown is increased, and lipolysis is activated. The net result is an increase in blood glucose levels. Renal effects include increased calcium excretion. The apparent half-life in premature infants is 9 hours.

SPECIAL CONSIDERATIONS/PREPARATION: Hydrocortisone sodium succinate is available as powder for injection in 2-mL vials containing 100 mg. Reconstitute using preservative-free sterile water for injection to 50 mg/mL (reconstituted solution contains 9 mg/mL benzyl alcohol). Also available in 2-, 4-, and 8-mL vials with a concentration of 125 mg/mL after reconstitution. Dilute with preservative-free normal saline or D_5W to a final concentration of 1 mg/mL. Dilution stable for 3 days refrigerated.

Solution Compatibility: D_5W, $D_{10}W$, and NS.

Terminal Injection Site Compatibility: Dex/AA solutions, fat emulsion. Acyclovir, amikacin, aminophylline, amphotericin B, ampicillin, atropine, aztreonam, calcium chloride, calcium gluconate, cefepime, chloramphenicol, clindamycin, dexamethasone, digoxin, dopamine, enalaprilat, epinephrine, erythromycin lactobionate, esmolol, famotidine, fentanyl, furosemide, heparin, hydralazine, insulin, isoproterenol, lidocaine, linezolid, lorazepam, magnesium, methicillin, metoclopramide, metronidazole, morphine, neostigmine, netilmicin, nicardipine, oxacillin, pancuronium, penicillin G, piperacillin, piperacillin-tazobactam, potassium chloride, procainamide, propofol, propranolol, prostaglandin E_1, remifentanil, sodium bicarbonate, vecuronium and vitamin K_1.

Incompatibility: Ciprofloxacin, midazolam, nafcillin, pentobarbital, phenobarbital, and phenytoin.

SELECTED REFERENCES

• Watterberg KL, Shaffer ML, Mishefske MJ, et al: Growth and neurodevelopmental outcomes after early low-dose hydrocortisone treatment in extremely low birth weight infants. *Pediatrics* 2007;120:40-48.
• Ng PC, Lee CH, Bnur FL, et al: A double-blind, randomized, controlled study of a "stress dose" of hydrocortisone for rescue treatment of refractory hypotension in preterm infants. *Pediatrics* 2006;117:367-375.

- Watterberg KL, Gerdes JS, Cole CH, et al: Prophylaxis of early adrenal insufficiency to prevent bronchopulmonary dysplasia: a multicenter trial. *Pediatrics* 2004;114:1649-1657.
- Fernandez E, Schrader R, Watterberg K: Prevalence of low cortisol values in term and near-term infants with vasopressor-resistant hypotension. *J Perinatol* 2004;25:114-118.
- Seri I, Tan R, Evans J: Cardiovascular effects of hydrocortisone in preterm infants with pressor-resistant hypotension. *Pediatrics* 2001;107:1070-1074.
- Botas CM, Kurlat I, Young SM, Sola A: Disseminated candidal infections and intravenous hydrocortisone in preterm infants. *Pediatrics* 1995;95:883.
- Briars GL, Bailey BJ: Surface area estimation: pocket calculator versus nomogram. *Arch Dis Child* 1994;70:246-247.
- Product Information, Pharmacia and Upjohn. 2003

IBUPROFEN LYSINE

DOSE & ADMINISTRATION: First dose: 10 mg/kg. **Second and third** doses: 5 mg/kg. Administer IV by syringe pump over 15 minutes at 24 hour intervals.

USES: Closure of Patent Ductus Arteriosus. Not indicated for IVH prophylaxis.

MONITORING: Assess for ductal closure. Monitor urine output. Assess for signs of bleeding.

ADVERSE EFFECTS/PRECAUTIONS: NeoProfen® is contraindicated in preterm neonates with 1) infection, 2) active bleeding, 3) thrombocytopenia or coagulation defects, 4) NEC, 5) significant renal dysfunction, and 6) congenital heart disease with ductal-dependent systemic blood flow. Decreased urine output is less severe and occurs less frequently than with indomethacin. Although the available (and few) data suggest that the displacement of bilirubin from albumin is minimal with an ibuprofen dosing regimen of 10-, 5-, 5-mg/kg (q24hr), a more significant increase in unbound bilirubin can be expected in those infants with a high unconjugated bilirubin/albumin ratio and those in whom high ibuprofen concentrations are achieved. There is one recent case report of pulmonary hypertension in a 32 week gestation infant in Italy who received ibuprofen lysine (not NeoProfen) for treatment of PDA. Several studies have demonstrated an increased risk of oxygen dependency at 28 days postnatal age, but not 36 weeks PMA. Ibuprofen, like other nonsteroidal anti-inflammatory drugs, can inhibit platelet aggregation.

PHARMACOLOGY: NeoProfen® is a lysine salt solution of racemic ibuprofen, an inhibitor of prostaglandin synthesis. In adults (no data in neonates) metabolism is primarily via hydroxylation by hepatic CYP 2C9 and 2C8, with renal elimination of unchanged drug (10-15%) and metabolites. The mean half-life in premature neonates is approximately 43 hours, with large interpatient variability. Clearance increases rapidly with postnatal age and PDA closure.

SPECIAL CONSIDERATIONS/PREPARATION: Supplied as a 10 mg/mL sterile solution for injection in 2 mL single use vials. Should be diluted prior to administration in an appropriate volume of dextrose or saline. Contains no preservatives and is not buffered. Administer within 30 minutes of preparation. The pH is adjusted to 7. Store at room temperature. **Protect from light**.

Solution Compatibility: NS, 0.45% NS, D_5W, $D_{10}W$, and LR.

Terminal Injection Site Compatibility: No data available.

SELECTED REFERENCES

- Aranda JV, et al. Multicentre randomized double-blind placebo controlled trial of ibuprofen L-lysine intravenous solution (IV ibuprofen) in premature infants for the early treatment of patent ductus arteriosus (PDA). Late-breaker Abstract presented at the Pediatric Academic Societies Annual Meeting, 2005.
- Capparelli EV, et al. Population pharmacokinetics of ibuprofen L-lysine during early treatment of patent ductus arteriosus in premature infants. Abstract 2863.253, Pediatric Academic Societies Annual Meeting, 2006.
- Ohlsson A, Walia R, Shah S. Ibuprofen for the treatment of patent ductus arteriosus in preterm and/or low birth weight infants. The Cochrane Database of Systematic Reviews 2005, Issue 4. Art. No.: CD003481. DOI: 10.1002/14651858.CD003481.pub2.
- Thomas RL, Parker GC, Van Overmeire B, Aranda JV. A meta-analysis of ibuprofen versus indomethacin for closure of patent ductus arteriosus. *Eur J Pediatr* 2005;164:135-140.
- Desfrere L, Zohar S, Morville P, et al. Dose-finding study of ibuprofen in patent ductus arteriosus using the continual reassessment method. *J Clin Pharm Ther* 2005;30:121-132.
- Van Overmeire B, Touw D, Schepens PJC, et al. Ibuprofen pharmacokinetics in preterm infants with patent ductus arteriosus. *Clin Pharmacol Ther* 2001;70:336-343.

- Bellini C, Campone F, Serra G. Pulmonary hypertension following L-lysine ibuprofen therapy in a preterm infant with patent ductus arteriosus. *CMAJ* 2006;174:1843-44.
- Product Information, Ovation, 2007

IMIPENEM / CILASTATIN

DOSE & ADMINISTRATION: 20 to 25 mg/kg per dose Q12 hours IV infusion over 30 minutes.

USES: Restricted to treatment of non-CNS infections caused by bacteria, primarily Enterobacteriaceae and anaerobes, resistant to other antibiotics.

MONITORING: Periodic CBC and hepatic transaminases. Assess IV site for signs of phlebitis.

ADVERSE EFFECTS/PRECAUTIONS: Seizures occur frequently in patients with meningitis, preexisting CNS pathology, and severe renal dysfunction. Local reactions at the injection site and increased platelet counts are the most frequent adverse effects. Others including eosinophilia, elevated hepatic transaminases, and diarrhea also occur in more than 5% of patients.

PHARMACOLOGY: Imipenem is a broad-spectrum carbapenem antibiotic combined in a 1:1 ratio with cilastatin, a renal dipeptidase inhibitor with no intrinsic antibacterial activity. Bactericidal activity is due to inhibition of cell wall synthesis. Clearance is directly related to renal function. Serum half-life of imipenem in neonates is 2.5 hours; the half-life of cilastatin is 9 hours.

SPECIAL CONSIDERATIONS/PREPARATION: Available as powder for injection in 250-mg, and 500-mg vials. Reconstitute with 10 mL of compatible diluent. When reconstituted with compatible diluent, solution is stable for 4 hours at room temperature, 24 hours refrigerated. Maximum concentration for infusion is 5 mg/mL.

Solution Compatibility: D_5W, $D_{10}W$, and NS.

Terminal Injection Site Compatibility: Fat emulsion. Acyclovir, aztreonam, cefepime, famotidine, insulin, linezolid, midazolam, propofol, remifentanil, and zidovudine.

Incompatibility: Amikacin, amiodarone, azithromycin, fluconazole, gentamicin, lorazepam, milrinone, sodium bicarbonate, and tobramycin.

SELECTED REFERENCES
- Garges HP, Alexander KA: Newer antibiotics: imipenem/cilastatin and meropenem. *NeoReviews* 2003;4:e364-68.
- Stuart RL, Turnidge J, Grayson ML: Safety of imipenem in neonates. *Pediatr Infect Dis J* 1995;14:804.
- Reed MD, Kliegman RM, Yamashita TS, et al: Clinical pharmacology of imipenem and cilastatin in premature infants during the first week of life. *Antimicrob Agents Chemother* 1990;34:1172.
- Ahonkhai VI, Cyhan GM, Wilson SE, Brown KR: Imipenem-cilastatin in pediatric patients: an overview of safety and efficacy in studies conducted in the United States. *Pediatr Infect Dis J* 1989;8:740.
- Nalin DR, Jacobsen CA: Imipenem/cilastatin therapy for serious infections in neonates and infants. *Scand J Infect Dis* 1987;Suppl.2:46.
- Product Information, Merck, 2006

INDOMETHACIN

DOSE & ADMINISTRATION: IV infusion by syringe pump over at least 30 minutes to minimize adverse effects on cerebral, GI, and renal blood flow velocities. Usually three doses per course, maximum two courses. Give at 12- to 24-hour intervals with close monitoring of urine output. If anuria or severe oliguria occurs, subsequent doses should be delayed. Longer treatment courses may be used: 0.2 mg/kg Q24 hours for a total of 5 to 7 days. **Prevention of IVH:** 0.1 mg/kg Q24 hours for 3 doses, beginning at 6 to 12 hours of age.

PDA CLOSURE DOSE (MG/KG)

Age at 1st dose	1st	2nd	3rd
< 48 h	0.2	0.1	0.1
2 to 7 d	0.2	0.2	0.2
> 7 d	0.2	0.25	0.25

USES: Closure of ductus arteriosus. Prevention of intraventricular hemorrhage.

MONITORING: Monitor urine output, serum electrolytes, glucose, creatinine and BUN, and platelet counts. Assess murmur, pulse pressure. Assess for GI bleeding by guaiacing stools and gastric aspirate. Observe for prolonged bleeding from puncture sites.

ADVERSE EFFECTS/PRECAUTIONS: If oliguria occurs, observe for hyponatremia and hypokalemia, and consider prolonging the dosing interval of renally excreted drugs (e.g. gentamicin). Consider withholding feedings. Hypoglycemia is common, usually preventable by increasing the glucose infusion rate by 2 mg/kg per minute. Causes platelet dysfunction. Contraindicated in active bleeding, significant thrombocytopenia or coagulation defects, necrotizing enterocolitis, and/or significantly impaired renal function. Rapid (<5-minute) infusions are associated with reductions in organ blood flow. Gastrointestinal perforations occur frequently if used concurrently with corticosteroids.

PHARMACOLOGY: Inhibitor of prostaglandin synthesis. Decreases cerebral, renal and GI blood flow. Metabolized in the liver to inactive compounds and excreted in the urine and feces. Serum half-life is approximately 30 hours, with a range of 15 to 50 hours, partially dependent on postnatal age. In most studies, the response of the ductus and adverse effects of indomethacin are only weakly correlated with plasma concentration.

SPECIAL CONSIDERATIONS/PREPARATION: Supplied as a lyophilized powder in 1-mg single dose vials. Indomethacin sodium trihydrate salt is not buffered, and is insoluble in solutions with pH <6; the manufacturer therefore recommends against continuous infusion in typical IV solutions. Reconstitute using 1 to 2 mL of preservative-free NS or sterile water for injection. Reconstituted indomethacin is stable in polypropylene syringes and glass vials for 12 days when stored at room temperature or refrigerated. Observe for precipitation.

Solution Compatibility: Sterile water for injection. (No visual precipitation in 24 hours): $D_{2.5}W$, D_5W, and NS.

Terminal Injection Site Compatibility: Furosemide, insulin, nitroprusside, potassium chloride, and sodium bicarbonate.

Incompatibility: $D_{7.5}W$, $D_{10}W$, Dex/AA. Calcium gluconate, cimetidine, dobutamine, dopamine, gentamicin, and, tobramycin.

SELECTED REFERENCES

- Fowlie PW, Davis PG: Prophylactic indomethacin for preterm infants: a systematic review and meta-analysis. *Arch Dis Child Fetal Neonatal Ed* 2003;88:F464-66.
- Itabashi K, Ohno T, Nishida H: Indomethacin responsiveness of patent ductus arteriosus and renal abnormalities in preterm infants treated with indomethacin. *J Pediatr* 2003;143:203-7.
- Clyman RI: Recommendations for the postnatal use of indomethacin: an analysis of four separate treatment strategies. *J Pediatr* 1996;128:601.
- Hammerman C, Aramburo MJ: Prolonged indomethacin therapy for the prevention of recurrences of patent ductus arteriosus. *J Pediatr* 1990;117:771.
- Hosono S, Ohono T, Kimoto H: Preventative management of hypoglycemia in very low-birthweight infants following indomethacin therapy for patent ductus arteriosus. *Pediatr Internat* 2001;43:465-468.
- Coombs RC, Morgan MEI, Durbin GM, et al: Gut blood flow velocities in the newborn: Effects of patent ductus arteriosus and parenteral indomethacin. *Arch Dis Child* 1990;65:1067.
- Colditz P, Murphy D, Rolfe P, Wilkinson AR: Effect of infusion rate of indomethacin on cerebrovascular responses in preterm infants. *Arch Dis Child* 1989;64:8.
- Walker SE, Gray S, Schmidt B: Stability of reconstituted indomethacin sodium trihydrate in original vials and polypropylene syringes. *Am J Health-Syst Pharm* 1998;15:154.
- Ishisaka DY, Van Vleet J, Marquardt E: Visual compatibility of indomethacin sodium trihydrate with drugs given to neonates by continuous infusion. *Am J Hosp Pharm* 1991;48:2442.
- Gersony WM, Peckham GJ, Ellison RC, et al: Effects of indomethacin in premature infants with patent ductus arteriosus: Results of a national collaborative study. *J Pediatr* 1983;102:895.
- Brash AR, Hickey DE, Graham TP, et al: Pharmacokinetics of indomethacin in the neonate: Relation of plasma indomethacin levels to response of the ductus arteriosus. *N Engl J Med* 1981;305:67.
- Yaffe SJ, Friedmann WF, Rogers D, et al: The disposition of indomethacin in preterm babies. *J Pediatr* 1980;97:1001.
- Schmidt B, Davis P, Moddeman D, et al: Long-term effects of indomethacin prophylaxis in extremely-low-birth-weight infants. *N Engl J Med* 2001; 344:1966-1972.
- Ment LR, Oh W, Ehrenkranz RA, et al: Low-dose indomethacin and prevention of intraventricular hemorrhage: A multicenter randomized trial. *Pediatrics* 1994;93:543.
- Product Information, Ovation Pharmaceuticals, 2006

Infasurf®

(CALFACTANT) INTRATRACHEAL SUSPENSION

DOSE & ADMINISTRATION: Initial dose is 3 mL/kg per dose intratracheally, divided into 2 aliquots followed by up to three subsequent doses of 3 mL/kg per dose administered at 12-hour intervals if needed.

Clear the trachea of secretions. Shorten a 5F end-hole catheter so the tip of the catheter will protrude just beyond end of ET tube above infant's carina. Slowly withdraw entire contents of vial into a plastic syringe through a large (greater than 20 gauge) needle. Do not filter or shake. Attach shortened catheter to syringe. Fill catheter with surfactant. Discard excess through catheter so only total dose to be given remains in syringe. Administer in two to four aliquots with the infant in different positions to enhance distribution in the lungs. The catheter can be inserted into the infant's endotracheal tube without interrupting ventilation by passing the catheter through a neonatal suction valve attached to the endotracheal tube. Alternatively, surfactant can be instilled through the catheter by briefly disconnecting the endotracheal tube from the ventilator. After administration of each aliquot, the dosing catheter is removed from the ET tube and the infant is ventilated for at least 30 seconds until stable.

PHARMACOLOGY: Pulmonary lung surfactants are essential for effective ventilation by modifying alveolar surface tension thereby stabilizing the alveoli. Infasurf® is a sterile, non-pyrogenic natural surfactant extracted from calf lungs containing phospholipids, neutral lipids, fatty acids, and surfactant-associated proteins B and C. Preservative free. Each mL of Infasurf® contains 35 mg of total phospholipids (26 mg of phosphatidylcholine of which 16 mg is disaturated phosphatidylcholine) and 0.65 mg of proteins including 0.26 mg of SP-B.

SPECIAL CONSIDERATIONS/PREPARATION: Available in 3-mL and 6-mL single-use vials. Refrigerate (2 °C to 8 °C (36 °F to 46 °F)) and protect from light. Inspect Infasurf® for discoloration; normal color is off-white. If settling occurs during storage, gently swirl vial in order to uniformly suspend. **Do not shake.** Used vials with residual drug should be discarded. Unopened vials that have been warmed to room temperature one time may be refrigerated within 24 hours and stored for future use. Should not be warmed and returned to the refrigerator more than once.

SELECTED REFERENCES

• Bloom BT, Kattwinkel J, Hall RT, et al: Comparison of Infasurf® (calf lung surfactant extract) to Survanta (beractant) in the treatment and prevention of respiratory distress syndrome. *Pediatrics* 1997;100:31-38.
• Hudak ML, Farrell EE, Rosenberg AA, et al: A multicenter randomized, masked comparison trial of natural versus synthetic surfactant for the treatment of respiratory distress syndrome. *J Pediatr* 1996;128:396-406.
• Kendig JW, Ryan RM, Sinkin RA, et al: Comparison of two strategies for surfactant prophylaxis in very premature infants: A multicenter randomized trial. *Pediatrics* 1998;101:1006-1012.
• Product Information, Forest Pharmaceuticals, 2003

INFUVITE® Pediatric

MULTIPLE VITAMINS FOR INFUSION

DOSE & ADMINISTRATION: IV administration: Infuvite® *Pediatric* is a sterile product consisting of two vials: a 4 mL vial labeled **Vial 1** and a 1 mL vial labeled **Vial 2**. The daily dose is a function of infant weight as indicated in the following table. **Do not exceed this daily dose.**

Infuvite Dosing

	< 1 kg	≥ 1 kg and < 3 kg	≥ 3 kg
Vial 1	1.2 mL	2.6 mL	4 mL
Vial 2	0.3 mL	0.65 mL	1 mL

ADVERSE EFFECTS/PRECAUTIONS: Warnings: INFUVITE® *Pediatric* is administered in intravenous solutions, which may contain aluminum that may be toxic. Aluminum may reach toxic levels with prolonged parenteral administration if kidney function is

impaired. Premature neonates are particularly at risk because their kidneys are immature, and they require large amounts of calcium and phosphate solution, which contain aluminum. Research indicates that patients with impaired kidney function,
including premature neonates who receive parenteral levels of aluminum at greater
than 4 to 5 mcg/kg per day accumulate aluminum at levels associated with central
nervous system and bone toxicity. Tissue loading may occur at even lower rates of
administration.

PHARMACOLOGY:

INFUVITE® PEDIATRIC

Vial 1 (4 mL)	Amt*
Vitamin A** (as palmitate)	2300 IU (0.7 mg)
Vitamin D** (IU) (cholecalciferol)	400 IU (10 mcg)
Ascorbic Acid (vitamin C)	80 mg
Vitamin E** (dl-alpha tocopheryl acetate)	7 IU (7 mg)
Thiamine (as hydrochloride) B_1	1.2 mg
Riboflavin (as phosphate) B_2	1.4 mg
Niacinamide B_3	17 mg
Pyridoxine hydrochloride B_6	1 mg
d-Panthenol	5 mg
Vitamin K_1 **	0.2 mg

Vial 2 (1 mL)	
Biotin	20 mcg
Folic Acid	140 mcg
Vitamin B_{12} (cyanocobalamin)	1 mcg

* Amounts based upon guidelines published by the American Medical.
Association Department of Foods and Nutrition, JPEN 3(4);25862:1979.
Vial 1 (4 mL) Inactive ingredients: 50 mg polysorbate 80, sodium hydroxide
and/or hydrochloric acid for pH adjustment and water for injection.

** Polysorbate 80 is used to water solubilize the oil-soluble vitamins A, D, E, and
K.
Vial 2 (1 mL) Inactive ingredients: 75 mg mannitol, citric acid and/or sodium
citrate for pH adjustment and water for injection.

SPECIAL CONSIDERATIONS/PREPARATION: After INFUVITE® *Pediatric* is diluted in an intravenous infusion, the resulting solution is ready for immediate use. Inspect visually for
particulate matter and discoloration prior to administration, whenever solution and
container permit. Exposure to light should be minimized. Discard any unused portion.
Store between 2-8 °C (36-46 °F).

Incompatibility: Alkaline solutions or moderately alkaline drugs: acetazolamide, aminophylline, ampicillin, and chlorothiazide. Direct addition to intravenous fat emulsions
is not recommended.

SELECTED REFERENCES

• Product Information, Baxter Clinitec 2001

INSULIN

DOSE & ADMINISTRATION: Continuous IV infusion: 0.01 to 0.1 unit/kg per hour. (Only
regular insulin for injection may be administered intravenously.) To saturate plastic tubing binding sites, fill IV tubing with insulin solution and wait for at least 20 minutes before
infusing . The use of higher insulin concentrations and longer wait times will shorten the
time to steady-state. Titrate using blood glucose concentration/reagent strips. **Intermittent dose:** 0.1 to 0.2 unit/kg Q6 to 12 hours subQ.

USES: Treatment of VLBW hyperglycemic infants with persistent glucose intolerance.
Adjuvant therapy for hyperkalemia.

MONITORING: Follow blood glucose concentration frequently (Q15 to 30 minutes) after
starting insulin infusion and after changes in infusion rate.

ADVERSE EFFECTS/PRECAUTIONS: May rapidly induce hypoglycemia. Insulin resistance may develop, causing a larger dose requirement. Euglycemic hyperinsulinemia due to exogenous insulin administration may cause metabolic acidosis.

PHARMACOLOGY: Degraded in liver and kidney. Enhances cellular uptake of glucose, conversion of glucose to glycogen, amino acid uptake by muscle tissue, synthesis of fat, and cellular uptake of potassium. Inhibits lipolysis and conversion of protein to glucose. Plasma half-life in adults is 9 minutes.

SPECIAL CONSIDERATIONS/PREPARATION: Regular human insulin (rDNA origin) is available as 100 units/mL concentration in 10-mL vials. For subcutaneous administration, dilute with sterile water or NS to a concentration of 0.5 or 1 unit/mL. For IV administration, make a 10 units/mL dilution with sterile water, then further dilute in compatible solution to a concentration of 0.05 to 1 unit/mL. **Keep refrigerated.**

Solution Compatibility: D_5W, and $D_{10}W$, and NS.

Terminal Injection Site Compatibility: Dex/AA solutions, fat emulsion. Amiodarone, ampicillin, aztreonam, cefazolin, cefoxitin, cimetidine, digoxin, dobutamine, esmolol, famotidine, gentamicin, heparin, hydrocortisone succinate, imipenem, indomethacin, lidocaine, meropenem, metoclopramide, midazolam, milrinone, morphine, nitroglycerin, pentobarbital, potassium chloride, propofol, ranitidine, sodium bicarbonate, sodium nitroprusside, ticarcillin/clavulanate, tobramycin, and vancomycin.

Incompatibility: Aminophylline, dopamine, nafcillin, phenobarbital, and phenytoin.

SELECTED REFERENCES

- Mena P, Llanos A, Uauy R: Insulin homeostasis in the extremely low birth weight infant. *Semin Perinatol* 2001;25:436-446.
- Fuloria M, Friedberg MA, DuRant RH, Aschner JL: Effect of flow rate and insulin priming on the recovery of insulin from microbore infusion tubing. *Pediatrics* 1998;102:1401-1406.
- Poindexter BB, Karn CA, Denne SC: Exogenous insulin reduces proteolysis and protein synthesis in extremely low birth weight infants. *J Pediatr* 1998;132:948-953.
- Ostertag SG, Jovanovic L, Lewis B, Auld PAM: Insulin pump therapy in the very low birth weight infant. *Pediatrics* 1986;78:625.
- Product Information, Novo Nordisk, 2005

INTRAVENOUS IMMUNE GLOBULIN (HUMAN)

DOSE & ADMINISTRATION: Usual dosage: 500 to 750 mg/kg per dose over 2 to 6 hours. For neonatal alloimmune thrombocytopenia, doses have ranged from 400 mg/kg to 1 gram/kg. Most studies have used a single dose, although additional doses have been given at 24 hour intervals. See "*Special Considerations/Preparation*" for product-specific information.

USES: Adjuvant treatment of fulminant neonatal sepsis, hemolytic jaundice, and neonatal alloimmune thrombocytopenia.

MONITORING: Frequent monitoring of heart rate and blood pressure. Check IV site for signs of phlebitis.

ADVERSE EFFECTS/PRECAUTIONS: Rare cases of hypoglycemia, transient tachycardia, and hypotension that resolved after stopping the infusion have been reported. No short-term or long-term adverse effects have been reported in neonates. Animal studies have demonstrated reticuloendothelial system blockade when higher doses (>1 g/kg) have been used. All donor units are nonreactive to HBsAg and HIV. The manufacturing process of these products now includes a solvent/detergent treatment to inactivate hepatitis C and other membrane-enveloped viruses.

PHARMACOLOGY: IVIG is a plasma-derived, concentrated form of IgG antibodies present in the donor population. Significant lot-to-lot variation of specific antibodies may occur with all products. No significant differences in clinical outcomes using the different products have been seen. All preparations are reported to contain more than 92% IgG monomers and a normal distribution of IgG subclasses. Total IgG titers in treated, septic neonates remain elevated for approximately 10 days.

SPECIAL CONSIDERATIONS/PREPARATION: Reconstitute lyophilized products with supplied diluent. All products are preservative-free. Shelf life varies, but is at least 2 years when stored properly.

IVIG Preparations

Brand	Form	Storage	Preparation*
Gamunex 10% (Talecris)	10, 25, 50, 100, and 200 mL vials	Refrigerate	Allow to come to room temperature
Flebogamma 5% (Grifols)	10, 50, 100, and 200 mL vials 50 mg/mL, 5% solution	Room temperature	Rotate gently. Preservative-free.
Octagam (Octapharma)	1, 2.5, 5, and 10 g vials 5% solution	Room temperature	5% solution. Do not shake.
Carimune NF (ZLB Behring)	1, 3, 6, and 12 g lyophilized vials	Room temperature	Preservative-free.
Polygam®, S/D (American Red Cross)	2.5, 5, and 10 g lyophilized vials 5% glucose, pH 6.8	Room temperature	5% and 10% solution. Preservative-free.
Panglobulin NF (American Red Cross)	1, 3, 6, and 12 g lyophilized vials	Room temperature	Preservative-free.
Gammagard S/D (Baxter)	0.5, 2.5, 5, and 10 g lyophilized vials	Room temperature	5% and 10% solution
Gammagard Liquid 10% (Baxter)	1, 2.5, 5, 10, and 20 g liquid vials	Refrigerate or Room temperature	10% solution

* Reconstitute lyophilized products with supplied diluent. All products are preservative free. Shelf life varies, but is at least 2 years, when stored properly.

Solution Compatibility: D_5W, $D_{15}W$, and Dex/AA.

Terminal Injection Site Compatibility: Fluconazole.

SELECTED REFERENCES

- Kreymann KG, de Heer G, Nierhaus A, Kluge S: Use of polyclonal immunoglobulins as adjunctive therapy for sepsis or septic shock. *Crit Care Med* 2007;35:2677-2685.
- Sandberg K, Fasth A, Berger A, et al: Preterm infants with low immunoglobulin G levels have increased risk for neonatal sepsis but do not benefit from prophylactic immunoglobulin G. *J Pediatr* 2000;137:623-628.
- Jensen HB, Pollock BH: Meta-analyses of the effectiveness of intravenous immune globulin for prevention and treatment of neonatal sepsis. *Pediatrics* 1997;99(2):e2.
- Blanchette VS, Rand ML: Platelet disorders in newborn infants: diagnosis and management. *Semin Perinatol* 1997;21:53-62.
- Weisman LE, Stoll BJ, Kueser TJ: Intravenous immunoglobulin therapy for early-onset sepsis in premature neonates. *J Pediatr* 1992;121:434.
- Christensen RD, Brown MS, Hall DC, et al: Effect on neutrophil kinetics and serum opsonic capacity of intravenous administration of immune globulin to neonates with clinical signs of early-onset sepsis. *J Pediatr* 1991;118:606.
- Gottstein R, Cooke RWI: Systematic review of intravenous immunoglobulin in haemolytic disease of the newborn. *Arch Dis Child Fetal Neonatal Ed* 2003;88:F6-F10.
- Tanyer G, Suklar Z, Dallar Y, et al: Multiple dose IVIG treatment of neonatal immune hemolytic jaundice. *J Trop Pediatr* 2001;47:50-53.

IPRATROPIUM

DOSE & ADMINISTRATION: Administer Q6 to 8 hours as nebulized solution. Doses studied in intubated neonates range from 36 to 72 mcg via metered dose inhaler (MDI) with spacer, and 75 to 175 mcg via jet nebulizer. Studies in adults indicate that approximately 10% of an MDI dose, versus 1 to 2% of a nebulizer dose, is delivered to the lung. MDI devices are not recommended for use in infants with tidal volumes less than 100 mL because of safety concerns: Potentially hypoxic mixture of ventilator gas and propellant, and unknown hazards of exposure to chlorofluorocarbons. Optimal dose in neonates has yet to be determined due to differences in aerosol drug delivery techniques, although the therapeutic margin appears to be wide.

USES: Anticholinergic bronchodilator for primary treatment of chronic obstructive pulmonary diseases and adjunctive treatment of acute bronchospasm. Ipratropium is not useful in the treatment of bronchiolitis.

MONITORING: Assess degree of bronchospasm.

ADVERSE EFFECTS/PRECAUTIONS: Temporary blurring of vision, precipitation of narrow-angle glaucoma, or eye pain may occur if solution comes into direct contact with the eyes.

PHARMACOLOGY: Ipratropium bromide is a quaternary ammonium derivative of atropine. It produces primarily large airway bronchodilation by antagonizing the action of acetylcholine at its receptor site. It is relatively bronchospecific when administered by inhalation because of limited absorption through lung tissue. Peak effect occurs 1 to 2 hours after administration. Duration of effect is 4 to 6 hours in children. The combination of ipratropium with a beta-agonist produces more bronchodilation than either drug individually.

SPECIAL CONSIDERATIONS/PREPARATION: Inhalation solution is supplied in 2.5-mL vials, containing ipratropium bromide 0.02% (200 mcg/mL) in a sterile, preservative-free, isotonic saline solution that is pH-adjusted to 3.4 with hydrochloric acid. It may be mixed with albuterol or metaproterenol if used within 1 hour. Compatibility data are not currently available with other drugs. Store at room temperature in foil pouch provided. Protect from light.

SELECTED REFERENCES

• Lee H, Arnon S, Silverman M: Bronchodilator aerosol administered by metered dose inhaler and spacer in subacute neonatal respiratory distress syndrome. *Arch Dis Child* 1994;70:F218.
• Consensus Conference in Aerosol Delivery: Aerosol Consensus Statement. *Respir Care* 1991;36:916.
• Brundage KL, Mohsini KJ Froese AB, Fisher JT: Bronchodilator response to ipratropium bromide in infants with bronchopulmonary dysplasia. *Am Rev Respir Dis* 1990;142:1137.
• Gross NJ: Ipratropium bromide. *N Engl J Med* 1988;319:486.
• Product Information, Dey, 2006

IRON DEXTRAN

DOSE & ADMINISTRATION: 0.4 to 1 mg/kg (400 to 1000 mcg/kg) per day IV continuous infusion in Dex/AA solutions containing at least 2% amino acids.

USES: Iron supplementation in patients unable to tolerate oral iron, especially those also being treated with erythropoietin.

MONITORING: Periodic CBC and reticulocyte count. Observe Dex/AA solution for rust-colored precipitates.

ADVERSE EFFECTS/PRECAUTIONS: No adverse effects have been observed in patients who have received low doses infused continuously. Large (50 mg) intramuscular doses administered to infants were associated with increased risk of infection. Retrospective reviews of adult patients who received larger doses injected over a few minutes report a 0.7% risk of immediate serious allergic reactions, and a 5% risk of delayed such as myalgia, arthralgia, phlebitis, and lymphadenopathy.

PHARMACOLOGY: Iron dextran for intravenous use is a complex of ferric hydroxide and low molecular mass dextran. The dextran serves as a protective lipophilic colloid. Radiolabeled iron dextran injected into adult subjects localized to the liver and spleen before being incorporated into RBC hemoglobin. Complete clearance occurred by 3 days. Approximately 40% of the labeled iron was bound to transferrin within 11 hours. The addition of iron dextran to Dex/AA solutions inhibits the spontaneous generation of peroxides.

SPECIAL CONSIDERATIONS/PREPARATION: Available as a 50 mg/mL concentration in 2-mL single-dose vials. Store at room temperature. ***Mix only in Dex/AA solutions containing at least 2% amino acids.

SELECTED REFERENCES

• Mayhew SL, Quick MW: Compatibility of iron dextran with neonatal parenteral nutrition solutions. *Am J Health-Syst Pharm* 1997;54:570-1.
• Lavoie J-C, Chessex P: Bound iron admixture prevents the spontaneous generation of peroxides in total parenteral nutrition solutions. *J Pediatr Gastroenterol Nutr* 1997;25:307-11.
• Friel JK, Andrews WL, Hall MS, et al: Intravenous iron administration to very-low-birth-weight newborns receiving total and partial parenteral nutrition. *JPEN* 1995;19:114-18.
• Burns DL, Mascioli EA, Bistrian BR: Parenteral iron dextran therapy: a review. *Nutrition* 1995;11:163-68.

• Kanakakorn K, Cavill I, Jacobs A: The metabolism of intravenously administered iron-dextran. *Br J Haematol* 1973;25:637-43.
• Product Information, Watson, 2006

ISOPROTERENOL

DOSE & ADMINISTRATION: 0.05 to 0.5 mcg/kg per minute continuous IV infusion. Maximum dose 2 mcg/kg per minute. Dosage often titrated according to heart rate. Acidosis should be corrected before infusion.

Solution Preparation Calculations To calculate the AMOUNT of drug needed per defined final fluid volume:

Desired final concentration (mg/mL) × defined final fluid volume (mL) = AMOUNT of drug to add to final infusion solution (mg).

To calculate the VOLUME of drug needed per defined final fluid volume:

$$\frac{\text{*AMOUNT of drug to add (mg)}}{\text{drug (vial) concentration (mg/mL)}} = \text{VOLUME of drug to add (mL)}$$

Example (for Isoproterenol): Mix 50 mL of 10 mcg/mL solution using isoproterenol concentration of 0.2 mg/mL.
10 mcg/mL = 0.01 mg/mL
0.01 mg/mL x 50 mL = 0.5 mg isoproterenol

$$\frac{\text{*0.5 mg}}{\text{0.2 mg/mL}} = \text{2.5 mL of isoproterenol}$$

Add 2.5 mL of isoproterenol (0.2 mg/mL) to 47.5 mL of compatible solution (eg, D_5W) to yield 50 mL of infusion solution with a concentration of 10 mcg/mL. Maximum concentration 20 mcg/mL.

ISOPROTERENOL TITRATION CHART

Concentration (mcg/mL)	Dose (mcg/kg/min)	IV Rate (mL/kg/hour)
5	0.05 0.1 0.5 1	0.6 1.2 6 12
10	0.05 0.1 0.5 1	0.3 0.6 3 6
15	0.05 0.1 0.5 1	0.2 0.4 2 4
20	0.05 0.1 0.5 1	0.15 0.3 1.5 3

USES: Increases cardiac output in patients with cardiovascular shock. Pulmonary vasodilator (older infants).

MONITORING: Continuous vital signs, intra-arterial blood pressure, CVP monitoring preferable. Periodic blood glucose reagent strips.

ADVERSE EFFECTS/PRECAUTIONS: Cardiac arrhythmias. Tachycardia severe enough to cause CHF. Decreases venous return to heart. Systemic vasodilation. May cause hypoxemia by increasing intrapulmonary shunt. Hypoglycemia.

PHARMACOLOGY: β-receptor stimulant, sympathomimetic. Increases cardiac output by 1) increasing rate (major) and 2) increasing strength of contractions (minor). Insulin secretion is stimulated. Afterload reduction via β_2 effects on arterioles.

SPECIAL CONSIDERATIONS/PREPARATION: Supplied as 0.2-mg/mL (1:5000) solution in 1-mL and 5-mL ampuls.

Solution Compatibility: D_5W, $D_{10}W$, and NS.

Terminal Injection Site Compatibility: Dex/AA solutions, fat emulsion. Aminophylline, amiodarone, caffeine citrate, calcium chloride, calcium gluceptate, calcium gluconate, cimetidine, dobutamine, famotidine, heparin, hydrocortisone succinate, milrinone, netilmicin, nitroprusside, pancuronium bromide, potassium chloride, propofol, prostaglandin E_1, ranitidine, remifentanil, and vecuronium.

Incompatibility: Furosemide and sodium bicarbonate.

SELECTED REFERENCES

• Cabal LA, Devaskar U, Siassi B, et al: Cardiogenic shock associated with perinatal asphyxia in preterm infants. J Pediatr 1980;96:705.
• Daoud FS, Reeves JT, Kelly DB: Isoproterenol as a potential pulmonary vasodilator in primary pulmonary hypertension. Am J Cardiol 1978;42:817.
• Product Information, Hospira, 2006

LAMIVUDINE (3TC)

DOSE & ADMINISTRATION: PO: 2 mg/kg per dose Q12 hours for one week following birth.

USES: Prevention of mother-to-child HIV transmission in resource-limited settings. Use only in combination with zidovudine for treatment of neonates born to HIV-infected women who have had no therapy during pregnancy (has received intrapartum therapy only). The zidovudine plus lamivudine regimen is considered an alternative to the preferred regimen of single-dose nevirapine plus zidovudine for 4 weeks in resource-limited settings. Treatment of infected infants with combination antiretroviral therapy should be done in consultation with a pediatric infectious disease expert.

MONITORING: Specific monitoring unnecessary due to short treatment course.

ADVERSE EFFECTS/PRECAUTIONS: Generally well tolerated - limited data in neonates.

PHARMACOLOGY: Lamivudine (3TC) is a synthetic nucleoside analog "prodrug" that inhibits HIV replication by interfering with viral reverse transcriptase. It is intracellularly converted in several steps to the active compound, then renally excreted. Poor CNS penetration, CSF:plasma ratio is 1:100. The oral solution is well-absorbed, with 66% bioavailability in children. The serum half-life in preterm infants less than 33 weeks gestation is approximately 14 hours. Viral resistance develops rapidly to monotherapy with lamivudine (3TC). TMP-SMX increases lamivudine blood levels (significance unknown).

SPECIAL CONSIDERATIONS/PREPARATION: Available as an oral solution in concentrations of 5 mg/mL (Epivir-HBV®) and 10 mg/mL (Epivir®). Store at room temperature.

SELECTED REFERENCES

• World Health Organization. Antiretroviral drugs for treating pregnant women and preventing HIV infection in infants: Toward universal access. 2006 version. Available at http://www.who.int/hiv/pub/guidelines/pmtctguidelines3.pdf.
• Mueller BU, Lewis LL, Yuen GJ, et al: Serum and cerebrospinal fluid pharmacokinetics of intravenous and oral lamivudine in human immunodeficiency virus-infected children. Antimicrob Agents Chemother 1998;42:3187-3192.
• Moodley J, Moodley D, Pillay K, et al: Pharmacokinetics and antiretroviral activity of lamivudine alone or when coadministered with zidovudine in human immunodeficiency virus type 1-infected pregnant women and their offspring. J Infect Dis 1998;178:1327-1333.
• Paediatric European Network for Treatment of AIDS: A randomized double-blind trial of the addition of lamivudine or matching placebo to current nucleoside analogue reverse transcriptase inhibitor therapy in HIV-infected children: the PENTA-4 trial. AIDS 1998;12:F151-F160.
• Horneff G, Adams O, Wahn V: Pilot study of zidovudine-lamivudine combination therapy in vertically HIV-infected antiretroviral-naive children. AIDS 1998;12:489-494.
• Product Information, GlaxoSmithKline, 2008

LANSOPRAZOLE

DOSE & ADMINISTRATION: 0.73 to 1.66 mg/kg per dose PO, once a day. See Special Considerations/Preparation for preparation.

USES: Treatment of reflux esophagitis.

MONITORING: Observe for symptomatic improvement within 3 days. Consider intraesophageal pH monitoring to assess for efficacy (pH >4.0). Measure AST and ALT if duration of therapy is greater than 8 weeks.

ADVERSE EFFECTS/PRECAUTIONS: Hypergastrinemia and mild transaminase elevations are the only Adverse Effects reported in children who received lansoprazole for extended periods of time. Available data are limited to small studies of infants and children.

PHARMACOLOGY: Lansoprazole inhibits gastric acid secretion by inhibition of hydrogen-potassium ATPase, the enzyme responsible for the final step in the secretion of hydrochloric acid by the gastric parietal cell ("proton pump"). Extensively metabolized in the liver by CYP 2C19 and 3A4. Onset of action is within one hour of administration, maximal effect is at approximately 1.5 hours. Average elimination half-life is 1.5 hours. Inhibition of acid secretion is about 50% of maximum at 24 hours and the duration of action is approximately 72 hours. The absorption of weakly acidic drugs (e.g., digoxin, furosemide) is enhanced. The absorption of weakly basic drugs (e.g., ketoconazole) is inhibited.

SPECIAL CONSIDERATIONS/PREPARATION: Prevacid® is supplied in packets for oral suspension containing either 15 mg or 30 mg lansoprazole as enteric-coated granules and delayed-release capsules. Also available in 15 mg and 30 mg orally disintegrating tablets and 30 mg IV injection. For patients able to drink, prepare the oral suspension as follows: empty the packet contents into a container containing 30 mL of water. Stir well. Draw up the patient-specific dose and administer immediately after mixing. Do not administer the oral suspension via enteral tubes. For administration via nasogastric tube, use the capsules or orally disintegrating tablets. For capsules, open the capsule and mix thoroughly in 30 mL of apple, orange, or tomato juice. Do not use other liquids. Immediately draw up the patient-specific dose and inject through the NG tube into the stomach. After administering the granules, flush the NG tube with additional juice to clear the tube. For orally disintegrating tablets, place the 15 mg tablet in a syringe and draw up 4 mL of water or 30 mg tablet in a syringe and draw up 10 mL of water. Shake gently and allow dispersal. Inject patient-specific dose into the NG tube within 15 minutes. Refill the syringe with approximately 5 mL of water and flush the NG tube.

SELECTED REFERENCES
- Gibbons TE, Gold BD: The use of proton pump inhibitors in children: a comprehensive review. *Paediatr Drugs* 2003;5:25-40.
- Scott LJ: Lansoprazole in the management of gastroesophageal reflux disease in children. *Paediatr Drugs* 2003;5:57-61.
- Tran A, Rey E, Pons G, Pariente-Khayat A, et al: Pharmacokinetic-pharmacodynamic study of oral lansoprazole in children. *Clin Pharmacol Ther* 2002;71:359-67.
- Franco M, Salvia G, Terrin G, Spadaro R, et al: Lansoprazole in the treatment of gastro-oesophageal reflux disease in childhood. *Dig Liver Dis* 2000;32:660-6.
- Product information, TAP Pharmaceuticals, 2007.

LEVETIRACETAM

DOSE & ADMINISTRATION: Initial dose: 10 mg/kg per dose Q24 hours IV or PO in the neonatal period, Q12 hours later in infancy. Adjust dosage upward as needed every 1 to 2 weeks to a maximum of 30 mg/kg per dose. **Frequency:** Administer every 24 hours in the immediate neonatal period, every 12 hours later in infancy. Administer IV slowly over 15 minutes. Dilute to a concentration of 5 mg/mL with a compatible diluent prior to administration.

USES: Anticonvulsant. In the neonatal period, it has been used as a second line of therapy for seizures refractory to phenobarbital and other anticonvulsants.

MONITORING: Serum trough concentrations are not routinely monitored, although they may be useful when determining the magnitude of dosing adjustments. Therapeutic concentrations are approximately 10 to 40 mcg/mL.

ADVERSE EFFECTS/PRECAUTIONS: Data in neonates are limited to case reports and abstracts. Sedation and irritability have been reported in neonates and young infants. When discontinuing therapy, wean the dose gradually to minimize the potential of increased seizure frequency.

PHARMACOLOGY: Rapidly and completely absorbed after oral administration, with the onset of action by 30 minutes and peak concentration within 2 hours. Bioavailability is not affected by food. Half-life in the immediate neonatal period is approximately 18 hours, decreasing to 6 hours by 6 months of age. Minimal protein binding. Linear pharmacokinetics. Primarily (66%) excreted unchanged in the urine, with some metabolism via enzymatic hydrolysis to inactive metabolites (no cytochrome p450 involvement). Dose should be adjusted in patients with renal impairment. The precise mechanism of action is unknown. Levetiracetam inhibits burst firing without affecting normal neuronal excitability, suggesting that levetiracetam may selectively prevent hypersynchronization of epileptiform burst firing and propagation of seizure activity. There are no known significant drug interactions.

SPECIAL CONSIDERATIONS/PREPARATION: Keppra® Injection for intravenous use is available in single-use 5 mL vials containing 500 mg (100 mg/mL). Keppra® Oral Solution is available in a concentration of 100 mg/mL (dye- and alcohol-free). Store both products at controlled room temperature.

Solution Compatibility: NS, Lactated Ringer's, and D$_5$W.

Terminal Injection Site Compatibility: Lorazepam.

SELECTED REFERENCES

- Shoemaker MT, Rotenberg JS: Levetiracetam for the treatment of neonatal seizures. *J Child Neurol* 2007;22:95-98.
- Grosso S, Cordelli DM, Franzoni E, et al: Efficacy and safety of levetiracetam in infants and young children with refractory epilepsy. *Seizure* 2007;16:345-350.
- Striano P, Coppola A, Pezzella M, et al: An open-label trial of levetiracetam in severe myoclonic epilepsy of infancy. *Neurology* 2007;69:250-254.
- Allegaert K, Lewi L, Naulaers G, et al: Levetiracetam pharmacokinetics in neonates at birth. *Epilepsia* 2006;47:1068-1069.
- Glauser TA, Mitchell WG, Weinstock A, et al: Pharmacokinetics of levetiracetam in infants and children with epilepsy. Epilepsia 2007;48:1117-22.
- Tomson T, Palm R, Kallen K, et al: Pharmacokinetics of levetiracetam during pregnancy, delivery, in the neonatal period, and lactation. *Epilepsia* 2007;48:1111-1116.
- De Smedt T, Raedt R, Vonck K, Boon P: Levetiracetam: Part II, the clinical profile of a novel anticonvulsant drug. CNS Reviews 2007;13:57-78.
- Product information, UCB, 2008.

LEVOTHYROXINE (T$_4$)

DOSE & ADMINISTRATION: Initial oral dose: 10 to 14 mcg/kg per dose PO Q24 hours. (37.5 to 50 mcg/dose for an average term infant). Dosage is adjusted in 12.5-mcg increments. Always round upward. **Initial IV dose:** 5 to 8 mcg/kg per dose Q24 hours.

USES: Treatment of hypothyroidism.

MONITORING: After 2 weeks of treatment, serum levothyroxine (T$_4$) concentration should be in the high normal range—10 to 16 mcg/dL—and should be maintained in this range for the first year of life. Serum triiodothyronine (T$_3$) concentration should be normal (70 to 220 ng/dL), and TSH should have declined from initial value. After 12 weeks of treatment, serum TSH concentration should be in the normal range, less than 15 mU/L. Serum T$_4$ and TSH concentrations should be measured at two weeks of age, then every 1 to 2 months, or 2 weeks after any change in dosage. Assess for signs of hypothyroidism: Lethargy, poor feeding, constipation, intermittent cyanosis, and prolonged neonatal jaundice. Assess for signs of thyrotoxicosis: hyperreactivity, altered sleep pattern, tachycardia, tachypnea, fever, exophthalmos, and goiter. Periodically assess growth, development, and bone-age advancement.

ADVERSE EFFECTS/PRECAUTIONS: Prolonged overtreatment can produce premature craniosynostosis and acceleration of bone age.

PHARMACOLOGY: Tissue deiodination converts T$_4$ to T$_3$, the active metabolite. Elimination of both T$_4$ and T$_3$ is equally in the urine and feces. Clinical effects will persist for 1 week after discontinuation of the drug. Levothyroxine prepared as an oral suspension is 50% to 80% bioavailable. Oral dosing produces effects within 3 to 5 days, while IV dosing produces effects in 6 to 8 hours.

SPECIAL CONSIDERATIONS/PREPARATION: Oral suspension is not commercially available. Available as scored tablets ranging from 25 to 300 mcg per tablet. Prepare oral dosage form by crushing tablet(s) and suspending in a small amount of sterile water, breast milk, or non-soy formula. **Use immediately.** Monitor patients closely when switching brand of drug, due to some differences in bioavailability. **The injectable form should not be given orally,** as it crystallizes when exposed to acid. Injectable form is available as lyophilized powder in vials containing 200 or 500 mcg. **Use only NS for reconstitution.** Manufacturer's suggested final concentrations are 40 mcg/mL or 100 mcg/mL; however, suggested dilution is a final concentration of 20 mcg/mL. **Use immediately. Do not add to any other IV solution.**

SELECTED REFERENCES

- Selva KA, Mandel SH, Rien L, et al: Initial treatment of L-thyroxine in congenital hypothyroidism. *J Pediatr* 2002;141:786-92.
- AAP Section on Endocrinology and Committee on Genetics, and Committee on Public Health, American Thyroid Association: Newborn screening for congenital hypothyroidism: Recommended guidelines. *Pediatrics* 1993;91:1203-1209.
- Germak JA, Foley TP: Longitudinal assessment of L-thyroxine therapy for congenital hypothyroidism. *J Pediatr* 1990;117:211.
- Product Information, Bedford, 2003

LIDOCAINE - ANTIARRHYTHMIC

DOSE & ADMINISTRATION: Initial bolus dose: 0.5 to 1 mg/kg IV push over 5 minutes. Repeat Q10 minutes as necessary to control arrhythmia. Maximum total bolus dose should not exceed 5 mg/kg. **Maintenance IV infusion:** 10 to 50 mcg/kg per minute. Premature neonates should receive lowest dosage.

LIDOCAINE TITRATION CHART

Concentration (mcg/mL)	Dose (mcg/kg/min)	IV Rate (mL/kg/hour)
800	10	0.75
	20	1.5
	30	2.25
	40	3
	50	3.75
1600	10	0.375
	20	0.75
	30	1.125
	40	1.5
	50	1.875
2400	10	0.25
	20	0.5
	30	0.75
	40	1
	50	1.25
4000	10	0.15
	20	0.3
	30	0.45
	40	0.6
	50	0.75
6000	10	0.1
	20	0.2
	30	0.3
	40	0.4
	50	0.5
8000	10	0.075
	20	0.15
	30	0.225
	40	0.3
	50	0.375

Solution Preparation Calculations To calculate the AMOUNT of drug needed per defined final fluid volume:

Desired final concentration (mg/mL) × defined final fluid volume (mL) = AMOUNT of drug to add to final infusion solution (mg).

To calculate the VOLUME of drug needed per defined final fluid volume:

$$\frac{\text{*AMOUNT of drug to add (mg)}}{\text{drug (vial) concentration (mg/mL)}} = \text{VOLUME of drug to add (mL)}$$

Example (for Lidocaine): Mix 50 mL of 2400 mcg/mL solution using lidocaine concentration of 20 mg/mL.

2400 mcg/mL = 2.4 mg/mL

2.4 mg/mL x 50 mL = 120 mg lidocaine

$$\frac{*120 \text{ mg}}{20 \text{ mg/mL}} = 6 \text{ mL of lidocaine}$$

Add 6 mL of lidocaine (20 mg/mL) to 44 mL of compatible solution (eg, D_5W) to yield 50 mL of infusion solution with a concentration of 2400 mcg/mL. Maximum concentration is 8000 mcg/mL.

USES: Short-term control of ventricular arrhythmias, including ventricular tachycardia, premature ventricular contractions, and arrhythmias resulting from digitalis intoxication.

MONITORING: Continuous monitoring of EKG, heart rate, and blood pressure. Assess level of consciousness. Observe for seizure activity. Therapeutic total lidocaine serum concentrations are 1 to 5 mcg/mL.

ADVERSE EFFECTS/PRECAUTIONS: Early signs of CNS toxicity are drowsiness, agitation, vomiting, and muscle twitching. Later signs include seizures, loss of consciousness, respiratory depression, and apnea. Cardiac toxicity is associated with excessive doses and includes bradycardia, hypotension, heart block, and cardiovascular collapse. **Contraindicated in infants with cardiac failure and heart block.** Serum lidocaine concentrations increase when using either cimetidine or propranolol in combination.

PHARMACOLOGY: Lidocaine is a Type 1b antiarrhythmic agent used intravenously. Onset of action is 1 to 2 minutes after bolus administration. Plasma half-life in neonates is 3 hours. Free drug fraction in both term and premature neonates is approximately twice that found in older children because of significantly reduced protein binding by α_1-acid glycoprotein. Transformed in the liver to metabolites with antiarrhythmic activity; approximately 30% is excreted unchanged in neonates.

SPECIAL CONSIDERATIONS/PREPARATION: Use only preservative-free lidocaine without epinephrine. Available in multiple concentrations ranging from 1% to 20%. To make a dilution for bolus dosing, dilute 10 mg lidocaine (0.5 mL of 2% solution) in 9.5 mL NS or D_5W, yielding a 1 mg/mL final concentration.

Solution Compatibility: D_5W, $D_{10}W$, and NS.

Terminal Injection Site Compatibility: Dex/AA solutions, fat emulsion. Alteplase, aminophylline, amiodarone, ampicillin, caffeine citrate, calcium chloride, calcium gluconate, cefazolin, cefoxitin, ceftriaxone, chloramphenicol, cimetidine, dexamethasone, digoxin, dobutamine, dopamine, enalaprilat, erythromycin lactobionate, esmolol, famotidine, fentanyl, flumazenil, furosemide, glycopyrrolate, heparin, hydrocortisone succinate, insulin, linezolid, methicillin, metoclopramide, morphine, nafcillin, nicardipine, nitroglycerin, penicillin G, pentobarbital, potassium chloride, procainamide, prostaglandin E_1, ranitidine, sodium bicarbonate, and sodium nitroprusside.

Incompatibility: Phenytoin.

SELECTED REFERENCES

• Lerman J, Strong A, LeDez KM, et al: Effects of age on the serum concentration of α_1-acid glycoprotein and the binding of lidocaine in pediatric patients. *Clin Pharmacol Ther* 1989;46:219.
• Mihaly GW, Moore RG, Thomas J: The pharmacokinetics and metabolism of the anilide local anesthetics in neonates. I. Lignocaine. *Eur J Clin Pharmacol* 1978;13:143.
• Gelband H, Rosen MR: Pharmacologic basis for the treatment of cardiac arrhythmias. *Pediatrics* 1975;55:59.

LIDOCAINE - ANTICONVULSANT

DOSE & ADMINISTRATION: Loading dose: 2 mg/kg IV over 10 minutes, followed immediately by a **Maintenance infusion:** 6 mg/kg per hour. Begin to taper infusion after 12 to 24 hours, as drug accumulation will occur.

USES: Treatment of severe recurrent or prolonged seizures that do not respond to first-line therapies.

MONITORING: Continuous monitoring of EKG, heart rate, and blood pressure. Observe for worsening of seizure activity. Measuring blood concentrations is not clinically useful except when accumulation is suspected.

ADVERSE EFFECTS/PRECAUTIONS: Do not use concurrently with phenytoin due to cardiac effects. Stop infusion immediately if significant cardiac arrhythmia occurs. Arrhythmias and significant bradycardia have occurred in 5% of reported cases. Slowing of the heart rate is common.

PHARMACOLOGY: The mode of action for lidocaine as an anticonvulsant drug is unknown. Lidocaine is metabolized in the liver into 2 active metabolites: monoethylglycinexylidide (MEGX) and glycinxylidide (GX). Approximately 30% is excreted unchanged in the urine. The half-life in neonates is at least 3 hours, and clearance is dose-dependent. The clinically effective dose of 6 mg/kg/hr will lead to accumulation of both lidocaine and metabolites within several hours. Free drug fraction in both term and premature neonates is approximately twice that found in older children because of significantly reduced protein binding by alpha 1-acid glycoprotein.

SPECIAL CONSIDERATIONS/PREPARATION: Use only preservative-free lidocaine without epinephrine. Available in multiple concentrations ranging from 1% to 20%. To make a dilution for bolus dosing, dilute 10 mg lidocaine (0.5 mL of 2% solution) in 9.5 mL NS or D_5W, yielding a 1 mg/mL final concentration.

Solution Compatibility: D_5W, $D_{10}W$, and NS.

Terminal Injection Site Compatibility: Dex/AA solutions, fat emulsion. Alteplase, aminophylline, amiodarone, ampicillin, caffeine citrate, calcium chloride, calcium gluconate, cefazolin, cefoxitin, ceftriaxone, chloramphenicol, cimetidine, dexamethasone, digoxin, dobutamine, dopamine, enalaprilat, erythromycin lactobionate, famotidine, fentanyl, flumazenil, furosemide, glycopyrrolate, heparin, hydrocortisone succinate, insulin, linezolid, methicillin, metoclopramide, morphine, nafcillin, nicardipine, nitroglycerin, penicillin G, pentobarbital, potassium chloride, procainamide, prostaglandin E_1, ranitidine, sodium bicarbonate, and sodium nitroprusside.

Incompatibility: Phenytoin.

SELECTED REFERENCES

- Van Rooij LGM, Toet MC, Rademaker KMA, et al: Cardiac arrhythmias in neonates receiving lidocaine as anticonvulsive treatment. *Eur J Pediatr* 2004;163:637-641.
- Hellstrom-Westas L, Svenningsen NW, Westgren U, et al: Lidocaine for treatment of severe seizures in newborn infants. II. Blood concentrations of lidocaine and metabolites during intravenous infusion. *Acta Paediatr* 1992;81:35-39.
- Hellstrom-Westas L, Westgren U, Rosen I, Svenningsen NW: Lidocaine for treatment of severe seizures in newborn infants. I. Clinical effects and cerebral electrical activity monitoring. *Acta Paediatr Scand* 1988;77:79-84.
- Rey E, Radvanyi-Bouvet MF, Bodiou C, et al: Intravenous lidocaine in the treatment of convulsions in the neonatal period: Monitoring plasma levels. *Ther Drug Monit* 1990;12:316-320.

LINEZOLID

DOSE & ADMINISTRATION: 10 mg/kg per dose Q8 hours by IV infusion over 30 to 120 minutes. Preterm newborns < 1 week of age: 10 mg/kg per dose Q12 hours. Oral dosing is the same as IV.

USES: Limited to treatment of non-CNS infections, including endocarditis, caused by gram positive organisms resistant to other antibiotics, e.g. methicillin-resistant *Staph. aureus*, penicillin-resistant *Strep. pneumoniae*, and vancomycin-resistant *Enterococcus faecium*. Treatment of VRE endocarditis that has failed conventional therapy. Do not use as empiric treatment or in any patient with infections caused by gram-negative organisms.

MONITORING: Weekly CBC, AST, ALT. Blood pressure if receiving sympathomimetics.

ADVERSE EFFECTS/PRECAUTIONS: Elevated transaminases and diarrhea occur in 6 to 10% of treated patients; thrombocytopenia, anemia, and rash occur in 1 to 2%. The FDA issued an alert regarding Zyvox (linezolid) on March 16, 2007. Patients in an open-label, randomized trial comparing linezolid to vancomycin, oxacillin, or dicloxacillin in the treatment of seriously ill patients with intravascular catheter-related bloodstream infections had a higher chance of death than did patients treated with any comparator antibiotic, and the chance of death was related to the type of organism causing the infection. Patients with Gram positive infections had no difference in mortality according to their antibiotic treatment. In contrast, mortality was higher in patients treated with linezolid who were infected with Gram negative organisms alone, with both Gram positive and Gram negative organisms, or who had no infection when they entered the study. See "http://www.fda.gov/cder/drug/InfoSheets/HCP/linezolidHCP.htm"

PHARMACOLOGY: Linezolid is an oxazolidinone agent that has a unique mechanism of inhibition of bacterial protein synthesis. It is usually bacteriostatic, although it may be bactericidal against *S. pneumoniae, B. fragilis,* and *C. perfringens.* Rapidly penetrates osteoarticular tissues and synovial fluid. CSF concentrations were 70% of plasma concentrations in older patients with non-inflamed meninges. Completely and rapidly absorbed when administered orally to adults and children. Metabolized by oxidation without cytochrome CYP induction. Excreted in the urine as unchanged drug (30%) and two inactive metabolites. Serum half-life in most neonates is 2 to 3 hours, with the exception of preterm neonates less than one week of age, who have a serum half-life of 5 to 6 hours.

SPECIAL CONSIDERATIONS/PREPARATION: Linezolid IV injection is supplied as a 2 mg/mL solution in single-use, ready-to-use 100-mL, 200-mL, and 300-mL plastic infusion bags in a foil laminate overwrap. Keep in the overwrap until use. Store at room temperature. Protect from freezing. IV injection may exhibit a yellow color that can intensify over time without affecting potency. An oral suspension is available, 100 mg per 5 mL. Store at room temperature. Use within 21 days after reconstitution. Protect from light.

Solution Compatibility: D_5W, NS, Lactated Ringers.

Terminal Injection Site Compatibility: Dex/AA. Acyclovir, amikacin, aminophylline, ampicillin, aztreonam, calcium gluconate, cefazolin, cefoxitin, ceftazidime, ceftriaxone, cefuroxime, cimetidine, clindamycin, dexamethasone, digoxin, dobutamine, dopamine, enalaprilat, esmolol, famotidine, fentanyl, fluconazole, furosemide, ganciclovir, gentamicin, heparin, hydrocortisone succinate, imipenem/cilastatin, lidocaine, lorazepam, magnesium, meropenem, methylprednisolone, metoclopramide, metronidazole, mezlocillin, midazolam, morphine, naloxone, netilmicin, nicardipine, nitroglycerin, pentobarbital, phenobarbital, piperacillin, piperacillin-tazobactam, potassium chloride, propranolol, ranitidine, remifentanil, sodium bicarbonate, theophylline, ticarcillin, tobramycin, trimethoprim-sulfamethoxazole, vancomycin, vecuronium, and zidovudine.

Incompatibility: Amphotericin B, chlorpromazine, diazepam, erythromycin lactobionate, pentamidine isethionate, and phenytoin.

SELECTED REFERENCES

- Tan TQ: Update on the use of linezolid: a pediatric perspective. *Pediatr Infect Dis J* 2004;23:955-956.
- Jungbluth GL, Welshman IR, Hopkins NK: Linezolid pharmacokinetics in pediatric patients: an overview. *Pediatr Infect Dis J* 2003;23:S153-157.
- Kearns GL, Jungbluth GL, Abdel-Rahman SM, et al: Impact of ontogeny on linezolid disposition in neonates and infants. *Clin Pharmacol Ther* 2003;74:413-22.
- DeVille JG, Adler S, Azimi PH: Linezolid versus vancomycin in the treatment of known or suspected resistant Gram-positive infections in neonates. *Pediatr Infect Dis J* 2003;22:S158-63.
- Saiman L, Goldfarb J, Kaplan SA, et al: Safety and tolerability of linezolid in children. *Pediatr Infect Dis J* 2003;22:S193-200.
- Garges HP, Alexander KA: Newer antibiotics: Linezolid. *NeoReviews* 2003;4:e128-32.
- Trissel LA, Williams KY, Gilbert DL: Compatibility screening of linezolid injection during simulated Y-site administration with other drugs and infusion solutions. *J Amer Pharm Assoc* 2000;40:515-519.
- Product information, Pfizer (Pharmacia & UpJohn), 2007.

LORAZEPAM

DOSE & ADMINISTRATION: 0.05 to 0.1 mg/kg per dose IV slow push. Repeat doses based on clinical response.

USES: Anticonvulsant—acute management of patients with seizures refractory to conventional therapy.

MONITORING: Monitor respiratory status closely. Observe IV site for signs of phlebitis or extravasation.

ADVERSE EFFECTS/PRECAUTIONS: Respiratory depression. Rhythmic myoclonic jerking has occurred in premature neonates receiving lorazepam for sedation.

PHARMACOLOGY: Dose-dependent CNS depression. Onset of action within 5 minutes; peak serum concentration within 45 minutes. Duration of action is 3 to 24 hours. Mean half-life in term neonates is 40 hours. Metabolized to an inactive glucuronide, which is excreted by the kidneys. Highly lipid-soluble. Phenobarbital serum concentrations may increase after lorazepam administration.

SPECIAL CONSIDERATIONS/PREPARATION: Limited data are available for neonates. Available in 2-mg/mL and 4-mg/mL concentrations (1 mL preservative free vial) and 2 mg/mL multidose vial (10 mL). Some available products contain 2% (20 mg/mL) benzyl alcohol and 18% polyethylene glycol 400 in propylene glycol. A dilution of 0.4 mg/mL may be prepared by adding 1 mL of 4 mg/mL concentration in 9 mL of preservative-free sterile water for injection. This will make it easier to measure the dose and decrease the benzyl alcohol content to 0.5 mg/kg per dose. Solutions should not be used if they are discolored or contain a precipitate.

Solution Compatibility: D_5W, NS, and sterile water for injection.

Terminal Injection Site Compatibility: Dex/AA solutions. Acyclovir, amikacin, amiodarone, bumetanide, cefepime, cefotaxime, cimetidine, dexamethasone, dobutamine, dopamine, epinephrine, erythromycin lactobionate, famotidine, fentanyl, fluconazole, fosphenytoin, furosemide, gentamicin, heparin, hydrocortisone succinate, labetalol, levetiracetam, linezolid, metronidazole, midazolam, milrinone, morphine, nicardipine, nitroglycerin, pancuronium bromide, piperacillin, piperacillin-tazobactam, potassium chloride, propofol, ranitidine, remifentanil, trimethoprim-sulfamethoxazole, vancomycin, vecuronium, and zidovudine.

Incompatibility: Fat emulsion. Aztreonam, caffeine citrate, imipenem/cilastatin, and omeprazole.

SELECTED REFERENCES

- Sexson WR, Thigpen J, Stajich GV: Stereotypic movements after lorazepam administration in premature neonates: a series and review of the literature. *J Perinatol* 1995;15:146-49.
- McDermott CA, Kowalczyk AL, Schnitzler ER, et al: Pharmacokinetics of lorazepam in critically ill neonates with seizures. *J Pediatr* 1992;120:479.
- Deshmukh A, Wittert W, Schnitzler E, Mangurten HH: Lorazepam in the treatment of refractory neonatal seizures. *Am J Dis Child* 1986;140:1042.
- Product Information, Bedford, 2004

MEROPENEM

DOSE & ADMINISTRATION: Sepsis: 20 mg/kg per dose Q12 hours IV infusion over 30 minutes. **Meningitis and infections caused by Pseudomonas species:** 40 mg/kg per dose Q8 hours IV infusion over 30 minutes.

USES: Limited to treatment of pneumococcal meningitis and other serious infections caused by susceptible gram-negative organisms resistant to other antibiotics, especially extended-spectrum beta-lactamase producing *Klebsiella pneumoniae*.

MONITORING: Periodic CBC (for thrombocytosis and eosinophilia) and hepatic transaminases. Assess IV site for signs of inflammation.

ADVERSE EFFECTS/PRECAUTIONS: Diarrhea (4%), nausea/vomiting (1%) and rash (2%). May cause inflammation at the injection site. The use of carbapenem antibiotics can result in the development of cephalosporin resistance in *Enterobacter, Pseudomonas, Serratia, Proteus, Citrobacter,* and *Acinetobacter* species. The risks of pseudomembranous colitis and fungal infections are also increased.

PHARMACOLOGY: Meropenem is a broad-spectrum carbapenem antibiotic that penetrates well into the CSF and most body tissues. It is relatively stable to inactivation by human renal dehydropeptidase. Plasma protein binding is minimal. Clearance is directly related to renal function, and 70% of a dose is recovered intact in the urine. Hepatic function does not affect pharmacokinetics. Serum half-life of meropenem is 3 hours in preterm and 2 hours in full term neonates.

SPECIAL CONSIDERATIONS/PREPARATION: Available (USA) as powder for injection in 500-mg, and 1000-mg vials. Reconstitute with 10 mL of compatible diluent (500 mg vial) or 20 mL (1000 mg vial). When reconstituted with sterile water for injection, stable for up to 2 hours at room temperature or up to 12 hours when refrigerated. When reconstituted with NS to a final concentration between 2.5-50 mg/mL, the solution is stable for up to 2 hours at room temperature or 18 hours when refrigerated. When reconstituted with D_5W to final concentration between 2.5-50 mg/mL, the solution is stable for up to 1 hour at room temperature or 8 hours when refrigerated. Solutions prepared in sterile water for injection or NS at concentrations of 1-20 mg/mL are stable in plastic syringes for up to 48 hours when refrigerated. Solutions prepared in D_5W at concentrations of 1-20 mg/mL are stable in plastic syringes for up to 6 hours when refrigerated. Solutions prepared for infusion in NS at concentrations of 1-20 mg/mL are stable in plastic IV bags for 4 hours at room temperature or 24 hours when refrigerated. Solutions prepared for infusion in D_5W at concentrations of 1-20 mg/mL are stable in plastic IV bags for 1 hour at room temperature or 4 hours when refrigerated.

Solution Compatibility: D_5W, $D_{10}W$, and NS.

Terminal Injection Site Compatibility: Dex/AA and fat emulsion. Acyclovir, aminophylline, atropine, calcium gluconate, cimetidine, dexamethasone, digoxin, dobutamine, dopamine, enalaprilat, fluconazole, furosemide, gentamicin, heparin, insulin, linezolid, metoclopramide, milrinone, morphine, norepinephrine, phenobarbital, ranitidine, sodium bicarbonate, vancomycin, and zidovudine.

Incompatibility: Amphotericin B and metronidazole.

SELECTED REFERENCES

- Garges HP, Alexander KA: Newer antibiotics: imipenem/cilastatin and meropenem. *NeoReviews* 2003;4:e364-68.
- Bradley JS: Meropenem: a new, extremely broad spectrum β-lactam antibiotic for serious infections in pediatrics. *Pediatr Infect Dis J* 1997;16:263-68.
- Blumer JL: Pharmacokinetic determinants of carbapenem therapy in neonates and children. *Pediatr Infect Dis J* 1996;15:733-37.
- Patel PR: Compatibility of meropenem with commonly used injectable drugs. *Am J Health-Syst Pharm* 1996;53:2853-55.
- Blumer JL, Reed MD, Kearns GL, et al: Sequential, single-dose pharmacokinetic evaluation of meropenem in hospitalized infants and children. *Antimicrob Agents Chemother* 1995;39:1721-25.
- Hurst M, Lamb HM: Meropenem: a review of its use in patients in intensive care. *Drugs* 2000;59:653-680.
- Product Information, Astra-Zeneca, 2007

METHADONE

DOSE & ADMINISTRATION: Initial dose: 0.05 to 0.2 mg/kg per dose Q12 to 24 hours PO. Reduce dose by 10 to 20% per week over 4 to 6 weeks. Adjust weaning schedule based on signs and symptoms of withdrawal.

USES: Treatment of opiate withdrawal.

MONITORING: Monitor respiratory and cardiac status closely. Assess for gastric residuals, abdominal distention, and loss of bowel sounds.

ADVERSE EFFECTS/PRECAUTIONS: Respiratory depression in excessive doses. Ileus and delayed gastric emptying.

PHARMACOLOGY: Long-acting narcotic analgesic. Oral bioavailability is 50%, with peak plasma levels obtained in 2 to 4 hours. Metabolized extensively via hepatic N-demethylation. Highly protein bound (90% adults). Serum half-life ranges from 16 to 25 hours in neonates and is prolonged in patients with renal failure. Rifampin and phenytoin accelerate the metabolism of methadone and can precipitate withdrawal symptoms.

SPECIAL CONSIDERATIONS/PREPARATION: Available as oral solutions in 1- and 2-mg/mL concentrations containing 8% alcohol, and a 10-mg/mL alcohol-free solution. May dilute 1 mL of the 10-mg/mL concentrated solution with 19 mL of sterile water to provide an oral dilution with a final concentration of 0.5 mg/mL. Stable for 24 hours refrigerated. Also available as 5- and 10-mg tablets.

SELECTED REFERENCES

- Guo J, Greenberg M, Finer NN, Heldt GP: Methadone is a superior detoxification agent compared to tincture opium for treatment of neonatal narcotic abstinence syndrome (NAS). Abstract 4850.230, 2006 Pediatric Academic Societies Annual Meeting.
- Tobias JD, Schleien CL, Haun SE: Methadone as treatment for iatrogenic narcotic dependency in pediatric intensive care unit patients. *Crit Care Med* 1990;18:1292.
- Koren G, Maurice L: Pediatric uses of opioids. *Ped Clin North Am* 1989;36:1141.
- Rosen TS, Pippenger CE: Pharmacologic observations on the neonatal withdrawal syndrome. *J Pediatr* 1976;88:1044.
- Product Information, Roxane, 2007

METOCLOPRAMIDE

DOSE & ADMINISTRATION: 0.033 to 0.1 mg/kg per dose PO or IV slow push Q8 hours.

USES: To facilitate gastric emptying and GI motility. May improve feeding intolerance. Use in GE reflux patients is controversial. (Also used to enhance lactation—10 mg Q8 hours.)

MONITORING: Measure gastric residuals. Observe for increased irritability or vomiting.

ADVERSE EFFECTS/PRECAUTIONS: Intended for short-term use (several weeks). Dystonic reactions and extrapyramidal symptoms are seen frequently at higher doses and with prolonged use; children are more susceptible than adults.

PHARMACOLOGY: Derivative of procainamide. Exact mode of action is unknown; however, metoclopramide has both dopamine-receptor blocking activity and peripheral cholinergic effects. Well absorbed from GI tract. Variable first-pass metabolism by liver. Significant fraction excreted unchanged in urine. Lipid-soluble, large volume of distribution. Serum half-life in adults is 4 hours; prolonged in patients with renal failure.

SPECIAL CONSIDERATIONS/PREPARATION: Available as a 5-mg/mL injectable solution (osmolarity 280 mOsm/kg). **Protect from light.** A 0.1 mg/mL dilution may be made by adding 0.4 mL of the 5-mg/mL concentration to 19.6 mL of preservative-free NS. Dilution is stable for 24 hours at room temperature. Oral preparation available in 1-mg/mL concentration. A 0.1 mg/mL oral dilution may be made by adding 1 mL of the 1 mg/mL concentration to 9 mL simple syrup. Stable for 4 weeks at room temperature.

Solution Compatibility: D_5W, and NS.

Terminal Injection Site Compatibility: Dex/AA solutions, fat emulsion. Acyclovir, aminophylline, atropine, aztreonam, caffeine citrate, cimetidine, ciprofloxacin, clindamycin, dexamethasone, famotidine, fentanyl, fluconazole, heparin, hydrocortisone, insulin, lidocaine, linezolid, meropenem, midazolam, morphine, multivitamins, piperacillin-tazobactam, potassium chloride, potassium phosphate, prostaglandin E_1, quinupristin-dalfopristin, ranitidine, remifentanil, and zidovudine.

Incompatibility: Ampicillin, calcium chloride, calcium gluconate, cefepime, chloramphenicol, erythromycin lactobionate, furosemide, penicillin G, propofol, and sodium bicarbonate.

SELECTED REFERENCES

- Meadow WL, Bui K, Strates E, et al: Metoclopramide promotes enteral feeding in preterm infants with feeding intolerance. *Dev Pharmacol Ther* 1989;13:38.
- Machida HM, Forbes DA, Gall DG, et al: Metoclopramide in gastroesophageal reflux of infancy. *J Pediatr* 1988;112:483.
- Ehrenkranz RA, Ackerman BA: Metoclopramide effect on faltering milk production by mothers of premature infants. *Pediatrics* 1986;78:614.
- Sankaran K, Yeboah E, Bingham WT, Ninan A: Use of metoclopramide in premature infants. *Dev Pharmacol Ther* 1982;5:114.
- Product Information, Baxter, 2004

METRONIDAZOLE

DOSE & ADMINISTRATION: Loading dose: 15 mg/kg PO or IV infusion by syringe pump over 60 minutes. **Maintenance dose:** 7.5 mg/kg per dose PO or IV infusion over 60 minutes. Begin one dosing interval after initial dose. To use dosing chart, please refer to explanatory note in "How to Use This Book."

DOSING INTERVAL CHART

PMA (weeks)	Postnatal (days)	Interval (hours)
≤29	0 to 28	48
	>28	24
30 to 36	0 to 14	24
	>14	12
37 to 44	0 to 7	24
	>7	12
≥45	ALL	8

USES: Reserved for treatment of meningitis, ventriculitis, and endocarditis caused by *Bacteroides fragilis* and other anaerobes resistant to penicillin; treatment of serious intra-abdominal infections; and treatment of infections caused by *Trichomonas vaginalis*. Treatment of *C. difficile* colitis.

MONITORING: Measure CSF drug concentrations when treating CNS infections. Trough drug concentration should be greater than minimum inhibitory concentration for organism.

ADVERSE EFFECTS/PRECAUTIONS: Metronidazole has been shown to be carcinogenic in mice and rats, and therefore has not been approved for pediatric use. Seizures and sensory polyneuropathy have been reported in a few adult patients receiving high doses over a prolonged period. Drug metabolites may cause brownish discoloration of the urine.

PHARMACOLOGY: Metronidazole is bactericidal for many anaerobic organisms. It is well absorbed after oral administration, with peak serum concentrations attained in 1 to 3 hours. Distribution in all tissues throughout the body is excellent. It is less than 20% protein bound. Hydroxylation in the liver occurs in term infants and premature infants exposed to antenatal betamethasone. Unchanged drug and the active metabolite are excreted renally. Elimination half-life is strongly related to gestational age, ranging from 22 to 109 hours.

SPECIAL CONSIDERATIONS/PREPARATION: Available in 5 mg/mL concentration in 100 mL single-dose plastic ready-to-use solution containers. Store at controlled room temperature. **Do not refrigerate** (crystals form, but redissolve on warming to room temperature). Osmolarity is 310 mOsm/L, pH is 5 to 7. Each container contains 14 mEq of sodium. Supplied as 250 mg and 500 mg for oral administration. Suspension may be prepared by crushing five 250-mg tablets (1250 mg), dissolving powder in 10 mL purified water, then adding cherry syrup to make a total volume of 83 mL. Final concentration is 15 mg/mL. **Protect from light.** Shake well. Suspension is stable for 30 days refrigerated.

Solution Compatibility: D_5W, and NS.

Solution Incompatibility: Manufacturer recommends that if metronidazole is used with a primary IV fluid system, the primary solution should be discontinued during metronidazole infusion.

Terminal Injection Site Compatibility: Dex/AA solutions, fat emulsion. Acyclovir, amikacin, aminophylline, amiodarone, ampicillin, cefazolin, cefepime, cefotaxime, cefoxitin, ceftazidime, ceftriaxone, chloramphenicol, clindamycin, dopamine, enalaprilat, esmolol, fluconazole, gentamicin, heparin, hydrocortisone succinate, linezolid, lorazepam, magnesium sulfate, midazolam, milrinone, morphine, netilmicin, nicardipine, penicillin G, piperacillin-tazobactam, prostaglandin E_1, remifentanil, and tobramycin.

Incompatibility: Aztreonam, and meropenem.

SELECTED REFERENCES

- Wenisch C, Parschalk B, Hasenhundl M, et al: Comparison of vancomycin, teicoplanin, metronidazole, and fusidic acid for the treatment of *Clostridium difficile* - associated diarrhea. *Clin Infect Dis* 1996;22:813.
- Allen LV, Errickson MA: Stability of ketoconazole, metolazone, metronidazole, procainamide hydrochloride, spironolactone in extemporaneously compounded oral liquids. *Am J Health Syst Pharm* 1996;53:2073-2078.
- Feder HM Jr: *Bacteroides fragilis* meningitis. *Rev Infect Dis* 1987;9:783.
- Roberts RJ: *Drug Therapy in Infants.* Philadelphia: WB Saunders Co, 1984, p 76.
- Hall P, Kaye CM, McIntosh N, Steele J: Intravenous metronidazole in the newborn. *Arch Dis Child* 1983;58:529.
- Oldenburg B, Speck WT: Metronidazole. *Pediatr Clin North Am* 1983;30:71.
- Jager-Roman E, Doyle PE, Baird-Lambert J, et al: Pharmacokinetics and tissue distribution of metronidazole in the newborn infant. *J Pediatr* 1982;100:651.
- Product Information, BBraun, 2004

MIDAZOLAM

DOSE & ADMINISTRATION: IV: 0.05 to 0.15 mg/kg **over at least 5 minutes.** Repeat as required, usually Q2 to 4 hours. May also be given IM. Dosage requirements are decreased by concurrent use of narcotics. **Continuous IV infusion:** 0.01 to 0.06 mg/kg per hour (10 to 60 mcg/kg/hour). Dosage may need to be increased after several days of therapy because of development of tolerance and/or increased clearance. **Intranasal:** 0.2 to 0.3 mg/kg per dose using 5-mg/mL injectable form. **Sublingual:** 0.2 mg/kg per dose using 5-mg/mL injectable form mixed with a small amount of flavored syrup. **Oral:** 0.25 mg/kg per dose using Versed® oral syrup.

USES: Sedative/hypnotic. Anesthesia induction. Treatment of refractory seizures.

MIDAZOLAM

MONITORING: Follow respiratory status and blood pressure closely, especially when used concurrently with narcotics. Assess hepatic function. Observe for signs of withdrawal after discontinuation of prolonged therapy.

ADVERSE EFFECTS/PRECAUTIONS: Respiratory depression and hypotension are common when used in conjunction with narcotics, or following rapid bolus administration. Seizure-like myoclonus has been reported in 8% of premature infants receiving continuous infusions - this also may occur following rapid bolus administration and in patients with underlying CNS disorders. Nasal administration may be uncomfortable because of a burning sensation.

PHARMACOLOGY: Relatively short-acting benzodiazepine with rapid onset of action. Sedative and anticonvulsant properties related to GABA accumulation and occupation of benzodiazepine receptor. Antianxiety properties related to increasing the glycine inhibitory neurotransmitter. Metabolized by hepatic CYP 3A4 to a less active hydroxylated metabolite, then glucuronidated before excretion in urine. Drug accumulation may occur with repeated doses, prolonged infusion therapy, or concurrent administration of cimetidine, erythromycin or fluconazole. Highly protein bound. Duration of action is 2 to 6 hours. Elimination half-life is approximately 4 to 6 hours in term neonates, and quite variable, up to 22 hours, in premature babies and those with impaired hepatic function. Bioavailability is approximately 36% with oral administration and 50% with sublingual and intranasal administration. Midazolam is water soluble in acidic solutions and becomes lipid soluble at physiologic pH.

SPECIAL CONSIDERATIONS/PREPARATION: A preservative-free preparation is available as 1- and 5-mg/mL concentrations in 1-, 2-, and 5-mL vials. Versed® is available in an injectable form as 1- and 5-mg/mL concentrations in 1-, 2-, 5-, and 10-mL vials. Contains 1% (10mg/mL) benzyl alcohol as a preservative. To decrease benzyl alcohol content, a 0.5 mg/mL dilution may be made by adding 1 mL of the 5-mg/mL concentration to 9 mL preservative-free sterile water for injection. Dilution stable for 24 hours refrigerated. Versed® oral syrup is available in a 2 mg/mL concentration. Store at room temperature.

Solution Compatibility: D_5W, NS, and sterile water for injection.

Terminal Injection Site Compatibility: Dex/AA solutions. Amikacin, aminophylline, amiodarone, atropine, calcium gluconate, cefazolin, cefotaxime, cimetidine, clindamycin, digoxin, dobutamine, dopamine, epinephrine, erythromycin lactobionate, esmolol, famotidine, fentanyl, fluconazole, gentamicin, glycopyrrolate, heparin, imipenem/cilastatin, insulin, linezolid, lorazepam, methadone, metoclopramide, metronidazole, milrinone, mivacurium, morphine, nicardipine, nitroglycerin, nitroprusside, pancuronium bromide, piperacillin, potassium chloride, propofol, prostaglandin E $_1$, ranitidine, remifentanil, sodium nitroprusside, theophylline, tobramycin, vancomycin, and vecuronium.

Incompatibility: Fat emulsion. Albumin, ampicillin, bumetanide, ceftazidime, dexamethasone, fosphenytoin, furosemide, hydrocortisone succinate, nafcillin, omeprazole, pentobarbital, phenobarbital, and sodium bicarbonate.

SELECTED REFERENCES

- de Wildt SN, Kearns GL, Hop WCJ, et al: Pharmacokinetics and metabolism of intravenous midazolam in preterm infants. *Clin Pharmacol Ther* 2001;70:525-531.
- Coté CJ, Cohen IT, Suresh S, et al: A comparison of three doses of a commercially prepared oral midazolam syrup in children. *Anesth Analg* 2002;94:37-43.
- Sheth RD, Buckley DJ, Gutierrez AR: Midazolam in the treatment of refractory neonatal seizures. *Clin Neuropharmacol* 1996;2:165-70.
- Olkkola KT, Ahonen J, Neuvonen PJ: The effect of the systemic antimycotics, itraconazole and fluconazole, on the pharmacokinetics and pharmacodynamics of intravenous and oral midazolam. *Anesth Analg* 1996;82:511.
- Jacqz-Aigrain E, Daoud P, Burtin P, et al: Placebo-controlled trial of midazolam sedation in mechanically ventilated newborn babies. *Lancet* 1994;344:646-50.
- Magnyn JF, d'Allest AM, Nedelcoux H, et al: Midazolam and myoclonus in neonate. *Eur J Pediatr* 1994;153:389.
- Karl HW, Rosenberger JL, Larach MG, Ruffie JM: Transmucosal administration of midazolam for premedication of pediatric patients: Comparison of the nasal and sublingual routes. *Anesthesiology* 1993;78:885.
- Jacqz-Aigrain E, Daoud P, Burtin P, et al: Pharmacokinetics of midazolam during continuous infusion in critically ill neonates. *Eur J Clin Pharmacol* 1992;42:329.
- van Straaten HLM, Rademaker CMA, de Vries LS: Comparison of the effect of midazolam or vecuronium on blood pressure and cerebral blood flow velocity in the premature newborn. *Dev Pharmacol Ther* 1992;19:191.
- Product Information, Hospira, 2004

MILRINONE

DOSE & ADMINISTRATION: Loading dose: 75 mcg/kg IV infused over 60 minutes, immediately followed by **Maintenance infusion:** 0.5 to 0.75 mcg/kg per minute. Note: Above doses are from studies of older infants and children. Adjust infusion rate based upon hemodynamic and clinical response. **Premature infants < 30 weeks GA: Loading dose:** 0.75 mcg/kg per minute for 3 hours, immediately followed by **Maintenance infusion:** 0.2 mcg/kg per minute. (Preliminary data from pilot study referenced below)

USES: Short term (<72 hours) treatment of acute low cardiac output after cardiac surgery or due to septic shock.

MONITORING: Continuous monitoring of blood pressure, heart rate and rhythm. Assess signs of cardiac output. Carefully monitor fluid and electrolyte changes and renal function during therapy. Monitor platelet counts.

ADVERSE EFFECTS/PRECAUTIONS: Assure adequate vascular volume prior to initiating therapy. Blood pressure will likely fall 5 to 9% after the loading dose, but should gradually return to baseline by 24 hours. Heart rate increases of 5 to 10% are also common. Thrombocytopenia was reported frequently in some studies and rarely in others. Arrhythmias occur occasionally.

PHARMACOLOGY: Milrinone improves cardiac output by enhancing myocardial contractility, enhancing myocardial diastolic relaxation and decreasing vascular resistance. It acts via selective phosphodiesterase III inhibition that leads to increased intracellular cyclic AMP, increased myocardial intracellular calcium, and increased reuptake of calcium after systole. Vasodilatation is related to increased levels of cyclic GMP in vascular smooth muscle. Unlike catecholamines, myocardial oxygen consumption is not increased. Elimination is primarily via renal mechanisms. Half-life is quite variable, ranging from approximately 10 hours in ELBW neonates to approximately 3 hours in older and more mature infants.

SPECIAL CONSIDERATIONS/PREPARATION: Available in 1 mg/mL solution for injection in 10-, 20-, and 50-mL single-dose vials. Dilute with compatible diluent prior to administration. Maximum concentration for infusion is 200 mcg/mL. Also available as premixed solution for injection, 200 mcg/mL in 5% Dextrose. pH of 3.2 to 4.

Solution Compatibility: D_5W, NS, and LR.

Terminal Injection Site Compatibility: Dex/AA. Acyclovir, amikacin, aminophylline, amiodarone, ampicillin, atracurium, atropine, bumetanide, calcium chloride, calcium gluconate, cefazolin, cefepime, cefotaxime, ceftazidime, cimetidine, clindamycin, dexamethasone, digoxin, dobutamine, dopamine, epinephrine, fentanyl, gentamicin, heparin, insulin, isoproterenol, lorazepam, meropenem, methylprednisolone, metronidazole, midazolam, morphine, nicardipine, nitroglycerin, norepinephrine, oxacillin, pancuronium, piperacillin, piperacillin-tazobactam, potassium chloride, propofol, propranolol, ranitidine, sodium bicarbonate, sodium nitroprusside, theophylline, ticarcillin, ticarcillin-clavulanate, tobramycin, vancomycin, and vecuronium.

Incompatibility: Furosemide, imipenem-cilastatin and procainamide.

SELECTED REFERENCES

• Paradisis M, Jiang X, McLachlan AJ, et al: Population pharmacokinetics and dosing regimen of milrinone in preterm infants. *Arch Dis Child Fetal Neonatal Ed* 2007;92:F204-209.
• Hoffman TM, Wernovsky G, Atz AM, et al: Efficacy and safety of milrinone in preventing low cardiac output syndrome in infants and children after corrective surgery for congenital heart disease. *Circulation* 2003;107:996-1002.
• Lindsay CA, Barton P, Lawless S, et al: Pharmacokinetics and pharmacodynamics of milrinone in pediatric patients with septic shock. *J Pediatr* 1998;132:329-34.
• Chang AC, Atz AM, Wernovsky G, et al: Milrinone: Systemic and pulmonary hemodynamic effects in neonates after cardiac surgery. *Crit Care Med* 1995;23:1907-14.
• Veltri MA, Conner KG: Physical compatibility of milrinone lactate injection with intravenous drugs commonly used in the pediatric intensive care unit. *Am J Health-Syst Pharm* 2002;59: 452-54.
• Akkerman SR, Zhang H, Mullins RE, Vaughn K: Stability of milrinone lactate in the presence of 29 critical care drugs and 4 i.v. solutions. *Am J Health-Syst Pharm* 1999;56:63-68.
• Paradisis M, Evans N, Kluckow M, et al: Pilot study of milrinone for prevention of low systemic blood flow in very preterm infants. *J Pediatr* 2006;148:306-313.
• Product Information, Sanofi, 2007

MIVACURIUM

DOSE & ADMINISTRATION: 0.2 mg/kg IV push over 30 seconds.

USES: Skeletal muscle relaxation/paralysis in infants requiring endotracheal intubation.

MONITORING: Assess vital signs frequently, and blood pressure continuously if possible.

ADVERSE EFFECTS/PRECAUTIONS: Hypotension may occur, most likely caused by mast cell activation and histamine release. There are also occasional reports of broncho-spasm in children with asthma. Inherited plasma cholinesterase deficiency may cause prolonged neuromuscular blockade. The mild form, affecting 1 in 25, results in ≈50% prolongation which is unlikely to be clinically significant. The severe form, affecting 1 in 2500, results in prolongation of paralysis for several hours.

PHARMACOLOGY: Mivacurium is a short-acting, nondepolarizing skeletal muscle relax-ant for IV administration. Competitive binding to cholinergic receptors occurs on the motor end-plate to antagonize the action of acetylcholine, resulting in a block of neu-romuscular transmission. Onset of action is usually 80 to 120 seconds. Duration of action is usually 15 to 20 minutes. Data in neonates are limited. Skeletal relaxation/paralysis may be reversed by acetylcholinesterase inhibitors such as neostigmine. The drug is a mixture of isomers that are extensively metabolized by plasma cholinesterase. This pro-cess appears to be fully active in most neonates. Renal and biliary excretion of unchanged mivacurium are minor elimination pathways; urine and bile are important elimination pathways for the two relatively inactive metabolites. Sensation remains intact. Analgesia should be used for painful procedures.

SPECIAL CONSIDERATIONS/PREPARATION: Available in 5-and 10-mL single-use vials (2 mg/mL) in Water for Injection and 20 mL and 50 mL multidose vials. pH 3.5 to 5. Diluted solutions should be used within 24 hrs of preparation. Multidose vials contain 0.9% w/v benzyl alcohol. Protect from light.

> **Solution Compatibility:** D₅W, NS, LR, and D₅NS.
>
> **Solution Incompatibility:** No data.
>
> **Terminal Injection Site Compatibility:** Fentanyl and midazolam.
>
> **Incompatibility:** Alkaline solutions having a pH greater than 8.5, barbiturates, pheny-toin, and sodium bicarbonate.

SELECTED REFERENCES

- McCluskey A, Meakin G: Dose-response and minimum time to satisfactory intubation conditions after mivacurium in children. *Anaesthesia* 1996;51:438-41.
- Cook DR, Gronert BJ, Woelfel SK: Comparison of the neuromuscular effects of mivacurium and suxa-methonium in infants and children. *Acta Anaesthesiol Scand* 1995;39:Suppl 106:35-40.
- Meretoja OA, Taivainen T, Wirtavuori K: Pharmacodynamics of mivacurium in infants. *Br J Anaesth* 1994;73:490-93.
- Product Information, Abbott, 2005

MORPHINE

DOSE & ADMINISTRATION: 0.05 to 0.2 mg/kg per dose IV over at least 5 minutes, IM, or SC. Repeat as required (usually Q4 hours). **Continuous infusion:** Give a loading dose of 100 to 150 mcg/kg over 1 hour followed by 10 to 20 mcg/kg per hour. **Treatment of opioid dependence:** Begin at most recent IV morphine dose equivalent. Taper 10 to 20% per day as tolerated. Oral dose is approximately 3 to 5 times IV dose. **Initial treat-ment of neonatal narcotic abstinence:** 0.03 to 0.1 mg/kg per dose PO Q3 to 4 hours. Wean dose by 10 to 20% every 2 to 3 days based on abstinence scoring. (The Finnegan score should be < 9). Use a 0.4-mg/mL dilution made from a concentrated oral morphine sulfate solution.

USES: Analgesia. Sedation. Treatment of opioid withdrawal and abstinence.

MONITORING: Monitor respiratory and cardiovascular status closely. Observe for abdominal distention and loss of bowel sounds. Consider urine retention if output is decreased.

ADVERSE EFFECTS/PRECAUTIONS: Naloxone should be readily available to reverse adverse effects. Marked respiratory depression (decreases the responsiveness of the respiratory center to CO_2 tension). Hypotension and bradycardia. Transient hypertonia.

Ileus and delayed gastric emptying. Urine retention. Tolerance may develop after prolonged use—wean slowly. Seizures reported in two infants who received bolus plus infusion.

PHARMACOLOGY: Narcotic analgesic—stimulates brain opioid receptors. Increases venous capacitance, caused by release of histamine and central suppression of adrenergic tone. GI secretions and motility decreased. Increases smooth muscle tone. Morphine is converted in the liver to two glucuronide metabolites (morphine-6-glucuronide and morphine-3-glucuronide) that are renally excreted. Morphine-6-glucuronide (M6G) is a potent respiratory-depressant and analgesic. Morphine-3-glucuronide (M3G) is an antagonist to the effects of morphine and morphine-6-glucuronide. Morphine is 20 to 40% bioavailable when administered orally. Pharmacokinetics are widely variable. Elimination half-life is approximately 9 hours for morphine and 18 hours for morphine-6-glucuronide. Steady state concentrations of morphine are reached by 24 to 48 hours.

SPECIAL CONSIDERATIONS/PREPARATION: Injectable solutions are available in dosage strengths ranging from 0.5- to 50-mg/mL. Oral morphine sulfate solutions are available in concentrations of 2, 4, and alcohol-free 20 mg/mL. A 0.4-mg/mL oral morphine dilution may be made by adding 1 mL of the 4-mg/mL injectable solution to 9 mL preservative-free normal saline. Stable for 7 days refrigerated. **Protect from light.**

Solution Compatibility: D_5W, $D_{10}W$, and NS. For continuous infusions of morphine **containing heparin:** Use only NS; maximum morphine concentration 5 mg/mL.

Terminal Injection Site Compatibility: Dex/AA solutions, fat emulsion. Acyclovir, alteplase, amikacin, aminophylline, amiodarone, ampicillin, atropine, aztreonam, bumetanide, caffeine citrate, calcium chloride, cefotaxime, cefoxitin, ceftazidime, ceftriaxone, chloramphenicol, cefazolin, cimetidine, clindamycin, dexamethasone, digoxin, dobutamine, dopamine, enalaprilat, epinephrine, erythromycin lactobionate, esmolol, famotidine, fentanyl, fluconazole, furosemide, gentamicin, glycopyrrolate, heparin, hydrocortisone succinate, insulin, lidocaine, linezolid, lorazepam, meropenem, metoclopramide, metronidazole, mezlocillin, midazolam, milrinone, nafcillin, nicardipine, nitroglycerin, oxacillin, pancuronium bromide, penicillin G, phenobarbital, piperacillin, piperacillin-tazobactam, potassium chloride, propofol, propranolol, prostaglandin E_1, ranitidine, remifentanil, sodium bicarbonate, sodium nitroprusside, ticarcillin/clavulanate, tobramycin, trimethoprim-sulfamethoxazole, vancomycin, vecuronium, and zidovudine.

Incompatibility: Azithromycin, cefepime, pentobarbital, and phenytoin.

SELECTED REFERENCES

- Langenfeld S, Birkenfeld L, Herkenrath P, et al: Therapy of the neonatal abstinence syndrome with tincture of opium or morphine drops. *Drug Alcohol Depend* 2005;77:31-36.
- Oei J, Lui K: Management of the newborn infant affected by maternal opiates and other drugs of dependency. *J Paediatr Child Health* 2007;43:9-18.
- Saarenmaa E, Neuvonen PJ, Rosenberg P, Fellman V: Morphine clearance and effects in newborn infants in relation to gestational age. *Clin Pharmacol Ther* 2000;68:160-166.
- American Academy of Pediatrics Committee on Drugs: Neonatal drug withdrawal. *Pediatrics* 1998;101:1079-1088.
- Yaster M, Kost-Byerly S, Berde C, Billet C: The management of opioid and benzodiazepine dependence in infants, children, and adolescents. *Pediatrics* 1996;98:135-40.
- Barrett DA, Barker DP, Rutter N, et al: Morphine, morphine-6-glucuronide and morphine-3-glucuronide pharmacokinetics in newborn infants receiving diamorphine infusions. *Br J Clin Pharmacol* 1996;41:531.
- Hartley R, Green M, Quinn M, Levene MI: Pharmacokinetics of morphine infusion in premature neonates. *Arch Dis Child* 1993;69:55.
- Chay PCW, Duffy BJ, Walker JS: Pharmacokinetic-pharmacodynamic relationships of morphine in neonates. *Clin Pharmacol Ther* 1992;51:334.
- Koren G, Butt W, Chinyanga H, et al: Postoperative morphine infusion in newborn infants: Assessment of disposition characteristics and safety. *J Pediatr* 1985;107:963.
- Product Information, Mayne, 2004

MUPIROCIN

DOSE & ADMINISTRATION: Cutaneous infections: Apply small amounts topically to affected areas 3 times daily. **Decolonization:** Apply small amounts to anterior nares twice daily for 5 to 7 days.

NAFCILLIN

USES: Topical use for skin infections caused by *Staphylococcus aureus, S epidermidis, S saprophyticus,* and *Streptococcus pyogenes.* As part of multiple interventions for infection control during MRSA outbreaks in the NICU. Routine use for decolonization is not recommended.

MONITORING: Assess affected area for continued infection.

ADVERSE EFFECTS/PRECAUTIONS: Use only on the skin. No adverse effects reported from topical administration. Routine use may lead to selective bacterial resistance.

PHARMACOLOGY: Topical antibacterial produced by fermentation of the organism *Pseudomonas fluorescens.* Inhibits protein synthesis by bonding to bacterial isoleucyl-transfer-RNA synthetase. Highly protein bound. Not absorbed into the systemic circulation after topical administration (older infants and children). Metabolized in the skin to an inactive compound and excreted.

SPECIAL CONSIDERATIONS/PREPARATION: Available in unit-dose packets and 15 and 30-g tubes as a 2% ointment and cream (20 mg/g).

SELECTED REFERENCES

- American Academy of Pediatrics. Staphylococcal Infections. In: Pickering LK, Baker CJ, Long SS, McMillan JA, eds. *Red Book: 2006 Report of the Committee on Infectious Diseases.* 27th ed. Elk Grove Village, IL: American Academy of Pediatrics 2006: pp 608-610.
- Khoury J, Jones M, Grim A, et al: Eradication of methicillin-resistant *Staphylococcus aureus* from a neonatal intensive care unit by active surveillance and aggressive infection control measures. *Infect Control Hosp Epidemiol* 2005;26:616-621.
- Saiman L, Cronquist A, Wu F, et al: An outbreak of methicillin-resistant *Staphylococcus aureus* in a neonatal intensive care unit. *Infect Control Hosp Epidemiol* 2003;24:317-321.
- Zakrzewska-Bode A, Muytjens HL, Liem KD, Hoogkamp-Korstanje JAA: Mupirocin resistance in coagulase-negative staphylococci, after topical prophylaxis for the reduction of colonization of central venous catheters. *J Hosp Infect* 1995;31:189.
- Pappa KA: The clinical development of mupirocin. *J Am Acad Dermatol* 1990;22:873.
- Leyden JJ: Mupirocin: A new topical antibiotic. *Semin Dermatol* 1987;6:48.
- Davies EA, Emmerson AM, Hogg GM, et al: An outbreak of infection with a methicillin-resistant *Staphylococcus aureus* in a special care baby unit: Value of topical mupirocin and of traditional methods of infection control. *J Hosp Infect* 1987;10:120.
- Product Information, OrthoNeutrogena, 2006

NAFCILLIN

DOSE & ADMINISTRATION: Usual dosage: 25 mg/kg per dose IV over 15 minutes. **Meningitis:** 50 mg/kg per dose. To use dosing chart, please refer to explanatory note in "How to Use This Book."

DOSING INTERVAL CHART

PMA (weeks)	PostNatal (days)	Interval (hours)
≤29	0 to 28 >28	12 8
30 to 36	0 to 14 >14	12 8
37 to 44	0 to 7 >7	12 8
≥45	ALL	6

USES: Treatment of infections caused by penicillinase-producing staphylococci, particularly if evidence of renal dysfunction.

MONITORING: Periodic CBC. Observe IV site for signs of extravasation.

ADVERSE EFFECTS/PRECAUTIONS: Increase dosing interval in patients with hepatic dysfunction. Irritating to veins—watch for phlebitis. Cases of granulocytopenia have been reported.

PHARMACOLOGY: Inhibits synthesis of bacterial cell wall. Better penetration into CSF than methicillin. Excreted via hepatic clearance.

SPECIAL CONSIDERATIONS/PREPARATION: Available in 1 and 2-g vials. Reconstitute 1-g vial with 3.4 mL of sterile water for injection to provide a final volume of 4 mL and a concentration of 250 mg/mL. Also available in 1-g in 50-mL and 2-g in 100-mL frozen single-dose bags. Thaw bags at room temperature or under refrigeration. Do not force thaw by immersing into water baths or microwaving. pH of resulting solution 6 to 8.5. Thawed solution stable for 3 days at room temperture, 21 days refrigerator. Reconstituted solution stable for 3 days at room temperature, 7 days refrigerated. Osmolality was determined to be 709 mOsm/kg of water. For direct intravenous injection, dilute in 15 to 30 ml of NS.

Solution Compatibility: D_5W, $D_{10}W$, and NS.

Terminal Injection Site Compatibility: Dex/AA solutions, fat emulsion. Acyclovir, aminophylline, atropine, chloramphenicol, cimetidine, dexamethasone, enalaprilat, esmolol, famotidine, fentanyl, fluconazole, heparin, lidocaine, morphine, nicardipine, potassium chloride, propofol, sodium bicarbonate, zidovudine.

Incompatibility: Amikacin, aztreonam, gentamicin, hydrocortisone succinate, insulin, methylprednisolone, midazolam, netilmicin, tobramycin, and vancomycin.

SELECTED REFERENCES

• Prober CG, Stevenson DK, Benitz WE: The use of antibiotics in neonates weighing less than 1200 grams. *Pediatr Infect Dis J* 1990;9:111.
• Kitzing W, Nelson JD, Mohs E: Comparative toxicities of methicillin and nafcillin. *Am J Dis Child* 1981;135:52.
• Banner W, Gooch WM, Burckart G, Korones SB: Pharmacokinetics of nafcillin in infants with low birth weights. *Antimicrob Agents Chemother* 1980;17:691.
• Product Information, Sandoz, 2004

NALOXONE

DOSE & ADMINISTRATION: Suggested dose: 0.1 mg/kg IV push. Doses needed to reverse narcotic-induced depression may be as low as 0.01 mg/kg. May give IM if adequate perfusion. Tracheal administration is not recommended. There are no studies to support or refute the current dosing recommendations.

USES: Narcotic antagonist. Adjuvant therapy to customary resuscitation efforts for narcotic-induced respiratory (CNS) depression. Naloxone is not recommended as part of the initial resuscitation of newborns with respiratory depression in the delivery room. Before naloxone is given, providers should restore heart rate and color by supporting ventilation.

MONITORING: Assess respiratory effort and neurologic status.

ADVERSE EFFECTS/PRECAUTIONS: No short-term toxicity observed. One case report of seizures secondary to acute opioid withdrawal after administration to an infant born to an opioid abuser. Long-term safety has not been investigated.

PHARMACOLOGY: Reverses respiratory depression by competing for CNS narcotic receptor sites. Onset of action is variable, but usually within minutes after IV administration, and approximately 1 hour after IM administration. Half-life in neonates is approximately 70 minutes. Metabolized by the liver and excreted in the urine. Increases circulating catecholamines.

SPECIAL CONSIDERATIONS/PREPARATION: Do not mix in an alkaline solution. Available in 0.4 mg/mL and 1 mg/mL concentrations. **Store at room temperature and protect from light.**

Solution Compatibility: No data are currently available on Dex/AA.

Terminal Injection Site Compatibility: Heparin, linezolid, and propofol. No data are currently available on potassium chloride and other medications.

SELECTED REFERENCES

• The International Liaison Committee on Resuscitation: The International Liaison Committee on Resuscitation (ILCOR) Consensus on Science With Treatment Recommendations for Pediatric and Neonatal Patients: Neonatal Resuscitation. *Pediatrics* 2006(5). http://www.pediatrics.org/cgi/content/full/117/5/e978.
• Guinsburg R, Wyckoff MH. Naloxone during neonatal resuscitation: acknowledging the unknown. *Clin Perinatol* 2006;33:121132.
• Herschel M, Khoshnood B, Lass N. Role of naloxone in newborn resuscitation. *Pediatrics* 2000;106:831-834.
• McGuire W, Fowlie PW. Naloxone for narcotic exposed newborn infants: systematic review. *Arch Dis Child Fetal Neonatal Ed* 2003;88:F308F311.
• Product Information, Hospira, 2005

NEOSTIGMINE

DOSE & ADMINISTRATION: Myasthenia gravis: 0.1 mg IM (give 30 minutes before feeding). 1 mg PO (give 2 hours before feeding). Dose may have to be increased and should be titrated. **Reversal of neuromuscular blockade:** 0.04 to 0.08 mg/kg IV, in addition to atropine 0.02 mg/kg.

USES: Neonatal transient myasthenia gravis. Neonatal persistent (congenital) myasthenia gravis. Reversing effects of neuromuscular blocking drugs.

MONITORING: Monitor respiratory and cardiovascular status closely.

ADVERSE EFFECTS/PRECAUTIONS: Contraindicated in presence of intestinal or urinary obstruction, bradycardia, or hypotension. Use cautiously in patients with bronchospasm or cardiac arrhythmia. Adverse effects include muscle weakness, tremors, bradycardia, hypotension, respiratory depression, bronchospasm, diarrhea, and excessive salivation.

PHARMACOLOGY: Inhibits acetylcholinesterase at the neuromuscular junction, allowing accumulation of acetylcholine and thus restoring activity.

SPECIAL CONSIDERATIONS/PREPARATION: Available as injectable solution in 1-mL ampules and 10-mL vials in concentrations of 1:1000 (1 mg/mL) and 1:2000 (0.5 mg/mL). **Protect from light.**

    Solution Compatibility: No data.

    Terminal Injection Site Compatibility: Glycopyrrolate, heparin, hydrocortisone succinate, netilmicin, pentobarbital and potassium chloride.

SELECTED REFERENCES

- Fisher DM, Cronnelly R, Miller RD, Sharma M: The neuromuscular pharmacology of neostigmine in infants and children. *Anesthesiology* 1983;59:220.
- Goudsouzian NG, Crone RK, Todres ID: Recovery from pancuronium blockade in the neonatal intensive care unit. *Br J Anaesth* 1981;53:1303.
- Sarnat HB: Neuromuscular disorders in the neonatal period, in Korobken R, Guillemenault C (eds): *Advances in Perinatal Neurology.* New York: Spectrum Publications, 1979, p 153.
- Product Information, Abraxis, 2006

NETILMICIN

DOSE & ADMINISTRATION: IV infusion by syringe pump over 30 minutes. Administer as a separate infusion from penicillin-containing compounds. IM injection is associated with variable absorption, especially in the very small infant. To use dosing chart, please refer to explanatory note in "How to Use This Book."

DOSING CHART

PMA (weeks)	Postnatal (days)	Dose (mg/kg)	Interval (hours)
≤29*	0 to 7	5	48
	8 to 28	4	36
	≥29	4	24
30 to 34	0 to 7	4.5	36
	≥8	4	24
≥35	ALL	4	24
* or significant asphyxia, PDA, or treatment with indomethacin			

USES: Treatment of infections caused by aerobic gram-negative bacilli (e.g. *Pseudomonas, Klebsiella, E coli*). Usually used in combination with a β-lactam antibiotic.

MONITORING: Measure serum concentrations when treating for more than 48 hours. Obtain peak concentration 30 minutes after end of infusion, and trough concentration just prior to the next dose. When treating patients with serious infections or significantly changing fluid or renal status consider measuring the serum concentration 24 hours after a dose, and use the chart below for the suggested dosing interval. Blood samples obtained to monitor serum drug concentrations should be spun and refrigerated or frozen as soon as possible. Therapeutic serum concentrations: **Peak:** 5 to 12 mcg/mL (or C_{max}/MIC ratio greater than 8:1) **Trough:** 0.5 to 1 mcg/mL

SUGGESTED DOSING INTERVALS

Level at 24 hours (mcg/mL)	Half-life (hours)	Suggested Dosing Interval (hours)
≤1	≈8	24
1.1 to 2.3	≈12	36
2.4 to 3.2	≈15	48
≥3.3		Measure level in 24 hours

ADVERSE EFFECTS/PRECAUTIONS: Transient and reversible renal tubular dysfunction may occur, resulting in increased urinary losses of sodium, calcium, and magnesium. Vestibular and auditory ototoxicity. The addition of other nephrotoxic and/or ototoxic medications (e.g. furosemide, vancomycin) may increase these adverse effects. Increased neuromuscular blockade (i.e. neuromuscular weakness and respiratory failure) may occur when used with pancuronium or other neuromuscular blocking agents and in patients with hypermagnesemia.

PHARMACOLOGY: Dosing recommendations are based on: (1) Higher peak concentrations increase concentration-dependent bacterial killing; (2) There is a post-antibiotic effect on bacterial killing, especially when treating concurrently with a β-lactam antibiotic; (3) There may be more toxicity with less frequent dosing, due to less renal drug accumulation. Volume of distribution is increased and clearance is decreased in patients with PDA. Serum half-life is prolonged in premature and asphyxiated newborns. Inactivation of netilmicin by penicillin-containing compounds appears to be a time-, temperature-, and concentration-dependent process. This is probably clinically significant only when penicillin-containing compounds are mixed in IV solutions or when the blood is at room temperature for several hours before the assay is performed.

SPECIAL CONSIDERATIONS/PREPARATION: Available in a concentration of 100 mg/mL in 1.5 mL vials. A 10 mg/mL dilution may be made by adding 1 mL of this solution to 9 mL of sterile water for injection. Dilution is stable for 72 hours refrigerated. Do not freeze. **No longer available in the US.**

Solution Compatibility: D_5W, $D_{10}W$, and NS.

Terminal Injection Site Compatibility: Dex/AA solutions, fat emulsion. Aminophylline, atropine, aztreonam, calcium gluconate, cefuroxime, clindamycin, dexamethasone, heparin (concentrations ≤ 1 unit/mL), hydrocortisone succinate, iron dextran, isoproterenol, linezolid, metronidazole, neostigmine, norepinephrine, pancuronium bromide, potassium chloride, procainamide, remifentanil, sodium bicarbonate, and vitamin K_1.

Incompatibility: Amphotericin B, ampicillin, cefepime, furosemide, heparin (concentrations >1 unit/mL), methicillin, mezlocillin, nafcillin, oxacillin, penicillin G, propofol, and ticarcillin/clavulanate.

SELECTED REFERENCES

- Contopoulos-Ioannidis DG, Giotis ND, Baliatsa DV, Ioannidis JPA: Extended-interval aminoglycoside administration for children: a meta-analysis. *Pediatrics* 2004;114:e111-e118.
- Stolk LML, Degraeuwe PLJ, Nieman FHM, et al: Population pharmacokinetics and relationship between demographic and clinical variables and pharmacokinetics of gentamicin in neonates. *Ther Drug Monit* 2002;24:527-31.
- Avent ML, Kinney JS, Istre GR, Whitfield JM: Gentamicin and tobramycin in neonates: comparison of a new extended dosing regimen with a traditional multiple daily dosing regimen. *Am J Perinatol* 2002;8:413-19.
- Giapros VI, Andronikou S, Cholevas VI, Papadopoulou ZL: Renal function in premature infants during aminoglycoside therapy. *Pediatr Nephrol* 1995;9:163.
- Daly JS, Dodge RA, Glew RH, et al: Effect of time and temperature on inactivation of aminoglycosides by ampicillin at neonatal dosages. *J Perinatol* 1997;17:42-45.

NEVIRAPINE

DOSE & ADMINISTRATION: PO: 2 mg/kg single dose at 48 to 72 hours of age. If the mother did not receive intrapartum single-dose nevirapine, administer 2 mg/kg as soon as possible after birth.

NICARDIPINE

USES: Used **only** in combination with zidovudine in the treatment of neonates born to HIV-infected women who have had no therapy during pregnancy (mother receives zidovudine plus a single 200-mg oral dose of nevirapine during labor). Dosing guidelines above are for prophylactic treatment of neonates born to HIV-infected women. Treatment of infected infants with combination antiretroviral therapy should be done in consultation with a pediatric infectious disease expert.

MONITORING: Specific monitoring unnecessary due to short treatment course.

ADVERSE EFFECTS/PRECAUTIONS: Limited data on toxicity—none reported in neonates.

PHARMACOLOGY: Nevirapine is a non-nucleoside antiretroviral agent that inhibits HIV-1 replication by selectively interfering with viral reverse transcriptase without requiring intracellular metabolism. It also inactivates cell-free virions in the genital tract and breast milk. Synergistic antiviral activity occurs when administered with zidovudine. Nevirapine is rapidly absorbed after oral administration to pregnant women and is highly lipophilic, resulting in therapeutic concentrations being readily transferred across the placenta to the fetus. Serum half-life in the neonates is approximately 44 hours. With the maternal/newborn regimen described above, serum concentrations are above 100 mcg/L throughout the first week of life. Nevirapine is extensively metabolized by, and an inducer of, hepatic CYP3A4 and CYP2B6 isoenzymes. Concomitant administration of phenobarbital or phenytoin, CYP3A inducers, may affect plasma concentrations.

SPECIAL CONSIDERATIONS/PREPARATION: Available as an oral suspension in a concentration of 10 mg/mL. Store at room temperature. Shake suspension gently prior to administration.

SELECTED REFERENCES

- Perinatal HIV Guidelines Working Group. Public Health Service Task Force Recommendations for Use of Antiretroviral Drugs in Pregnant HIV-1 Infected Women for Maternal Health and Interventions to Reduce Perinatal HIV-1 Transmission in the United States. November 2, 2007. Available at http://aidsinfo.nih.gov/ContentFiles/PerinatalGL.pdf.
- Mirochnick M, Dorenbaum A, Blanchard S, et al: Predose infant nevirapine concentration with the two-dose intrapartum neonatal nevirapine regimen: association with timing of maternal intrapartum nevirapine dose. *JAIDS* 2003;33:153-56.
- Mirochnick M, Clarke DF, Dorenbaum A: Nevirapine: pharmacokinetic considerations in children and pregnant women. *Drugs* 2000;39:281-293.
- Product Information, Boehringer Ingelheim, 2007

NICARDIPINE

DOSE & ADMINISTRATION: Initial dose: 0.5 mcg/kg per minute continuous IV infusion. Titrate dose to response. Blood pressure will begin to decrease within minutes of starting the infusion, reaching half of its ultimate decrease in approximately 45 minutes. Blood pressure equilibrium will not be achieved for approximately 50 hours (adult data). Maintenance doses are usually 0.5 to 2 mcg/kg per minute.

USES: Treatment of acute severe hypertension.

MONITORING: Continuous monitoring of blood pressure, heart rate and rhythm during initiation of therapy, and frequently thereafter. Observe IV site for signs of irritation.

ADVERSE EFFECTS/PRECAUTIONS: No adverse effects have been reported in neonates (small numbers). Hypotension and tachycardia are dose-dependent in adults. Headache, nausea, and vomiting were the other common effects reported.

PHARMACOLOGY: Nicardipine is a dihydropyridine calcium channel blocker that significantly decreases systemic vascular resistance. Unlike other calcium channel blockers, it has limited effects on the myocardium. It is extensively metabolized by the liver, and is highly protein bound. Following infusion in adults, nicardipine plasma concentrations decline tri-exponentially, with a rapid early distribution phase (alpha half-life of 2.7 minutes), an intermediate phase (beta half-life of 44.8 minutes), and a slow terminal phase (gamma half-life of 14.4 hours) that can only be detected after long-term infusions. Experience in neonates is limited, and there are no reported pharmacokinetic data.

SPECIAL CONSIDERATIONS/PREPARATION: Available as 2.5 mg/mL solution for injection in 10-mL ampuls. **Dilute prior to administration to a concentration of 0.1 mg/mL.** Dilution is stable at room temperature for 24 hours. Store ampuls at controlled room temperature. Freezing does not adversely affect the product, but exposure to elevated temperatures should be avoided. Protect from light. Store ampuls in carton until used.

Solution Compatibility: D_5W, NS, and D_5NS.

Solution Incompatibility: Lactated Ringers.

Terminal Injection Site Compatibility: No data available for Dex/AA solutions or fat emulsions. Amikacin, aminophylline, aztreonam, calcium gluconate, cefazolin, ceftizoxime, chloramphenicol, cimetidine, clindamycin, dobutamine, dopamine, enalaprilat, epinephrine, erythromycin lactobionate, esmolol, famotidine, fentanyl, gentamicin, heparin (concentrations ≤ 1 unit/mL), hydrocortisone, lidocaine, linezolid, lorazepam, magnesium sulfate, metronidazole, midazolam, milrinone, morphine, nafcillin, nitroglycerin, norepinephrine, penicillin G potassium, piperacillin, potassium chloride, potassium phosphate, ranitidine, sodium acetate, sodium nitroprusside, tobramycin, trimethoprim-sulfamethoxazole, vancomycin, and vecuronium.

Incompatibility: Ampicillin, cefoperazone, ceftazidime, furosemide, heparin (concentrations > 1 unit/mL), sodium bicarbonate and thiopental.

SELECTED REFERENCES

• McBride BF, White CM, Campbell M, Frey BM: Nicardipine to control neonatal hypertension during extracorporeal membrane oxygen support. *Am Pharmacother* 2003;37:667-670.
• Tobias JD: Nicardipine to control mean arterial pressure after cardiothoracic surgery in infants and children. *Am J Ther* 2001;8:3-6.
• Milou C, Debuche-Benouachkou V, Semama DS et al: Intravenous nicardipine as a first-line antihypertensive drug in neonates. *Intensive Care Med* 2000;26:956-958.
• Gouyon JB, Geneste B, Semama DS, et al: Intravenous nicardipine in hypertensive preterm infants. *Arch Dis Child Fetal Neonatal Ed* 1997;76:F126-127.
• Product Information, ESP Pharma, 2005.

NITRIC OXIDE

DOSE & ADMINISTRATION: Nitric oxide inhalation therapy (iNO) should be used only after mechanical ventilatory support has been optimized, including the use of surfactant. **Begin at 20 ppm.** If within 4 hours PaO_2 increases to at least 60 torr, decrease to 5 ppm. Continue at 5 ppm and wean fiO_2 as tolerated. When fiO_2 is less than 0.6 and ventilatory support has been decreased, wean iNO in 1 ppm increments at approximately 4 hour intervals as tolerated. Discontinue when stable on 1 ppm for 4 hours. The usual length of treatment is less than 4 days. Infants who cannot be weaned off after 4 days should undergo further diagnostic testing for other diseases. Administer via an FDA/EMEA approved delivery system designed to accurately deliver NO uninterrupted into the ventilator system in parts-per-million concentrations that are constant throughout the respiratory cycle, while limiting NO_2 production (e.g., INOvent™).

USES: Treatment of term and near-term infants (≥34 weeks GA) with hypoxic respiratory failure (Oxygenation Index > 25) associated with clinical or echocardiographic evidence of pulmonary hypertension. It is usually not effective in infants with congenital diaphragmatic hernia. Do not use in infants dependent on right-to-left cardiac blood flow.

MONITORING: Continuous monitoring of oxygenation, blood pressure and heart rate are mandatory. Measure blood methemoglobin concentration 4 hours after initiation of therapy and at 24 hour intervals thereafter. Monitoring of inspired gas must provide for continuous measurement of both NO and NO_2 concentrations, with a feedback mechanism that cuts off delivery if NO or NO_2 exceed acceptable limits.

ADVERSE EFFECTS/PRECAUTIONS: Abrupt discontinuation may result in worsening oxygenation and increased pulmonary artery pressures. The risks of methemoglobinemia and elevated NO_2 levels increase significantly at doses > 20 ppm. Methemoglobin has very high affinity for oxygen and has a profound effect on oxygen content. Small increases in methemoglobin cause significant decreases in available oxygen content. Normal methemoglobin levels are < 1%. In most neonatal studies, methemoglobinemia was defined as levels of 5 to 7%. Cyanosis develops at levels of 10%, although the patients generally remain asymptomatic. At methemoglobin levels approaching 30%, patients begin to experience respiratory distress, and cardiac, gastrointestinal, and neurologic symptoms. A methemoglobin level greater than 50% is usually lethal. Avoid concomitant use of acetaminophen, metoclopramide, sulfa drugs, topical anesthetics (EMLA, benzocaine, lidocaine, prilocaine). Congenital deficiencies in the methemoglobin reductase enzyme system occur but are rare. The environmental exposure limit set by the Occupational Safety and Health Administration is 25 ppm for NO and 5 ppm for NO_2.

PHARMACOLOGY: Inhaled nitric oxide (iNO) is a selective pulmonary vasodilator that decreases extrapulmonary right-to-left shunting. It activates guanyl cyclase by binding to its heme component leading to production of cyclic GMP, with subsequent relaxation of pulmonary vascular smooth muscle. Oxygenation is also improved due to the redirecting of blood from poorly aerated to better aerated distal air spaces. In addition, iNO appears to have both anti-oxidant and anti-inflammatory activities.

SPECIAL CONSIDERATIONS/PREPARATION: Nitric oxide for inhalation is supplied in medical grade gas cylinders. Store vertically in well-ventilated areas at room temperature. All cylinders should be returned to the supplier for disposal. Hospital personnel should receive specific training in the administration of iNO.

SELECTED REFERENCES

- Finer NN, Barrington KJ: Nitric oxide for respiratory failure in infants born at term or near term (Cochrane Review). In: *The Cochrane Library*, Issue 2, 2002. Oxford. Update Software.
- Clark RH, Huckaby JL, Kueser TJ, et al. Low-dose nitric oxide therapy for persistent pulmonary hypertension: 1-year follow-up. *J Perinatol* 2003; 23(4):300-303.
- Lipkin PH, Davidson D, Spivak L, et al. Neurodevelopmental and medical outcomes of persistent pulmonary hypertension in term newborns treated with nitric oxide. *J Pediatr* 2002;140(3):306-310.
- Finer NN, Sun JW, Rich W, et al: Randomized, prospective study of low-dose versus high-dose inhaled nitric oxide in the neonate with hypoxic respiratory failure. *Pediatrics* 2001;108:948-55.
- Clark RH, Kueser TJ, Walker MW, et al: Low-dose nitric oxide therapy for persistent pulmonary hypertension of the newborn. *N Engl J Med* 2000;342:469-74.
- Kinsella JP, Abman SH: Clinical approach to inhaled nitric oxide therapy in the newborn with hypoxemia. *J Pediatr* 2000;136:717-26.
- The Neonatal Inhaled Nitric Oxide Study Group: Inhaled nitric oxide in term and near-term infants: Neurodevelopmental follow-up of the The Neonatal Inhaled Nitric Oxide Study Group (NINOS). *J Pediatr* 2000;136:611-17.
- Davidson D, Barefield ES, Kattwinkel J, et al: Safety of withdrawing inhaled nitric oxide therapy in persistent pulmonary hypertension of the newborn. *Pediatrics* 1999;104:231-36.
- The Neonatal Inhaled Nitric Oxide Study Group: Inhaled nitric oxide in full-term and nearly full-term infants with hypoxic respiratory failure. *N Engl J Med* 1997;336:597-604.
- Product Information, Ino, 2006

NIZATIDINE

DOSE & ADMINISTRATION: PO: 2 to 5 mg/kg per dose Q12 hours orally.

USES: Prevention and treatment of stress ulcers and GI hemorrhage aggravated by gastric acid secretion.

MONITORING: Gastric pH may be measured to assess efficacy.

ADVERSE EFFECTS/PRECAUTIONS: Limited data in neonatal patients. One case report of thrombocytopenia. No other adverse effects have been reported in infants or children. Elevations in hepatic enzymes and asymptomatic ventricular tachycardia have been reported in adults.

PHARMACOLOGY: Inhibits gastric acid secretion by histamine H_2-receptor antagonism. Peak serum concentration occurs 0.5 to 3 hours after oral administration and is not influenced by food. Bioavailability is quite variable. Greater than 90% eliminated in the urine within 12 hours with 60% excreted unchanged. Elimination half-life in neonates is 3 to 7 hours, and is prolonged in preterm infants and patients with renal insufficiency.

SPECIAL CONSIDERATIONS/PREPARATION: Axid® alcohol-free oral solution (15 mg/mL) is supplied in 480 mL bottles. Store at room temperature.

SELECTED REFERENCES

- Orenstein SR, Gremse DA, Pantaleon CD, et al: Nizatidine for the treatment of pediatric gastroesophageal reflux symptoms: An open-label, multiple-dose, randomized, multicenter clinical trial in 210 children. *Clin Therapeutics* 2005;27:472-483.
- Hamamoto N, Hashimoto T, Adachi K, et al: Comparative study of nizatidine and famotidine for maintenance therapy of erosive esophagitis. *J Gastroenterol Hepatol* 2005 ;20:281-286.
- Abdel-Rahman SM, Johnson FK, Connor JD, et al: Developmental pharmacokinetics and pharmacodynamics of nizatidine. *JPGN 2004* ;38:442-451.
- Abdel-Rahman SM, Johnson FK, Gauthier-Dubois G, et al: The bioequivalence of nizatidine (Axid®) in two extemporaneously and two commercially prepared oral liquid formulations compared with capsule. *J Clin Pharmacol* 2003;43:148-153.
- Abdel-Rahman SM, Johnson FK, Manowitz N, et al: Single-dose pharmacokinetics of nizatidine (Axid®) in children. *J Clin Pharmacol* 2002;42:1089-1096.
- Product information, Braintree Laboratories, Inc., 2005.

NYSTATIN

DOSE & ADMINISTRATION: Topical: Apply ointment or cream to affected area Q6 hours. Continue treatment for 3 days after symptoms have subsided. **PO:** 1 mL (preterm) to 2 mL (term) of 100,000-units/mL suspension divided and applied with swab to each side of mouth Q6 hours. Continue treatment for 3 days after symptoms have subsided. **Prophylaxis:** 1 mL of 100,000 units/mL suspension orally or instilled into stomach via oro/nasogastic tube 3 times per day.

USES: Treatment of mucocutaneous candidal infections. Prophylaxis against invasive fungal infections in high risk VLBW infants.

MONITORING: Assess response to drug.

ADVERSE EFFECTS/PRECAUTIONS: Possible skin rash caused by vehicle in ointment/cream.

PHARMACOLOGY: Polyene antifungal similar in structure to amphotericin B. May be fungicidal or fungistatic. Binds to the fungal cell membrane causing disruption of the cell structure. Not absorbed well from the GI tract, skin, or mucous membranes.

SPECIAL CONSIDERATIONS/PREPARATION: Topical ointment/cream: 100,000 units/g in 15- and 30-g tubes. Ointment dissolved in polyethylene and mineral-oil-gel base. **Topical powder:** 100,000 units/g in 15- and 30-g plastic sqeeze bottles. **Oral suspension:** 100,000 units/mL in 5-, 60-, and 480-mL bottles. Shake well before applying to mouth. Appears to work best when not mixed with formula. Contains <1% alcohol, saccharin, and 50% sucrose.

SELECTED REFERENCES

- Ozturk MA, Gunes T, Koklu E, et al: Oral nystatin prophylaxis to prevent invasive candidiasis in neonatal intensive care unit. *Mycoses* 2006;49:484-492.
- Hoppe JE: Treatment of oropharyngeal candidiasis and candidal diaper dermatitis in neonates and infants: review and reappraisal. *Ped Inf Dis J* 1997;16:885-94.
- Faix RG, Kovarik SM, Shaw TR, Johnson RV: Mucocutaneous and invasive candidiasis among very low birth weight (<1500 grams) infants in intensive care nurseries: A prospective study. *Pediatrics* 1989;83:101.
- Roberts RJ: *Drug Therapy in Infants.* Philadelphia: WB Saunders Co, 1984, p 81.
- Munz D, Powell KR, Pai CH: Treatment of candidal diaper dermatitis: A double-blind placebo-controlled comparison of topical nystatin with topical plus oral nystatin. *J Pediatr* 1982;101:1022.
- Product Information, Actavis, 2006

OCTREOTIDE

DOSE & ADMINISTRATION: Treatment of hyperinsulinemic hypoglycemia: Initial dose: 1 mcg/kg per dose Q6h subQ or IV. Titrate upward to desired effect. Initial response should occur within 8 hours; tachyphylaxis may occur within several days. **Maximum dose:** 10 mcg/kg per dose Q6h. **Treatment of chylothorax:** Begin at 1 mcg/kg per hour continuous infusion, subQ or IV. Titrate upward as necessary; chyle production should significantly decrease within 24 hours. **Maximum dose:** 7 mcg/kg per hour.

USES: Treatment of refractory hyperinsulinemic hypoglycemia. Adjunctive treatment of congenital and post-operative chylothorax.

MONITORING: Monitor blood glucose closely.

ADVERSE EFFECTS/PRECAUTIONS: Vomiting, diarrhea, abdominal distention and steatorrhea may occur. Pulmonary hypertension has been reported in treated former premature infants with chronic lung disease. Hyperglycemia may occur in patients being treated for chylothorax.

PHARMACOLOGY: Octreotide is a long-acting analog of the natural hormone somatostatin. It is an even more potent inhibitor of growth hormone, glucagon, and insulin than somatostatin. Like somatostatin, it also suppresses LH response to GnRH, decreases splanchnic blood flow, and inhibits release of serotonin, gastrin, vasoactive intestinal peptide, secretin, motilin, and pancreatic polypeptide. After subcutaneous injection, octreotide is absorbed rapidly and completely from the injection site. The elimination half-life of octreotide from plasma is approximately 1.7 hours in adults, compared with 1-3 minutes for the natural hormone. Excreted unchanged into the urine.

SPECIAL CONSIDERATIONS/PREPARATION: Available in 1-mL single-dose ampules for injection containing 50-, 100-, or 500-mcg, and in 5-mL multiple-dose vials in concentrations of 200 and 1000 mcg/mL. pH 3.9 to 4.5. Osmolarity is 279 mOsm/kg. Refrigerate and protect from light. Do not warm artificially. After initial use, multiple dose vials should be discarded within 14 days. Ampuls should be opened just prior to administration and the unused portion discarded. For SC injection use undiluted drug unless dose volume is not accurately measurable. For continuous IV administration consider making a dilution of 10 to 25 mcg/mL using D_5W or NS.

Solution Compatibility: D_5W and NS.

Solution Incompatibility: Do not add directly to Dex/AA bag because of the formation of glycosyl octreotide conjugate.

Terminal Injection Site Compatibility: Dex/AA and heparin.

Incompatibility: Fat emulsion.

SELECTED REFERENCES

- Young S, Dalgleish S, Eccleston A, et al: Severe congenital chylothorax treated with octreotide. *J Perinatol* 2004;24:200-202.
- de Lonlay P, Touati G, Robert J-J, Saudubray J-M: Persistent hyperinsulinemic hypoglycaemia, *Semin Neonatol* 2002;7:95-100.
- Schwitzgebel VM, Gitelman SE: Neonatal hyperinsulinism. *Clin Perinatol* 1998;25:1015-38.
- Cheung Y-F, Leung MP, Yip M-M: Octreotide for treatment of postoperative chylothorax. *J Pediatr* 2001;139:157-59.
- Product Information, Novartis, 2005

OMEPRAZOLE

DOSE & ADMINISTRATION: 0.5 to 1.5 mg/kg per dose PO, once a day. See Special Considerations/Preparation section for oral preparation.

USES: Short-term (less than 8 weeks) treatment of documented reflux esophagitis or duodenal ulcer refractory to conventional therapy.

MONITORING: Observe for symptomatic improvement within 3 days. Consider intraesophageal pH monitoring to assess for efficacy (pH >4.0). Measure AST and ALT if duration of therapy is greater than 8 weeks.

ADVERSE EFFECTS/PRECAUTIONS: Hypergastrinemia and mild transaminase elevations are the only Adverse Effects reported in children who received omeprazole for extended periods of time. Available data are limited to small studies of infants and children.

PHARMACOLOGY: Omeprazole inhibits gastric acid secretion by inhibition of hydrogen-potassium ATPase, the enzyme responsible for the final step in the secretion of hydrochloric acid by the gastric parietal cell ("proton pump"). Onset of action is within one hour of administration, maximal effect is at approximately 2 hours. Inhibition of acid secretion is about 50% of maximum at 24 hours and the duration of action is approximately 72 hours.

SPECIAL CONSIDERATIONS/PREPARATION: Zegerid® (omeprazole/sodium bicarbonate) is supplied as a 20 mg powder for suspension packet. A 2 mg/mL concentration can be prepared by reconstituting with 10 mL of water. The appropriate dose can be administered through a nasogastric or orogastric tube. The suspension should be flushed through the tube with water or normal saline. A stability study of a 2-mg/mL concentration showed stability for 45 days in refrigerator. Prilosec® is supplied as 2.5-mg and 10-mg unit dose packets for delayed-release oral suspension (omeprazole magnesium) and as delayed-release capsules containing 10, 20, or 40-mg omeprazole as enteric-coated granules. To prepare the delayed-release suspension, empty the 2.5 mg packet into a container containing 5 mL of water (or the 10 mg packet into a container containing 15 mL of water). Stir and leave 2 to 3 minutes to thicken. Stir and administer appropriate patient-specific dose within 30 minutes. For nasogastric or gastric tube administration, add 5 mL of water to a catheter-tipped syringe then add contents of 2.5 mg packet (or add 15 mL of water to syringe for adding 10 mg packet). Shake syringe immediately and leave 2 to 3 minutes to thicken. Shake syringe and inject patient-specific dose through the tube within 30 minutes. Flush tube with an appropriate amount of water.

SELECTED REFERENCES

- Johnson CE, Cober MP, Ludwig JL: Stability of partial doses of omeprazole-sodium bicarbonate oral suspension. *Ann Pharmacother* 2007;41;1954-61.
- Alliet P, Raes M, Bruneel E, Gillis P: Omeprazole in infants with cimetidine-resistant peptic esophagitis. *J Pediatr* 1998;132:352-354.

• Quercia RA, Fan C, Liu X, et al: Stability of omeprazole in an extemporaneously prepared oral liquid. *Am J Health-Syst Pharm* 1997;54:1833-1836.
• Kato S, Ebina K, Fujii K, et al: Effect of omeprazole in the treatment of refractory acid-related diseases in childhood: endoscopic healing and twenty-four-hour intragastric acidity. *J Pediatr* 1996;128:415-421.
• Faure C, Michaud L, Shaghagi EK, Popon M, et al: Intravenous omeprazole in children: pharmacokinetics and effect on 24-hour intragastric pH. *J Pediatr Gastroenterol Nutr* 2001;33:144-8.
• Product Information, Santarus, 2008
• Product Information, AstraZeneca, 2008

OXACILLIN

DOSE & ADMINISTRATION: Usual dosage: 25 mg/kg per dose IV over at least 10 minutes. **Meningitis:** 50 mg/kg per dose. To use dosing chart, please refer to explanatory note in "How to Use This Book."

DOSING INTERVAL CHART

PMA (weeks)	PostNatal (days)	Interval (hours)
≤29	0 to 28 >28	12 8
30 to 36	0 to 14 >14	12 8
37 to 44	0 to 7 >7	12 8
≥45	ALL	6

USES: Treatment of infections caused by penicillinase-producing staphylococci.

MONITORING: Periodic CBC and urinalysis. AST, ALT. Irritating to veins—watch for phlebitis. Observe IV site for signs of extravasation.

ADVERSE EFFECTS/PRECAUTIONS: Interstitial nephritis associated with hematuria, albuminuria, and casts in urine. Bone marrow depression. Elevated AST and ALT. Hypersensitivity in the form of a rash. Tolerant strains of staphylococci have been reported.

PHARMACOLOGY: Inhibits synthesis of bacterial cell wall. Rapidly excreted renally unchanged. Poor CSF penetration. Good penetration of pleural, pericardial, and synovial fluids.

SPECIAL CONSIDERATIONS/PREPARATION: Available as powder injection in 250-mg, 500-mg, 1-g, 2-g, and 10-g vials. Reconstitute 250 mg vial with 5 mL of sterile water for injection to make a concentration of 50 mg/mL. Reconstituted solution is stable for 4 days at room temperature, 7 days refrigerated. Dilute further using sterile water or NS to a concentration less than or equal to 40 mg/mL. Dilution stable for 4 days refrigerated.

Solution Compatibility: D_5W, $D_{10}W$, and NS.

Terminal Injection Site Compatibility: Dex/AA solutions, fat emulsion. Acyclovir, chloramphenicol, dopamine, famotidine, fluconazole, heparin, hydrocortisone succinate, milrinone, morphine, potassium chloride, and zidovudine.

Incompatibility: Amikacin, caffeine citrate, gentamicin, netilmicin, sodium bicarbonate, and tobramycin.

SELECTED REFERENCES

• Maraqa NF, Gomez MM, Rathore MH, Alvarez AM: Higher occurrence of hepatotoxicity and rash in patients treated with oxacillin, compared with those treated with nafcillin and other commonly used antimicrobials. *Clin Infect Dis* 2002;34:50-54.
• Prober CG, Stevenson DK, Benitz WE: The use of antibiotics in neonates weighing less than 1200 grams. *Pediatr Infect Dis J* 1990;9:111.
• Nahata MC, Debolt SL, Powell DA: Adverse effects of methicillin, nafcillin, and oxacillin in pediatric patients. *Dev Pharmacol Ther* 1982;4:117.
• Axline SG, Yaffe SJ, Simon HJ: Clinical pharmacology of antimicrobials in premature infants: II. Ampicillin, methicillin, oxacillin, neomycin, and colistin. *Pediatrics* 1967;39:97.
• Product Information, Sandoz, 2005

PALIVIZUMAB

DOSE & ADMINISTRATION: 15 mg/kg per dose IM, preferably in the anterolateral aspect of the thigh. Repeat monthly during RSV season.

USES: Immunoprophylaxis against severe RSV lower respiratory tract infections in high risk infants:

- up to 24 months of age, hemodynamically significant acyanotic and cyanotic congenital heart disease,
- less than 24 months of age, chronic lung disease of prematurity (CLD) who have required medical therapy for CLD within 6 months before the start of the RSV season,
- up to 12 months of age, born at 28 weeks gestation or earlier,
- up to 6 months of age, born at 29 to 32 weeks gestation,
- less than 6 months of age, born between 32 to 35 weeks gestation with at least 2 additional risk factors.

Risk factors include child care attendance, school-aged siblings, exposure to environmental air pollutants, congenital abnormalities of the airways, or severe neuromuscular disease. Once an infant qualifies for initiation of prophylaxis, it should continue throughout the RSV season. Palivizumab is not effective for treatment of established RSV disease.

MONITORING: Observe injection site for induration and swelling.

ADVERSE EFFECTS/PRECAUTIONS: In clinical trials, upper respiratory infection, otitis media, fever, and rhinitis occurred slightly more frequently in palivizumab recipients. Cyanosis and arrhythmia were also seen slightly more frequently in patients with CHD. There are rare reports (<1 per 100,000 patients) of anaphylaxis, and hypersensitivity reactions have been reported. Do not administer to patients with a history of a prior severe reaction.

PHARMACOLOGY: Synagis® is a humanized monoclonal antibody produced by recombinant DNA technology. This composite of human (95%) and murine (5%) antibody sequences inhibits RSV replication. The mean half-life of Synagis® is approximately 20 days. Adequate antibody titers are maintained in most infants for one month following a 15-mg/kg dose. Due to a faster metabolic rate, some hospitalized VLBW infants (<500 g) may not maintain optimal RSV titers for the entire initial month until after the second dose. Palivizumab does not interfere with the response to other vaccines and as such, they can be administered concurrently.

SPECIAL CONSIDERATIONS/PREPARATION: Synagis® is supplied as 50-mg and 100-mg single-dose vials in ready-to-use, **NO RECONSTITUTION required** , liquid solution. Do not add any diluent to the liquid solution and use one dose per vial. Do not re-enter vial after initial withdrawal and discard any unused portions. Administer as soon as possible after withdrawal from the vial. **Do not FREEZE or SHAKE**. The liquid solution should be stored **refrigerated between 2 to 8°C (36 to 46°F).** Synagis® contains no preservatives, thiomersol, or other mercury salts.

SELECTED REFERENCES

- American Academy of Pediatrics. Respiratory Syncytial Virus (RSV) Infections. In: Pickering LK, Baker CJ, Long SS, McMillan JA, eds. *Red Book: 2006 Report of the Committee on Infectious Diseases.* 27th ed. Elk Grove Village, IL: American Academy of Pediatrics 2006:560-566.
- Meissner HC, Long SS, Committee on Infectious Diseases and Committee on Fetus and Newborn: Revised indications for the use of palivizumab and respiratory syncytial virus immune globulin intravenous for the prevention of respiratory syncytial virus infections. Policy Statement and Technical Report. *Pediatrics* 2003;122:1442-46 and 1447-52.
- Romero JR: Palivizumab prophylaxis of respiratory syncytial virus disease from 1998 to 2002: results from four years of palivizumab usage. *Pediatr Infect Dis J* 2003;22:S46-54.
- The Impact-RSV Study Group: Palivizumab, a humanized respiratory syncytial virus monoclonal antibody, reduces hospitalization from respiratory syncytial virus infection in high-risk infants. *Pediatrics* 1998;102:531-537.
- Groothuis JR: Safety and tolerance of palivizumab administration in a large northern hemisphere trial. *Pediatr Infect Dis J* 2001;20:628-629.
- Wu S-Y, Bonaparte J, Pyati S: Palivizumab use in very premature infants in the neonatal intensive care unit. *Pediatrics* 2004;114:e554-e556.
- Product Information, MedImmune, 2007.

PANCURONIUM

DOSE & ADMINISTRATION: 0.1 mg/kg (0.04 to 0.15 mg/kg) IV push, as needed for paralysis. Usual dosing interval is 1 to 2 hours. Adjust dose as needed based on duration of paralysis.

USES: Skeletal muscle relaxation/paralysis in infants requiring mechanical ventilation. Proposed desirable effects are improved oxygenation/ ventilation, reduced barotrauma, and reduced fluctuations in cerebral blood flow.

MONITORING: Monitor vital signs frequently, blood pressure continuously. Use some form of eye lubrication.

ADVERSE EFFECTS/PRECAUTIONS: Hypoxemia may occur because of inadequate mechanical ventilation and deterioration in pulmonary mechanics. Tachycardia and blood pressure changes (both hypotension and hypertension) occur frequently. Increased salivation.

PHARMACOLOGY: Nondepolarizing muscle-relaxant that competitively antagonizes autonomic cholinergic receptors and also causes sympathetic stimulation. Partially hydroxylated by the liver, 40% excreted unchanged in urine. Onset of action is 1 to 2 minutes; duration varies with dose and age. Reversed by neostigmine and atropine. Factors affecting duration of neuromuscular blockade: **Potentiation:** Acidosis, hypothermia, neuromuscular disease, hepatic disease, renal failure, cardiovascular disease, younger age, aminoglycosides, hypermagnesemia, and hypokalemia. **Antagonism:** Alkalosis, epinephrine, and hyperkalemia. Sensation remains intact; analgesia should be used for painful procedures.

SPECIAL CONSIDERATIONS/PREPARATION: Available in concentrations of 1-mg/mL (10 mL vials) and 2-mg/mL (2- and 5-mL vials). Products contain 1% (10 mg/mL) benzyl alcohol. **Refrigerate.**

Solution Compatibility: D_5W and NS.

Terminal Injection Site Compatibility: Dex/AA. Aminophylline, caffeine citrate, cefazolin, cimetidine, dobutamine, dopamine, epinephrine, esmolol, fentanyl, fluconazole, gentamicin, heparin, hydrocortisone succinate, isoproterenol, lorazepam, midazolam, milrinone, morphine, netilmicin, nitroglycerin, nitroprusside, propofol, prostaglandin E_1, ranitidine, trimethoprim-sulfamethoxazole, and vancomycin.

Incompatibility: Pentobarbital and phenobarbital.

SELECTED REFERENCES

- Bhutani VK, Abbasi S, Sivieri EM: Continuous skeletal muscle paralysis: Effect on neonatal pulmonary mechanics. *Pediatrics* 1988;81:419.
- Costarino AT, Polin RA: Neuromuscular relaxants in the neonate. *Clin Perinatol* 1987;14:965.
- Cabal LA, Siassi B, Artal R, et al: Cardiovascular and catecholamine changes after administration of pancuronium in distressed neonates. *Pediatrics* 1985;75:284.
- Product Information, Sicor, 2003

PAPAVERINE

DOSE & ADMINISTRATION: 30 mg per 250 mL of arterial catheter infusion solution.

USES: Prolongation of peripheral arterial catheter patency.

ADVERSE EFFECTS/PRECAUTIONS: Use with caution in VLBW infants in the first days after birth due to potential of developing or extending an intracranial hemorrhage. Chronic hepatitis, as evidenced by an increase in serum bilirubin and serum glutamic transaminase, has been reported in three adults following long-term papaverine therapy. One patient had jaundice, and another had abnormal liver function on biopsy.

PHARMACOLOGY: Papaverine directly relaxes the tonus of various smooth muscle, especially when it has been spasmodically contracted. It relaxes the smooth musculature of the larger blood vessels, especially coronary, systemic peripheral and pulmonary arteries. Vasodilation may be related to its ability to inhibit cyclic nucleotide phosphodiesterase, thus increasing levels of intracellular cyclic AMP. During administration, the muscle cell is not paralyzed and still responds to drugs and other stimuli causing contraction. Possibly because of its direct vasodilating action on cerebral blood vessels, papaverine increases cerebral blood flow and decreases cerebral vascular resistance in healthy subjects; oxygen consumption is unaltered. Papaverine is metabolized in the liver and excreted in the urine in an inactive form.

SPECIAL CONSIDERATIONS/PREPARATION: Supplied as 30 mg/mL solution for injection in 2 mL preservative-free vials and 10-mL multiple dose vials containing 0.5% chlorobutanol.

Solution Compatibility: N S, 0.45 NS, both with 1 unit/mL heparin

Solution Incompatibility: Lactated Ringers (precipitate forms)

Terminal Injection Site Compatibility: Phentolamine.

SELECTED REFERENCES

- Griffin MP, Siadaty MS: Papaverine prolongs patency of peripheral arterial catheters in neonates. *J Pediatr* 2005;146:62-65.
- Heulitt MJ, Farrington EA, O'Shea TM, et al: Double-blind randomized controlled trial of papaverine-containing solutions to prevent failure of arterial catheters in pediatric patients. *Crit Care Med* 1993;21:825-829.
- Product Information, Parenta Pharmaceuticals, Inc., 2006

PENICILLIN G

DOSE & ADMINISTRATION: »Use only aqueous crystalline penicillin G for IV administration« **Meningitis:** 75,000 to 100,000 units/kg per dose IV infusion over 30 minutes, or IM. **Bacteremia:** 25,000 to 50,000 units/kg per dose IV infusion over 15 minutes, or IM. **Group B streptococcal infections:** Some experts recommend using 200,000 units/kg per day for bacteremia and 450,000 units/kg per day for meningitis, in divided doses at more frequent intervals than those listed above. Consider adding aminoglycoside if tolerance is suspected or confirmed. **Gonococcal infection (only with proven penicillin-susceptible isolate):** Use higher doses listed for meningitis and bacteremia. **Congenital syphilis:** Aqueous crystalline penicillin G: 50,000 units/kg per dose IV over 15 minutes, given Q12 hours during the first 7 days of life, and Q8 hours thereafter, irrespective of gestational age; or **Procaine penicillin G:** 50,000 units/kg per dose IM, once daily. Treat for 10 to 14 days. **Procaine and benzathine penicillin G are for IM administration only.** To use dosing chart, please refer to explanatory note in "How to Use This Book."

DOSING INTERVAL CHART

PMA (weeks)	PostNatal (days)	Interval (hours)
≤29	0 to 28 >28	12 8
30 to 36	0 to 14 >14	12 8
37 to 44	0 to 7 >7	12 8
≥45	ALL	6

USES: Treatment of infections caused by susceptible organisms—congenital syphilis, gonococci, streptococci (non enterococcal).

MONITORING: Follow serum sodium and potassium when using high doses and in patients with renal failure. Observe IV site for signs of extravasation.

ADVERSE EFFECTS/PRECAUTIONS: Cardiac arrest has been reported in patients who received high doses infused rapidly. Significant CNS toxicity has been reported in adults with renal failure who developed CSF concentrations >10 mcg/mL. Bone marrow depression, granulocytopenia, and hepatitis are rare. Hypersensitivity has not been seen in neonates.

PHARMACOLOGY: Inhibits synthesis of bacterial cell wall. Excreted unchanged in the urine. CSF penetration is poor, except in inflamed meninges. Concentrates in joint fluid and urine.

SPECIAL CONSIDERATIONS/PREPARATION: Aqueous penicillin G is available as powder for injection in two salt forms: penicillin G potassium and penicillin G sodium. Penicillin G potassium contains 1.68 mEq (65.6 mg) potassium per 1 million units, and 0.3 mEq (6.8 mg) sodium per 1 million units. Penicillin G sodium contains 2 mEq (46 mg) sodium per 1 million units. Reconstitute the 5-million unit vial with 8 mL sterile water for injection to make a final concentration of 500,000 units/mL. Reconstituted solution good for 7 days refrigerated. A 100,000 unit/mL dilution may be made by adding 10 mL of reconstituted solution to 40 mL sterile water for injection. Dilution stable for 7 days refrigerated. Penicillin G sodium reconstituted solution stable for 3 days in refrigerator. Penicillin G potassium is also available as a premixed frozen iso-osmotic solution containing 1, 2 or 3 million units in 50 mL. Procaine and benzathine penicillin G for IM injection are available in multiple dosage strengths in vials and Tubex® syringes. **Note: Penicillin G is also known as benzylpenicillin - do not confuse with benzathine penicillin used for only IM injections. 1 million units is the equivalent of 600 mg.**

Solution Compatibility: D_5W, $D_{10}W$, and NS.

Terminal Injection Site Compatibility: Dex/AA solutions, fat emulsion. Acyclovir, amiodarone, caffeine citrate, calcium chloride, calcium gluconate, chloramphenicol, cimetidine, clindamycin, dopamine, enalaprilat, erythromycin lactobionate, esmolol, fluconazole, furosemide, heparin, hydrocortisone succinate, lidocaine, methicillin, metronidazole, morphine, nicardipine, pentobarbital, potassium chloride, prostaglandin E_1, ranitidine and sodium bicarbonate.

Incompatibility: Amikacin, aminophylline, amphotericin B, gentamicin, metoclopramide, netilmicin, and tobramycin.

SELECTED REFERENCES

- American Academy of Pediatrics. Syphilis. In: Pickering LK, Baker CJ, Long SS, McMillan JA, eds. *Red Book: 2006 Report of the Committee on Infectious Diseases.* 27th ed. Elk Grove Village, IL: American Academy of Pediatrics; 2006: pp 637-638.
- Centers for Disease Control and Prevention: Sexually transmitted diseases treatment guidelines 2006. *MMWR* 2006;55(No. RR-11).
- Stoll BJ: Congenital syphilis: evaluation and management of neonates born to mothers with reactive serologic tests for syphilis. *Pediatr Infect Dis J* 1994;13:845.
- Prober CG, Stevenson DK, Benitz WE: The use of antibiotics in neonates weighing less than 1200 grams. *Pediatr Infect Dis J* 1990;9:111.
- Roberts RJ: *Drug Therapy in Infants.* Philadelphia: WB Saunders Co, 1984, p45.
- Pyati SP, Pildes RS, Jacobs NM, et al: Penicillin in infants weighing two kilograms or less with early onset group B streptococcal disease. *N Engl J Med* 1983;308:1383.
- McCracken GH Jr, Ginsburg C, Chrane DF, et al: Clinical pharmacology of penicillin in newborn infants. *J Pediatr* 1973;82:692.
- Product Information, Pfizer, 2005

PENTOBARBITAL

DOSE & ADMINISTRATION: 2 to 6 mg/kg IV slow push.

USES: Sedative/hypnotic, for short-term use.

MONITORING: Monitor respiratory status and blood pressure closely. Serum concentration for sedation: 0.5 to 3 mcg/mL.

ADVERSE EFFECTS/PRECAUTIONS: Respiratory depression. Tolerance, dependence, and cardiovascular depression occur with continued use. Enhances metabolism of phenytoin, sodium valproate, and corticosteroids by microsomal enzyme induction.

PHARMACOLOGY: Short-acting barbiturate. Pentobarbital has no analgesic effects. Serum half-life is dose-dependent (15 to 50 hours in adults) and unknown in neonates. Metabolized by hepatic microsomal enzyme system.

SPECIAL CONSIDERATIONS/PREPARATION: Available as a 50-mg/mL solution in 20 mL and 50 mL multidose vials. Solution contains propylene glycol 40%, and alcohol 10%. Irritating to veins—pH is 9.5. A 5-mg/mL dilution may be made by adding 1 mL of the 50-mg/mL solution to 9 mL of preservative-free normal saline. Use immediately.

Solution Compatibility: D_5W, $D_{10}W$, and NS. No data are currently available on Dex/AA.

Terminal Injection Site Compatibility: Acyclovir, amikacin, aminophylline, atropine, calcium chloride, chloramphenicol, erythromycin lactobionate, hyaluronidase, insulin, lidocaine, linezolid, neostigmine, penicillin G, propofol, and sodium bicarbonate.

Incompatibility: Fat emulsion. Cefazolin, cimetidine, clindamycin, fentanyl, hydrocortisone succinate, midazolam, mivacurium, morphine, pancuronium bromide, phenytoin, ranitidine, and vancomycin. No data are currently available on heparin and potassium chloride.

SELECTED REFERENCES

- Strain JD, Harvey LA, Foley LC, Campbell JB: Intravenously administered pentobarbital sodium for sedation in pediatric CT. *Radiology* 1986;161:105.
- Product Information, Ovation, 2005

PHENOBARBITAL

DOSE & ADMINISTRATION: Loading dose: 20 mg/kg IV, given slowly over 10 to 15 minutes. Refractory seizures: Additional 5-mg/kg doses, up to a total of 40 mg/kg. **Maintenance:** 3 to 4 mg/kg **per day** beginning 12 to 24 hours after the load. **Frequency/Route:** Daily (Q12 hours probably unnecessary). IV slow push (most rapid control of seizures), IM, PO, or PR.

USES: Anticonvulsant. May improve outcomes in severely asphyxiated infants (40 mg/kg IV infusion over 1 hour, prior to onset of seizures). May enhance bile excretion in patients with cholestasis before ^{99}Tc-IDA scanning.

MONITORING: Phenobarbital monotherapy will control seizures in 43 to 85% of affected neonates - adding a second drug (phenytoin or lorazepam) is often needed. Therapeutic serum concentration is 15 to 40 mcg/mL. Drug accumulation may occur using recommended maintenance dose during the first two weeks of life. Altered (usually increased) serum concentrations may occur in patients also receiving phenytoin or valproate. Observe IV site for signs of extravasation and phlebitis.

ADVERSE EFFECTS/PRECAUTIONS: Sedation at serum concentrations above 40 mcg/mL. Respiratory depression at concentrations above 60 mcg/mL. Irritating to veins - pH is approximately 10 and osmolality is approximately 15,000 mOsm/kg H_2O.

PHARMACOLOGY: Phenobarbital limits the spread of seizure activity, possibly by increasing inhibitory neurotransmission. Approximately 30% protein bound. Primarily metabolized by liver, then excreted in the urine as p-hydroxyphenobarbital (no anticonvulsant activity). Serum half-life in neonates is 40 to 200 hours.

SPECIAL CONSIDERATIONS/PREPARATION: Injectable solution available in concentrations of 60-, 65-, and 130-mg/mL, all containing 10% (100 mg/mL) alcohol and 67.8% propylene glycol. Oral elixir is available in 20 mg/5 mL concentration.

Solution Compatibility: D_5W, $D_{10}W$, and NS. No data are currently available on neonatal Dex/AA solutions.

Terminal Injection Site Compatibility: Amikacin, aminophylline, caffeine citrate, calcium chloride, calcium gluconate, enalaprilat, fentanyl, fosphenytoin, heparin, linezolid, meropenem, morphine, propofol, prostaglandin E_1, and sodium bicarbonate.

Incompatibility: Fat emulsion. Cimetidine, clindamycin, hydralazine, hydrocortisone succinate, insulin, methadone, midazolam, pancuronium, ranitidine, and vancomycin.

SELECTED REFERENCES

• Volpe JJ: *Neurology of the Newborn*, ed 4. Philadelphia: WB Saunders Co, 2001, p 203-204.
• Hall RT, Hall FK, Daily SK: High-dose phenobarbital therapy in term newborn infants with severe perinatal asphyxia: A randomized, prospective study with three-year follow-up. *J Pediatr* 1998;132:345-348.
• Product Information, PAI, 2005
• Product Information, Hospira, 2004

PHENTOLAMINE

DOSE & ADMINISTRATION: Inject a 1-mg/mL solution of phentolamine subcutaneously into the affected area. Usual amount needed is 1 to 5 mL, depending on the size of the infiltrate. May be repeated if necessary.

USES: Prevention of dermal necrosis and sloughing caused by extravasation of vasoconstrictive agents, e.g. dopamine.

MONITORING: Assess affected area for reversal of ischemia. Monitor blood pressure.

ADVERSE EFFECTS/PRECAUTIONS: Hypotension could potentially occur if a very large dose is administered. Consider using topical 2% nitroglycerin ointment if affected extremity is significantly swollen.

PHARMACOLOGY: Alpha-adrenergic blocking agent that produces peripheral vasodilation, thereby reversing ischemia produced by vasopressor infiltration. The effect should be seen almost immediately. Biological half-life when injected subcutaneously is less than 20 minutes.

SPECIAL CONSIDERATIONS/PREPARATION: Available in 5-mg vial as a lyophilized powder. To prepare:

1) Reconstitute one vial with 1 mL of Sterile Water for Injection.

2) Dilute to a concentration of 1 mg/mL with 4 mL Sterile Water for Injection. Use immediately.

Do not use if solution is discolored or contains particulate contamination.

Terminal Injection Site Compatibility: Amiodarone, dobutamine, and papaverine.

SELECTED REFERENCES

- Subhani M, Sridhar S, DeCristofaro JD: Phentolamine use in a neonate for the prevention of dermal necrosis caused by dopamine: A case report. *J Perinatol* 2001;21:324-326.
- Denkler KA, Cohen BE: Reversal of dopamine extravasation injury with topical nitroglycerin ointment. *Plast Reconstr Surg* 1989;84:811.
- Siwy BK, Sadove AM: Acute management of dopamine infiltration injury with Regitine. *Plast Reconstr Surg* 1987;80:610.
- Product Information, Bedford, 1999

PHENYLEPHRINE (OPHTHALMIC)

DOSE & ADMINISTRATION: 1 drop instilled in the eye at least 10 minutes prior to funduscopic procedures. Use **only** the 2.5% ophthalmic solution in neonates. Apply pressure to the lacrimal sac during and for 2 minutes after instillation to minimize systemic absorption.

USES: Induction of mydriasis and cycloplegia for diagnostic and therapeutic ophthalmic procedures.

MONITORING: Monitor heart rate and oxygen saturation in babies with BPD.

ADVERSE EFFECTS/PRECAUTIONS: May cause decreased pulmonary compliance, tidal volume, and peak airflow in babies with BPD. Do not use in patients receiving beta-blocker medications (e.g. propranolol). The use of 10% solutions has caused systemic hypertension and tachycardia in infants.

PHARMACOLOGY: Alpha-adrenergic. Mydriasis begins within 5 minutes of instillation and lasts for 60 minutes. Without lacrimal sac occlusion, approximately 80% of each drop may pass through the nasolacrimal system and be available for rapid systemic absorption by the nasal mucosa.

SPECIAL CONSIDERATIONS/PREPARATION: Supplied as ophthalmic solution in 0.12%, 2.5%, and 10% concentrations in 2 to 15 mL quantities. Do not use solution that becomes discolored or contains precipitate. Refer to specific product or manufacturer's recommendation for storage. A preparation containing cyclopentolate 0.2% and phenylephrine 1% (Cyclomydril®) is commercially available in 2- and 8-mL Drop-tainers. A combination eye drop solution ("Caputo drops") may be prepared in a 15-mL bottle with 3.75 mL of cyclopentolate 2%, 7.5 mL of tropicamide 1%, and 3.75 mL of phenylephrine 10%. The final solution contains cyclopentolate 0.5%, tropicamide 0.5%, and phenylephrine 2.5%. Use within 24 hours, as the solution contains no preservatives.

SELECTED REFERENCES

- Wallace DK, Steinkuller PG: Ocular medications in children. *Clin Pediatr* 1998;37:645-652.
- Laws DE, Morton C, Weindling M, Clark D: Systemic effects of screening for retinopathy of prematurity. *Br J Ophthalmol* 1996;80:425-428.
- McGregor MLK: Adrenergic agonists, in Mauger TF, Craig EL (eds): *Havener's Ocular Pharmacology*, ed 6. St. Louis: Mosby-YearBook, 1994, pp 70-72.
- Mirmanesh SJ, Abbasi S, Bhutani VK: Alpha-adrenergic bronchoprovocation in neonates with bronchopulmonary dysplasia. *J Pediatr* 1992;121:622-625.
- Isenberg S, Everett S: Cardiovascular effects of mydriatics in low-birth-weight infants. *J Pediatr* 1984;105:111-112
- Caputo AR, Schnitzer RE, Lindquist TD, Sun S: Dilation in neonates: a protocol. *Pediatrics* 1982;69:77-80.
- Borromeo-McGrail V, Bordiuk JM, Keitel H: Systemic hypertension following ocular administration of 10% phenylephrine in the neonate. *Pediatrics* 1973;51:1032-1036.
- Product Information, Alcon, 2005

PHENYTOIN

DOSE & ADMINISTRATION: Loading dose: 15 to 20 mg/kg IV infusion over at least 30 minutes. **Maintenance dose:** 4 to 8 mg/kg Q24 hours IV slow push, or PO. (Up to 8 mg/kg per dose Q8 to 12 hours after 1 week of age). Maximum rate of infusion 0.5 mg/kg per minute. Flush IV with saline before and after administration. **Phenytoin is highly unstable in any IV solution. Avoid using in central lines because of the risk of precipitation. IM route not acceptable; drug crystallizes in muscle.** Oral absorption is erratic.

PIPERACILLIN

USES: Anticonvulsant often used to treat seizures refractory to phenobarbital.

MONITORING: Monitor for bradycardia, arrhythmias, and hypotension during infusion. Observe IV site for extravasation. Follow serum concentration closely: therapeutic range is 6 to 15 mcg/mL in the first weeks, then 10 to 20 mcg/mL due to changes in protein binding. Obtain initial trough level 48 hours after IV loading dose.

ADVERSE EFFECTS/PRECAUTIONS: Extravasation causes tissue inflammation and necrosis due to high pH and osmolality. High serum concentrations are associated with seizures. Drowsiness may be difficult to identify. Hypersensitivity reactions have been reported in infants. Toxicities with long-term therapy include cardiac arrhythmias, hypotension, gingivitis, nystagmus, rickets, hyperglycemia, and hypoinsulinemia. Phenytoin interacts with carbamazepine, cimetidine, corticosteroids, digoxin, furosemide, phenobarbital, and valproate.

PHARMACOLOGY: Hepatic metabolism capacity is limited—saturation may occur within therapeutic range. Pharmacokinetics are dose-dependent. Elimination rate is increased during first few weeks of life. Serum half-life is 18 to 60 hours. 85% to 90% protein bound. Bilirubin displaces phenytoin from protein-binding sites, resulting in increased free drug.

SPECIAL CONSIDERATIONS/PREPARATION: Injectable solution available in a concentration of 50 mg/mL. Contains 40% propylene glycol and 10% alcohol (100 mg/mL). Oral suspension available in a concentration of 25 mg/mL.

Solution Compatibility: Phenytoin is highly unstable in any IV solution.

Solution Incompatibility: D_5W and $D_{10}W$.

Terminal Injection Site Compatibility: Esmolol, famotidine, fluconazole, sodium bicarbonate.

Incompatibility: Dex/AA solutions, fat emulsion. Amikacin, aminophylline, chloramphenicol, ciprofloxacin, clindamycin, dobutamine, enalaprilat, fentanyl, heparin, hyaluronidase, hydrocortisone succinate, insulin, lidocaine, linezolid, methadone, mivacurium, morphine, nitroglycerin, pentobarbital, potassium chloride, procainamide, propofol, ranitidine, and vitamin K_1.

SELECTED REFERENCES

• Volpe JJ: *Neurology of the Newborn*, ed 4. Philadelphia: WB Saunders Co, 2001, p 204-205.
• Wheless JW: Pediatric use of intravenous and intramuscular phenytoin: lessons learned. *J Child Neurol* 1998;13(Suppl 1): S11-14.
• Product Information, Hospira, 2004
• Product Information, Pfizer, 2006

PIPERACILLIN

DOSE & ADMINISTRATION: 50 to 100 mg/kg per dose IV infusion by syringe pump over 30 minutes, or IM. To use dosing chart, please refer to explanatory note in "How to Use This Book."

DOSING INTERVAL CHART

PMA (weeks)	PostNatal (days)	Interval (hours)
≤29	0 to 28<	12
	>28	8
30 to 36	0 to 14	12
	>14	8
37 to 44	0 to 7	12
	>7	8
≥45	ALL	6

USES: Semisynthetic penicillin with increased activity against *Pseudomonas aeruginosa* and many strains of *Klebsiella*, *Serratia*, *E coli*, *Enterobacter*, *Citrobacter*, and *Proteus*. Also effective against group B *Streptococcus*.

MONITORING: Desired peak serum concentration is approximately 150 mcg/mL. Desired trough concentration ranges from 15 to 50 mcg/mL (available as bioassay). Peak serum concentration is lower with IM administration. Observe IV site for signs of extravasation.

ADVERSE EFFECTS/PRECAUTIONS: Eosinophilia. Hyperbilirubinemia. Elevations in ALT, AST, BUN, and serum creatinine.

PHARMACOLOGY: Piperacillin is a potent, broad-spectrum, semi-synthetic, ureidopenicillin possessing high activity against gram-negative bacteria. Inactivation by beta-lactamase-producing bacteria. Synergistic with aminoglycosides. Good penetration into bone; CSF penetration similar to that of other penicillins. Serum half-life depends on gestational age and postnatal age. Primarily excreted renally unchanged.

SPECIAL CONSIDERATIONS/PREPARATION: Available as powder for injection in 2-g, 3-g, 4-g, and 40-g vials. Reconstitute 2-g vial with 10 mL of sterile water for injection to make a final concentration of 200 mg/mL. Reconstituted solution stable for 24 hours at room temperature, 2 days refrigerated. A 50 mg/mL dilution may be made by adding 2.5 mL of reconstituted solution to 7.5 mL sterile water for injection. Dilution stable for 2 days refrigerated. **IM Administration:** Use 400 mg/mL concentration.

Solution Compatibility: D_5W, $D_{10}W$, and NS.

Terminal Injection Site Compatibility: Dex/AA solutions, fat emulsion. Acyclovir, aminophylline, aztreonam, clindamycin, enalaprilat, esmolol, famotidine, heparin, hydrocortisone succinate, linezolid, lorazepam, midazolam, milrinone, morphine, nicardipine, potassium chloride, propofol, ranitidine, remifentanil, and zidovudine.

Incompatibility: Amikacin, amiodarone, gentamicin, netilmicin, fluconazole, tobramycin, and vancomycin.

SELECTED REFERENCES

- Kacet N, Roussel-Delvallez M, Gremillet C, et al: Pharmacokinetic study of piperacillin in newborns relating to gestational and postnatal age. *Pediatr Infect Dis J* 1992;11:365.
- Prober CG, Stevenson DK, Benitz WE: The use of antibiotics in neonates weighing less than 1200 grams. *Pediatr Infect Dis J* 1990;9:111.
- Reed MD, Myers CM, Yamashita TS, Blumer JL: Developmental pharmacology and therapeutics of piperacillin in gram-negative infections. *Dev Pharmacol Ther* 1986;9:102.
- Placzek M, Whitelaw A, Want S, et al: Piperacillin in early neonatal infection. *Arch Dis Child* 1983;58:1006-1009.
- Product Information, Abraxis Pharmaceutical Products, 2006

PIPERACILLIN-TAZOBACTAM

DOSE & ADMINISTRATION: 50 to 100 mg/kg per dose (as piperacillin component) IV infusion by syringe pump over 30 minutes. To use dosing chart, please refer to explanatory note in "How to Use This Book."

DOSING INTERVAL CHART

PMA (weeks)	PostNatal (days)	Interval (hours)
≥29	0 to 28 >28	12 8
30 to 36	0 to 14 >14	12 8
37 to 44	0 to 7 >7	12 8
≥45	ALL	8

USES: Treatment of non-CNS infections, caused by susceptible beta-lactamase producing bacteria, including many strains of *E. coli, Enterobacter, Klebsiella, Haemophilus influenzae, Proteus mirabilis, Pseudomonas spp.,* and *Staph. aureus.* Also effective against group *B Streptococcus.*

MONITORING: Observe IV site for signs of extravasation.

ADVERSE EFFECTS/PRECAUTIONS: Eosinophilia. Hyperbilirubinemia. Elevations in ALT, AST, BUN, and serum creatinine.

PHARMACOLOGY: Zosyn® combines the extended-spectrum antibiotic piperacillin with the beta-lactamase inhibitor tazobactam in a 8:1 ratio. Piperacillin is primarily eliminated unchanged by renal mechanisms, whereas tazobactam undergoes significant hepatic metabolism. The mean half-life of piperacillin and tazobactam in neonates is approximately 1.5 hours. CNS penetration is modest (limited data). Sodium content is 2.35 mEq per gram of piperacillin.

SPECIAL CONSIDERATIONS/PREPARATION: Available as powder for injection (containing EDTA and sodium citrate) in 2.25-g, 3.375-g, and 4.5-g vials. Reconstitute 2.25-g vial with 10 mL of sterile water for injection to make a concentration of 200 mg/mL pipercillin. Reconstituted solution stable for 24 hours at room temperature, 48 hours refrigerated. pH 4.5 to 6.8. Each 2.25-g vial contains 2.79 mEq (64 mg) of sodium per gram of piperacillin. Dilute reconstituted solution further to a final concentration of 50 mg/mL (some sources recommend 20 mg/mL) using compatible solution.

Solution Compatibility: D_5W, $D_{10}W$, NS and LR.

Terminal Injection Site Compatibility: Dex/AA solutions, fat emulsion. Aminophylline, aztreonam, bumetanide, calcium gluconate, cefepime, cimetidine, clindamycin, dexamethasone, dopamine, enalaprilat, esmolol, fluconazole, furosemide, heparin, hydrocortisone succinate, linezolid, lorazepam, metoclopramide, metronidazole, milrinone, morphine, potassium chloride, ranitidine, remifentanil, sodium bicarbonate, trimethoprim-sulfamethoxazole, and zidovudine.

Incompatibility: Acyclovir, amikacin, amiodarone, amphotericin B, azithromycin, dobutamine, famotidine, ganciclovir, gentamicin, netilmicin, tobramycin, and vancomycin.

SELECTED REFERENCES

- Pillay T, Pillay DG, Adhikari M, Sturn AW: Piperacillin/tazobactam in the treatment of Klebsiella pneumoniae infections in neonates. *Am J Perinatol* 1998;15:47-51.
- Reed MD, Goldfarb J, Yamashita TS, Blumer JL: Single dose pharmacokinetics of piperacillin and tazobactam in infants and children. *Antimicrob Agents Chemother* 1994;38:2817-26.
- Schoonover L, Occhipinti D, Rodvold K, et al: Piperacillin/tazobactam: A new beta-lactam/beta-lactamase inhibitor combination. *Ann Pharmacother* 1995;29:501-14.
- Prober CG, Stevenson DK, Benitz WE: The use of antibiotics in neonates weighing less than 1200 grams. *Pediatr Infect Dis J* 1990;9:111.
- Product Information, Wyeth, 2007

PNEUMOCOCCAL 7-VALENT CONJUGATE VACCINE

DOSE & ADMINISTRATION: 0.5 mL IM in the anterolateral thigh. Please refer to the most recent AAP/ACIP immunization schedule. Shake vial vigorously before withdrawing dose. **Do not mix with other vaccines. When giving multiple vaccines, use a separate syringe for each and give at different sites.** Care should be taken to draw back on the plunger of the syringe before injection to be certain the needle is not in a blood vessel.

USES: Immunoprophylaxis against invasive disease caused by *S. pneumoniae*.

MONITORING: Observe injection site for erythema, induration (common), palpable nodule (uncommon), or sterile abscess (rare). Fever (common) may be treated with acetaminophen. Other common, self-limiting, systemic effects are drowsiness, fretfulness, and anorexia.

ADVERSE EFFECTS/PRECAUTIONS: Hypersensitivity to any component of the vaccine, including diphtheria toxoid, is a contraindication to the vaccine.

PHARMACOLOGY: Prevnar® is a sterile solution of saccharides of the capsular antigens of *Streptococcus pneumoniae* serotypes 4, 6B, 9V, 14, 18C, 19F, and 23F individually conjugated to diphtheria CRM $_{197}$ protein. The seven serotypes account for over 80% of invasive pneumococcal disease in children in the United States. Eighty percent of penicillin-nonsusceptible strains in the United States are one of these 7 serotypes. Each dose contains 0.125 mg aluminum as aluminum phosphate adjuvant.

SPECIAL CONSIDERATIONS/PREPARATION: Prevnar® is supplied in 0.5-mL single-dose vials and single-dose syringes. After being shaken vigorously, it should appear as a homogeneous white suspension. The vaccine should not be used if it cannot be resuspended. Store refrigerated at 2 °C to 8 °C (36 °F to 46 °F). **Do not freeze.**

SELECTED REFERENCES

- American Academy of Pediatrics. Pneumococcal Infections. In: Pickering LK, Baker CJ, Long SS, McMillan JA, eds. *Red Book: 2006 Report of the Committee on Infectious Diseases.* 27th ed. Elk Grove Village, IL: American Academy of Pediatrics; 2006: pp 532-534.

- Advisory Committee on Immunization Practices: Recommendations of the ACIP. Most recent updates available on the National Immunization Program website: http://www.cdc.gov/nip/publications/acip-list.htm
- American Academy of Pediatrics, Committee on Infectious Diseases: Recommendations for the prevention of pneumococcal infections, including the use of pneumococcal conjugate vaccine (Prevnar®), pneumococcal polysaccharide vaccine, and antibiotic prophylaxis. *Pediatrics* 2000;106:362-366.
- Shinefield H, Black S, Ray P, et al: Efficacy, immunogenicity and safety of heptavalent pneumococcal conjugate vaccine in low birth weight and preterm infants. *Pediatr Infect Dis J* 2002;21:182-186.
- Product information, Wyeth Pharmaceuticals, 2007.

POLIOVIRUS VACCINE ENHANCED-INACTIVATED

DOSE & ADMINISTRATION: 0.5 mL injected **subcutaneously** in the midlateral thigh or IM in the anterolateral thigh. Immunize premature infants according to their postnatal age. Please refer to the most recent immunization schedule. **When giving multiple vaccines, use a separate syringe for each and give at different sites.** Care should be taken to draw back on the plunger of the syringe before injection to be certain the needle is not in a blood vessel.

USES: Inactivated poliovirus vaccine is now the only poliovirus vaccine available in the United States. Indications in other countries include hospitalized infants, and infants with contraindications for OPV (e.g. immunodeficiency, HIV-positive, those with immunodeficient contacts).

MONITORING: No specific monitoring required.

ADVERSE EFFECTS/PRECAUTIONS: Occasional reactions include erythema and tenderness at the injection site. Trace components may infrequently cause allergic reactions.

PHARMACOLOGY: Sterile suspension of types 1, 2, and 3 poliovirus inactivated with formaldehyde. The vaccine produced using a microcarrier culture technique of monkey kidney cells has enhanced potency. Contains traces of streptomycin, neomycin, and polymyxin B.

SPECIAL CONSIDERATIONS/PREPARATION: IPOL® (Sanofi Pasteur) is a clear, colorless suspension, available in 0.5 mL single-dose syringes and multidose vial. Do not use if the vaccine is turbid or discolored. Refrigerate at 2 °C to 8 °C (36 °F to 46 °F). **Do not freeze.**

SELECTED REFERENCES

- American Academy of Pediatrics. Poliovirus Infections. In: Pickering LK, Baker CJ, Long SS, McMillan JA, eds. *Red Book: 2006 Report of the Committee on Infectious Diseases.* 27th ed. Elk Grove Village, IL: American Academy of Pediatrics; 2006: pp 544-545.
- Advisory Committee on Immunization Practices: Recommendations of the ACIP. Most recent updates available on the National Immunization Program website: http://www.cdc.gov/nip/publications/acip-list.htm
- American Academy of Pediatrics, Committee on Infectious Diseases: Poliomyelitis prevention: recommendations for use of inactivated poliovirus vaccine and live oral poliovirus vaccine. *Pediatrics* 1997;99:300.
- Product information, Sanofi Pasteur, 2005

POTASSIUM CHLORIDE

DOSE & ADMINISTRATION: Initial oral replacement therapy: 0.5 to 1 mEq/kg per day divided and administered with feedings (small, more frequent aliquots preferred). Adjust dosage based on monitoring of serum potassium concentrations.

$$1 \text{ g KCl} = 13.4 \text{ mEq K}^+ \qquad 1 \text{ mEq K}^+ = 74.6 \text{ mg KCl}$$

Acute treatment of symptomatic hypokalemia: Begin with 0.5 to 1 mEq/kg IV over 1 hour, then reassess. Maximum concentration: 40 mEq/L for peripheral, 80 mEq/L for central venous infusions.

MONITORING: Continuous EKG monitoring is mandatory if administering by the IV route, especially for central infusions. Observe IV site closely for signs of extravasation when using concentrated solutions. Monitor serum potassium concentration. Assess for GI intolerance.

ADVERSE EFFECTS/PRECAUTIONS: Rapid IV infusions, especially those through central lines, may cause arrhythmias including heart block and cardiac arrest. Peripheral IV administration of concentrated potassium solutions is associated with thrombophlebitis and pain at the injection site. GI irritation is common—most commonly diarrhea, vomiting, and bleeding—minimized by dividing oral doses and administering with feedings. Use with caution (if at all) in patients receiving potassium-sparing diuretics, e.g. spironolactone.

PHARMACOLOGY: Potassium is the major intracellular cation. Hypokalemia in critically ill neonates is usually the result of diuretic (furosemide, thiazides) therapy or diarrhea. Other causes include congenital adrenal hyperplasia and renal disorders. Alkalosis, as well as insulin infusions, will lower serum potassium concentrations by driving the ion intracellularly. Symptoms of hypokalemia include neuromuscular weakness and paralysis, ileus, urine retention, and EKG changes (ST segment depression, low-voltage T wave, and appearance of U wave). Hypokalemia increases digitalis toxicity. Oral potassium preparations are completely absorbed.

SPECIAL CONSIDERATIONS/PREPARATION: Potassium chloride for injection is supplied as 2-mEq/mL solution. **Always dilute before administration.** Hyperosmolar - 4355 mOsm/kg determined by freezing-point depression. pH ranges from 4 to 8 depending on buffering. Various oral solutions are available, with concentrations ranging from 10 to 40 mEq per 15 mL. Other oral forms available include powder packets, tablets, and sustained-release capsules.

Solution Compatibility: Most standard IV solutions.

Terminal Injection Site Compatibility: Most drugs.

Incompatibility: Amphotericin B, diazepam, and phenytoin.

SELECTED REFERENCES

• Satlin LM, Schwartz GJ: Disorders of potassium metabolism, in Ichikawa I (ed): *Pediatric Textbook of Fluids and Electrolytes.* Baltimore: Williams & Wilkins, 1990, p 227.
• Morgan BC: Rapidly infused potassium chloride therapy in a child. *JAMA* 1981;245:2446.
• DeFronzo RA, Bia M: Intravenous potassium chloride therapy. *JAMA* 1981;245:2446.

Procainamide

DOSE & ADMINISTRATION: Initial bolus dose: 7 to 10 mg/kg IV over 1 hour via syringe pump. **Maintenance IV infusion:** 20 to 80 mcg/kg per minute. Premature neonates should receive the lowest dose.

USES: Acute treatment of supraventricular tachycardia (SVT) refractory to vagal maneuvers and adenosine. Acute treatment of ventricular tachycardia unresponsive to cardioversion and adenosine. Ectopic tachycardia, junctional ectopic tachycardia, and atrial flutter. Consider obtaining expert consultation before use.

MONITORING: Continuous monitoring of the EKG, blood pressure and heart rate. Measure procainamide and N-acetyl procainamide (NAPA) concentrations at 2, 12, and 24 hours after starting the loading dose infusion. **Therapeutic concentrations:** Procainamide: 4-10 mcg/mL, NAPA 6 to 20 mcg/mL. Sum of procainamide and NAPA: 10-30 mcg/mL.

ADVERSE EFFECTS/PRECAUTIONS: Severe hypotension with rapid infusion, bradycardia, A-V block, and ventricular fibrillation have been reported in adult patients. Normal procainamide concentrations widen the QRS complex due to slowing of conduction in the Purkinje system and ventricular muscle. The drug should be discontinued if the QRS duration increases by more than 35 to 50 percent to avoid serious toxicity. Adverse effects are reversible with discontinuation of drug.

PHARMACOLOGY: Procainamide is a class IA antiarrhythmic agent that increases the effective refractory period of the atria and the ventricles of the heart. Onset of action occurs within minutes of starting the loading dose. Half-life is approximately 5 hours in the term neonate, and longer in preterms. Metabolized primarily in the liver to N-acetylprocainamide (NAPA), an active metabolite. The rate of acetylation is primarily genetically determined in adults and children. Preterm neonates have a higher NAPA:procainamide ratio than term infants presumably due to delayed excretion of NAPA. Renal function is a significant determinant of procainamide clearance. Cimetidine and amiodarone interact when given with procainamide, increasing procainamide serum levels.

SPECIAL CONSIDERATIONS/PREPARATION: Available in 10-mL vials providing 100 mg/mL or 2-mL vials providing 500 mg/mL. Store at room temperature. **DO NOT FREEZE.** Dilute initial bolus dose to a final concentration of 20 mg/mL and administer over 1 hour. Maintenance infusion should be diluted to 2 mg/mL before administration.

Solution Compatibility: 0.45% NaCl and NS.

Solution Incompatibility: All dextrose containing solutions.

Terminal Injection Site Compatibility: Amiodarone, dobutamine, famotidine, flumazenil, heparin, hydrocortisone, lidocaine, netilmicin, ranitidine, and sodium nitroprusside.

Incompatibility: Esmolol, milrinone, and phenytoin.

SELECTED REFERENCES

• Moffett BS, Cannon BC, Friedman RA, Kertesz NJ: Therapeutic levels of intravenous procainamide in neonates: A retrospective assessment. *Pharmacotherapy* 2006;26:1687-1693.

• Wong KK, Potts JE, Ethridge SP, Sanatani S: Medications used to manage supraventricular tachycardia in the infant: a North American survey. *Pediatr Cardiol* 2006;27:199-203.

• Bryson SM, Leson CL, Irwin DB, et al: Therapeutic monitoring and pharmacokinetic evaluation of procainamide in neonates. *DICP* 1991;25:68-71.

• Product Information, Hospira, 2004

PROPRANOLOL

DOSE & ADMINISTRATION: Starting oral dose: 0.25 mg/kg per dose Q6 hours. Increase as needed to maximum of 3.5 mg/kg per dose Q6 hours. **Starting IV dose:** 0.01 mg/kg Q6 hours over 10 minutes. Increase as needed to maximum of 0.15 mg/kg per dose Q6 hours. Effective dosage requirements will vary significantly.

USES: Treatment of tachyarrhythmias and hypertension. Preferred therapy for SVT if associated with Wolff-Parkinson-White syndrome. Palliation of tetralogy of Fallot and hypertrophic obstructive cardiomyopathy. Adjunctive treatment of neonatal thyrotoxicosis.

MONITORING: Continuous EKG monitoring during acute treatment of arrhythmias and during IV therapy. Measure systemic blood pressure frequently. Measure blood glucose during initiation of treatment and after dosage changes. Assess for increased airway resistance.

ADVERSE EFFECTS/PRECAUTIONS: Adverse effects are related to beta-receptor blockade: Bradycardia, bronchospasm, and hypoglycemia are most frequently reported. Hypotension occurs in patients with underlying myocardial dysfunction. Contraindicated in patients with reactive airway disease or diminished myocardial contractility. A withdrawal syndrome (nervousness, tachycardia, sweating, hypertension) has been associated with sudden cessation of the drug.

PHARMACOLOGY: Propranolol is the most widely used nonselective β-adrenergic-receptor blocking agent. Peak serum concentration is reached approximately 2 hours after an oral dose. Propranolol undergoes significant first-pass hepatic metabolism, resulting in 30% to 40% bioavailability. Protein binding is 70% in neonates. Serum half-life is prolonged in patients with liver disease. Elimination is by renal excretion of metabolites.

SPECIAL CONSIDERATIONS/PREPARATION: Oral solutions are available in concentrations of 4 mg/mL and 8 mg/mL. Injectable form is available in 1-mL ampules containing 1 mg. Make a 0.1 mg/mL dilution by adding 1 ampul to 9 mL preservative-free normal saline. **Protect from light.** Store at room temperature.

Solution Compatibility: D_5W and NS.

Terminal Injection Site Compatibility: Alteplase, dobutamine, heparin, hydrocortisone succinate, linezolid, milrinone, morphine, potassium chloride, and propofol.

SELECTED REFERENCES

• Schneeweiss A: Neonatal cardiovascular pharmacology, in Long WA (ed): *Fetal and Neonatal Cardiology.* Baltimore: WB Saunders Co, 1990, p 675.

• Pickoff AS, Zies L, Ferrer PL, et al: High-dose propranolol therapy in the management of supraventricular tachycardia. *J Pediatr* 1979;94:144.

• Gillette P, Garson A, Eterovic E, et al: Oral propranolol treatment in infants and children. *J Pediatr* 1978;92:141.

• Product Information, Roxane, 2007

PROTAMINE

DOSE & ADMINISTRATION: Time since last heparin dose in minutes and protamine dose: < 30 min: 1 mg/100 units heparin received. 30 to 60 min: 0.5 to 0.75 mg/100 units heparin received. 60 to 120 min: 0.375 to 0.5 mg/100 units heparin received. > 120 min: 0.25 to 0.375 mg/100 units heparin received. **Maximum dose:** 50 mg **Infusion rate:** should not exceed 5 mg/min

USES: Heparin antagonist.

MONITORING: Monitor vital signs, clotting functions, and blood pressure continuously. Observe for bleeding.

ADVERSE EFFECTS/PRECAUTIONS: Excessive doses can cause serious bleeding problems. Hypotension, bradycardia, dyspnea, and transitory flushing have been reported in adults. Risk factors for severe protamine adverse reactions include high doses, rapid administration, repeated doses, previous exposure to protamine or protamine-containing insulins, severe left ventricular dysfunction, and abnormal preoperative pulmonary hemodynamics.

PHARMACOLOGY: Anticoagulant when given alone. Combines ionically with heparin to form a stable complex devoid of anticoagulant activity. Rapid action after IV use (5 minutes).

SPECIAL CONSIDERATIONS/PREPARATION: Available as a 10-mg/mL concentration preservative-free in 5- and 25-mL vials. Store at room temperature. Can be diluted in D_5W or NS.

    Solution Compatibility: D_5W and NS. No data are currently available on Dex/AA.

    Terminal Injection Site Compatibility: Cimetidine and ranitidine.

SELECTED REFERENCES

• Monagle P, Chan A, Massicotte P, et al: Antithrombotic therapy in children: the seventh ACCP conference on antithrombotic and thrombolytic therapy. *Chest* 2004;126:645-687.
• Product Information, Abraxis, 2007

PYRIDOXINE

DOSE & ADMINISTRATION: Initial diagnostic dose: 50 to 100 mg IV push, or IM. **Maintenance dose:** 50 to 100 mg PO Q24 hours. High doses may be required during periods of intercurrent illness.

USES: Diagnosis and treatment of pyridoxine-dependent seizures.

MONITORING: When possible, initial administration of pyridoxine should be accompanied by EEG monitoring.

ADVERSE EFFECTS/PRECAUTIONS: Risk of profound sedation. Ventilator support may be necessary.

PHARMACOLOGY: Pyridoxine-dependent seizures are a result of defective binding of pyridoxine in the formation of GABA (an inhibitory neurotransmitter). Administration of pharmacologic doses of pyridoxine will correct this GABA deficiency.

SPECIAL CONSIDERATIONS/PREPARATION: Injectable form available in concentration of 100 mg/mL (1 mL in 2-mL vial). May use injectable form orally; mix in simple syrup if desired. **Protect from light.**

    Solution Incompatibility: Alkaline solutions. No data are currently available on Dex/AA.

    Terminal Injection Site Compatibility: Fat emulsion.

    Incompatibility: Iron salts and oxidizing agents. No data are currently available on heparin and potassium chloride.

SELECTED REFERENCES

• Gospe SM: Current perspectives on pyridoxine-dependent seizures. *J Pediatr* 1998;132:919-923.
• Gordon N: Pyridoxine dependency: An update. *Dev Med Child Neurol* 1997;39:63.
• Mikati MA, Trevathan E, Krishnamoorthy KS, Lombroso CT: Pyridoxine-dependent epilepsy: Investigations and long-term followup. *Electroencephalogr Clin Neurophysiol* 1991;78:215
• Kroll JS: Pyridoxine for neonatal seizures: An unexpected danger. *Dev Med Child Neurol* 1985;27:369.
• Bankier A, Turner M, Hopkins IJ: Pyridoxine-dependent seizures: A wider clinical spectrum. *Arch Dis Child* 1983;58:415.
• Product Information, Abraxis, 2006

QUINUPRISTIN/DALFOPRISTIN

DOSE & ADMINISTRATION: 7.5 mg/kg/dose Q12 hours by IV infusion over 60 minutes. Administration via a central catheter is recommended.

USES: Limited to treatment of infections caused by gram positive organisms resistant to other antibiotics, e.g. methicillin-resistant *Staph. aureus* and vancomycin-resistant *Enterococcus faecium* (not *E faecalis*).

MONITORING: Periodic measurement of serum bilirubin and transaminases. Assess peripheral IV site for signs of inflammation.

ADVERSE EFFECTS/PRECAUTIONS: Myalgias and arthralgias occur frequently in adults with hepatic or renal failure. Elvations in serum bilirubin and transaminases are common. Diarrhea and rash occur infrequently.

PHARMACOLOGY: No data are available for infants. Synercid® is a parenteral antimicrobial agent which consists of two streptogramin antibiotics (quinupristin and dalfopristin in a 30:70 ratio) that inhibit bacterial protein synthesis by binding to separate sites on the bacterial ribosome. Serum half-life of quinupristin in adults ranges from 1 to 3 hours, and of dalfopristin ranges from 5 to 9 hours. 75% is excreted via the biliary route.

SPECIAL CONSIDERATIONS/PREPARATION: Synercid® is supplied as a lyophilized powder in single-dose, 10-mL vials containing 500 mg. Store refrigerated. Reconstitute under aseptic conditions by adding 5 mL of Sterile Water for Injection or D_5W. Before administration, dilute with D_5W to a concentration not exceeding 2 mg/mL. Diluted solution is stable for 5 hours at room temperature, or 54 hours if stored under refrigeration. **Do not freeze.**

   Solution Compatibility: D_5W.

   Solution Incompatibility: NS.

   Terminal Injection Site Compatibility: Aztreonam, ciprofloxacin, fluconazole, metoclopramide, and potassium chloride.

SELECTED REFERENCES
- Loeffler AM, Drew RH, Perfect JR, et al: Safety and efficacy of quinupristin/dalfopristin for treatment of invasive Gram-positive infections in pediatric patients. *Pediatr Infect Dis J* 2002;21:950-56.
- Gray JW, Darbyshire PJ, Beath SV, et al: Experience with quinupristin/dalfopristin in treating infections with vancomycin-resistant *Enterococcus faecium* in children. *Pediatr Infect Dis J* 2000;19:234-238.
- Lamb HM, Figgitt DP, Faulds D; Quinupristin/Dalfopristin: A review of its use in the management of serious gram-positive infections. *Drugs* 1999;58:1061-1097.
- Product Information, Monarch Pharmaceuticals, 2004.

RANITIDINE

DOSE & ADMINISTRATION: PO: 2 mg/kg per dose Q8 hours. **IV:** Term: 1.5 mg/kg per dose Q8 hours slow push. Preterm: 0.5 mg/kg per dose Q12 hours slow push. **Continuous IV infusion:** 0.0625 mg/kg per hour.

USES: Prevention and treatment of stress ulcers and GI hemorrhage aggravated by gastric acid secretion.

MONITORING: Gastric pH may be measured to assess efficacy.

ADVERSE EFFECTS/PRECAUTIONS: One case report of thrombocytopenia. No other adverse effects have been reported in infants or children. Elevations in hepatic enzymes, leukopenia, and bradycardia have been reported in adults.

PHARMACOLOGY: Inhibits gastric acid secretion by histamine H_2-receptor antagonism. Peak serum concentration occurs 1 to 3 hours after oral administration and is not influenced by food. Bioavailability is quite variable. Hepatic biotransformation predominates after oral absorption, with 30% excreted unchanged in the urine. In contrast, 70% of an IV dose is excreted unchanged in the urine. Elimination half-life in neonates is 3 to 7 hours, and is prolonged in preterm infants and patients with renal or hepatic insufficiency.

SPECIAL CONSIDERATIONS/PREPARATION: Available as a 1 mg/mL preservative-free solution for injection in 50 mL single-dose plastic containers, and a 25 mg/mL injectable solution in 2- and 6-mL vials. A 2 mg/mL dilution may be made by adding 0.8 mL of the 25 mg/mL concentration to 9.2 mL preservative-free sterile water or normal saline for injection. Stable for 48 hours at room temperature. May be given orally; absorption is equivalent to that of the oral solution. Manufacturer's oral solution (15 mg/mL) contains 7.5% alcohol. Also available as 150- and 300-mg tablets. May prepare oral solution by crushing a 150-mg tablet and dissolving in 30 mL of sterile water to yield a final concentration of 5 mg/mL. Stable for 28 days refrigerated.

Solution Compatibility: D_5W, $D_{10}W$, and NS.

Terminal Injection Site Compatibility: Dex/AA solutions, fat emulsion. Acyclovir, acetazolamide, amikacin, aminophylline, ampicillin, atropine, aztreonam, cefazolin, cefepime, cefoxitin, ceftazidime, chloramphenicol, clindamycin, dexamethasone, digoxin, dobutamine, dopamine, enalaprilat, epinephrine, erythromycin lactobionate, fentanyl, fluconazole, flumazenil, furosemide, gentamicin, glycopyrrolate, heparin, insulin, isoproterenol, lidocaine, linezolid, lorazepam, meropenem, metoclopramide, midazolam, milrinone, morphine, nicardipine, nitroprusside, pancuronium bromide, penicillin G, piperacillin, piperacillin-tazobactam, potassium chloride, propofol, prostaglandin E_1, protamine, remifentanil, tobramycin, vancomycin, vecuronium, vitamin K_1, and zidovudine.

Incompatibility: Amphotericin B, pentobarbital, phenobarbital, and phenytoin.

SELECTED REFERENCES

- Kuusela A-L: Long term gastric pH monitoring for determining optimal dose of ranitidine for critically ill preterm and term neonates. *Arch Dis Child Fetal Neonatal Ed* 1998;78:F151-F153.
- Kelly EJ, Chatfield SL, Brownlee KG, et al: The effect of intravenous ranitidine on the intragastric pH of preterm infants receiving dexamethasone. *Arch Dis Child* 1993;69:37.
- Fontana M, Massironi E, Rossi A, et al: Ranitidine pharmacokinetics in newborn infants. *Arch Dis Child* 1993;68:602.
- Sutphen JL, Dillard VL: Effect of ranitidine on twenty-four-hour gastric acidity in infants. *J Pediatr* 1989;114:472.
- Grant SM, Langtry HD, Brogden RN: Ranitidine: An updated review of its pharmacodynamic and pharmacokinetic properties and therapeutic use in peptic ulcer disease and other allied diseases. *Drugs* 1989;37:801.
- Product Information, GlaxoSmithKline, 2007

RIFAMPIN

DOSE & ADMINISTRATION: PO: 10 to 20 mg/kg per dose Q24 hours. May administer with feedings. **IV:** 5 to 10 mg/kg per dose Q12 hours, given via syringe pump over 30 minutes. **Do not administer IM or SC. Prophylaxis for high-risk contacts of invasive meningococcal disease:** 5 mg/kg per dose PO Q12 hours, for 2 days. **Prophylaxis for high-risk contacts of invasive H influenzae type b disease:** 10 mg/kg per dose PO Q24 hours, for 4 days.

USES: Used in combination with vancomycin or aminoglycosides for treatment of persistent staphylococcal infections. Prophylaxis against infections caused by N meningitidis and H influenzae type b.

MONITORING: Monitor hepatic transaminases and bilirubin. Periodic CBC for thrombocytopenia. Observe IV site for signs of extravasation.

ADVERSE EFFECTS/PRECAUTIONS: Causes orange/red discoloration of body secretions (e.g. sweat, urine, tears, sputum). Extravasation may cause local irritation and inflammation. Rifampin in a potent inducer of several cytochrome P450 enzymes. If administered concomitantly, the following drugs may have decreased pharmacologic effects due to increased metabolism: aminophylline, amiodarone, ecimetidine, corticosteroids, digoxin, enalapril, fluconazole, midazolam, morphine, phenobarbital, phenytoin, propranolol, and zidovudine.

PHARMACOLOGY: Rifampin is a semisynthetic antibiotic with a wide spectrum of antibacterial activity against staphylococci, most streptococci, H influenzae, Neisseria sp., Legionella, Listeria, some Bacteroides species, Mycobacterium tuberculosis, and certain atypical mycobacterium. Enterococci and aerobic gram-negative bacilli are generally resistant. Not used as monotherapy because resistance may develop during therapy. Inhibits transcription of DNA to RNA by binding to the beta subunit of bacterial RNA-polymerase. Well absorbed orally. Rapidly deacetylated to desacetylrifampin (active metabolite) and undergoes enterohepatic circulation. Nearly all of the rifampin excreted into the bile is deacetylated within 6 hours. Serum half-life ranges from 1 to 3 hours.

SPECIAL CONSIDERATIONS/PREPARATION: Available as a lyophilized powder for injection in 600-mg vials. Reconstitute with 10 mL of sterile water for injection to make a final concentration of 60 mg/mL. Reconstituted solution is stable for 24 hours at room temperature. Further dilution is required - maximum concentration for infusion is 6 mg/mL. A 3 mg/mL dilution may be made by adding 0.5 mL of reconstituted solution to 9.5 mL of NS or D_5W. Dilution made with NS is stable for 24 hours at room temperature. Dilution made with D_5 W is stable for 4 hours at room temperature. Do not use if solution precipitates. A neonatal suspension may be prepared by mixing 5 mL (300 mg) of the reconstituted IV solution with 25 mL of simple syrup to make a final concentration of 10 mg/mL. Shake well before use. Suspension is stable for 4 weeks at room temperature or refrigerated. Also available in 150- and 300-mg capsules. Preparation of oral suspension using capsules yields variable dosage bioavailability.

Solution Compatibility: D_5W and NS. No data available on Dex/AA or fat emulsion.

Terminal Injection Site Compatibility: No data available.

SELECTED REFERENCES

- Sharma A, Patole SK, Whitehall JS: Intravenous rifampicin in neonates with persistent staphylococcal bacteraemia. *Acta Paediatr* 2002;91:670-673.
- Fernandez M, Rench MA, Albanyan EA, Edwards MS: Failure of rifampin to eradicate group B streptococcal colonization in infants. *Pediatr Infect Dis J* 2001;20:371-376.
- Tan TQ, Mason EO, Ou C-N, et al: Use of intravenous rifampin in neonates with persistent staphylococcal bacteremia, *Antimicrob Agents Chemother* 1993;37:2401.
- Koup JR, William-Warren J, Viswanathan CT, et al: Pharmacokinetics of rifampin in children. II. Oral bioavailability. *Ther Drug Monit* 1986;8:17.
- Koup JR, William-Warren J, Weber A, et al: Pharmacokinetics of rifampin in children. I. Multiple dose intravenous infusion. *Ther Drug Monit* 1986;8:11.
- McCracken GH, Ginsburg CM, Zweighaft TC, et al: Pharmacokinetics of rifampin in infants and children: relevance to prophylaxis against Haemophilus influenzae type B disease. *Pediatrics* 1980;66:17
- Nahata MC, Morosco RS, Hipple TF: Effect of preparation method and storage on rifampin concentration in suspensions. *Ann Pharmacother* 1994;28:182.
- Product Information, Bedford, 2004

ROTAVIRUS VACCINE

DOSE & ADMINISTRATION: 2 mL per dose. FOR ORAL USE ONLY. NOT FOR INJECTION. To administer the vaccine: 1) Tear open the pouch and remove the dosing tube. 2) Clear the fluid from the dispensing tip by holding tube vertically and tapping cap. 3) Puncture the dispensing tip by screwing cap *clockwise* unitl it becomes tight, then remove the cap by turning it *counterclockwise*. 4) Administer dose by gently squeezing liquid into infant's mouth toward the inner cheek until dosing tube is empty. If for any reason an incomplete dose is administered (e.g., infant spits or regurgitates the vaccine), a replacement dose is NOT recommended, since this was not studied in the clinical trials.The first dose should be given between 6 and 12 weeks of age, and the 2 subsequent doses at 4 to 10 weeks intervals. The third dose should be given at no later than 32 weeks of age due to lack of safety and efficacy data in infants after this age. Please refer to the most recent AAP/ACIP immunization schedule.

USES: Immunoprophylaxis against rotavirus gastroenteritis caused by serotypes G1, G2, G3, and G4.

ADVERSE EFFECTS/PRECAUTIONS: Data from the phase III efficacy trials (n = 71725) did not suggest an increased risk of intussusception relative to placebo. However, the Food and Drug Administration (FDA) notified health care providers and consumers on February 13, 2007 about 28 post-marketing reports of intussusception following administration of RotaTeq®. According to the FDA, approximately 3.5 million doses of RotaTeq® were distributed in the United States as of February 1, 2007. Intussusception can occur spontaneously in the absence of vaccination and its cause is usually unknown. Of the 28 reported cases of intussusception, it is not known how many, if any, were vaccine-related. However, the number of intussusception cases reported to date after RotaTeq® administration does not exceed the number expected based on background rates of 18-43 per 100,000 per year for an unvaccinated population of children ages 6 to 35 weeks. RotaTeq® or placebo was administered to 2,070 pre-term infants (25 to 36 weeks gestational age, median 34 weeks) according to their age in weeks since birth. Safety and efficacy were similar as for full term infants.

PHARMACOLOGY: RotaTeq® is a bovine-based pentavalent vaccine containing 5 live reassortant rotaviruses. The rotavirus parent strains of the reassortants were isolated from human and bovine hosts. Four reassortant rotaviruses express 1 of the outer capsid proteins (G1, G2, G3, or G4) from the human rotavirus parent strain and the attachment protein (P7(5)) from the bovine rotavirus parent strain. The fifth reassortant virus expresses the attachment protein (P1A(8)) from the human rotavirus parent strain and the outer capsid protein G6 from the bovine rotavirus parent strain. The reassortants are suspended in a buffered stabilizer solution. Each vaccine dose contains sucrose, sodium citrate, sodium phosphate monobasic monohydrate, sodium hydroxide, polysorbate 80, cell-culture media, and trace amounts of fetal bovine serum. There are no preservatives or thimerosal. Fecal shedding of vaccine virus occurred in 32 (8.9%) of 360 subjects after dose 1, 0 (0%) of 249 subjects after dose 2, and 1 (0.3%) of 385 subjects after dose 3. In phase III studies, shedding was observed as early as 1 day and as late as 15 days after a dose. The potential for transmission of vaccine virus was not assessed through epidemiologic studies. RotaTeq® can be coadministered with other childhood vaccines. It has 98% efficacy for prevention of severe illness and 74% for prevention of rotavirus-induced diarrheal episodes.

SPECIAL CONSIDERATIONS/PREPARATION: RotaTeq® is supplied as a suspension for oral use in individually pouched single-dose tubes. Each dosage tube contains 2 mL. It is a pale yellow clear liquid that may have a pink tint. Store and transport refrigerated. Protect from light. Administer as soon as possible after being removed from refrigeration. Discard in approved biological waste containers.

SELECTED REFERENCES

- American Academy of Pediatrics, Committee on Infectious Diseases. Prevention of rotavirus disease: guidelines for use of rotavirus vaccine. *Pediatrics* 2007;119:171181.
- Centers for Disease Control and Prevention. Postmarketing monitoring of intussusception after RotaTeq® vaccination - United States, February 1, 2006-February 15, 2007. *MMWR* 2007; 56(10):218-222.
- Parashar UD, Alexander JP, Glass RI; Advisory Committee on Immunization Practices (ACIP), Centers for Disease Control and Prevention (CDC). Prevention of rotavirus gastroenteritis among infants and children: recommendations of the Advisory Committee on Immunization Practices. *MMWR Recomm Rep.* 2006;55(RR-12):113.
- Product information, Merck & Co., 2007.

SILDENAFIL

DOSE & ADMINISTRATION: 0.3 to 1 mg/kg per dose via orogastric tube every 6 to 12 hours. Some authors have successfully used doses of 2 mg/kg.

USES: Limited to treatment of patients with persistent pulmonary hypertension refractory to inhaled nitric oxide and other conventional therapies, those who are persistently unable to be weaned off of inhaled nitric oxide, or in situations where nitric oxide is not available. It has also been reported to improve pulmonary blood flow in patients with severe Ebstein's anomaly.

MONITORING: Continuous monitoring of blood pressure and oxygenation.

ADVERSE EFFECTS/PRECAUTIONS: Use in neonates should be restricted and considered experimental. Data in neonates are very limited. The most concerning short term adverse effects are worsening oxygenation and systemic hypotension. There is one case report of bleeding after circumcision in a neonate receiving chronic therapy. Use with caution in infants with sepsis. Sildenafil causes transient impairment of color discrimination in adults, and there is concern that it could increase the risk of severe retinopathy of prematurity.

PHARMACOLOGY: Sildenafil is a selective phosphodiesterase (PDE5) inhibitor. This inhibition leads to accumulation of cyclic GMP in pulmonary smooth muscle cells, causing pulmonary vascular relaxation. It may also potentiate the effect of inhaled nitric oxide. Oral absorption is rapid in adults with approximately 40% bioavailability; peak concentrations are reached in 30 to 120 minutes. It is metabolized primarily by hepatic CYP3A4 to an active metabolite (N-desmethyl sildenafil) that has PDE5 inhibitory activity. Both sildenafil and the metabolite have terminal half-lives of 4 hours in adults. Patients with significant hepatic or renal dysfunction have reduced clearance. Significant increases in sildenafil concentrations may occur when used concomitantly with drugs that are CYP3A4 inhibitors: e.g., erythromycin, amilodipine, and cimetidine.

SPECIAL CONSIDERATIONS/PREPARATION: Revatio® is supplied as 20 mg tablets; Viagra® is supplied as 25 mg, 50 mg, and 100 mg tablets. To prepare an oral suspension, thoroughly crush one tablet into a fine powder and add enough Ora-Plus to make a final concentration of 2 mg/mL. Suspension is stable for 1 month if refrigerated.

SELECTED REFERENCES

- Gamboa D, Robbins D, Saba Z: Bleeding after circumcision in a newborn receiving sildenafil. *Clin Pediatr* 2007;46:842-43.
- Noori S, Friedlich P, Wong P, et al: Cardiovascular effects of sildenafil in neonates and infants with congenital diaphragmatic hernia and pulmonary hypertension. *Neonatology* 2007;91:92-100.
- Baquero H, Soliz A, Neira F, et al: Oral sildenafil in infants with persistent pulmonary hypertension of the newborn: a pilot randomized blinded study. *Pediatrics* 2006;117:1077-1083.
- Nahata MC, Morosco RS, Brady MT: Extemporaneous sildenafil citrate oral suspensions for the treatment of pulmonary hypertension in children. *Am J Health-Syst Pharm* 2006;63:254-257.
- Baquero H, Neira F, Venegas V, et al: Outcome at 18 months of age after sildenafil therapy for refractory neonatal hypoxemia. Poster at 2005 PAS Annual Meeting, Abstract 2119.
- Pham P, Hoyer A, Shaughnessy R, Law YM: A novel approach incorporating sildenafil in the management of symptomatic neonates with Ebstein's anomaly. *Pediatr Cardiol* 2006;27:614-617.
- Travadi JN, Patole SK: Phosphodiesterase inhibitors for persistent pulmonary hypertension of the newborn: a review. *Pediatr Pulmonol* 2003;36:529-535.
- Atz AM, Wessel DL: Sildenafil ameliorates effects of inhaled nitric oxide withdrawal. *Anesthesiology* 1999;91:307-310.
- Product Information, Pfizer, 2008

SODIUM BICARBONATE

DOSE & ADMINISTRATION: Usual dosage: 1 to 2 mEq/kg IV over at least 30 minutes. **Dosage based on base deficit:** HCO_3 needed (mEq) = HCO_3 deficit (mEq/L) x (0.3 x body wt (kg)) Administer half of calculated dose, then assess need for remainder. **Maximum concentration used: 0.5 mEq/mL.** Dilute if desired. Can also be administered by continuous IV infusion or PO.

USES: Treatment of documented metabolic acidosis. Treatment of bicarbonate deficit caused by renal or GI losses. Use of sodium bicarbonate during brief CPR is discouraged, but may be useful during prolonged arrests after adequate ventilation is established and there is no response to other therapies.

MONITORING: Follow acid/base status, ABGs.

ADVERSE EFFECTS/PRECAUTIONS: Rationale against use in resuscitation:
1) Rapid infusion of hypertonic solution is linked to IVH.
2) When administered during inadequate ventilation, PCO_2 increases, thereby decreasing pH.
3) Carbon dioxide diffuses more readily across cell membranes than bicarbonate, thereby decreasing intracellular pH.

Other adverse effects: Local tissue necrosis, hypocalcemia, and hypernatremia.

PHARMACOLOGY: Rationale for use in prolonged resuscitation:
1) Decreases pulmonary vasculature resistance.
2) Improves myocardial function.
3) Increases response of myocardium to sympathomimetics.

SPECIAL CONSIDERATIONS/PREPARATION: Supplied by many manufacturers in multiple concentrations: 4% (0.48 mEq/mL), 4.2% (0.5 mEq/mL), 7.5% (0.9 mEq/mL) and 8.4% (1 mEq/mL). Maximum concentration used in neonates is 0.5 mEq/mL. May dilute with sterile water for injection. Do not infuse with calcium or phosphate containing solutions - precipitation will occur.

OSMOLARITY

Concentration (%)	Concentration (mEq/mL)	Approximate Osmolarity (mOsm/L)
8.4	1	1800
4.2	0.5	900
2.8	0.33	600
2.1	0.25	450

Solution Compatibility: D_5W, $D_{10}W$, and NS.

Terminal Injection Site Compatibility: Fat emulsion. Acyclovir, amikacin, aminophylline, amphotericin B, ampicillin, atropine, aztreonam, cefepime, cefoxitin, ceftazidime, ceftriaxone, chloramphenicol, cimetidine, clindamycin, dexamethasone, erythromycin lactobionate, esmolol, famotidine, fentanyl, furosemide, heparin, hyaluronidase, hydrocortisone succinate, indomethacin, insulin, lidocaine, linezolid, meropenem, milrinone, morphine, nafcillin, netilmicin, penicillin G, pentobarbital, phenobarbital, phenytoin, piperacillin-tazobactam, potassium chloride, propofol, remifentanil, vancomycin, and vitamin K_1.

Incompatibility: Dex/AA. Amiodarone, calcium chloride, calcium gluconate, cefotaxime, ciprofloxacin, dobutamine, dopamine, epinephrine, glycopyrrolate, imipenem/cilastatin, isoproterenol, magnesium sulfate, methadone, methicillin, metoclopramide, midazolam, mivacurium, nicardipine, norepinephrine, oxacillin, ticarcillin/clavulanate, and vecuronium.

SELECTED REFERENCES

• van Alfen-van der Velden AA, Hopman JC, Klaessens JH, et al: Effects of rapid versus slow infusion of sodium bicarbonate on cerebral hemodynamics and oxygenation in preterm infants. *Biol Neonate* 2006;90:122-127.
• Lokesh L, Kumar P, Murki S, Narang A. A randomized controlled trial of sodium bicarbonate in neonatal resuscitation - effect on immediate outcome. *Resuscitation* 2004;60:219-23.
• Murki M, Kumar P, Lingappa L, Narang A. Effect of a single dose of sodium bicarbonate given during neonatal resuscitation at birth on the acid-base status on first day of life. *Journal of Perinatology* 2004;24:696-9.
• Ammari AN, Schulze KF: Uses and abuses of sodium bicarbonate in the neonatal intensive care unit. *Curr Opin Pediatr* 2002;14:151-156.
• Wyckoff MH, Perlman J, Niermeyer S: Medications during resuscitation - what is the evidence? *Semin Neonatol* 2001;6:251-259.
• Howell JH: Sodium bicarbonate in the perinatal setting—revisited. *Clin Perinatol* 1987;14:807.

SODIUM NITROPRUSSIDE

DOSE & ADMINISTRATION: Initial Dose: 0.25 to 0.5 mcg/kg per minute continuous IV infusion by syringe pump. Use a large vein for IV. Titrate dose upward Q20 minutes until desired response is attained. Usual **maintenance dose** is < 2 mcg/kg per minute. For hypertensive crisis, may use up to 10 mcg/kg per minute, but for no longer than 10 minutes. Sodium thiosulfate has been coadministered with sodium nitroprusside to accelerate the metabolism of cyanide; however, this has not been extensively studied.

USES: Acute treatment of hypertensive emergencies. Acute afterload reduction in patients with refractory congestive heart failure.

MONITORING: Continuous heart rate and intra-arterial blood pressure monitoring is mandatory. Daily measurement of RBC cyanide (should be less than 200 ng/mL) and serum thiocyanate (should be less than 50 mcg/mL) concentrations. Assess frequently for development of metabolic acidosis. Daily assessment of renal and hepatic function. Monitor IV site closely.

ADVERSE EFFECTS/PRECAUTIONS: Severe hypotension and tachycardia. Cyanide toxicity may occur with prolonged treatment (> 3 days) and high (>3 mcg/kg per minute) doses. Use with caution in liver and renal failure patients due to possible impairment of the metabolism of cyanide to thiocyanate. Extravasation can cause tissue sloughing and necrosis.

PHARMACOLOGY: Direct-acting nonselective (arterial and venous) vasodilator. Immediately interacts with RBC oxyhemoglobin, dissociating and forming methemoglobin with release of cyanide and nitric oxide. Rapid onset of action with a serum half-life of 3 to 4 minutes in adults. Further metabolized to thiocyanate in the liver and kidney. Thiocyanate is renally eliminated with a half-life of 4 to 7 days.

SPECIAL CONSIDERATIONS/PREPARATION: Available as powder for injection in 2 mL single-dose 50 mg vials. Reconstitute contents of vial with 2 to 3 mL of D_5W or NS. **Do not administer reconstituted drug directly from vial.** Dilute entire vial contents to a final concentration less than or equal to 200 mcg/mL (0.2 mg/mL) in D_5W or NS. Use within 24 hours of preparation. **Protect from light** with aluminum foil or other opaque material. Blue, green or deep red discoloration indicates nitroprusside inactivation. Slight brownish discoloration is common and not significant.

Solution Compatibility: D_5W and NS only.

Terminal Injection Site Compatibility: Fat emulsion. Aminophylline, caffeine citrate, calcium chloride, cimetidine, dobutamine, dopamine, enalaprilat, epinephrine, esmolol, famotidine, furosemide, heparin, indomethacin, insulin, isoproterenol, lidocaine, magnesium, midazolam, milrinone, morphine, nicardipine, nitroglycerin, pancuronium, potassium chloride, procainamide, propofol, prostaglandin E$_1$, ranitidine, and vecuronium.

Incompatibility: Amiodarone.

SELECTED REFERENCES

- Seto W, Trope A, Carfrae L, et al: Visual compatibility of sodium nitroprusside with other injectable medications given to pediatric patients. *Am J Health-Syst Pharm* 2001;58:1422-6.
- Friederich JA, Butterworth JF: Sodium nitroprusside: Twenty years and counting. *Anesth Analg* 1995;81:152.
- Benitz WE, Malachowski N, Cohen RS, et al: Use of sodium nitroprusside in neonates: Efficacy and safety. *J Pediatr* 1985;106:102.
- Roberts RJ: *Drug Therapy in Infants.* Philadelphia: WB Saunders Co, 1984, p 184.
- Dillon TR, Janos GG, Meyer RA, et al: Vasodilator therapy for congestive heart failure. *J Pediatr* 1980;96:623.
- Product Information, Hospira, 2004

SOTALOL

DOSE & ADMINISTRATION: Initial dose: 1 mg/kg per dose PO Q12 hours. Gradually increase as needed every 3 to 5 days until stable rhythm is maintained. **Maximum dose:** 4 mg/kg per dose PO Q12 hours.

USES: Treatment of refractory ventricular and supraventricular tachyarrhythmias.

MONITORING: Frequent EKG during initiation of therapy.

ADVERSE EFFECTS/PRECAUTIONS: Proarrhythmic effects occur in 10% of pediatric patients: sinoatrial block, A-V block, torsades de pointes and ventricular ectopic activity. These effects usually occur in the first few days of treatment. Prolongation of the QT interval is dose-dependent. Other adverse effects include fatigue, dyspnea, and hypotension.

PHARMACOLOGY: Sotalol is an antiarrhythmic agent that combines Class II beta-blocking properties with Class III prolongation of cardiac action potential duration. Betapace® is a racemic mixture of d- and l-sotalol. Oral bioavailability is good, but absorption is decreased by 20 to 30% by food, especially milk. Sotalol does not bind to plasma proteins, is not metabolized, and is renally excreted as unchanged drug. Limited pharmacokinetic data in infants show a half-life of 8 hours, increasing significantly in elderly patients and those with renal dysfunction.

SPECIAL CONSIDERATIONS/PREPARATION: Supplied in 80-mg, 120-mg, 160-mg, and 240-mg tablets. A 5 mg/mL oral suspension may be made as follows: crush 5 (five) 120-mg tablets, slowly mix in 84 mL of 1% methylcellulose, then add enough simple syrup to make a total volume of 120 mL. Stable for 60 days when kept refrigerated.

SELECTED REFERENCES

- Saul JP, Schaffer MS, Karpawich PP, et al: Single dose pharmacokinetics of sotalol in a pediatric population with supraventricular and/or ventricular tachyarrhythmia. *J Clin Pharmacol* 2001;41:35-43.
- Pfammatter JP, Paul T, Lehmann C, Kallfelz HC: Efficacy and proarrhythmia of oral sotalol in pediatric patients. *J Am Coll Cardiol* 1995;26:1002.
- Tanel RE, Walsh EP, Lulu JA, and Saul JP: Sotalol for refractory arrhythmias in pediatric and young adult patients: Initial efficacy and long-term outcome. *Am Heart J* 1995;130:791.
- Hohnloser SH, Woosley RL: Sotalol. *N Engl J Med* 1994;331:31.
- Nappi JM, McCollam PL: Sotalol: A breakthrough antiarrhythmic? *Ann Pharmacother* 1993;27:1359.
- Maragnes P, Tipple M, Fournier A: Effectiveness of oral sotalol for treatment of pediatric arrhythmias. *Am J Cardiol* 1992;69:751.
- Product Information, Berlex, 2004

SPIRONOLACTONE

DOSE & ADMINISTRATION: 1 to 3 mg/kg per dose Q24 hours PO.

USES: Used in combination with other diuretics in the treatment of congestive heart failure and BPD (situations of increased aldosterone secretion).

MONITORING: Follow serum potassium closely during long-term therapy. Also, measuring urinary potassium is a useful indicator of effectiveness.

ADVERSE EFFECTS/PRECAUTIONS: Rashes, vomiting, diarrhea, paresthesias. Dose-dependent androgenic effects in females. Gynecomastia in males. Headaches, nausea, and drowsiness. Use with caution in patients with impaired renal function. May cause false positive ELISA screening tests for congenital adrenal hyperplasia.

SUCROSE

PHARMACOLOGY: Competitive antagonist of mineralocorticoids (e.g. aldosterone). Metabolized to canrenone and 7-a-thiomethylspironolactone, active metabolites with extended elimination half-lives. Decreases excretion of potassium. Highly protein bound. Increases excretion of calcium, magnesium, sodium, and chloride (small effect). Serum half-life with long term use is 13 to 24 hours. Addition of spironolactone to thiazide diuretic therapy in patients with BPD may yield little, if any, additional benefit.

SPECIAL CONSIDERATIONS/PREPARATION: Available in 25-mg, 50-mg, and 100-mg tablets. A simple syrup suspension can be made by crushing eight 25-mg spironolactone tablets and suspending the powder in 50 mL of simple syrup. Final concentration is 4 mg/mL; solution is stable for 1 month refrigerated.

SELECTED REFERENCES

* Brion LP, Primhak RA, Ambrosio-Perz I: Diuretics acting on the distal renal tubule for preterm infants with (or developing) chronic lung disease (Cochrane Review). In: The Cochrane Library Issue 1, 2003. Oxford: Update Software.
* Hoffman DJ, Gerdes JS, Abbasi S: Pulmonary function and electrolyte balance following spironolactone treatment in preterm infants with chronic lung disease: a double-blind, placebo-controlled randomized trial. J Perinatol 2000;20:41-45.
* Terai I, Yamano K, Ichihara N, et al: Influence of spironolactone on neonatal screening for congenital adrenal hyperplasia. Arch Dis Child Fetal Neonatal Ed 1999;81;F179.
* Mathur LK, Wickman A: Stability of extemporaneously compounded spironolactone suspensions. Am J Hosp Pharm 1989;46:2040.
* Overdiek HW, Hermens WA, Merkus FW: New insights into the pharmacokinetics of spironolactone. Clin Pharmacol Ther 1985;38:469.
* Karim A: Spironolactone: Disposition, metabolism, pharmacodynamics, and bioavailability. Drug Metab Rev 1978;8:151.
* Loggie JMH, Kleinman LI, Van Maanen EF: Renal function and diuretic therapy in infants and children. Part II. J Pediatr 1975;86:657.
* Product Information, Actavis, 2006

SUCROSE

DOSE & ADMINISTRATION: Administer orally 2 minutes prior to the painful procedure by using a pacifier dipped in the sweet solution, up to a maximum of 2 mL. 0.5 mL of 24% sucrose is equivalent to 0.12 grams of sucrose. Other solutions containing 50% sucrose and artificial sweetener have also been shown to be effective.

USES: Mild analgesia and behavioral comforting.

MONITORING: Assess for signs of pain and discomfort.

ADVERSE EFFECTS/PRECAUTIONS: Sucrose 24% has an osmolarity of ≈1000 mOsm/L. The adverse effects of repeated doses in premature infants are unknown.

SPECIAL CONSIDERATIONS/PREPARATION: Sweet-Ease®, a 24% sucrose and water solution, is aseptically packaged in an 15 ml cup with a peel off lid that is suitable for dipping a pacifier or for administration via a dropper.

SELECTED REFERENCES

* Stevens B, Yamada J, Ohlsson A: Sucrose for analgesia in newborn infants undergoing painful procedures (Cochrane Review). In: The Cochrane Library, Issue 1, 2003. Oxford Update Software.
* Abad F, Diaz-Gomez NM, Domenech E, et al: Oral sucrose compares favorably with lidocaine-prilocaine cream for pain relief during venepuncture in neonates. Acta Paediatr 2001;90:160-165.
* Blass EM, Watt LB: Suckling and sucrose-induced analgesia in human newborns. Pain 1999;83:611-623.
* Bucher H-U, Moser T, Von Siebenthal K, et al: Sucrose reduces pain reaction to heel lancing in preterm infants: A placebo-controlled, randomized and masked study. Pediatr Res 1995;38:332-335.
* Product Information, Sweetease® website: http://sweetease.respironics.com/

SURFACTANT (NATURAL, ANIMAL-DERIVED)

DOSE & ADMINISTRATION: See specific products (beractant, calfactant, or poractant alfa) for dosing and administration information.

USES: Prophylaxis of infants at high risk for RDS (those < 29 weeks gestation). **Rescue** treatment of infants with moderate to severe RDS. **Treatment of mature infants with respiratory failure** due to meconium aspiration syndrome, pneumonia, or persistent pulmonary hypertension.

MONITORING: Assess ET tube patency and position. Oxygen saturation, EKG, and blood pressure should be monitored continuously during dosing. Assess for impairment of gas exchange caused by blockage of the airway. After dosing, frequent assessments of oxygenation and ventilation should be performed to prevent postdose hyperoxia, hypocarbia, and overventilation.

ADVERSE EFFECTS/PRECAUTIONS: Administration of exogenous surfactants should be restricted to highly supervised clinical settings, with immediate availability of clinicians experienced with intubation, ventilator management, and general care of premature infants. Reflux of exogenous surfactant up the ET tube and falls in oxygenation occur frequently. If the infant becomes dusky or agitated, heart rate slows, oxygen saturation falls more than 15%, or surfactant backs up in the ET tube, dosing should be slowed or halted. If necessary, ventilator settings and/or FiO_2 should be turned up. Pulmonary hemorrhage occurs in 2% to 4% of treated infants, primarily the smallest patients with untreated PDA. This may be due to hemorrhagic pulmonary edema caused by the rapid fall in pulmonary vascular resistance and resulting increased pulmonary blood flow.

PHARMACOLOGY: In infants with RDS, exogenous surfactant therapy reverses atelectasis and increases FRC, with rapid improvements in oxygenation. All preparations reduce mortality from RDS. Natural surfactants are more effective than synthetics in reducing pulmonary air leak. There are no significant differences between preparations in chronic lung disease or other long term outcomes. All commercially available preparations contain surfactant apoprotein C (SP-C), none contain SP-A. The lung-mince extracts Survanta® and Curosurf® contain less than 10% of the SP-B contained in the lung-wash extract Infasurf®.

SELECTED REFERENCES
REVIEW REFERENCES

- Suresh GK, Soll RF: Current surfactant use in premature infants. *Clin Perinatol* 2001;28:671-694.
- Rodriguez RJ, Martin RJ: Exogenous surfactant therapy in newborns. *Resp Care Clin North Am* 1999;5:595-616.
- Kattwinkel J: Surfactant: Evolving issues. *Clin Perinatol* 1998; 25:17-32.
- Morley CJ: Systematic review of prophylactic vs rescue surfactant. *Arch Dis Child* 1997;77:F70-F74.
- Halliday HL: Natural vs synthetic surfactants in neonatal respiratory distress syndrome. *Drugs* 1996;51:226-237.

SELECTED REFERENCES FOR NON-RDS INDICATIONS

- Lotze A, Mitchell BR, Bulas DI, et al: Multicenter study of surfactant (Beractant) use in the treatment of term infants with severe respiratory failure. *J Pediatr* 1998;132:40.
- Findlay RD, Taeusch HW, Walther FJ: Surfactant replacement therapy for meconium aspiration syndrome. *Pediatrics* 1996;97:48.

SURVANTA®

(BERACTANT) INTRATRACHEAL SUSPENSION

DOSE & ADMINISTRATION: 4 mL/kg per dose intratracheally, divided into 4 aliquots. **Prophylaxis:** First dose is given as soon as possible after birth, with up to three additional doses in the first 48 hours of life, if indicated. **Rescue treatment of RDS:** Up to four doses in first 48 hours of life, no more frequently than Q6 hours. Before administration, allow to stand at room temperature for 20 minutes, or warm in the hand for at least 8 minutes. **Artificial warming methods should not be used.** Shorten a 5F end-hole catheter so tip of catheter will protrude just beyond end of ET tube above infant's carina. Slowly withdraw entire contents of vial into a plastic syringe through a large (greater than 20 gauge) needle. **Do not filter or shake.** Attach shortened catheter to syringe. Fill catheter with Survanta. Discard excess Survanta through catheter so only total dose to be given remains in syringe. Administer four quarter-doses with the infant in different positions to enhance distribution. The catheter can be inserted into the infant's endotracheal tube through a neonatal suction valve without interrupting ventilation. Alternatively, Survanta® can be instilled through the catheter by briefly disconnecting the endotracheal tube from the ventilator. After administration of each quarter-dose, the dosing catheter is removed from the ET tube and the infant is ventilated for at least 30 seconds until stable.

PHARMACOLOGY: Survanta® is a modified natural bovine lung extract containing phospholipids, neutral lipids, fatty acids, and surfactant-associated proteins B and C, to which colfosceril palmitate (DPPC), palmitic acid, and tripalmitin are added. Resulting drug provides 25 mg/mL phospholipids (including 11 to 15.5 mg/mL DPPC), 0.5 to 1.75 mg/mL triglycerides, 1.4 to 3.5 mg/mL fatty acids, and less than 1 mg/mL protein.

THAM ACETATE

Survanta® is suspended in NS and heat sterilized. Animal metabolism studies show that most of a dose becomes lung-associated within hours of administration, and lipids enter endogenous surfactant pathways of reuse and recycling.

SPECIAL CONSIDERATIONS/PREPARATION: Available in 4- and 8-mL single-use vials. Refrigerate (2 °C to 8 °C (36 °F to 46 °F)) and protect from light. Inspect Survanta® for discoloration; normal color is off-white to light-brown. If settling occurs during storage, **swirl** vial gently. **Do not shake.** Vials should be entered only once. Used vials with residual drug should be discarded. Unopened vials that have been warmed to room temperature one time may be refrigerated within 24 hours and stored for future use. Should not be warmed and returned to the refrigerator more than once.

SELECTED REFERENCES

- Zola EM, Overbach AM, Gunkel JH, et al: Treatment investigational new drug experience with Survanta (beractant). *Pediatrics* 1993;91:546.
- Hoekstra RE, Jackson JC, Myers TF, et al: Improved neonatal survival following multiple doses of bovine surfactant in very premature neonates at risk for respiratory distress syndrome. *Pediatrics* 1991;88:10.
- Liechty EA, Donovan E, Purohit D, et al: Reduction of neonatal mortality after multiple doses of bovine surfactant in low birth weight neonates with respiratory distress syndrome. *Pediatrics* 1991;88:19.
- Product Information, Ross, 2004

THAM ACETATE

(TROMETHAMINE)

DOSE & ADMINISTRATION: 1 to 2 mmol/kg (3.3 to 6.6 mL/kg) per dose IV. Infuse in a large vein over at least 30 minutes. Dose (of the 0.3 M solution) may be calculated from the following formula:

Dose (mL) = Weight (kg) × Base deficit (mEq/L)

Maximum dose in neonates with normal renal function is approximately 5 to 7 mmol/kg per 24 hours. Clinical studies support only short term use.

USES: Treatment of metabolic acidosis, primarily in mechanically ventilated patients with significant hypercarbia or hypernatremia. **Do not use in patients who are anuric or uremic.** THAM is not indicated for treatment of metabolic acidosis caused by bicarbonate deficiency.

MONITORING: Observe IV site closely for signs of extravasation. Follow blood-gas results to assess therapeutic efficacy. Follow urine output. Monitor for respiratory depression, hypoglycemia, and hyperkalemia when using several doses.

ADVERSE EFFECTS/PRECAUTIONS: Most reports of toxicity in neonates (hypoglycemia, hyperkalemia, liver necrosis) were related to rapid umbilical venous infusion of high doses of THAM base solutions that were more alkaline and hypertonic than the THAM acetate solution currently available from Abbott (pH 8.6; osmolarity 380 mOsm/L). **Irritating to veins**.

PHARMACOLOGY: THAM (Tris-Hydroxymethyl Aminomethane) is a proton acceptor that generates NH_3^+ and HCO_3^- without generating CO_2. The protonated R-NH_3^+ is eliminated by the kidneys. Unlike bicarbonate, THAM does not require an open system for CO_2 elimination in order to exert its buffering effect.

SPECIAL CONSIDERATIONS/PREPARATION: Supplied as a 0.3-M solution (1 mmol = 3.3 mL) in a 500-mL single-dose container with no bacteriostatic agent. Intended for single-dose use and unused portion should be disgarded. **Compatibilities:** No data are currently available on solutions and additives.

SELECTED REFERENCES

- Holmdahl MH, Wiklund L, Wetterberg T, et al: The place of THAM in the management of acidemia in clinical practice. *Acta Anaethesiol Scand* 2000;44:524-527.
- Nahas GG, Sutin KM, Fermon C, et al: Guidelines for the treatment of acidemia with THAM. *Drugs* 1998;55:191-224. (Errata published 1998;55:517).
- Baum JD, Robertson NRC: Immediate effects of alkaline infusion in infants with respiratory distress syndrome. *J Pediatr* 1975;87:255.
- Strauss J: Tris (hydroxymethyl amino-methane (THAM)): A pediatric evaluation. *Pediatrics* 1968;41:667.

- Gupta JM, Dahlenburg GW, Davis JW: Changes in blood gas tensions following administration of amine buffer THAM to infants with respiratory distress syndrome. *Arch Dis Child* 1967;42:416-427.
- Product Information, Hospira, 2006

TICARCILLIN / CLAVULANATE

DOSE & ADMINISTRATION: 75 to 100 mg/kg per dose IV infusion by syringe pump over 30 minutes. To use dosing chart, please refer to explanatory note in "How to Use This Book."

DOSING INTERVAL CHART

PMA (weeks)	PostNatal (days)	Interval (hours)
≤29	0 to 28 >28	12 8
30 to 36	0 to 14 >14	12 8
37 to 44	0 to 7 >7	12 8
≥45	ALL	6

USES: Treatment of non-CNS infections, caused by susceptible β-lactamase producing bacteria, including many strains of *E. coli, Enterobacter, Klebsiella, Haemophilus influenzae, Proteus mirabilis, Pseudomonas* spp., and *Staph. aureus.*

MONITORING: Serum concentrations are not routinely monitored. Assess renal function prior to therapy. Measure serum sodium concentrations and hepatic transaminases periodically. Observe IV site for signs of extravasation.

ADVERSE EFFECTS/PRECAUTIONS: Eosinophilia. Hyperbilirubinemia. Elevations in ALT, AST, BUN, and serum creatinine. Hypernatremia may be exacerbated in ELBW patients.

PHARMACOLOGY: Timentin® combines the extended-spectrum antibiotic ticarcillin with the β-lactamase inhibitor clavulanic acid in a 30:1 ratio. Ticarcillin is primarily eliminated unchanged by renal mechanisms, whereas clavulanate undergoes significant hepatic metabolism. As a result the mean half-life of ticarcillin in neonates is 4.2 hours compared to a mean half-life of 2 hours for clavulanate. CNS penetration is modest (limited data). Sodium content is 4.75 mEq per gram, therefore each dose will contain 0.35 to 0.48 mEq per kg body weight.

SPECIAL CONSIDERATIONS/PREPARATION: Available as powder for injection in 3.1-g vials. Reconstitute vial by adding 13 mL of sterile water for injection. Dilute further with a compatible solution to a concentration between 10 and 100 mg/mL. Dilutions are stable for 24 hours at room temperature, 3 days refrigerated (D_5W), and 7 days refrigerated (NS and LR). Frozen dilutions stable for 7 days for D_5W and 30 days for NS and LR.

Solution Compatibility: D_5W, LR, and NS.

Terminal Injection Site Compatibility: Dex/AA solutions, fat emulsion. Acyclovir, aminophylline, aztreonam, cefepime, famotidine, fluconazole, heparin, insulin, milrinone, morphine, propofol, remifentanil, and theophylline.

Incompatibility: Amikacin, azithromycin, gentamicin, netilmicin, sodium bicarbonate, tobramycin, and vancomycin.

SELECTED REFERENCES

- Rubino CM, Gal P, Ransom JL: A review of the pharmacokinetic and pharmacodynamic characteristics of β-lactam/β-lactamase inhibitor combination antibiotics in premature infants. *Pediatr Infect Dis J* 1998;17:1200-1210.
- Reed MD: A reassessment of ticarcillin/clavulanic acid dose recommendations for infants, children, and adults. *Pediatr Infect Dis J* 1998;17:1195-1199.
- Product Information, GlaxoSmithKline, 2007

TOBRAMYCIN

DOSE & ADMINISTRATION: IV infusion by syringe pump over 30 minutes. Administer as a separate infusion from penicillin-containing compounds. IM injection is associated with variable absorption, especially in the very small infant. To use dosing chart, please refer to explanatory note in "How to Use This Book."

DOSING CHART

PMA (weeks)	Postnatal (days)	Dose (mg/kg)	Interval (hours)
≤29*	0 to 7	5	48
	8 to 28	4	36
	≥29	4	24
30 to 34	0 to 7	4.5	36
	≥8	4	24
≥35	ALL	4	24
* or significant asphyxia, PDA, or treatment with indomethacin			

USES: Treatment of infections caused by aerobic gram-negative bacilli (e.g. *Pseudomonas, Klebsiella, E coli*). Usually used in combination with a β-lactam antibiotic.

MONITORING: Measure serum concentrations when treating for more than 48 hours. Obtain peak concentration 30 minutes after end of infusion, and trough concentration just prior to the next dose. When treating patients with serious infections or significantly changing fluid or renal status consider measuring the serum concentration 24 hours after a dose, and use the chart below for the suggested dosing interval. Blood samples obtained to monitor serum drug concentrations should be spun and refrigerated or frozen as soon as possible. Therapeutic serum concentrations: **Peak:** 5 to 12 mcg/mL (or C_{max}/MIC ratio greater than 8:1) **Trough:** 0.5 to 1 mcg/mL To use dosing chart, please refer to explanatory note in "How to Use This Book."

SUGGESTED DOSING INTERVALS

Level at 24 hours (mcg/mL)	Half-life (hours)	Suggested Dosing Interval (hours)
≤1	≈8	24
1.1 to 2.3	≈12	36
2.4 to 3.2	≈15	48
≥3.3		Measure level in 24 hours

ADVERSE EFFECTS/PRECAUTIONS: Transient and reversible renal tubular dysfunction may occur, resulting in increased urinary losses of sodium, calcium, and magnesium. Vestibular and auditory ototoxicity. The addition of other nephrotoxic and/or ototoxic medications (e.g. furosemide, vancomycin) may increase these adverse effects. Increased neuromuscular blockade (i.e. neuromuscular weakness and respiratory failure) may occur when used with pancuronium or other neuromuscular blocking agents and in patients with hypermagnesemia.

PHARMACOLOGY: Dosing recommendations are based on: (1) Higher peak concentrations increase concentration-dependent bacterial killing; (2) There is a post-antibiotic effect on bacterial killing, especially when treating concurrently with a β-lactam antibiotic; (3) There may be less toxicity with less frequent dosing, due to less renal drug accumulation. Volume of distribution is increased and clearance is decreased in patients with PDA. Serum half-life is prolonged in premature and asphyxiated newborns. Inactivation of tobramycin by penicillin-containing compounds appears to be a time-, temperature-, and concentration-dependent process. This is probably clinically significant only when penicillin-containing compounds are mixed in IV solutions or when the blood is at room temperature for several hours before the assay is performed.

SPECIAL CONSIDERATIONS/PREPARATION: Pediatric injectable solution available in a concentration of 10 mg/mL.

Solution Compatibility: D_5W, $D_{10}W$, and NS.

Terminal Injection Site Compatibility: Dex/AA solutions, fat emulsion. Acyclovir, aminophylline, amiodarone, aztreonam, calcium gluconate, cefoxitin, ceftazidime, ciprofloxacin, clindamycin, dopamine, enalaprilat, esmolol, fluconazole, furosemide, insulin, heparin (concentrations ≤1 unit/mL), linezolid, metronidazole, midazolam, milrinone, morphine, nicardipine, ranitidine, remifentanil, theophylline, and zidovudine.

Incompatibility: Amphotericin B, ampicillin, azithromycin, cefepime, imipenem/cilastatin, indomethacin, heparin (concentrations >1 unit/mL), methicillin, mezlocillin, nafcillin, oxacillin, penicillin G, propofol, and ticarcillin/clavulanate.

SELECTED REFERENCES

• Contopoulos-Ioannidis DG, Giotis ND, Baliatsa DV, Ioannidis JPA: Extended-interval aminoglycoside administration for children: a meta-analysis. *Pediatrics* 2004;114:e111-e118.
• Avent ML, Kinney JS, Istre GR, Whitfield JM: Gentamicin and tobramycin in neonates: comparison of a new extended dosing regimen with a traditional multiple daily dosing regimen. *Am J Perinatol* 2002;8:413-19.
• de Hoog M, Schoemaker RC, Mouton JW, van den Anker JN: Tobramycin population pharmacokinetics in neonates. *Clin Pharmacol Ther* 1997;62:392-399.
• Giapros VI, Andronikou S, Cholevas VI, Papadopoulou ZL: Renal function in premature infants during aminoglycoside therapy. *Pediatr Nephrol* 1995;9:163.
• Daly JS, Dodge RA, Glew RH, et al: Effect of time and temperature on inactivation of aminoglycosides by ampicillin at neonatal dosages. *J Perinatol* 1997;17:42-45.
• Williams BS, Ransom JL, Gal P, et al: Gentamicin pharmacokinetics in neonates with patent ductus arteriosus. *Crit Care Med* 1997;25:273-275.
• Product Information, Hospira, 2005

TROPICAMIDE (OPHTHALMIC)

DOSE & ADMINISTRATION: 1 drop instilled in the eye at least 10 minutes prior funduscopic procedures. Use **only** the 0.5% ophthalmic solution in neonates. Apply pressure to the lacrimal sac during and for 2 minutes after instillation to minimize systemic absorption.

USES: Induction of mydriasis and cycloplegia for diagnostic and therapeutic ophthalmic procedures.

MONITORING: Monitor heart rate and assess for signs of ileus prior to feeding.

ADVERSE EFFECTS/PRECAUTIONS: Feedings should be withheld for 4 hours following procedure. Systemic effects are those of anticholinergic drugs: Fever, tachycardia, vasodilatation, dry mouth, restlessness, decreased gastrointestinal motility, and urinary retention. The use of solutions with concentrations of 1% or greater have caused systemic toxicity in infants.

PHARMACOLOGY: Anticholinergic drug that produces pupillary dilation by inhibiting the sphincter pupillae muscle, and paralysis of accommodation. Mydriasis begins within 5 minutes of instillation, cycloplegia occurs in 20 to 40 minutes. Recovery of accommodation occurs in 6 hours. Without lacrimal sac occlusion, approximately 80% of each drop may pass through the nasolacrimal system and be available for rapid systemic absorption by the nasal mucosa.

SPECIAL CONSIDERATIONS/PREPARATION: Supplied as ophthalmic solution in 0.5%, and 1% concentrations in 2-, 3-, and 15-mL dropper bottles. Store away from heat. **Do not refrigerate.** A combination eye drop solution ("Caputo drops") may be prepared in a 15-mL bottle with 3.75 mL of cyclopentolate 2%, 7.5 mL of tropicamide 1%, and 3.75 mL of phenylephrine 10%. The final solution contains cyclopentolate 0.5%, tropicamide 0.5%, and phenylephrine 2.5%. Use within 24 hours, as the solution contains no preservatives.

SELECTED REFERENCES

• Wallace DK, Steinkuller PG: Ocular medications in children. *Clin Pediatr* 1998;37:645-652.
• Laws DE, Morton C, Weindling M, Clark D: Systemic effects of screening for retinopathy of prematurity. *Br J Ophthalmol* 1996;80:425-428.
• McGregor MLK: Anticholinergic agents, in Mauger TF, Craig EL (eds): *Havener's Ocular Pharmacology*, ed 6. St. Louis: Mosby-YearBook, 1994, pp 148-155.

• Caputo AR, Schnitzer RE, Lindquist TD, Sun S: Dilation in neonates: a protocol. *Pediatrics* 1982;69:77-80.
• Product Information, Alcon, 2004

URSODIOL

DOSE & ADMINISTRATION: 10 to 15 mg/kg per dose Q 12 hours PO.

USES: Treatment of cholestasis associated with parenteral nutrition, biliary atresia, and cystic fibrosis. Also used to dissolve cholesterol gallstones.

MONITORING: Hepatic transaminases and direct bilirubin concentration.

ADVERSE EFFECTS/PRECAUTIONS: Nausea/vomiting, abdominal pain, constipation, and flatulence.

PHARMACOLOGY: Ursodiol is a hydrophobic bile acid that decreases both the secretion of cholesterol from the liver and its intestinal absorption. It is well absorbed orally. After conjugation with taurine or glycine, it then enters the enterohepatic circulation where it is excreted into the bile and intestine. It is hydrolyzed back to the unconjugated form or converted to lithocholic acid which is excreted in the feces. Serum half-life is 3 to 4 days in adults. Dissolution of gallstones may take several months. Aluminum-containing antacids bind ursodiol and inhibit absorption.

SPECIAL CONSIDERATIONS/PREPARATION: Available in 300-mg capsules. A liquid suspension may be made by opening ten (10) 300-mg capsules into a glass mortar. Mix this powder with 10 mL of glycerin and stir until smooth. Add 60 mL of Ora-Plus® to the mixture and stir. Transfer the contents of the mortar to a glass amber bottle and shake well. Add a small amount of Orange Syrup to the mortar and rinse. Pour the remaining contents into the amber glass bottle, then add enough simple syrup to make the final volume 120 mL, with a final concentration of 25-mg/mL. Shake vigorously. Mixture is stable for 60 days stored at room temperature or refrigerated.

SELECTED REFERENCES

• Chen C-Y, Tsao P-N, Chen H-L, et al: Ursodeoxycholic acid (UDCA) therapy in very-low-birth-weight infants with parenteral nutrition-associated cholestasis. *J Pediatr* 2004;145:317-321.
• Levine A, Maayan A, Shamir R, et al: Parenteral nutrition-associated cholestasis in preterm neonates: Evaluation of ursodeoxycholic acid treatment. *J Pediatr Endocrinol Metab* 1999;12:549-553.
• Balisteri WF: Bile acid therapy in pediatric hepatobiliary disease: the role of ursodeoxycholic acid. *J Pediatr Gastroenterol Nutr* 1997;24:573-89.
• Teitelbaum DH: Parenteral nutrition-associated cholestasis. *Curr Opin Pediatr* 1997;9:270-75.
• Mallett MS Hagan RL, Peters DA: Stability of ursodiol 25mg/mL in an extemporaneously prepared oral liquid. *Am J Health-Syst Pharm* 1997;54:1401.
• Spagnuolo MI, Iorio R, Vegnente A, Guarino A: Ursodeoxycholic acid for treatment of cholestasis in children. *Gastroenterol* 1996;111:716-719.
• Ward A, Brogden RN, Heel RC, et al: Ursodeoxycholic acid: A review of its pharmacological properties and therapeutic efficacy. *Drugs* 1984;27:95.

VANCOMYCIN

DOSE & ADMINISTRATION: IV infusion by syringe pump over 60 minutes. **Meningitis:** 15 mg/kg per dose **Bacteremia:** 10 mg/kg per dose To use dosing chart, please refer to explanatory note in "How to Use This Book."

DOSING INTERVAL CHART

PMA (weeks)	PostNatal (days)	Interval (hours)
≤29	0 to 14 >14	18 12
30 to 36	0 to 14 >14	12 8
37 to 44	0 to 7 >7	12 8
≤45	ALL	6

USES: Drug of choice for serious infections caused by methicillin-resistant staphylococci (e.g. *S aureus* and *S epidermidis*) and penicillin-resistant pneumococci.

MONITORING: Serum trough concentrations should be followed in neonates because of changes in renal function related to maturation and severity of illness. Peak concentrations have not been clearly demonstrated to correlate with efficacy, but monitoring these has been recommended when treating meningitis. **Trough:** 5 to 10 mcg/mL for most infections. Many experts recommend 15 to 20 mcg/mL when treating MRSA pneumonia, endocarditis, or bone/joint infections. **Peak:** 30 to 40 mcg/mL when treating meningitis. (Draw 30 minutes after end of infusion.) Assess renal function. Observe IV site for signs of extravasation and phlebitis.

ADVERSE EFFECTS/PRECAUTIONS: Nephrotoxicity and ototoxicity: Enhanced by aminoglycoside therapy. **Rash and hypotension (red man syndrome):** Appears rapidly and resolves within minutes to hours. Lengthening infusion time usually eliminates risk for subsequent doses. **Neutropenia:** Reported after prolonged administration (more than 3 weeks). **Phlebitis:** May be minimized by slow infusion and dilution of the drug.

PHARMACOLOGY: Vancomycin is bactericidal for most gram-positive bacteria, but bacteriostatic for enterococci. It interferes with cell wall synthesis, inhibits RNA synthesis, and alters plasma membrane function. Killing activity is primarily a time-dependent process, not concentration-dependent. MICs for sensitive organisms are ≤ 1 mcg/mL. Diffusion into the lung and bone is variable. CSF concentrations in premature infants ranged from 26 to 68% of serum concentrations. Protein binding is as high as 50% in adults. Elimination is primarily by glomerular filtration, with a small amount of hepatic metabolism.

SPECIAL CONSIDERATIONS/PREPARATION: Available as powder for injection in 500-mg and 1-g vials. Reconstitute 500-mg vial with 10 mL sterile water for injection to make a final concentration of 50 mg/mL. Reconstituted solution stable for 14 days refrigerated. Dilute prior to administration using D_5W or NS to a maximum concentration of 5 mg/mL.

Solution Compatibility: D_5W, $D_{10}W$, and NS.

Terminal Injection Site Compatibility: Dex/AA solutions, fat emulsion. Acyclovir, amikacin, ampicillin, aminophylline, amiodarone, aztreonam, caffeine citrate, calcium gluconate, cimetidine, enalaprilat, esmolol, famotidine, fluconazole, heparin (concentrations ≤ 1 unit/mL), hydrocortisone succinate, insulin, linezolid, lorazepam, meropenem, midazolam, milrinone, morphine, nicardipine, pancuronium bromide, potassium chloride, propofol, ranitidine, remifentanil, sodium bicarbonate, vecuronium, and zidovudine.

Incompatibility: Cefazolin, cefepime, cefotaxime, cefoxitin, ceftazidime, ceftriaxone, chloramphenicol, dexamethasone, heparin (concentrations >1 unit/mL), methicillin, mezlocillin, nafcillin, pentobarbital, phenobarbital, piperacillin, piperacillin-tazobactam, ticarcillin, and ticarcillin/clavulanate.

SELECTED REFERENCES

• Hidayat LK, Hsu DI, Quist R, et al: High-dose vancomycin therapy for methicillin-resistant *Staphylococcus aureus* infections. *Arch Intern Med* 2006;166:2138-2144.
• de Hoog M, Schoemaker RC, Mouton JW, van den Anker JN: Vancomycin population pharmacokinetics in neonates. *Clin Pharmacol Ther* 2000;67:360-367.
• Ahmed A: A critical evaluation of vancomycin for treatment of bacterial meningitis. *Pediatr Infect Dis J* 1997;16:895-903.
• Trissel LA, Gilbert DL, Martinez JF: Concentration dependency of vancomycin hydrochloride compatibility with beta-lactam antibiotics during simulated y-site administration. *Hosp Pharm* 1998;33:1515-1520.
• Reiter PD, Doron MW: Vancomycin cerebrospinal fluid concentrations after intravenous administration in premature infants. *J Perinatol* 1996;16:331-335.
• Schilling CG, Watson DM, McCoy HG, Uden DL: Stability and delivery of vancomycin hydrochloride when admixed in a total parenteral nutrition solution. *JPEN* 1989;13:63.
• Lacouture PG, Epstein MF, Mitchell AA: Vancomycin-associated shock and rash in newborn infants. *J Pediatr* 1987;111:615.
• Schaible DH, Rocci ML, Alpert GA, et al: Vancomycin pharmacokinetics in infants: Relationships to indices of maturation. *Pediatr Infect Dis* 1986;5:304.
• Product Information, Abraxis Pharmaceutical Products, 2006

VECURONIUM

DOSE & ADMINISTRATION: 0.1 mg/kg (0.03 to 0.15 mg/kg) IV push, as needed for paralysis. Usual dosing interval is 1 to 2 hours. Adjust dose as needed based on duration of paralysis.

USES: Skeletal muscle relaxation/paralysis in infants requiring mechanical ventilation. Proposed desirable effects are improved oxygenation/ ventilation, reduced barotrauma, and reduced fluctuations in cerebral blood flow.

MONITORING: Monitor vital signs frequently, blood pressure continuously. Use some form of eye lubrication.

ADVERSE EFFECTS/PRECAUTIONS: Hypoxemia may occur because of inadequate mechanical ventilation and deterioration in pulmonary mechanics. When used alone, cardiovascular side effects are minimal; however, decreases in heart rate and blood pressure have been observed when used concurrently with narcotics.

PHARMACOLOGY: Nondepolarizing muscle-relaxant that competitively antagonizes autonomic cholinergic receptors. Sympathetic stimulation is minimal. Vecuronium is metabolized rapidly in the liver to 3-desacetyl-vecuronium, which is 50% to 70% active, and is excreted renally. Newborns, particularly premature infants, are especially sensitive to vecuronium; this sensitivity diminishes with age. Onset of action is 1 to 2 minutes; duration of effect is prolonged with higher doses and in premature infants. Skeletal relaxation/paralysis is reversed by neostigmine and atropine. **Potentiation:** Acidosis, hypothermia, neuromuscular disease, hepatic disease, renal failure, cardiovascular disease, younger age, aminoglycosides, hypermagnesemia, and hypokalemia. **Antagonism:** Alkalosis, epinephrine, and hyperkalemia.

Sensation remains intact; analgesia should be used for painful procedures.

SPECIAL CONSIDERATIONS/PREPARATION: Available as powder for injection in 10-mg and 20-mg vials. After reconstitution- 24 hrs stability in refrigerator. Single use only, discard unused portion. After dilution, use within 24 hours after admixing. A 0.4-mg/mL dilution may be made by diluting 1 mL of 1-mg/mL concentration with 1.5 mL of preservative-free normal saline. Dilution is stable for 24 hours in refrigerator.

Solution Compatibility: D_5W, LR, and NS.

Terminal Injection Site Compatibility: Dex/AA solutions. Aminophylline, amiodarone, cefazolin, cefoxitin, cimetidine, ciprofloxacin, dobutamine, dopamine, epinephrine, esmolol, fentanyl, fluconazole, gentamicin, heparin, hydrocortisone succinate, isoproterenol, linezolid, lorazepam, midazolam, milrinone, morphine, nicardipine, nitroglycerin, nitroprusside, propofol, ranitidine, trimethoprim-sulfamethoxazole, and vancomycin.

Incompatibility: Diazepam, furosemide, and sodium bicarbonate.

SELECTED REFERENCES

- Martin LD, Bratton SL, O'Rourke P: Clinical uses and controversies of neuromuscular blocking agents in infants and children. *Crit Care Med* 1999;27:1358-1368.
- Segredo V, Matthay MA, Sharma ML, et al: Prolonged neuromuscular blockage after long-term administration of vecuronium in two critically ill patients. *Anesthesiology* 1990;72:566.
- Bhutani VK, Abbasi S, Sivieri EM: Continuous skeletal muscle paralysis: Effect on neonatal pulmonary mechanics. *Pediatrics* 1988;81:419.
- Gravlee GP, Ramsey FM, Roy RC, et al: Rapid administration of a narcotic and neuromuscular blocker: A hemodynamic comparison of fentanyl, sufentanil, pancuronium, and vecuronium. *Anesth Analg* 1988;67:39.
- Meretoja OA, Wirtavuori K, Neuvonen PJ: Age-dependence of the dose-response curve of vecuronium in pediatric patients during balanced anesthesia. *Anesth Analg* 1988;67:21.
- Costarino AT, Polin RA: Neuromuscular relaxants in the neonate. *Clin Perinatol* 1987;14:965.
- Product Information, Hospira, 2005

VI-DAYLIN® MULTIVITAMIN PRODUCTS

DOSE & ADMINISTRATION: 1 dropperful (1 mL) Q24 hours, or as directed by physician. Percentages of the Reference Daily Intakes (%RDIs) listed in the table below are for infants.

VI-DAYLIN® MULTIVITAMIN PRODUCTS

	Vi-Daylin® ADC Vitamin Drops		Vi-Daylin® ADC Vitamins + Iron Drops		Vi-Daylin® Multivitamin Drops		Vi-Daylin® Multivitamin + Iron Drops	
	Amt	(%RDI)	Amt	(%RDI)	Amt	(%RDI)	Amt	(%RDI)
Vitamins								
A (IU)	1350	(90)	1350	(90)	1350	(90)	1350	(90)
D (IU)	400	(100)	400	(100)	360	(90)	360	(90)
C (mg)	32	(90)	32	(90)	32	(90)	32	(90)
E (IU)					5	(90)	5	(90)
Thiamine (B_1) (mg)					0.4	(80)	0.5	(89)
Riboflavin (B_2) (mg)					0.5	(90)	0.5	(90)
Niacin (mg)					7	(90)	7	(90)
B_6 (mg)					0.4	(90)	0.4	(90)
B_{12} (mcg)					1.4	(68)		
Minerals								
Iron (mg)			9	60			9	(60)

VI-SOL® MULTIVITAMIN PRODUCTS

DOSE & ADMINISTRATION: 1 dropperful (1 mL) Q24 hours, or as directed by physician. Percentages of the Reference Daily Intakes (%RDIs) listed in the table below are for infants.

VI-SOL® PRODUCTS

	Tri-Vi-Sol® Multivitamin Drops		Tri-Vi-Sol® Multivitamin with Iron Drops		Poly-Vi-Sol® Multivitamin Drops		Poly-Vi-Sol® Multivitamin with Iron Drops	
	Amt	(%RDI)	Amt	(%RDI)	Amt	(%RDI)	Amt	(%RDI)
Vitamins								
A (IU)	1500	(100)	1500	(100)	1500	(100)	1500	(100)
D (IU)	400	(100)	400	(100)	400	(100)	400	(100)
C (mg)	35	(100)	35	(100)	35	(100)	35	(100)
E (IU)					5	(100)	5	(100)
Thiamine (B_1) (mg)					0.5	(100)	0.5	(100)
Riboflavin (B_2) (mg)					0.6	(100)	0.6	(100)
Niacin (mg)					8	(100)	8	(100)
B_6 (mg)					0.4	(100)	0.4	(100)
B_{12} (mcg)					2	(100)	2	(100)
Minerals								
Iron (mg)			10	(67)			10	(67)

Vᴵᴛᴀᴍᴵɴ **A**

(RETINYL PALMITATE)

DOSE & ADMINISTRATION: Parenteral treatment of Vitamin A deficiency: 5000 IU IM 3 times weekly for 4 weeks. Administer using 29-g needle and insulin syringe. **DO NOT ADMINISTER IV.**

USES: To reduce the risk of Chronic Lung Disease in high risk premature neonates with Vitamin A deficiency. In the NICHD-sponsored trial, 14 infants needed to be treated to prevent 1 case of Chronic Lung Disease.

MONITORING: Assess regularly for signs of toxicity: full fontanel, lethargy, irritability, hepatomegaly, edema, mucocutaneous lesions, and bony tenderness. Consider measuring plasma retinol concentrations if available, especially if patient is also receiving glucocorticoid therapy. Desired concentrations are approximately 30 to 60 mcg/dL. Concentrations <20 mcg/dL indicate deficiency, while those >100 mcg/dL are potentially toxic.

ADVERSE EFFECTS/PRECAUTIONS: See monitoring section. Coincident treatment with glucocorticoids should be avoided, as it significantly raises plasma vitamin A concentrations.

PHARMACOLOGY: The pulmonary histopathologic changes of BPD and Vitamin A deficiency are remarkably similar. Vitamin A is the generic name for a group of fat soluble compounds which have the biological activity of the primary alcohol, retinol. Retinol metabolites exhibit potent and site-specific effects on gene expression and on lung growth and development. Retinol is supplied in the diet as retinyl esters.

SPECIAL CONSIDERATIONS/PREPARATION: Available as Aquasol A® Parenteral (watermiscible vitamin A palmitate) 50,000 IU per mL, equivalent to 15 mg retinol per mL, in 2 mL vials. **Protect from light.** Store refrigerated at 36 to 46 °F (2 to 8 °C). Do not freeze.

SELECTED REFERENCES

- Tyson JE, Wright LL, Oh W, Kennedy K, et al: Vitamin A supplementation for extremely-low-birth-weight infants. *N Engl J Med* 1999;340:1962-68.
- Darlow BA, Graham PJ. Vitamin A supplementation for preventing morbidity and mortality in very low birthweight infants (Cochrane Review). In: *The Cochrane Library*, Issue 1, 2004. Chichester, UK: John Wiley & Sons, Ltd.
- Shenai JP: Vitamin A supplementation in very low birthweight neonates: rationale and evidence. *Pediatrics* 1999;104:1369-74.
- Product information, Mayne, 2005

Vᴵᴛᴀᴍᴵɴ **E**

(DL-ALPHA-TOCOPHEROL ACETATE)

DOSE & ADMINISTRATION: 5 to 25 IU per day PO. Dilute with feedings. Do not administer simultaneously with iron—iron absorption is impaired.

USES: Prevention of vitamin E deficiency. May be indicated in babies receiving erythropoietin and high iron dosages. Higher doses used to reduce oxidant-induced injury (ROP, BPD, IVH) remain controversial.

MONITORING: Assess feeding tolerance. Signs of vitamin E deficiency include hemolytic anemia and thrombocytosis. Physiologic serum vitamin E concentrations are between 0.8 and 3.5 mg/dL.

ADVERSE EFFECTS/PRECAUTIONS: Feeding intolerance may occur due to hyperosmolarity of preparation. Pharmacologic doses of alpha tocopherol have been associated with increased rates of sepsis (antioxidant effect of drug) and NEC (osmolarity of oral formulation).

PHARMACOLOGY: Alpha-tocopherol is the most active antioxidant of the group of tocopherols known as Vitamin E. The amount required by the body is primarily dependent upon the dietary intake of fat, especially polyunsaturated fatty acids (PUFA). Human milk and currently available infant formulas contain adequate Vitamin E and have appropriate E:PUFA ratios to prevent hemolytic anemia. Infants receiving supplemental iron amounts above 2 mg/kg/day may also require additional Vitamin E. Oral absorption of vitamin E is dependent upon hydrolysis that requires bile salts and pancreatic esterases. This can be quite variable in very immature infants and those with fat malabsorption. Free tocopherol is absorbed in the small intestine, taken via chylomicrons into the gastrointestinal lymphatics, then carried via low-density lipoproteins to be incorporated into cell membranes. Significant tissue accumulation may occur with pharmacologic doses.

SPECIAL CONSIDERATIONS/PREPARATION: Available as liquid drops: Aquavit E® (Cypress Pharmaceutical), 15 IU (=15 mg) per 0.3 mL. Water solubilized with polysorbate 80. Also contains propylene glycol. Hyperosmolar (3620 mOsm/kg H_2O). Store at controlled room temperature.

SELECTED REFERENCES

- Gross SJ: Vitamin E. In Tsang RC, Lucas A, Uauy R, Zlotkin S (eds): *Nutritional Needs of the Preterm Infant: Scientific Basis and Practical Guidelines.* Pauling, New York: Caduceus Medical Publishers, 1993, pp 101-109.
- Roberts RJ, Knight ME: Pharmacology of vitamin E in the newborn. *Clin Perinatol* 1987;14:843-855.
- Raju TNK, Langenberg P, Bhutani V, Quinn GE: Vitamin E prophylaxis to reduce retinopathy of prematurity: A reappraisal of published trials. *J Pediatr* 1997;131:844-850.

VITAMIN K₁

DOSE & ADMINISTRATION: Recommended Prophylaxis: 0.5 to 1 mg IM at birth. **Preterm infants <32 weeks gestation: BW >1000 grams:** 0.5 mg IM. **BW <1000 grams:** 0.3 mg/kg IM. **Alternate strategy for healthy, term, exclusively breast-fed infants:** 2 mg PO with the first feed, at 1 week, 4 weeks, and 8 weeks of age. ***Note:** there is no approved oral formulation in the United States. Oral prophylaxis is contraindicated in infants who are premature, ill, on antibiotics, have cholestasis, or have diarrhea. There has been an increased number of cases of hemorrhagic disease of the newborn in countries that have changed to oral prophylaxis, primarily in patients who received only a single oral dose. Also: Maternal daily intake of 5 mg/day of phylloquinone significantly increases Vitamin K concentrations in breastmilk and infant plasma. **Treatment of severe hemorrhagic disease:** 1 to 10 mg IV slow push. (See Adverse Effects/Precautions for rate of administration.)

USES: Prophylaxis and therapy of hemorrhagic disease of the newborn. Treatment of hypoprothrombinemia secondary to factors limiting absorption or synthesis of vitamin K₁.

MONITORING: Check prothrombin time when treating clotting abnormalities. (A minimum of 2 to 4 hours is needed for measurable improvement.)

ADVERSE EFFECTS/PRECAUTIONS: Severe reactions, including death, have been reported with IV administration in adults. These reactions are extremely rare, and have resembled anaphylaxis and included shock and cardiac/respiratory arrest. **With IV administration, give very slowly, not exceeding 1 mg per minute, with physician present.** Pain and swelling may occur at IM injection site. Efficacy of treatment with vitamin K₁ is decreased in patients with liver disease. The risk of childhood cancer is not increased by IM administration of vitamin K₁. **Note:** A box warning statement in the AquaMEPHYTON® product information states that intramuscular administration "should be restricted to those situations where the subcutaneous route is not feasible and the serious risk is considered justified". However, this does not apply to newborns, and the American Academy of Pediatrics recommends the single intramuscular dose at birth as above. The product information labeling reflects this recommended newborn dosing.

PHARMACOLOGY: Vitamin K₁ (phytonadione) promotes formation of the following clotting factors in the liver: active prothrombin (factor II), proconvertin (factor VII), plasma thromboplastin component (factor IX), and Stuart factor (factor X). Vitamin K₁ does **not** counteract the anticoagulant action of heparin.

SPECIAL CONSIDERATIONS/PREPARATION: Available as a 2 mg/mL aqueous dispersion in 0.5-mL ampules and 10 mg/mL aqueous dispersion in 1-mL ampules and 2.5- and 5-mL vials. Contains 0.9% (9 mg/mL) benzyl alcohol as a preservative. *** **Efficacy with giving this preparation orally is uncertain.** *** **Protect from light.**

　Solution Compatibility: D_5W, $D_{10}W$, and NS.

　Terminal Injection Site Compatibility: Dex/AA. Amikacin, ampicillin, dobutamine, chloramphenicol, cimetidine, epinephrine, famotidine, heparin, hydrocortisone succinate, netilmicin, potassium chloride, ranitidine, and sodium bicarbonate.

　Incompatibility: Phenytoin.

ZIDOVUDINE (ZDV, AZT)

SELECTED REFERENCES

- American Academy of Pediatrics Committee on Nutrition: Vitamins. In: *Pediatric Nutrition Handbook.* 5th ed. Elk Grove Village, Il: American Academy of Pediatrics 2004: pp 350-51.
- Costakos DT, Greer FR, Love LA, et al: Vitamin K prophylaxis for premature infants: 1 mg versus 0.5 mg. *Am J Perinatol* 2003;20:485-90.
- American Academy of Pediatrics, Committee on Fetus and Newborn: Controversies concerning vitamin K and the newborn. *Pediatrics* 2003;112:191-92.
- Kumar D, Greer FR, Super DM, et al: Vitamin K status of premature infants: implications for current recommendations. *Pediatrics* 2001;108:1117-1122.
- Fiore LD, Scola MA, Cantillon CE, Brophy MT: Anaphylactoid reactions to Vitamin K. *J Thromb Thrombolysis* 2001;11:175-188.
- Zipursky AL: Prevention of vitamin K deficiency bleeding in newborns. *Br J Haematol* 1999;104:430-437.
- Greer FR: Vitamin K deficiency and hemorrhage in infancy. *Clin Perinatol* 1995;22:759.
- Greer FR, Marshall SP, Foley AL, Suttie JW: Improving the vitamin K status of breastfeeding infants with maternal vitamin K supplements. *Pediatrics* 1997;99:88.
- Product Information, Hospira, 2004.

ZIDOVUDINE (ZDV, AZT)

DOSE & ADMINISTRATION: IV: 1.5 mg/kg per dose, given via infusion pump over 1 hour. **PO:** 2 mg/kg per dose. **Do not administer IM.** May administer with food, although manufacturer recommends administration 30 minutes before or 1 hour after a meal. Begin treatment within 6 to 12 hours of birth, and continue for 6 weeks. Initiation of postexposure prophylaxis after the age of 2 days is not likely to be effective. Subsequent treatment is based on HIV culture results. To use dosing chart, please refer to explanatory note in "How to Use This Book."

DOSING INTERVAL CHART

Gestational Age (weeks)	Postnatal Age (days)	Interval (hours)
≤29	0 to 28	12
	>28	8
30 to 34	0 to 14	12
	>14	8
≥35	ALL	6

USES: Dosing guidelines above are for prophylactic treatment of neonates born to HIV-infected women. Treatment of infected infants with combination antiretroviral therapy should be done in consultation with a pediatric infectious disease expert.

MONITORING: CBC at the beginning of therapy, then every other week to assess for anemia, thrombocytopenia, and neutropenia.

ADVERSE EFFECTS/PRECAUTIONS: Anemia and neutropenia occur frequently, and are associated with serum concentrations greater than 3 micromol/L. Mild cases usually respond to a reduction in dose. Severe cases may require cessation of treatment and/or transfusion. Bone marrow toxicity may be increased by concomitant administration of acyclovir, ganciclovir, and TMP-SMX. Lactic acidemia is common in infants exposed to in utero highly active antiretroviral therapy. Concomitant treatment with fluconazole or methadone significantly reduces zidovudine metabolism - dosing interval should be prolonged.

PHARMACOLOGY: Zidovudine is a nucleoside analog that inhibits HIV replication by interfering with viral reverse transcriptase. It is converted intracellularly in several steps to a triphosphate derivative, metabolized via hepatic glucuronidation, then renally excreted. Protein binding is approximately 25%. Zidovudine distributes into cells by passive diffusion and is relatively lipophilic. The CSF: plasma ratio is 0.24. The relationship between serum concentration and clinical efficacy is unclear. The oral syrup is well-absorbed, but only 65% bioavailable due to significant first-pass metabolism. The serum half-life in term newborns is 3 hours, declining to 2 hours after 2 weeks of age. In preterm infants less than 33 weeks gestation, half-life during the first two weeks of life ranges from 5 to 10 hours, decreasing to 2 to 6 hours afterward.

SPECIAL CONSIDERATIONS/PREPARATION: Available as a syrup for oral use in a concentration of 10 mg/mL. The IV form is supplied in a concentration of 10 mg/mL in a 20 mL single-use vial. **Dilute before IV administration to a concentration not exceeding 4**

mg/mL. A dilution of 4 mg/mL may be prepared by adding 4 mL of the 10-mg/mL concentration to 6 mL D$_5$W. After dilution the drug is stable at room temperature for 24 hours. Both forms should be stored at room temperature and protected from light.

Solution Compatibility: D$_5$W and NS.

Terminal Injection Site Compatibility: Dex/AA solutions, fat emulsion. Acyclovir, amikacin, amphotericin B, aztreonam, cefepime, ceftazidime, ceftriaxone, cimetidine, clindamycin, dexamethasone, dobutamine, dopamine, erythromycin lactobionate, fluconazole, gentamicin, heparin, imipenem, linezolid, lorazepam, meropenem, metoclopramide, morphine, nafcillin, oxacillin, piperacillin, piperacillin-tazobactam, potassium chloride, ranitidine, remifentanil, tobramycin, trimethoprim-sulfamethoxazole, and vancomycin.

Incompatibility: Blood products and protein solutions.

SELECTED REFERENCES

• American Academy of Pediatrics. Human Immunodeficiency Virus Infection. In: Pickering LK, Baker CJ, Long SS, McMillan JA, eds. *Red Book: 2006 Report of the Committee on Infectious Diseases.* 27th ed. Elk Grove Village, IL: American Academy of Pediatrics; 2006: pp 393-394.
• Perinatal HIV Guidelines Working Group. Public Health Service Task Force Recommendations for Use of Antiretroviral Drugs in Pregnant HIV-1 Infected Women for Maternal Health and Interventions to Reduce Perinatal HIV-1 Transmission in the United States. November 2, 2007. Available at http://aidsinfo.nih.gov/ContentFiles/PerinatalGL.pdf.
• Capparelli EV, Mirochnick MH, Danker WM: Pharmacokinetics and tolerance of zidovudine in preterm infants. *J Pediatr* 2003;142:47-52.
• Alimenti A, Burdge DR, Ogilvie GS, et al: Lactic acidemia in human immunodeficiency virus-uninfected infants exposed to antiretroviral therapy. *Pediatr Infect Dis J* 2003;22:782-8.
• Mirochnick M, Capparelli E, Conner J: Pharmacokinetics of zidovudine in infants: A population analysis across studies. *Clin Pharmacol Ther* 1999;66:16-24.
• Acosta EP, Page LM, Fletcher CV: Clinical pharmacokinetics of zidovudine. *Drugs* 1996;30:251.
• Connor EM, Sperling RS, Gelber R, et al: Reduction of maternal-infant transmission of human immunodeficiency virus type 1 with zidovudine treatment. *N Engl J Med* 1994;331:1173.
• Boucher FD, Modlin JF, Weller S: Phase I evaluation of zidovudine administered to infants exposed at birth to the human immunodeficiency virus. *J Pediatr* 1993;122:137.
• Product Information, GlaxoSmithKline, 2006.

Indices

BRAND/GENERIC INDEX

Organized alphabetically, this index includes the brand and generic names of each product described in the PDR and NeoFax drug sections. PDR drug entries are capitalized; most use brand names but a few generic names are also used. NeoFax drug entries always use generic names. In addition, *NeoFax page numbers are shown in italics.* If more than one brand name is associated with a generic, each brand can be found under the generic entry.

THERAPEUTIC CLASS INDEX

Organized alphabetically, this index includes the therapeutic class for each drug described in the PDR concise drug section. Therapeutic class headings are based on information provided in the drug monographs. The drug entries listed under each bold therapeutic class are organized alphabetically by brand name or monograph title (shown in capitalized letters), followed by the generic name in parentheses. (Note: Does not include NeoFax drug monographs.)

B

C

OPIOID ANTITUSSIVE/ANTIHISTAMINE
TUSSIONEX PENNKINETIC
(Hydrocodone Polistirex) 453

OPIOID/ANTICHOLINERGIC
LONOX (Diphenoxylate HCl) 254

**ORGANOPHOSPHATE/CHOLINESTERASE
INHIBITOR**
OVIDE (Malathion) 321

ORNITHINE DECARBOXYLASE INHIBITOR
VANIQA (Eflornithine HCl) 465

OSMOTIC LAXATIVE
GENERLAC (Lactulose) 237
MIRALAX (Polyethylene Glycol 3350) 281

OXAZOLIDINONE CLASS ANTIBACTERIAL
ZYVOX (Linezolid) 512

P

PANCREATIC ENZYME SUPPLEMENT
CREON (Protease) 108
PANCREASE MT (Protease) 324
VIOKASE (Protease) 476
ZYMASE (Protease) 511

**PARTIAL D$_2$/5HT$_{1A}$ AGONIST/5HT$_{2A}$
ANTAGONIST**
ABILIFY DISCMELT (Aripiprazole) 1

**PARTIAL OPIOID AGONIST/OPIOID
ANTAGONIST**
SUBUTEX (Naloxone) 412

PENICILLIN
BICILLIN C-R (Penicillin G Procaine) 60
BICILLIN C-R 900/300 (Penicillin G
Procaine) 60
BICILLIN L-A (Penicillin G Benzathine) 61
PERMAPEN (Penicillin G Benzathine) 334
PFIZERPEN (Penicillin G Potassium) 335
VEETIDS (Penicillin V Potassium) 331

PENICILLIN (PENICILLINASE-RESISTANT)
DICLOXACILLIN (Dicloxacillin Sodium) 138

PENICILLIUM-DERIVED ANTIFUNGAL
GRIFULVIN V (Griseofulvin) 203
GRIS-PEG (Griseofulvin) 203

PEPTIDE SYNTHESIS INHIBITOR
TRECATOR (Ethionamide) 447

PERIPHERAL VASODILATOR
MINOXIDIL (Minoxidil) 279

PHENOTHIAZINE
CHLORPROMAZINE (Chlorpromazine) 84
PERPHENAZINE (Perphenazine) 334

PHENOTHIAZINE DERIVATIVE
PHENERGAN INJECTION
(Promethazine HCl) 336
PROCHLORPERAZINE
(Prochlorperazine) 355
PROMETHEGAN (Promethazine HCl) 359

PHENOTHIAZINE DERIVATIVE/ANTITUSSIVE
PROMETHAZINE DM (Promethazine
HCl) 359
PROMETHAZINE W/CODEINE
(Promethazine HCl) 362

**PHENOTHIAZINE DERIVATIVE/
SYMPATHOMIMETIC**
PROMETHAZINE VC (Promethazine
HCl) 360

**PHENOTHIAZINE DERIVATIVE/ANTITUSSIVE/
SYMPATHOMIMETIC**
PROMETHAZINE VC/CODEINE
(Promethazine HCl) 361

PHENYLTRIAZINE
LAMICTAL CD (Lamotrigine) 238

PIPERAZINE ANTIHISTAMINE
HYDROXYZINE HCL (Hydroxyzine HCl) 216
VISTARIL (Hydroxyzine Pamoate) 217

PIPERIDINE PHENOTHIAZINE
THIORIDAZINE (Thioridazine HCl) 435

**PLATELET-DERIVED GROWTH FACTOR
(RECOMBINANT HUMAN)**
REGRANEX (Becaplermin) 376

PLATELET-REDUCING AGENT
AGRYLIN (Anagrelide HCl) 15

PLEUROMUTILIN ANTIBACTERIAL
ALTABAX (Retapamulin) 24

POLYENE ANTIFUNGAL
ABELCET (Amphotericin B (Lipid
Complex)) 1
AMBISOME (Amphotericin B) 26
AMPHOTEC (Amphotericin B
Cholesteryl Sulfate) 29
NYSTATIN ORAL (Nystatin) 311
NYSTATIN TOPICAL (Nystatin) 311
NYSTOP (Nystatin) 312

POLYENE ANTIFUNGAL/CORTICOSTEROID
NYSTATIN/TRIAMCINOLONE
(Triamcinolone Acetonide) 312

PROSTAGLANDIN E$_1$
PROSTIN VR PEDIATRIC (Alprostadil) 365

PROTEASE INHIBITOR
INVIRASE (Saquinavir Mesylate) 227
KALETRA (Ritonavir) 230
LEXIVA (Fosamprenavir Calcium) 248
NORVIR (Ritonavir) 304
VIRACEPT (Nelfinavir Mesylate) 477

PROTEIN
PULMOZYME (Dornase Alfa) 368

PROTEIN SYNTHESIS INHIBITOR
ONCASPAR (Pegaspargase) 316

PROTEIN-TYROSINE KINASE INHIBITOR
GLEEVEC (Imatinib Mesylate) 200

PROTON PUMP INHIBITOR
ACIPHEX (Rabeprazole Sodium) 6
NEXIUM (Esomeprazole Magnesium) 299
PREVACID SOLUTAB (Lansoprazole) 348
PRILOSEC (Omeprazole) 351

PSORALEN
OXSORALEN (Methoxsalen) 323

PURIFIED NEUROTOXIN COMPLEX
BOTOX (Botulinum Toxin Type A) 64

PURINE ANALOG
PURINETHOL (Mercaptopurine) 368
THIOGUANINE (Thioguanine) 435

PYRETHROID PEDICULICIDE
NIX (Permethrin) 301

PYRETHROID SCABICIDAL AGENT
ACTICIN (Permethrin) 7
ELIMITE (Permethrin) 158

Appendix: Reference Tables

CDC GROWTH CHARTS

ABBREVIATIONS, ACRONYMS, AND SYMBOLS

ABBREVIATIONS	DESCRIPTIONS
- (eg, 6-8)	to (eg, 6 to 8)
/	per
<	less than
>	greater than
≤	less than or equal to
≥	greater than or equal to
α	alpha
β	beta
5-FU	5-fluorouracil
5-HT	5-hydroxytriptamine (serotonin)
ABECB	acute bacterial exacerbation of chronic bronchitis
aa	of each
a/A	arterial-alveolar (gradient)
a/ApO$_2$	arterial-alveolar oxygen tension ratio
ABGs	arterial blood gases
ACTH	adrenocorticotrophic hormone
ad	right ear
ADHD	attention-deficit/hyperactivity disorder
A-fib	atrial fibrillation
A-flutter	atrial flutter
AIDS	acquired immunodeficiency syndrome
ALT	alanine transaminase (SGPT)
am	morning
AMI	acute myocardial infarction
AMP	adenosine monophosphate
ANA	antinuclear antibodies
ANC	absolute neutrophil count
APAP	acetaminophen
APTT	activated partial thromboplastin time
as	left ear
ASA	aspirin
AST	aspartate transaminase (SGOT)
ATP	adenosine triphosphate
ATPase	adenosine triphosphatase
au	each ear
AUC	area under the curve
AV	atrioventricular
bid	twice daily
BMI	body mass index
BP	blood pressure
BPD	bronchopulmonary dysplasia

(Continued)

ABBREVIATIONS	DESCRIPTIONS
BPH	benign prostatic hypertrophy
bpm	beats per minute
BSA	body surface area
BUN	blood urea nitrogen
CABG	coronary artery bypass graft
CAD	coronary artery disease
Cap	capsule
CAP	community-acquired pneumonia
CBC	complete blood count
CF	cystic fibrosis
CHF	congestive heart failure
cm	centimeter
CMV	cytomegalovirus
C_{max}	peak plasma concentration
CNS	central nervous system
COPD	chronic obstructive pulmonary disease
CrCl	creatinine clearance
Cre	cream
CRF	chronic renal failure
CSF	cerebrospinal fluid
CVA	cerebrovascular accident
CVD	cardiovascular disease
CVP	central venous pressure
CYP450	cytochrome P450
D_5NS	5% dextrose in normal saline solution
D_5W	5% dextrose in water solution
$D_{10}W$	10% dextrose in water solution
$D_{15}W$	15% dextrose in water solution
$D_{20}W$	20% dextrose in water solution
d/c	discontinue
DHEA	dehydroepiandrosterone
DIC	disseminated intravascular coagulation
DM	diabetes mellitus
DNA	deoxyribonucleic acid
DPPC	dipalmitoyl phosphatidylcholine
DT	diphtheria, tetanus (vaccine)
DTP	diphtheria, tetanus, pertussis (vaccine)
DVT	deep vein thrombosis
ECG	electrocardiogram
EEG	electroencephalogram
EKG	electrocardiogram
eg	for example
EPS	extrapyramidal symptom
ESRD	end-stage renal disease

(Continued)

ABBREVIATIONS	DESCRIPTIONS
ET	endotracheal
FiO$_2$	fractional inspired oxygen concentration
FRC	functional residual capacity
FSH	follicle-stimulating hormone
g	gram
GABA	gamma-aminobutyric acid
GAD	general anxiety disorder
GCSF	granulocyte colony stimulating factor
GE	gastroesophageal
GERD	gastroesophageal reflux disease
GFR	glomerular filtration rate
GI	gastrointestinal
GnRH	gonadotropin-releasing hormone
GVHD	graft versus host disease
HBeAg	hepatitis B e antigen
HBIG	hepatitis B immune globulin
HBsAg	hepatitis B surface antigen
HCG	human chorionic gonadotropin
Hct	hematocrit
HCTZ	hydrochlorothiazide
HDL	high density lipoprotein
Hgb	hemoglobin
Hib	*Haemophilus influenzae* type b
HIV	human immunodeficiency virus
HMG-CoA	3-hydroxy-3-methylglutaryl-coenzyme A
HR	heart rate
hr or hrs	hour or hours
hs	bedtime
HSV	herpes simplex virus
HTN	hypertension
IBD	inflammatory bowel disease
IBS	irritable bowel syndrome
IC	intracardiac
ICH	intracranial hemorrhage
IgG	immunoglobulin G
IM	intramuscular
INH	isoniazid
Inj	injection
INR	international normalized ratio
IOP	intraocular pressure
IPV	inactivated polio vaccine (Salk)
IU	international units
IV	intravenous/intravenously
IVH	intraventricular hemorrhage

(Continued)

ABBREVIATIONS	DESCRIPTIONS
IVIG	intravenous immune globulin (human)
K+	potassium
kg	kilogram
KIU	kallikrein inhibitor unit
L	liter
lbs	pounds
LD	loading dose
LDL	low density lipoprotein
Lf	potency of a given weight of an internationally accepted standard
LFT	liver function test
LH	luteinizing hormone
LHRH	luteinizing-hormone releasing hormone
Lot	lotion
Loz	lozenge
LR	lactated Ringer's solution
LVH	left ventricular hypertrophy
M	molar
MAC	mycobacterium avium complex
Maint	maintenance
MAOI	monoamine oxidase inhibitor
Max	maximum
mcg	microgram
mEq	milli-equivalent
mg	milligram
MI	myocardial infarction
min	minute (usually as mL/min)
mL	milliliter
mm	millimeter
mM	millimolar
MRI	magnetic resonance imaging
MS	multiple sclerosis
msec	millisecond
MTX	methotrexate
Na	sodium
NaCl	sodium chloride
NEC	necrotizing enterocolitis
NG	nasogastric
NKA	no known allergies
NMS	neuroleptic malignant syndrome
NPO	nothing by mouth
NS	normal saline solution (0.9% sodium chloride)
NSAID	nonsteroidal anti-inflammatory drug

(Continued)

ABBREVIATIONS	DESCRIPTIONS
NV	nausea and vomiting
OA	osteoarthritis
OCD	obsessive-compulsive disorder
od	right eye
Oint	ointment
OPV	oral polio vaccine
os	left eye
ou	each eye
PAT	paroxysmal atrial tachycardia
pc	after meals
PCO_2	partial pressure of carbon dioxide in the blood
PCP	*Pneumocystis carinii* pneumonia
PD	Parkinson's disease
PDA	patent ductus arteriosus
PID	pelvic inflammatory disease
pkt, pkts	packet, packets
pm	evening
PMA	postmenstrual age
PO_2	partial pressure of oxygen in the blood
po	orally
PONV	postoperative nausea and vomiting
ppm	parts per million
pr	rectally
prn	as needed
PSA	prostate-specific antigen
PSVT	paroxysmal supraventricular tachycardia
pta	prior to admission
PT	prothrombin time
PTSD	post-traumatic stress disorder
PTT	partial thromboplastin time
PTU	propylthiouracil
PUD	peptic ulcer disease
PVC	premature ventricular contraction
PVD	peripheral vascular disease
q4h, q6h, q8h, etc.	every four hours, every six hours, every eight hours, etc.
qd	once daily
qh	every hour
qid	four times daily
qod	every other day
qs	a sufficient quantity
qs ad	a sufficient quantity up to
RA	rheumatoid arthritis

(Continued)

ABBREVIATIONS	DESCRIPTIONS
RBC	red blood cells
RDIs	reference daily intakes
RDS	respiratory distress syndrome
REM	rapid eye movement
RNA	ribonucleic acid
ROP	retinopathy of prematurity
SA	sinoatrial node
SAH	subarachnoid hemorrhage
SBP	systolic blood pressure
sec	second(s)
SGA	small for gestational age
SGOT	serum glutamic-oxaloacetic transaminase (AST)
SGPT	serum glutamic-pyruvic transaminase (ALT)
SIADH	syndrome of inappropriate antidiuretic hormone secretion
SLE	systemic lupus erythematosus
SOB	shortness of breath
Sol	solution
SQ	subcutaneous
SrCr	serum creatinine
SSRI	selective serotonin reuptake inhibitor
SSSI	skin and skin structure infection
STD	sexually transmitted disease
subQ	subcutaneously
Sup	suppository
Sus	suspension
SVT	supraventricular tachycardia
^{99}Tc-IDA	techneticum 99m-image display and analysis
$t_{1/2}$	half-life
Tab	tablet
Tab, SL	sublingual tablet
TB	tuberculosis
TBG	thyroxine binding globulin
tbl	tablespoon
TCA	tricyclic antidepressant
TD	tardive dyskinesia
TFT	thyroid function test
TG	triglyceride
tid	three times daily
T_{max}	time to maximum concentration
TNF	tumor necrosis factor
TPN	total parenteral nutrition

(Continued)

ABBREVIATIONS	DESCRIPTIONS
TSH	thyroid stimulating hormone
tsp	teaspoonful
TTP	thrombotic thrombocytopenic purpura
U	unit
UAC	umbilical artery catheter
ud	as directed
ULN	upper limit of normal
URTI/URI	upper respiratory tract infection
US RDAs	US Recommended Daily Allowances
UTI	urinary tract infection
UV	ultraviolet
WBC	white blood cell count
Vd	volume of distribution
VLBW	very low birth weight
VTE	venous thromboembolism
X	times (eg, >2X ULN)
yr or yrs	year or years

CALCULATIONS AND FORMULAS

WEIGHTS AND MEASURES

METRIC MEASURES

1 kilogram (kg)	1000 g
1 gram (g)	1000 mg
1 milligram (mg)	0.001 g
1 microgram (mcg or μg)	0.001 mg; 1 x 10^{-6} g
1 liter (L)	1000 mL
1 milliliter (mL)	0.001 L; 1 cc (cubic centimeter)

APOTHECARY MEASURES (AP)

1 scruple	20 grains (gr)
1 drachm	3 scruples; 60 gr
1 ounce (oz)	8 drachms; 24 scruples; 480 gr
1 pound (lb)	12 oz; 96 drachms; 288 scruples; 5760 gr

U.S. FLUID MEASURES

1 fluidrachm	60 minim
1 fluidounce	8 fluidrachm; 480 minim
1 pint (pt)	16 fl oz; 7680 minim
1 quart (qt)	2 pt; 32 fl oz
1 gallon (gal)	4 qt; 128 fl oz

AVOIRDUPOIS WEIGHT (AV)

1 ounce	437.5 gr
1 pound	16 oz

CONVERSION FACTORS

1 gram	15.4 gr
1 grain	64.8 mg
1 ounce (Av)	28.35 g; 437.5 gr
1 ounce (Ap)	31.1 g; 480 gr
1 pound (Av)	453.6 g; 2.68 lb (Ap); 2.20 lb (Av)
1 fluidounce	29.57 mL
1 fluidrachm	3.697 mL
1 minim	0.06 mL

COMMON MEASURES

1 teaspoonful	5 mL; 1/8 fl oz
1 tablespoonful	15 mL; 1/2 fl oz
1 wineglassful	60 mL; 2 fl oz
1 teacupful	120 mL; 4 fl oz
1 gallon	3800 mL; 128 fl oz
1 quart	960 mL; 32 fl oz
1 pint	480 mL; 16 fl oz (exactly 473.2 mL)
8 fluid ounces	240 mL
4 fluid ounces	120 mL
2.2 lb	1 kg

DOSE EQUIVALENTS

WEIGHT (METRIC)	WEIGHT (APOTHECARY)
30 g	1 ounce
15 g	4 drams
10 g	2 1/2 drams
7.5 g	2 drams
6 g	90 grains
5 g	75 grains
4 g	60 grains; 1 dram
3 g	45 grains
2 g	30 grains; 1/2 dram
1.5 g	22 grains
1 g	15 grains
750 mg	12 grains
600 mg	10 grains
500 mg	7 1/2 grains
400 mg	6 grains
300 mg	5 grains
250 mg	4 grains

(Continued)

A9

DOSE EQUIVALENTS *(Continued)*

WEIGHT (METRIC)	WEIGHT (APOTHECARY)
200 mg	3 grains
150 mg	2 ½ grains
125 mg	2 grains
100 mg	1 ½ grains
75 mg	1 ¼ grains
60 mg	1 grain
50 mg	¾ grain
40 mg	⅔ grain
30 mg	½ grain
25 mg	⅜ grain
20 mg	⅓ grain
15 mg	¼ grain
12 mg	⅕ grain
10 mg	⅙ grain
8 mg	⅛ grain
6 mg	¹/₁₀ grain
5 mg	¹/₁₂ grain
4 mg	¹/₁₅ grain
3 mg	¹/₂₀ grain
2 mg	¹/₃₀ grain
1.5 mg	¹/₄₀ grain
1.2 mg	¹/₅₀ grain
1 mg	¹/₆₀ grain

LIQUID MEASURES (METRIC)	LIQUID MEASURES (APOTHECARY)
1000 mL	1 quart
750 mL	1 ½ pints
500 mL	1 pint
230 mL	8 fluid ounces
200 mL	7 fluid ounces
100 mL	3 ½ fluid ounces
50 mL	1 ¾ fluid ounces
30 mL	1 fluid ounces
15 mL	4 fluid drams
10 mL	2 ½ fluid drams
8 mL	2 fluid drams
5 mL	1 ¼ fluid drams
4 mL	1 fluid dram
3 mL	45 minims
2 mL	30 minims
1 mL	15 minims
0.75 mL	12 minims
0.6 mL	10 minims
0.5 mL	8 minims
0.3 mL	5 minims
0.25 mL	4 minims
0.2 mL	3 minims
0.1 mL	1 ½ minims
0.06 mL	1 minim
0.05 mL	¾ minim
0.03 mL	½ minim

MILLIEQUIVALENT (mEq) AND MILLIMOLE (mmol)

CALCULATIONS

moles = $\dfrac{\text{weight of a substance (grams)}}{\text{molecular weight of that substance (grams)}}$	**OR**	= $\dfrac{\text{equivalent}}{\text{valence of ion}}$
millimoles = $\dfrac{\text{weight of a substance (milligrams)}}{\text{molecular weight of that substance (milligrams)}}$	**OR** = $\dfrac{\text{milliequivalents}}{\text{valence of ion}}$	**OR** = moles x 1000
equivalents = moles x valence of ion		
milliequivalents = millimoles x valence of ion	**OR**	= equivalents x 1000

(Continued)

CONVERSIONS

mg/100mL to mEq/L	$mEq/L = \dfrac{(mg/100mL) \times 10 \times valence}{atomic\ weight}$
mEq/L to mg/100mL	$mg/100mL = \dfrac{(mEq/L) \times atomic\ weight}{10 \times valence}$
mEq/L to volume percent of a gas	$volume\ \% = \dfrac{(mEq/L) \times 22.4}{10}$

ACID-BASE ASSESSMENT

DEFINITIONS

PIO_2	Oxygen partial pressure of inspired gas (mmHg); 150 mmHg in room air at sea level
FiO_2	Fractional pressure of oxygen in inspired gas (0.21 in room air)
PAO_2	Alveolar oxygen partial pressure
$PACO_2$	Alveolar carbon dioxide partial pressure
PaO_2	Arterial oxygen partial pressure
$PaCO_2$	Arterial carbon dioxide partial pressure
R	Respiratory exchange quotient (typically 0.8, increases with high carbohydrate diet, decreases with high fat diet)

HENDERSON-HASSELBALCH EQUATION

$pH = 6.1 + \log [HCO_3^- / (0.03)\ (pCO_2)]$

ALVEOLAR GAS EQUATION

$PIO_2 = FiO_2 \times$ (total atmospheric pressure - vapor pressure of H_2O at 37°C)
$\quad\quad = FiO_2 \times$ (760 mmHg - 47 mmHg)

$PaO_2 = PIO_2 - PaCO_2/R$

ALVEOLAR/ARTERIAL OXYGEN GRADIENT

$PAO_2 - PaO_2$

ACID-BASE DISORDERS

Disorder	pH	HCO₃⁻	PCO₂	Compensation
Metabolic acidosis	< 7.35	Primary decrease	Compensatory decrease	1.2-mmHg decrease in PCO_2 for every 1-mmol/L decrease in HCO_3^- **or** $PCO_2 = (1.5 \times HCO_3^-) + 8\ (\pm 2)$ **or** $PCO_2 = HCO_3^- + 15$ **or** $PCO_2 =$ last 2 digits of pH x 100
Metabolic alkalosis	> 7.45	Primary increase	Compensatory increase	0.6-0.75 mmHg increase in PCO_2 for every 1-mmol/L increase in HCO_3^-. PCO_2 should not rise above 60 mm Hg in compensation.
Respiratory acidosis	< 7.35	Compensatory increase	Primary increase	*Acute:* 1-2 mmol decrease in HCO_3^-. for every 10-mmHg decrease in PCO_2. *Chronic:* 3-4 mmol increase in HCO_3^-. for every 10-mmHg increase in PCO_2
Respiratory alkalosis	> 7.45	Compensatory decrease	Primary decrease	*Acute:* 1-2 mmol increase in HCO_3^-. for every 10-mmHg increase in PCO_2. *Chronic:* 4-5 mmol decrease in HCO_3^-. for every 10-mmHg decrease in PCO_2.

ACID-BASE EQUATION

H^+ (in mEq/L) = (24 x $PaCO_2$) divided by HCO_3^-

(Continued)

OTHER CALCULATIONS

ANION GAP

Anion gap = Na^+ - (Cl^- + HCO_3^- measured)

AA GRADIENT

Aa gradient [(713) (FiO_2 - ($PaCO_2$ divided by 0.8))] - PaO_2

OSMOLALITY

Definition:
Osmolality is a measure of the total number of particles in a solution.

U.S. units (sodium as mEq/L, BUN (blood urea nitrogen) and glucose as (mg/dL)
  Plasma osmolality (mOsm/kg) = 2([Na^+] + [K^+]) + ([BUN]/2.8) + ([glucose]/18)

SI units (all variables in mmol/L):
  Plasma osmolality (mOsm/kg) = 2[Na^+] + [urea] + [glucose]
  Normal range plasma osmolality: 280 - 303 mOsm/kg

Corrected Sodium
Corrected Na+ = measured Na^+ + [1.5 x (glucose - 150 divided by 100)]*
*Do not correct for glucose <150.

Total Serum Calcium Corrected for Albumin Level
[(Normal albumin - patient's albumin) x 0.8] + patient's measured total calcium

Water Deficit
Water deficit = 0.6 x body weight [1 - (140 divided by Na^+)]*
*Body weight is estimated weight in kg; Na^+ is serum or plasma sodium.

Bicarbonate Deficit
HCO_3^- deficit = [0.4 x weight (kg)] x (HCO_3^- desired - HCO_3^- measured)

CHILD-PUGH SCORE

The Child-Pugh classification used to assess the prognosis of chronic liver disease, mainly cirrhosis. Child-Pugh is also used to determine the required strength of treatment and the necessity of liver transplantation.

Score:
  The score employs five clinical measures of liver disease. Each measure is scored 1-3, with
  3 indicating most severe derangement.

Measure	1 point	2 points	3 points	Units
Bilirubin (total)*	<34 (<2)	34-50 (2-3)	>50 (>3)	mol/L (mg/dL)
Serum albumin	>3	528-35	<28	mg/L
INR*	<1.7	1.71-2.20	> 2.20	no unit
Ascites	None	Suppressed with medication	Refractory	no unit
Hepatic encephalopathy	None	Grade I-II (or suppressed with medication)	Grade III-IV (or refractory)	no unit

* In primary sclerosing cholangitis and primary biliary cirrhosis, the bilirubin references are changed to reflect the fact that these diseases feature high conjugated bilirubin levels. The upper limit for 1 point is 68 mol/L (4 mg/dL) and the upper limit for 2 points is 170 mol/L (10 mg/dL).

** Some older reference works substitute PT prolongation for INR.

Interpretation:
  Chronic liver disease is classified into Child-Pugh class A to C, employing the added score from above.

Points	Class	One year survival	Two year survival
5-6	A	100%	85%
7-9	B	81%	57%
10-15	C	45%	35%

CREATININE CLEARANCE

Clinically, creatinine clearance is a useful measure for estimating the glomerular filtration rate (GFR) of the kidneys.

Factors	Abbreviations
Creatinine clearance	Cl_{Cr}
Plasma creatinine concentration	P_{Cr}
Serum creatinine concentration	S_{Cr}
Urine creatinine concentration	U_{Cr}
Urine flow rate	V
Plasma creatinine concentration	P_{Cr}

(Continued)

CREATININE CLEARANCE *(Continued)*

Calculations:

$$Cl_{Cr} = \frac{U_{Cr} \times V}{P_{Cr}}$$

Example:
Patient with P_{Cr} 1 mg/dL, U_{Cr} 60 mg/dL, and V of 0.5 dL/hr.

$$Cl_{Cr} = \frac{60 \text{ mg/dL} \times 0.5 \text{ dL/hr}}{1 \text{ mg/dL}} = 30 \text{ dL/hr}$$

Cockcroft-Gault formula: Estimates creatinine clearance (mL/min).

Male:

$$Cl_{Cr} = \frac{(140 - \text{age}) \times \text{mass (kg)}}{72 \times S_{Cr} \text{ (mg/dL)}}$$

Example:
Male patient, 67 years of age, weight 75 kg, and S_{Cr} 1 mg/dL.

$$Cl_{Cr} = \frac{(140 - 67) \times 75}{72 \times 1} = 76 \text{ mL/min}$$

Female:

$$Cl_{Cr} = \frac{(140 - \text{age}) \times \text{mass (kg)}}{72 \times S_{Cr} \text{ (mg/dL)}} \times 0.85 \text{ if female}$$

Example:
Female patient, 67 years of age, weight 75 kg, and S_{Cr} 1 mg/dL.

$$Cl_{Cr} = \frac{(140 - 67) \times 75}{72 \times 1} \times 0.85 = 64.6 \text{ mL/min}$$

Note: Using actual body weight (ABW) in obese patients can significantly overestimate creatinine clearance. Adjusted ideal body weight (IBW) can provide more approximate estimate. Adjusted IBW = IBW + 0.4 (ABW - IBW).

BASAL ENERGY EXPENDITURE (BEE)

Basal energy expenditure: the amount of energy required to maintain the body's normal metabolic activity (ie, respiration, maintenance of body temperature, etc).

H = height (cm), W = weight (kg), A = age (years)

Male:
BEE = 66.67 + 13.75W + 5H - 6.76A

Female:
BEE = 665.1 + 9.56W + 1.85H - 4.68A

BODY MASS INDEX (BMI)

$$BMI = \frac{\text{weight (kg)}}{[\text{height (m)}]^2}$$

BODY SURFACE AREA (BSA)

$$BSA \text{ (m}^2) = \sqrt{\frac{\text{height (in)} \times \text{weight (lb)}}{3131}} \qquad \textbf{OR} \qquad BSA \text{ (m}^2) = \sqrt{\frac{\text{height (cm)} \times \text{weight (kg)}}{3600}}$$

IDEAL BODY WEIGHT (IBW)

Adults (18 years and older; IBW is in kg):
  IBW (male) = 50 + (2.3 x height [inches] over 5 feet)
  IBW (female) = 45.5 + (2.3 x height [inches] over 5 feet)

Children (IBW is in kg; height is in cm):
  1-18 years of age:
  $$IBW = \frac{(\text{height}^2 \times 1.65)}{100}$$

  5 feet and taller:
  IBW (male) = 39 + (2.27 x height [inches] over 5 feet)
  IBW (female) = 42.2 + (2.27 x height [inches] over 5 feet)

(Continued)

POUNDS/KILOGRAM CONVERSION

1 pound = 0.45359 kilogram				1 kilogram = 2.2 pounds			
lb	**kg**	**lb**	**kg**	**lb**	**kg**	**lb**	**kg**
1	0.45	105	47.63	210	95.25	315	142.88
5	2.27	110	49.89	215	97.52	320	145.15
10	4.54	115	52.16	220	99.79	325	147.42
15	6.80	120	54.43	225	102.06	330	149.68
20	9.07	125	56.70	230	104.33	335	151.95
25	11.34	130	58.97	235	106.59	340	154.22
30	13.61	135	61.23	240	108.86	345	156.49
35	15.88	140	63.50	245	111.13	350	158.76
40	18.14	145	65.77	250	113.40	355	161.02
45	20.41	150	68.04	255	115.67	360	163.29
50	22.68	155	70.31	260	117.93	365	165.56
55	24.95	160	72.57	265	120.20	370	167.83
60	27.22	165	74.84	270	122.47	375	170.10
65	29.48	170	77.11	275	124.74	380	172.36
70	31.75	175	79.38	280	127.01	385	174.63
75	34.02	180	81.65	285	129.27	390	176.90
80	36.29	185	83.91	290	131.54	395	179.17
85	38.56	190	86.18	295	133.81	400	181.44
90	40.82	195	88.45	300	136.08	405	183.70
95	43.09	200	90.72	305	138.34	405	183.70
100	45.36	205	92.99	310	140.61	415	188.24

TEMPERATURE CONVERSION

Fahrenheit to Celsius = (°F - 32) x 5/9 = °C				Celsius to Fahrenheit = (°C x 9/5) + 32 = °F			
°F	**°C**	**°F**	**°C**	**°C**	**°F**	**°C**	**°F**
0.0	-17.8	92.0	33.3	0.0	32.0	49.0	120.2
5.0	-15.0	93.0	33.9	5.0	41.0	50.0	122.0
10.0	-12.2	94.0	34.4	10.0	50.0	51.0	123.8
15.0	-9.4	95.0	35.0	15.0	59.0	85.0	185.0
20.0	-6.7	96.0	35.6	20.0	68.0	52.0	125.6
25.0	-3.9	97.0	36.1	25.0	77.0	53.0	127.4
30.0	-1.1	98.0	36.7	30.0	86.0	54.0	129.2
35.0	1.7	98.6	37.0	35.0	95.0	55.0	131.0
40.0	4.4	99.0	37.2	36.0	96.8	56.0	132.8
45.0	7.2	100.0	37.8	37.0	98.6	57.0	134.6
50.0	10.0	101.0	38.3	38.0	100.4	58.0	136.4
55.0	12.8	102.0	38.9	39.0	102.2	59.0	138.2
60.0	15.6	103.0	39.4	40.0	104.0	60.0	140.0
65.0	18.3	104.0	40.0	41.0	105.8	65.0	149.0
70.0	21.1	105.0	40.6	42.0	107.6	70.0	158.0
75.0	23.9	106.0	41.1	43.0	109.4	75.0	167.0
80.0	26.7	107.0	41.7	44.0	111.2	80.0	176.0
85.0	29.4	108.0	42.2	45.0	113.0	90.0	194.0
90.0	32.2	109.0	42.8	46.0	114.8	95.0	203.0
91.0	32.8	110.0	43.3	47.0	116.6	100.0	212.0
				48.0	118.4	105.0	221.0

(Continued)

PEDIATRIC DOSAGE ESTIMATION FORMULAS

The following formulas can be used to estimate the approximate pediatric dosage of a medication. These formulas are based on the adult dose and either the child's age or weight. These formulas should be used with caution as the response to any drug is not always directly proportional to the age or weight of the child relative to the usual adult dose. Dosage will also vary based on the formula used. Care should be taken when using any of these methods to calculate the child's dosage. Some products have FDA approved pediatric indications and dosages, always refer to full prescribing information first before calculating a pediatric dosage.

BASED ON WEIGHT

Augsberger's Rule:

$\frac{[(1.5 \times \text{weight [kg]}) + 10]}{100} \times \text{adult dose} = \text{approximate child's dose}$

Example: If the child's weight is 15 kg (33 lb) and the adult dose is 50 mg then the child's dose is 16.25 mg.
$\frac{[(1.5 \times 15 \text{ kg}) + 10]}{100} \times 50 \text{ mg} = 0.325 \times 50 \text{ mg} = 16.25 \text{ mg}$

Clark's Rule:

(weight [lb]/150) x adult dose = approximate child's dose

Example: If the child's weight is 15 kg (33 lb) and the adult dose is 50 mg then the child's dose is 11 mg.
(33/150) x 50 mg = 0.22 x 50 mg = 11 mg

Based on Age

Augsberger's Rule:

$\frac{[(4 \times \text{age [years]}) + 20]}{100} \times \text{adult dose} = \text{approximate child's dose}$

Example: If the child's age is 8 years and the adult dose is 50 mg then the child's dose is 26 mg.
[(4 x 8) + 20)/100] x 50 mg = 0.52 X 50 mg = 26 mg

Dilling's Rule:

(age [years]/20) x adult dose = approximate child's dose

Example: If the child's age is 8 years and the adult dose is 50 mg then the child's dose is 20 mg.
(8/20) x 50 mg = 0.40 x 50 mg = 20 mg

Cowling's Rule:

$\frac{[\text{age at next birthday (years)}]}{24} \times \text{adult dose} = \text{approximate child's dose}$

Example: If the child is going to turn 8 years old in few months and the adult dose is 50 mg then the child's dose is 16.7 mg. (8/24) x 50 mg = 0.33 x 50 mg = 16.7 mg

Younge's Rule:

$\frac{[\text{age (years)}]}{\text{age} + 12} \times \text{adult dose} = \text{approximate child's dose}$

Example: If the child's age is 8 years and the adult dose is 50 mg then the child's dose is 20 mg.
[8/(8+12)] x 50 mg = 0.4 x 50 mg = 20 mg

Fried's Rule (younger than 1 year):

$\frac{[\text{age (months)}]}{150} \times \text{adult dose} = \text{approximate infant's dose}$

Example: If the child's age is 10 months and the adult dose is 50 mg then the child's dose is 3.33 mg.
(10/150) x 50 mg = 0.067 x 50 mg = 3.33 mg

DRUG INFORMATION CENTERS

ALABAMA
BIRMINGHAM

Drug Information Service
University of Alabama
UAB Hospital Pharmacy

Drug Information-JT1720
619 S. 19th St.
Birmingham, AL 35249-6860
Mon.-Fri. 7 AM-4 PM
    205-934-2162
www.health.uab.edu/pharmacy

Global Drug
Information Service
Samford University
McWhorter School
of Pharmacy

800 Lakeshore Dr.
Birmingham, AL 35229-7027
Mon. 8 AM-9 PM
Tues.-Fri. 8 AM-4:30 PM
    205-726-2519 or 2891
www.samford.edu/schools/
pharmacy/dic/index.html

HUNTSVILLE

Huntsville Hospital Drug
Information Center

101 Sivley Rd.
Huntsville, AL 35801
Mon.-Fri. 8 AM-4:30 PM
    256-265-8284

ARIZONA
TUCSON

Arizona Poison and Drug
Information Center

1259 N. Martin Ave.
Drachman Hall B308
Tucson, AZ 85724
7 days/week, 24 hours
    520-626-6016
    800-222-1222 **(Emergency)**
www.pharmacy.arizona.edu

ARKANSAS
LITTLE ROCK

Arkansas Drug Information Center

4301 W. Markham St.
Slot 522-2
Little Rock, AR 72205
Mon.-Fri. 8:30 AM-5 PM
    501-686-6161
    (Little Rock area only -
    for healthcare
    professionals only)
    888-228-1233
    (AR only - **for healthcare**
    professionals only)

CALIFORNIA
LOS ANGELES

Los Angeles Regional
Drug Information Center
LAC & USC Medical Center

1200 N. State St.
Trailer 25
Los Angeles, CA 90033
Mon.-Fri. 8 AM-4 PM
Closed 12 PM to 1 PM
    323-226-7741

SAN DIEGO

Drug Information Service
University of California
San Diego Medical Center

200 West Arbor Dr.
MC 8925
San Diego, CA 92103-8925
Mon.-Fri. 9 AM-5 PM
    619-543-6971
    (for healthcare
    professionals only)

STANFORD

Drug Information Center
University of California
Stanford Hospital and Clinics

300 Pasteur Dr.
Room H-0301
Stanford, CA 94305
Mon.-Fri. 8 AM-4 PM
    650-723-6422

COLORADO
DENVER

Rocky Mountain Poison
and Drug Center

990 Bannock St.
(Physical address)
777 Bannock St.
(Mailing address)
Denver, CO 80264
    303-739-1100
    800-222-1222 **(Emergency)**
www.rmpdc.org

CONNECTICUT
FARMINGTON

Drug Information Service
University of Connecticut
Health Center

263 Farmington Ave.
Farmington, CT 06030
Mon.-Fri. 10 AM-2 PM
    860-679-2783

HARTFORD

Drug Information Center
Hartford Hospital

PO Box 5037
80 Seymour St.
Hartford, CT 06102
Mon.-Fri. 8:30 AM-5 PM
    860-545-2221
    860-545-2961 (After 5 PM)
www.hartfordhospital.org

NEW HAVEN

Drug Information Center
Yale-New Haven Hospital

20 York St.
New Haven, CT 06540-3202
Mon.-Fri. 9 AM-5 PM
    203-688-2248
www.ynhh.org

DISTRICT OF COLUMBIA

Drug Information Service
Howard University Hospital

2041 Georgia Ave. NW
Room BB06
Washington, DC 20060
Mon.-Fri. 8:30 AM-4 PM
    202-865-7413
www.huhosp.org/patientpublic/
pharmacy.htm

FLORIDA
FT. LAUDERDALE

Nova Southeastern University
College of Pharmacy
Drug Information Center

3200 S. University Dr.
Ft. Lauderdale, FL 33328
Mon.-Fri. 9 AM-5 PM
    954-262-3103
http://pharmacy.nova.edu

GAINESVILLE

Drug Information &
Pharmacy Resource Center
Shands Hospital at
University of Florida

PO Box 100316
Gainesville, FL 32610-0316
Mon.-Fri. 9 AM-5 PM
    352-265-0408
    (for healthcare
    professionals only)
http://shands.org/professional/drugs

JACKSONVILLE

Drug Information Service
Shands Jacksonville

655 W. 8th St.
Jacksonville, FL 32209
Mon.-Fri. 8:30 AM-5 PM
    904-244-4185
    (for healthcare
    professionals only)
Mon.-Fri. 9:30 AM-4 PM
    904-244-4700
    (for consumers)

http://jax.shands.org/
education/pharmacy/contact.asp

ORLANDO

Orlando Regional Drug Information
Service Orlando Regional
Healthcare System

1414 Kuhl Ave., MP 192
Orlando, FL 32806
Mon.-Fri. 8 AM-4 PM
    321-841-8717

TALLAHASSEE

Drug Information Education Center
Florida Agricultural and Mechanical
University College of Pharmacy and
Pharmaceutical Sciences

Tallahassee, FL 32307
Mon.-Fri. 9 AM-5 PM
    850-561-2688

WEST PALM BEACH

Drug Information Center
Nova Southeastern University,
West Palm Beach

3970 RCA Blvd.
Suite 7006A
Palm Beach Gardens, FL 33410
Mon.-Fri. 9 AM-5 PM
    561-622-0658
    (for healthcare
    professionals only)

GEORGIA

ATLANTA

Emory University Hospital
Dept. of Pharmaceutical Services-
Drug Information

1364 Clifton Rd. NE
Atlanta, GA 30322
Mon.-Fri. 9 AM-4 PM
    404-712-4644
    (for healthcare
    professionals only)

Drug Information Service
Northside Hospital

1000 Johnson Ferry Rd. NE
Atlanta, GA 30342
Mon.-Fri. 9 AM-4 PM
    404-851-8676 (GA only)

COLUMBUS

Columbus Regional Drug
Information Center

710 Center St.
Columbus, GA 31902
Mon.-Fri. 8 AM-5 PM
    706-571-1934
    (for healthcare
    professionals only)

IDAHO

POCATELLO

Drug Information Center
Idaho State University
School of Pharmacy

970 S. 5th St.
Campus Box 8092
Pocatello, ID 83209
Mon.-Thur. 8:30 AM-5 PM
Fri. 8:30 AM-3 PM
    208-282-4689
    800-334-7139 (ID only)
http://pharmacy.isu.edu

ILLINOIS

CHICAGO

Drug Information Center
Northwestern Memorial Hospital

Feinberg Pavilion, LC 700
251 E. Huron St.
Chicago, IL 60611
Mon.-Fri. 8:30 AM-5 PM
    312-926-7573

Drug Information Center
University of Illinois at Chicago

833 S. Wood St.
MC 886
Chicago, IL 60612-7231
Mon.-Fri. 8 AM-4 PM
    312-996-3681
    (for healthcare
    professionals only)
Mon.-Fri. 9 AM-12 PM
    312-996-5332
    (for consumers)
www.uic.edu/pharmacy/
services/di/index.html

HARVEY

Drug Information Center
Ingalls Memorial Hospital

1 Ingalls Dr.
Harvey, IL 60426
Mon.-Fri. 8 AM-7 PM

Sat. 9 AM-3:30 PM
    708-333-4300

HINES

Drug Information Service
Hines Veterans Administration
Hospital

Pharmacy Services
MC119
PO Box 5000
Hines, IL 60141-5000
Mon.-Fri. 8 AM-4:30 PM
    708-202-8387, ext. 23780

PARK RIDGE

Drug Information Center
Advocate Lutheran General Hospital

1775 Dempster St.
Park Ridge, IL 60068
Mon.-Fri. 7:30 AM-4 PM
    847-723-8128
    (for healthcare
    professionals only)

INDIANA

INDIANAPOLIS

Drug Information Center
St. Vincent Hospital
and Health Services

2001 W. 86th St.
Indianapolis, IN 46260
Mon.-Fri. 8 AM-4 PM
    317-338-3200
    (for healthcare
    professionals only)

Drug Information Service
Clarian Health Partners

Pharmacy Department I-65
at 21st St.
Room CG04
Indianapolis, IN 46202
Mon.-Fri. 8 AM-4:30 PM
    317-962-1750

MUNCIE

Drug Information Center
Ball Memorial Hospital

2401 University Ave.
Muncie, IN 47303
Mon.-Fri. 8 AM-4:30 PM
    765-747-3033

IOWA

DES MOINES

Regional Drug
Information Center
Mercy Medical Center-
Des Moines

1111 Sixth Ave.
Des Moines, IA 50314
Mon.-Fri. 8 AM-4:30 PM
    515-247-3286
    (regional service; in-house
    service answered 7 days/
    week, 24 hours)

IOWA CITY

Drug Information Center
University of Iowa
Hospitals and Clinics

200 Hawkins Dr.
Iowa City, IA 52242
Mon.-Fri. 8 AM-4:30 PM
319-356-2600

KANSAS
KANSAS CITY

Drug Information Center
University of Kansas
Medical Center

3901 Rainbow Blvd.
Kansas City, KS 66160
Mon.-Fri. 8:30 AM-4:30 PM
913-588-2328

KENTUCKY
LEXINGTON

University of Kentucky
Central Pharmacy
Chandler Medical Center

800 Rose St.
C-114
Lexington, KY 40536-0293
7 days/week, 24 hours
859-323-5642
859-323-6289

LOUISIANA
MONROE

Louisiana Drug and Poison
Information Center
University of Louisiana at Monroe
College of Pharmacy

Sugar Hall
Monroe, LA 71209-6430
Mon.-Thur. 8 AM-4:30 PM
Fri. 8 AM-11:30 AM
318-342-1710

NEW ORLEANS

Xavier University Drug
Information Center
Tulane University
Hospital and Clinic

1440 Canal St.
Suite 808
New Orleans, LA 70112
Mon.-Fri. 9 AM-5 PM
504-588-5670

MARYLAND
ANDREWS AFB

Drug Information Services

79 MDSS/SGQP
1050 W. Perimeter Rd.
Suite D1-119
Andrews AFB, MD 20762-6660
Mon.-Fri. 7:30 AM-5 PM
240-857-4565

BALTIMORE

Drug Information Service
Johns Hopkins Hospital

600 N. Wolfe St.
Carnegie 180
Baltimore, MD 21287-6180
Mon.-Fri. 8:30 AM-5 PM
410-955-6348

Drug Information Service
University of Maryland

School of Pharmacy
Hall Room 760
20 North Pine St.
Baltimore, MD 21201
Mon.-Fri. 8:30 AM-5 PM
410-706-7568
(consumers only)
410-706-0898
(for healthcare
professionals only)
www.pharmacy.umaryland.
edu/umdi

EASTON

Drug Information
Pharmacy Dept.
Memorial Hospital

219 S. Washington St.
Easton, MD 21601
7 days/week, 7 AM-5:30 PM
410-822-1000, ext. 5645

MASSACHUSETTS
BOSTON

Drug Information Services
Brigham and Women's Hospital

75 Francis St.
Boston, MA 02115
Mon.-Fri. 7 AM-3 PM
617-732-7166

WORCESTER

Drug Information Pharmacy
UMass Memorial
Medical Center
Healthcare Hospital

55 Lake Ave. North
Worcester, MA 01655
Mon.-Fri. 8:30 AM-5 PM
508-856-3456
508-856-2775 (24-hour)

MICHIGAN
ANN ARBOR

Drug Information Service Dept. of
Pharmacy Services
University of Michigan
Health System

1500 East Medical Center Dr.
UH B2D301
Box 0008
Ann Arbor, MI 48109-0008
Mon.-Fri. 8 AM-5 PM
734-936-8200

DETROIT

Drug Information Center
Dept. of Pharmacy Services
Detroit Receiving Hospital and
University Health Center

4201 St. Antoine Blvd.
Detroit, MI 48201
Mon.-Fri. 9 AM-5 PM
313-745-4556
www.dmcpharmacy.org

LANSING

Drug Information Services
Sparrow Hospital

1215 East Michigan Ave.
Lansing, MI 48912
7 days/week, 24 hours
517-364-2444

PONTIAC

Drug Information Center
St. Joseph Mercy Oakland

44405 Woodward Ave.
Pontiac, MI 48341
Mon.-Fri. 8 AM-4:30 PM
248-858-3055

ROYAL OAK

Drug Information Services
William Beaumont Hospital

3601 West 13 Mile Rd.
Royal Oak, MI 48073-6769
Mon.-Fri. 8 AM-4:30 PM
248-898-4077

SOUTHFIELD

Drug Information Service
Providence Hospital

16001 West 9 Mile Rd.
Southfield, MI 48075
Mon.-Fri. 8 AM-4 PM
248-849-3125

MISSISSIPPI
JACKSON

Drug Information Center
University of Mississippi
Medical Center

2500 N. State St.
Jackson, MS 39216
Mon.-Fri. 8 AM-4:30 PM
601-984-2060

MISSOURI
KANSAS CITY

University of Missouri-Kansas City
Drug Information Center

2464 Charlotte St.
Suite 1220
Kansas City, MO 64108
Mon.-Fri. 9 AM-4 PM
816-235-5490
http://druginfo.umkc.edu/

SPRINGFIELD

Drug Information Center
St. John's Hospital

1235 E. Cherokee St.
Springfield, MO 65804
Mon.-Fri. 8 AM-4:30 PM
417-820-3488

ST. JOSEPH

Regional Medical Center Pharmacy

5325 Faraon St.
St. Joseph, MO 64506
7 days/week, 24 hours
816-271-6141

MONTANA

MISSOULA

Drug Information Service
University of Montana School of
Pharmacy and Allied Health
Sciences

32 Campus Dr.
1522 Skaggs Bldg.
Missoula, MT 59812-1522
Mon.-Fri. 8 AM-5 PM
406-243-5254
800-501-5491
www.health.umt.edu/dis

NEBRASKA

OMAHA

Drug Informatics Service
School of Pharmacy
Creighton University

2500 California Plaza
Health Science Library
Room 204
Omaha, NE 68178
Mon.-Fri. 8:30 AM-4:30 PM
402-280-5101
http://druginfo.creighton.edu

NEW JERSEY

NEWARK

New Jersey Poison Information and
Education System

140 Bergen St.
Newark, NJ 07107
Mon.-Fri. 8 AM- 5 PM
973-972-9280
800-222-1222 (Emergency)
www.njpies.org

NEW BRUNSWICK

Drug Information Service
Robert Wood Johnson
University Hospital

Pharmacy Department
1 Robert Wood Johnson Pl.
New Brunswick, NJ 08901
Mon.-Fri. 8:30 AM-4:30 PM
732-937-8842

NEW MEXICO

ALBUQUERQUE

New Mexico Poison Center
University of New Mexico
Health Sciences Center

MSC09 5080
1 University of New Mexico
Albuquerque, NM 87131
7 days/week, 24 hours
505-272-4261
800-222-1222 (Emergency)
http://hsc.unm.edu/pharmacy/
poison

NEW YORK

BROOKLYN

International Drug
Information Center
Long Island University
Arnold & Marie Schwartz
College of Pharmacy &
Health Sciences

75 DeKalb Ave.
RM-HS509
Brooklyn, NY 11201
Mon.-Fri. 9 AM-5 PM
718-488-1064
www.liu.edu

NEW HYDE PARK

Drug Information Center
St. John's University at Long
Island Jewish Medical Center

270-05 76th Ave.
New Hyde Park, NY 11040
Mon.-Fri. 8 AM-3 PM
718-470-DRUG (3784)

NEW YORK CITY

Drug Information Center
Memorial Sloan-Kettering
Cancer Center

1275 York Ave.
RM S-702
New York, NY 10021
Mon.-Fri. 9 AM-5 PM
212-639-7552

Drug Information Center
Mount Sinai Medical Center

1 Gustave Levy Pl.
New York, NY 10029
Mon.-Fri. 9 AM-5 PM
212-241-6619
(for in-house healthcare
professionals only)

ROCHESTER

Finger Lakes
Poison and Drug
Information Center
University of Rochester

601 Elmwood Ave.
Rochester, NY 14642
Mon.-Fri. 8 AM-5 PM
585-275-3718

NORTH CAROLINA

BUIES CREEK

Drug Information Center
School of Pharmacy
Campbell University

PO Box 1090
Buies Creek, NC 27506
Mon.-Fri. 8:30 AM-4:30 PM
910-893-1200,
ext. 2701
800-760-9697 (Toll free),
ext. 2701
800-327-5467 (NC only)

CHAPEL HILL

University of North
Carolina Hospitals
Drug Information Center
Dept. of Pharmacy

101 Manning Dr.
Chapel Hill, NC 27514
Mon.-Fri. 8 AM-4:30 PM
919-966-2373

DURHAM

Drug Information Center
Duke University Health
Systems

DUMC Box 3089
Durham, NC 27710
Mon.-Fri. 8 AM-5 PM
919-684-5125

GREENVILLE

Eastern Carolina Drug
Information Center
Pitt County
Memorial Hospital
Dept. of Pharmacy Service

PO Box 6028
2100 Stantonsburg Rd.
Greenville, NC 27835
Mon.-Fri. 8 AM-5 PM
252-847-4257

WINSTON-SALEM

Drug Information
Service Center
Wake-Forest University
Baptist Medical Center

Medical Center Blvd.
Winston-Salem, NC 27157
Mon.-Fri. 8 AM-5 PM
336-716-2037
(for healthcare
professionals only)

OHIO

ADA

Drug Information Center
Raabe College of Pharmacy
Ohio Northern University

Ada, OH 45810
Mon.-Thurs. 8:30 AM-5 PM
Fri. 8:30 AM-4 PM
    419-772-2307
    www.onu.edu/pharmacy/druginfo

CINCINNATI

Drug and Poison
Information Center
Children's Hospital
Medical Center

3333 Burnet Ave.
Cincinnati, OH 45229
Mon.-Fri. 9 AM-5 PM
    513-636-5063
    (administration)
    513-636-5111
    (7 days/week, 24 hours)

CLEVELAND

Drug Information Service
Cleveland Clinic Foundation

9500 Euclid Ave.
Cleveland, OH 44195
Mon.-Fri. 8:30 AM-4:30 PM
    216-444-6456
    (for healthcare
    professionals only)

Columbus

Drug Information Center
Ohio State University Hospital
Dept. of Pharmacy

Doan Hall 368
410 W. 10th Ave.
Columbus, OH 43210-1228
Mon.-Fri. 8 AM-4:30 PM
    614-293-8679
    (for in-house healthcare
    professionals only)

Drug Information Center
Riverside Methodist Hospital

3535 Olentangy River Road
Columbus, OH 43214
7 days/week, 24 hours
    614-566-5425

TOLEDO

Drug Information Services
St. Vincent Mercy Medical Center

2213 Cherry St.
Toledo, OH 43608-2691
Mon.-Fri. 7 AM-5 PM
    419-251-4227
    www.rx.medctr.ohio-state.edu

OKLAHOMA

OKLAHOMA CITY

Drug Information Service
Integris Health

3300 Northwest Expressway
Oklahoma City, OK 73112
Mon.-Fri. 8 AM-4:30 PM
    405-949-3660

Drug Information Center
OU Medical Center

1200 Everett Dr.
Oklahoma City, OK 73104
Mon.-Fri. 8 AM-4:30 PM
    405-271-6226
Fax: 405-271-6281

TULSA

Drug Information Center
Saint Francis Hospital

6161 S. Yale Ave.
Tulsa, OK 74136
Mon.-Fri. 8 AM-4:30 PM
    918-494-6339
    (for healthcare
    professionals only)

PENNSYLVANIA

PHILADELPHIA

Drug Information Center
Temple University Hospital
Dept. of Pharmacy

3401 N. Broad St.
Philadelphia, PA 19140
Mon.-Fri. 8 AM-4:30 PM
    215-707-4644

Drug Information Service
Dept. of Pharmacy
Thomas Jefferson
University Hospital

111 S. 11th St.
Philadelphia, PA 19107-5089
Mon.-Fri. 8 AM-5 PM
    215-955-8877

University of Pennsylvania
Health System Drug Information
Service Hospital of the University
of Pennsylvania
Dept. of Pharmacy

3400 Spruce St.
Philadelphia, PA 19104
Mon.-Fri. 8:30 AM-4 PM
    215-662-2903

PITTSBURGH

Pharmaceutical
Information Center
Mylan School of Pharmacy
Duquesne University

431 Mellon Hall
Pittsburgh, PA 15282
Mon.-Fri. 8 AM-4 PM
    412-396-4600

UPLAND

Drug Information Center
Crozer-Chester Medical Center
Dept. of Pharmacy

1 Medical Center Blvd.
Upland, PA 19013
Mon.-Fri. 8 AM-4:30 PM
    610-447-2851
    (for in-house healthcare
    professionals only)

PUERTO RICO

PONCE

Centro Informacion
Medicamentos
Escuela de Medicina de Ponce

PO Box 7004
Ponce, PR 00732-7004
Mon.-Fri. 8 AM-4:30 PM
    787-840-2575

SAN JUAN

Centro de Informacion de
Medicamentos-CIM
Escuela de Farmacia-RCM

PO Box 365067
San Juan, PR 00936-5067
Mon.-Fri. 8 AM-4:30 PM
    787-758-2525, ext. 1516

SOUTH CAROLINA

CHARLESTON

Drug Information Service
Medical University of
South Carolina

150 Ashley Ave.
Rutledge Tower Annex
Room 604
PO Box 250584
Charleston, SC 29425-0810
Mon.-Fri. 9 AM-5:30 PM
    843-792-3896
    800-922-5250

SPARTANBURG

Drug Information Center
Spartanburg Regional
Healthcare System

101 E. Wood St.
Spartanburg, SC 29303
Mon.-Fri. 8 AM-4:30 PM
    864-560-6910

TENNESSEE

KNOXVILLE

Drug Information Center
University of Tennessee
Medical Center at Knoxville

1924 Alcoa Highway
Knoxville, TN 37920-6999
Mon.-Fri. 8 AM-4:30 PM
    865-544-9124

MEMPHIS

**South East Regional Drug
Information Center
VA Medical Center**

1030 Jefferson Ave.
Memphis, TN 38104
Mon.-Fri. 6:30 AM-4 PM
901-523-8990, ext. 6720

**Drug Information Center
University of Tennessee**

875 Monroe Ave.
Suite 109
Memphis, TN 38163
Mon.-Fri. 8 AM-5 PM
901-448-5556

TEXAS

AMARILLO

**Drug Information Center
Texas Tech Health
Sciences Center**

School of Pharmacy
1300 Coulter Rd.
Amarillo, TX 79106
Mon.-Fri. 8 AM-5 PM
806-356-4008

GALVESTON

**Drug Information Center
University of Texas
Medical Branch**

301 University Blvd.
Galveston, TX 77555-0701
Mon.-Fri. 8 AM-5 PM
409-772-2734

HOUSTON

**Drug Information Center
Ben Taub General Hospital
Texas Southern University/HCHD**

1504 Taub Loop
Houston, TX 77030
Mon.-Fri. 8:30 AM-5 PM
713-873-3710

LACKLAND A.F.B.

**Drug Information Center
Dept. of Pharmacy
Wilford Hall Medical Center**

2200 Bergquist Dr.
Suite 1
Lackland A.F.B., TX 78236
7 days/week, 24 hours
210-292-5414

LUBBOCK

**Drug Information and Consultation
Service
Covenant Medical Center**

3615 19th St.
Lubbock, TX 79410
7 days/week, 24 hours
806-725-0408

SAN ANTONIO

**Drug Information Service
University of Texas Health Science
Center at San Antonio
Dept. of Pharmacology**

7703 Floyd Curl Drive
San Antonio, TX 78229-3900
Mon.-Fri. 8 AM-4 PM
210-567-4280

TEMPLE

**Drug Information Center
Scott and White Memorial Hospital**

2401 S. 31st St.
Temple, TX 76508
Mon.-Fri. 8 AM-5 PM
254-724-4636

UTAH

SALT LAKE CITY

**Drug Information Service
University of Utah Hospital**

421 Wakara Way
Suite 204
Salt Lake City, UT 84108
Mon.-Fri. 7:30 AM-5 PM
801-581-2073

VIRGINIA

HAMPTON

**Drug Information Center
Hampton University School
of Pharmacy**

Hampton Harbors Annex
Hampton, VA 23668
Mon.-Fri. 9 AM-4 PM
757-728-6693

WEST VIRGINIA

MORGANTOWN

**West Virginia Center for
Drug and Health Information
West Virginia University
Robert C. Byrd
Health Sciences Center**

1124 HSN, PO Box 9520
Morgantown, WV 26506
Mon.-Fri. 8:30 AM-5 PM
304-293-6640
800-352-2501 (WV)
www.hsc.wvu.edu/SOP

WYOMING

LARAMIE

**Drug Information Center
University of Wyoming**

1000 East University Ave.
Dept. 3375
Laramie, WY 82071
Mon.-Fri. 8:30 AM-4:30 PM
307-766-6988

POISON CONTROL CENTERS

The American Association of Poison Control Centers (AAPCC) uses a single, nationwide emergency number to automatically link callers with their regional poison center. This toll-free number, **800-222-1222**, also works for **teletype lines (TTY)** for the hearing-impaired and **telecommunication devices (TTD)** for individuals who are deaf. However, a few local poison centers and the ASPCA/Animal Poison Control Center are not part of this nationwide system and continue to use separate numbers.

Most of the centers listed below are certified by the AAPCC. Certified centers are marked by an asterisk after the name. Each has to meet certain criteria. It must, for example, serve a large geographic area; it must be open 24 hours a day and provide direct-dial or toll-free access; it must be supervised by a medical director; and it must have registered pharmacists or nurses available to answer questions from the public.

Within each state, centers are listed alphabetically by city. Some state poison centers also list their original emergency numbers (including TTY/TDD), which only work within that state. For these listings, callers may use either the state number or the nationwide 800 number.

ALABAMA

BIRMINGHAM

Regional Poison Control Center, The Children's Hospital of Alabama (*)

1600 7th Ave. South
Birmingham, AL 35233-1711
Business: 205-939-9201
Emergency: 800-222-1222
www.chsys.org

TUSCALOOSA

Alabama Poison Center (*)

2503 Phoenix Dr.
Tuscaloosa, AL 35405
Business: 205-345-0600
Emergency: 800-222-1222
                800-462-0800 (AL)
www.alapoisoncenter.org

ALASKA

JUNEAU

Alaska Poison Control System

Section of Community
Health and EMS
410 Willoughby Ave.
Room 103
Box 110616
Juneau, AK 99811-0616
Business: 907-465-3027
Emergency: 800-222-1222
www.chems.alaska.gov

(PORTLAND, OR)

**Oregon Poison Center (*)
Oregon Health Sciences University**

3181 SW Sam Jackson Park Rd.
CB550
Portland, OR 97239
Business: 503-494-8968
Emergency: 800-222-1222
www.oregonpoison.com

ARIZONA

PHOENIX

**Banner Poison Control Center (*)
Banner Good Samaritan
Medical Center**

901 E. Willetta St.
Room 2701
Phoenix, AZ 85006
Business: 602-495-4884
Emergency: 800-222-1222
www.bannerpoisoncontrol.com

TUCSON

**Arizona Poison and Drug
Information Center**

1295 N. Martin Ave.
Drachman Hall B308
Tucson, AZ 85724
Business: 520-626-7899
Emergency: 800-222-1222

ARKANSAS

LITTLE ROCK

**Arkansas Poison and
Drug Information Center
College of Pharmacy - UAMS**

4301 West Markham St.
Mail Slot 522-2
Little Rock, AR 72205-7122
Business: 501-686-6161
Emergency: 800-222-1222
                800-376-4766 (AR)
TDD/TTY: 800-641-3805

ASPCA/Animal Poison Control Center

1717 South Philo Rd.
Suite 36
Urbana, IL 61802
Business: 217-337-5030
Emergency: 888-426-4435
                800-548-2423
www.napcc.aspca.org

CALIFORNIA

FRESNO/MADERA

**California Poison Control System-Fresno/Madera Div. (*)
Children's Hospital of Central California**

9300 Valley Children's Place
MB 15
Madera, CA 93638-8762
Business: 559-622-2300
Emergency: 800-222-1222
                800-876-4766 (CA)
TDD/TTY: 800-972-3323
www.calpoison.org

SACRAMENTO

**California Poison Control System-Sacramento Div.(*)
UC Davis Medical Center**

Room HSF 1024
2315 Stockton Blvd.
Sacramento, CA 95817
Business: 916-227-1400
Emergency: 800-222-1222
                800-876-4766 (CA)
TDD/TTY: 800-972-3323
www.calpoison.org

SAN DIEGO

**California Poison Control
System-San Diego Div. (*)
UC San Diego Medical Center**

200 West Arbor Dr.
San Diego, CA 92103-8925
Business: 858-715-6300
Emergency: 800-222-1222
                800-876-4766 (CA)
TDD/TTY: 800-972-3323
www.calpoison.org

SAN FRANCISCO

**California Poison Control
System-San Francisco Div. (*)
San Francisco General Hospital
University of California
San Francisco**

Box 1369
San Francisco, CA 94143-1369
Business: 415-502-6000
Emergency: 800-222-1222
                800-876-4766 (CA)
TDD/TTY: 800-972-3323
www.calpoison.org

A

COLORADO
DENVER

**Rocky Mountain Poison
and Drug Center (*)**

777 Bannock St.
Mail Code 0180
Denver, CO 80204-4507
Business: 303-739-1100
Emergency: 800-222-1222
TDD/TTY: 303-739-1127 (CO)
www.RMPDC.org

CONNECTICUT
FARMINGTON

**Connecticut Regional
Poison Control Center (*)
University of Connecticut Health
Center**

263 Farmington Ave.
Farmington, CT 06030-5365
Business: 860-679-4540
Emergency: 800-222-1222
TDD/TTY: 866-218-5372
http://poisoncontrol.uchc.edu

DELAWARE
(PHILADELPHIA, PA)

**The Poison Control Center (*)
Children's Hospital of Philadelphia**

34th St. & Civic Center Blvd.
Philadelphia, PA 19104-4303
Business: 215-590-2003
Emergency: 800-222-1222
TDD/TTY: 215-590-8789
www.poisoncontrol.chop.edu

DISTRICT OF COLUMBIA
WASHINGTON, DC

National Capital Poison Center (*)

3201 New Mexico Ave., NW
Suite 310
Washington, DC 20016
Business: 202-362-3867
Emergency: 800-222-1222
www.poison.org

FLORIDA
JACKSONVILLE

**Florida Poison Information Center-
Jacksonville (*)
SHANDS Hospital**

655 West 8th St.
Jacksonville, FL 32209
Business: 904-244-4465
Emergency: 800-222-1222
http://fpicjax.org

MIAMI

**Florida Poison Information Center-
Miami (*)
University of Miami–
Department of Pediatrics**

PO Box 016960 (R-131)
Miami, FL 33101
Business: 305-585-5250
Emergency: 800-222-1222
www.miami.edu/poison-center

TAMPA

**Florida Poison
Information Center-Tampa (*)
Tampa General Hospital**

PO Box 1289
Tampa, FL 33601-1289
Business: 813-844-7044
Emergency: 800-222-1222
www.poisoncentertampa.org

GEORGIA
ATLANTA

**Georgia Poison Center (*)
Hughes Spalding Children's
Hospital, Grady Health System**

80 Jesse Hill Jr. Dr., SE
PO Box 26066
Atlanta, GA 30303-3050
Business: 404-616-9237
Emergency: 800-222-1222
             404-616-9000
             (Atlanta)
TDD: 404-616-9287
www.georgiapoisoncenter.org

HAWAII
(DENVER, CO)

**Rocky Mountain Poison
and Drug Center (*)**

777 Bannock St.
Mail Code 0180
Denver, CO 80204-4507
Business: 303-739-1100
Emergency: 800-222-1222
www.RMPDC.org

IDAHO
(DENVER, CO)

**Rocky Mountain Poison
and Drug Center (*)**

777 Bannock St.
Mail Code 0180
Denver, CO 80204-4507
Business: 303-739-1100
Emergency: 800-222-1222
www.RMPDC.org

ILLINOIS
CHICAGO

Illinois Poison Center (*)

222 South Riverside Plaza
Suite 1900
Chicago, IL 60606
Business: 312-906-6136
Emergency: 800-222-1222
TDD/TTY: 312-906-6185
www.illinoispoisoncenter.org

INDIANA
INDIANAPOLIS

**Indiana Poison Control Center (*)
Clarian Health Partners Methodist
Hospital**

I-65 at 21st St.
Indianapolis, IN 46206-1367
Business: 317-962-2335
Emergency: 800-222-1222
             800-382-9097
             317-962-2323
             (Indianapolis)
TTY: 317-962-2336
www.clarian.org/poisoncontrol

IOWA
SIOUX CITY

**Iowa Statewide Poison Control
Center Iowa Health System and
the University of Iowa Hospitals
and Clinics**

401 Douglas St.
Suite 402
Sioux City, IA 51101
Business: 712-279-3710
Emergency: 800-222-1222
             712-277-2222 (IA)
www.iowapoison.org

KANSAS
KANSAS CITY

**University of Kansas
Poison Control
Medical Center**

3901 Rainbow Blvd.
Room B-400
Kansas City, KS 66160-7231
Business   913-588-6638
Emergency: 800-222-1222
             800-332-6633 (KS)
TDD: 913-588-6639
www.kumc.com/bodyside.cmf?2144

KENTUCKY
LOUISVILLE

**Kentucky Regional
Poison Center (*)**

PO Box 35070
Louisville, KY 40232-5070
Business: 502-629-7264
Emergency: 800-222-1222
www.krpc.com

LOUISIANA
MONROE

**Louisiana Drug and Poison
Information Center (*)
University of Louisiana at Monroe**

700 University Ave.
Monroe, LA 71209-6430
Business: 318-342-3648
Emergency: 800-222-1222
              800-256-9822
              (LA only)

www.lapcc.org

MAINE
PORTLAND

**Northern New England
Poison Center**

Maine Medical Center
22 Bramhall St.
Portland, ME 04102
Business: 207-662-0111
Emergency: 800-222-1222
              207-871-2879 (ME)
TDD/TTY: 207-662-4900 (ME)
www.nnepc.org

MARYLAND
BALTIMORE

**Maryland Poison Center (*)
University of Maryland at Baltimore
School of Pharmacy**

220 Arch St.
Office Level 1
Baltimore, MD 21201
Business: 410-706-7604
Emergency: 800-222-1222
TDD: 410-706-1858
www.mdpoison.com

(WASHINGTON, DC)

**National Capital
Poison Center (*)**

3201 New Mexico Ave., NW
Suite 310
Washington DC 20016
Business: 202-362-3867
Emergency: 800-222-1222
TDD/TTY: 202-362-8563 (MD)
www.poison.org

MASSACHUSETTS
BOSTON

**Regional Center for Poison Control
and Prevention (*)
(Serving Massachusetts and Rhode
Island)**

300 Longwood Ave.
Boston, MA 02115
Business: 617-355-6609
Emergency: 800-222-1222
TDD/TTY: 888-244-5313
www.maripoisoncenter.com

MICHIGAN
DETROIT

**Regional Poison
Control Center (*)
Children's Hospital of Michigan**

4160 John R. Harper
   Professional Office Bldg.
Suite 616
Detroit, MI 48201
Business: 313-745-5335
Emergency: 800-222-1222
TDD/TTY: 800-356-3232
www.mitoxic.org/pcc

GRAND RAPIDS

**DeVos Children's Hospital
Regional Poison Center (*)**

100 Michigan St., NE
Grand Rapids, MI 49503
Business: 616-391-3690
Emergency: 800-222-1222
http://poisoncenter.
    devoschildrens.org

MINNESOTA
MINNEAPOLIS

**Minnesota Poison Control System
(*) Hennepin County Medical Center**

701 Park Ave.
Mail Code RL
Minneapolis, MN 55415
Business: 612-873-3144
Emergency: 800-222-1222
www.mnpoison.org

MISSISSIPPI
JACKSON

**Mississippi Regional Poison Control
Center, University of Mississippi
Medical Center**

2500 North State St.
Jackson, MS 39216
Business: 601-984-1680
Emergency: 800-222-1222

MISSOURI
ST. LOUIS

**Missouri Regional
Poison Center (*)
Cardinal Glennon
Children's Hospital**

7980 Clayton Rd.
Suite 200
St. Louis, MO 63117
Business: 314-772-5200
Emergency: 800-222-1222
TDD/TTY: 314-612-5705
www.cardinalglennon.com

MONTANA
(DENVER, CO)

**Rocky Mountain Poison
and Drug Center (*)**

777 Bannock St.
Mail Code 0180
Denver, CO 80204-4507
Business: 303-739-1100
Emergency: 800-222-1222
TDD/TTY: 303-739-1127
www.RMPDC.org

NEBRASKA
OMAHA

**The Poison Center (*)
Children's Hospital**

8401 W. Dodge St.
Suite 115
Omaha, NE 68114
Business: 402-955-5555
Emergency: 800-222-1222
www.nebraskapoison.com

NEVADA
(DENVER, CO)

**Rocky Mountain Poison
and Drug Center (*)**

777 Bannock St.
Mail Code 0180
Denver, CO 80204-4507
Business: 303-739-1100
Emergency: 800-222-1222
www.RMPDC.org

(PORTLAND, OR)

**Oregon Poison Center (*)
Oregon Health
Sciences University**

3181 SW Sam Jackson Park Rd.
Portland, OR 97201
Business: 503-494-8600
Emergency: 800-222-1222
www.oregonpoison.com

A

NEW HAMPSHIRE
(PORTLAND, ME)

Northern New England Poison Center

Maine Medical Center
22 Bramhall St.
Portland, ME 04102
Business: 207-662-0111
Emergency: 800-222-1222
www.nnepc.org

NEW JERSEY
NEWARK

**New Jersey Poison Information and Education System (*)
UMDNJ**

65 Bergen St.
Newark, NJ 07101
Business: 973-972-9280
Emergency: 800-222-1222
TDD/TTY: 973-926-8008
www.njpies.org

NEW MEXICO
ALBUQUERQUE

New Mexico Poison and Drug Information Center (*)

MSC09-5080
1 University of New Mexico
Albuquerque, NM 87131-0001
Business: 505-272-4261
Emergency: 800-222-1222
http://HSC.UNM.edu/pharmacy/
poison

NEW YORK
BUFFALO

Western New York Regional Poison Control Center (*) Children's Hospital of Buffalo

219 Bryant St.
Buffalo, NY 14222
Business: 716-878-7654
Emergency: 800-222-1222
www.fingerlakespoison.org

MINEOLA

**Long Island Regional Poison and Drug Information Center (*)
Winthrop University Hospital**

259 First St.
Mineola, NY 11501
Business: 516-663-2650
Emergency: 800-222-1222
TDD: 516-747-3323
(Nassau)
631-924-8811
(Suffolk)
www.lirpdic.org

NEW YORK CITY

**New York City Poison Control Center (*)
NYC Dept. of Health**

455 First Ave.
Room 123
New York, NY 10016
Business: 212-447-8152
Emergency: 800-222-1222
(English) 212-340-4494
212-POISONS
(212-764-7667)
Emergency: 212-venenos
(Spanish) (212-836-3667)
TDD: 212-689-9014

ROCHESTER

**Finger Lakes Regional Poison and Drug Information Center(*)
University of Rochester
Medical Center**

601 Elmwood Ave.
Box 321
Rochester, NY 14642
Business: 585-273-4155
Emergency: 800-222-1222
TTY: 585-273-3854

SYRACUSE

**Central New York Poison Center (*)
SUNY Upstate Medical University**

750 East Adams St.
Syracuse, NY 13210
Business: 315-464-7078
Emergency: 800-222-1222
www.cnypoison.org

NORTH CAROLINA
CHARLOTTE

**Carolinas Poison Center (*)
Carolinas Medical Center**

PO Box 32861
Charlotte, NC 28232
Business: 704-512-3795
Emergency: 800-222-1222
www.ncpoisoncenter.org

NORTH DAKOTA
BISMARK

**ND Department of Health
Injury Prevention Program**

600 E. Boulevard Ave.
Bismark, ND 58505
Business: 612-873-3144
Emergency: 800-222-1222
www.ndpoison.org

OHIO
CINCINNATI

**Cincinnati Drug and Poison Information Center (*)
Regional Poison Control System**

3333 Burnet Ave.
Vernon Place, 3rd Floor
Cincinnati, OH 45229
513-636-5063
Emergency: 800-222-1222
TDD/TTY: 800-253-7955
www.cincinnatichildrens.org/dpic

CLEVELAND

Greater Cleveland Poison Control Center

11100 Euclid Ave.
MP 6007
Cleveland, OH 44106-6007
Business: 216-844-1573
Emergency: 800-222-1222
216-231-4455 (OH)

COLUMBUS

Central Ohio Poison Center (*)

700 Children's Dr.
Room L032
Columbus, OH 43205-2696
Business: 614-722-2635
Emergency: 800-222-1222
TTY: 614-228-2272
www.bepoisonsmart.com

OKLAHOMA
OKLAHOMA CITY

**Oklahoma Poison Control Center (*)
Children's Hospital at OU Medical Center**

940 Northeast 13th St.
Room 3510
Oklahoma City, OK 73104
Business: 405-271-5062
Emergency: 800-222-1222
www.oklahomapoison.org

OREGON
PORTLAND

**Oregon Poison Center (*)
Oregon Health Sciences University**

3181 S.W. Sam Jackson Park Rd.,
CB550
Portland, OR 97239
Business: 503-494-8968
Emergency: 800-222-1222
www.ohsu.edu/poison

PENNSYLVANIA
PHILADELPHIA

The Poison Control Center (*)
Children's Hospital of Philadelphia

34th Street & Civic Center Blvd.
Philadelphia, PA 19104-4399
Business: 215-590-2003
Emergency: 800-222-1222
                 215-386-2100 (PA)
TDD/TTY: 215-590-8789
www.poisoncontrol.chop.edu

PITTSBURGH

Pittsburgh Poison Center (*)
Children's Hospital of Pittsburgh

3705 Fifth Ave.
Pittsburgh, PA 15213
Business: 412-390-3300
Emergency: 800-222-1222
                 412-681-6669
www.chp.edu/clinical/03a_
    poison.php

RHODE ISLAND
(BOSTON, MA)

**Regional Center for Poison Control
and Prevention (*)**

**(Serving Massachusetts and Rhode
Island)**

300 Longwood Ave.
Boston, MA 02115
Business: 617-355-6609
Emergency: 800-222-1222
TDD/TTY: 888-244-5313
www.maripoisoncenter.com

SOUTH DAKOTA
(MINNEAPOLIS, MN)

**Hennepin Regional Poison Center
(*) Hennepin County Medical Center**

701 Park Ave.
Minneapolis, MN 55415
Business: 612-873-3144
Emergency: 800-222-1222
www.mnpoison.org

SIOUX FALLS

**Provides education only—Does not
manage exposure cases.**

**Sioux Valley Poison Control
Center (*)**

1305 W. 18th St.
Box 5039
Sioux Falls, SD 57117-5039
Business: 605-328-6670
www.sdpoison.org

TENNESSEE
NASHVILLE

**Tennessee
Poison Center (*)**

1161 21st Ave. South
501 Oxford House
Nashville, TN 37232-4632
Business: 615-936-0760
Emergency: 800-222-1222
www.poisonlifeline.org

TEXAS
AMARILLO

**Texas Panhandle
Poison Center (*)**
Northwest Texas Hospital

1501 S. Coulter Dr.
Amarillo, TX 79106
Business: 806-354-1630
Emergency: 800-222-1222
www.poisoncontrol.org

DALLAS

North Texas Poison Center (*)
Texas Poison Center Network
**Parkland Health and Hospital
System**

5201 Harry Hines Blvd.
Dallas, TX 75235
Business: 214-589-0911
Emergency: 800-222-1222
www.poisoncontrol.org

EL PASO

**West Texas Regional
Poison Center (*)**
Thomason Hospital

4815 Alameda Ave.
El Paso, TX 79905
Business   915-534-3800
Emergency: 800-222-1222
www.poisoncontrol.org

GALVESTON

**Southeast Texas
Poison Center (*)**
**The University of Texas
Medical Branch**

3.112 Trauma Bldg.
301 University Blvd.
Galveston, TX 77555-1175
Business: 409-772-9142
Emergency: 800-222-1222
www.poisoncontrol.org

SAN ANTONIO

South Texas Poison Center (*)
**The University of Texas Health
Science Center–San Antonio**

7703 Floyd Curl Dr., MSC 7849
San Antonio, TX 78229-3900
Business: 210-567-5762
Emergency: 800-222-1222
www.poisoncontrol.org

TEMPLE

Central Texas Poison Center (*)
Scott & White Memorial Hospital

2401 South 31st St.
Temple, TX 76508
Business: 254-724-7401
Emergency: 800-222-1222
www.poisoncontrol.org

UTAH
SALT LAKE CITY

Utah Poison Control Center (*)

585 Komas Dr.
Suite 200
Salt Lake City, UT 84108
Business: 801-587-0600
Emergency: 800-222-1222
http://uuhsc.utah.edu/poison

VERMONT
(PORTLAND, ME)

**Northern New England
Poison Center**

Maine Medical Center
22 Bramhall St.
Portland, ME 04102
Business: 207-662-7220
Emergency: 800-222-1222
www.nnepc.org

VIRGINIA
CHARLOTTESVILLE

Blue Ridge Poison Center (*)
University of Virginia Health System

PO Box 800774
Charlottesville, VA 22908-0774
Business: 434-924-0347
Emergency: 800-222-1222
www.healthsystem.virginia.edu.brpc

RICHMOND

Virginia Poison Center (*)
Virginia Commonwealth University

PO Box 980522
Richmond, VA 23298-0522
Business: 804-828-4780
Emergency: 800-222-1222
                 804-828-9123
www.vcu.edu/mcved/vpc

WASHINGTON
SEATTLE

Washington Poison Center (*)

155 NE 100th St.
Suite 400
Seattle, WA 98125-8011
Business: 206-517-2359
Emergency: 800-222-1222
www.wapc.org

WEST VIRGINIA
CHARLESTON

**West Virginia
Poison Center (*)**

3110 MacCorkle Ave. SE
Charleston, WV 25304
Business: 304-347-1212
Emergency: 800-222-1222
www.wvpoisoncenter.org

WISCONSIN
MILWAUKEE

Wisconsin Poison Center

Suite CC 660
PO Box 1997
Milwaukee, WI 53201
Business: 414-266-2952
Emergency: 800-222-1222
TDD/TTY: 414-266-2542
www.wisconsinpoison.org

WYOMING
(OMAHA, NE)

**The Poison Center (*)
Nebraska Regional Poison Center**

8401 W. Dodge St.
Suite 115
Omaha, NE 68114
Business: 402-955-5555
Emergency: 800-222-1222
www.nebraskapoison.com

PROFESSIONAL ORGANIZATIONS FOR PEDIATRICS

Ambulatory Pediatric Association
6728 Old McLean Village Dr.
McLean, VA 22101
703-556-9222
www.ambpeds.org

American Academy for Cerebral Palsy and Developmental Medicine
EDI - AACPDM
555 E. Wells St.
Suite 1100
Milwaukee, WI 53202
414-918-3014
www.aacpdm.org

American Academy of Child & Adolescent Psychiatry
3615 Wisconsin Ave., NW
Washington, DC 20016-3007
202-966-7300
www.aacap.org

American Academy of Pediatrics
141 Northwest Point Blvd.
Elk Grove Village, IL 60007
847-434-400
www.aap.org

American Academy of Pediatric Dentistry
211 East Chicago Ave.
Suite 1700
Chicago, IL 60611-2637
312-337-2169
www.aapd.org

American Association for Pediatric Ophthalmology & Strabismus
PO Box 193832
San Francisco, CA 94119-3832
415-561-8505
www.aapos.org

American Board of Genetic Counseling
PO Box 14216
Lenexa, KS 66285
913-895-4617
www.abgc.net

American Board of Medical Genetics
9650 Rockville Pike
Bethesda, MD 20814-3998
301-634-7315
www.abmg.org

American Board of Pediatrics
111 Silver Cedar Ct.
Chapel Hill, NC 27514
919-929-0461
www.abp.org

American Pediatric Society & Society for Pediatric Research
3400 Research Forest Dr.
Suite B-7
The Woodlands, TX 77381
281-419-0052
www.aps-spr.org

American Pediatric Surgical Association
111 Deer Lake Rd.
Suite 100
Deerfield, IL 60015
847-480-9576
www.eapsa.org

American Pediatric Surgical Nurses Association
PO Box 1605
Lansdale, PA 19446
614-722-3926
www.apsna.org

American Society for Adolescent Psychiatry
PO Box 570218
Dallas, TX 75357-0218
972-613-0985
www.adolpsych.org

American Society of Pediatric Hematology/Oncology
4700 W. Lake Ave.
Glenview, IL 60025
847-375-4716
www.aspho.org

American Society of Pediatric Nephrology
3400 Research Forest Dr.
Suite B-7
The Woodlands, TX 77381
281-419-0052
www.aspneph.com

Association of Children's Prosthetic-Orthotic Clinics
6300 N. River Rd.
Suite 727
Rosemont, IL 60018-4226
847-698-1637
www.acpoc.org

Association of Pediatric Oncology Nurses
4700 W. Lake Ave.
Glenview, IL 60025-1485
847-375-4724
www.apon.org

California Society of Pediatric Dentistry
PO Box 4977
Palos Verdes, CA 90274
310-465-1580
www.cspd.org

Child Neurology Society
1000 W. County Rd. E
Suite 290
St. Paul, MN 55126
651-486-9447
www.childneurologysociety.org

International Pediatric Endosurgery Group
11300 W. Olympic Blvd.
Suite 600
Los Angeles, CA 90064
310-437-0553
www.ipeg.org

March of Dimes
1275 Mamaroneck Ave.
White Plains, NY 10605
914-997-4488
www.marchofdimes.com

Midwest Society for Pediatric Research
3400 Research Forest Dr.
Suite B-7
The Woodlands, TX 77381
281-419-0052
www.aps-spr.org

National Association of Pediatric Nurse Practitioners
20 Brace Rd.
Suite 200
Cherry Hill, NJ 08034-2634
856-857-9700
www.napnap.org

National Childhood Cancer Foundation
4600 East-West Highway
Suite 600
Bethesda, MD 20814-3457
800-458-6223
www.nccf.org

North American Society for Pediatric Gastroenterology, Hepatology & Nutrition
PO Box 6
Flourtown, PA 19031
215-233-0808
www.naspghan.org

Society for Adolescent Medicine
1916 Copper Oaks Circle
Blue Springs, MO 64015
816-224-8010
www.adolescenthealth.org

Society for Developmental & Behavioral Pediatrics
6728 Old McLean Village Dr.
McLean, VA 22101
703-556-9222
www.sdbp.org

Society for Fetal Urology
University of Alabama
1600 7th Ave., South
ACC #318
Birmingham, AL 35233
205-939-9840
http://main.uab.edu

Society for Pediatric Dermatology
8365 Keystone Crossing
Suite 107
Indianapolis, IN 46240
317-202-0224
www.pedsderm.net

Society for Pediatric Radiology
1891 Preston White Dr.
Reston, VA 20191
703-648-0680
www.pedrad.org

Society of Pediatric Nurses
7794 Grow Dr.
Pensacola, FL 32514
850-494-9467
www.pedsnurses.org

Society for Pediatric Urology
900 Cummings Center
Suite 221-U
Beverly, MA 01915
978-927-8330
www.spuonline.org

Southern Society for Pediatric Research
Children's Hospital of the King's Daughters
601 Children's Lane
Norfolk, VA 23507
757-668-7456
www.aps-spr.org

Sudden Infant Death Syndrome (SIDS) Alliance
1314 Bedford Ave.
Suite 210
Baltimore, MD 21208
800-221-7437
www.sidsalliance.org

ACNE PRODUCTS

BRAND	INGREDIENT/STRENGTH	DOSE
BENZOYL PEROXIDE		
Clean & Clear Continuous Control Acne Cleanser	Benzoyl Peroxide 10%	**Adults & Peds:** Use bid.
Clean & Clear Persa-Gel 10, Maximum Strength	Benzoyl Peroxide 10%	**Adults & Peds:** Use qd-tid.
Clearasil Daily Acne Stay Clear Cream	Benzoyl Peroxide 10%	**Adults & Peds:** Use qd-tid.
Clearasil Total Acne Control	Benzoyl Peroxide 10%	**Adults & Peds:** Use qd-tid.
Clearasil Acne Treatment Tinted Cream	Benzoyl Peroxide 10%	**Adults & Peds:** Use up to tid.
Clearasil Ultra Acne Treatment Vanishing Cream	Benzoyl Peroxide 10%	**Adults & Peds:** Use up to tid.
Neutrogena Clear Pore Cleanser Mask	Benzoyl Peroxide 3.5%	**Adults & Peds:** Use biw-tiw.
Neutrogena On-the-Spot Acne Treatment Vanishing Cream	Benzoyl Peroxide 2.5%	**Adults & Peds:** Apply qd initially, then bid-tid.
Oxy Chill Factor Daily Wash	Benzoyl Peroxide 10%	**Adults & Peds:** Use qd.
Oxy Maximum Daily Wash	Benzoyl Peroxide 10%	**Adults & Peds:** Use qd.
Oxy Spot Treatment	Benzoyl Peroxide 10%	**Adults & Peds:** Use qd-tid.
PanOxyl Aqua Gel Maximum Strength gel	Benzoyl Peroxide 10%	**Adults & Peds:** Apply qd initially, then bid-tid.
PanOxyl Bar 10% Maximum Strength	Benzoyl Peroxide 10%	**Adults & Peds:** Apply qd initially, then bid-tid.
PanOxyl Bar 5%	Benzoyl Peroxide 5%	**Adults & Peds:** Use qd initially, then bid-tid.
ZAPZYT Maximum Strength Acne Treatment gel	Benzoyl Peroxide 10%	**Adults & Peds:** Use up to tid. If dryness occurs, use qd or qod.
ZAPZYT Treatment Bar	Benzoyl Peroxide 10%	**Adults & Peds:** Use qd initially, then bid-tid. If dryness occurs, use qd or qod.
SALICYLIC ACID		
Aveeno Clear Complexion Cleansing Bar	Salicylic Acid 0.5%	**Adults & Peds:** Use daily.
Aveeno Clear Complexion Foaming Cleanser	Salicylic Acid 0.5%	**Adults & Peds:** Use daily.
Aveeno Correcting Treatment, Clear Complexion	Salicylic Acid 1%	**Adults & Peds:** Use qd-tid.
Biore Blemish Fighting Cleansing Cloths	Salicylic Acid 2%	**Adults & Peds:** Use qd-tid.
Biore Blemish Fighting Ice Cleanser	Salicylic Acid 2%	**Adults & Peds:** Use qd.
Bye Bye Blemish Anti-Acne Serum	Salicylic Acid 1%	**Adults & Peds:** Use qd-tid.
Bye Bye Blemish Drying Lotion	Salicylic Acid 2%	**Adults & Peds:** Use pm.
Bye Bye Blemish Purifying Acne Mask	Salicylic Acid 0.5%	**Adults & Peds:** Use qd.
Clean & Clear Advantage Acne Cleanser	Salicylic Acid 2%	**Adults & Peds:** Use qd.
Clean & Clear Advantage Acne Spot Treatment	Salicylic Acid 2%	**Adults & Peds:** Use qd.
Clean & Clear Advantage Cleansing Pads	Salicylic Acid 2%	**Adults & Peds:** Use qd.
Clean & Clear Blackhead Clearing Astringent	Salicylic Acid 1%	**Adults & Peds:** Use qd.
Clean & Clear Blackhead Clearing Daily Cleansing Pads	Salicylic Acid 1%	**Adults & Peds:** Use qd.

(Continued)

BRAND	INGREDIENT/STRENGTH	DOSE
SALICYLIC ACID *(Continued)*		
Clean & Clear Blackhead Clearing Scrub	Salicylic Acid 2%	**Adults & Peds:** Use qd.
Clean & Clear Clear Advantage Daily Acne Control Moisturizer	Salicylic Acid 0.5%	**Adults & Peds:** Use qd.
Clean & Clear Continuous Control Acne Wash, Oil Free	Salicylic Acid 2%	**Adults & Peds:** Use qd-tid.
Clean & Clear Oil-Free Acne Moisturizer	Salicylic Acid 0.5%	**Adults & Peds:** Use qd-tid.
Clearasil Stay Clear Deep Cleanse Acne Fighting Cleansing Wipes	Salicylic Acid 2%	**Adults & Peds:** Use qd-tid.
Clearasil Stay Clear Skin Perfecting Wash	Salicylic Acid 2%	**Adults & Peds:** Use bid.
Clearasil Stay Clear Oil Free Gel Wash	Salicylic Acid 2%	**Adults & Peds:** Use bid.
Clearasil Stay Clear Daily Pore Cleansing Pads	Salicylic Acid 2%	**Adults & Peds:** Use qd-tid.
Clearasil Stay Clear Daily Facial Scrub	Salicylic Acid 2%	**Adults & Peds:** Use qd.
Clearasil Ultra Acne Clearing Gel Wash	Salicylic Acid 2%	**Adults & Peds:** Use qd.
Clearasil Ultra Daily Face Wash	Salicylic Acid 2%	**Adults & Peds:** Use qd.
Clearasil Ultra Acne Clearing Scrub	Salicylic Acid 2%	**Adults & Peds:** Use qd.
Clearasil Ultra Deep Pore Cleansing Pads	Salicylic Acid 2%	**Adults & Peds:** Use qd-tid.
L'Oreal Pure Pore-Clearing Cleanser	Salicylic Acid 1%	**Adults & Peds:** Use tid.
Neutrogena Advanced Solutions Acne Mark Fading Peel with CelluZyme	Salicylic Acid 2%	**Adults & Peds:** Use qw-tiw.
Neutrogena Blackhead Eliminating Astringent	Salicylic Acid 1%	**Adults & Peds:** Use qd-tid.
Neutrogena Blackhead Eliminating Daily Scrub	Salicylic Acid 2%	**Adults & Peds:** Use bid.
Neutrogena Blackhead Eliminating Foaming Pads	Salicylic Acid 0.5%	**Adults & Peds:** Use qd.
Neutrogena Body Clear Body Scrub	Salicylic Acid 2%	**Adults & Peds:** Use qd.
Neutrogena Oil Free Acne Wash Foam Cleanser	Salicylic Acid 2%	**Adults & Peds:** Use qd.
Neutrogena Clear Pore Oil-Eliminating Astringent	Salicylic Acid 2%	**Adults & Peds:** Use qd-tid.
Neutrogena Oil Free Acne Stress Control Power Clear Scrub	Salicylic Acid 2%	**Adults & Peds:** Use qd.
Neutrogena Oil Free Acne Stress Control Power Foam Wash	Salicylic Acid 0.5%	**Adults & Peds:** Use qd-tid.
Neutrogena Acne Stress Control 3-in-1 Hydrating Acne Treatment	Salicylic Acid 2%	**Adults & Peds:** Use qd-tid.
Neutrogena Oil Free Acne Wash Cleansing Cloths	Salicylic Acid 2%	**Adults & Peds:** Use qd.
Neutrogena Oil Free Acne Wash Cream Cleanser	Salicylic Acid 2%	**Adults & Peds:** Use qd-bid.
Neutrogena Rapid Clear Acne Defense Face Lotion	Salicylic Acid 2%	**Adults & Peds:** Use qd-tid.
Neutrogena Rapid Clear Acne Eliminating Spot Gel	Salicylic Acid 2%	**Adults & Peds:** Use qd-tid.
Neutrogena Skin Polishing Acne Cleanser	Salicylic Acid 0.5%	**Adults & Peds:** Use bid.

(Continued)

BRAND	INGREDIENT/STRENGTH	DOSE
SALICYLIC ACID (Continued)		
Neutrogena Oil-Free Anti-Acne Moisturizer	Salicylic Acid 0.5%	**Adults & Peds:** Use qd initially, then bid-tid. If dryness occurs, use qd or qod.
Noxzema Continuous Clean Deep Foaming Cleanser	Salicylic Acid 2%	**Adults & Peds:** Use qd.
Noxzema Triple Clean Anti-Blemish Astringent	Salicylic Acid 2%	**Adults & Peds:** Use qd-tid. If dryness occurs, use qd or qod.
Noxzema Triple Clean Anti-Blemish Pads	Salicylic Acid 2%	**Adults & Peds:** Use qd-tid.
Olay Daily Facials Lathering Cleansing Cloths-Clarifying for Combination/Oily Skin	Salicylic Acid (strength NA)	**Adults & Peds:** Apply qd.
Olay Regenerist Daily Regenerating Cleanser	Salicylic Acid	**Adults & Peds:** Use qd.
Olay Total Effects Plus Blemish Control Moisturizer	Salicylic Acid	**Adults & Peds:** Apply qd-tid.
Oxy Chill Cleansing Pads	Salicylic Acid 2%	**Adults & Peds:** Use qd-tid.
Oxy Chill Face Scrub	Salicylic Acid 2%	**Adults & Peds:** Use qd-tid.
Oxy Maximum Bar Soap	Salicylic Acid 0.5%	**Adults & Peds:** Use qd-tid.
Oxy Maximum Face Scrub	Salicylic Acid 2%	**Adults & Peds:** Use qd-tid.
Oxy Maximum Daily Cleansing Pads	Salicylic Acid 2%	**Adults & Peds:** Use qd-tid.
Oxy Body Wash	Salicylic Acid 2%	**Adults & Peds:** Use qd.
Phisoderm Anti-Blemish Body Wash	Salicylic Acid 2%	**Adults & Peds:** Use qd.
St. Ives Medicated Apricot Scrub	Salicylic Acid 2%	**Adults & Peds:** Use qd.
Stridex Facewipes to Go with Acne Medication	Salicylic Acid 0.5%	**Adults & Peds:** Use qd-tid.
Stridex Triple Action Acne Pads Maximum Strength, Alcohol Free	Salicylic Acid 2%	**Adults & Peds:** Use qd-tid.
Stridex Essential Care Pads with Salicylic Acid	Salicylic Acid 1%	**Adults & Peds:** Use qd-tid.
Stridex Triple Action Medicated Acne Pads, Sensitive Skin	Salicylic Acid 0.5%	**Adults & Peds:** Use qd-tid.
ZAPZYT Acne Wash Treatment For Face & Body	Salicylic Acid 2%	**Adults & Peds:** Use bid.
ZAPZYT Pore Treatment Gel	Salicylic Acid 2%	**Adults & Peds:** Use qd-tid.
TRICLOSAN		
Noxema Triple Clean Anti-Bacterial Cleanser	Triclosan 0.3%	**Adults & Peds ≥6 months:** Use qd each time skin is cleansed.

ANTIFUNGAL PRODUCTS

BRAND	INGREDIENT/STRENGTH	DOSE
BUTENAFINE		
Lotrimin Ultra Antifungal Cream	Butenafine HCl 1%	**Adults & Peds ≥12 yrs:** Use bid.
CLOTRIMAZOLE		
FungiCure Anti-Fungal Liquid Spray	Clotrimazole 1%	**Adults & Peds:** Use bid.
Lotrimin AF Antifungal Athlete's Foot Cream	Clotrimazole 1%	**Adults & Peds ≥2 yrs:** Use bid.
Lotrimin AF Antifungal Athlete's Foot Topical Solution	Clotrimazole 1%	**Adults & Peds ≥2 yrs:** Use bid.
Lotrimin AF For Her Antifungal Cream	Clotrimazole 1%	**Adults & Peds ≥2 yrs:** Use bid.
MICONAZOLE		
Clearly Confident Triple Action Fungus Treatment	Miconazole Nitrate 2%	**Adults:** Apply to affected area bid.
Desenex Antifungal Liquid Spray	Miconazole Nitrate 2%	**Adults:** Use bid.
Desenex Antifungal Powder	Miconazole Nitrate 2%	**Adults:** Use bid.
Desenex Antifungal Spray	Miconazole Nitrate 2%	**Adults:** Use bid.
DiabetAid Antifungal Foot Bath Tablets	Miconazole Nitrate 2%	**Adults & Peds ≥2 yrs:** Use prn.
Diabet-X Antifungal Skin Treatment Cream	Miconazole Nitrate 2%	**Adults & Peds ≥2 yrs:** Use prn.
Lotrimin AF Antifungal Aerosol Liquid Spray	Miconazole Nitrate 2%	**Adults & Peds ≥2 yrs:** Use bid.
Lotrimin AF Antifungal Jock Itch Aerosol Powder Spray	Miconazole Nitrate 2%	**Adults & Peds ≥2 yrs:** Use bid.
Lotrimin AF Antifungal Powder	Miconazole Nitrate 2%	**Adults & Peds ≥2 yrs:** Use bid.
Micatin Athlete's Foot Cream	Miconazole Nitrate 2%	**Adults:** Use bid.
Micatin Athlete's Foot Spray Liquid	Miconazole Nitrate 2%	**Adults:** Use bid.
Micatin Athlete's Foot Spray Liquid	Miconazole Nitrate 2%	**Adults:** Use bid.
Micatin Jock Itch Spray Powder	Miconazole Nitrate 2%	**Adults:** Use bid.
Micatin Jock Itch Antifungal Cream	Miconazole Nitrate 2%	**Adults:** Use bid.
Neosporin AF Antifungal Cream	Miconazole Nitrate 2%	**Adults & Peds ≥12 yrs:** Use bid.
Neosporin AF Athlete's Foot Antifungal Spray Liquid	Miconazole Nitrate 2%	**Adults & Peds ≥12 yrs:** Use bid.
Neosporin AF Athlete's Foot Antifungal Spray Powder	Miconazole Nitrate 2%	**Adults & Peds ≥12 yrs:** Use bid.
Neosporin AF Jock Itch Antifungal Cream	Miconazole Nitrate 2%	**Adults & Peds ≥12 yrs:** Use bid.
Zeasorb Super Absorbent Antifungal Powder	Miconazole Nitrate 2%	**Adults & Peds:** Use bid.
TERBINAFINE		
Lamisil AT Antifungal Cream	Terbinafine HCl 1%	**Adults & Peds ≥12 yrs:** Use bid.
Lamisil AT Antifungal Spray Pump	Terbinafine HCl 1%	**Adults & Peds ≥12 yrs:** Use qd or bid.
Lamisil AT Athlete's Foot Cream	Terbinafine HCl 1%	**Adults & Peds ≥12 yrs:** Use bid.
Lamisil AT Athlete's Foot Gel	Terbinafine HCl 1%	**Adults & Peds ≥12 yrs:** Use qd.
Lamisil AT Athlete's Foot Spray Pump	Terbinafine HCl 1%	**Adults & Peds ≥12 yrs:** Use bid.

(Continued)

BRAND	INGREDIENT/STRENGTH	DOSE
TERBINAFINE *(Continued)*		
Lamisil AT for Women Cream	Terbinafine HCl 1%	**Adults & Peds** ≥**12 yrs:** Use bid.
Lamisil AT Jock Itch Cream	Terbinafine HCl 1%	**Adults & Peds** ≥**12 yrs:** Use qd.
Lamisil AT Jock Itch Spray Pump	Terbinafine HCl 1%	**Adults & Peds** ≥**12 yrs:** Use qd.
TOLNAFTATE		
Aftate Antifungal Liquid Spray for Athlete's Foot	Tolnaftate 1%	**Adults:** Use qd-bid
FungiCure Anti-Fungal Gel	Tolnaftate 1%	**Adults & Peds:** Use bid.
Gold Bond Antifungal Foot Swabs	Tolnaftate 1%	**Adults & Peds:** Use bid.
Miracle of Aloe Miracure Anti-Fungal	Tolnaftate 1%	**Adults & Peds** ≥**12 yrs:** Use bid.
Swabplus Foot Care Fungus Relief Swabs	Tolnaftate 1%	**Adults & Peds:** Use bid.
Tinactin Antifungal Deodorant Powder Spray	Tolnaftate 1%	**Adults & Peds:** Use bid.
Tinactin Antifungal Liquid Spray	Tolnaftate 1%	**Adults & Peds:** Use bid.
Tinactin Antifungal Powder Spray	Tolnaftate 1%	**Adults & Peds:** Use bid.
Tinactin Antifungal Cream	Tolnaftate 1%	**Adults & Peds:** Use bid.
Tinactin Antifungal Absorbent Powder	Tolnaftate 1%	**Adults & Peds:** Use qd-tid.
Tinactin Antifungal Jock Itch Powder Spray	Tolnaftate 1%	**Adults & Peds:** Use qd-tid.
UNDECYLENIC ACID		
Fungi Nail Anti-fungal Solution	Undecylenic Acid 25%	**Adults & Peds:** Use bid.
FungiCure Anti-fungal Liquid	Undecylenic Acid 10%	**Adults & Peds:** Use bid.
Tineacide Antifungal Cream	Undecylenic Acid 10%	**Adults & Peds** ≥**12 yrs:** Use bid.

ANTISEBORRHEAL PRODUCTS

BRAND	INGREDIENT/STRENGTH	DOSE
COAL TAR		
DHS Tar Dermatological Hair & Scalp Shampoo	Coal Tar 0.5%	**Adults & Peds:** Use biw.
DHS Tar Shampoo	Coal Tar 0.5%	**Adults & Peds:** Use at least biw.
Neutrogena T/Gel Shampoo Original Formula	Coal Tar 0.5%	**Adults & Peds:** Use at least biw.
Neutrogena T/Gel Stubborn Itch Shampoo	Coal Tar 0.5%	**Adults & Peds:** Use at least biw.
Polytar Shampoo	Coal Tar 0.5%	**Adults & Peds:** Use at least biw.
Polytar Soap	Coal Tar 0.5%	**Adults & Peds:** Use prn.
Psoriasin Liquid Dab-on	Coal Tar 0.66%	**Adults:** Apply to affected area qd-qid.
Ionil-T Shampoo	Coal Tar 1%	**Adults & Peds:** Use at least biw.
Neutrogena T/Gel Shampoo Extra Strength	Coal Tar 1%	**Adults & Peds:** Use at least biw.
Psoriasin Gel	Coal Tar 1.25%	**Adults:** Apply to affected area qd-qid.
Ionil-T Plus Shampoo	Coal Tar 2%	**Adults & Peds:** Use at least biw.
MG217 Ointment	Coal Tar 2%	**Adults & Peds:** Apply to affected area qd-qid.
Denorex Therapeutic Protection 2-in-1 Shampoo	Coal Tar 2.5%	**Adults & Peds:** Use at least biw.
Denorex Therapeutic Protection Shampoo	Coal Tar 2.5%	**Adults & Peds:** Use at least biw.
MG217 Tar Shampoo	Coal Tar 3%	**Adults & Peds:** Use at least biw.
Ionil T Therapeutic Coal Tar Shampoo	Coal Tar 5%	**Adults & Peds:** Use biw.
CORTICOSTEROIDS		
Aveeno Hydrocortisone 1% Anti-Itch Cream	Hydrocortisone 1%	**Adults & Peds:** ≥2 yrs: Apply to affected area tid-qid.
Cortaid Advanced 12-Hour Anti-Itch Cream	Hydrocortisone 1%	**Adults & Peds:** ≥2 yrs: Apply to affected area tid-qid.
Cortaid Intensive Therapy Cooling Spray	Hydrocortisone 1%	**Adults & Peds:** ≥2 yrs: Apply to affected area tid-qid.
Cortaid Intensive Therapy Moisturizing Cream	Hydrocortisone 1%	**Adults & Peds:** ≥2 yrs: Apply to affected area tid-qid.
Cortaid Maximum Strength Cream	Hydrocortisone 1%	**Adults & Peds:** ≥2 yrs: Apply to affected area tid-qid.
Cortaid Maximum Strength Ointment	Hydrocortisone 1%	**Adults & Peds:** ≥2 yrs: Apply to affected area tid-qid.
Cortizone-10 Cream	Hydrocortisone 1%	**Adults & Peds:** ≥2 yrs: Apply to affected area tid-qid.
Cortizone-10 Maximum Strength Anti-Itch Ointment	Hydrocortisone 1%	**Adults & Peds:** ≥2 yrs: Apply to affected area tid-qid.
Cortizone-10 Ointment	Hydrocortisone 1%	**Adults & Peds:** ≥2 yrs: Apply to affected area tid-qid.
Cortizone-10 Intensive Healing Formula	Hydrocortisone 1%	**Adults & Peds:** ≥2 yrs: Apply to affected area tid-qid.
PYRITHIONE ZINC		
Denorex Dandruff Shampoo, Daily Protection	Pyrithione Zinc 2%	**Adults & Peds:** Use biw.
Garnier Fructis Fortifying Shampoo, Anti-Dandruff	Pyrithione Zinc 1%	**Adults & Peds:** Use biw.
Head & Shoulders Dry Scalp Care Dandruff Shampoo Plus Conditioner, Shampoo; Conditioner	Pyrithione Zinc 1%	**Adults & Peds:** Use biw.

(Continued)

BRAND	INGREDIENT/STRENGTH	DOSE
PYRITHIONE ZINC *(Continued)*		
Head & Shoulders Smooth & Silky Dandruff Shampoo Plus Conditioner; Shampoo; Conditioner	Pyrithione Zinc 1%	**Adults & Peds:** Use biw.
Head & Shoulders Citrus Breeze Dandruff Shampoo Plus Conditioner; Shampoo	Pyrithione Zinc 1%	**Adults & Peds:** Use biw.
Head & Shoulders Classic Clean Dandruff Shampoo Plus Conditioner; Shampoo; Conditioner	Pyrithione Zinc 1%	**Adults & Peds:** Use biw.
Head & Shoulders Extra Volume Dandruff Shampoo	Pyrithione Zinc 1%	**Adults & Peds:** Use biw.
Head & Shoulders Ocean Lift Dandruff Shampoo Plus Conditioner; Shampoo	Pyrithione Zinc 1%	**Adults & Peds:** Use biw.
Head & Shoulders Dandruff Refresh Shampoo Plus Conditioner; Shampoo	Pyrithione Zinc 1%	**Adults & Peds:** Use biw.
Head & Shoulders Restoring Shine Dandruff Shampoo Plus Conditioner; Shampoo	Pyrithione Zinc 1%	**Adults & Peds:** Use biw.
Head & Shoulders Sensitive Care Dandruff Shampoo Plus Conditioner; Shampoo	Pyrithione Zinc 1%	**Adults & Peds:** Use biw.
Head & Shoulders Intensive Solutions Dandruff Shampoo and Conditioner; Shampoo	Pyrithione Zinc 1%	**Adults & Peds:** Use biw.
L'Oreal VIVE Pro Anti-Dandruff for Men Shampoo	Pyrithione Zinc 1%	**Adults & Peds:** Use biw.
Neutrogena T-Gel Daily Control Dandruff Shampoo	Pyrithione Zinc 1%	**Adults & Peds:** Use biw.
Pantene Pro-V Shampoo + Conditioner, Anti-Dandruff	Pyrithione Zinc 1%	**Adults & Peds:** Use biw.
Pert Plus Shampoo Plus Conditioner, Dandruff Control	Pyrithione Zinc 0.45%	**Adults & Peds:** Use biw.
Selsun Salon 2-in-1 Pyrithione Zinc Shampoo	Pyrithione Zinc 1%	**Adults & Peds:** Use biw.
Suave for Men 2 in 1 Shampoo/ Conditioner, Dandruff	Pyrithione Zinc 0.5%	**Adults & Peds:** Use biw.
SALICYLIC ACID		
Neutrogena T/Gel Conditioner	Salicylic Acid 2%	**Adults & Peds:** Use at least tiw.
Psoriasin Therapeutic Shampoo and Body Wash	Salicylic Acid 3%	**Adults & Peds:** Use biw.
Neutrogena T/Sal Shampoo, Scalp Build-up Control	Salicylic Acid 3%	**Adults & Peds:** Use biw.
Scalpicin Anti-Itch Liquid Scalp Treatment (Combe)	Salicylic Acid 3%	**Adults:** Apply to affected area qd-qid.
SELENIUM SULFIDE		
Head & Shoulders Dandruff Shampoo, Intensive Treatment	Selenium Sulfide 1%	**Adults & Peds:** Use biw.
Selsun Blue Dandruff Shampoo, Medicated Treatment	Selenium Sulfide 1%	**Adults & Peds:** Use biw.
Selsun Blue Dandruff Shampoo Plus Conditioner	Selenium Sulfide 1%	**Adults & Peds:** Use biw.
Selsun Blue Dandruff Shampoo	Selenium Sulfide 1%	**Adults & Peds:** Use biw.
Selsun Blue Dandruff Shampoo, Moisturizing Treatment	Selenium Sulfide 1%	**Adults & Peds:** Use biw.
SULFUR/SALICYLIC ACID		
Sebulex Medicated Dandruff Shampoo	Sulfur/Salicylic Acid 2%-2%	**Adults & Peds:** Use qd.

CONTACT DERMATITIS PRODUCTS

BRAND	INGREDIENT/STRENGTH	DOSE
ANTIHISTAMINE		
Benadryl Extra Strength Gel	Diphenhydramine HCl 2%	**Adults & Peds ≥2 yrs:** Apply to affected area tid-qid.
ANTIHISTAMINE COMBINATION		
Benadryl Extra Strength Itch-Stopping Cream	Diphenhydramine HCl/Zinc Acetate 2%-0.1%	**Adults & Peds ≥2 yrs:** Apply to affected area tid-qid.
Benadryl Extra Strength Spray	Diphenhydramine HCl/Zinc Acetate 2%-0.1%	**Adults & Peds ≥12 yrs:** Apply to affected area tid-qid.
Benadryl Itch Relief Spray	Diphenhydramine HCl/Zinc Acetate 2%-0.1%	**Adults & Peds ≥2 yrs:** Apply to affected area tid-qid.
Benadryl Itch Relief Stick	Diphenhydramine HCl/Zinc Acetate 2%-0.1%	**Adults & Peds ≥2 yrs:** Apply to affected area tid-qid.
Benadryl Original Cream	Diphenhydramine HCl/Zinc Acetate 1%-0.1%	**Adults & Peds ≥2 yrs:** Apply to affected area tid-qid.
CalaGel Anti-Itch Gel	Diphenhydramine HCl/Zinc Acetate/Benzethonium Chloride 2%-0.215%-0.15%	**Adults & Peds ≥2 yrs:** Apply to affected area tid-qid.
Ivarest Anti-Itch Cream	Diphenhydramine HCl/Calamine 2%-14%	**Adults & Peds ≥2 yrs:** Apply to affected area tid-qid.
ASTRINGENT		
Domeboro Powder Packets	Aluminum Acetate/Aluminum Sulfate	**Adults & Peds:** Dissolve 1-2 packets and apply to affected area for 15-30 min tid.
Ivy-Dry Super Lotion Extra Strength	Zinc Acetate/Benzyl Alcohol/Camphor/Menthol 2%-10%-0.5%-0.25%	**Adults & Peds: ≥6 yrs:** Apply to affected area qd-tid.
ASTRINGENT COMBINATION		
Aveeno Calamine and Pramoxine HCl Anti-Itch Cream	Calamine/Pramoxine HCl 3%-1%	**Adults & Peds ≥2 yrs:** Apply to affected area tid-qid.
Aveeno Anti-Itch Concentrated Lotion	Calamine/Pramoxine HCl/Camphor 3%-1%-0.47%	**Adults & Peds ≥2 yrs:** Apply to affected area qid.
Caladryl Clear Lotion	Zinc Acetate/Pramoxine HCl 0.1%-1%	**Adults & Peds ≥2 yrs:** Apply to affected area tid-qid.
Caladryl Lotion	Calamine/Pramoxine HCl 8%-1%	**Adults & Peds ≥2 yrs:** Apply to affected area tid-qid.
Calamine Lotion (generic)	Calamine/Zinc Oxide	**Adults & Peds:** Apply to affected area prn.
CLEANSER		
Ivy-Dry Scrub	Polyethylene, sodium lauryl sulfoacetate, cetearyl alcohol, nonoxynol-9, camellia sinensis oil, phenoxyethanol, methylparaben, propylparaben, triethanolamine, carbomer, erythorbic acid, aloe barbadensis extract, tocopheryl acetate extract, tetrasodium EDTA	**Adults & Peds:** Wash affected area prn.
Cortaid Poison Ivy Care Toxin Removal Cloths	Water, lauroyl sarcosinate, glycerin, DMDM, hydantoin, methylparaben, tetrasodium EDTA, Aloe barnadenis leaf extract, citric acid	**Adults & Peds:** Wash affected area prn.
CORTICOSTEROID		
Aveeno 1% Hydrocortisone Anti-Itch Cream	Hydrocortisone 1%	**Adults & Peds ≥2 yrs:** Apply to affected area tid-qid.
Cortaid Advanced 12-Hour Anti-Itch Cream	Hydrocortisone 1%	**Adults & Peds ≥2 yrs:** Apply to affected area tid-qid.
Cortaid Intensive Therapy Cooling Spray	Hydrocortisone 1%	**Adults & Peds ≥2 yrs:** Apply to affected area tid-qid.
Cortaid Intensive Therapy Moisturizing Cream	Hydrocortisone 1%	**Adults & Peds ≥2 yrs:** Apply to affected area tid-qid.
Cortaid Maximum Strength Cream	Hydrocortisone 1%	**Adults & Peds ≥2 yrs:** Apply to affected area tid-qid.

(Continued)

BRAND	INGREDIENT/STRENGTH	DOSE
CORTICOSTEROID *(Continued)*		
Cortaid Maximum Strength Ointment	Hydrocortisone 1%	**Adults & Peds ≥2 yrs:** Apply to affected area tid-qid.
Cortizone-10 Cream	Hydrocortisone 1%	**Adults & Peds ≥2 yrs:** Apply to affected area tid-qid.
Cortizone-10 Maximum Strength Anti-Itch Ointment	Hydrocortisone 1%	**Adults & Peds ≥2 yrs:** Apply to affected area tid-qid.
Cortizone-10 Ointment	Hydrocortisone 1%	**Adults & Peds ≥2 yrs:** Apply to affected area tid-qid.
Cortizone-10 Plus Intensive Healing Formula	Hydrocortisone 1%	**Adults & Peds ≥2 yrs:** Apply to affected area tid-qid.
IvyStat!	Hydrocortisone 1%	**Adults & Peds ≥2 yrs:** Apply to affected area tid-qid.
Dermarest Eczema Lotion	Hydrocortisone 1%	**Adults & Peds ≥2 yrs:** Apply to affected area tid-qid.
COUNTERIRRITANT		
Gold Bond First Aid Quick Spray	Menthol/Benzethonium Chloride 1%-0.13%	**Adults & Peds ≥2 yrs:** Apply to affected area tid-qid.
Gold Bond Medicated Maximum Strength Anti-Itch Cream	Menthol/Pramoxine HCl 1%-1%	**Adults & Peds ≥2 yrs:** Apply to affected area tid-qid.
Ivy Block Lotion	Bentoquatam 5%	**Adults & Peds ≥2 yrs:** Apply q4h for continued protection.
LOCAL ANESTHETIC		
Solarcaine Aloe Extra Burn Relief Gel	Lidocaine HCl 0.5%	**Adults & Peds ≥2 yrs:** Apply to affected area tid-qid.
Solarcaine Aloe Extra Spray	Lidocaine HCl 0.5%	**Adults & Peds ≥2 yrs:** Apply to affected area tid-qid.
Solarcaine First Aid Medicated Spray	Benzocaine/Triclosan 20%-0.13%	**Adults & Peds ≥2 yrs:** Apply to affected area qd-tid.
LOCAL ANESTHETIC COMBINATION		
Bactine First Aid Liquid	Lidocaine HCl/Benzalkonium Chloride 2.5%-0.13%	**Adults & Peds ≥2 yrs:** Apply to affected area qd-tid.
Lanacane Maximum Strength Cream	Benzocaine/Benzethonium Chloride 20%-0.2%	**Adults & Peds ≥2 yrs:** Apply to affected area qd-tid.
Lanacane Maximum Strength Spray	Benzocaine/Benzethonium Chloride 20%-0.2%	**Adults & Peds ≥2 yrs:** Apply to affected area qd-tid.
Lanacane Original Formula Cream	Benzocaine/Benzethonium Chloride 6%-0.2%	**Adults & Peds ≥2 yrs:** Apply to affected area qd-tid.
SKIN PROTECTANT		
Aveeno Skin Relief Moisturizing Cream	Dimethicone 2.5%	**Adults & Peds ≥2 yrs:** Apply to affected area tid-qid.
SKIN PROTECTANT COMBINATION		
Aveeno Itch Relief Lotion	Dimethicone/Menthol	**Adults & Peds ≥2 yrs:** Apply to affected area tid-qid.
Gold Bond Extra Strength Medicated Body Lotion Triple Action Relief	Dimethicone/Menthol 5%-0.5%	**Adults & Peds:** Apply to affected area tid-qid.
Gold Bond Medicated Body Lotion	Dimethicone/Menthol 5%-0.15%	**Adults & Peds:** Apply to affected area prn.
Gold Bond Medicated Extra Strength Powder	Zinc Oxide/Menthol 0.5%-0.8%	**Adults & Peds ≥2 yrs:** Apply to affected area tid-qid.
Vaseline Intensive Care Lotion Advanced Healing	Dimethicone 1%-White Petrolatum	**Adults & Peds:** Apply to affected area prn.

DANDRUFF PRODUCTS

BRAND	INGREDIENT/STRENGTH	DOSE
COAL TAR		
Denorex Therapeutic Protection 2-in-1 Shampoo	Coal Tar 2.5%	**Adults & Peds:** Use biw.
DHS Tar Dermatological Hair & Scalp Shampoo	Coal Tar 0.5%	**Adults & Peds:** Use biw.
Ionil T Shampoo	Coal Tar 1%	**Adults & Peds:** Use biw.
Ionil T Plus Shampoo	Coal Tar 2%	**Adults & Peds:** Use biw.
Neutrogena T-Gel Shampoo Original Formula	Coal Tar 0.5%	**Adults & Peds:** Use biw.
Neutrogena T-Gel Shampoo, Extra Strength	Coal Tar 1%	**Adults & Peds:** Use biw.
Neutrogena T-Gel Stubborn Itch Shampoo	Coal Tar 0.5%	**Adults & Peds:** Use biw.
KETOCONAZOLE		
Nizoral Anti-Dandruff Shampoo	Ketoconazole 1%	**Adults & Peds ≥12:** Use q3-4d prn.
PYRITHIONE ZINC		
Denorex Dandruff Shampoo, Daily Protection	Pyrithione Zinc 2%	**Adults & Peds:** Use biw.
Garnier Fructis Fortifying Shampoo, Anti-Dandruff	Pyrithione Zinc 1%	**Adults & Peds:** Use biw.
Head & Shoulders Dry Scalp Care Dandruff Shampoo Plus Conditioner; Shampoo; Conditioner	Pyrithione Zinc 0.5%	**Adults & Peds:** Use biw.
Head & Shoulders Smooth & Silky Dandruff Shampoo Plus Conditioner; Shampoo; Conditioner	Pyrithione Zinc 1%	**Adults & Peds:** Use biw.
Head & Shoulders Citrus Breeze Dandruff Shampoo Plus Conditioner; Shampoo	Pyrithione Zinc 1%	**Adults & Peds:** Use biw.
Head & Shoulders Classic Clean Dandruff Shampoo Plus Conditioner; Shampoo; Conditioner	Pyrithione Zinc 1%	**Adults & Peds:** Use biw.
Head & Shoulders Extra Volume Dandruff Shampoo	Pyrithione Zinc 1%	**Adults & Peds:** Use biw.
Head & Shoulders Ocean Lift Dandruff Shampoo Plus Conditioner; Shampoo	Pyrithione Zinc 1%	**Adults & Peds:** Use biw.
Head & Shoulders Dandruff Refresh Shampoo Plus Conditioner; Shampoo	Pyrithione Zinc 1%	**Adults & Peds:** Use biw.
Head & Shoulders Restoring Shine Dandruff Shampoo Plus Conditioner; Shampoo	Pyrithione Zinc 1%	**Adults & Peds:** Use biw.
Head & Shoulders Sensitive Care Dandruff Shampoo Plus Conditioner; Shampoo	Pyrithione Zinc 1%	**Adults & Peds:** Use biw.
Head & Shoulders Intensive Solutions Dandruff Shampoo and Conditioner; Shampoo	Pyrithione Zinc 2%	**Adults & Peds:** Use biw.
L'Oreal VIVE Pro Anti-Dandruff for Men Shampoo	Pyrithione Zinc 1%	**Adults & Peds:** Use biw.
Neutrogena T-Gel Daily Control Dandruff Shampoo	Pyrithione Zinc 1%	**Adults & Peds:** Use biw.
Pantene Pro-V Shampoo + Conditioner, Anti-Dandruff	Pyrithione Zinc 1%	**Adults & Peds:** Use biw.

(Continued)

BRAND	INGREDIENT/STRENGTH	DOSE
PYRITHIONE ZINC *(Continued)*		
Pert Plus Shampoo Plus Conditioner, Dandruff Control	Pyrithione Zinc 0.45%	**Adults & Peds:** Use biw.
Selsun Salon 2-in-1 Pyrithione Zinc Shampoo	Pyrithione Zinc 1%	**Adults & Peds:** Use biw.
Suave for Men 2 in 1 Shampoo/ Conditioner, Dandruff	Pyrithione Zinc 0.5%	**Adults & Peds:** Use biw.
SALICYLIC ACID		
Denorex Dandruff Shampoo, Extra Strength	Salicylic Acid 3%	**Adults & Peds:** Use biw.
Neutrogena T/Sal Shampoo, Scalp Build-up Control	Salicylic Acid 3%	**Adults & Peds:** Use biw.
Scalpicin Anti-Itch Liquid Scalp Treatment	Salicylic Acid 3%	**Adults & Peds:** Apply to affected area qd-qid.
SELENIUM SULFIDE		
Head & Shoulders Dandruff Shampoo, Intensive Treatment	Selenium Sulfide 1%	**Adults & Peds:** Use biw.
Selsun Blue Dandruff Shampoo, Medicated Treatment	Selenium Sulfide 1%	**Adults & Peds:** Use biw.
Selsun Blue Dandruff Shampoo Plus Conditioner	Selenium Sulfide 1%	**Adults & Peds:** Use biw.
Selsun Blue Dandruff Shampoo	Selenium Sulfide 1%	**Adults & Peds:** Use biw.
Selsun Blue Dandruff Shampoo, Moisturizing Treatment	Selenium Sulfide 1%	**Adults & Peds:** Use biw.
SULFUR/SALICYLIC ACID		
Sebulex Medicated Dandruff Shampoo	Sulfur/Salicylic Acid 2%-2%	**Adults & Peds ≥12yrs:** Use qd.

DIAPER RASH PRODUCTS

BRAND	INGREDIENT/STRENGTH	DOSE
WHITE PETROLATUM		
Balmex Extra Protective Clear Ointment	White Petrolatum 51%	**Peds:** Apply prn.
Vaseline Baby, Baby Fresh Scent	White Petrolatum 100%	**Peds:** Apply prn.
Vaseline Petroleum Jelly	White Petrolatum 100%	**Peds:** Apply prn.
ZINC OXIDE		
Aveeno Baby Soothing Relief Diaper Rash Cream	Zinc Oxide 13%	**Peds:** Apply prn.
Balmex Diaper Rash Ointment with Aloe & Vitamin E	Zinc Oxide 11.3%	**Peds:** Apply prn.
Boudreaux's Butt Paste, Diaper Rash Ointment	Zinc Oxide 16%	**Peds:** Apply prn.
California Baby Diaper Rash Cream	Zinc Oxide 12%	**Peds:** Apply prn.
Canus Li'l Goat's Milk Ointment	Zinc Oxide 40%	**Peds:** Apply prn.
Desitin Diaper Rash Ointment, Creamy	Zinc Oxide 10%	**Peds:** Apply prn.
Desitin Original Diaper Rash Ointment	Zinc Oxide 40%	**Peds:** Apply prn.
Huggies Diaper Rash Cream	Zinc Oxide 10%	**Peds:** Apply prn.
Johnson's Baby Diaper Rash Cream with Zinc Oxide	Zinc Oxide 13%	**Peds:** Apply prn.
Mustela Bebe Vitamin Barrier Cream	Zinc Oxide 10%	**Peds:** Apply prn.
COMBINATION PRODUCTS		
A+D Original Ointment, Diaper Rash and All-Purpose Skincare Formula	Petrolatum/Lanolin 53.4%-15.5%	**Peds:** Apply prn.
A+D Zinc Oxide Diaper Rash Cream with Aloe	Dimethicone/Zinc Oxide 1%-10%	**Peds:** Apply prn.

DRY SKIN PRODUCTS

BRAND	INGREDIENTS	DOSE
AmLactin Moisturizing Cream	Water, Lactic Acid, Ammonium Hydroxide, Light Mineral Oil, Glyceryl Stearate, PEG-100 Stearate, Glycerin, Propylene Glycol, Magnesium Aluminum Silicate, Laureth 4, Polyoxyl 40 Stearate, Cetyl Alcohol, Methylcellulose, Methyl Paraben, Propylparaben, Methylcellulose	**Adults & Peds:** Apply bid.
AmLactin Moisturizing Lotion	Water, Lactic Acid, Ammonium Hydroxide, Light Mineral Oil, Glyceryl Stearate, PEG-100 Stearate, Glycerin, Propylene Glycol, Magnesium Aluminum Silicate, Laureth 4, Polyoxyl 40 Stearate, Cetyl Alcohol, Methylcellulose, Methylparaben, Propylparaben, Methylcellulose	**Adults & Peds:** Apply bid.
AmLactin XL Moisturizing Lotion Ultraplex	Water, Ammonium Lactate, Potassium Lactate, Sodium Lactate, Emulsifying Wax, Light Mineral Oil, White Petrolatum, Glycerin, Propylene Glycol, Stearic Acid, Xanthum Gum, Methyl and Propylparabens	**Adults & Peds:** Apply bid.
Aquaphor Baby Healing Ointment	Petrolatum, Mineral Oil, Ceresin, Lanolin Alcohol, Panthenol, Glycerin, Bisabolol	**Adults & Peds:** Apply prn.
Aquaphor Original Ointment	Petrolatum, Mineral Oil, Ceresin, Lanolin Alcohol, Panthenol, Glycerin, Bisabolol	**Adults & Peds:** Apply to affected area prn.
Aveeno Baby Moisture Soothing Relief Cream	Water, Glycerin, Petrolatum, Mineral Oil, Cetyl Alcohol, Dimethicone, Avena Sativa (Oat) Kernel Flour, Carbomer, Sodium Hydroxide, Ceteareth-6, Hydrolyzed Milk Protein, Hydrolyzed Oats, PEG-25 Soya Sterol, Tetrasodium EDTA, Methylparaben, Citric Acid, Sodium Citrate, Benzalkonium Chloride, Benzaldehyde, Butylene Glycol, Butylparaben, Ethylparaben, Ethyl Alcohol, Isobutylparaben, Phenoxyethanol, Propylparaben, Stearyl Alcohol	**Adults & Peds:** Apply prn.
Aveeno Baby Soothing Bath Treatment Packets	Colloidal Oatmeal 43%, Calcium Silicilate, Laureth-4 Mineral Oil	**Adults & Peds:** Bathe in 1 packet for 15-20 min qd-bid.
Aveeno Daily Baby Lotion	Dimethicone 1.2%, Glycerin Distearyldimonium Chloride, Petrolatum, Isopropyl Palmitate, Cetyl Alcohol, Oat Flour Avena Sativa, Allontoin, Benzyl Alcohol, Sodium Chloride	**Peds:** Apply prn.
Aveeno Daily Moisturizer, Ultra-Calming SPF 15	Avobenzone/Octinoxate/Octisalate (3%-7.5%-2) Avena Sativa Kernel Flour (Oat), Benzalkonium Chloride, C12-15 Alkyl Benzoate, Cetyl Alcohol, Diethylhexyl 2,6-Naphthalate, Dimethicone, Disodium EDTA, Distearyl-dimonium Chloride, Glycerin, Methylparaben, Steareth 21, Water	**Adults:** Apply qd.
Aveeno Daily Moisturizing Lotion	Dimethicone 1.25%, Avena Sativa (Oat) Kernal, Benzyl Alcohol, Cetyl Alcohol, Distearyldimonium Chloride, Glycerin, Isopropyl Palmitate, Petrolatum, Sodium Chloride, Water	**Adults:** Apply prn.
Aveeno Intense Relief Hand Cream	Water, Glycerin, Distearyldimonium Chloride, Petrolatum, Isopropyl Palmitate, Cetyl Alcohol, Aluminum Starch Octenyl Succinate, Dimethicone, Avena Sativa (Oat) Kernel Flour, Benzyl Alcohol, Sodium Chloride	**Adults & Peds:** Apply prn.
Aveeno Moisturizing Bar for Dry Skin	Avena Stativa (Oat) Flour, Water, Cetearyl Alcohol, Stearic Acid, Sodium Cocoyl Isethionate, Water, Disodium Lauryl Sulfosuccinate, Glycerin, Hydrogenated Vegetable Oil, Titanium Dioxide, Citric Acid, Sodium Trideceth Sulfate, Hydrogenated Castor Oil	**Adults & Peds:** Use qd.
Aveeno Moisturizing Lotion, Skin Relief	Dimethicone 1.25%, Allantoin, Avena Sativa Kernel Flour (Oat), Benzyl Alcohol, Cetyl Alcohol, Distearyldimonium Chloride, Glycerin, Isopropyl Palmitate, Menthol, Petrolatum, Sodium Chloride, Triticum Vulgare Germ Protein (Wheat), Water	**Adult & Peds:** ≥2 yrs: Apply qd.

(Continued)

BRAND	INGREDIENTS	DOSE
Aveeno Positively Radiant Moisturizing Lotion	Water, Glycerin, Emulsifying Wax, Ethylhexyl Isononanoate, Glycine Soja (Soybean) Seed Extract, Propylene Glycol Isoceteth-3 Acetate, Dimethicone, Polyacrylamide, Cyclomethicone, Stearic Acid, Phenoxyethanol, c13-14 Isoparaffin, Dimethicone Copolyol, Benzyl Alcohol, TItanium Dioxide, Fragrance, Iodopropynyl Butylcarbamate, Tocopherol Acetate, Panthenol, Panthenyl Ethylether, Glyceryl Laurate, Laureth-7, Methylparaben, Silica, Mica, Polymethyl Methacrylate, Cetearyl Alcohol, Tetrasodium EDTA, Butylparaben, Ethylparaben, Isobutylparaben, Propylparaben, DMDM Hydantoin, Panthenol, BHT, Citric Acid	**Adults:** Apply qd.
Aveeno Positively Radiant Daily Moisturizer SPF 15	Avobenzone/Octinoxate/Octisalate Arachidyl Alcohol (3%-7.5%-2%), Arachidyl Glucoside, Behenyl Alcohol, Benzalkonium Chloride, Benzyl Alcohol, BHT, Bisphenylpropyl Dimethicone, Butylparaben, c12-15 Alkyl Benzoate, c13-14 Isoparaffin, Cetearyl Alcohol, Cetearyl Glucoside, Dimethicone, Disodium EDTA, Ethylene/Acrylic Acid Copolymer, Ethylparaben, Fragrance, Glycerin, Glycine Soja (Soybean) Seed Extract, Iodopropyl Butylcarbamate, Isobutylparaben, Laureth-7, Methylparaben, Mica, Panthenol, Phenoxyethanol, Polyacrylamide, Polymethyl Methacrylate, Propylparaben, Silica, Stearath-2, Stearath-21, Titanium Dioxide, Water, Sodium Hydroxide, Citric Acid	**Adults:** Use daily.
Aveeno Positively Radiant Daily Cleansing Pads	Water, Cocamidopropyl Betaine, Decyl Glucoside, Glycerin, Disodium Lauroamphodiacetate, PEG-16 Soy Sterol, Polysorbate 20, PPG-2 Hydroxyethyl Cocamide, Phenoxyethanol, Tetrasodium EDTA, Butylene Glycol, Sodium Coco PG-dimonium Chloride Phosphate, Sodium Citrate, Glycine Soja (Soybean) Protein, Citric Acid, PEG-14m, Methylparaben, Butylparaben, Ethylparaben, Isobutylparaben, Propylparaben, Fragrance	**Adults:** Use daily.
Aveeno Positively Smooth Facial Moisturizer	Water, C12-15 Alkyl Benzoate, Cetearyl Alcohol, Bisphenylpropyl Dimethicone, Glycine, Soja Seed Extract, Butylene Glycol, Arachidyl Alcohol, Glycine Soja Protein, Dimethicone, Glycerin, Panthenol, Polyacrylamide, Phenoxyethanol, Cetearyl Glucoside, Behenyl Alcohol, Benzyl Alcohol, C13-14 Isoparaffin, DMDM Hydantoin, Arachidyl Glucoside, Disodium EDTA, Methylparaben, Laureth 7, BHT, Ethylparaben, Butylparaben, Propylparaben, Isobutylparaben, Fragrance, Iodopropynyl Butylcarbamate	**Adults:** Apply prn.
Aveeno Positively Smooth Moisturizing Lotion	Water, Glycerin, Emulsifying Wax, Isononanoate, Gylcine Soja Seed Extract, Propylene Glycol Isoceteth-3 Acetate, Dimethicone, Cyclomethicone, Polyacrylamide, Stearic Acid, Panthenyl Ethyl Ether, Tocopheryl Acetate, Panthenol, Phenoxyethanol, C13-14 Isoparaffin, Dimethicone Copolyol, Benzyl Alcohol, DMDM Hydantoin, Glyceryl Laurate, Laureth 7, Methylparaben, Cetearyl Alcohol, Disodium EDTA, Butylparaben, Ethylparaben, BHT, Propylparaben, Isobutylparaben, Fragrance, Iodopropyl Butylcarbamate, Glycine Soja Seed Extract, Panthenyl Ethyl Ether, Tocopherol Acetate, Panthenol BHT, Sodium Hydroxide, Citric Acid	**Adults:** Apply prn.
Aveeno Radiant Skin Daily Moisturizer with SPF 15	Octinoxate (Octyl Methoxycinnamate)/Avobenzone / Octisalate (Octyl Salicylate) 7.5%-3%-2%; Arachidyl Alcohol, Arachidyl Glucoside, Behenyl Alcohol, Benzalkonium Chloride, Benzyl Alcohol, BHT, Bisphenylpropyl Dimethicone, Butylparaben, C12-15 AlkylBenzoate, C13-14 Isoparaffin, Cetearyl Alcohol, Cetearyl Glucoside, Dimethicone, Disodium EDTA, Ethylene/Acrylic Acid Copolymer, Ethylparaben, Fragrance, Glycerin, Glycine Soja (Soybean) Seed Extract, Iodopropynyl Butylcarbamate, Isobutylparaben, Laureth-7, Methylparaben, Mica, Panthenol, Phenoxyethanol, Polyacrylamide, Polymethylmethacrylate, Propylparaben, Silica, Stearath-2, Stearath-21, Titanium Dioxide, Water, Sodium Hydroxide, Citric Acid	**Adults:** Apply prn.

(Continued)

BRAND	INGREDIENTS	DOSE
Aveeno Body Wash, Fragrance Free	Water, Glycerin, Cocomidopropyl Betaine, Sodium Laureth Sulfate, Decyl Glucoside, Avena Sativa (Oat) Kernel Flour, Glycine Soja (Soybean) Seed Oil, Helianthus Annuus (Sunflower) Seed Oil, Citric Acid, Sodium Lauroampho PG-Acetate Phosphate, Guar Hydroxypropyltrimonium Chloride, PEG-120 Methyl Glucose Trioleate, PEG-150 Pentaerythrityl Tetrastearate, Hydroxypropyltrimonium Hydrolyzed Wheat Protein, Hydroxypropyltrimonium Wheat Starch, Tetrasodium EDTA, Quaternium-15, Fragrance	**Adults:** Use prn.
Carmol-10 Lotion	Urea 10%, Carbomer 940, Cetyl Alcohol, Isopropyl Palmitate, PEG 8 Doleate, PEG 8 Distearate, Propylene Glycol, Propylene Glycol Dipelargonate, Sodium Laureth Sulfate, Stearic Acid, Trolamine, Xanthan Gum	**Adults & Peds:** Apply qd-bid.
Carmol-20 Cream	Urea 20%, Water, Isopropyl Myristate, Isopropyl Palmitate, Stearic Acid, Propylene Glycol, Trolamine, Sodium Laureth, Carbomer, Xanthan Gum, Fragrance	**Adults & Peds:** Apply qd-bid.
Cetaphil Daily Facial Moisturizer SPF 15	Avobenzone 3%, Octocrylene 10%, Water, Diisopropyl Adipate, Cyclomethicone, Glyceryl Stearate, PEG-100 Stearate, Glycerin, Polymethyl Methacrylate, Phenoxyethanol, Benzyl Alcohol, Acrylates/C10-30 Alkyl Acrylate Crosspolymer, Tocopheryl Acetate, Carbomer 940, Disodium EDTA, Triethanolamine	**Adults & Peds:** Apply prn.
Cetaphil Moisturizing Cream	Water, Glyceryl Polyglycerylmethacrylate, Propylene Glycol, Petrolatum, Dicaprylyl Ether, PEG-5 Glyceryl Stearate, Glycerin, Dimethicone, Dimethiconol, Cetyl Alcohol, Sweet Almond Oil, Acrylates/C10-30 Alkylacrylate Crosspolymer, TocopherylAcetate, Phenoxyethanol, Benzyl Alcohol, Disodium EDTA, Sodium Hydroxide, Lactic Acid	**Adults & Peds:** Apply prn.
Cetaphil Moisturizing Lotion	Water, Glycerin, Hydrogenated Polyisobutene, Cetearyl Alcohol, Ceteareth-20, Macadamia Nut Oil, Dimethicone, Tocopheryl Acetate, Stearoxytrimethylsilane, Stearyl Alcohol, Panthenol, Farnesol, Benzyl Alcohol, Phenoxyethanol, Acrylates/C10-30Alkyl Acrylate Crosspolymer, Sodium Hydroxide, Citric Acid	**Adults & Peds:** Apply prn.
Cetaphil Therapeutic Hand Cream	Water, Glycerin, Cetearyl Alcohol, Oleth-2, PEG-2 Stearate, ButyrospermumParkii, Ethylhexyl Methoxycinnamate, Dimethicone, Stearyl Alcohol, Glyceryl Stearate, PEG-100 Stearate, Methylparaben,Tocopherol, Arginine PCA, Chlorhexidine Digluconate	**Adults & Peds:** Apply prn.
Corn Huskers Lotion	Water, Glycerin, SD Alcohol 40, Sodium Calcium Alginate, Oleyl Sarcosin, Methylparaben, Guar Gum, Triethanolamine, Calcium Sulfate, Calcium Chloride, Fumaric Acid, Boric Acid, Fragrance	**Adults & Peds:** Apply prn.
Curel Continuous Comfort Original Formula	Water, Glycerin, Distearyldimonium Chloride, Petrolatum, Isopropyl Palmitate, Cetyl Alcohol, Butyrospermum Park II (Shea Butter), Acacia Senegal Gum, Dimethicone, Fragrance, Sodium Chloride, Gelatin, Methylparaben, Propylparaben	**Adults:** Apply to skin prn.
Curel Continuous Comfort Fragrance Free	Water, Glycerin, Distearyldimonium Chloride, Petrolatum, Isopropyl Palmitate, Cetyl Alcohol, Acacia Senegal Gum, Dimethicone, Sodium Chloride, Gelatin, Methylparaben, Propylparaben	**Adults:** Apply to skin prn.
Curel Natural Healing Soothing Lotion	Water, Glycerin, Distearyldimonium Chloride, Petrolatum, Isopropryl Palmitate, Cetyl Alcohol, Lavandula Angustifolia (Lavender) Flower Extract, Anthemis Nobilis (Chamomile) Flower Extract, Avena Sativa (Oat) Meal Extract, Propylene Glycol, Pentylene Glycol, Dimethicone, Fragrance, Sodium Chloride, Methylparaben, Propylparaben, Caramel	**Adults:** Apply to skin prn.
Curel Natural Healing Nourishing Lotion	Water, Glycerin, Distearyldimonium Chloride, Petrolatum, Isopropryl Palmitate, Cetyl Alcohol, Butyrospermum Parkii (Shea Butter), Vanilla Planifolia Fruit Extract, Honey (Mel), Propylene Glycol, Butylene Glycol, Dipropylene Glycol, Dimethicone, Fragrance, Sodium Chloride, Methylparaben, Propylparaben, Caramel	**Adults:** Apply to skin prn.

(Continued)

BRAND	INGREDIENTS	DOSE
Curel Natural Healing Revitalizing Lotion	Water, Glycerin, Distearyldimonium Chloride, Petrolatum, Isopropyl Palmitate, Cetyl Alcohol, Camellia Sinensis (Green Tea) Leaf Extract, Aloe Barbadensis Leaf Extract, Cucumis Sativus (Cucumber) Fruit Extract, Propylene Glycol, Dimethicone, Fragrance, Sodium Chloride, Methylparaben, Propylparaben, Caramel	**Adults:** Apply to skin prn.
Curel Ultra Healing Intensive Moisture Lotion	Water, Glycerin, Petrolatum, Cetearyl Alcohol, Benhentrimonium Chloride, Cetyl-PG Hydroxyethyl Palmitamide, Isopropyl Palmitate, Butyrospermum Park II (Shea Butter), Avena Sativa (Oat) Meal Extract, Eucalyptus Globulus Leaf Extract, Citrus Aurantium Dulcis (orange) Peel Oil, Cyclopentasiloxane, Dimethicone, Acacia Senegal Gum, Gelatin, DMDM Hydantoin	**Adults:** Apply to skin prn.
Eucerin Creme Original	Water, Petrolatum, Mineral Oil, Ceresin, Lanolin Alcohol Methylchloroisothiazolinone, Methylisothiazolinone	**Adults & Peds:** Apply prn.
Eucerin Dry Skin Therapy Calming Cream	Water, Glycerin, Cetyl Palmitate, Mineral Oil, Caprylic/Capric Triglyceride, Octyldodecanol, Cetyl Alcohol, Glycerly Stearate, Colloidal Oatmeal, Dimethicone, PEG-40 Stearate, Phenoxyethanol, DMDM Hydantoin, Iodopropynyl Butylcarbamate	**Adults & Peds: >2 yrs:** Apply prn.
Eucerin Dry Skin Therapy Plus Intensive Repair Lotion	Water, Mineral Oil, PEG-7 Hydrogenated Castor Oil, Isohexadecane, Sodium Lactate, Urea, Glycerin, Isopropyl Palmitate, Panthenol, Microcrystalline Wax, Magnesium Sulfate, Lanolin Alcohol, Bisabolol, Methylchloroisothiazolinone, Methylisothiazolinone	**Adults:** Apply prn.
Eucerin Sensitive Facial Skin Gentle Hydrating Cleanser	Water, Sodium Laureth Sulfate, Cocamidopropyl Betaine, Disodium Cocamphodiacetate, Glycol Distearate, PEG 7 Glyceryl Cocoate, PEG 5 Lanolate, Cocamide MEA, Laureth 10, Citric Acid, PEG 120 Methyl Glucose Dioleate, Lanolin Alcohol, Imidazolidinyl Urea	**Adults:** Use qd.
Eucerin Plus Hand Creme Extensive Repair	Water, Glycerin, Urea, Glyceryl Stearate, Stearyl Alcohol, Dicaprylyl Ether, Sodium Lactate, Dimethicone, PEG-40 Stearate, Cyclopentasiloxane, Cyclohexasiloxane, Auminum Starch Octenylsuccinate, Lactic Acid, Xanthan Gum, Phenoxyethanol, Methylparaben, Propylparaben	**Adults & Peds:** Apply qd.
Eucerin Lotion Daily Replenishing	Water, Sunflower Seed Oil, Petrolatum, Glycerin, Glyceryl Stearate SE, Octyldodecanol, Caprylic/Capric Triglyceride, Stearic Acid, Dimethicone, Cetearyl Alcohol, Lanolin Alcohol, Panthenol, Tocopheryl Acetate, Cholesterol, Carbomer, Disodium EDTA, Sodium Hydroxide, Phenoxyethanol, Methylparaben, Ethylparaben, Propylparaben, Butylparaben, Isobutylparaben, BHT	**Adults & Peds:** Apply qd.
Eucerin Lotion Original	Water, Mineral Oil, Isopropyl Myristate, PEG-40 Sorbitan Peroleate, Glyceryl Lanolate, Sorbitol, Propylene Glycol, Cetyl Palmitate, Magnesium Sulfate, Aluminum Stearate, Lanolin Alcohol, BHT, Methylchloroisothiazolinone, Methylisothiazolinone	**Adults & Peds:** Apply prn.
Eucerin Lotion Plus Intensive Repair	Mineral Oil, PEG-7 Hydrogenated Castor Oil, Isohexadecane, Sodium Lactate, Urea, Glycerin, Isopropyl Palmitate, Panthenol, Microcrystalline Wax, Magnesium Sulfate, Lanolin Alcohol, Bisabolol, Methylchloroisothiazolinone, Methylisothiazolinone	**Adults & Peds:** Apply prn.
Eucerin Redness Relief Daily Perfecting Lotion	Octinoxate, Octisalate, Titanium Dioxide, Water, Glycerine, Dimethicone, Polyglyceryl-3 Methylglucose Distearate, Butyrospermum Parkii (Shea Butter), Lauroyl Lysine, Squalane, Alcohol Denat., Sorbitan Stearate, Phenoxyethanol, Butylene Glycol, Magnesium Aluminum Silicate, Glycyrrhiza Inflata Root Extract, Xanthan Gum, Methylparaben, Propylparaben, Ethylparaben, Iodopropynyl Butylcarbamate, Trimethoxycaprylylsilane, Chromium Oxide Greens, Chromium Hydroxide Green, Ultramarines	**Adults & Peds:** Apply prn.
Eucerin Redness Relief Soothing Cleanser	Water, Glycerin, Sodium Laureth Sulfate, Carbomer, Phenoxyethanol, PEG-40 Hydrogenated Castor Oil, Sodium Methyl Cocoyl Taurate, PEG-7 Glyceryl Cocoate, Decyl Glucoside, Glycyrrhiza Inflata Root Extract, Xanthan Gum, Sodium Hydroxide, Methylparaben, Butylparaben, Ethylparaben, Isobutylparaben, Propylparaben, Benzophenone-4	**Adults & Peds:** Use qam and qpm.

(Continued)

BRAND	INGREDIENTS	DOSE
Eucerin Redness Relief Soothing Moisture Lotion	Cyclopentasiloxane, Titanium Dioxide, Water, Glycerin, Propylene Glycol Dicaprylate/Dicaprate, Dimethicone Crosspolymer, Polyglyceryl-3 diisostearate Methylmethacrylate Crosspolymer, Mica, Glyceral Oleate, Microcrystalline Wax, Copernicia Cerifa (Carnauba Wax), Euphoria Cerifera (Candelilla) Wax, Acrylates/Octylacrylamide Copolymer, Panthenol, Butylene Glycol, Glycyrrhiza Inflata Root Extract, Disodium EDTA, PEG/PPG-18/18 Demethicone, Diazolidinyl Urea, Phenoxyethanol, Iodopropynyl Butylcarbamate, Chromium Oxide Greens, Iron Oxide	**Adults & Peds:** Apply qam and qpm.
Eucerin Redness Relief Soothing Night Crème	Water, Glycerin, Panthenol, Caprylic/Capric Triglyceride, Dicaprylyl Carbonate, Octyldodecanol, C12-15 Alkyl Benzoate, Dimethicone, Squalane, Tapioca Starch, Cetearyl Alcohol, Glyceryl Stearate Citrate, Myristyl Myristate, Butylene Glycol, Benzyl Alcohol, Glycyrrhiza Inflata Root Extract, Carbomer, Phenoxyethanol, Ammonium Acryloyldimethyltaurate/VP Copolymer, Sodium Hydroxide, Methylparaben, Propylparaben, Iodopropynyl Butylcarbamate	**Adults & Peds:** Apply qpm.
Gold Bond Ultimate Healing Skin Therapy Lotion, Aloe	Glycerin, Dimethicone, Petrolatum, Jojoba Esters, Cetyl Alcohol, Aloe Barbadensis Leaf Juice, Stearyl Alcohol, Distearyldimonium Chloride, Cetearyl Alcohol, Steareth-21, Steareth-2, Propylene Glycol, Chamomilla Recutita Flower Extract, Polysorbate 60, Stearamidopropyl PG-Dimonium Chloride Phosphate, Methyl Gluceth 20, Tocopheryl Acetate, Magnesium Ascorbyl Phosphate, Hydrolyzed Collagen, Hydrolyzed Elastin, Retinyl Palmitate, Hydrolyzed Jojoba Esters, Glyceryl Stearate, Dipotassium EDTA, Fragrance, Potassium Hydroxide, Diazolidinyl Urea, Methylparaben, Propylparaben	**Adults & Peds:** Apply prn.
Gold Bond Ultimate Healing Skin Therapy Powder	Corn Starch, Sodium Bicarbonate, Silica, Fragrance, Ascrobyl Palmitate, Aloe Barbadensis Leaf Extract, Lavandula Angustifolia Extract, Chamomilla Recutita Flower Extract, Rosmarinus Officinalis Leaf Extract, Acacia Farnesiana Extract, Tocopheryl Acetate, Retinyl Palmitate, Polyoxymethylene Urea, Isopropyl Myristate, Benzethonium Chloride	**Adults & Peds:** Apply prn.
Keri Moisture Therapy Advance Extra Dry Skin Lotion	Water; Glycerin, Stearic Acid, Hydrogenated Polyisobutene, Petrolatum, Cetyl Alcohol, Aloe Barbadensis Leaf Juice, Tocopheryl Acetate, Cyclopentasiloxane, Dimethicone Copolyol, Glyceryl Stearate, PEG-100 Stearate, Dimethicone, Carbomer, Methylparaben, PEG-5 Soya Sterol, Magnesium Aluminum Silicate, Propylparaben, Phenoxyethanol, Disodium EDTA, Diazolidinyl Urea, Sodium Hydroxide, Fragrance	**Adults & Peds:** Apply prn.
Keri Moisture Therapy Lotion, Sensitive Skin	Water, Glycerin, Stearic Acid, Hydrogenated Polyisobutene, Petrolatum, Cetyl Alcohol, Aloe Barbadensis Leaf Juice, Tocopheryl Acetate (Vitamin E Acetate), Cyclopenta Siloxane, Dimethicone Copolyol, Glyceryl Stearate, PEG 100 Stearate, Dimethicone, Carbomer, Methylparaben, PEG 5 Soy Sterol, Magnesium Aluminum Silicate, Propylparaben, Phenoxyethanol, Disodium EDTA, Diazolidinyl Urea, Sodium Hydroxide	**Adults:** Apply prn.
Keri Original Formula Lotion	Water, Mineral Oil, Glycerin, PEG 40 Stearate, Glyceryl Stearate, PEG 100 Stearate, PEG 4 Dilaurate, Laureth 4, Aloe Barbadensis Leaf Juice, Sunflower (Helianthus Annuus) Seed Oil, Tocopheryl Acetate (Vitamin E Acetate), Carborner, Methylparaben, Propylparaben, Fragrance, DMDM Hydantoin, Iodopropynyl Butylcarbamate, Sodium Hydroxide, Disodium EDTA	**Adults & Peds:** Apply prn.
Keri Shea Butter Moisture Therapy Lotion	Water, Mineral Oil, Glycerin, Butyrospermum Parkii, PEG-40 Stearate, Glyceryl Stearate, PEG-4 Dilaurate, Laureth 4, Aloe Barbadensis Leaf Juice, Helianthus Annuus Seed Oil, Tocopheryl Acetate, Carbomer, Methylparaben, Propylparaben, DMDM Hydantoin, Iodopropynyl Butylcarbamate, Sodium Hydroxide, Disodium EDTA, Fragrance	**Adults & Peds:** Apply prn.

(Continued)

BRAND	INGREDIENTS	DOSE
Lac-Hydrin Five Lotion	Water, Lactic Acid, Ammonium Hydroxide, Glycerin, Petrolatum, Squalane, Steareth-2, POE-21-Stearyl Ether, Propylene Glycol Dioctanoate, Cetyl Alcohol, Dimethicone, Methylchloroisothiazoline, Methylisothiazolinone	**Adults & Peds:** Apply bid.
Lubriderm Advanced Therapy Lotion	Water, Cetyl Alcohol, Glycerin, Mineral Oil, Cyclomethicone, Propylene Glycol Dicaprylate/Dicaprate, PEG-40 Stearate, Isopropyl Isostearate, Emulsifying Wax, Lecithin, Carbomer, Diazolidinyl Urea, Titanium Dioxide, Sodium Benzoate, BHT, TriPPG-3 Myristyl Ether Citrate, Disodium EDTA, Retinyl Palmitate, Tocopheryl Acetate, Sodium Pyruvate, Fragrance, Sodium Hydroxide, Xanthan Gum, Iodopropynyl Butylcarbamate, Cyclotetrasiloxane Cetearyl Alcohol, Polysorbate 60, Cyclopentasiloxane, Trifluoro-methylC 1-4, alkyl dimethicone, Aluminum Stearate	**Adults & Peds:** Apply prn.
Lubriderm Daily Moisture Fragrance Free Lotion	Water, Mineral Oil, Petrolatum, Sorbitol Stearic Acid, Lanolin, Lanolin Alcohol, Cetyl Alcohol, Glyceryl Stearate/PEG-100 Stearate, Triethanolamine, Dimethicone, Propylene Glycol, Microcrystalline Wax, Tri-PPG-3 Myristyl Ether Citrate, Disodium EDTA, Methylparaben, Ethylparaben, Propylparaben, Xanthan Gum, Butylparaben, Methyldibromoglutaronitrile	**Adults & Peds:** Apply prn.
Lubriderm Daily Moisture Lotion	Water, Mineral Oil, Petrolatum, Sorbitol Stearic Acid, Lanolin, Lanolin Alcohol, Cetyl Alcohol, Glyceryl Stearate/PEG-100 Stearate, Triethanolamine, Dimethicone, Propylene Glycol, Microcrystalline Wax, PPG-3 Myristyl Ether Citrate, Disodium EDTA, Methylparaben, Ethylparaben, Propylparaben, Xanthan Gum, Butylparaben, Methyldibromoglutaronite, Fragrance, PEG-4 Laurate	**Adults & Peds:** Apply prn.
Lubriderm Sensitive Skin Lotion	Water, Butylene Glycol, Mineral Oil, Petrolatum, Glycerin, Cetyl Alcohol, Propylene Glycol Dicaprylate/Dicaprate, PEG-40 Stearate, C11-13 Isoparaffin, Glyceryl Stearate, Tri-PPG-3 Myristyl Ether Citrate, Emulsifying Wax, Dimethicone, DMDM Hydantoin, Methylparaben, Carbomer, Ethylparaben, Propylparaben, Titanium Dioxide, Disodium EDTA, Sodium Hydroxide, Butylparaben, Xanthan Gum	**Adults & Peds:** Apply prn.
Lubriderm Daily UV Moisturizer Lotion, SPF 15	Octyl Methoxycinnamate/Octyl Salicylate/Oxybenzone (7.5%-4%-3%), Purified Water, C 12-15 Alkyl Benzoate, Cetearyl Alcohol, Ceteareth-20, Cetyl Alcohol, Glyceryl Monostearate, Propylene Glycol, White Petrolatum, Diazolidinyl Urea, Trolamine, Edetate Disodium, Xanthan Gum, Acrylates/C 10-30 Alkyl Acrylate Crosspolymer, Vitamin E, Iodopropynyl Butylcarbamate, Fragrance, Carbomer	**Adults & Peds: >6 mo:** Apply prn.
Lubriderm Skin Nourishing Moisturizing Lotion with Premium Oat Extract	Water, Caprylic/Capric Triglycerides, Glycerin, Glyceryl Stearate SE, Petrolatum, Castor Oil, Cocoa Butter, Polysorbate 60, Cetyl Alcohol, wax, Glyceryl Stearate, PEG 100 Stearate, Diazolidinyl Urea, Xanthan Gum, Disodium EDTA, Fragrance, Iodopropynyl Butylcarbamate	**Adults:** Apply prn.
Lubriderm Skin Nourishing Moisturizing Lotion with Shea and Cocoa Butters	Water, Glycerin, Cetyl Alcohol, Glyceryl Stearate SE, Petrolatum, Emulsifying Wax, Caprylic/Capric Triglyceride, Castor Oil, Octyldodecanol, Shea Butter, Cocoa Butter, Dimethicone, Tocopheryl Acetate, Diazolidinyl Urea, Xanthan Gum, Disodium EDTA, Fragrance, Iodopropynyl Butylcarbamate	**Adults:** Apply prn.
Lubriderm Skin Nourishing Moisturizing Lotion with Sea Kelp Extract	Water, Glycerin, Glyceryl Stearate SE, Cetyl Alcohol, Emulsifying Wax, Petrolatum, Caprylic/Capric Triglyceride, Castor Oil, Octyldodecanol, Dimethicone, Diazolidinyl Urea, Propylene Glycol, Xanthan Gum, Disodium EDTA, Fragrance, Giant Kelp Leaf Extract, Iodopropynyl Butylcarbamate	**Adults:** Apply prn.
Neutrogena Body Moisturizer Cream, Norwegian Formula	Water, Glycerin, Emulsifying Wax, Octyl Isononanoate, Dimethicone, Propylene Glycol Isoceteth-3 Acetate, Cyclomethicone, Stearic Acid, Aloe Extract, Matricaria Extract, Tocopheryl Acetate, Dimethicone Copolyol, Acrylates/C10-30 Alkyl Acrylate Crosspolymer, Cetearyl Alcohol, Sodium Cetearyl Sulfate, Sodium Sulfate, Hydrogenated Lanolin, Glyceryl Laurate, Tetrasodium EDTA, Triethanolamine, BHT, Propylene Glycol, Methylparaben, Ethylparaben, Propylparaben, Diazolidinyl Urea, Benzalkonium Chloride, Fragrance	**Adults & Peds:** Apply prn.

(Continued)

BRAND	INGREDIENTS	DOSE
Neutrogena Comforting Butter Body Cream	Water, Glycerin, Distearyldimonium Chloride, Petrolatum, Isopropyl Palmitate, Cetyl Alcohol, Dimethicone, Panthenol, Butyrospermum Parkii, Cocoa (Theobroma Cacao) Seed Butter, Mango (Mangifera Indica) Seed Butter, Benzyl Alcohol, BHT, Sodium Chloride, Yellow 5, Yellow 6, Fragrance	**Adults & Peds:** Apply prn.
Neutrogena Norwegian Formula Body/Hand Cream	Water (Purified), Glycerin, Emulsifying Wax, Octyl Isononanoate, Dimethicone, Propylene Glycol Isoceteth 3 AcetateCyclomethicone, Stearic Acid, Aloe Extract, Matricaria Extract, Tocopheryl Acetate, Dimethicone Copolyol, Acrylates C10-30 Alkyl Acrylate Crosspolymer, Cetearyl Alcohol, Sodium Cetearyl Sulfate, Sodium Sulfate, Hydrogenated Lanolin, Glyceryl Laurate, Tetrasodium EDTA, triethanolamine, BHT, Propylene Glycol, Methylparaben, Ethylparaben, Propylparaben, Diazolidinyl Urea, Benzalkonium Chloride, Fragrance	**Adults & Peds:** Apply qd.
Neutrogena Summer Glow Moisturizer	Avobenzone, Octisalate, Oxybenzone, Water, Glycerin, Dimethicone, Dihydroxyacetone, Silica, Diethylhexyl 2,6-Naphthalate, C12-15 Alkyl Benzoate, Potassium Cetyl Phosphate, Hydroxypropyl Starch Phosphate, Glyceryl Stearate, PEG 100 Stearate, Hydrogenated Palm Glycerides, Cetyl Alcohol, BHT, Magnesium Aluminum Silicate, Chlorphenesin, Tetrasodium EDTA, Citric Acid, Sodium Citrate, Phenoxyethanol, Methylparaben, Fragrance	**Adults & Peds:** Apply qd.
Nivea Body Age Defying Moisturizer For Body	Water, Glycerin, Mineral Oil, Caprylic/Capric Triglycerides, Cetyl Alcohol, Dimethicone, Glyceryl Stearate, Cyclopentasiloxane, Cyclohexasiloxane, PEG-40 Stearate, Creatine, 1-Methylhydantoin-2-Imide, Ubiquinone, Fragrance, Carbomer, Sodium Hydroxide, Phenoxyethanol, Methylparaben, Propylparaben	**Adults:** Apply to damp skin prn.
Nivea Essentially Enriched Lotion	Water, Mineral Oil, C13-16 Isoparaffin, Glycerin, Isopropyl Palmitate, Petrolatum, PEG-40, Sorbitan Perisostearate, Polyglyceryl-3 Diisostearate, Prunus Amygdalus Dulcis (Sweet Almond) Oil, Tocopheryl Acetate, Taurine, Sea Salt, Magnesium Sulfate, Fragrance, Citric Acid, Sodium Citrate, Potassium Sorbate	Apply prn.
Nivea Body Original Lotion, Dry Skin	Water, Mineral Oil, Glycerin, Isopropyl Palmitate, Glyceryl Stearate SE, Cetearyl Alcohol, Tocopheryl Acetate, Lanolin Alcohol, Isopropyl Myristate, Simethicone, Fragrance, Carbomer, Hydroxypropyl Methylcellulose, Sodium Hydroxide, Methylcellulose, Sodium Hydroxide, Methylchloroisothiazolinone, Methylisothiazolinone	**Adults:** Apply to damp skin prn.
Nivea Smooth Sensation Body Oil	Mineral oil, Caprylic/Capric Triglycerides, Persea Gratissima Oil (Avocado), Fragrance	**Adults:** Apply to damp skin prn.
Nivea Smooth Sensation Daily Lotion, Dry Skin	Water, Glycerin, Mineral Oil, Caprylic/Capric Triglycerides, Cetyl Alcohol, Dimethicone, Glyceryl Stearate, Cyclopentasiloxane, Cyclohexasiloxane, PEG-40 Stearate, Ginkgo Bilbo Leaf Extract, Tocopheryl Acetate, Butyrospermum Parkii (Shea Butter), Phenoxyethanol, Fragrance, Carbomer, Sodium Hydroxide, EDTA, Methylparaben, Propylparaben	**Adults:** Apply to damp skin prn.
Nivea Creme	Mineral Oil, Petrolatum, Glycerin, Microcrystalline Wax, Lanolin Alcohol, Paraffin, Panthenol, Magnesium Sulfate, Decyl Oleate, Octyldodecanol, Aluminum Stearate, Methylchloroisothiazolinone, Methylisothiazolinone, Citric Acid, Magnesium Stearate, Fragrance	**Adults & Peds:** Apply prn.
Pacquin Hand & Body Cream	Water, Glycerin, Stearic Acid, Potassium Stearate, Sodium Stearate, Cetyl Alcohol, Fragrance, Diisopropyl Sebacate, Carbomer 940, Methylparaben Propylparaben, Cetyl Esters Wax, Lanolin, Myristallactate	**Adults & Peds:** Apply qd.
Pacquin Plus Hand & Body Cream	Water, Glycerin, Stearic Acid, Potassium Stearate, Carbomer 940, Cetyl Alcohol, Cetyl Esters wax, Diisopropyl propyl Sebacate, Lanolin, Myristyl Lactate, Sodium Stearate, Methyl- and Propylparabens	**Adults & Peds:** Apply qd.

(Continued)

BRAND	INGREDIENTS	DOSE
Vaseline Intensive Care Skin Protectant Lotion for Extra Dry Skin, Fragrance Free	Water, Glycerin, Petrolatum, Stearic Acid, Glycol Stearate, Dimethicone, Isopropyl Isostearate, Tapioca Starch, Cetyl Alcohol, Glyceryl Stearate, Magnesium Aluminum Silicate, Carbomer, Ethylene Brassylate, Triethanolamine, Disodium EDTA, Phenoxyethanol, Methylparaben, Propylparaben, Titanium Dioxide	**Adults & Peds:** Apply prn.
Vaseline Intensive Care Cocoa Butter Deep Conditioning Lotion	Water, Petrolatum, Glycerin, Stearic Acid, Isopropyl Palmitate, Glycol Stearate, Dimethicone, Theobroma Cacao Seed Butter (Cocoa), Butyrospermum Parkii (Shea Butter), Helianthus Annuus Seed Oil or Glycine Soja Oil (Sunflower, Soybean), Glycine Soja Sterol (Soybean), Tocopheryl Acetate (Vitamin E Acetate), Retinyl Palmitate (Vitamin A Palmitate), Sodium Stearoyl-2-Lactylate, Collagen Amino Acids, Urea, Glyceryl Stearate, Cetyl Alcohol, Magnesium Aluminum Silicate, Carbomer, Lecithin, Mineral Water, Sodium PCA, Potassium Lactate, Lactic Acid, Fragrance, Stearamide AMP, Triethanolamine, Methylparaben, DMDM Hydantoin, Disodium EDTA, Caramel, Titanium Dioxide	**Adults & Peds:** Apply prn.
Vaseline Intensive Care Healthy Body Complexion Nourishing Body Lotion	Water, Glycerin, Dimethicone, Potassium Lactate, Stearic Acid, Sodium Hydroxypropyl Starch Phosphate, Mineral Oil, Glycol Stearate, Lactic Acid, Glycine Soja Sterol (Soybean), Lecithin, Petrolatum, Tocopheryl Acetate (Vitamin E Acetate), Retinyl Palmitate (Vitamin A Palmitate), Helianthus Annuus Seed Acid (Sunflower), Sodium PCA, Sodium Stearoyl Lactate, Urea, Collagen Amino Acids, Mineral Water, Glyceryl Stearate, Cetyl Alcohol, Magnesium Aluminum Silicate, Fragrance, Stearamide AMP, Ethylhexyl Methoxycinnamate, Corn Oil, Methylparaben, DMDM Hydantoin, Disodium EDTA, Xanthan Gum, BHT	**Adults & Peds:** Apply prn.
Vaseline Intensive Care Healthy Hand & Nail Lotion	Water, Potassium Lactate, Sodium Hydroxypropyl Starch Phosphate, Glycerin, Stearic Acid, Mineral Oil, Dimethicone, Lactic Acid, Glycol Stearate, PEG 100 Stearate, Keratin, Glycine Soja Sterol (Soybean), Lecithin, Tocopheryl Acetate (Vitamin E Acetate), Retinyl Palmitate (Vitamin A Palmitate), Healianthus Annuus Seed Oil (Sunflower), Sodium PCA, Sodium Stearoyl Lactate, Urea, Collagen Amino Acids, Ethylhexyl Methoxycinnamate, Petrolatum, Mineral Water, Cetyl Alcohol, Stearamide AMP, Cyclomethicone, Magnesium Aluminum Silicate, Glyceryl Stearate, Fragrance, XanthanGum,Corn Oil, BHT, Disodium EDTA, Methylparaben, DMDM Hydantoin	**Adults & Peds:** Apply prn.
Vaseline Intensive Care Aloe Cool & Fresh Moisturizing Lotion	Water, Glycerin, Stearic Acid, Glycol Stearate, Aloe Barbadensis Leaf Juice (Aloe Vera), Cucumis Sativus Extract (Cucumber), Helianthus Annuus Seed Oil (Sunflower), Glycine Soja Oil (Soybean), Glycine Soja Sterol (Soybean), Sodium Stearoyl-2 Lactylate, Tocopheryl Acetate (Vitamin E Acetate), Retinyl Palmitate (Vitamin A Palmitate), Sodium Acrylate/Acryloyldimethyl Taurate Copolymer, Dimethicone, Glyceryl Stearate, Cetyl Alcohol, Lecithin, Mineral Water, Sodium PCA, Potassium Lactate, Lactic Acid, Collagen Amino Acids, Urea, Fragrance, Triethanolamine, DMDM Hydantoin, Iodopropynyl Butylcarbamate, Disodium EDTA, Titanium Dioxide	**Adults & Peds:** Apply prn.
Vaseline Intensive Care Lotion Total Moisture	Water, Glycerin, Stearic Acid, Glycol Stearate, Petrolatum, Isopropyl Palmitate, Glycine Soja Sterol (Soybean), Helianthus Annuus Seed Oil (Sunflower), Glycine Soja Oil (Soybean), Avena Sativa Kernel Protein (Oat), Sodium Stearoyl-2 Lactylate, Tocopheryl Acetate (Vitamin E Acetate), Retinyl Palmitate (Vitamin A Palmitate), Panthenol (Provitamin B5), Carbomer, Lecithin, Keratin, Dimethicone, Glyceryl Stearate, Cetyl Alcohol, Sodium PCA, Potassium Lactate, Lactic Acid, Collagen Amino Acids, Mineral Water, Fragrance, Triethanolamine, Magnesium Aluminum Silicate, Urea, Methylparaben, DMDM Hydantoin, Iodopropynyl Butylcarbamate, Disodium EDTA, Titanium dioxide	**Adults & Peds:** Apply prn.

(Continued)

BRAND	INGREDIENTS	DOSE
Vaseline Intensive Care Nightly Renewal Light Body Lotion	Water, Glycerin, Isopropyl Myristate, Dimethicone, Cyclopentasiloxane, Stearic Acid, Tapioca Starch, Glycol Stearate, Helianthus Annuus Seed Oil (Sunflower), Glycine Soja Oil, Glycine Soja Sterol (Soybean), Vitis VInefera Seed Extract (Grape), Lavendula Angustifolia Extract (Lavendar), Lecithin, Tocopheryl Acetate (Vitamin E Acetate) , Retinyl Palmitate (Vitamin A Palmitate), Urea, Collagen Amino Acids, Sodium PCA, Potassium Lactate, Lactic Acid, Cetyl Alcohol, Glyceryl Stearate, Magnesium Aluminum Silicate, Carbomer, Methyl Methacrylate Crosspolymer, Fragrance	**Adults & Peds:** Apply prn.
Vaseline Intensive Rescue Moisture Locking Lotion	Water, Glycerin, Petrolatum, Stearic Acid, Glycol Stearate, Dimethicone, Cyclopenta, Siloxane, Hydrogenated Polyiso-butene, Ethylhexyl Cocoate, Hydrogenated Didecene, Glycol Stearate, Paraffin, Theobroma Cacao (Cocoa) Seed Butter, Butyrospermum Parkii (Shea Butter), Potato Starch Modified, PEG 90 Diisostearate, Dimethiconol, Disteareth 75 IPDI, Glyceryl Stearate, Sodium Acrylate/Sodium Acryloyldimethyl Taurate Copolymer, Microcrystal-line Wax, Xanthan Gum, Triethanolamine, Polysorbate 80, Dimethicone Copolyol, Cetyl Alcohol, Isohexadecane, Phenoxyethanol, Disodium EDTA, Propylene Glycol, Ethylene Brassylate, Methylparaben, Propylparaben	**Adults & Peds:** Apply prn.
Vaseline Jelly	White Petrolatum	**Adults & Peds:** Apply prn.
Vaseline Petroleum Jelly Cream Deep Moisture	White Petrolatum, Water, Caprylic/Capric Triglyceride; Stearic Acid, Glycerin, Glycol Stearate, Sodium Hydroxy-propyl Starch Phosphate, PEG-100 Stearate, Glyceryl Stearate, Cetyl Alcohol, Tocopheryl Acetate (Vitamin E Acetate), Acrylates/C10-30 Alkyl Acrylate Crosspolymer	**Adults & Peds:** Apply prn.
Vaseline Intensive Care Cocoa Butter Deep Conditioning Lotion	Water, Petrolatum, Glycerin, Stearic Acid, Isopropyl Pal-mitate, Glycol Stearate, Dimethicone, Theobroma Cacao (Cocoa) Seed Butter, Butyrospermum Parkii (Shea Butter), Helianthus Annuus (Sunflower) Seed Oil or Glycine Soja (Soybean) Sterol, Tocopheryl Acetate (Vitamin E Acetate), Retinyl Palmitate (Vitamin A Palmitate), Sodium Stearoyl-2-Lactylate, Collagen Amino Acids, Urea, Glyceryl Stearate, Cetyl Alcohol, Magnesium Aluminum Silicate, Carbomer, Lecithin, Mineral Water, Sodium PCA, Potassium Lactate, Lactic Acid, Fragrance, Stearamide AMP, Triethanolamine, Methylparaben, DMDM Hydantoin, Disodium EDTA, Caramel, Titanium Dioxide	**Adults & Peds:** Apply prn.

PSORIASIS PRODUCTS

BRAND	INGREDIENT/ STRENGTH	DOSE
COAL TAR		
Denorex Therapeutic Protection 2-in-1 shampoo	Coal Tar 2.5%	**Adults & Peds:** Use at least biw.
Denorex Therapeutic Protection shampoo	Coal Tar 2.5%	**Adults & Peds:** Use at least biw.
DHS tar Shampoo	Coal Tar 0.5%	**Adults & Peds:** Use at least biw.
Ionil-T Plus Shampoo	Coal Tar 2%	**Adults & Peds:** Use at least biw.
Ionil-T Shampoo	Coal Tar 1%	**Adults & Peds:** Use at least biw.
MG217 Ointment	Coal Tar 2%	**Adults & Peds:** Apply to affected area qd-qid.
MG217 tar Shampoo	Coal Tar 3%	**Adults & Peds:** Use at least biw.
Neutrogena T/Gel Shampoo Extra Strength	Coal Tar 1%	**Adults & Peds:** Use at least biw.
Neutrogena T/Gel Shampoo Original Formula	Coal Tar 0.5%	**Adults & Peds:** Use at least biw.
Neutrogena T/Gel Stubborn Itch Shampoo	Coal Tar 0.5%	**Adults & Peds:** Use at least biw.
Polytar Shampoo	Coal Tar 0.5%	**Adults & Peds:** Use at least biw.
Polytar soap	Coal Tar 0.5%	**Adults & Peds:** Apply to affected area prn.
Psoriasin Multi-Symptom Psoriasis Relief Gel	Coal Tar 1.25%	**Adults & Peds:** Apply to affected area qd-qid.
Psoriasin Multi-Symptom Psoriasis Relief Ointment	Coal Tar 2%	**Adults & Peds:** Apply to affected area qd-qid.
CORTICOSTEROIDS		
Aveeno Hydrocortisone 1% Anti-Itch Cream	Hydrocortisone 1%	**Adults & Peds:** ≥2 yrs: Apply to affected area tid-qid.
Cortaid Advanced 12-Hour Anti-Itch Cream	Hydrocortisone 1%	**Adults & Peds:** ≥2 yrs: Apply to affected area tid-qid.
Cortaid Intensive Therapy Cooling Spray	Hydrocortisone 1%	**Adults & Peds:** ≥2 yrs: Apply to affected area tid-qid.
Cortaid Intensive Therapy Moisturizing Cream	Hydrocortisone 1%	**Adults & Peds:** ≥2 yrs: Apply to affected area tid-qid.
Cortaid Maximum Strength Cream	Hydrocortisone 1%	**Adults & Peds:** ≥2 yrs: Apply to affected area tid-qid.
Cortaid Maximum Strength Ointment	Hydrocortisone 1%	**Adults & Peds:** ≥2 yrs: Apply to affected area tid-qid.
Cortizone-10 Cream	Hydrocortisone 1%	**Adults & Peds:** ≥2 yrs: Apply to affected area tid-qid.
Cortizone-10 Maximum Strength Anti-Itch Ointment	Hydrocortisone 1%	**Adults & Peds:** ≥2 yrs: Apply to affected area tid-qid.
Cortizone-10 Ointment	Hydrocortisone 1%	**Adults & Peds:** ≥2 yrs: Apply to affected area tid-qid.
Cortizone-10 Plus Intensive Healing Formula	Hydrocortisone 1%	**Adults & Peds:** ≥2 yrs: Apply to affected area tid-qid.
SALICYLIC ACID		
Dermarest Psoriasis Overnight Treatment	Salicylic Acid 3%	**Adults & Peds:** Apply to affected area qhs. **Max:** qid.
Dermarest Psoriasis Medicated Moisturizer	Salicylic Acid 2%	**Adults & Peds:** Apply to affected area qd-qid.
Dermarest Psoriasis Medicated Scalp Treatment	Salicylic Acid 3%	**Adults & Peds:** Apply to affected area qd-qid.
Dermarest Psoriasis Medicated Shampoo/Conditioner	Salicylic Acid 3%	**Adults & Peds:** Apply to affected area at least biw.
Dermarest Psoriasis Skin Treatment	Salicylic Acid 3%	**Adults & Peds:** Apply to affected area qd-qid.
Neutrogena T/Gel Conditioner	Salicylic Acid 2%	**Adults & Peds:** Use at least biw.
Psoriasin Therapeutic Shampoo and Body Wash	Salicylic Acid 3%	**Adults & Peds:** Use biw.
Psoriasin Therapeutic Shampoo With Panthenol	Salicylic Acid 3%	**Adults & Peds:** Use biw.

WOUND CARE PRODUCTS

BRAND	INGREDIENT/STRENGTH	DOSE
NEOMYCIN/POLYMYXIN B/BACITRACIN COMBINATIONS		
Bacitracin Ointment	Bacitracin 500 U	**Adults & Peds:** Apply to affected area qd-tid.
Bactine Pain Relieving Protective Antibiotic	Neomycin/polymyxin B/bacitracin/pramoxine 3.5mg-10,000 U- 500 U- 1%	**Adults & Peds:** Apply to affected area qd-tid.
Neosporin Ointment	Neomycin/polymyxin B/bacitracin 3.5mg-5,000 U-400 U	**Adults & Peds:** Apply to affected area qd-tid.
Neosporin Plus Pain Relief Cream	Neomycin/polymyxin B/pramoxine 3.5mg-10,000 U-10mg	**Adults & Peds:** Apply to affected area qd-tid.
Neosporin Plus Pain Relief Ointment	Neomycin/polymyxin B/bacitracin/pramoxine 3.5mg-10,000 U-500 U-10mg	**Adults & Peds:** Apply to affected area qd-tid.
Neosporin To Go Ointment	Neomycin/polymyxin B/bacitracin 3.5mg-5,000 U-400 U	**Adults & Peds:** Apply to affected area qd-tid.
Polysporin Ointment	Polymyxin B/bacitracin 10,000 U-500 U	**Adults & Peds:** Apply to affected area qd-tid.
BENZALKONIUM CHLORIDE COMBINATIONS		
Bactine First Aid Liquid	Lidocaine HCl/benzalkonium chloride 2.5%-0.13%	**Adults & Peds:** ≥2 yrs: Apply to affected area qd-tid.
Bactine Pain Relieving Cleansing Spray	Lidocaine HCl/benzalkonium chloride 2.5%-0.13%	**Adults & Peds:** ≥2 yrs: Apply to affected area qd-tid.
BENZETHONIUM CHLORIDE COMBINATIONS		
Gold Bond First Aid Quick Spray	Menthol/benzethonium chloride 1%-0.13%	**Adults & Peds:** ≥2 yrs: Apply to affected area tid-qid.
Lanacane Maximum Strength Cream	Benzocaine/benzethonium chloride 20%-2%	**Adults & Peds:** ≥2 yrs: Apply to affected area tid-qid.
CHLORHEXIDINE GLUCONATE		
Hibiclens	Chlorhexidine gluconate 4%	**Adults & Peds:** Apply sparingly to affected area prn.
IODINE		
Betadine Skin Cleanser	Povidone-iodine 7.5%	**Adults & Peds:** Apply to affected area. Wash vigorously for 15 seconds and rinse.
Betadine Solution	Povidone-iodine 10%	**Adults & Peds:** Apply to affected area qd-tid.
MISCELLANEOUS		
Aquaphor Healing Ointment	Petrolatum, mineral oil, ceresin, lanolin	**Adults & Peds:** Apply to affected area prn.
Proxacol Hydrogen Peroxide	Hydrogen peroxide 3%	**Adults:** Apply to affected area qd-tid.
Wound Wash Sterile Saline Spray	Sterile sodium chloride solution 0.9%	**Adults & Peds:** Apply to affected area prn.

ANTACID AND HEARTBURN PRODUCTS

BRAND	INGREDIENT/STRENGTH	DOSE
ANTACID		
Alka-Seltzer Gold Tablets	Citric Acid/Potassium Bicarbonate/ Sodium Bicarbonate 1000mg-344mg-1050mg	**Adults:** ≥**60 yrs:** 2 tabs q4h prn. **Max:** 6 tabs q24h. **Adults & Peds:** ≥**12 yrs:** 2 tabs q4h prn. **Max:** 8 tabs q24h. **Peds:** ≤**12 yrs:** 1 tab q4h prn. **Max:** 4 tabs q24h.
Alka-Seltzer Heartburn Relief Tablets	Citric Acid/Sodium Bicarbonate 1000mg-1940mg	**Adults:** ≥**60 yrs:** 2 tabs q4h prn. **Max:** 4 tabs q24h. **Adults & Peds:** ≥**12 yrs:** 2 tabs q4h prn. **Max:** 8 tabs q24h.
Alka-Seltzer Tablets, Original	Aspirin/Sodium Bicarbonate/Citric Acid 325mg-1916mg-1000mg	**Adults:** ≥**60 yrs:** 2 tabs q4h prn. **Max:** 4 tabs q24h. **Adults & Peds:** ≥**12 yrs:** 2 tabs q4h prn. **Max:** 8 tabs q24h.
Alka-Seltzer Tablets, Extra-Strength	Aspirin/Sodium Bicarbonate/Citric Acid 500mg-1985mg-1000mg	**Adults:** ≥**60 yrs:** 2 tabs q6h prn. **Max:** 3 tabs q24h. **Adults & Peds:** ≥**12 yrs:** 2 tabs q6h prn. **Max:** 7 tabs q24h.
Brioschi Powder	Sodium Bicarbonate/Tartaric Acid 2.69g-2.43g/dose	**Adults & Peds:** ≥**12 yrs:** 1 capful (6g) dissolved in 4-6 oz water q1h. **Max:** 6 doses q24h.
Gaviscon Extra Strength Liquid	Aluminum Hydroxide/Magnesium Carbonate 254mg-237.5mg/5mL	**Adults:** 2-4 tsp (10-20mL) qid.
Gaviscon Extra Strength Tablets	Aluminum Hydroxide/Magnesium Carbonate 160mg-105mg	**Adults:** 2-4 tabs qid. **Max:** 16 doses q24h.
Gaviscon Regular Strength Chewable Tablets	Aluminum Hydroxide/Magnesium Carbonate 80mg-20mg	**Adults:** 2-4 tabs qid. **Max:** 16 tabs q24h.
Gaviscon Regular Strength Liquid	Aluminum Hydroxide/Magnesium Carbonate 95mg-358mg/15mL	**Adults:** 1-2 tbl (15-30mL) qid.
Gaviscon Acid Breakthrough, Chewable Tablets	Calcium Carbonate 500mg	**Adults:** 2 tabs prn. **Max:** 15 tabs q24h.
Maalox Antacid Barrier Chewable Tablets	Calcium Carbonate 500mg	**Adults:** 2-4 tabs qid. **Max:** 16 tabs q24h.
Maalox Quick Dissolve Regular Strength Chewable Tablets	Calcium Carbonate 600mg	**Adults:** 1-2 tabs prn. **Max:** 12 tabs q24h.
Mylanta, Children's	Calcium Carbonate 400mg	**Peds: 6-11 yrs (48-95 lbs):** Take 2 tab prn. **Max:** 6 tabs q24h. **Peds: 2-5 yrs (24-47 lbs):** Take 1 tab prn **Max:** 3 tabs q24h.
Mylanta Ultimate Strength Liquid	Aluminum Hydroxide/Magnesium Hydroxide 500mg-500mg/5mL	**Adults & Peds** ≥**12 yrs:** 2-4 tsp (10-20mL) qid (between meals & hs). **Max:** 9 tsp (45mL) q24h for ≤2 weeks.
Mylanta Supreme Antacid Liquid	Calcium Carbonate/Magnesium Hydroxide 400mg-135mg/5mL	**Adults:** 2-4 tsp (10-20mL) qid. **Max:** 18 tsp (90mL) q24h.
Mylanta Ultimate Strength Chewable Tablets	Calcium Carbonate/Magnesium Hydroxide 700mg-300mg	**Adults:** 2-4 tabs qid. (between meals & hs). **Max:** 10 tabs q24h for ≤2 weeks.
Phillips Milk of Magnesia Liquid	Magnesium Hydroxide 400mg/5mL	**Adults & Peds:** ≥**12 yrs:** 30-60mL qd. **Peds: 6-11 yrs:** 15-30mL qd. **2-5 yrs:** 5-15mL qd.
Rolaids Extra Strength Softchews	Calcium Carbonate 1177mg	**Adults:** 2-3 chews q1h prn. **Max:** 6 chews q24h.
Rolaids Extra Strength Tablets	Calcium Carbonate/Magnesium Hydroxide 675mg-135mg	**Adults:** 2-4 tabs q1h prn. **Max:** 10 tabs q24h.
Rolaids Tablets	Calcium Carbonate/Magnesium Hydroxide 550mg-110mg	**Adults:** 2-4 tabs q1h prn. **Max:** 12 tabs q24h.
Titralac Chewable Tablets	Calcium Carbonate 420mg	**Adults:** 2 tabs q2-3h prn. **Max:** 19 tabs q24h.

(Continued)

BRAND	INGREDIENT/STRENGTH	DOSE
ANTACID *(Continued)*		
Tums Chewable Tablets	Calcium Carbonate 500mg	**Adults:** 2-4 tabs q1h prn. **Max:** 15 tabs q24h.
Tums E-X Chewable Tablets	Calcium Carbonate 750mg	**Adults:** 2-4 tabs prn. **Max:** 10 tabs q24h.
Tums E-X Sugar Free Chewable Tablets	Calcium Carbonate 750mg	**Adults:** 2-4 tabs prn. **Max:** 10 tabs q24h.
Tums Kids Chewable Tablets	Calcium Carbonate 750mg	**Peds: >4 yrs (>49 lbs):** Take 1 tab tid. **Max:** 4 tabs q24h. **Peds: 2-4 yrs (24-47 lbs):** Take ½ tab bid. **Max:** 2 tabs q24h.
Tums Smoothies Tablets	Calcium Carbonate 750mg	**Adults:** 2-4 tabs prn. **Max:** 10 tabs q24h.
Tums Ultra 1000 Chewable Tablets	Calcium Carbonate 1000mg	**Adults:** 2-4 tabs prn. **Max:** 7 tabs q24h for ≤2 weeks.
ANTACID/ANTIFLATULENT		
Gas-X with Maalox Capsules	Calcium Carbonate/Simethicone 250mg-62.5mg	**Adults:** 2-4 caps prn. **Max:** 8 caps q24h.
Gas-X Extra Strength with Maalox Capsules	Calcium Carbonate/Simethicone 500mg-125mg	**Adults:** 1-2 caps prn. **Max:** 4 caps q24h.
Gelusil Chewable Tablets	Aluminum Hydroxide/Magnesium Hydroxide/Simethicone 200mg-200mg-20mg	**Adults:** 2-4 tabs qid.
Maalox Max Liquid	Aluminum Hydroxide/Magnesium Hydroxide/Simethicone 400mg-400mg-40mg/5mL	**Adults & Peds: ≥12 yrs:** 2-4 tsp (10-20mL) qid. **Max:** 12 tsp (60mL) q24h.
Maalox Max Chewable Tablets	Calcium Carbonate/Simethicone 100mg-60mg	**Adults:** 1-2 tabs prn. **Max:** 8 tabs q24h.
Maalox Regular Strength Liquid	Aluminum Hydroxide/Magnesium Hydroxide/Simethicone 200mg-200mg-20mg/5mL	**Adults & Peds: ≥12 yrs:** 2-4 tsp (10-20mL) qid. **Max:** 12 tsp (60mL) q24h.
Mylanta Maximum Strength Liquid	Aluminum Hydroxide/Magnesium Hydroxide/Simethicone 400mg-400mg-40mg/5mL	**Adults & Peds: ≥12 yrs:** 2-4 tsp (10-20mL) qid. **Max:** 12 tsp (60mL) q24h.
Mylanta Regular Strength Liquid	Aluminum Hydroxide/Magnesium Hydroxide/Simethicone 200mg-200mg-20mg/5mL	**Adults & Peds: ≥12 yrs:** 2-4 tsp (10-20mL) qid. **Max:** 12 tsp (60mL) q24h.
Rolaids Multi-Symptom Chewable Tablets	Calcium Carbonate/Magnesium Hydroxide/Simethicone 675mg-135mg-60mg	**Adults:** 2 tabs qid prn. **Max:** 8 tabs q24h.
Titralac Plus Chewable Tablets	Calcium Carbonate/Simethicone 420mg-21mg	**Adults:** 2 tabs q2-3h prn. **Max:** 19 tabs q24h.
BISMUTH SUBSALICYLATE		
Maalox Total Stomach Relief Maximum Strength Liquid	Bismuth Subsalicylate 525mg/15mL	**Adults & Peds: ≥12 yrs:** 2 tbl (30mL) q1/2-1h. **Max:** 8 tbl (120mL) q24h.
Pepto Bismol Chewable Tablets	Bismuth Subsalicylate 262mg	**Adults & Peds: ≥12 yrs:** 2 tabs q1/2-1h. **Max:** 8 doses q24h.
Pepto Bismol Caplets	Bismuth Subsalicylate 262mg	**Adults & Peds: ≥12 yrs:** 2 tabs q1/2-1h. **Max:** 8 doses q24h.
Pepto Bismol Liquid	Bismuth Subsalicylate 262mg/15mL	**Adults & Peds: ≥12 yrs:** 2 tbl (30mL) q1/2-1h. **Max:** 8 doses (240mL) q24h.
Pepto Bismol Maximum Strengtth Liquid	Bismuth Subsalicylate 525mg/15mL	**Adults & Peds: ≥12 yrs:** 2 tbl (30mL) q1h. **Peds: 9-12 yrs:** 1 tbl (15mL) q1h. **6-9 yrs:** 2 tsp (10mL) q1h. **3-6 yrs:** 1 tsp (5mL). **Max:** 8 doses (240mL) q24h.

(Continued)

BRAND	INGREDIENT/STRENGTH	DOSE
H₂-RECEPTOR ANTAGONIST		
Pepcid AC Chewable Tablets	Famotidine 10mg	**Adults & Peds:** ≥**12 yrs:** 1 tab qd. **Max:** 2 tabs q24h.
Pepcid AC Gelcaps	Famotidine 10mg	**Adults & Peds:** ≥**12 yrs:** 1 tab qd. **Max:** 2 tabs q24h.
Pepcid AC Maximum Strength EZ Chews	Famotidine 20mg	**Adults & Peds:** ≥**12 yrs:** 1 tab qd. **Max:** 2 tabs q24h.
Pepcid AC Maximum Strength Tablets	Famotidine 20mg	**Adults & Peds:** ≥**12 yrs:** 1 tab qd. **Max:** 2 tabs q24h.
Pepcid AC Tablets	Famotidine 10mg	**Adults & Peds:** ≥**12 yrs:** 1 tab qd. **Max:** 2 tabs q24h.
Tagamet HB Tablets	Cimetidine 200mg	**Adults & Peds:** ≥**12 yrs:** 1 tab qd. **Max:** 2 tabs q24h.
Zantac 150 Tablets	Ranitidine 150mg	**Adults & Peds:** ≥**12 yrs:** 1 tab qd. **Max:** 2 tabs q24h.
Zantac 75 Tablets	Ranitidine 75mg	**Adults & Peds:** ≥**12 yrs:** 1 tab qd. **Max:** 2 tabs q24h.
H₂-RECEPTOR ANTAGONIST/ANTACID		
Pepcid Complete Chewable Tablets	Famotidine/Calcium Carbonate/ Magnesium Hydroxide 10mg-800mg-165mg	**Adults & Peds:** ≥**12 yrs:** 1 tab qd. **Max:** 2 tabs q24h.
PROTON PUMP INHIBITOR		
Prilosec OTC Tablets	Omeprazole 20mg	**Adults:** 1 tab qd x 14 days. May repeat 14 day course q 4 months.

ANTIDIARRHEAL PRODUCTS

BRAND	INGREDIENT/STRENGTH	DOSE
ABSORBENT AGENTS		
Equalactin Chewable Tablets	Calcium Polycarbophil 625mg	**Adults:** ≥**12 yrs:** 2 tabs q30min prn. **Max:** 8 tabs q24h. **Peds: 6-12 yrs:** 1 tab q30min. **Max:** 4 tabs q24h. **2 to** ≤**6 yrs:** 1 tab q30min. **Max:** 2 tabs q24h.
Fibercon Caplets	Calcium Polycarbophil 625mg	**Adults:** ≥**12 yrs:** 2 tabs qd. **Max:** 8 tabs q24h.
Konsyl Fiber Caplets	Calcium Polycarbophil 625mg	**Adults:** ≥**12 yrs:** 2 tabs qd. **Max:** 8 tabs q24h. **Peds: 6-12 yrs:** 1 tab qd. **Max:** 3 tabs q24h.
ANTIPERISTALTIC AGENTS		
Imodium A-D Caplet	Loperamide HCl 2mg	**Adults:** ≥**12 yrs:** 2 caplets after first loose stool; 1 caplet after each subsequent loose stool. **Max:** 4 caplets q24h. **Peds: 9-11 yrs (60-95 lbs):** 1 caplet after first loose stool; ½ caplet after each subsequent loose stool. **Max:** 3 caplets q24h. **6-8 yrs (48-59 lbs):** 1 caplet after first loose stool; ½ caplet after each subsequent loose stool. **Max:** 2 caplets q24h.
Imodium A-D E-Z Chews	Loperamide HCl 2mg	**Adults:** ≥**12 yrs:** 2 caplets after first loose stool; 1 caplet after each subsequent loose stool. **Max:** 4 caplets q24h. **Peds: 9-11 yrs (60-95 lbs):** 1 caplet after first loose stool; ½ caplet after each subsequent loose stool. **Max:** 3 caplets q24h. **6-8 yrs (48-59 lbs):** 1 caplet after first loose stool; 1/2 caplet after each subsequent loose stool. **Max:** 2 caplets q24h.
Imodium A-D Liquid	Loperamide HCl 1mg/7.5mL	**Adults:** ≥**12 yrs:** 30mL (6 tsp) after first loose stool; 15mL (3 tsp) after each subsequent loose stool. **Max:** 60mL (12 tsp) q24h. **Peds: 9-11 yrs (60-95 lbs):** 15mL (3 tsp) after first loose stool; 7.5mL (1½ tsp) after each subsequent loose stool. **Max:** 45mL (9 tsp) q24h. **6-8 yrs (48-59 lbs):**15mL (3 tsp) after first loose stool; 7.5mL (1½ tsp) after each subsequent loose stool. **Max:** 30mL (6 tsp) q24h.
ANTIPERISTALTIC/ANTIFLATULENT AGENTS		
Imodium Advanced Caplet	Loperamide HCl/Simethicone 2mg-125mg	**Adults:** ≥**12 yrs:** 2 caplets after first loose stool; 1 caplet after each subsequent loose stool. **Max:** 4 caplets q24h. **Peds: 9-11 yrs (60-95 lbs):** 1 caplet after first loose stool; 1/2 caplet after each subsequent loose stool. **Max:** 3 caplets q24h. **6-8 yrs (48-59 lbs):** 1 caplet after first loose stool; ½ caplet after each subsequent loose stool. **Max:** 2 caplets q24h.

(Continued)

BRAND	INGREDIENT/STRENGTH	DOSE
ANTIPERISTALTIC/ANTIFLATULENT AGENTS *(Continued)*		
Imodium Advanced Chewable Tablet	Loperamide HCl/Simethicone 2mg-125mg	**Adults: ≥12 yrs:** 2 caplets after first loose stool; 1 caplet after each subsequent loose stool. **Max:** 4 caplets q24h. **Peds: 9-11 yrs (60-95 lbs):** 1 caplet after first loose stool; ½ caplet after each subsequent loose stool. **Max:** 3 caplets q24h. **6-8 yrs (48-59 lbs):** 1 caplet after first loose stool; ½ caplet after each subsequent loose stool. **Max:** 2 caplets q24h.
BISMUTH SUBSALICYLATE		
Kaopectate Caplets	Bismuth Subsalicylate 262mg	**Adults & Peds: ≥12 yrs:** 2 caplets q½-1h prn. **Max:** 8 doses q24h.
Kaopectate Extra Strength Liquid	Bismuth Subsalicylate 525mg/15mL	**Adults: ≥12 yrs:** 2 tbl (30mL). **Peds: 9-12 yrs:** 1 tbl (15mL) q1h prn. **6-9 yrs:** 2 tsp (10mL) q1h prn. **3-6 yrs:** 1 tsp (5mL) q1h prn. **Max:** 8 doses q24h.
Kaopectate Liquid	Bismuth Subsalicylate 262mg/15mL	**Adults: ≥12 yrs:** 2 tbl (30mL). **Peds: 9-12 yrs:** 1 tbl (15mL) q1h prn. **6-9 yrs:** 2 tsp (10mL) q1h prn. **3-6 yrs:** 1 tsp (5mL) q1h prn. **Max:** 8 doses q24h.
Pepto Bismol Chewable Tablets	Bismuth Subsalicylate 262mg	**Adults & Peds: ≥12 yrs:** 2 tabs q½-1h. **Max:** 8 doses (16 tabs) q24h.
Pepto Bismol Caplets	Bismuth Subsalicylate 262mg	**Adults & Peds: ≥12 yrs:** 2 tabs q½-1h. **Max:** 8 doses (16 caps) q24h.
Pepto Bismol Liquid	Bismuth Subsalicylate 262mg/15mL	**Adults & Peds: ≥12 yrs:** 2 tbl (30mL) q½-1h prn. **Max:** 8 doses (16 tbl) q24h.
Pepto Bismol Maximum Strength	Bismuth Subsalicylate 525mg/15mL	**Adults: ≥12 yrs:** 2 tbl (30mL) q1h prn. **Max:** 4 doses (8 tbl) q24h.

ANTIFLATULANT PRODUCTS

BRAND	INGREDIENT/STRENGTH	DOSE
ALPHA-GALACTOSIDASE		
Beano Food Enzyme Dietary Supplement Drops	Alpha-Galactosidase Enzyme 150 GalU	**Adults:** Add 5 drops before meals.
Beano Food Enzyme Dietary Supplement Tablets	Alpha-Galactosidase Enzyme 150 GalU	**Adults:** Take 3 tabs before meals.
ANTACID/ANTIFLATULENCE		
Gas-X with Maalox Capsules	Calcium Carbonate/Simethicone 250mg-62.5mg	**Adults:** 2-4 caps prn. **Max:** 8 caps q24h.
Gas-X Extra Strength with Maalox Capsules	Calcium Carbonate/Simethicone 500mg-125mg	**Adults:** 1-2 caps prn. **Max:** 4 caps q24h.
Gelusil Chewable Tablets	Aluminum Hydroxide/Magnesium Hydroxide/Simethicone 200mg-200mg-20mg	**Adults:** 2-4 tabs qid.
Maalox Max Liquid	Aluminum Hydroxide/Magnesium Hydroxide/Simethicone 400mg-400mg-40mg/5mL	**Adults & Peds: ≥12 yrs:** 2-4 tsp (10-20mL) qid. **Max:** 12 tsp (60mL) q24h.
Maalox Max Chewable Tablets	Calcium Carbonate/Simethicone 100mg-60mg	**Adults:** 1-2 tabs prn. **Max:** 8 tabs q24h.
Maalox Regular Strength Liquid	Aluminum Hydroxide/Magnesium Hydroxide/Simethicone 200mg-200mg-20mg/5mL	**Adults & Peds: ≥12 yrs:** 2-4 tsp (10-20mL) qid. **Max:** 12 tsp (60mL) q24h.
Mylanta Maximum Strength Liquid	Aluminum Hydroxide/Magnesium Hydroxide/Simethicone 400mg-400mg-40mg/5mL	**Adults & Peds: ≥12 yrs:** 2-4 tsp (10-20mL) qid. **Max:** 12 tsp (60mL) q24h.
Mylanta Regular Strength Liquid	Aluminum Hydroxide/Magnesium Hydroxide/Simethicone 200mg-200mg-20mg/5mL	**Adults & Peds: ≥12 yrs:** 2-4 tsp (10-20mL) qid. **Max:** 24 tsp (120mL) q24h.
Rolaids Antacid & Antigas Soft Chews	Calcium Carbonate/Simethicone 1177mg-80mg	**Adults:** 2-3 chews hourly prn.
Titralac Plus Chewable Tablets	Calcium Carbonate/Simethicone 420mg-21mg	**Adults:** 2 tabs q2-3h prn. **Max:** 19 tabs q24h.
SIMETHICONE		
GasAid Maximum Strength Anti-Gas Softgels	Simethicone 125mg	**Adults:** Take 1-2 caps prn and qhs. **Max:** 4 caps q24h.
Gas-X Infant Drops	Simethicone 20mg/0.3mL	**Peds: ≥2 yrs (≥24 lbs):** 0.6mL prn. **Peds: <2 yrs (<24 lbs):** 0.3mL prn. **Max:** 6 doses q24h.
Gas-X Children's Thin Strips	Simethicone 40mg	**Peds: 2-12 yrs:** 1 strip prn and hs. **Max:** 6 strips q24h.
Gas-X Thin Strips	Simethicone 62.5mg	**Adults:** Allow 2-4 strips to dissolve prn. **Max:** 8 strips q24h.
Gas-X Antigas Chewable Tablets	Simethicone 80mg	**Adults:** Take 1-2 caps prn and qhs. **Max:** 6 caps q24h.
Gas-X Extra Strength Antigas Softgels	Simethicone 125mg	**Adults:** Take 1-2 caps prn and qhs. **Max:** 4 caps q24h.
Gas-X Maximum Strength Antigas Softgels	Simethicone 166mg	**Adults:** Take 1-2 caps prn and qhs. **Max:** 3 caps q24h.
Little Tummys Gas Relief Drops	Simethicone 20mg/0.3mL	**Peds: ≥2 yrs (≥24 lbs):** 0.6mL prn (after meals & hs). **Peds: <2 yrs (<24 lbs):** 0.3mL prn (after meals & hs). **Max:** 12 doses q24h.
Mylanta Gas Maximum Strength Softgels	Simethicone 125mg	**Adults:** Chew 1-2 tabs (after meals & hs). **Max:** 4 tabs q24h.
Mylanta Gas Maximum Strength Chewable Tablets	Simethicone 125mg	**Adults:** Chew 1-2 tabs (after meals & hs). **Max:** 4 tabs q24h.
Mylicon Infant's Gas Relief Drops	Simethicone 20mg/0.3mL	**Peds: ≥2 yrs (≥24 lbs):** 0.6mL (after meals & hs). **Peds: <2 yrs (<24 lbs):** 0.3mL (after meals & hs). **Max:** 12 doses q24h.

LAXATIVE PRODUCTS

BRAND	INGREDIENT/STRENGTH	DOSE
BULK-FORMING		
Citrucel Caplets	Methylcellulose 500mg	**Adults: ≥12 yrs:** 2 caps qd prn. **Max:** 12 tabs q24h. **Peds: 6-12 yrs:** 1 cap qd prn. **Max:** 6 tabs q24h.
Citrucel Powder	Methylcellulose 2g/tbl	**Adults: ≥12 yrs:** 1 tbl (11.5g) qd tid. **Peds: 6-12 yrs:** ½ tbl (5.75g) qd.
Equalactin Chewable Tablet	Calcium Polycarbophil 625mg	**Adults & Peds: ≥12 yrs:** 2 tabs qd. **Max:** 8 tabs qd. **Peds: 6-12 yrs:** 1 tab qd. **Max:** 2 tabs qd. **2 to <6 yrs:** 1 tab qd. **Max:** 2 tabs qd.
Fibercon Caplets	Calcium Polycarbophil 625mg	**Adults & Peds: ≥12 yrs:** 2 tabs qd. **Max:** 8 tabs qd. **Peds: 6-12 yrs:** 1 tab qd. **Max:** 4 tabs qd. **2 to <6 yrs:** 1 tab qd. **Max:** 2 tabs qd.
Konsyl Easy Mix Powder	Psyllium 6g/tsp	**Adults: ≥12 yrs:** 1 tsp qd-tid. **Peds: 6-12 yrs:** ½ tsp qd-tid.
Konsyl Fiber Caplets	Calcium Polycarbophil 625mg	**Adults & Peds: ≥12 yrs:** 2 tabs qd. **Max:** 8 tabs qd.
Konsyl Orange Powder	Psyllium 3.4g	**Adults: ≥12 yrs:** 1 tsp qd-tid. **Peds: 6-12 yrs:** ½ tsp qd-tid.
Konsyl Original Powder	Psyllium 6g/tsp	**Adults: ≥12 yrs:** 1 tsp qd-tid. **Peds: 6-12 yrs:** ½ tsp qd-tid.
Konsyl-D Powder	Psyllium 3.4g/tsp	**Adults: ≥12 yrs:** 1 tsp qd-tid. **Peds: 6-12 yrs:** ½ tsp qd-tid.
Metamucil Capsules	Psyllium 0.52g	**Adults & Peds: ≥12 yrs:** 5 caps qd-tid.
Metamucil Original Texture Powder	Psyllium 3.4g/tbs	**Adults: ≥12 yrs:** 1 tbs qd-tid. **Peds: 6-12 yrs:** ½ tsp qd-tid.
Metamucil Smooth Texture Powder	Psyllium 3.4g/tbs	**Adults: ≥12 yrs:** 1 tbs qd-tid. **Peds: 6-12 yrs:** ½ tsp qd-tid.
Metamucil Wafers	Psyllium 3.4 g/dose	**Adults: ≥12 yrs:** 2 wafers qd-tid. **Peds: 6-12 yrs:** 1 wafer qd-tid.
HYPEROSMOTICS		
Fleet Children's Babylax Suppositories	Glycerin 2.3g	**Peds: 2-5 yrs:** 1 supp. ud.
Fleet Glycerin Suppositories	Glycerin 2g	**Adults & Peds: ≥6 yrs:** 1 supp ud.
Fleet Liquid Glycerin Suppositories	Glycerin 5.6g	**Adults & Peds: ≥6 yrs:** 1 supp ud.
Fleet Mineral Oil Enema	Mineral Oil 133mL	**Adults: ≥12 yrs:** 1 bottle (133mL). **Peds: 2-12 yrs:** ½ bottle (66.5mL)
HYPEROSMOTIC COMBINATION		
Fleet Pain Relief Pre-Moistened Anorectal Pads	Glycerin/Pramoxine HCl 12%-1%	**Adults & Peds: ≥12 yrs:** Apply to affected area up to five times daily.
OSMOTIC		
MiraLAX	Polyethylene Glycol 3350	**Adults & Peds: ≥17 yrs:** Stir and dissolve 17g in 4-8 oz of beverage and drink qd. Use no more than 7 days.
SALINES		
Ex-Lax Milk of Magnesia Liquid	Magnesium Hydroxide 400mg/5mL	**Adults & Peds: ≥12 yrs:** Take 2-4 tbs hs. **Peds: 6-11 yrs:** 1-2 tbs hs. **2-5 yrs:** 1-3 tbs hs.

(Continued)

BRAND	INGREDIENT/STRENGTH	DOSE
SALINES *(Continued)*		
Fleet Children's Enema	Monobasic Sodium Phosphate/Dibasic Sodium Phosphate 9.5g-3.5g/66mL	**Peds: 5-11 yrs:** 1 bottle (66mL). **2-5 yrs:** ½ bottle (33mL).
Fleet Enema	Monobasic Sodium Phosphate/Dibasic Sodium Phosphate 19g-7g/133mL	**Adults & Peds: ≥12 yrs:** 1 bottle (133mL).
Fleet Phospho-Soda	Monobasic Sodium Phosphate/Dibasic Sodium Phosphate 2.4g-0.9g/5mL	**Adults: ≥12 yrs:** 1 tbl in 8 oz of water. **Max:** 3 tbl. **Peds: 10-11 yrs:** 1 tbl in 8 oz of water. **Max:** 1 tbl. **5-9 yrs:** ½ tbl in 8 oz of water. **Max:** ½ tbl.
Magnesium Citrate Solution	Magnesium Citrate 1.75gm/30mL	**Adults: ≥12 yrs:** 300mL. **Peds: 6-12 yrs:** 90-210mL. **2-6 yrs:** 60-90mL.
Phillips Antacid/Laxative Chewable Tablets	Magnesium Hydroxide 311mg	**Adults: ≥12 yrs:** 6-8 tabs qd. **Peds: 6-11 yrs:** 3-4 tabs qd. **2-5 yrs:** 1-2 tabs qd.
Phillips Soft Chews, Laxative	Magnesium/Sodium 500mg-10 mg	**Adults & Peds: ≥12 yrs:** Take 2-4 tab qd. **Max:** 4 tab q24h.
Phillips Cramp-Free Laxative Caplets	Magnesium 500 mg	**Adults & Peds: ≥12 yrs:** Take 2-4 tabs qd. **Max:** 4 tabs q24h.
Phillips Milk of Magnesia Concentrated Liquid	Magnesium Hydroxide 800mg/5mL	**Adults: ≥12 yrs:** 15-30mL qd. **Peds: 6-11 yrs:** 7.5-15mL qd. **2-5 yrs:** 2.5-7.5mL qd.
Phillips Milk of Magnesia Liquid	Magnesium Hydroxide 400mg/5mL	**Adults: ≥12 yrs:** 30-60mL qd. **Peds: 6-11 yrs:** 15-30mL qd. **2-5 yrs:** 5-15mL qd.
SALINE COMBINATION		
Phillips M-O Liquid	Magnesium Hydroxide/Mineral Oil 300mg-1.25mL/5mL	**Adults: ≥12 yrs:** 30-60mL qd. **Peds: 6-11 yrs:** 5-15mL qd.
STIMULANTS		
Alophen Enteric Coated Stimulant Laxative Pills	Bisacodyl 5mg	**Adults: ≥12 yrs:** Take 1-3 tabs qd. **Peds: 6-12 yrs:** Take 1 tab qd.
Carter's Laxative, Sodium Free Pills	Bisacodyl 5mg	**Adults:** qd.**12 yrs:** Take 1-3 tabs (usually 2 tabs) qd. **Peds: 6-12 yrs:** Take 1 tab qd.
Castor Oil	Castor Oil	**Adults: ≥12 yrs:** 15-60mL. **Peds: 2-12 yrs:** 5-15mL.
Correctol Stimulant Laxative Tablets For Women	Bisacodyl 5mg	**Adults: ≥12 yrs:** Take 1-3 tabs qd. **Peds: 6-12 yrs:** Take 1 tab qd.
Doxidan Capsules	Bisacodyl 5mg	**Adults: ≥12 yrs:** 1-3 caps (usually 2) qd. **Peds: 6-12 yrs:** 1 cap qd.
Dulcolax Overnight Relief Laxative Tablets	Bisacodyl 5mg	**Adults: ≥12 yrs:** 1-3 tabs (usually 2) qd. **Peds: 6-12 yo:** 1 tab qd.
Dulcolax Suppository	Bisacodyl 10mg	**Adults: ≥12 yrs:** 1 supp qd. **Peds: 6-12 yrs:** ½ supp qd.
Dulcolax Tablets	Bisacodyl 5mg	**Adults: ≥12 yrs:** 1-3 tabs (usually 2) qd. **Peds: 6-12 yrs:** 1 tab qd.
Ex-Lax Maximum Strength Tablets	Sennosides 25mg	**Adults: ≥12 yrs:** 2 tabs qd-bid. **Peds: 6-12 yrs:** 1 tab qd-bid.
Ex-Lax Tablets	Sennosides 15mg	**Adults: ≥12 yrs:** 2 tabs qd-bid. **Peds: 6-12 yrs:** 1 tab qd-bid.
Ex-Lax Ultra Stimulant Laxative Tablets	Bisacodyl 5mg	**Adults: ≥12 yrs:** 1-3 tabs qd. **Peds: 6-12 yrs:** 1 tab qd.
Fleet Bisacodyl Suppositories	Bisacodyl 10mg	**Adults: ≥12 yrs:** 1 supp. qd. **Peds: 6-12 yrs:** ½ supp. qd.

(Continued)

BRAND	INGREDIENT/STRENGTH	DOSE
STIMULANTS *(Continued)*		
Fleet Stimulant Laxative Tablets	Bisacodyl 5mg	**Adults:** ≥**12 yrs:** 1-3 tabs (usually 2) qd. **Peds: 6-12 yrs:** 1 tab qd.
Nature's Remedy Caplets	Aloe/Cascara Sagrada 100mg-150mg	**Adults:** ≥**12 yrs:** 2 tabs qd-bid. **Max:** 4 tabs bid. **Peds: 6-12 yrs:** 1 tab qd-bid. **Max:** 2 tabs bid. **2-6 yrs:** ½ tab qd-bid. **Max:** 1 tab bid.
Perdiem Overnight Relief Tablets	Sennosides 15mg	**Adults:** ≥**12 yrs:** 2 tabs qd-bid. **Peds: 6-12 yrs:** 1 tab qd-bid.
Senokot Tablets	Sennosides 8.6mg	**Adults:** ≥**12 yrs:** 2 tabs qd. **Max** 4 tabs bid. **Peds: 6-12 yrs:** 1 tab qd. **Max:** 2 tabs bid. **2-6 yrs:** ½ tab qd. **Max:** 1 tab bid.
STIMULANT COMBINATIONS		
Peri-Colace Tablets	Sennosides/Docusate 8.6mg-50mg	**Adults:** ≥**12 yrs:** 2-4 tabs qd. **Peds: 6-12 yrs:** 1-2 tabs qd. **2-6 yrs:** 1 tab qd.
Senokot S Tablets	Sennosides/Docusate 8.6mg-50mg	**Adults:** ≥**12 yrs:** 2 tabs qd. **Max:** 4 tabs bid. **Peds: 6-12 yrs:** 1 tab qd. **Max:** 2 tabs bid. **2-6 yrs:** ½ tab qd. **Max:** 1 tab bid.
SURFACTANTS (STOOL SOFTENERS)		
Colace Capsules	Docusate Sodium 100mg	**Adults:** ≥**12 yrs:** 1-3 caps qd. **Peds: 2-12 yrs:** 1 cap qd.
Colace Capsules	Docusate Sodium 50mg	**Adults:** ≥**12 yrs:** 1-6 caps qd. **Peds: 2-12 yrs:** 1-3 caps qd.
Colace Liquid	Docusate Sodium 10mg/mL	**Adults:** ≥**12 yrs:** 5-15mL qd-bid. **Peds: 2-12 yrs:** 5-15mL qd.
Colace Syrup	Docusate Sodium 60mg/15mL	**Adults:** ≥**12 yrs:** 15-90mL qd. **Peds: 2-12 yrs:** 5-37.5mL qd.
Correctol Stool Softener Laxative Soft-Gels	Docusate Sodium 100mg	**Adults:** ≥**12 yrs:** Take 2 caps qd. **Peds: 2-12 yrs:** Take 1 cap qd
Docusol Constipation Relief, Mini Enemas	Docusate Sodium 283mg	**Adults:** ≥12 yrs: Take 1-3 units qd. **Peds: 6-12 yrs:** Take 1 unit qd
Dulcolax Stool Softener Capsules	Docusate Sodium 100mg	**Adults:** ≥**12 yrs:** 1-3 caps qd. **Peds: 2-12 yrs:** 1 cap qd.
Ex-Lax Stool Softener Tablets	Docusate Sodium 100mg	**Adults:** ≥**12 yrs:** 1-3 caps qd. **Peds: 2-12 yrs:** 1 cap qd.
Kaopectate Liqui-Gels	Docusate Calcium 240mg	**Adults & Peds:** ≥**12 yrs:** 1 cap qd until normal bowel movement.
Phillips Stool Softener Capsules	Docusate Sodium 100mg	**Adults:** ≥**12 yrs:** 1-3 caps qd. **Peds: 6-12 yrs:** 1 cap qd.
Kaopectate Liqui-Gels	Docusate Calcium 240mg	**Adults & Peds:** ≥**12 yrs:** 1 cap qd until normal bowel movement.
Phillips Stool Softener Capsules	Docusate Sodium 100mg	**Adults:** ≥**12 yrs:** 1-3 caps qd. **Peds: 2-12 yrs:** 1 cap qd.

ALLERGIC RHINITIS PRODUCTS

BRAND	INGREDIENT/STRENGTH	DOSE
ANTIHISTAMINE		
Alavert Oral Disintegrating Tablets	Loratadine 10mg	**Adults & Peds:** ≥6 yrs: 1 tab qd. **Max:** 1 tab q24h.
Alavert 24-Hour Allergy Tablets	Loratadine 10mg	**Adults & Peds:** ≥6 yrs: 1 tab qd. **Max:** 1 tab q24h.
Benadryl Allergy Quick Dissolve Strips	Diphenhydramine HCl 25mg	**Adults & Peds:** ≥12 yrs: Dissolve 1-2 strips on tongue q4-6h. **Max:** 6 doses q24h.
Benadryl Allergy Capsules	Diphenhydramine HCl 25mg	**Adults & Peds:** ≥12 yrs: 1-2 caps q4-6h. **Peds: 6-12 yrs:** 1 cap q4-6h. **Max:** 6 doses q24h.
Benadryl Allergy Chewable Tablets	Diphenhydramine HCl 12.5mg	**Adults & Peds:** ≥12 yrs: 2-4 tabs q4-6h. **Peds: 6-12 yrs:** 1-2 tabs q4-6h. **Max:** 6 doses q24h.
Benadryl Allergy Liquid	Diphenhydramine HCl 12.5mg/5mL	**Adults & Peds:** ≥12 yrs: 2-4 tsp (10-20mL) q4-6h. **Peds: 6-12 yrs:** 1-2 tsp (5-10mL) q4-6h. **Max:** 6 doses q24h.
Benadryl Allergy Ultratab	Diphenhydramine HCl 25mg	**Adults & Peds:** ≥12 yrs: 1-2 tabs q4-6h. **Peds: 6-12 yrs:** 1 tab q4-6h. **Max:** 6 doses q24h.
Benadryl Children's Quick Dissolve Strips	Diphenhydramine HCl 12.5mg	**Adults & Peds:** ≥12 yrs: Dissolve 1 or 2 strips on tongue q4-6h. Allow first strip to dissolve before placing second strip on tongue. **Max:** 6 doses q24h.
Chlor-Trimeton 4-Hour Allergy Tablets	Chlorpheniramine Maleate 4mg	**Adults & Peds:** ≥12 yrs: 1 tab q4-6h. **Max:** 6 tabs q24h. **Peds: 6-12 yrs:** ½ tab q4-6h. **Max:** 3 tabs q24h.
Claritin 24 Hour Allergy Tablets	Loratadine 10mg	**Adults & Peds:** ≥6 yrs: 1 tab qd. **Max:** 1 tab q24h.
Claritin Children's Syrup	Loratadine 5mg/5mL	**Adults & Peds:** ≥6 yrs: 2 tsp qd. **Max:** 2 tsp q24h. **Peds: 2-6 yrs:** 1 tsp qd. **Max:** 1 tsp q24h.
Claritin RediTabs	Loratadine 10mg	**Adults & Peds:** ≥6 yrs: 1 tab qd. **Max:** 1 tab q24h.
Dimetapp ND Children's Allergy Tablets	Loratadine 10mg	**Adults & Peds:** ≥6 yrs: 1 tab qd. **Max:** 1 tab q24h.
Zyrtec Tablets	Cetirizine 10mg	**Adults: 18 yrs-64 yrs & Peds:** ≥6 yrs: 1 tab q24h. **Max:** 1 tab q24h.
Zyrtec Children's Syrup	Cetirizine 5mg/5mL	**Adults** ≥65: 1 tsp q24h. **Peds: 2-6 yrs:** ½ tsp (2.5mL) qd or bid. ≥**6 to 12:** 1 or 2 tsp (5-10mL) qd. **Max: Adults:** ≥**65 & Peds: 2-6 yrs:** 1 tsp (5mL) q24h ≥**6 to 12yrs:** 2 tsp (10mL) qd
Zyrtec Children's Chewables 5mg	Cetirizine 5mg	**Adults & Peds** ≥6 yrs-64 yrs: 1 tab q24h. **Adults** ≥65 yrs: 1 tab q24h. **Max:** 1 tab q24h.
Zyrtec Children's Chewables 10mg	Cetirizine 10mg	**Adults & Peds** ≥6 yrs: 1 tab q24h. **Adults** ≥65 yrs: Ask doctor. **Max:** 1 tab qd
Zyrtec Children's Hive Relief Syrup	Cetirizine 5mg/5mL	**Adults & Peds** ≥6 yrs-64yrs: 1-2 tsp (5-10ml) q24h. **Max:** 2 tsp (10ml) q24h. **Adults** >65: 1 tsp q24h. **Max:** 1 tsp (5ml) q24h.

(Continued)

BRAND	INGREDIENT/STRENGTH	DOSE
ANTIHISTAMINE COMBINATIONS		
Advil Allergy Sinus Caplets	Chlorpheniramine Maleate/ Ibuprofen/Pseudoephedrine 2mg-200mg-30mg	**Adults & Peds: ≥12 yrs:** 1 tab q4-6h. **Max:** 6 tabs q24h.
Alavert D-12 Hour Allergy and Sinus Tablets	Loratadine/Pseudoephedrine Sulfate 5mg-120mg	**Adults & Peds: ≥12 yrs:** 1 tab q12h. **Max:** 2 tabs q24h.
Benadryl Allergy & Sinus Headache Caplets	Diphenhydramine HCl/ Acetaminophen/Phenylephrine HCl/ 12.5mg-325mg-5mg	**Adults & Peds: ≥12 yrs:** 2 caps q4h. **Max:** 12 caps q24h.
Benadryl Severe Allergy & Sinus Headache Caplets	Diphenhydramine HCl/ Acetaminophen/Phenylephrine HCl 25mg-325mg-5mg	**Adults & Peds: ≥12 yrs:** 2 tabs q4h. **Max:** 12 tabs q24h.
Benadryl-D Allergy & Sinus Liquid	Diphenhydramine HCl/ Phenylephrine 12.5mg-5mg/5mL	**Adults & Peds: ≥12 yrs:** 2 tsp q4h. **Peds: 6-12 yrs:** 1 tsp q4h. **Max:** 6 doses q24h.
Claritin-D 12 Hour Allergy & Congestion Tablets	Loratadine/Pseudoephedrine Sulfate 5mg-120mg	**Adults & Peds: ≥12 yrs:** 1 tab q12h. **Max:** 2 tabs q24h.
Claritin-D 24 Hour Allergy & Congestion Tablets	Loratadine/Pseudoephedrine Sulfate 10mg-240mg	**Adults & Peds: ≥12 yrs:** 1 tab q12h. **Max:** 1 tab q24h.
Drixoral Cold & Allergy Sustained Action Tablets	Dexbrompheniramine Maleate/Pseudoephedrine HCl 6mg-120mg	**Adults & Peds: ≥12 yrs:** 1 tabs q12h. **Max:** 2 tabs q24h.
Dimetapp Elixir Cold & Allergy	Brompheniramine/Phenylephrine 1mg-2.5mg/5ml	**Adults & Peds: ≥12 yrs:** 4 tsp (20mL) q4h. **Peds: 6-12 yrs:** 2 tsp (10mL) q4h. **Max:** 6 doses q24h.
Dimetapp Children's Chewable Tablets	Brompheniramine/Phenylephrine 1mg-2.5mg	**Peds: ≥6-12 yrs:** 2 tabs q4h. **Max:** 6 doses q24h
Sudafed Sinus & Allergy Tablets	Chlorpheniramine/ Pseudoephedrine 4mg-60mg	**Adults: ≥12 yrs:** 1 tab q4-6h. **Peds: 6-12 yrs:** 1/2 tab q4h-6h. **Max:** 4 doses q24h.
Tylenol Allergy Complete Multi-Symptom Cool Burst Caplets	Chlorpheniramine Maleate/ Acetaminophen/Phenylephrine HCl 2mg-325mg-5mg	**Adults & Peds: ≥12 yrs:** 2 tabs q4h. **Max:** 12 tabs q24h.
Tylenol Allergy Complete Nighttime Cool Burst Caplets	Diphenhydramine HCl/ Acetaminophen/Phenylephrine HCl 25mg-325mg-5mg	**Adults & Peds: ≥12 yrs:** 2 tabs q4h. **Max:** 12 tabs q24h.
Tylenol Severe Allergy Caplets	Diphenhydramine HCl/ Acetaminophen 12.5mg-500mg	**Adults & Peds: ≥12 yrs:** 2 tabs q4-6h. **Max:** 8 tabs q24h.
TOPICAL NASAL DECONGESTANTS		
4-Way Fast Acting Nasal Decongestant Spray	Phenylephrine HCl 1%	**Adults & Peds: ≥12 yrs:** Instill 2-3 sprays per nostril q4h.
4-Way Mentholated Nasal Decongestant Spray	Phenylephrine HCl 1%	**Adults & Peds: ≥12 yrs:** Instill 2-3 sprays per nostril q4h.
Afrin No Drip Extra Moisturizing Nasal Spray	Oxymetazoline HCl 0.05%	**Adults & Peds: ≥6 yrs:** Instill 2-3 sprays per nostril q10-12h. **Max:** 2 doses q24h.
Afrin No Drip Sinus Nasal Spray	Oxymetazoline HCl 0.05%	**Adults & Peds: ≥6 yrs:** Instill 2-3 sprays per nostril q10-12h. **Max:** 2 doses q24h.
Afrin Original Nasal Spray	Oxymetazoline HCl 0.05%	**Adults & Peds: ≥6 yrs:** Instill 2-3 sprays per nostril q10-12h.
Afrin No Drip Original Pump Mist Nasal Spray	Oxymetazoline HCl 0.05%	**Adults & Peds: ≥6 yrs:** Instill 2-3 sprays per nostril q10-12h. **Max:** 2 doses q24h.
Afrin No Drip All Night 12 Hour Pump Mist	Oxymetazoline HCl 0.05%	**Adults & Peds: ≥6 yrs:** Instill 2-3 sprays per nostril q10-12h.
Benzedrex Inhaler	Propylhexedrine 250mg	**Adults & Peds: ≥6 yrs:** Inhale 2 sprays per nostril q2h

(Continued)

BRAND	INGREDIENT/STRENGTH	DOSE
TOPICAL NASAL DECONGESTANTS *(Continued)*		
Dristan 12 Hour Nasal Spray	Oxymetazoline HCl 0.05%	**Adults & Peds: ≥12 yrs:** Instill 2-3 sprays per nostril q10-12h. **Max:** 2 doses q24h.
Neo-Synephrine 12 Hour Extra Moisturizing Nasal Spray	Oxymetazoline HCl 0.05%	**Adults & Peds: ≥6 yrs:** Instill 2-3 sprays per nostril q10-12h. **Max:** 2 doses per 24 hours.
Neo-Synephrine 12 Hour Nasal Decongestant Spray	Oxymetazoline HCl 0.05%	**Adults & Peds: ≥6 yrs:** Instill 2-3 sprays per nostril q10-12h.
Neo-Synephrine Extra Strength Nasal Decongestant Drops	Phenylephrine HCl 1%	**Adults & Peds: ≥12 yrs:** Instill 2-3 drops per nostril q4h.
Neo-Synephrine Extra Strength Nasal Spray	Phenylephrine HCl 1%	**Adults & Peds: ≥6 yrs:** Instill 2-3 sprays per nostril q4h.
Neo-Synephrine Mild Formula Nasal Spray	Phenylephrine HCl 0.25%	**Adults & Peds: ≥6 yrs:** Instill 2-3 sprays per nostril q4h.
Neo-Synephrine Regular Strength Nasal Decongestant Spray	Phenylephrine HCl 0.5%	**Adults & Peds: ≥12 yrs:** Instill 2-3 sprays per nostril q4h.
Nostrilla 12 Hour Nasal Decongestant	Oxymetazoline HCl 0.05%	**Adults & Peds: ≥6 yrs:** Instill 2-3 sprays per nostril q10-12h. **Max:** 2 doses q24h.
Vicks Sinex 12 Hour Ultra Fine Mist For Sinus Relief	Oxymetazoline HCl 0.05%	**Adults & Peds: ≥6 yrs:** Instill 2-3 sprays per nostril q10-12h. **Max:** 2 doses q24h.
Vicks Sinex Long Acting Nasal Spray For Sinus Relief	Oxymetazoline HCl 0.05%	**Adults & Peds: ≥6 yrs:** Instill 2-3 sprays per nostril q10-12h. **Max:** 2 doses per day.
Vicks Sinex Nasal Spray For Sinus Relief	Phenylephrine HCl 0.5%	**Adults & Peds: ≥12 yrs:** Instill 2-3 sprays per nostril q4h.
Zicam Extreme Congestion Relief	Oxymetazoline HCl 0.05%	**Adults & Peds: ≥6 yrs:** Instill 2-3 sprays per nostril q10-12h. **Max:** 2 doses q24h.
Zicam Intense Sinus Relief	Oxymetazoline HCl 0.05%	**Adults & Peds: ≥12 yrs:** Instill 2-3 sprays per nostril q10-12h. **Max:** 2 doses q24h.
TOPICAL NASAL MOISTURIZERS		
4-Way Saline Moisturizing Mist	Water, Boric Acid, Glycerin, Sodium Chloride, Sodium Borate, Eucalyptol, Menthol, Polysorbate 80, Benzalkonium Chloride	**Adults & Peds: ≥2 yrs:** Instill 2-3 sprays per nostril prn.
Ayr Baby's Saline Nose Spray, Drops	Sodium Chloride 0.65%	**Peds:** Instill 2 to 6 drops in each nostril.
Ayr Saline Nasal Gel With Soothing Aloe	Water, Methyl Gluceth 10, Propylene Glycol, Glycerin, Glyceryl Polymethacrylate, Triethanolamine, Aloe Barbadensis Leaf Juice (Aloe Vera Gel), PEG/PPG 18/18 Dimethicone, Carbomer, Poloxamer 184, Sodium Chloride, Xanthan Gum, Diazolidinyl Urea, Methylparaben, Propylparaben, Glycine Soja Oil (Soybean), Geraniuim Maculatum Oil, Tocopheryl Acetate, Blue 1	**Adults & Peds: ≥12 yrs:** Apply to nostril prn.

(Continued)

BRAND	INGREDIENT/STRENGTH	DOSE
TOPICAL NASAL MOISTURIZERS *(Continued)*		
Ayr Saline Nasal Gel, No-Drip Sinus Spray	Water, Sodium Carbomethyl Starch, Propylene Glycol, Glycerin, Aloe Barbadensis Leaf Juice (Aloe Vera Gel), Sodium Chloride, Cetyl Pyridinium Chloride, Citric Acid, Disodium EDTA, Glycine Soja (Soybean Oil), Tocopheryl Acetate, Benzyl Alcohol, Benzalkonium Chloride, Geranium Maculatum Oil	**Adults & Peds:** ≥12 yrs: Instill 1 spray in each nostril prn.
Ayr Saline Nasal Mist	Sodium Chloride 0.65%	**Adults & Peds:** ≥12 yrs: Instill 2 sprays per nostril prn.
ENTSOL Mist, Buffered Hypertonic Nasal Irrigation Mist	Purified Water, Sodium Chloride, Sodium Phosphate Dibasic Edetate Disodium, Potassium Phosphate Monobasic, Benzalkonium Chloride	**Adults & Peds:** ≥12 yrs: Instill 1-2 sprays per nostril prn.
ENTSOL Single Use, Pre-Filled Nasal Wash Squeeze Bottle	Purified Water, Sodium Chloride, Sodium Phosphate Dibasic, Potassium Phosphate Monobasic	**Adults & Peds:** ≥12 yrs: Use as directed.
ENTSOL Spray, Buffered Hypertonic Saline Nasal Spray	Purified Water, Sodium Chloride Phosphate Dibasic, Potassium Phosphate Monobasic	**Adults & Peds:** ≥12 yrs: Instill 1 spray per nostril bid, 2-6 times daily
ENTSOL Nasal Gel with Aloe and Vitamin E	Water (Purified), Propylene Glycol, Aloe, Glycerin, Dimethicone Copolyol, Poloxamer 184, Methyl Gluceth 10, Triethanolamine, Carbomer, Sodium Chloride, Vitamin E, Disodium EDTA, Xanthan Gum, Benzalkonium Chloride	**Adults & Peds:** Use prn.
Little Noses Saline Spray/Drops, Non-Medicated	Sodium Chloride 0.65%	**Peds:** 2-6 drops or sprays per nostril as directed.
Ocean Premium Saline Nasal Spray	Sodium Chloride 0.65%	**Adults & Peds:** ≥6 yrs: Instill 2 sprays per nostril prn.
Simply Saline Sterile Saline Nasal Mist	Sodium Chloride 0.9%	**Adults & Peds:** ≥12 yrs: Use prn as directed.
SinoFresh Moisturizing Nasal & Sinus Spray	Purified water, Propylene Glycol, Monobasic Sodium Phosphate, Dibasic Sodium Phosphate, Sodium Chloride, Polysorbate 80, Sorbitol Solution, Essential Oil Blend (Wintergreen Oil, Spearmint Oil, Peppermint Oil, Eucalyptus Oil) Cetylpyridinium Chloride, Benzalkonium Chloride	**Adults & Peds:** ≥12 yrs: Instill 1-3 sprays per nostril bid.
MISCELLANEOUS		
NasalCrom Nasal Allergy Symptom Prevention and Controller, Nasal Spray	Cromolyn Sodium 5.2mg	**Adults & Peds:** ≥2 yrs: Instill 1 spray per nostril q4-6h. **Max:** 6 doses q24h.
Similasan Hay Fever Relief, Non-Drowsy Formula, Nasal Spray	Cardiospermum HPUS 6X, Galphimia Glauca HPUS 6X, Luffa Operculata HPUS 6X, Sabadilla HPUS 6x	**Adults & Peds:** Instill 1 to 3 sprays in each nostril prn.
Zicam Allergy Relief, Homeopathic Nasal Solution, Pump	Luffa Operculata 4x, 12x, 30x, Galphimia Glauca 12x, 30x, Histaminum Hydrochloricum 12x, 30x, 200x, Sulphur 12x, 30x, 200x	**Adults & Peds:** ≥6 yrs: Instill 1 spray per nostril q4h.

IS IT A COLD, THE FLU, OR AN ALLERGY?

	COLD	FLU	AIRBORNE ALLERGY
SYMPTOMS			
Chest discomfort	Mild to moderate	Common; can become severe	Sometimes
Cough	Common (hacking cough)	Sometimes	Sometimes
Duration	3-14 days	Days to weeks	Weeks (eg, 6 weeks for ragweed or grass pollen seasons)
Extreme exhaustion	Never	Early and prominent	Never
Fatigue, weakness	Sometimes	Can last up to 2-3 weeks	Sometimes
Fever	Rare	Characteristic, high (100-102°F); lasts 3-4 days	Never
General aches, pains	Slight	Usual; often severe	Never
Headache	Rare	Prominent	Sometimes
Itchy eyes	Rare or never	Rare or never	Common
Runny nose	Common		Common
Sneezing	Usual	Sometimes	Usual
Sore throat	Common	Sometimes	Sometimes
Stuffy nose	Common	Sometimes	Common
TREATMENT*			
	Antihistamines	Amantadine	Antihistamines
	Decongestants	Rimantadine	Nasal steroids
	Nonsteroidal anti-inflammatories	Oseltamivir	Decongestants
		Zanamavir	
PREVENTION			
	Wash your hands often; avoid close contact with anyone with a cold	Annual vaccination Amantadine Rimantadine Oseltamivir	Avoid allergens such as pollen, house flies, dust mites, mold, pet dander, cockroaches
COMPLICATIONS			
	Sinus infection	Bronchitis	Sinus infections
	Middle ear infection	Pneumonia	Asthma
	Asthma	Can be life-threatening	

Adapted from the National Institute of Allergy and Infectious Diseases, September 2005.

*Used only for temporary relief of cold symptoms.

COUGH-COLD-FLU PRODUCTS

BRAND NAME	ANALGESIC	ANTIHISTAMINE	DECONGESTANT	COUGH SUPPRESSANT	EXPECTORANT	DOSE
ANTIHISTAMINE + DECONGESTANT						
Actifed Cold & Allergy Tablets		Chlorpheniramine Maleate 4mg	Phenylephrine HCl 10mg			**Adults:** ≥**12 yrs:** 1 tab q4-6h. **Max:** 6 doses q24h. **Peds: 6-12 yrs:** ½ tab q4-6h. **Max:** 2 tabs q24h.
Benadryl Children's Allergy & Cold Fastmelt Tablets		Diphenhydramine HCl 19mg	Pseudoephedrine HCl 30mg			**Adults:** ≥**12 yrs:** 2 tabs q4h. **Peds: 6-12 yrs:** 1 tab q4h. **Max:** 4 tabs q24h.
Benadryl-D Allergy/Sinus Tablets		Diphenhydramine HCl 25mg	Phenylephrine HCl 10mg			**Adults & Peds:** ≥**12 yrs:** 1 tab q4h. **Max:** 6 tab q24h.
Children's Benadryl-D Allergy & Sinus Liquid		Diphenhydramine HCl 12.5mg/5mL	Phenylephrine HCl 5mg/5mL			**Adults:** ≥**12 yrs:** 2 tsp (10mL) q4h. **Peds: 6-12 yrs:** 1 tsp (5mL) q4h. **Max:** 6 doses q24h.
Dimetapp Children's Cold & Allergy Elixir		Brompheniramine Maleate 1mg/5mL	Phenylephrine HCl 2.5mg/5mL			**Adults & Peds:** ≥**12 yrs:** 2 tabs q4h. **Max:** 8 tabs q24h. **Peds: 6-12 yrs:** 1 tab q4h. **Max:** 6 doses q24h.
Dimetapp Children's Cold & Allergy Chewable Tablets		Brompheniramine Maleate 1mg	Phenylephrine HCl 2.5mg			**Peds: 6-12 yrs:** 2 tabs q4h. **Max:** 6 doses q24h.
Pedicare Children's NightRest Multi-Symptom Cold Liquid		Diphenhydramine HCl 12.5mg/5mL	Phenylephrine HCl 5mg/5mL			**Peds: 6-12 yrs:** 1 tsp (5mL) q4h. **Max:** 6 doses q24h.
Robitussin Night Time Cough & Cold Liquid		Diphenhydramine HCl 6.25mg/5mL	Phenylephrine HCl 2.5mg/5mL			**Adults & Peds:** ≥**12 yrs:** 4 tsp (20mL) q4h. **Peds: 6-12 yrs:** 2 tsp (10mL) q4h. **Max:** 6 doses q24h.
Robitussin Pediatric Night Time Cough & Cold Liquid		Diphenhydramine HCl 6.25mg/5mL	Phenylephrine HCl 2.5mg/5mL			**Adults & Peds:** ≥**12 yrs:** 4 tsp (20mL) q4h. **Peds: 6-12 yrs:** 2 tsp (10mL) q4h. **Max:** 6 doses q24h.
Sudafed Sinus & Allergy Tablets		Chlorpheniramine Maleate 4mg	Pseudoephedrine HCl 60mg			**Adults:** ≥**12 yrs:** 1 tab q4-6h. **Peds: 6-12 yrs:** ½ tab q4-6h. **Max:** 4 doses q24h.
Sudafed Sinus Nighttime Tablets		Triprolidine HCl 2.5mg	Pseudoephedrine HCl 60mg			**Adults & Peds:** ≥**12 yrs:** 1 tab q4-6h. **Peds: 6-12 yrs:** ½ tab q4-6h. **Max:** 4 doses q24h.

BRAND NAME	ANALGESIC	ANTIHISTAMINE	DECONGESTANT	COUGH SUPPRESSANT	EXPECTORANT	DOSE
Theraflu Nighttime Cold & Cough Thin Strips		Diphenhydramine HCl 25mg/strips	Phenylephrine HCl 10mg/strip			**Adults: ≥12 yrs:** 1 strip q4h. **Max:** 6 strips q24h.
Triaminic Cold & Allergy Liquid		Chlorpheniramine Maleate 1mg/5mL	Phenylephrine HCl 2.5mg/5mL			**Peds: 6-12 yrs:** 2 tsp (10mL) q4h. **Max:** 6 doses q24h.
Triaminic Nighttime Cough & Cold Liquid		Diphenhydramine HCl 6.25mg/5mL	Phenylephrine HCl 2.5mg/5mL			**Peds: 6-12 yrs:** 2 tsp (10mL) q4h **Max:** 6 doses q24h.
Triaminic Nighttime Cough & Cold Thin Strips		Diphenhydramine HCl 12.5mg/strip	Phenylephrine HCl 5mg/strip			**Peds: 6-12 yrs:** 1 strip q4h. **Max:** 6 strips q24h.
ANTIHISTAMINE + DECONGESTANT + ANALGESIC						
Actifed Cold & Sinus Caplets	Acetaminophen 500mg	Chlorpheniramine Maleate 2mg	Pseudoephedrine HCl 30mg			**Adults & Peds: ≥12 yrs:** 2 tabs q6h. **Max:** 8 tabs q24h.
Advil Multi-Symptom Cold Caplets	Ibuprofen 200mg	Chlorpheniramine Maleate 2mg	Pseudoephedrine HCl 30mg			**Adults & Peds: ≥12 yrs:** 1 tab q4-6h. **Max:** 6 tabs q24h.
Advil Allergy Sinus Caplets	Ibuprofen 200mg	Chlorpheniramine Maleate 2mg	Pseudoephedrine HCl 30mg			**Adults & Peds: ≥12 yrs:** 1 tab q4-6h. **Max:** 6 tabs q24h.
Advil Allergy Sinus Children's Liquid	Ibuprofen 100mg	Chlorpheniramine Maleate 1mg	Pseudoephedrine HCl 15mg			**Peds: 6-11 yrs (48-95 lbs):** 2 tsp q6h. **Max:** 8 tsp q24h.
Alka-Seltzer Plus Cold Effervescent Tablets	Acetaminophen 325mg	Chlorpheniramine Maleate 2mg	Phenylephrine HCl 5mg			**Adults & Peds: ≥12 yrs:** 2 tabs q4h. **Max:** 8 tabs q24h.
Alka-Seltzer Plus Cold Cherry Burst Formula Effervescent Tablets	Acetaminophen 250mg	Chlorpheniramine Maleate 2mg	Phenylephrine HCl 5mg			**Adults & Peds: ≥12 yrs:** 2 tabs q4h. **Max:** 8 tabs q24h.
Alka-Seltzer Plus Cold Orange Zest Formula Effervescent Tablets	Acetaminophen 250mg	Chlorpheniramine Maleate 2mg	Phenylephrine HCl 5mg			**Adults & Peds: ≥12 yrs:** 2 tabs q4h. **Max:** 8 tabs q24h.
Alka-Seltzer Plus Regular Seltzer Multi-Symptom Cold Relief Effervescent Tablets	Acetaminophen 250mg	Chlorpheniramine Maleate 2mg	Phenylephrine HCl 5mg			**Adults & Peds: ≥12 yrs:** 2 tabs q4h. **Max:** 8 tabs q24h.
Benadryl Allergy & Cold Caplets	Acetaminophen 325mg	Diphenhydramine HCl 12.5mg	Phenylephrine HCl 5mg			**Adults & Peds: ≥12 yrs:** 2 tabs q4h. **Max:** 12 tabs q24h. **Peds: 6-12 yrs:** 1 tab q4h. **Max:** 5 tabs q24h.
Benadryl Allergy & Sinus Headache Caplets	Acetaminophen 325mg	Diphenhydramine HCl 12.5mg	Phenylephrine HCl 5mg			**Adults & Peds: ≥12 yrs:** 2 tabs q4h. **Max:** 12 tabs q24h. **Peds: 6-12 yrs:** 1 tab q4h. **Max:** 5 tabs q24h.

(Continued)

BRAND NAME	ANALGESIC	ANTIHISTAMINE	DECONGESTANT	COUGH SUPPRESSANT	EXPECTORANT	DOSE
ANTIHISTAMINE + DECONGESTANT + ANALGESIC *(Continued)*						
Benadryl Severe Allergy & Sinus Headache Caplets	Acetaminophen 325mg	Diphenhydramine HCl 25mg	Phenylephrine HCl 5mg			**Adults & Peds: ≥12 yrs:** 2 tabs q4h. **Max:** 12 tabs q24h.
Comtrex Day & Night Severe Cold & Sinus Caplets	Acetaminophen 325mg	Chlorpheniramine Maleate 2mg (nighttime dose only)	Phenylephrine HCl 5mg			**Adults & Peds: ≥12 yrs:** *Daytime:* 2 daytime tabs q4h. **Max:** 8 daytime tabs q24h. *Nighttime:* 2 nighttime tabs q24h. **Max:** 4 nighttime tabs q24h.
Contac Cold & Flu Maximum Strength Caplets	Acetaminophen 500mg	Chlorpheniramine Maleate 2mg	Phenylephrine HCl 5mg			**Adults & Peds: ≥12 yrs:** 2 tabs q4-6h **Max:** 8 tabs q24h.
Dristan Cold Multi-Symptom Tablets	Acetaminophen 325mg	Chlorpheniramine Maleate 2mg	Phenylephrine HCl 5mg			**Adults & Peds: ≥12 yrs:** 2 tabs q4h. **Max:** 12 tabs q24h.
Robitussin Cold & Congestion Tablets	Acetaminophen 325mg	Chlorpheniramine Maleate 2mg	Phenylephrine HCl 5mg			**Adults & Peds: ≥12 yrs:** 2 tabs q4h. **Max:** 12 tabs q24h.
Sudafed Sinus PE Nighttime Cold Caplets	Acetaminophen 325mg	Diphenhydramine HCl 25mg	Phenylephrine HCl 5mg			**Adults & Peds: ≥12 yrs:** 2 tabs q4h. **Max:** 12 tabs q24h.
Sudafed PE Nighttime Cold Caplets	Acetaminophen 325mg	Diphenhydramine HCl 12.5mg	Phenylephrine HCl 5mg			**Adults & Peds: ≥12 yrs:** 2 tabs q4h. **Max:** 12 tabs q24h. **Peds: 6-12 yrs:** 1 tab q4h. **Max:** 5 tabs q24h.
Sudafed PE Severe Cold Caplets	Acetaminophen 325mg	Diphenhydramine HCl 12.5mg	Phenylephrine HCl 5mg			**Adults & Peds: ≥12 yrs:** 2 tabs q4h. **Max:** 12 tabs q24h. **Peds: 6-12 yrs:** 1 tab q4h. **Max:** 5 tabs q24h.
Theraflu Cold & Sore Throat Hot Liquid	Acetaminophen 325mg/packet	Pheniramine Maleate 20mg/packet	Phenylephrine HCl 10mg/packet			**Adults & Peds: ≥12 yrs:** 1 packet q4h. **Max:** 6 packets q24h.
Theraflu Nighttime Severe Hot Liquid	Acetaminophen 650mg/packet	Pheniramine Maleate 20mg/packet	Phenylephrine HCl 10mg/packet			**Adults & Peds: ≥12 yrs:** 1 packet q4h. **Max:** 6 packets q24h.
Theraflu Flu & Sore Throat Liquid	Acetaminophen 650mg/packet	Pheniramine Maleate 20mg/packet	Phenylephrine HCl 10mg/packet			**Adults & Peds: ≥12 yrs:** 1 packet q4h. **Max:** 6 packets q24h.
Theraflu Nighttime Warming Relief Syrup	Acetaminophen 325mg/15mL	Diphenhydramine HCl 12.5mg/15mL	Phenylephrine HCl 5mg/15mL			**Adults & Peds: ≥12 yrs:** 2 tbl (30mL) q4h. **Max:** 6 doses (12 tbl) q24h.
Theraflu Flu & Sore Throat Relief Syrup	Acetaminophen 325mg/15mL	Diphenhydramine HCl 12.5mg/15mL	Phenylephrine HCl 5mg/15mL			**Adults & Peds: ≥12 yrs:** 2 tbl (30mL) q4h. **Max:** 6 doses (12 tbl) q24h.
Tylenol Children's Plus Cold Liquid	Acetaminophen 160mg/5mL	Chlorpheniramine Maleate 1mg/5mL	Phenylephrine HCl 2.5mg/5mL			**Peds: 6-11 yrs (48-95 lbs):** 2 tsp (10mL) q4h. **Max:** 5 doses q24h.

BRAND NAME	ANALGESIC	ANTIHISTAMINE	DECONGESTANT	COUGH SUPPRESSANT	EXPECTORANT	DOSE
ANTIHISTAMINE + DECONGESTANT + ANALGESIC *(Continued)*						
Tylenol Children's Plus Cold & Allergy Liquid	Acetaminophen 160mg/5mL	Diphenhydramine HCl 12.5mg/5mL	Phenylephrine HCl 2.5mg/5mL			**Peds: 6-11 yrs (48-95 lbs):** 2 tsp (10mL) q4-6h. **Max:** 4 doses q24h.
Tylenol Children's Plus Cold & Allergy Liquid	Acetaminophen 160mg/5mL	Diphenhydramine HCl 12.5mg/5mL	Pseudoephedrine HCl 15mg/5mL			**Peds: 6-11 yrs (48-95 lbs):** 2 tsp (10mL) q4-6h. **Max:** 4 doses q24h.
Tylenol Sinus Congestion & Pain Nighttime Caplets	Acetaminophen 325mg	Chlorpheniramine Maleate 2mg	Phenylephrine HCl 5mg			**Adults & Peds:** ≥12 yrs: 2 tabs q4h. **Max:** 12 tabs q24h.
Tylenol Allergy Multi-Symptom Caplets	Acetaminophen 325mg	Chlorpheniramine Maleate 2mg	Phenylephrine HCl 5mg			**Adults & Peds:** ≥12 yrs: 2 tabs q4h. **Max:** 12 tabs q24h.
Tylenol Allergy Multi-Symptom Nighttime Caplets	Acetaminophen 325mg	Diphenhydramine HCl 25mg	Phenylephrine HCl 5mg			**Adults & Peds:** ≥12 yrs: 2 tabs q4h. **Max:** 12 tabs q24h.
Vicks NyQuil Sinus Liquicaps	Acetaminophen 325mg	Doxylamine Succinate 6.25 mg	Phenylephrine HCl 5mg			**Adults & Peds:** ≥12 yrs: 2 tabs q4h. **Max:** 6 doses q24h.
COUGH SUPPRESSANT						
Delsym 12 Hour Cough Relief Liquid				Dextromethorphan Polistrex 30mg/5mL		**Adults:** ≥12 yrs: 2 tsp (10mL) q12h. **Max:** 4 doses q24h. **Peds: 6-12 yrs:** 1 tsp (5mL) q12h. **Max:** 2 doses q24h. **2-6 yrs:** ½ tsp (2.5mL) q12h. **Max:** 1 dose q24h.
PediaCare Long-Acting Cough Liquid				Dextromethorphan HBr 7.5mg/5mL		**Peds: 6-12 yrs:** 2 tsp q6-8h. **2-6 yrs:** 1 tsp q6-8h. **Max:** 4 doses q24h.
Robitussin Cough Long-Acting Liquid				Dextromethorphan HBr 15mg/5mL		**Adults & Peds:** ≥12 yrs: 2 tsp (10mL) q6-8h. **Max:** 8 tsp (40mL) q24h.
Robitussin CoughGels Liqui-gels				Dextromethorphan HBr 15mg		**Adults & Peds:** ≥12 yrs: 2 caps q6-8h. **Max:** 8 caps q24h.
Robitussin Pediatric Cough Liquid				Dextromethorphan HBr 7.5mg/5mL		**Adults:** ≥12 yrs (≥96 lbs): 4 tsp (20mL) q6-8h. **Peds: 6-12 yrs (48-95 lbs):** 2 tsp (10mL) q6-8h. **2-6 yrs:** 1 tsp (5mL) q6-8h. **Max:** 4 doses q24h.
Triaminic Long-Acting Cough Liquid				Dextromethorphan HBr 7.5mg/5mL		**Peds: 6-12 yrs:** 2 tsp (10mL) q6-8h. **2-6 yrs:** 1 tsp (5mL) q6-8h. **Max:** 4 doses q24h.

(Continued)

BRAND NAME	ANALGESIC	ANTIHISTAMINE	DECONGESTANT	COUGH SUPPRESSANT	EXPECTORANT	DOSE
COUGH SUPPRESSANT *(Continued)*						
Triaminic Long Acting Cough Thin Strips				Dextromethorphan 5.5mg/strip		**Peds: 6-12 yrs:** 2 strips q6-8h. **Max:** 8 strips q24h.
Vicks DayQuil Cough Liquid				Dextromethorphan HBr 15mg/15mL		**Adults & Peds: ≥12 yrs:** 2 tbl (30mL) q6-8h. **Peds: 6-12 yrs:** 1 tbl (15mL) q6-8h. **Max:** 4 doses q24h.
Vicks 44 Liquid				Dextromethorphan HBr 30mg/15mL		**Adults & Peds: ≥12 yrs:** 1 tbl (15mL) q6-8h. **Peds: 6-12 yrs:** 1.5 tsp (7.5mL) q6-8h. **Max:** 4 doses q24h.
Vicks BabyRub				Eucalyptus, petrolatum, fragrance, aloe extract, eucalyptus oil, lavender oil, rosemary oil		**Peds:** Gently massage on the chest, neck, and back to help soothe and comfort.
Vicks Casero Cough Suppressant/Topical Analgesic				Camphor 4.7%, Menthol 2.6%, Eucalyptus 1.2%		**Adults & Peds: ≥2 yrs:** Apply 3 times q24h.
Vicks Cough Drops Cherry Flavor				Menthol 1.7mg		**Adults & Peds: ≥5 yrs:** 3 drops q1-2h.
Vicks Cough Drops Original Flavor				Menthol 3.3mg		**Adults & Peds: ≥5 yrs:** 2 drops q1-2h.
Vicks VapoRub Cream				Camphor 5.2%, Menthol 2.8%, Eucalyptus 1.2%		**Adults & Peds: ≥2 yrs:** Apply q8h.
Vicks VapoRub Ointment				Camphor 4.8%, Menthol 2.6%, Eucalyptus 1.2%		**Adults & Peds: ≥2 yrs:** Apply q8h.
Vicks VapoSteam				Camphor 6.2%		**Adults & Peds: ≥2 yrs:** 1 tbl/quart q8h.
COUGH SUPPRESSANT + ANTIHISTAMINE						
Coricidin HBP Cough & Cold Tablets		Chlorpheniramine Maleate 4mg		Dextromethorphan HBr 30mg		**Adults & Peds: ≥12 yrs:** 1 tab q6h. **Max:** 4 tabs q24h.
Dimetapp Long-Acting Cold Plus Cough Elixir		Chlorpheniramine Maleate 1mg/5mL		Dextromethorphan HBr 7.5mg/5mL		**Peds: ≥12 yrs:** 4 tsp (20mL) q6h. **6-12 yrs:** 2 tsp (10 mL) q6h. **Max:** 4 doses q24h.

BRAND NAME	ANALGESIC	ANTIHISTAMINE	DECONGESTANT	COUGH SUPPRESSANT	EXPECTORANT	DOSE
COUGH SUPPRESSANT + ANTIHISTAMINES (Continued)						
Robitussin Cough & Cold Long-Acting Liquid		Chlorpheniramine Maleate 2mg/5mL		Dextromethorphan HBr 15mg/5mL		**Adults: ≥12 yrs:** 2 tsp (10mL) q6h. **Max:** 4 doses q24h.
Robitussin Pediatric Cough & Cold Long-Acting Liquid		Chlorpheniramine Maleate 1mg/5mL		Dextromethorphan HBr 7.5mg/5mL		**Adults & Peds: ≥12 yrs:** 4 tsp (20mL) q6h. **Peds: 6-12 yrs:** 2 tsp (10mL) q6h. **Max:** 4 doses q24h.
Triaminic Softchews Cough & Runny Nose		Chlorpheniramine Maleate 1mg		Dextromethorphan HBr 5mg		**Peds: 6-12 yrs:** 2 tabs q4-6h. **Max:** 6 doses q24h.
Vicks Children's NyQuil Liquid		Chlorpheniramine Maleate 2mg/15mL		Dextromethorphan HBr 15mg/15mL		**Adults: ≥12 yrs:** 2 tbl (30mL) q6h. **Peds: 6-11 yrs:** 1 tbl (15mL) q6h. **Max:** 4 doses q24h.
Vicks NyQuil Cough Liquid		Doxylamine Succinate 6.25mg/15mL		Dextromethorphan HBr 15mg/15mL		**Adults & Peds: ≥12 yrs:** 2 tbl (30mL) q6h. **Max:** 8 tbl (120mL) q24h.
Vicks Pediatric Formula 44M Cough & Cold Relief		Chlorpheniramine Maleate 2mg/15mL		Dextromethorphan HBr 15mg/15mL		**Adults & Peds: ≥12 yrs:** 2 tbl (30mL) q6h. **Peds: 6-12 yrs:** 1 tbl (15mL) q6h. **Max:** 4 doses q24h.
COUGH SUPPRESSANT + ANALGESIC						
Triaminic Cough & Sore Throat Liquid	Acetaminophen 160mg/5mL			Dextromethorphan HBr 5mg/5mL		**Peds: 6-12 yrs:** 2 tsp (10mL) q4h. **2-6 yrs:** 1 tsp (5mL) q4h. **Max:** 5 doses q24h.
Triaminic Softchews Cough & Sore Throat Tablets	Acetaminophen 160mg			Dextromethorphan HBr 5mg		**Peds: 6-12 yrs:** 2 tabs q4h. **2-6 yrs:** 1 tab q4h. **Max:** 5 doses q24h.
Tylenol Children's Plus Cough & Sore Throat Liquid	Acetaminophen 160mg/5mL			Dextromethorphan HBr 5mg/5mL		**Peds: 6-11 yrs: (48-95 lbs):** 2 tsp (10mL) q4h. **2-5 yrs (24-47 lbs):** 1 tsp (5mL) q4h. **Max:** 5 doses q24h.
Tylenol Cough & Sore Throat Daytime Liquid	Acetaminophen 1000mg/30mL			Dextromethorphan HBr 30mg/30mL		**Adults & Peds: ≥12 yrs:** 2 tbl (30mL) q6h. **Max:** 8 tbl q24h.
COUGH SUPPRESSANT + ANTIHISTAMINES + ANALGESIC						
Alka-Seltzer Plus Flu Effervescent Tablets	Aspirin 500mg	Chlorpheniramine Maleate 2mg		Dextromethorphan HBr 15mg		**Adults & Peds: ≥12 yrs:** 2 tabs q6h. **Max:** 8 tabs q24h.
Alka-Seltzer Plus Nighttime Liquid Gels	Acetaminophen 325mg	Doxylamine Succinate 6.25mg		Dextromethorphan HBr 15mg		**Adults & Peds: ≥12 yrs:** 2 tabs q6h. **Max:** 12 tabs q24h.

(Continued)

BRAND NAME	ANALGESIC	ANTIHISTAMINE	DECONGESTANT	COUGH SUPPRESSANT	EXPECTORANT	DOSE
COUGH SUPPRESSANT + ANTIHISTAMINES + ANALGESIC *(Continued)*						
Tylenol Children's Plus Cough & Runny Nose Liquid	Acetaminophen 160mg/5mL	Chlorpheniramine Maleate 1mg/5mL		Dextromethorphan HBr 5mg/5mL		**Peds: 6-11 yrs (48-95 lbs):** 2 tsp (10mL) q4h. **Max:** 5 doses q24h.
Coricidin HBP Maximum Strength Flu Tablets	Acetaminophen 500mg	Chlorpheniramine Maleate 2mg		Dextromethorphan HBr 15mg		**Adults & Peds: ≥12 yrs:** 2 tabs q6h. **Max:** 8 tabs q24h.
Triaminic Flu Cough & Fever Liquid	Acetaminophen 160mg/5mL	Chlorpheniramine Maleate 1mg/5mL		Dextromethorphan HBr 7.5mg/5mL		**Peds: 6-12 yrs:** 2 tsp (10mL) q6h. **Max:** 4 doses (20mL) q24h.
Tylenol Nighttime Cough & Sore Throat Cool Burst Liquid	Acetaminophen 1000mg/30mL	Doxylamine 12.5mg/30mL		Dextromethorphan HBr 30mg/30mL		**Adults & Peds: ≥12 yrs:** 2 tbl (30mL) q6h. **Max:** 8 tbl (120mL) q24h.
Vicks 44M Liquid	Acetaminophen 162.5mg/5mL	Chlorpheniramine Maleate 1mg/5mL		Dextromethorphan HBr 7.5mg/5mL		**Adults & Peds: ≥12 yrs:** 4 tsp (20mL) q6h. **Max:** 16 tsp (80mL) q24h.
Vicks NyQuil Liquicaps	Acetaminophen 325mg	Doxylamine Succinate 6.25mg		Dextromethorphan HBr 15mg		**Adults & Peds: ≥12 yrs:** 2 caps q6h. **Max:** 8 caps q24h.
Vicks NyQuil Liquid	Acetaminophen 500mg/15mL	Doxylamine Succinate 6.25mg/15mL		Dextromethorphan HBr 15mg/15mL		**Adults & Peds: ≥12 yrs:** 2 tbl (30mL) q6h. **Max:** 8 tbl (120mL) q24h.
COUGH SUPPRESSANT + ANTIHISTAMINES + ANALGESIC + DECONGESTANT						
Alka-Seltzer Plus Cough & Cold Liquid Gels	Acetaminophen 325mg	Chlorpheniramine Maleate 2mg	Phenylephrine HCl 5mg	Dextromethorphan HBr 10mg		**Adults & Peds: ≥12 yrs:** 2 caps q4h. **Max:** 12 caps q24h.
Alka-Seltzer Plus Effervescent Tablets	Acetaminophen 250mg	Doxylamine Succinate 6.25mg	Phenylephrine HCl 5mg	Dextromethorphan HBr 10mg		**Adults & Peds: ≥12 yrs:** 2 tabs q4h. **Max:** 8 tabs q24h.
Alka-Seltzer Plus Cough & Cold Effervescent Tablets	Acetaminophen 250mg	Chlorpheniramine Maleate 2mg	Phenylephrine HCl 5mg	Dextromethorphan HBr 10mg		**Adults & Peds: ≥12 yrs:** 2 tabs q4h. **Max:** 8 tabs q24h.
Alka-Seltzer Plus Cough & Cold Liquid	Acetaminophen 162.5mg/5mL	Chlorpheniramine Maleate 1mg/5mL	Phenylephrine HCl 2.5mg/5mL	Dextromethorphan HBr 5mg/5mL		**Adults & Peds: ≥12 yrs:** 4 tsp q4h. **Max:** 24 tsp q24h.
Alka-Seltzer Plus Night Cold Liquid	Acetaminophen 162.5mg/5mL	Doxylamine Succinate 3.125/5mL	Phenylephrine HCl 2.5mg/5mL	Dextromethorphan HBr 5mg/5mL		**Adults & Peds: ≥12 yrs:** 4 tsp q4h. **Max:** 24 tsp q24h.
Comtrex Nighttime Cold & Cough Caplets	Acetaminophen 325mg	Chlorpheniramine Maleate 2mg	Phenylephrine HCl 5mg	Dextromethorphan HBr 10mg		**Adults & Peds: ≥12 yrs:** 2 tabs q6h. **Max:** 8 tabs q24h.
Dimetapp Children's Nighttime Flu Liquid	Acetaminophen 160mg/5mL	Chlorpheniramine Maleate 1mg/5mL	Phenylephrine HCl 2.5mg/5mL	Dextromethorphan HBr 5mg/5mL		**Adults: ≥12 yrs:** 4 tsp (20mL) q4h. **Peds: 6-12 yrs:** 2 tsp (10mL) q4h. **Max:** 5 doses q24h.
Robitussin Nighttime Cold Cough & Flu Liquid	Acetaminophen 160mg/5mL	Chlorpheniramine Maleate 1mg/5mL	Phenylephrine HCl 2.5mg/5mL	Dextromethorphan HBr 5mg/5mL		**Adults & Peds: ≥12 yrs:** 4 tsp (20mL) q4h. **Peds: 6-12 yrs:** 2 tsp (10mL) q4h. **Max:** 5 doses q24h.

BRAND NAME	ANALGESIC	ANTIHISTAMINE	DECONGESTANT	COUGH SUPPRESSANT	EXPECTORANT	DOSE
COUGH SUPPRESSANT + ANTIHISTAMINE + ANALGESIC + DECONGESTANT *(Continued)*						
Theraflu Nighttime Severe Cold Caplets	Acetaminophen 325mg	Chlorpheniramine Maleate 2mg	Phenylephrine HCl 5mg	Dextromethorphan HBr 10mg		**Adults & Peds: ≥12 yrs:** 2 tabs q6h. **Max:** 8 tabs q24h.
Tylenol Children's Plus Multisymptom Cold Liquid	Acetaminophen 160mg/5mL	Chlorpheniramine Maleate 1mg/5mL	Phenylephrine HCl 2.5mg/5mL	Dextromethorphan HBr 5mg/5mL		**Peds: 6-11 yrs (48-95 lbs):** 2 tsp (10mL) q4h. **Max:** 5 doses q24h.
Tylenol Children's Plus Flu Liquid	Acetaminophen 160mg/5mL	Chlorpheniramine Maleate 1mg/5mL	Phenylephrine HCl 2.5mg/5mL	Dextromethorphan HBr 5mg/5mL		**Peds: 6-11 yrs (48-95 lbs):** 2 tsp (10mL) q6-8h. **Max:** 4 doses q24h.
Tylenol Children's Plus Flu Liquid	Acetaminophen 160mg/5mL	Chlorpheniramine Maleate 1mg/5mL	Pseudoephedrine HCl 15mg/5mL	Dextromethorphan HBr 7.5mg/5mL		**Peds: 6-11 yrs (48-95 lbs):** 2 tsp (10mL) q6-8h. **Max:** 4 doses q24h.
Tylenol Cold Head Congestion Nighttime Caplets	Acetaminophen 325mg	Chlorpheniramine Maleate 2mg	Phenylephedrine HCl 5mg	Dextromethorphan HBr 10mg		**Adults & Peds: ≥12 yrs:** 2 tabs q4h. **Max:** 12 tabs q24h.
Tylenol Cold Multi-Symptom Nighttime Caplets	Acetaminophen 325mg	Chlorpheniramine Maleate 2mg	Phenylephedrine HCl 5mg	Dextromethorphan HBr 10mg		**Adults & Peds: ≥12 yrs:** 2 tabs q4h. **Max:** 12 tabs q24h.
Tylenol Cold Multi-Symptom Nighttime Liquid	Acetaminophen 325mg/15mL	Doxylamine 6.25mg/30mL	Phenylephedrine HCl 5mg/15mL	Dextromethorphan HBr 10mg/15mL		**Adults & Peds: ≥12 yrs:** 2 tbl (30mL) q4h. **Max:** 12 tbl (180mL) q24h.
Vicks NyQuil D Liquid	Acetaminophen 500mg/15mL	Doxylamine 6.25mg/15mL	Phenylephedrine HCl 30mg/15mL	Dextromethorphan HBr 15mg/15mL		**Adults & Peds: ≥12 yrs:** 2 tbl (30mL) q6h. **Max:** 4 doses q24h.
COUGH SUPPRESSANT + ANTIHISTAMINE + DECONGESTANT						
Dimetapp DM Children's Cold & Cough Elixir		Brompheniramine Maleate 1mg/5mL	Phenylephrine HCl 2.5mg/5mL	Dextromethorphan HBr 5mg/5mL		**Adults: ≥12 yrs:** 4 tsp (20mL) q4h. **Peds: 6-12 yrs:** 2 tsp (10mL) q4h. **Max:** 6 doses q24h.
Robitussin Allergy & Cough Liquid		Chlorpheniramine Maleate 2mg/5mL	Phenylephrine HCl 5mg/5mL	Dextromethorphan HBr 10mg/5mL		**Adults: ≥12 yrs:** 2 tsp (10mL) q4h. **Peds: 6-12 yrs:** 1 tsp (5mL) q4h. **Max:** 6 doses q24h.
Theraflu Cold & Cough Hot Liquid		Pheniramine Maleate 20mg/packet	Phenylephrine HCl 10mg/packet	Dextromethorphan HBr 20mg/packet		**Adults & Peds: ≥12 yrs:** 1 packet q4h. **Max:** 6 packets q24h.
COUGH SUPPRESSANT + DECONGESTANT						
Dimetapp Toddler's Decongestant Plus Cough Drops			Phenylephrine HCl 1.25mg/0.8mL	Dextromethorphan HBr 2.5mg/0.8mL		**Peds: 2-6 yrs:** 1.6mL q4h. **Max:** 6 doses q24h.
PediaCare Children's Multi-Symptom Cold Liquid			Phenylephrine HCl 2.5mg/5mL	Dextromethorphan HBr 5mg/5mL		**Peds: 6-12 yrs:** 2 tsp (10mL) q4h. **2-6 yrs:** 1 tsp (5mL) q4h. **Max:** 6 doses q24h.

(Continued)

COUGH-COLD-FLU PRODUCTS

BRAND NAME	ANALGESIC	ANTIHISTAMINE	DECONGESTANT	COUGH SUPPRESSANT	EXPECTORANT	DOSE
COUGH SUPPRESSANT + DECONGESTANT *(Continued)*						
Sudafed Children's Cold & Cough Liquid			Pseudoephedrine HCl 15mg/5mL	Dextromethorphan HBr 5mg/5mL		**Adults & Peds: ≥12 yrs:** 4 tsp (20mL) q4h. **Peds: 6-12 yrs:** 2 tsp (10mL) q4h. **2-6 yrs:** 1 tsp (5mL) q4h. **Max:** 4 doses q24h.
Theraflu Daytime Cold & Cough Thin Strips			Phenylephrine HCl 10mg/strip	Dextromethorphan HBr 20mg/strip		**Adults & Peds: ≥12 yrs:** 1 strip q4h. **Max:** 6 strips q24h.
Triaminic Daytime Cold & Cough Liquid			Phenylephrine HCl 2.5mg/5mL	Dextromethorphan HBr 5mg/5mL		**Peds: 6-12 yrs:** 2 tsp (10mL) q4h. **2-6 yrs:** 1 tsp (5mL) q4h. **Max:** 6 doses q24h.
Triaminic Daytime Cold & Cough Thin Strips			Phenylephrine HCl 2.5mg/strip	Dextromethorphan HBr 3.67mg/strip		**Peds: 6-12 yrs:** 2 strips q4h. **2-6 yrs:** 1 strip q4h. **Max:** 6 doses q24h.
Vicks 44D Cough & Congestion Relief Liquid			Phenylephrine HCl 10mg/15mL	Dextromethorphan HBr 20mg/15mL		**Adults: ≥12 yrs:** 1 tbl (15mL) q4h. **Peds: 6-12 yrs:** 1.5 tsp (7.5mL) q4h. **Max:** 6 doses q24h.
COUGH SUPPRESSANT + DECONGESTANT + ANALGESIC						
Alka-Seltzer Plus Day Cold Liquid Gels	Acetaminophen 325mg		Phenylephrine HCl 5mg	Dextromethorphan HBr 10mg		**Adults & Peds: ≥12 yrs:** 2 caps q4h. **Max:** 12 caps q24h.
Alka-Seltzer Plus Day & Night Liquid Gels	Acetaminophen 325mg		Phenylephrine HCl 5mg	Dextromethorphan HBr 10mg		**Adults & Peds: ≥12 yrs:** 2 caps q4h. **Max:** 12 caps q24h.
Alka-Seltzer Plus Day & Night Effervescent Tablets	Acetaminophen 250mg		Phenylephrine HCl 5mg	Dextromethorphan HBr 10mg		**Adults & Peds: ≥12 yrs:** 2 tabs q4h. **Max:** 8 tabs q24h.
Alka-Seltzer Plus Day Cold Liquid	Acetaminophen 162.5mg/5mL		Phenylephrine HCl 2.5mg/5mL	Dextromethorphan HBr 5mg/5mL		**Adults & Peds: ≥12 yrs:** 4 tsps q4h. **Max:** 6 doses q24h.
Comtrex Cold & Cough Caplets	Acetaminophen 325mg		Phenylephrine HCl 5mg	Dextromethorphan HBr 10mg		**Adults & Peds: ≥12 yrs:** 2 tabs q4h. **Max:** 12 tabs q24h.
Theraflu Daytime Warming Relief Syrup	Acetaminophen 325mg/15mL		Phenylephrine HCl 5mg/15mL	Dextromethorphan HBr 10mg/15mL		**Adults & Peds: ≥12 yrs:** 2 tbl (30mL) q4h. **Max:** 6 doses (12 tbl) q24h.
Theraflu Daytime Severe Cold Caplets	Acetaminophen 325mg		Phenylephrine HCl 5mg	Dextromethorphan HBr 15mg		**Adults & Peds: ≥12 yrs:** 2 tabs q6h. **Max:** 8 tabs q24h.
Tylenol Cold Head Congestion Daytime Capsules	Acetaminophen 325mg		Phenylephrine HCl 5mg	Dextromethorphan HBr 10mg		**Adults & Peds: ≥12 yrs:** 2 caps q4h. **Max:** 12 caps q24h.
Tylenol Cold Head Congestion Day/Night Pack	Acetaminophen 325mg		Phenylephrine HCl 5mg	Dextromethorphan HBr 10mg		**Adults & Peds: ≥12 yrs:** 2 tabs q4h. **Max:** 12 tabs q24h.

BRAND NAME	ANALGESIC	ANTIHISTAMINE	DECONGESTANT	COUGH SUPPRESSANT	EXPECTORANT	DOSE
COUGH SUPPRESSANT + DECONGESTANT + ANALGESIC *(Continued)*						
Tylenol Cold Multi-Symptom Daytime Capsules	Acetaminophen 325mg		Phenylephrine HCl 5mg	Dextromethorphan HBr 10mg		**Adults & Peds: ≥12 yrs:** 2 caps q4h. **Max:** 12 caps q24h.
Tylenol Cold Multi-Symptom Daytime Cool Burst Liquid	Acetaminophen 325mg/15mL		Phenylephrine HCl 5mg/15mL	Dextromethorphan HBr 10mg/15mL		**Adults & Peds: ≥12 yrs:** 2 tbl (30mL) q4h. **Max:** 6 doses (12 tbl) q24h.
Tylenol Cold Multi-Symptom Day/Night Pack	Acetaminophen 325mg		Phenylephrine HCl 5mg	Dextromethorphan HBr 10mg		**Adults & Peds: ≥12 yrs:** 2 caps q4h. **Max:** 12 caps q24h.
Tylenol Flu Daytime Gelcaps	Acetaminophen 500mg		Pseudoephedrine HCl 30mg	Dextromethorphan HBr 15mg		**Adults & Peds: ≥12 yrs:** 2 caps q6h. **Max:** 8 caps q24h.
Vicks DayQuil Liquicaps	Acetaminophen 325mg		Phenylephrine HCl 5mg	Dextromethorphan HBr 10mg		**Adults & Peds: ≥12 yrs:** 2 caps q4h. **Max:** 6 caps q24h.
Vicks DayQuil Liquid	Acetaminophen 325mg/15mL		Phenylephrine HCl 5mg/15mL	Dextromethorphan HBr 10mg/15mL		**Adults & Peds: ≥12 yrs:** 2 tbl (30mL) q4h. **Max:** 12 tbl (120mL) q24h.
COUGH SUPPRESSANT + DECONGESTANT + EXPECTORANT						
Robitussin CF Liquid			Phenylephrine HCl 5mg/5mL	Dextromethorphan HBr 10mg/5mL	Guaifenesin 100mg/5mL	**Adults: ≥12 yrs:** 2 tsp (10mL) q4h. **Peds: 6-12 yrs:** 1 tsp (5mL) q4h. **2-6 yrs:** ½ tsp (2.5mL) q4h. **Max:** 6 doses q24h.
COUGH SUPPRESSANT + DECONGESTANT + EXPECTORANT + ANALGESIC						
Sudafed Cold & Cough Capsules	Acetaminophen 250mg		Pseudoephedrine HCl 30mg	Dextromethorphan HBr 10mg	Guaifenesin 100mg	**Adults & Peds: ≥12 yrs:** 2 caps q4h. **Max:** 8 caps q24h.
Sudafed PE Cold & Cough Caplets	Acetaminophen 325mg		Phenylephrine HCl 5mg	Dextromethorphan HBr 10mg	Guaifenesin 100mg	**Adults & Peds: ≥12 yrs:** 2 tabs q4h. **Max:** 12 tabs q24h.
Tylenol Cold Multi-Symptom Severe Liquid	Acetaminophen 325mg/15mL		Phenylephrine HCl 5mg/15mL	Dextromethorphan HBr 10mg/15mL	Guaifenesin 200mg/15mL	**Adults & Peds: ≥12 yrs:** 2 tbs q4h. **Max:** 12 tbs q24h.
Tylenol Cold Multi-Symptom Severe Caplets	Acetaminophen 325mg		Phenylephrine HCl 5mg	Dextromethorphan HBr 10mg	Guaifenesin 200mg	**Adults & Peds: ≥12 yrs:** 2 tabs q4h. **Max:** 12 tabs q24h.
Tylenol Cold Head Congestion Severe Caplets	Acetaminophen 325mg		Phenylephrine HCl 5mg	Dextromethorphan HBr 10mg	Guaifenesin 200mg	**Adults & Peds: ≥12 yrs:** 2 tabs q4h. **Max:** 12 tabs q24h.
Tylenol Cold Severe Congestion Daytime Caplets	Acetaminophen 325mg		Pseudoephedrine HCl 30mg	Dextromethorphan HBr 15mg	Guaifenesin 200mg	**Adults & Peds: ≥12 yrs:** 2 tabs q6h. **Max:** 8 tabs q24h.

(Continued)

BRAND NAME	ANALGESIC	ANTIHISTAMINE	DECONGESTANT	COUGH SUPPRESSANT	EXPECTORANT	DOSE
COUGH SUPPRESSANT & EXPECTORANT						
Alka-Seltzer Plus Mucus & Congestion Effervescent Tablets				Dextromethorphan HBr 10mg	Guaifenesin 200mg	**Adults & Peds: ≥12 yrs:** 2 tabs q4h. **Max:** 8 tabs q24h.
Coricidin HBP Chest Congestion & Cough Softgels				Dextromethorphan HBr 10mg	Guaifenesin 200mg	**Adults & Peds: ≥12 yrs:** 1-2 caps q4h. **Max:** 12 caps q24h.
Mucinex DM Extended-Release Tablets				Dextromethorphan HBr 30mg	Guaifenesin 600mg	**Adults & Peds: ≥12 yrs:** 1-2 tabs q12h. **Max:** 4 tabs q24h.
Mucinex Liquid Cherry				Dextromethorphan HBr 5mg	Guaifenesin 100mg	**Peds: 6-12 yrs:** 1-2 tsp q4h. **2-6 yrs:** ½-1 tsp q4h. **Max:** 6 doses q24h.
Robitussin Cough & Congestion Liquid				Dextromethorphan HBr 10mg/5mL	Guaifenesin 200mg/5mL	**Adults: ≥12 yrs:** 2 tsp (10mL) q4h. **Peds: 6-12 yrs:** 1 tsp (5mL) q4h. **2-6 yrs:** ½ tsp (2.5mL) q4h. **Max:** 6 doses q24h.
Robitussin DM Liquid				Dextromethorphan HBr 10mg/5mL	Guaifenesin 100mg/5mL	**Adults: ≥12 yrs:** 2 tsp (10mL) q4h. **Peds: 6-12 yrs:** 1 tsp (5mL) q4h. **2-6 yrs:** ½ tsp (2.5mL) q4h. **Max:** 6 doses q24h.
Robitussin Sugar-Free Cough Liquid				Dextromethorphan HBr 10mg/5mL	Guaifenesin 100mg/5mL	**Adults: ≥12 yrs:** 2 tsp (10mL) q4h. **Peds: 6-12 yrs:** 1 tsp (5mL) q4h. **2-6 yrs:** ½ tsp (2.5mL) q4h. **Max:** 6 doses q24h.
Vicks 44E Liquid				Dextromethorphan HBr 20mg/15mL	Guaifenesin 200mg/15mL	**Adults: ≥12 yrs:** 1 tbl (15mL) q4h. **Peds: 6-12 yrs:** 1.5 tsp (7.5mL) q4h. **Max:** 6 doses q24h.
Vicks 44E Pediatric Liquid				Dextromethorphan HBr 10mg/15mL	Guaifenesin 100mg/15mL	**Adults: ≥12 yrs:** 2 tbl (30mL) q4h. **Peds: 6-12 yrs:** 1 tbl (15mL) q4h. **2-5 yrs:** ½ tbl (7.5mL) q4h. **Max:** 6 doses q24h.
DECONGESTANT						
Contac-D Cold Decongestant Tablets			Phenylephrine HCl 10mg			**Adults & Peds: ≥12 yrs:** 1 tabs q4h. **Max:** 6 tabs q24h.
Dimetapp Toddler's Drops Decongestant			Phenylephrine HCl 1.25mg/0.8mL			**Peds: 2-6 yrs:** 1.6mL q4h. **Max:** 6 doses q24h.

BRAND NAME	ANALGESIC	ANTIHISTAMINE	DECONGESTANT	COUGH SUPPRESSANT	EXPECTORANT	DOSE
DECONGESTANT (Continued)						
PediaCare Children's Decongestant Liquid			Phenylephrine HCl 2.5mg/5mL			**Peds: 6-12 yrs:** 2 tsp (10mL) q4h. **2-6 yrs:** 1 tsp (5mL) q4h. **Max:** 6 doses q24h.
Sudafed 12-Hour Tablets			Pseudoephedrine HCl 120mg			**Adults & Peds: ≥12 yrs:** 1 tab q12h. **Max:** 2 tabs q24h.
Sudafed 24-Hour Tablets			Pseudoephedrine HCl 240mg			**Adults & Peds: ≥12 yrs:** 1 tab q24h. **Max:** 1 tab q24h.
Sudafed Children's Chewable Tablets			Pseudoephedrine HCl 15mg			**Adults: ≥12 yrs:** 4 tabs q4-6h. **Peds: 6-12 yrs:** 2 tabs q4-6h. **2-6 yrs:** 1 tab q4-6h. **Max:** 4 doses q24h.
Sudafed Children's Liquid			Pseudoephedrine HCl 15mg/5mL			**Adults: ≥12 yrs:** 4 tsp (20mL) q4-6h. **Peds: 6-12 yrs:** 2 tsp (10mL) q4-6h. **2-6 yrs:** 1 tsp (5mL) q4-6h. **Max:** 4 doses q24h.
Sudafed PE Tablets			Phenylephrine HCl 10mg			**Adults & Peds: ≥12 yrs:** 1 tab q4h. **Max:** 6 tabs q24h.
Sudafed PE Quick Dissolve Strips			Phenylephrine HCl 10mg			**Adults & Peds: ≥12 yrs:** 1 film q4h. **Max:** 6 films q24h.
Sudafed Nasal Decongestant Tablets			Pseudoephedrine HCl 30mg			**Adults: ≥12 yrs:** 2 tabs q4-6h. **Peds: 6-12 yrs:** 1 tab q4-6h. **Max:** 4 doses q24h.
Triaminic Cold with Stuffy Nose Thin Strips			Phenylephrine HCl 2.5mg/strip			**Peds: 6-12 yrs:** 2 strips q4h. **2-6 yrs:** 1 strip q4h. **Max:** 6 doses q24h.
Vicks Sinex 12-Hour Nasal Spray			Oxymetazoline HCl 0.05%			**Adults & Peds: ≥6 yrs:** 2-3 sprays q10-12h. **Max:** 2 doses q24h.
Vicks Sinex Nasal Spray			Phenylephrine HCl 0.5%			**Adults & Peds: ≥12 yrs:** 2-3 sprays q4h. **Max:** 18 sprays q24h.
Vicks Sinex UltraFine Mist			Phenylephrine HCl 0.5%			**Adults & Peds: ≥12 yrs:** 2-3 sprays q4h. **Max:** 18 sprays q24h.
Vicks Sinex 12-Hour UltraFine Mist			Oxymetazoline HCl 0.05%			**Adults & Peds: ≥6 yrs:** 2-3 sprays q10-12h. **Max:** 2 doses q24h.

(Continued)

BRAND NAME	ANALGESIC	ANTIHISTAMINE	DECONGESTANT	COUGH SUPPRESSANT	EXPECTORANT	DOSE
DECONGESTANT (Continued)						
Vicks Vapor Inhaler			Levmetamfetamine 50mg			**Adults:** ≥12 yrs: 2 inhalations q2h. **Max:** 24 inhalations q24h. **Peds:** 6-12 yrs: 1 inhalation q2h. **Max:** 12 inhalations q24h.
DECONGESTANT + ANALGESIC						
Advil Children's Cold Liquid	Ibuprofen 100mg/5mL		Pseudoephedrine HCl 15mg/5mL			**Peds: 6-11 yrs (48-95 lbs):** 2 tsp (10mL) q6h. **2-5 yrs (24-47 lbs):** 1 tsp (5mL) q6h. **Max:** 4 doses q24h
Advil Cold & Sinus Caplets	Ibuprofen 200mg		Pseudoephedrine HCl 30mg			**Adults & Peds:** ≥12 yrs: 1-2 tabs q4-6h. **Max:** 6 tabs q24h.
Advil Cold & Sinus Liqui-gels	Ibuprofen 200mg		Pseudoephedrine HCl 30mg			**Adults & Peds:** ≥12 yrs: 1-2 caps q4-6h. **Max:** 6 caps q24h.
Alka-Seltzer Plus Cold & Sinus Tablets	Acetaminophen 250mg		Phenylephrine HCl 5mg			**Adults & Peds:** ≥12 yrs: 2 tabs q4h. **Max:** 8 tab q24h.
Alka-Seltzer Plus Sinus Effervescent Tablets	Acetaminophen 250mg		Phenylephrine HCl 5mg			**Adults & Peds:** ≥12 yrs: 2 tabs q4h. **Max:** 8 tab q24h.
Contac Cold & Flu Day & Night Caplets	Acetaminophen 500mg		Phenylephrine HCl 5mg			**Adults & Peds:** ≥12 yrs: 2 tabs q4-6h. **Max:** 8 tabs q24h.
Contac Cold & Flu Non-Drowsy Maximum Strength Caplets	Acetaminophen 500mg		Phenylephrine HCl 5mg			**Adults & Peds:** ≥12 yrs: 2 tabs q4-6h. **Max:** 8 tabs q24h.
Motrin Children's Cold Suspension	Ibuprofen 100mg/5mL		Pseudoephedrine HCl 15mg/5mL			**Peds: 6-12 yrs (48-95 lbs):** 2 tsp (10mL) q6h. **2-6 yrs (24-47 lbs):** 1 tsp (5mL) q6h. **Max:** 4 doses q24h.
Sinutab Sinus Tablets	Acetaminophen 500mg		Phenylephrine HCl 5mg			**Adults & Peds:** ≥12 yrs: 2 tabs q6h. **Max:** 8 tabs q24h.
Sudafed PE Sinus Headache Caplets	Acetaminophen 325mg		Phenylephrine HCl 5mg			**Adults & Peds:** ≥12 yrs: 2 tabs q4h. **Max:** 12 tabs q24h.
Sudafed Sinus & Cold Liquid Capsules	Acetaminophen 325mg		Pseudoephedrine HCl 30mg			**Adults & Peds:** ≥12 yrs: 2 caps q4-6h. **Max:** 8 caps q24h.
Theraflu Daytime Severe Cold Hot Liquid	Acetaminophen 650mg		Phenylephrine HCl 10mg			**Adults & Peds:** ≥12 yrs: 1 packet q4h. **Max:** 6 packets q24h.

BRAND NAME	ANALGESIC	ANTIHISTAMINE	DECONGESTANT	COUGH SUPPRESSANT	EXPECTORANT	DOSE
DECONGESTANT + ANALGESIC *(Continued)*						
Tylenol Sinus Congestion & Pain Daytime Caplets	Acetaminophen 325 mg		Phenylephrine HCl 5mg			**Adults & Peds: ≥12 yrs:** 2 tabs q4h. **Max:** 12 tabs q24h.
Tylenol Sinus Congestion & Pain Daytime Gelcaps	Acetaminophen 325 mg		Phenylephrine HCl 5mg			**Adults & Peds: ≥12 yrs:** 2 caps q4h. **Max:** 12 caps q24h.
Tylenol Sinus Congestion & Pain Daytime Rapid Release Gelcaps	Acetaminophen 325 mg		Phenylephrine HCl 5mg			**Adults & Peds: ≥12 yrs:** 2 caps q4h. **Max:** 12 caps q24h.
Vicks DayQuil Sinus Liquicaps	Acetaminophen 325 mg		Phenylephrine HCl 5mg			**Adults & Peds: ≥12 yrs:** 2 caps q4h. **Max:** 6 caps q24h.
DECONGESTANT + EXPECTORANT						
Dimetapp Children's Cold & Chest Congestion Syrup			Phenylephrine HCl 5mg/5mL		Guaifenesin 100mg/5mL	**Adults: ≥12 yrs:** 2 tsp (10mL) q4h. **Peds: 6-12 yrs:** 1 tsp (5mL) q4h. 2-6 yrs: ½ tsp (2.5mL) 14 h. **Max:** 6 doses q24h.
Mucinex D Extended-Release Tablets			Pseudoephedrine HCl 60mg		Guaifenesin 600mg	**Adults & Peds: ≥12 yrs:** 2 tabs q12h. **Max:** 4 tabs q24h.
Robitussin PE Head & Chest Liquid			Phenylephrine HCl 5mg/5mL		Guaifenesin 100mg/5mL	**Adults: ≥12 yrs:** 2 tsp (10mL) q4h. **Peds: 6-12 yrs:** 1 tsp (5mL) q4h. **Max:** 6 doses q24h.
Sudafed Non-Drying Sinus Liquid Caps			Pseudoephedrine HCl 30mg		Guaifenesin 200mg	**Adults & Peds: ≥12 yrs:** 2 caps q4h. **Max:** 8 caps q24h.
Sudafed PE Non-Drying Sinus Caplets			Phenylephrine HCl 5mg		Guaifenesin 200mg	**Adults & Peds: ≥12 yrs:** 2 tabs q4h. **Max:** 12 tabs q24h.
Triaminic Chest & Nasal Liquid			Phenylephrine HCl 2.5mg/5mL		Guaifenesin 50mg/5mL	**Adults & Peds: ≥12 yrs:** 1 tsp q 4h. **Max:** 6 doses q24h. **Peds: 6-12 yrs:** 2 tsp (10mL), **2-6 yrs:** 1 tsp (5mL).
DECONGESTANT + EXPECTORANT + ANALGESIC						
Tylenol Sinus Congestion & Severe Pain Caplets	Acetaminophen 325 mg		Phenylephrine HCl 5mg		Guaifenesin 200mg	**Adults & Peds: ≥12 yrs:** 2 tabs q4h. **Max:** 12 tabs q24h.

BRAND NAME	ANALGESIC	ANTIHISTAMINE	DECONGESTANT	COUGH SUPPRESSANT	EXPECTORANT	DOSE
EXPECTORANT						
Mucinex Extended-Release Tablets					Guaifenesin 600mg	**Adults & Peds: ≥12 yrs:** 1-2 tabs q12h. **Max:** 4 tabs q24h.
Mucinex Liquid Grape					Guaifenesin 100mg/5mL	**Peds: 6-12 yrs:** 1-2 tsp q4h. **2-6 yrs:** ½-1 tsp q4h. **Max:** 6 doses 24h.
Mucinex Mini-Melts Bubble Gum Packets					Guaifenesin 100mg	**Adults & Peds: ≥12 yrs:** 2-4 packets q4h. **Peds: 6-12 yrs:** 1-2 packets q4h. **2-6 yrs:** 1 packet q4h. **Max:** 6 doses q24h.
Mucinex Mini-Melts Grape Packets					Guaifenesin 50mg	**Peds: 6-12 yrs:** 2-4 packets q4h. **2-6 yrs:** 1-2 packets q4h. **Max:** 6 doses 24h.
Robitussin Chest Congestion Liquid					Guaifenesin 100mg/5mL	**Adults: ≥12 yrs:** 2-4 tsp (10-20mL) q4h. **Peds: 6-12 yrs:** 1-2 tsp (5-10mL) q4h. **2-6 yrs:** ½-1 tsp (2.5-5mL) q4h. **Max:** 6 doses q24h.
Vicks Casero Chest Congestion Relief Liquid					Guaifenesin 100mg/6.25mL	**Adults & Peds: ≥12 yrs:** 2.5 tsp (12.5mL) q4h. **Peds: 6-12 yrs:** 1.25 tsp (6.25mL) q4h. **2-6 yrs:** 3.12mL q4h. **Max:** 6 doses q24h.
EXPECTORANT + ANALGESIC						
Comtrex Deep Chest Cold Caplets	Acetaminophen 325mg				Guaifenesin 200mg	**Adults & Peds: ≥12 yrs:** 2 tabs q4-6h. **Max:** 12 tabs q24h.
Tylenol Chest Congestion Caplets	Acetaminophen 325mg				Guaifenesin 200mg	**Adults & Peds: ≥12 yrs:** 2 tabs q4-6h. **Max:** 12 tabs q24h.

BRAND NAME	ANALGESIC	ANTIHISTAMINE	DECONGESTANT	COUGH SUPPRESSANT	EXPECTORANT	DOSE
EXPECTORANT + ANALGESIC *(Continued)*						
Tylenol Chest Congestion Liquid	Acetaminophen 500mg/15mL				Guaifenesin 200mg/15mL	**Adults & Peds:** ≥**12 yrs:** 2 tbl (30mL) q4-6h. **Max:** 8 tbl (120mL) q24h.
Theraflu Flu & Chest Liquid	Acetaminophen 1000mg/packet				Guaifenesin 400mg/packet	**Adults & Peds:** ≥**12 yrs:** 1 packet q6h. **Max:** 4 packets q24h.
EXPECTORANT + DECONGESTANT + COUGH SUPPRESSANT						
Robitussin Cold & Cough CF Liquid			Phenylephrine HCl 5mg/5mL	Dextromethorphan HBr 10mg/5mL	Guaifenesin 100mg/5mL	**Adults & Peds:** ≥**12 yrs:** 2 tsp (10mL) q4h. **Peds: 6-12 yrs:** 1 tsp (5mL) q4h. **2-6 yrs:** ½ tsp (2.5mL) q4h. **Max:** 6 doses q24h.
Robitussin Pediatric Cold & Cough CF Liquid			Phenylephrine HCl 2.5mg/5mL	Dextromethorphan HBr 5mg/2.5mL	Guaifenesin 100mg/2.5mL	**Peds: 2-6 yrs:** 2.5mL q4h. **Max:** 6 doses q24h.
EXPECTORANT + DECONGESTANT + ANALGESIC						
Tylenol Sinus Congestion & Severe Pain Caplets	Acetaminophen 325mg		Phenylephrine HCl 5mg		Guaifenesin 200mg	**Adults & Peds:** ≥**12 yrs:** 2 tabs q4h. **Max:** 12 tabs q24h.
Tylenol Sinus Severe Congestion Daytime Caplets	Acetaminophen 325mg		Pseudoephedrine HCl 30mg		Guaifenesin 200mg	**Adults & Peds:** ≥**12 yrs:** 2 tabs q6h. **Max:** 8 tabs q24h.
ANTIHISTAMINE + ANALGESIC						
Coricidin Cold & Flu Tablets	Acetaminophen 325mg	Chlorpheniramine Maleate 2mg				**Adults & Peds:** ≥**12 yrs:** 2 tabs q4-6h. **Max:** 12 tabs q24h.
Tylenol Sore Throat Nighttime Liquid	Acetaminophen 1000mg/30mL	Diphenhydramine HCl 50mg/30mL				**Adults & Peds:** ≥**12 yrs:** 2 tbl (30mL) q4-6h. **Max:** 8 tbl (120mL) q24h.

NASAL DECONGESTANT/MOISTURIZING PRODUCTS

BRAND	INGREDIENT/STRENGTH	DOSE
PSEUDOEPHEDRINE		
Sudafed 12 Hour Tablets	Pseudoephedrine HCl 120mg	**Adults & Peds:** ≥**12 yrs:** 1 tab q12h. **Max:** 2 tabs/day.
Sudafed 24 Hour Tablets	Pseudoephedrine HCl 240mg	**Adults & Peds:** ≥**12 yrs:** 1 tab q24h. **Max:** 1 tab/day.
Sudafed Children's Nasal Decongestant Chewable Tablets	Pseudoephedrine HCl 15mg	**Peds: 6-12 yrs:** 2 tabs q4-6h. **Max:** 4 doses/day.
Sudafed Children's Nasal Decongestant Liquid	Pseudoephedrine HCl 15mg/5mL	**Adults:** ≥**12 yrs:** 4 tsp (20mL) q4-6h. **Peds: 6-12 yrs:** 2 tsp (10mL) q4h. **2-6 yrs:** 1 tsp (5mL) q4-6h. **Max:** 4 doses/day.
Sudafed Nasal Decongestant Tablets	Pseudoephedrine HCl 30mg	**Adults:** ≥**12 yrs:** 2 tabs q4-6h. **Peds: 6-12 yrs:** 1 tab q4-6h. **Max:** 4 doses/day.
PHENYLEPHRINE		
Pediacare Children's Decongestant Liquid	Phenylephrine 2.5/5mL	**Peds: 6-12 yrs:** 2 tsp (10mL) q4h. **2-6 yrs:** 1 tsp (5mL) q4-6h. **Max:** 4 doses/day.
Sudafed PE	Phenylephrine 10mg	**Adults & Peds:** ≥**12 yrs:** 1 tablet every 4 hours. **Max:** 6 tabs per day.
Sudafed PE Quick Dissolve Strips	Phenylephrine 10mg	**Adults & Peds:** ≥**12 yrs:** Dissolve 1 strip on tongue every 4 hours. **Max:** 6 doses per day.
TOPICAL NASAL DECONGESTANTS		
4-Way Fast Acting Nasal Decongestant Spray	Phenylephrine HCl 1%	**Adults & Peds:** ≥**12 yrs:** Instill 2-3 sprays per nostril q4h.
4-Way Mentholated Nasal Decongestant Spray	Phenylephrine HCl 1%	**Adults & Peds:** ≥**12 yrs:** Instill 2-3 sprays per nostril q4h.
4-Way No Drip Nasal Decongestant Spray	Oxymetazoline HCl 0.05%	**Adults & Peds:** ≥**6 yrs:** Instill 2-3 sprays per nostril q10-12h.
Afrin No Drip Extra Moisturizing Nasal Spray	Oxymetazoline HCl 0.05%	**Adults & Peds:** ≥**6 yrs:** Instill 2-3 sprays per nostril q10-12h. **Max:** 2 doses q24h.
Afrin No Drip Sinus Nasal Spray	Oxymetazoline HCl 0.05%	**Adults & Peds:** ≥**6 yrs:** Instill 2-3 sprays per nostril q10-12h.
Afrin Original Nasal Spray	Oxymetazoline HCl 0.05%	**Adults & Peds:** ≥**6 yrs:** Instill 2-3 sprays per nostril q10-12h.
Afrin No-Drip Original Pump Mist Nasal Spray	Oxymetazoline HCl 0.05%	**Adults & Peds:** ≥**6 yrs:** Instill 2-3 sprays per nostril q10-12h.
Afrin No Drip Severe Congestion Nasal Spray	Oxymetazoline HCl 0.05%	**Adults & Peds:** ≥**6 yrs:** Instill 2-3 sprays per nostril q10-12h.
Afrin No Drip All Night 12 Hour Pump Mist	Oxymetazoline HCl 0.05%	**Adults & Peds:** ≥**6 yrs:** Instill 2-3 sprays per nostril q10-12h.
Benzedrex Inhaler	Propylhexedrine 250 mg	**Adults & Peds:** ≥**6 yrs:** Inhale 2 sprays per nostril q2h.
Dristan 12 Hour Nasal Spray	Oxymetazoline HCl 0.05%	**Adults & Peds:** ≥**6 yrs:** Instill 2-3 sprays per nostril q10-12h. **Max:** 2 doses q24h.
Neo-Synephrine 12 Hour Extra Moisturizing Nasal Spray	Oxymetazoline HCl 0.05%	**Adults & Peds:** ≥**6 yrs:** Instill 2-3 sprays per nostril q10-12h. **Max:** 2 doses q24h.
Neo-Synephrine 12 Hour Nasal Decongestant Spray	Oxymetazoline HCl 0.05%	**Adults & Peds:** ≥**6 yrs:** Instill 2-3 sprays per nostril q10-12h.
Neo-Synephrine Extra Strength Nasal Decongestant Drops	Phenylephrine HCl 1%	**Adults & Peds:** ≥**12 yrs:** Instill 2-3 drops per nostril q4h.
Neo-Synephrine Extra Strength Nasal Spray	Phenylephrine HCl 1%	**Adults & Peds:** ≥**6 yrs:** Instill 2-3 sprays per nostril q4h.
Neo-Synephrine Mild Formula Nasal Spray	Phenylephrine HCl 0.25%	**Adults & Peds:** ≥**6 yrs:** Instill 2-3 sprays per nostril q4h.

(Continued)

BRAND	INGREDIENT/STRENGTH	DOSE
TOPICAL NASAL DECONGESTANTS *(Continued)*		
Neo-Synephrine Regular Strength Nasal Decongestant Spray	Phenylephrine HCl 0.5%	**Adults & Peds: ≥12 yrs:** Instill 2-3 sprays per nostril q4h.
Nostrilla 12 Hour Nasal Decongestant	Oxymetazoline HCl 0.05%	**Adults & Peds: ≥6 yrs:** Instill 2-3 sprays per nostril q10-12h. **Max:** 2 doses q24h.
Vicks Sinex 12 Hour Ultra Fine Mist For Sinus Relief	Oxymetazoline HCl 0.05%	**Adults & Peds: ≥12 yrs:** Instill 2-3 sprays per nostril q10-12h.
Vicks Sinex Long Acting Nasal Spray For Sinus Relief	Oxymetazoline HCl 0.05%	**Adults & Peds: ≥12 yrs:** Instill 2-3 sprays per nostril q10-12h. **Max:** 2 doses q24h.
Vicks Sinex Nasal Spray For Sinus Relief	Phenylephrine HCl 0.5%	**Adults & Peds: ≥12 yrs:** Instill 2-3 sprays per nostril q4h.
Zicam Extreme Congestion Relief	Oxymetazoline HCl 0.05%	**Adults & Peds: ≥12 yrs:** Instill 2-3 sprays per nostril q10-12h. **Max:** 2 doses q24h.
Zicam Intense Sinus Relief	Oxymetazoline HCl 0.05%	**Adults & Peds: ≥12 yrs:** Instill 2-3 sprays per nostril q10-12h. **Max:** 2 doses q24h.
TOPICAL NASAL MOISTURIZERS		
4-Way Saline Moisturizing Mist	Water, Boric Acid, Glycerin, Sodium Chloride, Sodium Borate, Eucalyptol, Menthol, Polysorbate 80, Benzalkonium Chloride	**Adults & Peds: ≥2 yrs:** Instill 2-3 sprays per nostril prn.
Ayr Baby's Saline Nose Spray, Drops	Sodium Chloride 0.65%	**Peds:** Instill 2 to 6 drops in each nostril.
Ayr Saline Nasal Gel With Soothing Aloe	Water, Methyl Gluceth 10, Propylene Glycol, Glycerin, Glyceryl Polymethacry-late, Triethanolamine, Aloe Barbadensis Leaf Juice (Aloe Vera Gel), PEG/PPG 18/18 Dimethicone, Carbomer, Poloxamer 184, Sodium Chloride, Xanthan Gum, Diazolidinyl Urea, Methylparaben, Propyl-paraben, Glycine Soja Oil (Soybean), Geranium Maculatum Oil, Tocopheryl Acetate, Blue 1	**Adults & Peds:** Apply to nostril prn.
Ayr Saline Nasal Gel, No-Drip Sinus Spray	Water, Sodium Carbomethyl Starch, Propylene Glycol, Glycerin, Aloe Barbadensis Leaf Juice (Aloe Vera Gel), Sodium Chloride, Cetyl Pyridinium Chloride, Citric Acid, Disodium EDTA, Glycine Soja (Soybean Oil), Tocopheryl Acetate, Benzyl Alcohol, Benzalkonium Chloride, Geranium Maculatum Oil	**Adults & Peds: ≥12 yrs:** Instill 1 spray in each nostril as directed.
Ayr Saline Nasal Mist	Sodium Chloride 0.65%	**Adults & Peds: ≥12 yrs:** Instill 2 sprays per nostril prn.
ENTSOL Mist, Buffered Hypertonic Nasal Irrigation Mist	Purified Water, Sodium Chloride, Sodium Phosphate Dibasic Edetate Disodium, Potassium Phosphate Monobasic, Benzalkonium Chloride	**Adults & Peds:** Instill 1-2 sprays per nostril prn.
ENTSOL Single Use, Pre-Filled Nasal Wash Squeeze Bottle	Purified Water, Sodium Chloride, Sodium Phosphate Dibasic, Potassium Phosphate Monobasic	**Adults & Peds: ≥12 yrs:** Use as directed.
ENTSOL Spray, Buffered Hypertonic Saline Nasal Spray	Purified Water, Sodium Chloride Phosphate Dibasic, Potassium Phosphate Monobasic	**Adults & Peds: ≥12 yrs:** Instill 1 spray per nostril bid, 6 times daily
ENTSOL Nasal Gel with Aloe and Vitamin E	Water (Purified), Propylene Glycol, Aloe, Glycerin, Dimethicone Copolyol, Poloxamer 184, Methyl Gluceth 10, Triethanolamine, Carbomer, Sodium Chlor-ide, Vitamin E, Disodium EDTA, Xanthan Gum, Benzalkonium Chloride	**Adults & Peds:** Use prn.

(Continued)

BRAND	INGREDIENT/STRENGTH	DOSE
TOPICAL NASAL MOISTURIZERS *(Continued)*		
Little Noses Saline Spray/Drops, Non-Medicated	Sodium Chloride 0.65%	**Peds:** 2-6 drops per nostril as directed.
Ocean Premium Saline Nasal Spray	Sodium Chloride 0.65%	**Adults & Peds:** ≥**6 yrs:** Instill 2 sprays per nostril prn.
Simply Saline Sterile Saline Nasal Mist	Sodium Chloride 0.9%	**Adults & Peds:** ≥**12 yrs:** Use prn as directed.
SinoFresh Moisturizing Nasal & Sinus Spray	Purified Water, Propylene Glycol, Monobasic Sodium Phosphate, Dibasic Sodium Phosphate, Sodium Chloride, Polysorbate 80, Sorbitol Solution, Essential Oil Blend (Wintergreen Oil, Spearmint Oil, Peppermint Oil, Eucalyptus Oil) Cetylpyridinium Chloride, Benzalkonium Chloride	**Adults & Peds:** ≥**12 yrs:** Instill 1-3 sprays per nostril bid.

ANALGESIC PRODUCTS

BRAND	INGREDIENT/STRENGTH	DOSE
ACETAMINOPHEN		
Anacin Extra Strength Aspirin Free Tablets	Acetaminophen 500mg	**Adults & Peds:** ≥**12 yrs:** 2 tabs q6h. **Max:** 8 tabs q24h.
Feverall Childrens' Suppositories	Acetaminophen 120mg	**Peds: 3-6 yrs:** 1-2 Supp. q4-6h. **Max:** 6 supp. q24h.
Feverall Infants' Suppositories	Acetaminophen 80mg	**Peds: 3-11 months:** 1 supp. q6h. **12-36 months:** 1 supp. q4h. **Max:** 6 supp. q24h.
Feverall Jr. Strength Suppositories	Acetaminophen 325mg	**Peds: 6-12 yrs:** 1 supp. q4-6h. **Max:** 6 supp. q24h.
Tylenol 8 Hour Caplets	Acetaminophen 650mg	**Adults & Peds:** ≥**12 yrs:** 2 tabs q8h prn. **Max:** 6 tabs q24h.
Tylenol 8 Hour Geltabs	Acetaminophen 650mg	**Adults & Peds:** ≥**12 yrs:** 2 tabs q8h prn. **Max:** 6 tabs q24h.
Tylenol Arthritis Caplets	Acetaminophen 650mg	**Adults:** 2 tabs q8h prn. **Max:** 6 tabs q24h.
Tylenol Arthritis Geltabs	Acetaminophen 650mg	**Adults:** 2 tabs q8h prn. **Max:** 6 tabs q24h.
Tylenol Children's Meltaways Tablets	Acetaminophen 80mg	**Peds: 2-3 yrs (24-35 lbs):** 2 tabs **4-5 yrs (36-47 lbs):** 3 tabs. **6-8 yrs (48-59 lbs):** 4 tabs. **9-10 yrs (60-71 lbs):** 5 tabs. **11 yrs (72-95 lbs):** 6 tabs. May repeat q4h. **Max:** 5 doses q24h.
Tylenol Children's Suspension	Acetaminophen 160mg/5mL	**Peds: 2-3 yrs (24-35 lbs):** 1 tsp (5mL). **4-5 yrs (36-47 lbs):** 1.5 tsp (7.5mL). **6-8 yrs (48-59 lbs):** 2 tsp (10mL). **9-10 yrs (60-71 lbs):** 2.5 tsp (12.5mL). **11 yrs (72-95 lbs):** 3 tsp (15mL). May repeat q4h. **Max:** 5 doses q24h.
Tylenol Extra Strength Caplets	Acetaminophen 500mg	**Adults & Peds:** ≥**12 yrs:** 2 tabs q4-6h prn. **Max:** 8 tabs q24h.
Tylenol Extra Strength Cool Caplets	Acetaminophen 500mg	**Adults & Peds:** ≥**12 yrs:** 2 tabs q4-6h prn. **Max:** 8 tabs q24h.
Tylenol Extra Strength Gelcaps	Acetaminophen 500mg	**Adults & Peds:** ≥ **12 yrs:** 2 caps q4-6h prn. **Max:** 8 caps q24h.
Tylenol Rapid Blast Liquid	Acetaminophen 500mg/15mL	**Adults & Peds:** ≥**12 yrs:** 2 tbl (30mL) q4-6h prn. **Max:** 8 tbl (120mL) q24h.
Tylenol Extra Strength EZ Tablets	Acetaminophen 500mg	**Adults & Peds:** ≥**12 yrs:** 2 tabs q4-6h prn. **Max:** 8 tabs q24h.
Tylenol Extra Strength Go Tablets	Acetaminophen 500mg	**Adults & Peds:** ≥**12 yrs:** 2 tabs q4-6h prn. **Max:** 8 tabs q24h.
Tylenol Infants' Suspension	Acetaminophen 80mg/0.8mL	**Peds: 2-3 yrs (24-35 lbs):** 1.6 mL q4h prn. **Max:** 5 doses (8mL) q24h.
Tylenol Junior Meltaways Tablets	Acetaminophen 160mg	**Peds: 6-8 yrs (48-59 lbs):** 2 tabs. **9-10 yrs (60-71 lbs):** 2.5 tabs. **11 yrs (72-95 lbs):** 3 tabs. **12 yrs (≥96 lbs):** 4 tabs. May repeat q4h. **Max:** 5 doses q24h.
Tylenol Regular Strength Tablets	Acetaminophen 325mg	**Adults & Peds:** ≥**12 yrs:** 2 tabs q4-6h prn. **Max:** 12 tabs q24h. **Peds: 6-11 yrs:** 1 tab q4-6h. **Max:** 5 tabs q24h.
ACETAMINOPHEN COMBINATIONS		
Anacin Advanced Headache Tablets	Acetaminophen/Aspirin/Caffeine 250mg-250mg-65mg	**Adults & Peds:** ≥**12 yrs:** 2 tabs q6h. Max: 8 tabs q24h.

(Continued)

BRAND	INGREDIENT/STRENGTH	DOSE
ACETAMINOPHEN COMBINATIONS *(Continued)*		
Excedrin Back & Body Caplets	Acetaminophen/Aspirin Buffered 250mg-250mg	**Adults & Peds:** ≥**12 yrs:** 2 tabs q6h **Max:** 8 tabs q24h.
Excedrin Extra Strength Caplets	Acetaminophen/Aspirin/Caffeine 250mg-250mg-65mg	**Adults & Peds:** ≥**12 yrs:** 2 tabs q6h. **Max:** 8 tabs q24h.
Excedrin Extra Strength Geltabs	Acetaminophen/Aspirin/Caffeine 250mg-250mg-65mg	**Adults & Peds:** ≥**12 yrs:** 2 tabs q6h. **Max:** 8 tabs q24h.
Excedrin Extra Strength Tablets	Acetaminophen/Aspirin/Caffeine 250mg-250mg-65mg	**Adults & Peds:** ≥**12 yrs:** 2 tabs q6h. **Max:** 8 tabs q24h.
Excedrin Migraine Caplets	Acetaminophen/Aspirin/Caffeine 250mg-250mg-65mg	**Adults:** 2 tabs prn. **Max:** 2 tabs q24h.
Excedrin Migraine Geltabs	Acetaminophen/Aspirin/Caffeine 250mg-250mg-65mg	**Adults:** 2 tabs prn. **Max:** 2 tabs q24h.
Excedrin Migraine Tablets	Acetaminophen/Aspirin/Caffeine 250mg-250mg-65mg	**Adults:** 2 tabs prn. **Max:** 2 tabs q24h.
Excedrin Sinus Headache Caplets	Acetaminophen/Phenylephrine HCl 325mg-5mg	**Adults & Peds:** ≥**12 yrs:** 2 tabs q4h. **Max:** 12 tabs q24h.
Excedrin Sinus Headache Tablets	Acetaminophen/Phenylephrine HCl 325mg-5mg	**Adults & Peds:** ≥**12 yrs:** 2 tabs q4h. **Max:** 12 tabs q24h.
Excedrin Tension Headache Caplets	Acetaminophen/Caffeine 500mg-65mg	**Adults & Peds:** ≥**12 yrs:** 2 tabs q6h. **Max:** 8 tabs q24h.
Excedrin Tension Headache Geltabs	Acetaminophen/Caffeine 500mg-65mg	**Adults & Peds:** ≥**12 yrs:** 2 tabs q6h. **Max:** 8 tabs q24h.
Excedrin Tension Headache Tablets	Acetaminophen/Caffeine 500mg-65mg	**Adults & Peds:** ≥**12 yrs:** 2 tabs q6h. **Max:** 8 tabs q24h.
Goody's Extra Strength Headache Powders	Acetaminophen/Aspirin/Caffeine 260mg-520mg-32.5mg	**Adults & Peds:** ≥**12 yrs:** 1 powder q4-6h. **Max:** 4 powders q24h.
Midol Menstrual Headache Caplets	Acetaminophen/Caffeine 500mg-65g	**Adults & Peds:** ≥**12 yrs:** 2 tabs q6h. **Max:** 8 tabs q24h.
Midol Menstrual Complete Caplets	Acetaminophen/Caffeine/Pyrilamine Maleate 500mg-60mg-15mg	**Adults & Peds:** ≥**12 yrs:** 2 tabs q6h. **Max:** 8 tabs q24h.
Midol Menstrual Complete Gelcaps	Acetaminophen/Caffeine/Pyrilamine Maleate 500mg-60mg-15mg	**Adults & Peds:** ≥**12 yrs:** 2 tabs q6h. **Max:** 8 tabs q24h.
Midol Teen Formula Caplets	Acetaminophen/Pamabrom 500mg-25mg	**Adults & Peds:** ≥**12 yrs:** 2 tabs q6h. **Max:** 8 tabs q24h.
Pamprin Multi-Symptom Caplets	Acetaminophen/Pamabrom/Pyrilamine 500mg-25mg-15mg	**Adults & Peds:** ≥**12 yrs:** 2 tabs q4-6h. **Max:** 8 tabs q24h.
Premsyn PMS Caplets	Acetaminophen/Pamabrom/Pyrilamine 500mg-25mg-15mg	**Adults & Peds:** ≥**12 yrs:** 2 tabs q4-6h. **Max:** 8 tabs q24h.
Tylenol Women's Menstrual Relief	Acetaminophen/Pamabrom 500mg-25mg	**Adults & Peds:** ≥**12 yrs:** 2 tabs q4-6h. **Max:** 8 tabs q24h.
Vanquish Caplets	Acetaminophen/Aspirin/Caffeine 194mg-227mg-33mg	**Adults & Peds:** ≥**12 yrs:** 2 tabs q6h. **Max:** 8 tabs q24h.
ACETAMINOPHEN/SLEEP AIDS		
Excedrin PM Caplets	Acetaminophen/Diphenhydramine 500mg-38mg	**Adults & Peds:** ≥**12 yrs:** 2 tabs qhs.
Excedrin PM Geltabs	Acetaminophen/Diphenhydramine citrate 500mg-38 mg	**Adults & Peds:** ≥**12 yrs:** 2 tabs qhs.
Excedrin PM Tablets	Acetaminophen/Diphenhydramine citrate 500mg-38 mg	**Adults & Peds:** ≥**12 yrs:** 2 tabs qhs.
Goody's PM Powder	Acetaminophen/Diphenhydramine 1000mg-76mg/dose	**Adults & Peds:** ≥**12 yrs:** 1 packet (2 powders) qhs.
Tylenol PM Caplets	Acetaminophen/Diphenhydramine 500mg-25mg	**Adults & Peds:** ≥**12 yrs:** 2 tabs qhs.
Tylenol PM Rapid Release Gels	Acetaminophen/Diphenhydramine 500mg-25mg	**Adults & Peds:** ≥**12 yrs:** 2 caps qhs.
Tylenol PM Geltabs	Acetaminophen/Diphenhydramine 500mg-25mg	**Adults & Peds:** ≥**12 yrs:** 2 tabs qhs.
Tylenol PM Vanilla Liquid	Acetaminophen/Diphenhydramine 1000mg-50mg/30 mL	**Adults & Peds:** ≥**12 yrs:** 2 tbl (30mL) qhs. **Max:** 8 tbl (120mL) q24h.

(Continued)

BRAND	INGREDIENT/STRENGTH	DOSE
NSAIDs		
Advil Caplets	Ibuprofen 200mg	**Adults & Peds:** ≥12 yrs: 1-2 tabs q4-6h. **Max:** 6 tabs q24h.
Advil Children's Chewable Tablets	Ibuprofen 50mg	**Peds: 2-3 yr (24-35 lb):** 2 tabs q6-8h. **4-5 yr (36-47 lb):** 3 tabs q6-8h. **6-8 yr (48-59 lb):** 4 tabs q6-8h. **9-10 yr (60-71 lb):** 5 tabs q6-8h. **11 yr (72-95 lb):** 6 tabs q6-8h. **Max:** 4 doses q24h
Advil Children's Suspension	Ibuprofen 100mg/5mL	**Peds: 2-3 yrs (24-35 lbs)** (5mL). **4-5 yrs (36-47 lbs):** 1.5 tsp (7.5mL). **6-8 yrs (48-59 lbs):** 2 tsp (10mL). **9-10 yrs (60-71 lbs):** 2.5 tsp (12.5mL). **11 yrs (72-95 lbs):** 3 tsp (15mL). May repeat q6-8h. **Max:** 4 doses q24h.
Advil Gel Caplets	Ibuprofen 200mg	**Adults & Peds:** ≥12 yrs: 1-2 caps q4-6h. **Max:** 6 caps q24h.
Advil Infants' Concentrated Drops	Ibuprofen 50mg/1.25mL	**Peds: 6-11 months (12-17 lbs):** 1.25mL. **12-23 months (18-23 lbs):** 1.875mL. May repeat q6-8h. **Max:** 4 doses q24h.
Advil Junior Strength Swallow Tablets	Ibuprofen 100mg	**Peds: 6-10 yrs (48-71 lbs):** 2 tabs. **11 yrs (72-95 lbs):** 3 tabs. May repeat q6-8h. **Max:** 4 doses q24h.
Advil Junior Strength Chewable Tablets	Ibuprofen 100mg	**Peds: 6-8 yrs (48-59 lbs):** 2 tabs. **9-10 yrs (60-71 lbs):** 2.5 tabs. **11 yrs (72-95 lbs):** 3 tabs. May repeat q6-8h. **Max:** 4 doses q24h.
Advil Liqui-Gels	Ibuprofen 200mg	**Adults & Peds:** ≥12 yrs: 1-2 caps q4-6h. **Max:** 6 caps q24h.
Advil Migraine Capsules	Ibuprofen 200mg	**Adults:** 2 caps prn. **Max:** 2 caps q24h.
Advil Tablets	Ibuprofen 200mg	**Adults & Peds:** ≥12 yrs: 1-2 tabs q4-6h. **Max:** 6 tabs q24h.
Aleve Caplets	Naproxen Sodium 220mg	**Adults:** ≥65 yrs: 1 tab q12h. **Max:** 2 tabs q24h. **Adults & Peds:** ≥12 yrs: 1 tab q8-12h. **Max:** 3 tabs q24h.
Aleve Liquid Gels	Naproxen Sodium 220mg	**Adults & Peds:** ≥12 yrs: 1 cap q8-12h. May take 1 additional tab within 1 hour of first dose. **Max:** 3 caps q24h.
Aleve Smooth Gels	Naproxen Sodium 220mg	**Adults & Peds:** ≥12 yrs: 1 cap q8-12h. May take 1 additional tab within 1 hour of first dose. **Max:** 3 caps q24h.
Aleve Tablets	Naproxen Sodium 220mg	**Adults & Peds:** ≥12 yrs: 1 tab q8-12h. May take 1 additional tab within 1 hour of first dose. **Max::** 3 tabs q24h.
Midol Cramps and Body	Ibuprofen 200mg	**Adults & Peds:** ≥12 yrs: 1-2 tabs q4-6h. **Max:** 6 tabs q24h.
Midol Extended Relief Caplets	Naproxen Sodium 220mg	**Adults & Peds:** ≥12 yrs: 1-2 tabs q8-12h. **Max:** 3 tabs q24h.
Motrin Children's Suspension	Ibuprofen 100mg/5mL	**Peds: 2-3 yrs (24-35 lbs):** 1 tsp (5mL). **4-5 yrs (36-47 lbs):** 1.5 tsp (7.5mL). **6-8 yrs (48-59 lbs):** 2 tsp (10mL). **9-10 yrs (60-71 lbs):** 2.5 tsp (12.5mL). **11 yrs (72-95 lbs):** 3 tsp (15mL). May repeat q6-8h. **Max:** 4 doses q24h.

(Continued)

BRAND	INGREDIENT/STRENGTH	DOSE
NSAIDs *(Continued)*		
Motrin IB Caplets	Ibuprofen 200mg	**Adults & Peds:** ≥**12 yrs:** 1-2 tabs q4-6h. **Max:** 6 tabs q24h.
Motrin IB Gelcaps	Ibuprofen 200mg	**Adults & Peds:** ≥**12 yrs:** 1-2 tabs q4-6h. **Max:** 6 tabs q24h.
Motrin IB Tablets	Ibuprofen 200mg	**Adults & Peds:** ≥**12 yrs:** 1-2 tabs q4-6h. **Max:** 6 tabs q24h.
Motrin Infants' Drops	Ibuprofen 50mg/1.25mL	**Peds: 6-11 months (12-17 lbs):** 1.25mL. **12-23 months (18-23 lbs):** 1.875mL. May repeat q6-8h. **Max:** 4 doses q24h.
Motrin Junior Strength Caplets	Ibuprofen 100mg	**Peds: 6-8 yrs (48-59 lbs):** 2 tabs. **9-10 yrs (60-71 lbs):** 2.5 tabs. **11 yrs (72-95 lbs):** 3 tabs. May repeat q6-8h. **Max:** 4 doses q24h.
Motrin Junior Strength Chewable Tablets	Ibuprofen 100mg	**Peds: 6-8 yrs (48-59 lbs):** 2 tabs. **9-10 yrs (60-71 lbs):** 2.5 tabs. **11 yrs (72-95 lbs):** 3 tabs. May repeat q6-8h. **Max:** 4 doses q24h.
Pamprin All Day Caplets	Naproxen Sodium 220mg	**Adults & Peds:** ≥**12 yrs:** 1-2 tabs q8-12h. **Max:** 3 tabs q24h.
SALICYLATES		
Anacin 81 Tablets	Aspirin 81mg	**Adults & Peds:** ≥**12 yrs:** 2 tabs q6h. **Max:** 8 tabs q24h.
Aspergum Chewable Tablets	Aspirin 227mg	**Adults & Peds:** ≥**12 yrs:** 2 tabs q4h. **Max:** 16 tabs q24h.
Bayer Aspirin Extra Strength Caplets	Aspirin 500mg	**Adults & Peds:** ≥**12 yrs:** 1-2 tabs q4-6h. **Max:** 8 tabs q24h.
Bayer Aspirin Safety Coated Caplets	Aspirin 325mg	**Adults & Peds:** ≥**12 yrs:** 1-2 tabs q4h. **Max:** 12 tabs q24h.
Bayer Children's Aspirin Chewable Tablets	Aspirin 81mg	**Adults & Peds:** ≥**12 yrs:** 4-8 tabs q4h. **Max:** 48 tabs q24h.
Bayer Low Dose Aspirin Tablets	Aspirin 81mg	**Adults & Peds:** ≥**12 yrs:** 4-8 tabs q4h. **Max:** 48 tabs q24h.
Bayer Sugar Free Low Dose Aspirin Tablets	Aspirin 81mg	**Adults & Peds:** ≥**12 yrs:** 4-8 tabs q4h. **Max:** 48 tabs q24h.
Bayer Genuine Aspirin Tablets	Aspirin 325mg	**Adults & Peds:** ≥**12 yrs:** 1-2 tabs q4h or 3 tabs q6h. **Max:** 12 tabs q24h.
Bayer Extra-Strength Plus Caplets	Aspirin 500mg Buffered with Calcium Carbonate 500mg	**Adults & Peds:** ≥**12 yrs:** 1-2 tabs q4-6h. **Max:** 8 tabs q24h.
Doan's Caplets	Magnesium Salicylate Tetrahydrate 580mg	**Adults & Peds:** ≥**12 yrs:** 2 tabs q4h. **Max:** 12 tabs q24h.
Ecotrin Low Strength Tablets	Aspirin 81mg	**Adults:** 4-8 tabs q4h. **Max:** 48 tabs q24h.
Ecotrin Regular Strength Tablets	Aspirin 325mg	**Adults & Peds:** ≥**12 yrs:** 1-2 tabs q4h. **Max:** 12 tabs q24h.
Ecotrin Maximum Strength Tablets	Aspirin 500mg	**Adults & Peds:** ≥**12 yrs:** 2 tabs q6h. **Max:** 8 tabs q24h.
Halfprin 162mg Tablets	Aspirin 162mg	**Adults & Peds:** ≥**12 yrs:** 2-4 tabs q4h. **Max:** 24 tabs q24h.
Halfprin 81mg Tablets	Aspirin 81mg	**Adults & Peds:** ≥**12 yrs:** 4-8 tabs q4h. **Max:** 48 tabs q24h.
St. Joseph Chewable Aspirin Tablets	Aspirin 81mg	**Adults & Peds:** ≥**12 yrs:** 4-8 tabs q4h. **Max:** 48 tabs q24h.
St. Joseph Enteric Safety-Coated Tablets	Aspirin 81mg	**Adults & Peds:** ≥**12 yrs:** 4-8 tabs q4h. **Max:** 48 tabs q24h.

(Continued)

BRAND	INGREDIENT/STRENGTH	DOSE
SALICYLATES, BUFFERED		
Alka-Seltzer Original Effervescent Tablets	Aspirin/Citric Acid/Sodium Bicarbonate 325mg-1000mg-1916mg	**Adults & Peds:** ≥**12 yrs:** 2 tabs q4h. **Max:** 8 tabs q24h.
Alka-Seltzer Extra Strength Effervescent Tablets	Aspirin/Citric Acid/Sodium Bicarbonate 500mg-1000mg-1985mg	**Adults & Peds:** ≥**12 yrs:** 2 tabs q6h. **Max:** 7 tabs q24h.
Ascriptin Regular Strength Tablets	Aspirin Buffered with Maalox/Calcium Carbonate 325mg	**Adults & Peds:** ≥**12 yrs:** 2 tabs q4h. **Max:** 12 tabs q24h.
Bayer Extra Strength Plus Caplets	Aspirin Buffered with Calcium Carbonate 500mg	**Adults & Peds:** ≥**12 yrs:** 1-2 tabs q4-6h. **Max:** 8 tabs q24h.
Bufferin Extra Strength Tablets	Aspirin Buffered with Calcium Carbonate/Magnesium Oxide/Magnesium Carbonate 500mg	**Adults & Peds:** ≥**12 yrs:** 2 tabs q6h. **Max:** 8 tabs q24h.
Bufferin Tablets	Aspirin Buffered with Calcium Carbonate/Magnesium Oxide/Magnesium Carbonate 325mg	**Adults & Peds:** ≥**12 yrs:** 2 tabs q4h. **Max:** 12 tabs q24h.
SALICYLATE COMBINATIONS		
Alka-Seltzer Morning Relief Effervescent Tablets	Aspirin/Caffeine 500mg-65mg	**Adults & Peds:** ≥**12 yrs:** 2 tabs q6h. **Max:** 8 tabs q24h. ≥**60 yrs: Max:** 4 tabs q24h.
Anacin Max Strength Tablets	Aspirin/Caffeine 500mg-32mg	**Adults & Peds:** ≥**12 yrs:** 2 tabs q6h. **Max:** 8 tabs q24h.
Anacin Tablets	Aspirin/Caffeine 400mg-32mg	**Adults & Peds:** ≥**12 yrs:** 2 tabs q6h. **Max:** 8 tabs q24h.
Bayer Back & Body Pain Caplets	Aspirin/Caffeine 500mg-32.5mg	**Adults & Peds:** ≥**12 yrs:** 2 tabs q6h. **Max:** 8 tabs q24h.
BC Arthritis Strength Powders	Aspirin/Caffeine/Salicylamide 742mg-38mg-222mg	**Adults & Peds:** ≥**12 yrs:** 1 powder q3-4h. **Max:** 4 powders q24h.
BC Original Formula Powders	Aspirin/Caffeine/Salicylamide 650mg-33.3mg-195mg	**Adults & Peds:** ≥**12 yrs:** 1 powder q3-4h. **Max:** 4 powders q24h.
SALICYLATE/SLEEP AID		
Alka-Seltzer PM Effervescent Tablets	Aspirin/Diphenhydramine Citrate 325mg-38 mg	**Adults & Peds:** ≥**12 yrs:** 2 tabs qhs.
Bayer PM Caplets	Aspirin/Diphenhydramine 500mg-38.3mg	**Adults & Peds:** ≥**12 yrs:** 2 tabs qhs.
Doan's Extra Strength PM Caplets	Magnesium Salicylate Tetrahydrate/Diphenhydramine 580mg-25mg	**Adults & Peds:** ≥**12 yrs:** 2 tabs qhs.

ANTIPYRETIC PRODUCTS

BRAND	INGREDIENT/STRENGTH	DOSE
ACETAMINOPHEN		
Anacin Aspirin Free Extra Strength Tablets	Acetaminophen 500mg	**Adults & Peds:** ≥12 yrs: 2 tabs q6h. **Max:** 8 tabs q24h.
Feverall Childrens' Suppositories	Acetaminophen 120mg	**Peds: 3-6 yrs:** 1-2 supp. q4-6h. **Max:** 6 supp q24h.
Feverall Infants' Suppositories	Acetaminophen 80mg	**Peds: 3-11 months:** 1 supp q6h. **12-36 months:** 1 supp q4h. **Max:** 6 supp q24h.
Feverall Jr. Strength Suppositories	Acetaminophen 325mg	**Peds: 6-12 yrs:** 1 supp q4-6h. **Max:** 6 supp q24h.
Tylenol 8 Hour Caplets	Acetaminophen 650mg	**Adults & Peds:** ≥12 yrs: 2 tabs q8h prn. **Max:** 6 tabs q24h.
Tylenol 8 Hour Geltabs	Acetaminophen 650mg	**Adults & Peds:** ≥12 yrs: 2 tabs q8h prn. **Max:** 6 tabs q24h.
Tylenol Arthritis Caplets	Acetaminophen 650mg	**Adults:** 2 tabs q8h prn. **Max:** 6 tabs q24h.
Tylenol Arthritis Geltabs	Acetaminophen 650mg	**Adults:** 2 tabs q8h prn. **Max:** 6 tabs q24h.
Tylenol Children's Meltaways Tablets	Acetaminophen 80mg	**Peds: 2-3 yrs (24-35 lbs):** 2 tabs. **4-5 yrs (36-47 lbs):** 3 tabs. **6-8 yrs (48-59 lbs):** 4 tabs. **9-10 yrs (60-71 lbs):** 5 tabs. **11 yrs (72-95 lbs):** 6 tabs. May repeat q4h. **Max:** 5 doses q24h.
Tylenol Children's Suspension	Acetaminophen 160mg/5mL	**Peds: 2-3 yrs (24-35 lbs):** 1 tsp (5mL). **4-5 yrs (36-47 lbs):** 1.5 tsp (7.5mL). **6-8 yrs (48-59 lbs):** 2 tsp (10mL). **9-10 yrs (60-71 lbs):** 2.5 tsp (12.5mL). **11 yrs (72-95 lbs):** 3 tsp (15mL). May repeat q4h. **Max:** 5 doses q24h.
Tylenol Extra Strength Caplets	Acetaminophen 500mg	**Adults & Peds:** ≥12 yrs: 2 tabs q4-6h prn. **Max:** 8 tabs q24h.
Tylenol Extra Strength Cool Caplets	Acetaminophen 500mg	**Adults & Peds:** ≥12 yrs: 2 tabs q4-6h prn. **Max:** 8 tabs q24h.
Tylenol Extra Strength Gelcaps	Acetaminophen 500mg	**Adults & Peds:** ≥12 yrs: 2 caps q4-6h prn. **Max:** 8 caps q24h.
Tylenol Extra Strength Geltabs	Acetaminophen 500mg	**Adults & Peds:** ≥12 yrs: 2 tabs q4-6h prn. **Max:** 8 tabs q24h.
Tylenol Extra Strength Liquid	Acetaminophen 1000mg/30mL	**Adults & Peds:** ≥12 yrs: 2 tbl (30mL) q4-6h prn. **Max:** 8 tbl (120mL) q24h.
Tylenol Extra Strength Tablets	Acetaminophen 500mg	**Adults & Peds:** ≥12 yrs: 2 tabs q4-6h prn. **Max:** 8 tabs q24h.
Tylenol Infants' Suspension	Acetaminophen 80mg/0.8mL	**Peds: 2-3 yrs (24-35 lbs):** 1.6 mL q4h prn. **Max:** 5 doses (8mL) q24h.
Tylenol Junior Meltaways Tablets	Acetaminophen 160mg	**Peds: 6-8 yrs (48-59 lbs):** 2 tabs. **9-10 yrs (60-71 lbs):** 2.5 tabs. **11 yrs (72-95 lbs):** 3 tabs. **12 yrs (≥96 lbs):** 4 tabs. May repeat q4h. **Max:** 5 doses q24h.
Tylenol Regular Strength Tablets	Acetaminophen 325mg	**Adults & Peds:** ≥12 yrs: 2 tabs q4-6h prn. **Max:** 12 tabs q24h. **Peds: 6-11 yrs:** 1 tab q4-6h. **Max:** 5 tabs q24h.

(Continued)

BRAND	INGREDIENT/STRENGTH	DOSE
NONSTEROIDAL ANTI-INFLAMMATORY DRUGS (NSAIDs)		
Advil Children's Chewable Tablets	Ibuprofen 50mg	**Peds: 2-3 yrs (24-35 lbs):** 2 tabs q6-8h. **4-5 yrs (36-47 lbs):** 3 tabs q6-8h. **6-8 yrs (48-59 lbs):** 4 tabs q6-8h. **9-10 yrs (60-71 lbs):** 5 tabs q6-8h. **11 yrs (72-95 lbs):** 6 tabs q6-8h. **Max:** 4 doses q24h.
Advil Children's Suspension	Ibuprofen 100mg/5mL	**Peds: 2-3 yrs (24-35 lbs):** 1 tsp (5mL). **4-5 yrs (36-47 lbs):** 1.5 tsp (7.5mL). **6-8 yrs (48-59 lbs):** 2 tsp (10mL). **9-10 yrs (60-71 lbs):** 2.5 tsp (12.5mL). **11 yrs (72-95 lbs):** 3 tsp (15mL). May repeat q6-8h. **Max:** 4 doses q24h.
Advil Gel Caplets	Ibuprofen 200mg	**Adults & Peds: ≥12 yrs:** 1-2 caps q4-6h. **Max:** 6 caps q24h.
Advil Infants' Concentrated Drops	Ibuprofen 50mg/1.25mL	**Peds: 6-11 months (12-17 lbs):** 1.25mL. **12-23 months (18-23 lbs):** 1.875mL. May repeat q6-8h. **Max:** 4 doses q24h.
Advil Junior Strength Chewable Tablets	Ibuprofen 100mg	**Peds: 6-8 yrs (48-59 lbs):** 2 tabs. **9-10 yrs (60-71 lbs):** 2.5 tabs. **11 yrs (72-95 lbs):** 3 tabs. May repeat q6-8h. **Max:** 4 doses q24h.
Advil Junior Strength Swallow Tablets	Ibuprofen 100mg	**Peds: 6-10 yrs (48-71 lbs):** 2 tabs **11 yrs (72-95 lbs):** 3 tabs. May repeat q6-8h. **Max:** 4 doses q24h.
Advil Liqui-Gels	Ibuprofen 200mg	**Adults & Peds: ≥12 yrs:** 1-2 caps q4-6h. **Max:** 6 caps q24h.
Advil Tablets	Ibuprofen 200mg	**Adults & Peds: ≥12 yrs:** 1-2 tabs q4-6h. **Max:** 6 tabs q24h.
Aleve Caplets	Naproxen Sodium 220mg	**Adults & Peds: ≥12 yrs:** 1 tab q8-12h. May take 1 additional tab within 1 hour of first dose. **Max:** 3 tabs q24h.
Aleve Liquid Gels	Naproxen Sodium 220mg	**Adults & Peds: ≥12 yrs:** 1 cap q8-12h. May take 1 additional tab within 1 hour of first dose. **Max:** 3 caps q24h.
Aleve Smooth Gels	Naproxen Sodium 220mg	**Adults & Peds: ≥12 yrs:** 1 cap q8-12h. May take 1 additional tab within 1 hour of first dose. **Max:** 3 caps q24h.
Aleve Tablets	Naproxen Sodium 220mg	**Adults & Peds: ≥12 yrs:** 1 tab q8-12h. May take 1 additional tab within 1 hour of first dose. **Max:** 3 caps q24h.
Motrin Children's Suspension	Ibuprofen 100mg/5mL	**Peds: 2-3 yrs (24-35 lbs):** 1 tsp (5mL). **4-5 yrs (36-47 lbs):** 1.5 tsp (7.5mL). **6-8 yrs (48-59 lbs):** 2 tsp (10mL). **9-10 yrs (60-71 lbs):** 2.5 tsp (12.5mL). **11 yrs (72-95 lbs):** 3 tsp (15mL). May repeat q6-8h. **Max:** 4 doses q24h.
Motrin IB Caplets	Ibuprofen 200mg	**Adults & Peds: ≥12 yrs:** 1-2 tabs q4-6h. **Max:** 6 tabs q24h.
Motrin IB Tablets	Ibuprofen 200mg	**Adults & Peds: ≥12 yrs:** 1-2 tabs q4-6h. **Max:** 6 tabs q24h.
Motrin Infants' drops	Ibuprofen 50mg/1.25mL	**Peds: 6-11 months (12-17 lbs):** 1.25mL. **12-23 months (18-23 lbs):** 1.875mL. May repeat q6-8h. **Max:** 4 doses q24h.

(Continued)

BRAND	INGREDIENT/STRENGTH	DOSE
NONSTEROIDAL ANTI-INFLAMMATORY DRUGS (NSAIDs) *(Continued)*		
Motrin Junior Strength Caplets	Ibuprofen 100mg	**Peds: 6-8 yrs (48-59 lbs):** 2 tabs. **9-10 yrs (60-71 lbs):** 2.5 tabs. **11 yrs (72-95 lbs):** 3 tabs. May repeat q6-8h. **Max:** 4 doses q24h.
Motrin Junior Strength Chewable Tablets	Ibuprofen 100mg	**Peds: 6-8 yrs (48-59 lbs):** 2 tabs. **9-10 yrs (60-71 lbs):** 2.5 tabs. **11 yrs (72-95 lbs):** 3 tabs. May repeat q6-8h. **Max:** 4 doses q24h.
SALICYLATES		
Anacin 81 Tablets	Aspirin 81mg	**Adults & Peds: ≥12 yrs:** 2 tabs q6h. **Max:** 8 tabs q24h.
Aspergum Chewable Tablets	Aspirin 227mg	**Adults & Peds: ≥12 yrs:** 2 tabs q4h. **Max:** 16 tabs q24h.
Bayer Aspirin Extra Strength Caplets	Aspirin 500mg	**Adults & Peds: ≥12 yrs:** 1-2 tabs q4-6h. **Max:** 8 tabs q24h.
Bayer Genuine Aspirin Caplets	Aspirin 325mg	**Adults & Peds: ≥12 yrs:** 1-2 tabs q4h or 3 tabs q6h. **Max:** 12 tabs q24h.
Bayer Aspirin Safety Coated Caplets	Aspirin 325mg	**Adults & Peds: ≥12 yrs:** 1-2 tabs q4h or 3 tabs q6h. **Max:** 12 tabs q24h.
Bayer Children's Aspirin Chewable Tablets	Aspirin 81mg	**Adults & Peds: ≥12 yrs:** 4-8 tabs q4h. **Max:** 48 tabs q24h.
Bayer Low Dose Aspirin Tablets	Aspirin 81mg	**Adults & Peds: ≥12 yrs:** 4-8 tabs q4h. **Max:** 48 tabs q24h.
Ecotrin Low Strength Tablets	Aspirin 81mg	**Adults:** 4-8 tabs q4h. **Max:** 48 tabs q24h.
Ecotrin Enteric Regular Strength Tablets	Aspirin 325mg	**Adults & Peds: ≥12 yrs:** 1-2 tabs q4h. **Max:** 12 tabs q24h.
Ecotrin Maximum Strength Tablets	Aspirin 500mg	**Adults & Peds: ≥12 yrs:** 2 tabs q6h. **Max:** 8 tabs q24h.
Halfprin 162mg Tablets	Aspirin 162mg	**Adults & Peds: ≥12 yrs:** 2-4 tabs q4h. **Max:** 24 tabs q24h.
Halfprin 81mg Tablets	Aspirin 81mg	**Adults & Peds: ≥12 yrs:** 4-8 tabs q4h. **Max:** 48 tabs q24h.
St. Joseph Aspirin Chewable Tablets	Aspirin 81mg	**Adults & Peds: ≥12 yrs:** 4-8 tabs q4h. **Max:** 48 tabs q24h.
St. Joseph Enteric Safety-Coated Tablets	Aspirin 81mg	**Adults & Peds: ≥12 yrs:** 4-8 tabs q4h. **Max:** 48 tabs q24h.
SALICYLATES, BUFFERED		
Bayer Extra Strength Plus Caplets	Aspirin Buffered with Calcium Carbonate 500mg	**Adults & Peds: ≥12 yrs:** 1-2 tabs q4-6h. **Max:** 8 tabs q24h.
Bufferin Extra Strength Tablets	Aspirin Buffered with Calcium Carbonate/Magnesium Oxide/Magnesium Carbonate 500mg	**Adults & Peds: ≥12 yrs:** 2 tabs q6h. **Max:** 8 tabs q24h.
Bufferin Tablets	Aspirin Buffered with Calcium Carbonate/Magnesium Oxide/Magnesium Carbonate 325mg	**Adults & Peds: ≥12 yrs:** 2 tabs q4h. **Max:** 12 tabs q24h.

ACNE MANAGEMENT: SYSTEMIC THERAPIES

DRUG (BRAND)	HOW SUPPLIED	DOSAGE	SIDE EFFECTS
ANTIBIOTICS			
Doxycycline hyclate (Doryx, Vibramycin)	Cap: 75mg, 100mg	100mg q12h on 1st day, followed by 100mg qd.	Anorexia, nausea, vomiting, diarrhea, dysphagia, enterocolitis, rash, exfoliative dermatitis, renal toxicity, hypersensitivity reactions, blood dyscrasias
Doxycycline monohydrate (Monodox)	Cap: 50mg, 100mg	100mg q12h or 50mg q6h for 1 day, then 100mg/day.	GI effects, photosensitivity, rash, blood dyscrasias, hypersensitivity reactions
Doxycyline, USP (Oracea)	Cap: 40mg	40mg qd am.	Anorexia, nausea, sinusitis, diarrhea, abdominal pain
Minocycline HCl (Dynacin, Minocin)	Cap: 50mg, 75mg, 100mg; Tab: 50mg, 75mg, 100mg	200mg initially, then 100mg q12h; alternative is 100-200mg initially, then 50mg qid.	Anorexia, nausea, vomiting, diarrhea, dysphagia, enterocolitis, pancreatitis, increased LFTs, hepatitis, liver failure, renal toxicity, rash, exfoliative dermatitis, Stevens-Johnson syndrome, skin and mucous membrane pigmentation, blood dyscrasias, headache, tooth discoloration
Minocycline HCl (Solodyn)	Tab, Extended-Release: 45mg, 90mg, 135mg	1mg/kg qd for 12 weeks.	Headache, fatigue, dizziness, pruritus, malaise, mood alteration
Tetracycline hydrochloride (Sumycin)	Sus: 125mg/5mL; Tab: 250mg, 500mg	Mild-Moderate: 250mg qid or 500mg bid. Severe: 500mg qid. Severe Acne: Initial: 1g/day in divided doses. Maint: After improvement, 125-500mg/day.	GI effects, photosensitivity, increased BUN, hypersensitivity reactions, blood dyscrasias, dizziness, headache
ORAL CONTRACEPTIVES			
Ethinyl Estradiol and Drospirenone (YAZ)	Tab: (Ethinyl Estradiol-Drospirenone) 0.02mg-3mg	1 tab qd for 28 days, then repeat. Start on first Sunday of menses or begin 1st day of menses.	Nausea, vomiting, breakthrough bleeding, spotting, amenorrhea, migraine, vaginal candidiasis, edema, weight changes, depression, urticaria, angioedema, circulatory symptoms, dysmenorrhea
Ethinyl Estradiol and Norgestimate (Ortho Tri-Cyclen)	Tab: (Ethinyl Estradiol-Norgestimate) 0.035mg-0.18mg, 0.035mg-0.215mg, 0.035mg-0.25mg	1 tab qd for 28 days, then repeat. Start on first Sunday of menses or begin 1st day of menses.	Nausea, vomiting, breakthrough bleeding, spotting, amenorrhea, migraine, depression, vaginal candidiasis, edema, weight changes
Ethinyl Estradiol and Norethindrone (Estrostep Fe)	Tab: (Ethinyl Estradiol-Norethindrone) 0.035mg-1mg, 0.030mg-1mg, 0.020mg-1mg and 75mg ferrous fumarate	1 tab qd for 28 days, then repeat. Start on first Sunday of menses or begin 1st day of menses.	Nausea, vomiting, breakthrough bleeding, spotting, amenorrhea, migraine, depression, vaginal candidiasis, edema, weight changes
RETINOID			
Isotretinoin (Accutane, Amnesteem, Claravis, Sotret)	Accutane, Amnesteem, Claravis: (Cap) 10mg, 20mg, 40mg Sotret: (Cap) 10mg, 20mg, 30mg, 40mg	0.5-1mg/kg/day given bid for 15-20 weeks.	Cheilitis, dry skin and mucous membranes, conjunctivitis, blood dyscrasias, epistaxis, decreased HDL, elevated cholesterol and TG, elevated blood sugar, arthralgias, back pain, hearing/vision impairment, rash, photosensitivity reactions, psychiatric disorders

(Continued)

DRUG (BRAND)	HOW SUPPLIED	DOSAGE	SIDE EFFECTS
VITAMIN/MINERAL			
Nicotinamide/ Folic acid/Zinc (Nicomide)	Tab: (Nicotinamide-Folic acid-Zinc) 750mg-500mcg-25m	1 tab qd-bid.	Nausea, vomiting, transient LFT elevations, allergic sensitization

References:
FDA-Approved Product Labeling.

ACNE MANAGEMENT: TOPICAL THERAPIES

DRUG (BRAND)	HOW SUPPLIED	DOSAGE	SIDE EFFECTS
ANTIBACTERIAL/KERATOLYTIC AGENTS & COMBINATIONS			
Benzoyl peroxide (Benzac AC, Benzagel, Triaz)	Benzac AC: (Gel) 5%, 10% [60g], (Wash) 10% [60g]; Benzagel: (Gel) 5%, 10% [42.5g], (Wash) 10% [60g]; Triaz: (Gel) 3%, 6%, 9% [42.5g], (Cleanser) 3%, 6%, 9% [170.3g, 240.2g], (Pads) 3%, 6%, 9% [30g]	(Benzac) Apply qd-bid. (Benzagel) Apply wash qd-bid; apply gel qd initially or qhs for light skin. (Triaz) Apply gel/ wash qd-bid.	Erythema, peeling, contact dermatitis, dryness
Benzoyl peroxide/ Sulfur (Sulfoxyl Lotion Regular/Strong)	Lot: (Regular) 10%-2% [59mL]; (Strong) 10%-5% [59mL]	Apply initially once daily for the first week then twice daily, as tolerated.	Erythema, peeling, contact, dermatitis, dryness, irritation, itching, redness
Clindamycin/ Benzoyl peroxide (Benzaclin, Duac)	Benzaclin: (Gel) 1%-5% [25g, 50g]; Duac: (Gel) 1%-5% [45g]	(Benzaclin) Apply qd. (Duac) Apply once in the evening.	Dry skin, erythema, peeling, and burning
Benzoyl peroxide/ Erythromycin (Benzamycin)	Gel: 5%-3% [46.6g, 60s]	Apply bid.	Dryness, urticaria, skin irritation, skin discoloration, oiliness
Benzoyl peroxide (Brevoxyl, Zoderm)	Brevoxyl: (Gel) 4%, 8% [42.5g, 90g], (Lot, Cleanser) 4%, 8% [297g], (Lot, Creamy Wash) 4%, 8% [170g]; Zoderm: (Cleanser) 4.5%, 6.5%, 8.5% [400mL], (Cre/Gel) 4.5%, 6.5%, 8.5% [125mL]	(Brevoxyl) Apply gel qd-bid; apply lotion qd for first week then bid as tolerated. (Zoderm) Apply qd-bid.	Erythema, peeling, contact dermatitis, dryness
ANTIBIOTICS & COMBINATIONS			
Clindamycin (Cleocin T, Clindagel, Clindets, Evoclin Foam)	Cleocin T: (Gel) 1% [30g, 60g], (Lot) 1% [60mL], (Sol) 1% [30mL, 60mL], (Swab, Pledgets) 1% [60s]; Clindagel: 1% [40, 75mL]; Clindets: (Swab) 1% [69]; Evoclin: (Foam) 1% [50g, 100g]	(Cleocin T) Apply bid. (Clindagel) Apply qd. (Clindets) Apply bid. (Evoclin Foam) Apply qd.	Local irritation, stains clothing
Clindamycin/ Tretinoin (Ziana)	Gel: 1.2%-0.025% [2g, 30g, 60g]	Apply qd at bedtime.	Nasopharyngitis, erythema, scaling, itching, burning
Erythromycin (A/T/S, Erygel Erythromycin Topical Swabs)	A/T/S: (Gel) 2% [30g], (Sol) 2% [60mL]; Erycette: (Swab) 2% [60g]; Erygel: 2% [30g, 60g]; Erythromycin Topical Swabs: 2% [60g]	(A/T/S) Apply gel qd-bid; apply solution bid. (Erygel) Apply qd-bid. Erythromycin Topical Swabs: Apply bid	Local irritation, stains clothing, peeling, dryness, itching, erythema, oiliness.
Sulfacetamide (Klaron)	Lot: 10% [118mL]	Apply bid.	Itching, redness, irritation
Sulfacetamide/ Sulfur (Plexion TS, Sulfacet-R, Zetacet)	Plexion TS: (Lot) 10%-5% [30g]; Sulfacet-R/Zetacet: (Lot) 10%-5% [25g]	Apply qd-tid.	Itching, redness, irritation
Sulfacetamide/ Sulfur (Plexion SCT, Rosac)	Plexion SCT: (Cre) 10%-5% [120g]; Rosac: (Cre) 10%-5% [45g]	Apply qd-tid.	Local irritation
Sulfacetamide/ Sulfur (Clenia, Plexion, Rosula)	Clenia: (Cleanser) 10%-5% [170g, 340g], Cre: 10%-5% [28g]; Plexion: (Cleanser) 10%-5% [170.3g, 340.2g]; Rosula: (Cleanser) 10%-5% [355mL], Gel 10%-5% [45mL]	Apply cream qd initially then titrate to bid-tid prn. (Plexion) Apply qd-bid. (Rosula) Apply cleanser qd-bid; apply gel qd-tid.	Local irritation
Sulfacetamide/ Urea (Rosula NS Dicarboxylic Acids)	(Swab) 10%-10% [30ˢ]	Apply qd-bid.	Local hypersensitivity, instances of Stevens-Johnson syndrome

(Continued)

DRUG (BRAND)	HOW SUPPLIED	DOSAGE	SIDE EFFECTS
ANTIBIOTICS & COMBINATIONS *(Continued)*			
Azelaic acid (Azelex, Finevin)	(Cre) 20% [30g, 50g]	Apply bid.	Dryness, scaling, erythema, burning, irritation, pruritus; rarely, hypopigmentation
Azelaic acid (Finacea, Retinoids)	(Gel) 15% [30g]	Apply bid.	Burning, stinging, tingling, pruritus, scaling, dry skin
Adapalene (Differin)	(Cre, Gel) 0.1% [45g]; (Sol) 0.1% [30mL]	Apply hs.	Erythema, scaling, dryness, pruritus, burning, sunburn, acne flares
Tazarotene (Tazorac)	(Cre) 0.05%, 0.1% [30g, 60g]; (Gel) 0.05%, 0.1% [30g, 100g]	Apply hs.	Pruritus, burning/stinging; erythema, irritation, skin pain, desquamation, dry skin, rash
Tretinoin (Atralin, Avita, Retin-A)	(Cre) 0.025%, 0.05%, 0.1% [20g, 45g]; (Gel) 0.05%, 0.01%, 0.025% [15g, 45g]; (Sol) 0.05% [28mL]	Apply hs.	Local skin reactions (red, edematous, blistered, crusted), photosensitivity, temporary skin pigmentation changes
Tretinoin microsphere (Retin-A-Micro)	(Gel) 0.04%, 0.1% [20g, 45g]	Apply hs.	

Source: FDA-approved product labeling.

TOPICAL CORTICOSTEROIDS

STEROID	DOSAGE FORM(S)	STRENGTH (%)	POTENCY	FREQUENCY
Alclometasone Dipropionate (Aclovate)	Cre, Oint	0.05	Low	bid/tid
Amcinonide (Cyclocort)	Cre, Oint	0.05, 0.005	Medium	bid/tid
Augmented Betamethasone Dipropionate (Diprolene, Diprolene AF)	Cre, Oint	0.05	Very High	qd/bid
	Cre, Lot	0.05	High	qd/bid
Betamethasone Dipropionate	Cre, Lot, Oint	0.05	High	qd/bid
Betamethasone Valerate (Luxiq)	Foam	0.12	Medium	bid
Clobetasol Propionate (Clobevate, Clobex, Cormax, Embeline E, Olux, Olux E, Temovate, Temovate-E)	Cre, Foam (Olux)	0.05	Very High	bid
	Cream (Embeline E), Foam, Gel (Clobevate), Lotion (Clobex), Oint, Shampoo (Clobex), Sol	0.05	Very High	qd (shampoo)
Clocortolone Pivalate (Cloderm)	Cre	0.1	Low	tid
Desonide (Desonate, DesOwen, Verdeso)	Cre, Foam, Gel (Desonate), Lot, Oint	0.05	Low	bid/tid
Desoximetasone (Topicort, Topicort LP)	Cre	0.05	Medium	bid
	Cre, Oint	0.25	High	bid
	Gel	0.05	High	bid
Diflorasone Diacetate (Psorcon)	Oint (Psorcon)	0.05	Very High	qd/qid
Fluocinolone Acetonide (Capex, Derma-Smoothe/FS, Synalar)	Cre, Oint	0.025	Medium	bid/qid
	Sol	0.01	Medium	bid/qid
	Oil (Derma-Smoothe/FS)	0.01	Medium	qd/tid
	Shampoo (Capex)	0.01	Medium	qd
Fluocinonide (Lidex, Lidex-E, Vanos)	Cre, Gel, Oint, Sol	0.05	High	bid/qid
	Cre	0.1	Very High	qd/bid
Flurandrenolide (Cordran, Cordran SP)	Cre, Oint	0.025	Medium	bid/tid
	Cre, Lot, Oint	0.05	Medium	bid/tid
	Tape	4mcg/cm^2	Medium	qd/bid
Fluticasone Propionate (Cutivate)	Cre, Lot	0.05	Medium	qd/bid
	Oint	0.005	Medium	bid
Halcinonide (Halog, Halog-E)	Cre, Oint, Sol	0.1	High	qd/tid
Halobetasol Propionate (Ultravate)	Cre, Oint	0.05	Very High	qd/bid
Hydrocortisone (Anusol HC, Hytone)	Lot	2	Low	tid/qid
	Cre, Lot, Oint	2.5	Low	tid/qid
Hydrocortisone Butyrate (Locoid, Locoid Lipo Cream)	Cre, Lot, Oint, Sol	0.1	Medium	bid/tid
Hydrocortisone Probutate (Pandel)	Cre	0.1	Medium	qd/bid
Hydrocortisone Valerate (Westcort)	Cre, Oint	0.2	Medium	bid/tid
Mometasone Furoate (Elocon)	Cre, Lot, Oint	0.1	Medium	qd
Prednicarbate (Dermatop)	Cre, Oint	0.1	Medium	bid
Triamcinolone Acetonide (Kenalog, Triderm)	Cre, Lot, Oint	0.025	Medium	bid/qid
	Cre, Lot, Oint	0.1	Medium	bid/tid
	Cre, Oint	0.5	High	bid/tid
	Spray	0.147	Medium	tid/qid

INSULIN FORMULATIONS

TYPE OF INSULIN	BRAND	ONSET* (hrs)	PEAK* (hrs)	DURATION* (hrs)	COMMON PITFALLS**
Rapid-acting Insulin Glulisine Insulin Lispro Insulin Aspart	Apidra Humalog Novolog	– <0.25 <0.25	0.5 to 1.7 0.5 to 1.5 0.5 to 1	1 to 3 3 to 5 3 to 5	See individual comments. Hypoglycemia occurs if lag time is too long or the patient exercises within 1 hr of dose; with high-fat meals, the dose should be adjusted downward.
Short-acting Regular Insulin	Humulin R† Novolin R	0.5 to 1 0.5 to 1	2 to 4 2 to 5	4 to 12 8	Lag time is not used appropriately; the insulin should be given 20 to 30 minutes before the patient eats.
Intermediate-acting NPH (Isophane)	Humulin N Novolin R	1 to 3	6 to 12	18 to 24	In many patients, breakfast injection does not last the evening until the evening meal; administration with the evening meal does not meet insulin needs on awakening.
Long-acting Insulin glargine Insulin detemir	Lantus Levemir	1 –	Flat 6 to 8	24 24	Administer once daily at the same time every day. See individual comments.
Combinations Isophane insulin suspension (70%)/regular insulin (30%)	Humulin 70/30 Novolin 70/30	0.5 to 1	4 to 6	24	See individual comments.
Isophane insulin suspension (50%)/regular insulin (50%)	Humulin 50/50	0.5 to 1	3 to 5	24	See individual comments.
Insulin lispro protamine (75%)/insulin lispro (25%)	Humalog Mix 75/25	≤0.25	0.5 to 4	24	See individual comments.
Insulin aspart protamine (70%)/insulin aspart (30%)	Novolog Mix 70/30	≤0.25	1 to 4	24	See individual comments.

*Approximate parameters following SC injection of an average patient dose; insulin concentration: 100U/mL. (Not applicable for inhalation insulin.)

**Source: Hirsch, IB. Type 1 Diabetes Mellitus and the Use of Flexible Insulin Regimens. *Am Fam Physician.* November 1999;60(8):2343-2352,2355-2356.

†Also available 500 U/mL for insulin resistant patients (rapid onset; up to 24 hour duration).

ANTIBIOTIC SENSITIVITY – AMINOGLYCOSIDES*

ORGANISMS	Amikacin	Gentamicin	Streptomycin	Tobramycin
ANAEROBES				
Actinomyces				
Bacillus anthracis				
Bacteroides fragilis				
Clostridium difficile				
Clostridium species				
GRAM-NEGATIVE AEROBES				
Acinetobacter baumannii	++	+		++
Aeromonas hydrophila	++	++		++
Bartonella henselae		++		
Bordetella species				
Burkholderia cepacia				
Campylobacter jejuni		+		
Citrobacter species	++	+++		+++
Coxiella burnetti				
Enterobacter species	+++	+++		+++
Escherichia coli	+	++		++

+++ = excellent activity (1st line recommendation). ++ = good activity (2nd line recommendation). + = moderate activity (acceptable in vitro data suggesting some isolates may be sensitive).

Blank = no or insufficient activity, or unknown.

†† 2nd line against *S. typhi*. † Penicillin sensitive; MIC ≤1.0 mcg/mL. §§ Penicillin resistant; MIC ≥2.0 mcg/mL.

*These are generalizations. There are major differences among countries, areas, and hospitals depending on antibiotic usage patterns.

ORGANISMS	Amikacin	Gentamicin	Streptomycin	Tobramycin
GRAM-NEGATIVE AEROBES *(Continued)*				
Francisella tularensis		+++	+++	+
Haemophilus influenzae	+	+		+
Klebsiella species	++	++		++
Legionella species				
Moraxella catarrhalis	+	+		+
Morganella morganii	++	++		++
Neisseria gonorrhoeae				
Neisseria meningitidis				
Pasturella multocida				
Proteus mirabilis	++	+++		++
Proteus vulgaris	++	+++		++
Providencia stuartii	++	++		++
Pseudomonas aeruginosa	+++	+++		+++
Rickettsia species				
Salmonella species				
Serratia species	++	++		++
Shigella species	+	+		+
Stenotrophomonas maltophilia				

+++ = excellent activity (1st line recommendation). ++ = good activity (2nd line recommendation). + = moderate activity (acceptable in vitro data suggesting some isolates may be sensitive).
Blank = no or insufficient activity, or unknown.
†† 2nd line against *S. typhi*. † Penicillin sensitive; MIC ≤1.0 mcg/mL. §§ Penicillin resistant; MIC ≥2.0 mcg/mL.
* These are generalizations. There are major differences among countries, areas, and hospitals depending on antibiotic usage patterns.

AMINOGLYCOSIDES (CONTINUED)

ORGANISMS	Amikacin	Gentamicin	Streptomycin	Tobramycin
GRAM-NEGATIVE AEROBES *(Continued)*				
Vibrio vulnificus				
Yersinia enterocolitica	++	++		++
Yersinia pestis		++	+++	+
GRAM-POSITIVE AEROBES				
Enterococcus faecalis		++	++	
Enterococcus faecium		+	+	
Enterococcus faecium (VRE)		+	+	
Listeria monocytogenes	+	+		+
Nocardia	++			
Staphylococcus aureus (MSSA)				
Staphylococcus aureus (MRSA)				
Staphylococcus epidermidis		+		
Staphylococcus epidermidis (MRSE)		+		
Streptococcus pneumoniae†				
Streptococcus pneumoniae§§				

+++ = excellent activity (1st line recommendation). ++ = good activity (2nd line recommendation). + = moderate activity (acceptable in vitro data suggesting some isolates may be sensitive).

Blank = no or insufficient activity, or unknown. † Penicillin sensitive; MIC ≤1.0 mcg/mL. §§ Penicillin resistant; MIC ≥2.0 mcg/mL.

†† 2nd line against *S. typhi*. † Penicillin sensitive; MIC ≤1.0 mcg/mL.

*These are generalizations. There are major differences among countries, areas, and hospitals depending on antibiotic usage patterns.

ORGANISMS	Amikacin	Gentamicin	Streptomycin	Tobramycin
GRAM-POSITIVE AEROBES *(Continued)*				
Streptococcus (Group A,B,C,FG)				
Streptococcus species		+		
MISCELLANEOUS				
Chlamydia pneumoniae				
Chlamydia trachomatis				
Ehrlichia/Anaplasma species				
MYCOBACTERIA				
Mycobacterium avium (MAI) *(non-HIV)*	++		+	
Mycoplasma pneumoniae				
SPIROCHETES				
Leptospira interrogans				
Treponema pallidum (syphilis)				

+++ = excellent activity (1st line recommendation).   ++ = good activity (2nd line recommendation).   + = moderate activity (acceptable in vitro data suggesting some isolates may be sensitive).

Blank = no or insufficient activity, or unknown.

†† 2nd line against *S. typhi*.   † 2nd line against *S. typhi*.   §§ Penicillin resistant; MIC ≥2.0 mcg/mL.

† Penicillin sensitive; MIC ≤1.0 mcg/mL.

*These are generalizations. There are major differences among countries, areas, and hospitals depending on antibiotic usage patterns.

ANTIBIOTIC SENSITIVITY – CARBAPENEMS/MONOBACTAMS*

ORGANISMS	Aztreonam	Ertapenem	Imipenem/Cilastatin	Meropenem
ANAEROBES				
Actinomyces			++	++
Bacillus anthracis				
Bacteroides fragilis		+++	+++	+++
Clostridium difficile				
Clostridium species		++	++	++
GRAM-NEGATIVE AEROBES				
Acinetobacter baumannii	+		+++	+++
Aeromonas hydrophila	++	+	++	++
Bartonella henselae				
Bordetella species		+	+	+
Burkholderia cepacia		+	+	++
Campylobacter jejuni		+	+	+
Citrobacter species	++	+++	+++	+++
Coxiella burnetii				
Enterobacter species	++	++	+++	+++
Escherichia coli	++	++	++	++

+++ = excellent activity (1st line recommendation). ++ = good activity (2nd line recommendation). + = moderate activity (acceptable in vitro data suggesting some isolates may be sensitive).

Blank = no or insufficient activity, or unknown. † Penicillin sensitive; MIC ≤1.0 mcg/mL. §§ Penicillin resistant; MIC ≥2.0 mcg/mL.

†† 2nd line against S. typhi. ‡ Penicillin sensitive; MIC ≤1.0 mcg/mL.

*These are generalizations. There are major differences among countries, areas, and hospitals depending on antibiotic usage patterns.

ORGANISMS	Aztreonam	Ertapenem	Imipenem/Cilastatin	Meropenem
GRAM-NEGATIVE AEROBES (Continued)				
Francisella tularensis				
Haemophilus influenzae	++	++	++	++
Klebsiella species	++	++	++	++
Legionella species				
Moraxella catarrhalis	++	++	++	++
Morganella morganii	++	++	++	++
Neisseria gonorrhoeae	+		+	+
Neisseria meningitidis	++		++	++
Pasturella multocida			++	++
Proteus mirabilis	++	++	++	++
Proteus vulgaris	++	++	++	++
Providencia stuartii	++	++	++	++
Pseudomonas aeruginosa	+++		+++	+++
Rickettsia species				
Salmonella species	++	++	++	++
Serratia species	++	++	++	++
Shigella species	++	++	++	++
Stenotrophomonas maltophilia				

+++ = excellent activity (1st line recommendation). ++ = good activity (2nd line recommendation). + = moderate activity (acceptable in vitro data suggesting some isolates may be sensitive).

Blank = no or insufficient activity or unknown.

† Penicillin sensitive: MIC ≤1.0 mcg/mL;   §§ Penicillin resistant: MIC ≥2.0 mcg/mL.

†† 2nd line against S. typhi.   † Penicillin sensitive: MIC ≤1.0 mcg/mL.

* These are generalizations. There are major differences among countries, areas, and hospitals depending on antibiotic usage patterns.

CARBAPENEMS/MONOBACTAMS (CONTINUED)

ORGANISMS	Aztreonam	Ertapenem	Imipenem/Cilastatin	Meropenem
GRAM-NEGATIVE AEROBES *(Continued)*				
Vibrio vulnificus				
Yersinia enterocolitica	++			
Yersinia pestis				
GRAM-POSITIVE AEROBES				
Enterococcus faecalis		+	++	+
Enterococcus faecium			+	
Enterococcus faecium (VRE)				
Listeria monocytogenes			+	+
Nocardia			++	
Staphylococcus aureus (MSSA)		++	++	++
Staphylococcus aureus (MRSA)				
Staphylococcus epidermidis		++	++	++
Staphylococcus epidermidis (MRSE)				
Streptococcus pneumoniae†		++	++	++
Streptococcus pneumoniae§§		++	++	++

+++ = excellent activity (1st line recommendation). ++ = good activity (2nd line recommendation). + = moderate activity (acceptable in vitro data suggesting some isolates may be sensitive).

Blank = no or insufficient activity, or unknown.   § Penicillin resistant; MIC ≥2.0 mcg/mL.

†† 2nd line against *S. typhi*.   † Penicillin sensitive; MIC ≤1.0 mcg/mL.   §§ Penicillin resistant; MIC ≥2.0 mcg/mL.

*These are generalizations. There are major differences among countries, areas, and hospitals depending on antibiotic usage patterns.

ORGANISMS	Aztreonam	Ertapenem	Imipenem/Cilastatin	Meropenem
GRAM-POSITIVE AEROBES *(Continued)*				
Streptococcus (Group A,B,C,F,G)		++	++	++
Streptococcus species		++	++	++
MISCELLANEOUS				
Chlamydia pneumoniae				
Chlamydia trachomatis				
Ehrlichia/Anaplasma species				
MYCOBACTERIA				
Mycobacterium avium (MAI) (non-HIV)				
Mycoplasma pneumoniae				
SPIROCHETES				
Leptospira interrogans				
Treponema pallidum (syphilis)				

+++ = excellent activity (1st line recommendation).   ++ = good activity (2nd line recommendation).   + = moderate activity (acceptable in vitro data suggesting some isolates may be sensitive).

Blank = no or insufficient activity, or unknown.

† 2nd line against *S. typhi*.   † Penicillin sensitive: MIC ≤1.0 mcg/mL.   §§ Penicillin resistant: MIC ≥2.0 mcg/mL.

*These are generalizations. There are major differences among countries, areas, and hospitals depending on antibiotic usage patterns.

ANTIBIOTIC SENSITIVITY – CEPHALOSPORINS*

ORGANISMS	Cefaclor	Cefadroxil	Cefazolin	Cefdinir	Cefepime	Cefixime	Cefotaxime	Cefoxitin	Cefpodoxime Proxetil	Cefprozil	Ceftazidime	Ceftibuten	Ceftizoxime	Ceftriaxone	Cefuroxime Axetil	Cephalexin
ANAEROBES																
Actinomyces							+						+	++		
Bacillus anthracis																
Bacteroides fragilis								++					+			
Clostridium difficile																
Clostridium species	+		+		+		+	++		+	+		+	+	+	
GRAM-NEGATIVE AEROBES																
Acinetobacter baumannii					++		+				++		+	+		
Aeromonas hydrophila					++	++	++	+			++		++	++	+	
Bartonella henselae																
Bordetella species																
Burkholderia cepacia					+						++		+			
Campylobacter jejuni					+		+							+		
Citrobacter species					+++		++				++		++	++	+	
Coxiella burnetti																
Enterobacter species					+++		+				++		++	++		
Escherichia coli	++	+++	+++	++	++	++	+++	++	++	+++	++	++	++	+++	++	+++

+++ = excellent activity (1st line recommendation). ++ = good activity (2nd line recommendation). + = moderate activity (acceptable in vitro data suggesting some isolates may be sensitive).

Blank = no or insufficient activity, or unknown.

† Penicillin sensitive; MIC ≤1.0 mcg/mL.   §§ Penicillin resistant; MIC ≥2.0 mcg/mL.

†† 2nd line against *S. typhi*.

*These are generalizations. There are major differences among countries, areas, and hospitals depending on antibiotic usage patterns.

ORGANISMS	Cefaclor	Cefadroxil	Cefazolin	Cefdinir	Cefepime	Cefixime	Cefotaxime	Cefoxitin	Cefpodoxime Proxetil	Cefprozil	Ceftazidime	Ceftibuten	Ceftizoxime	Ceftriaxone	Cefuroxime Axetil	Cephalexin
GRAM-NEGATIVE AEROBES *(Continued)*																
Francisella tularensis																
Haemophilus influenzae	++			+++	++	++	+++	++	+++	++	++	++	+++	+++	++	
Klebsiella species	+	++	++	++	++	++	+++	++	++	++	++	++	+++	+++	++	++
Legionella species																
Moraxella catarrhalis	+++	+	+	+++	++	++	+++	+	+++	+++	+	+++	+++	+++	+++	+
Morganella morganii					++	+++	+++	+			++	++	+++	+++	+	
Neisseria gonorrhoeae	+				++	+	++	++	++	+	+	++	++	+++	+	
Neisseria meningitidis					++	++	++				+	++	++	++	++	
Pasturella multocida			+	++	++	++	++		++		++	++	++	++	++	+
Proteus mirabilis	++	++	++	+++	++	++	+++	++	+++	+++	++	+++	+++	+++	+++	++
Proteus vulgaris					++	++	+++	+	+		++	+	+++	+++	++	
Providencia stuartii					+++	++	+++	+	+		+++	+	++	+++	+	
Pseudomonas aeruginosa					+++						+++					
Rickettsia species																
Salmonella species							+++††						+++	+++		
Serratia species				+	+++	+	+++	+	+		++		+++	+++		

+++ = excellent activity (1st line recommendation). ++ = good activity (2nd line recommendation). + = moderate activity (acceptable in vitro data suggesting some isolates may be sensitive).

Blank = no or insufficient activity, or unknown.

†† 2nd line against *S. typhi*. † Penicillin sensitive; MIC ≤1.0 mcg/mL. §§ Penicillin resistant; MIC ≥2.0 mcg/mL.

*These are generalizations. There are major differences among countries, areas, and hospitals depending on antibiotic usage patterns.

CEPHALOSPORINS (CONTINUED)

ORGANISMS	Cefaclor	Cefadroxil	Cefazolin	Cefdinir	Cefepime	Cefixime	Cefotaxime	Cefoxitin	Cefpodoxime Proxetil	Cefprozil	Ceftazidime	Ceftibuten	Ceftizoxime	Ceftriaxone	Cefuroxime Axetil	Cephalexin
GRAM-NEGATIVE AEROBES *(Continued)*																
Shigella species				+	++		++	+	++	+	++	+	++	++	++	
Stenotrophomonas maltophilia											+					
Vibrio vulnificus							++				+++					
Yersinia enterocolitica				++	++	++	++	+	++		++	++	++	++	+	
Yersinia pestis							+							+		
GRAM-POSITIVE AEROBES																
Enterococcus faecalis																
Enterococcus faecium																
Enterococcus faecium (VRE)																
Listeria monocytogenes							++									
Nocardia												+		++	+	
Staphylococcus aureus (MSSA)	+	+++	+++	++	++		++	+	++	+	+		++	++	++	++
Staphylococcus aureus (MRSA)																

+++ = excellent activity (1st line recommendation). ++ = good activity (2nd line recommendation). + = moderate activity (acceptable in vitro data suggesting some isolates may be sensitive).

Blank = no or insufficient activity, or unknown.

†† 2nd line against *S. typhi.* † Penicillin sensitive; MIC ≤1.0 mcg/mL. §§ Penicillin resistant; MIC ≥2.0 mcg/mL.

• These are generalizations. There are major differences among countries, areas, and hospitals depending on antibiotic usage patterns.

ORGANISMS	Cefaclor	Cefadroxil	Cefazolin	Cefdinir	Cefepime	Cefixime	Cefotaxime	Cefoxitin	Cefpodoxime Proxetil	Cefprozil	Ceftazidime	Ceftibuten	Ceftizoxime	Ceftriaxone	Cefuroxime Axetil	Cephalexin
GRAM-POSITIVE AEROBES *(Continued)*																
Staphylococcus epidermidis	+	++	++		+		+	+	+	++			+	+	++	++
Staphylococcus epidermidis (MRSE)																
Streptococcus pneumoniae†	++	++	++	++	++	++	++	+	++	++	+	+	++	++	++	++
Streptococcus pneumoniae§§					+		+++		+				++	+++		
Streptococcus (Group A,B,C,F,G)	++	++	++	++	++	++	++	+	++	++	+	+	++	++	++	++
Streptococcus species	++	++	++	++	++	++	++	+	++	++	+	+	+	++	++	++
MISCELLANEOUS																
Chlamydia pneumoniae																
Chlamydia trachomatis																
Ehrlichia/Anaplasma species																
MYCOBACTERIA																
Mycobacterium avium (MAI) (non-HIV)																

+++ = excellent activity (1st line recommendation).   ++ = good activity (2nd line recommendation).   + = moderate activity (acceptable in vitro data suggesting some isolates may be sensitive).

Blank = no or insufficient activity, or unknown.

†† 2nd line against *S. typhi*.   † Penicillin sensitive; MIC ≤1.0 mcg/mL.   §§ Penicillin resistant; MIC ≥2.0 mcg/mL.

*These are generalizations. There are major differences among countries, areas, and hospitals depending on antibiotic usage patterns.

CEPHALOSPORINS (CONTINUED)

ORGANISMS	Cefaclor	Cefadroxil	Cefazolin	Cefdinir	Cefepime	Cefixime	Cefotaxime	Cefoxitin	Cefpodoxime Proxetil	Cefprozil	Ceftazidime	Ceftibuten	Ceftizoxime	Ceftriaxone	Cefuroxime axetil	Cephalexin
MYCOBACTERIA *(Continued)*																
Mycoplasma pneumoniae														++		
SPIROCHETES																
Leptospira interrogans							++									
Treponema pallidum (syphilis)													+	++		

+++ = excellent activity (1st line recommendation). ++ = good activity (2nd line recommendation). + = moderate activity (acceptable in vitro data suggesting some isolates may be sensitive).

Blank = no or insufficient activity, or unknown.

†† 2nd line against *S. typhi.*   † Penicillin sensitive; MIC <1.0 mcg/mL.   §§ Penicillin resistant; MIC ≥2.0 mcg/mL.

* These are generalizations. There are major differences among countries, areas, and hospitals depending on antibiotic usage patterns.

ORGANISMS	Ciprofloxacin	Gemifloxacin	Levofloxacin	Moxifloxacin	Norfloxacin	Ofloxacin
ANAEROBES						
Actinomyces				+		
Bacillus anthracis	+++		++	++		++
Bacteroides fragilis				+		
Clostridium difficile						
Clostridium species				+		
GRAM-NEGATIVE AEROBES						
Acinetobacter baumannii	++		++	+		+
Aeromonas hydrophila	+++		+++	+++	+	+++
Bartonella henselae	+					
Bordetella species	+		+	+		
Burkholderia cepacia	++		+	+		
Campylobacter jejuni	+++		++	+++	++	++
Citrobacter species	++		++	+	+	+
Coxiella burnetii	++		++			++
Enterobacter species	++		++	++	++	++
Escherichia coli	++		++	++	+++	++

+++ = excellent activity (1st line recommendation).   ++ = good activity (2nd line recommendation).   + = moderate activity (acceptable in vitro data suggesting some isolates may be sensitive).
Blank = no or insufficient activity or unknown.
†† 2nd line against *S. typhi*.   † Penicillin sensitive; MIC ≤1.0 mcg/mL.   §§ Penicillin resistant; MIC ≥2.0 mcg/mL.
*These are generalizations. There are major differences among countries, areas, and hospitals depending on antibiotic usage patterns.

FLUOROQUINOLONES (CONTINUED)

ORGANISMS	Ciprofloxacin	Gemifloxacin	Levofloxacin	Moxifloxacin	Norfloxacin	Ofloxacin
GRAM-NEGATIVE AEROBES *(Continued)*						
Francisella tularensis	++					
Haemophilus influenzae	++	++	++	++		++
Klebsiella species	++	+	++	++	++	++
Legionella species	+++	++	+++	+++		+++
Moraxella catarrhalis	++	++	++	++		++
Morganella morganii	++		++	+	++	+
Neisseria gonorrhoeae	+++		+++	++	+	+++
Neisseria meningitidis	++		++	++		++
Pasturella multocida	++		+	+		+
Proteus mirabilis	++		++	++	+++	++
Proteus vulgaris	++		++	++	+++	++
Providencia stuartii	++		++	+	++	+
Pseudomonas aeruginosa	+++		+++	++	++	++
Rickettsia species	++		++	+		++
Salmonella species	+++	++††	+++	+++	+++	+++
Serratia species	+++		+++	++	++	++
Shigella species	+++		+++	+++	+++	+++
Stenotrophomonas maltophilia	+		+	++	+	+

+++ = excellent activity (1st line recommendation). ++ = good activity (2nd line recommendation). + = moderate activity (acceptable in vitro data suggesting some isolates may be sensitive).

Blank = no or insufficient activity, or unknown.   §§ Penicillin resistant: MIC ≥2.0 mcg/mL.

†† 2nd line against *S. typhi*.   † Penicillin sensitive; MIC ≤1.0 mcg/mL.   § Penicillin resistant: MIC ≥2.0 mcg/mL.

*These are generalizations. There are major differences among countries, areas, and hospitals depending on antibiotic usage patterns.

ORGANISMS	Ciprofloxacin	Gemifloxacin	Levofloxacin	Moxifloxacin	Norfloxacin	Ofloxacin
GRAM-NEGATIVE AEROBES (Continued)						
Vibrio vulnificus	+		+	+		
Yersinia enterocolitica	++		++	++	++	++
Yersinia pestis	+		+			
GRAM-POSITIVE AEROBES						
Enterococcus faecalis	+		++	++	+	+
Enterococcus faecium	+		+	+		+
Enterococcus faecium (VRE)						
Listeria monocytogenes						
Nocardia						
Staphylococcus aureus (MSSA)	+	++	++	++	+	+
Staphylococcus aureus (MRSA)			+	+		
Staphylococcus epidermidis (MSSA)	+		+	+	+	+
Staphylococcus epidermidis (MRSE)	+		+	+		+
Streptococcus pneumoniae†	+	++	++	++		+
Streptococcus pneumoniae§§	+	+++	+++	+++		+

+++ = excellent activity (1st line recommendation). ++ = good activity (2nd line recommendation). + = moderate activity (acceptable in vitro data suggesting some isolates may be sensitive).

Blank = no or insufficient activity, or unknown.

†† 2nd line against *S. typhi.*   † Penicillin sensitive; MIC ≤1.0 mcg/mL.   §§ Penicillin resistant; MIC ≥2.0 mcg/mL.

*These are generalizations. There are major differences among countries, areas, and hospitals depending on antibiotic usage patterns.

FLUOROQUINOLONES (CONTINUED)

ORGANISMS	Ciprofloxacin	Gemifloxacin	Levofloxacin	Moxifloxacin	Norfloxacin	Ofloxacin
GRAM-POSITIVE AEROBES *(Continued)*						
Streptococcus (Group A,B,C,F,G)	+	+	+	+		+
Streptococcus species	+	++	++	++	+	+
MISCELLANEOUS						
Chlamydia pneumoniae	++	++	++	++		++
Chlamydia trachomatis			++	++		++
Ehrlichia/Anaplasma species	+		+			+
MYCOBACTERIA						
Mycobacterium avium (MAI) (non-HIV)	++	++	++	++		++
Mycoplasma pneumoniae	++	++	++	++		++
SPIROCHETES						
Leptospira interrogans						
Treponema pallidum (syphilis)						

+++ = excellent activity (1st line recommendation).   ++ = good activity (2nd line recommendation).   + = moderate activity (acceptable in vitro data suggesting some isolates may be sensitive).

Blank = no or insufficient activity, or unknown.

† Penicillin sensitive; MIC ≤1.0 mcg/mL.   §§ Penicillin resistant; MIC ≥2.0 mcg/mL.

* 2nd line against *S. typhi.*   †† 2nd line against *S. typhi.*

*These are generalizations. There are major differences among countries, areas, and hospitals depending on antibiotic usage patterns.

ANTIBIOTIC SENSITIVITY – MACROLIDES & CLINDAMYCIN*

ORGANISMS	Azithromycin	Clarithromycin	Clindamycin	Erythromycin	Telithromycin
ANAEROBES					
Actinomyces	++	++	++	++	
Bacillus anthracis		+	++	+	
Bacteroides fragilis			++		
Clostridium difficile			++		
Clostridium species					
GRAM-NEGATIVE AEROBES					
Acinetobacter baumannii					
Aeromonas hydrophila					
Bartonella henselae	+++	+++		+++	
Bordetella species	+++	+++		+++	++
Burkholderia cepacia					
Campylobacter jejuni	+++	+++	++	+++	
Citrobacter species					
Coxiella burnetii				+	
Enterobacter species					
Escherichia coli					

+++ = excellent activity (1st recommendation).   ++ = good activity (2nd line recommendation).   + = moderate activity (acceptable in vitro data suggesting some isolates may be sensitive).

Blank = no or insufficient activity, or unknown.

† Penicillin sensitive; MIC ≤1.0 mcg/mL.   §§ Penicillin resistant; MIC ≥2.0 mcg/mL.

†† 2nd line against S. typhi.

*These are generalizations. There are major differences among countries, areas, and hospitals depending on antibiotic usage patterns.

MACROLIDES & CLINDAMYCIN (CONTINUED)

ORGANISMS	Azithromycin	Clarithromycin	Clindamycin	Erythromycin	Telithromycin
GRAM-NEGATIVE AEROBES *(Continued)*					
Francisella tularensis					
Haemophilus influenzae	++	++		+	++
Klebsiella species					
Legionella species	+++	+++		++	++
Moraxella catarrhalis	+++	+++		++	++
Morganella morganii					
Neisseria gonorrhoeae	++			+	
Neisseria meningitidis					
Pasturella multocida	+				
Proteus mirabilis					
Proteus vulgaris					
Providencia stuartii					
Pseudomonas aeruginosa					
Rickettsia species				+	+
Salmonella species	++				
Serratia species					
Shigella species	+				
Stenotrophomonas maltophilia					

+++ = excellent activity (1st line recommendation). ++ = good activity (2nd line recommendation). + = moderate activity (acceptable in vitro data suggesting some isolates may be sensitive).
Blank = no or insufficient activity, or unknown. † Penicillin sensitive; MIC ≤1.0 mcg/mL. §§ Penicillin resistant; MIC ≥2.0 mcg/mL.
†† 2nd line against *S. typhi*.
*These are generalizations. There are major differences among countries, areas, and hospitals depending on antibiotic usage patterns.

ORGANISMS	Azithromycin	Clarithromycin	Clindamycin	Erythromycin	Telithromycin
GRAM-NEGATIVE AEROBES *(Continued)*					
Vibrio vulnificus					
Yersinia enterocolitica					
Yersinia pestis					
GRAM-POSITIVE AEROBES					
Enterococcus faecalis					
Enterococcus faecium					
Enterococcus faecium (VRE)					
Listeria monocytogenes				++	
Nocardia	++	++	++	+	++
Staphylococcus aureus (MSSA)			++		
Staphylococcus aureus (MRSA)	+	+	++	+	
Staphylococcus epidermidis	+	+	++	+	
Staphylococcus epidermidis (MRSE)	++	++	++	++	++
Streptococcus pneumoniae†			++		+++
Streptococcus pneumoniae§§	++	++	++	++	++

+++ = excellent activity (1st line recommendation). ++ = good activity (2nd line recommendation). + = moderate activity (acceptable in vitro data suggesting some isolates may be sensitive).
Blank = no or insufficient activity, or unknown.
†† 2nd line against *S. typhi*.   † Penicillin sensitive; MIC ≤1.0 mcg/mL.   §§ Penicillin resistant; MIC ≥2.0 mcg/mL.
* These are generalizations. There are major differences among countries, areas, and hospitals depending on antibiotic usage patterns.

A133

MACROLIDES & CLINDAMYCIN (CONTINUED)

ORGANISMS	Azithromycin	Clarithromycin	Clindamycin	Erythromycin	Telithromycin
GRAM-POSITIVE AEROBES (Continued)					
Streptococcus (Group A,B,C,F,G)	++	++	++	++	
Streptococcus species					
MISCELLANEOUS					
Chlamydia pneumoniae	+++	+++		+++	++
Chlamydia trachomatis	+++	++	++	++	
Ehrlichia/Anaplasma species	++	+++			
MYCOBACTERIA					
Mycobacterium avium (MAI) (non-HIV)	+++	+++		+++	++
Mycoplasma pneumoniae				++	
SPIROCHETES					
Leptospira interrogans	+				
Treponema pallidum (syphilis)				+	

+++ = excellent activity (1st line recommendation).   ++ = good activity (2nd line recommendation).   + = moderate activity (acceptable in vitro data suggesting some isolates may be sensitive).

Blank = no or insufficient activity, or unknown.

†† 2nd line against *S. typhi.*   † Penicillin-sensitive, MIC ≤1.0 mcg/mL.   §§ Penicillin resistant; MIC ≥2.0 mcg/mL.

*These are generalizations. There are major differences among countries, areas, and hospitals depending on antibiotic usage patterns.

ANTIBIOTIC SENSITIVITY – PENICILLINS*

ORGANISMS	Amoxicillin	Amoxicillin + Clavulanate	Ampicillin	Ampicillin + Sulbactam	Dicloxacillin	Nafcillin/ Oxacillin	Penicillin	Piperacillin	Piperacillin + Tazobactam	Ticarcillin + Clavulanic Acid
ANAEROBES										
Actinomyces	+++	++	+++	++			+++			
Bacillus anthracis	++	+	++	+			++			
Bacteroides fragilis		+++		+++				+	+++	+++
Clostridium difficile										
Clostridium species	++	++	++	++			+++	++	++	++
GRAM-NEGATIVE AEROBES										
Acinetobacter baumannii				++				+	++	++
Aeromonas hydrophila								+	+	+
Bartonella henselae										
Bordetella species										
Burkholderia cepacia								+	+	+
Campylobacter jejuni	++	+								+
Citrobacter species								++	++	++
Coxiella burnetti										
Enterobacter species								++	++	++
Escherichia coli	+++	++	+++	++				++	++	++

+++ = excellent activity (1st line recommendation).   ++ = good activity (2nd line recommendation).   + = moderate activity (acceptable in vitro data suggesting some isolates may be sensitive).

Blank = no or insufficient activity, or unknown.

†† 2nd line against *S. typhi*.   † Penicillin sensitive; MIC ≤1.0 mcg/mL.   §§ Penicillin resistant; MIC ≥2.0 mcg/mL.

* These are generalizations. There are major differences among countries, areas, and hospitals depending on antibiotic usage patterns.

PENICILLINS (CONTINUED)

ORGANISMS	Amoxicillin	Amoxicillin + Clavulanate	Ampicillin	Ampicillin + Sulbactam	Dicloxacillin	Nafcillin/ Oxacillin	Penicillin	Piperacillin	Piperacillin + Tazobactam	Ticarcillin + Clavulanic Acid
GRAM-NEGATIVE AEROBES (Continued)										
Francisella tularensis										
Haemophilus influenzae	+	+++	+	++						++
Klebsiella species		++		++				++	++	++
Legionella species										
Moraxella catarrhalis		+++		++					++	++
Morganella morganii		++						++	++	++
Neisseria gonorrhoeae		++		++					++	++
Neisseria meningitidis	+	++	++	++			++	++	++	++
Pasteurella multocida	++	+++	++	++			+++	++	++	++
Proteus mirabilis	+++	++	+++	++				++	++	++
Proteus vulgaris								++	++	++
Providencia stuartii								++	++	++
Pseudomonas aeruginosa								+++	+++	++
Rickettsia species										
Salmonella species	+	++	+	++				++	++	++
Serratia species		++						++	++	++
Shigella species	++	++	++					+	+	+

+++ = excellent activity (1st line recommendation).   ++ = good activity (2nd line recommendation).   + = moderate activity (acceptable in vitro data suggesting some isolates may be sensitive).

Blank = no or insufficient activity, or unknown.

† Penicillin sensitive; MIC ≤1.0 mcg/mL.   §§ Penicillin resistant; MIC ≥2.0 mcg/mL.

†† 2nd line against *S. typhi*.   ‡ Penicillin sensitive; MIC ≤1.0 mcg/mL.

*These are generalizations. There are major differences among countries, areas, and hospitals depending on antibiotic usage patterns.

ORGANISMS	Amoxicillin	Amoxicillin + Clavulanate	Ampicillin	Ampicillin + Sulbactam	Dicloxacillin	Nafcillin/ Oxacillin	Penicillin	Piperacillin	Piperacillin + Tazobactam	Ticarcillin + Clavulanic Acid
GRAM-NEGATIVE AEROBES (Continued)										
Stenotrophomonas maltophilia								+	+	++
Vibrio vulnificus				++					++	
Yersinia enterocolitica		+		++				++	++	++
Yersinia pestis	+		+							
GRAM-POSITIVE AEROBES										
Enterococcus faecalis	+++	++	+++	++			+++	++	++	++
Enterococcus faecium	+	+	+	+			+	+	+	
Enterococcus faecium (VRE)										
Listeria monocytogenes	+++	++	+++	++			++	++	++	++
Nocardia	+	++	+	++						
Staphylococcus aureus (MSSA)		++		++	+++	+++			++	++
Staphylococcus aureus (MRSA)										
Staphylococcus epidermidis		++		++	+++	+++			++	++
Staphylococcus epidermidis (MRSE)										
Streptococcus pneumoniae†	+++	++	++	++	+	+	+++	++	++	++
Streptococcus pneumoniae§§	++	++	++	++			++	+	+	+

+++ = excellent activity (1st line recommendation).   ++ = good activity (2nd line recommendation).   + = moderate activity (acceptable in vitro data suggesting some isolates may be sensitive).

Blank = no or insufficient activity, or unknown.

†† 2nd line against S. typhi.   † Penicillin sensitive; MIC ≤1.0 mcg/mL.   §§ Penicillin resistant; MIC ≥2.0 mcg/mL.

*These are generalizations. There are major differences among countries, areas, and hospitals depending on antibiotic usage patterns.

PENICILLINS (CONTINUED)

ORGANISMS	Amoxicillin	Amoxicillin + Clavulanate	Ampicillin	Ampicillin + Subbactam	Dicloxacillin	Nafcillin/ Oxacillin	Penicillin	Piperacillin	Piperacillin + Tazobactam	Ticarcillin + Clavulanic Acid
GRAM-POSITIVE AEROBES (Continued)										
Streptococcus (Group A,B,C,F,G)	+++	+	+++	+	+	+	+++	+	+	+
Streptococcus species	+++	+	++	+	+	+	+++	++	+	+
MISCELLANEOUS										
Chlamydia pneumoniae										
Chlamydia trachomatis										
Ehrlichia/Anaplasma species										
MYCOBACTERIA										
Mycobacterium avium (MAI) (non-HIV)										
Mycoplasma pneumoniae										
SPIROCHETES										
Leptospira interrogans	++		+++				+++			
Treponema pallidum (syphilis)	++		++				+++			

+++ = excellent activity (1st line recommendation).   ++ = good activity (2nd line recommendation).   + = moderate activity (acceptable in vitro data suggesting some isolates may be sensitive).

Blank = no or insufficient activity, or unknown.

†† 2nd line against *S. typhi.*   † Penicillin sensitive; MIC ≤1.0 mcg/mL.   §§ Penicillin resistant; MIC ≥2.0 mcg/mL.

*These are generalizations. There are major differences among countries, areas, and hospitals depending on antibiotic usage patterns.

ANTIBIOTIC SENSITIVITY – SULFONAMIDES*

ORGANISMS	Trimethoprim + Sulfamethoxazole
ANAEROBES	
Actinomyces	
Bacillus anthracis	
Bacteroides fragilis	
Clostridium difficile	
Clostridium species	
GRAM-NEGATIVE AEROBES	
Acinetobacter baumannii	+
Aeromonas hydrophila	++
Bartonella henselae	
Bordetella species	++
Burkholderia cepacia	+++
Campylobacter jejuni	
Citrobacter species	++
Coxiella burnetti	
Enterobacter species	++

ANTIBIOTIC SENSITIVITY – TETRACYCLINES*

ORGANISMS	Doxycycline	Minocycline	Tetracycline
ANAEROBES			
Actinomyces	++	++	++
Bacillus anthracis	++		++
Bacteroides fragilis	+		+
Clostridium difficile			
Clostridium species	+		+
GRAM-NEGATIVE AEROBES			
Acinetobacter baumannii	++	++	++
Aeromonas hydrophila	++	++	++
Bartonella henselae	+++	++	++
Bordetella species	+		+
Burkholderia cepacia		++	
Campylobacter jejuni	++	++	++
Citrobacter species			
Coxiella burnetti	+++	+++	+++
Enterobacter species			

+++ = excellent activity (1st line recommendation). ++ = good activity (2nd line recommendation). + = moderate activity (acceptable in vitro data suggesting some isolates may be sensitive).
Blank = no or insufficient activity, or unknown.
†† 2nd line against *S. typhi.*   † Penicillin sensitive; MIC ≤1.0 mcg/mL.   §§ Penicillin resistant; MIC ≥2.0 mcg/mL.
*These are generalizations. There are major differences among countries, areas, and hospitals depending on antibiotic usage patterns.

SULFONAMIDES (CONTINUED)

ORGANISMS	Trimethoprim + Sulfamethoxazole
GRAM-NEGATIVE AEROBES (Continued)	
Escherichia coli	+++
Francisella tularensis	
Haemophilus influenzae	+++
Klebsiella species	+++**
Legionella species	++
Moraxella catarrhalis	+++
Morganella morganii	
Neisseria gonorrhoeae	
Neisseria meningitidis	
Pasturella multocida	++
Proteus mirabilis	++
Proteus vulgaris	++
Providencia stuartii	++
Pseudomonas aeruginosa	
Rickettsia species	
Salmonella species	++
Serratia species	+

TETRACYCLINES (CONTINUED)

ORGANISMS	Doxycycline	Minocycline	Tetracycline
GRAM-NEGATIVE AEROBES (Continued)			
Escherichia coli	+	+	+
Francisella tularensis	++	++	++
Haemophilus influenzae	++	++	++
Klebsiella species	+	+	
Legionella species	++	++	++
Moraxella catarrhalis	++	++	++
Morganella morganii	++	++	++
Neisseria gonorrhoeae	+	+	+
Neisseria meningitidis	+	+	+
Pasturella multocida	++	++	++
Proteus mirabilis	+	+	+
Proteus vulgaris	+	+	+
Providencia stuartii			
Pseudomonas aeruginosa			
Rickettsia species	+++	+++	+++
Salmonella species	+	+	+
Serratia species			

+++ = excellent activity (1st line recommendation).   ++ = good activity (2nd line recommendation).   + = moderate activity (acceptable in vitro data suggesting some isolates may be sensitive).

Blank = no or insufficient activity, or unknown.   §§ Penicillin resistant; MIC ≥2.0 mcg/mL.

†† 2nd line against S. typhi.   † Penicillin sensitive; MIC ≤1.0 mcg/mL.

*These are generalizations. There are major differences among countries, areas, and hospitals depending on antibiotic usage patterns.

ORGANISMS	Trimethoprim + Sulfamethoxazole	Doxycycline	Minocycline	Tetracycline
GRAM-NEGATIVE AEROBES (Continued)				
Shigella species	++	+	+	+
Stenotrophomonas maltophilia	+++		+	
Vibrio vulnificus		+++	+++	+++
Yersinia enterocolitica	+++			
Yersinia pestis	+	++	++	++
GRAM-POSITIVE AEROBES				
Enterococcus faecalis		+	+	+
Enterococcus faecium				
Enterococcus faecium (VRE)		+	+	+
Listeria monocytogenes	++	+	+	+
Nocardia	+++	++	++	+
Staphylococcus aureus (MSSA)	++	++	++	+
Staphylococcus aureus (MRSA)	++	++	++	+
Staphylococcus epidermidis	++	++	++	+
Staphylococcus epidermidis (MRSE)	++	++	++	++
Streptococcus pneumoniae†	++	++	++	++

+++ = excellent activity (1st line recommendation). ++ = good activity (2nd line recommendation). + = moderate activity (acceptable in vitro data suggesting some isolates may be sensitive).

Blank = no or insufficient activity, or unknown.

†† 2nd line against *S. typhi.*   † Penicillin sensitive; MIC ≤1.0 mcg/mL.   §§ Penicillin resistant; MIC ≥2.0 mcg/mL.

*These are generalizations. There are major differences among countries, areas, and hospitals depending on antibiotic usage patterns.

ANTIBIOTIC SENSITIVITY – SULFONAMIDES AND TETRACYCLINES

SULFONAMIDES (CONTINUED)

ORGANISMS	Trimethoprim + Sulfamethoxazole
GRAM-POSITIVE AEROBES *(Continued)*	
Streptococcus pneumoniae§§	
Streptococcus (Group A,B,C,F,G)	++
Streptococcus species	++
MISCELLANEOUS	
Chlamydia pneumoniae	
Chlamydia trachomatis	+
Ehrlichia/Anaplasma species	
MYCOBACTERIA	
Mycobacterium avium (MAI) (non-HIV)	
Mycoplasma pneumoniae	
SPIROCHETES	
Leptospira interrogans	
Treponema pallidum (syphilis)	

TETRACYCLINES (CONTINUED)

ORGANISMS	Doxycycline	Minocycline	Tetracycline
GRAM-POSITIVE AEROBES *(Continued)*			
Streptococcus pneumoniae§§	+	+	+
Streptococcus (Group A,B,C,F,G)	+	+	+
Streptococcus species	+	+	+
MISCELLANEOUS			
Chlamydia pneumoniae	+++	+++	+++
Chlamydia trachomatis	+++	+++	+++
Ehrlichia/Anaplasma species	+++	+++	+++
MYCOBACTERIA			
Mycobacterium avium (MAI) (non-HIV)			
Mycoplasma pneumoniae	++	++	++
SPIROCHETES			
Leptospira interrogans	++	++	++
Treponema pallidum (syphilis)	++	++	++

+++ = excellent activity (1st line recommendation). ++ = good activity (2nd line recommendation). + = moderate activity (acceptable in vitro data suggesting some isolates may be sensitive).
Blank = no or insufficient activity, or unknown.
†† 2nd line against *S. typhi.*   † Penicillin sensitive; MIC ≤1.0 mcg/mL.   §§ Penicillin resistant; MIC ≥2.0 mcg/mL.
*These are generalizations. There are major differences among countries, areas, and hospitals depending on antibiotic usage patterns.

ANTIBIOTIC SENSITIVITY – MISCELLANEOUS*

ORGANISMS	Chloramphenicol	Colistin	Daptomycin	Fosfomycin	Linezolid	Metronidazole	Nitrofurantoin	Quinupristin + Dalfopristin	Rifampin	Vancomycin
ANAEROBES										
Actinomyces										+
Bacillus anthracis	++							+	++	++
Bacteroides fragilis	++					+++		+		
Clostridium difficile					+	+++			+	++
Clostridium species	++				+	++		+		+
GRAM-NEGATIVE AEROBES										
Aeromonas hydrophila	+									
Bartonella henselae	+								++	
Bordetella species	+								+	
Burkholderia cepacia	++								+	
Campylobacter jejuni	++									
Citrobacter species		+		+			++			
Coxiella burnetti	+								++	
Enterobacter species		+		+						
Escherichia coli	+	+		++			++		+	
Francisella tularensis	++									

+++ = excellent activity (1st line recommendation). ++ = good activity (2nd line recommendation). + = moderate activity (acceptable in vitro data suggesting some isolates may be sensitive).

Blank = no or insufficient activity, or unknown.

†† 2nd line against S. typhi.   † Penicillin Sensitive; MIC ≤1.0 mcg/mL.   §§ Penicillin resistant; MIC ≥2.0 mcg/mL.

*These are generalizations. There are major differences among countries, areas, and hospitals depending on antibiotic usage patterns.

MISCELLANEOUS (CONTINUED)

ORGANISMS	Chloramphenicol	Colistin	Daptomycin	Fosfomycin	Linezolid	Metronidazole	Nitrofurantoin	Quinupristin + Dalfopristin	Rifampin	Vancomycin
GRAM-NEGATIVE AEROBES (Continued)										
Haemophilus influenzae	++								+	
Klebsiella species	+	+								
Legionella species				+					++	
Moraxella catarrhalis	++							+	+	
Morganella morganii				+			+			
Neisseria gonorrhoeae	++			+				+	++	
Neisseria meningitidis	++							+	++	
Pasturella multocida									+	
Proteus mirabilis				++			++		+	
Proteus vulgaris				+			+		+	
Providencia stuartii				+			++			
Pseudomonas aeruginosa	+	++								
Rickettsia species	++								+	
Salmonella species	++	+								
Serratia species	+			+			+		+	
Shigella species	++	+								
Stenotrophomonas maltophilia	+	+								

+++ = excellent activity (1st line recommendation). ++ = good activity (2nd line recommendation). + = moderate activity (acceptable in vitro data suggesting some isolates may be sensitive).
Blank = no or insufficient activity, or unknown.
†† 2nd line against *S. typhi*.   † Penicillin sensitive; MIC ≤1.0 mcg/mL.   §§ Penicillin resistant; MIC ≥2.0 mcg/mL.
*These are generalizations. There are major differences among countries, areas, and hospitals depending on antibiotic usage patterns.

ORGANISMS	Chloramphenicol	Colistin	Daptomycin	Fosfomycin	Linezolid	Metronidazole	Nitrofurantoin	Quinupristin + Dalfopristin	Rifampin	Vancomycin
GRAM-NEGATIVE AEROBES *(Continued)*										
Vibrio vulnificus										
Yersinia enterocolitica	++									
Yersinia pestis	++									
GRAM-POSITIVE AEROBES										
Enterococcus faecalis	+			++	++		++			++
Enterococcus faecium	++		++	++	+++		++	++	+	+++
Enterococcus faecium (VRE)	++		++	+	+++		++	+++	+	
Listeria monocytogenes	++				+			+		+
Nocardia					+					
Staphylococcus aureus (MSSA)	+		++		++		++	++	++	++
Staphylococcus aureus (MRSA)	+		++		++		+	++	++	+++
Staphylococcus epidermidis	+		++		++		++	++	++	+++
Staphylococcus epidermidis (MRSE)	+		++		++		+	++		+++
Streptococcus pneumoniae†	+		++		++			++	++	++
Streptococcus pneumoniae§§	+		++		++			++	++	+++

+++ = excellent activity (1st line recommendation). ++ = good activity (2nd line recommendation). + = moderate activity (acceptable in vitro data suggesting some isolates may be sensitive).

Blank = no or insufficient activity, or unknown.

†† 2nd line against *S. typhi.*   † Penicillin sensitive; MIC ≤1.0 mcg/mL.   §§ Penicillin resistant; MIC ≥2.0 mcg/mL.

*These are generalizations. There are major differences among countries, areas, and hospitals depending on antibiotic usage patterns.

MISCELLANEOUS (CONTINUED)

ORGANISMS	Chloramphenicol	Colistin	Daptomycin	Fosfomycin	Linezolid	Metronidazole	Nitrofurantoin	Quinupristin + Dalfopristin	Rifampin	Vancomycin
GRAM-POSITIVE AEROBES (Continued)										
Streptococcus (Group A,B,C,F,G)	+		+		++			++	+	++
Streptococcus species	++		+		++			+	+	++
MISCELLANEOUS										
Chlamydia pneumoniae								+	+	
Chlamydia trachomatis							+		+	
Ehrlichia/Anaplasma species	++								++	
MYCOBACTERIA										
Mycobacterium avium (MAI) (non-HIV)					+				++	
Mycoplasma pneumoniae								+		
SPIROCHETES										
Leptospira interrogans										
Treponema pallidum (syphilis)	++									

+++ = excellent activity (1st line recommendation).   ++ = good activity (2nd line recommendation).   + = moderate activity (acceptable in vitro data suggesting some isolates may be sensitive).

Blank = no or insufficient activity, or unknown.

†† 2nd line against S. typhi.   † Penicillin sensitive; MIC ≤1.0 mcg/mL.   §§ Penicillin resistant; MIC ≥2.0 mcg/mL.

*These are generalizations. There are major differences among countries, areas, and hospitals depending on antibiotic usage patterns.

ANTIBIOTICS: NEONATAL RECOMMENDED CONCENTRATIONS FOR ADMINISTRATION

| GENERIC NAME | ROUTE | UNITS | CONCENTRATION | | | |
			AVAILABLE	DEFAULT	HIGH	LOW
Acyclovir	IV	mg/mL	50*	7	7	5
Amikacin	IV	mg/mL	50*	10	10	5
Amikacin	IM	mg/mL	50	50	50	10
Amphotericin B	IV	mg/mL	5*	0.1	0.1	0.05
Amphotericin B Lipid Complex	IV	mg/mL	5*	2	2	0.5
Amphotericin B Liposome	IV	mg/mL	4*	2	2	1
Ampicillin	IV	mg/mL	125 or 250*	50	100	20
Ampicillin	IM	mg/mL	250	250	250	125
Azithromycin	IV	mg/mL	100*	2	2	2
Aztreonam	IV	mg/mL	50	50	66	20
Aztreonam	IM	mg/mL	125 or 250	167	333	83
Caspofungin	IV	mg/mL	5.2*	0.2	0.5	0.2
Cefepime	IV	mg/mL	100	100	160	100
Cefepime	IM	mg/mL	280	280	280	160
Cefazolin	IV	mg/mL	225*	100	125	20
Cefazolin	IM	mg/mL	225	330	330	100
Cefotaxime	IV	mg/mL	50 or 100	50	100	25
Cefotaxime	IM	mg/mL	230 or 300	300	330	100
Cefoxitin	IV	mg/mL	100*	40	100	20
Ceftazidime	IV	mg/mL	50	100	200	50
Ceftazidime	IM	mg/mL	200	200	100	50
Ceftriaxone	IV	mg/mL	40 or 100*	40	40	20
Ceftriaxone	IM	mg/mL	250	250	250	100
Chloramphenicol	IV	mg/mL	100*	10	100	5
Clindamycin	IV	mg/mL	150*	10	18	6
Erythromycin Lactobionate	IV	mg/mL	50*	5	5	1
Fluconazole	IV	mg/mL	2	2	2	2
Ganciclovir	IV	mg/mL	50*	5	10	5
Gentamicin	IV	mg/mL	10	10	10	2
Gentamicin	IM	mg/mL	40	10	40	10
Imipenem - Cilastatin	IV	mg/mL	2.5 or 5	5	5	2.5
Linezolid	IV	mg/mL	2	2	2	2
Meropenem	IV	mg/mL	50	50	50	25
Metronidazole	IV	mg/mL	5	5	5	5
Nafcillin	IV	mg/mL	250*	40	40	20
Netilmicin	IM	mg/mL	100*	5	100	2.5
Oxacillin	IV	mg/mL	50	25	100	25
Penicillin G	IV	U/mL	500,000	100,000	500,000	50,000
Piperacillin	IV	mg/mL	200	100	200	50
Piperacillin	IM	mg/mL	400	300	400	100
Piperacillin - Tazobactam	IV	mg/mL	200	100	200	50
Rifampin	IV	mg/mL	60*	3	6	3
Ticarcillin -Clavulanate	IV	mg/mL	200	50	100	10
Tobramycin	IV	mg/mL	10	10	10	2
Tobramycin	IM	mg/mL	40	40	40	10
Vancomycin	IV	mg/mL	50*	5	5	2.5
Zidovudine (ZDV, AZT)	IV	mg/mL	10*	4	4	2

* See Special Considerations/Preparation section in the NeoFax drug profile for dilution details.
Adapted from *NeoFax 2008*.

ANTIBIOTICS: ORAL

DRUG	BRAND	FORMULATIONS (mg or mg/5mL)*
CEPHALOSPORINS		
Cefaclor	Cefaclor	**Cap:** 250, 500 **Sus:** 125, 187, 250, 375
	Cefaclor ER	**Tab, ER:** 500
Cefadroxil	Duricef	**Cap:** 500 **Sus:** 125, 250, 500 **Tab:** 1g
Cefdinir	Omnicef	**Cap:** 300 **Sus:** 125, 250
Cefditoren	Spectracef	**Tab:** 200
Cefixime	Suprax	**Sus:** 100
Cefpodoxime	Vantin	**Sus:** 50, 100 **Tab:** 100, 200
Cefprozil	Cefzil	**Sus:** 125, 250 **Tab:** 250, 500
Ceftibuten	Cedax	**Cap:** 400 **Sus:** 90
Cefuroxime	Ceftin	**Sus:** 125, 250 **Tab:** 125, 250, 500
Cephalexin	Keflex	**Cap:** 250, 500, 750
	Panixine	**Tab, Dispersible:** 125mg, 250mg
FLUOROQUINOLONES		
Ciprofloxacin**	Cipro	**Sus:** 250, 500 **Tab:** 100, 250, 500, 750
	Cipro XR	**Tab, ER:** 500, 1000
	ProQuin XR	**Tab, ER:** 500
Gemifloxacin	Factive	**Tab:** 320
Levofloxacin**	Levaquin	**Sol:** 125 **Tab:** 250, 500, 750
Lomefloxacin	Maxaquin	**Tab:** 400mg
Moxifloxacin	Avelox	**Tab:** 400
Norfloxacin	Noroxin	**Tab:** 400
Ofloxacin	Floxin	**Tab:** 200, 300, 400
MACROLIDES		
Azithromycin**	Zithromax	**Sus:** 100, 200, 1g/pkt **Tab:** 250, 500, 600
	Zmax	**Sus, ER:** 2g
Clarithromycin	Biaxin	**Sus:** 125, 250 **Tab:** 250, 500
	Biaxin XL	**Tab, ER:** 500
Dirithromycin		**Tab:** 250
Erythromycin ethylsuccinate	E.E.S.	**Sus:** 200, 400 **Tab:** 400
	EryPed	**Sus:** 100, 200, 400 **Tab, Chewable Tab:** 200
	Eryc	**Cap, DR:** 250
	Ery-Tab	**Tab, DR:** 250, 333, 500
	Erythromycin Base	**Tab:** 250mg, 500mg
	Erythromycin Delayed-Release	**Cap: Delayed-Release:** 250mg
	PCE	**Tab:** 333, 500
PENICILLINS		
Amoxicillin	Amoxil	**Cap:** 250, 500 **Chew, Tab:** 200, 400 **Drops:** 50mg/mL **Sus:** 125, 200, 250, 400 **Tab:** 500, 875

(Continued)

DRUG	BRAND	FORMULATIONS (mg or mg/5mL)*
PENICILLINS *(Continued)*		
	DisperMox	**Tab, Dispersible:** 200, 400, 600
Ampicillin	Principen	**Cap:** 250, 500 **Sus:** 125, 250
Carbenicillin	Geocillin	**Tab:** 382
Dicloxacillin	Dicloxacillin Sodium	**Cap:** 125, 250, 500 **Sus:** 62.5
Penicillin V	Veetids	**Sus:** 125, 250 **Tab:** 250, 500
TETRACYCLINES		
Demeclocycline	Declomycin	**Tab:** 150, 300
Doxycycline	Doryx	**Cap:** 75, 100
	Monodox	**Cap:** 50, 100
	Periostat	**Tab:** 20
	Vibramycin	**Cap:** 50, 100 **Syr:** 50 **Sus:** 25
	Vibra-Tabs	**Tab:** 100
Minocycline**	Minocin	**Cap:** 50, 100
	Dynacin	**Cap:** 50, 75, 100 **Tab:** 50, 75, 100
	Solodyn	**Tab, Extended Release:** 45, 90, 135
Tetracycline	Sumycin	**Sus:** 125 **Tab:** 250, 500
OTHER		
Clindamycin**	Cleocin	**Cap:** 75, 150, 300 **Sus:** 75
Dapsone	Dapsone	**Tab:** 25, 100
Fosfomycin	Monurol	**Powder:** 3g/packet
Linezolid**	Zyvox	**Sus:** 100 **Tab:** 400, 600
Methanamine	Hiprex	**Tab:** 1g
Metronidazole	Flagyl	**Cap:** 375 **Tab:** 250, 500
	Flagyl ER	**Tab, ER:** 750
Nitrofurantoin	Furadantin	**Sus:** 25
	Macrobid	**Cap:** 100
	Macrodantin	**Cap:** 25, 50, 100
Telithromycin	Ketek	**Tab:** 300, 400
Trimethoprim	Primsol	**Sol:** 50
Vancomycin**	Vancocin	**Cap:** 125, 250
COMBINATIONS		
Erythromycin ethylsuccinate/ Sulfisoxazole	Pediazole	**Sus:** 200/600
Amoxicillin/Clavulanate	Augmentin	**Chew, Tab:** 125/31.25, 250/62.5, 200/28.5, 400/57 **Sus:** 125/31.2, 200/28.5, 400/57, 250/62.5 **Tab:** 250/125, 500/125, 875/125
	Augmentin ES 600	**Sus:** 600/42.9
	Augmentin XR	**Tab, ER:** 1000/62.5
Sulfamethoxazole/ Trimethoprim	Bactrim, Septra**	**Tab:** 400/80 **Sus:** (Septra) 200/40
	Bactrim DS, Septra DS	**Tab, DS:** 800/160
* Unless otherwise indicated.	**Injection formulation available.	

ANTIBIOTICS: SYSTEMIC

BRAND NAME (Generic)	DOSAGE FORM/ STRENGTH	INDICATIONS	ADULT DOSE	PEDIATRIC DOSE
AMINOGLYCOSIDES				
Amikacin (amikacin sulfate)	**Inj:** 50mg/mL, 250mg/mL	Short-term treatment of serious infections caused by gram-negative bacteria such as septicemia, and respiratory tract, bone/joint, CNS (including meningitis), skin and soft tissue, and intra-abdominal infections; burns and postoperative infections; complicated and recurrent urinary tract infections (UTI); and staphylococcal disease.	(IM/IV)15mg/kg/day given q8h or q12h. Max: 15mg/kg/day. Heavier Weight Patients: Max: 1.5g/day. Recurrent Uncomplicated UTI: 250mg bid. Duration: 7-10 days. Stop therapy if no response after 3-5 days. Reduce dose if suspect renal dysfunction. Discontinue if azotemia increases or if a progressive decrease in urinary output occurs.	15mg/kg/day given bid-tid. Newborns: LD: 10mg/kg. MD: 7.5mg/kg q12h. Duration: 7-10 days.
Amikacin Pediatric (amikacin sulfate)	**Inj:** 50mg/mL	Short-term treatment of serious infections caused by gram-negative bacteria such as septicemia, and respiratory tract, bone/joint, CNS (including meningitis), skin and soft tissue, and intra-abdominal infections; burns and postoperative infections; complicated and recurrent urinary tract infections (UTI); and staphylococcal disease.		15mg/kg/day given bid-tid. Newborns: LD: 10mg/kg. MD: 7.5mg/kg q12h. Duration: 7-10 days.
Gentamicin sulfate	**Inj:** 10mg/mL, 40mg/mL	Treatment of bacterial neonatal sepsis, bacterial septicemia, and serious bacterial infections of the CNS (meningitis), urinary tract, respiratory tract, gastrointestinal tract (including peritonitis), skin, bone and soft tissue (including burns) caused by susceptible strains of microorganisms.	(IM/IV) Serious Infections: 3mg/kg/day given q8h. Life-Threatening Infections: 5mg/kg/day tid-qid; reduce to 3mg/kg/day as soon as clinically indicated. Treat for 7-10 days; may need longer course in difficult and complicated infections. Renal Impairment: Reduced dose given q8h or usual dose given at prolonged intervals based on either CrCl or serum creatinine. Dialysis: 1-1.7mg/kg, depending on severity of infection, at end of each dialysis period. Obese Patients: Calculate dose based on estimated lean body mass.	6-7.5mg/kg/day (2-2.5mg/kg given q8h). Infants and Neonates: 7.5mg/kg/day (2.5mg/kg given q8h). Premature and Full-Term Neonates 1 week: 5mg/kg/day (2.5mg/kg given q12h). Treat for 7-10 days; may need longer course in difficult and complicated infections. Renal Impairment: Reduced dose given q8h or usual dose given at prolonged intervals based on either CrCl or serum creatinine. Dialysis: 2mg/kg at end of each dialysis period. Obese Patients: Calculate dose based on estimated lean body mass.

(Continued)

BRAND NAME (Generic)	DOSAGE FORM/ STRENGTH	INDICATIONS	ADULT DOSE	PEDIATRIC DOSE
Tobramycin (tobramycin sulfate)	Inj: 10mg/mL, 40mg/mL, 1.2g	Treatment of serious lower respiratory tract, CNS (eg, meningitis), intra-abdominal, bone, skin and skin structure, and complicated/recurrent urinary tract infections; and septicemia.	(IM/IV) Serious Infections: 3mg/kg/day given q8h. Life-Threatening Infections: Up to 5mg/kg/day given tid-qid. Reduce to 3mg/kg/day as soon as clinically indicated. Max: 5mg/kg/day unless serum levels monitored. Treat for 7-10 days; may need longer course in difficult and complicated infections. Severe Cystic Fibrosis: Initial: 10mg/kg/day given qid. Measure levels to determine subsequent doses. Renal Impairment: Initial: 1mg/kg, followed by reduced doses given q8h or normal doses given at prolonged intervals based on either CrCl or serum creatinine. Do not use either method during dialysis. Obese Patients: Calculate dose based on estimated lean body weight plus 40% of the excess as the basic weight on which to figure mg/kg. ADD-Vantage vials are not for IM use.	>1 week: (IM/IV) 6-7.5mg/kg/day given tid-qid (eg, 2-2.5mg/kg q8h or 1.5-1.89mg/kg q6h). 1 week: Up to 2mg/kg q12h. Treat for 7-10 days; may need longer course in difficult and complicated infections. Severe Cystic Fibrosis: Initial: 10mg/kg/day given qid. Measure levels to determine subsequent doses. Renal Impairment: LD: 1mg/kg, followed by reduced doses given q8h or normal doses given at prolonged intervals based on either CrCl or serum creatinine. Do not use either method during dialysis. Obese Patients: Calculate dose based on estimated lean body weight plus 40% of the excess as the basic weight on which to figure mg/kg. ADD-Vantage vials are not for IM use.
Streptomycin sulfate	Inj: 1g	Treatment of moderate to severe infections such as mycobacterium tuberculosis (TB) and non-TB infections (eg, plague, tularemia, chancroid, granuloma inguinale, H.influenzae and K.pneumoniae infections, UTI, gram-negative bacillary bacteremia, endocardial infections).	IM only. TB: 15mg/kg/day (Max: 1g), or 25-30mg/kg twice weekly (Max: 1.5g), or 25-30mg/kg three times weekly (Max: 1.5g). Do not exceed a total dose of 120g over the course of therapy unless no other therapeutic options exist. Elderly (>60 yrs): Reduce dose. Treat for minimum of 1 year if possible. Tularemia: 1-2g/day in divided doses for 7-14 days until afebrile for 5-7 days. Plague: 1g bid for minimum of 10 days. Streptococcal Endocarditis: With PCN, 1g bid for week 1, then 500mg bid for week 2. Elderly (>60 yrs): 500mg bid for 2 weeks. Enterococcal Endocarditis: With PCN, 1g bid for 2 weeks, then 500mg bid for 4 weeks. Renal Impairment: Reduce dose. Moderate/Severe Infections: 1-2g/day in divided doses q6-12h. Max: 2g/day.	IM only. TB: 20-40mg/kg/day (Max: 1g), or 25-30 mg/kg twice weekly (Max: 1.5g), or 25-30mg/kg three times weekly (Max: 1.5g). Do not exceed a total dose of 120g over the course of therapy unless no other therapeutic options exist. Treat for minimum of 1 year if possible. Moderate/Severe Infections: 20-40mg/kg/day (8-20mg/lb/day) in divided doses q6-12h.
TOBI (tobramycin)	Sol: 60mg/mL (300mg/ampule)	Management of cystic fibrosis patients with P.aeruginosa.	Inhale via nebulizer 300mg q12h for 28 days, then stop for 28 days. Resume therapy for next 28-day on/28-day off cycle.	≥6 yrs: Inhale via nebulizer 300mg q12h for 28 days, then stop for 28 days. Resume therapy for next 28-day on/28-day off cycle.

BRAND NAME (Generic)	DOSAGE FORM/ STRENGTH	INDICATIONS	ADULT DOSE	PEDIATRIC DOSE
CARBAPENEMS				
Doribax (doripenem)	Inj: 500mg	Treatment of complicated intra-abdominal and urinary tract infections, including pyelonephritis, caused by susceptible microorganisms.	500 mg IV q8h for 5-14 days (intra-abdominal) or 10 days (UTI). Infuse over 1 hr. Renal impairment: CrCl >50mL/min: No dose adjustment. CrCl 30-50mL/min: 250mg IV q8h. CrCl >10 to <30mL/min: 250mg IV q12h.	
Invanz (ertapenem sodium)	Inj: 1g	Treatment of complicated intra-abdominal infections; skin and skin structure infections (SSSI), including diabetic foot infections without osteomyelitis; community acquired pneumonia (CAP); complicated urinary tract infections (UTI) including pyelonephritis; acute pelvic infections including postpartum endomyometritis, septic abortion, and post surgical gynecologic infections; prophylaxis of surgical site infection following elective colorectal surgery.	Treatment: 1g IM/IV qd. Duration: Intra-Abdominal Infections: 5-14 days. SSSI: 7-14 days. CAP/UTI: 10-14 days. Pelvic Infection: 3-10 days. May administer IV for up to 14 days and IM for up to 7 days. CrCl ≤30mL/min/1.73m²: 500mg IM/IV qd. Hemodialysis: Give 150mg IM/IV after dialysis only if 500mg dose was given within 6 hrs prior to dialysis. Prophylaxis: 1g IV as single dose given 1 hr prior to surgical incision.	≥13 yrs: 1g IM/IV qd. 3 mo-12 yrs: 15mg/kg IM/IV bid (not to exceed 1g/day). Treatment Duration: Intra-Abdominal Infections: 5-14 days. SSSI: 7-14 days. CAP/UTI: 10-14 days. Pelvic Infections: 3-10 days. May administer IV for up to 14 days and IM for up to 7 days. CrCl ≤30mL/min/1.73 m²:
Merrem (meropenem)	Inj: 500mg, 1g	Treatment of intra-abdominal infections, bacterial meningitis, and complicated skin and skin structure infections (cSSSI) caused by susceptible strains of microorganisms.	Intra-Abdominal: 1g q8h. CrCl 26-50mL/min: 1 g q12h. CrCl 10-25mL/min: 500mg q12h. CrCl <10mL/min: 500mg q24h. cSSSI: 500mg q8h. CrCl 26-50mL/min: 500mg q12h. CrCl 10-25mL/min: 250mg q12h. CrCl <10mL/min: 250mg q24h.	3 months >50kg: Intra-Abdominal: 1g q8h. Meningitis: 2g q8h. cSSSI: 500mg q8h. 50kg: Intra-Abdominal: 20mg/kg q8h. Max: 1g q8h. Meningitis: 40mg/kg q8h. Max: 2g q8h. cSSSI: 10mg/kg q8h. Max: 500mg q8h.
CEPHALOSPORINS, FIRST GENERATION				
Cefazolin (cefazolin)	Inj: 500mg, 1g, 10g, 20g	Treatment of respiratory tract, urinary tract (UTI), skin and skin structure, biliary tract, bone and joint, and genital infections, septicemia, and endocarditis caused by susceptible strains of microorganisms. Perioperative prophylaxis for surgical procedures classified as contaminated or potentially contaminated.	Moderate-Severe Infections: 500mg-1g q6-8h. Mild Gram-Positive Cocci Infection: 250-500mg q8h. Acute, Uncomplicated UTI: 1g q12h. Pneumococcal Pneumonia: 500mg q12h. Severe Life-Threatening Infection (eg, Endocarditis, Septicemia): 1-1.5g q6h. Max: 12g/day (rare). Perioperative Prophylaxis: 1g IM/IV 0.5-1 hr before surgery. For Procedures ≥2 hrs: 500mg-1g IM/IV during surgery. Maint: 500mg-1g IV/IV q6-8h for 24 hrs post-op. Continue for 3-5 days post-op for devastating procedures (eg, open-heart surgery and prosthetic arthroplasty). Renal Impairment: CrCl 35-54 mL/min: Full dose q8h. CrCl 11-34 mL/min ½ usual dose q12h. CrCl <10mL/min: ½ usual dose q18-24h. Apply reduced dosage recommendations after initial LT is given.	Mild-Moderately Severe Infection: 25-50mg/kg/day in 3-4 equal doses. Severe Infection: 100mg/kg/day in divided doses. Renal impairment: CrCl 40-70mL/min: 60% of normal daily dose in equally divided doses q12h. CrCl 20-40mL/min: 25% of normal daily dose in equally divided doses q12h. CrCl 5-20mL/min: 10% of normal daily dose q24h. Apply reduced dosage recommendations after initial LD is given.

(Continued)

BRAND NAME (Generic)	DOSAGE FORM/ STRENGTH	INDICATIONS	ADULT DOSE	PEDIATRIC DOSE
Duricef (cefadroxil monohydrate)	**Cap:** 500mg; **Sus:** 250mg/5mL [50mL, 100mL], 500mg/5mL [50mL, 75mL, 100mL]; **Tab:** 1g	Skin and skin structure infections (SSSI) and urinary tract infections (UTI), pharyngitis, and tonsillitis.	Uncomplicated Lower UTI: 1-2g/day given qd or bid. Other UTI: 1gm bid. SSSI: 1g qd or 500mg bid. Group A β-hemolytic Strep Pharyngitis/ Tonsillitis: 1g qd or 500mg bid for 10 days. CrCl ≤50mL/min: Initial: 1g. Maint: CrCl 25-50mL/min: 500mg q12h; CrCl 10-25mL/min: 500mg q24h; CrCl 0-10mL/min: 500mg q36h.	UTI/SSSI: 15mg/kg q12h. Pharyngitis/Tonsillitis/ Impetigo: 30mg/kg qd or 15mg/kg q12h. Treat β-hemolytic strep infections for at least 10 days.
Keflex (cephalexin)	**Cap:** 250mg, 333mg 500mg, 750mg; **Sus:** 125mg/5mL, 250mg/5mL [100mL, 200mL]	Treatment of otitis media and skin and skin structure infections (SSSI); bone, genitourinary tract, and respiratory tract infections.	Usual: 25-50mg/kg/day in divided doses. Streptococcal Pharyngitis/SSSI/Uncomplicated Cystitis (>15 yrs): 500mg q12h. Treat cystitis for 7-14 days. Max: 4g/day.	Usual: 25-50mg/kg/day in divided doses. Streptococcal Pharyngitis (>1 yr)/SSSI: May divide dose and give q12h. Otitis Media: 75-100mg/kg/day in divided doses. Administer for ≥10 days in, β-hemolytic streptococcal infections.
Panixine (cephalexin)	**Tab. Dispersible:** 125mg, 250mg	Skin and skin structure (SSSI), bone genitourinary and respiratory tract infections, otitis media, acute prostatitis.	Usual: 25-50mg/kg/day in divided doses. Streptococcal Pharyngitis/SSSI/Uncomplicated Cystitis (>15 yrs): 500mg q12h. Treat cystitis for 7-14 days. Max: 4g/day.	Usual: 25-50mg/kg/day in divided doses. Streptococcal Pharyngitis (>1 yr)/SSSI: May divide dose and give q12h. Otitis Media: 75-100mg/kg/day in divided doses. Administer for ≥10 days in, β-hemolytic streptococcal infections.
CEPHALOSPORINS, SECOND GENERATION				
Cefaclor	**Cap:** 250mg, 500mg; **Sus:** 125mg/5mL [75mL, 150mL], 187mg/5mL [50mL, 100mL], 250mg/5mL [75mL, 150mL], 375mg/5mL [50mL, 100mL]	Treatment of otitis media, pharyngitis, tonsillitis, lower respiratory tract, urinary tract, and skin and skin structure infections caused by susceptible strains of microorganisms.	Usual: 250mg q8h. Severe Infections/Pneumonia: 500mg q8h. Treat β-hemolytic strep for 10 days.	≥1 mo: Usual: 20mg/kg/day given q8h. Otitis Media/Serious Infections: 40mg/kg/day. Max: 1g/day. May administer q12h for otitis media and pharyngitis. Treat β-hemolytic strep for 10 days.
Cefaclor ER	**Tab. Extended-Release:** 375mg, 500mg	Acute bacterial exacerbation of chronic bronchitis (ABECB), secondary bacterial infections of acute bronchitis, pharyngitis, tonsillitis, and uncom- plicated skin and skin structure infections (SSSI) caused by susceptible strains of microorganisms.	ABECB/Acute Bronchitis: 500mg q12h for 7 days. Pharyngitis/Tonsillitis: 375mg q12h for 10 days. SSSI: 375mg q12h for 7-10 days. Take with meals. Do not crush, cut or chew tab.	≥16 yrs: ABECB/Acute Bronchitis: 500mg q12h for 7 days. Pharyngitis/Tonsillitis: 375mg q12h for 10 days. SSSI: 375mg q12h for 7-10 days. Take with meals. Do not crush, cut or chew tab.

BRAND NAME (Generic)	DOSAGE FORM/ STRENGTH	INDICATIONS	ADULT DOSE	PEDIATRIC DOSE
CEPHALOSPORINS, SECOND GENERATION *(Continued)*				
Cefoxitin (cefoxitin sodium)	**Inj:** 1g/50mL, 2g, 2g/50mL, 10g	Treatment of lower respiratory tract, urinary tract, intra-abdominal, gynecological, skin and skin structure, and bone and joint infections, and septicemia. For surgical prophylaxis.	Usual: 1-2g IV q6-8h. Uncomplicated Infections: 1g IV q6-8h. Moderate-Severe: 1g IV q4h or 2g IV q6-8h. Gas Gangrene/Other Infections Requiring Higher Dose: 2g IV q4h or 3g IV q6h. Renal Insufficiency: LD: 1-2g IV. Maint: CrCl 30-50mL/min: 1-2g IV q8-12h. CrCl 10-29mL/min: 1-2g IV q12-24h. CrCl 5-9mL/min: 0.5-1g IV q12-24h. CrCl <5mL/min: 0.5-1g IV q24-48h. Hemodialysis: LD: 1-2g IV after dialysis. Maint: See renal insufficiency doses above. Prophylaxis: Uncontaminated GI Surgery/Hysterectomy: 2g IV 0.5-1 hr prior to surgery, then 2g IV q6h after first dose up to 24 hrs. C-Section: 2g IV single dose after umbilical cords is clamped, or 2g IV after umbilical cordis clamped followed by 2g IV 4 and 8 hrs after initial dose.	≥3 mo: 80-160mg/kg/day divided into 4-6 equal doses. Max: 12g/day. Prophylaxis: Uncontaminated GI Surgery/Hysterectomy: 30-40mg/kg IV 0.5-1 hr prior to surgery, then 30-40mg/kg IV q6h after first dose up to 24 hrs.
Ceftin (cefuroxime axetil)	**Sus:** 125mg/5mL [100mL], 250mg/ 5mL [50mL, 100mL]; **Tab:** 125mg, 250mg, 500mg	(Sus/Tab) Pharyngitis/tonsillitis, acute otitis media, and impetigo. (Tab) Uncomplicated skin and skin structure (SSSI), and urinary tract infection (UTI), gonorrhea, early lyme disease, acute bacterial maxillary sinusitis, acute bacterial exacerbations of chronic bronchitis (ABECB) and secondary bacterial infections of acute bronchitis.	(Tab) Pharyngitis/Tonsillitis/Sinusitis: 250mg bid for 10 days. ABECB/SSSI: 250-500mg bid for 10 days. Acute Bronchitis: 250-500mg bid for 5-10 days. UTI: 125-250mg bid for 7-10 days. Gonorrhea: 1000mg single dose. Lyme Disease: 500mg bid for 20 days.	≥13 yrs: (Tab) Pharyngitis/Tonsillitis/Sinusitis: 250mg bid for 10 days. ABECB/SSSI: 250-500mg bid for 10 days. Acute Bronchitis: 250-500mg bid for 5-10 days. UTI: 125-250mg bid for 7-10 days. Gonorrhea: 1000mg single dose. 3 mo-12 yrs: (Sus) Pharyngitis/Tonsillitis: 10mg/kg bid for 10 days. Max: 500mg/day. Otitis Media/Sinusitis/Impetigo: 15mg/kg bid for 10 days. Max: 1000mg/day. (Tab-If can swallow whole) Pharyngitis/Tonsillitis: 125mg bid for 10 days. Otitis Media/Sinusitis: 250mg bid for 10 days.
Cefzil (cefprozil)	**Sus:** 125mg/5mL, 250mg/5mL [50mL, 75mL, 100mL]; **Tab:** 250mg, 500mg	Mild to moderate pharyngitis/tonsillitis, otitis media, acute sinusitis, secondary bacterial infection of acute bronchitis, acute bacterial exacerbation of chronic bronchitis (ABECB), and uncomplicated skin and skin structure infections (SSSI).	≥13 yrs: Pharyngitis/Tonsillitis: 500mg q24h for 10 days. Acute Sinusitis: 250-500mg q12h for 10 days. ABECB/Acute Bronchitis: 500mg q12h for 10 days. SSSI: 250-500mg q12h or 500mg q24h. CrCl <30mL/min: 50% of standard dose.	2-12 yrs: Pharyngitis/Tonsillitis: 7.5mg/kg q12h for 10 days. SSSI: 20mg/kg q24h for 10 days. 6 mos-12 yrs: Otitis Media: 15mg/kg q12h for 10 days. Acute Sinusitis: 7.5-15mg/kg q12h for 10 days. Do not exceed adult dose. CrCl <30mL/min: 50% of standard dose.

(Continued)

BRAND NAME (Generic)	DOSAGE FORM/ STRENGTH	INDICATIONS	ADULT DOSE	PEDIATRIC DOSE
Mefoxin (cefoxitin sodium)	**Inj:** 1g, 1g/50mL, 2g, 2g/50mL, 10g	Treatment of lower respiratory tract, urinary tract, intra-abdominal, gynecological, skin and skin structure, and bone and joint infections, and septicemia. For surgical prophylaxis.	Usual: 1-2g IV q6-8h. Uncomplicated Infections: 1g IV q6-8h. Moderate-Severe: 1g IV q4h or 2g IV q6-8h. Gas Gangrene/Other Infections Requiring Higher Dose: 2g IV q4h or 3g IV q6h. Renal Insufficiency: LD: 1-2g IV. Maint: CrCl 30-50mL/ min: 1-2g IV q8-12h. CrCl 10-29mL/min: 1-2g IV q12-24h. CrCl 5-9mL/min: 0.5-1g IV q12-24h. CrCl <5mL/min: 0.5-1g IV q24-48h. Hemodialysis: LD: 1-2g IV after dialysis. Maint: See renal insufficiency doses above. Prophylaxis: Uncontaminated GI Surgery/Hysterectomy: 2g IV 0.5-1 hr prior to surgery, then 2g IV q6h after first dose up to 24 hrs. C-Section: 2g IV single dose after umbilical cord is clamped, or 2g IV after umbilical cord is clamped followed by 2g IV 4 and 8 hrs after initial dose.	≥3 mos: 80-160mg/kg/day divided into 4-6 equal doses. Max: 12g/day. Prophylaxis: Uncontaminated GI Surgery/Hysterectomy: 30-40mg/kg IV 0.5-1 hr prior to surgery, then 30- 40mg/kg IV q6h after first dose up to 24 hrs.
Zinacef (cefuroxime)	**Inj:** 750mg, 1.5g, 7.5g, 750mg/50mL, 1.5g/50mL	Treatment of septicemia; meningitis; gonorrhea; lower respiratory tract, urinary tract, skin and skin structure (SSSI), and bone and joint infections caused by susceptible strains of microorganisms. For preoperative and perioperative surgical prophylaxis.	Usual: 750mg-1.5g q8h for 5-10 days. Uncomplicated Pneumonia and UTI/SSSI/Disseminated Gonococcal Infections: 750mg q8h. Severe/ Complicated Infections: 1.5g q8h. Bone and Joint Infections: 1.5g q8h. Life-Threatening Infections/ Infections With Susceptible Organisms: 1.5g q6h. Meningitis: Max 3g q8h. Uncomplicated Gonococcal Infection: 1.5g IM single dose at 2 different sites with 1g PO probenecid. Surgical Prophylaxis: 1.5g IV 0.5-1 hr before incision, then 750mg IM/IV q8h with prolonged procedure. Open Heart Surgery (Perioperative): 1.5g IV at induction of anesthesia and q12h thereafter, for total of 6g. Renal impairment: CrCl 10-20mL/min: 750mg q12h. CrCl <10mL/min: 750mg q24h. Hemodialysis: Give further dose at end of dialysis.	>3 months: Usual: 50-100 mg/kg/day in divided doses q6-8h. Severe infections: 100mg/kg/day (not to exceed max adult dose). Bone and Joint Infections: 150mg/kg/day in divided doses q8h (not to exceed max adult dose). Meningitis: 200-240mg/kg/ day IV in divided doses q6-8h. Renal Dysfunction: Modify dosing frequency consistent with adult recommendations.

BRAND NAME (Generic)	DOSAGE FORM/ STRENGTH	INDICATIONS	ADULT DOSE	PEDIATRIC DOSE
CEPHALOSPORINS, THIRD GENERATION				
Cedax (ceftibuten)	**Cap:** 400mg; **Sus:** 90mg/5mL [30mL, 60mL, 90mL, 120mL]	Acute bacterial exacerbations of chronic bronchitis (ABECB), acute bacterial otitis media, pharyngitis and tonsillitis.	ABECB/Otitis Media/Pharyngitis/Tonsillitis: 400mg qd for 10 days. Max: 400mg/day. CrCl 30-49mL/min: 4.5mg/kg or 200mg qd. CrCl 5-29mL/min: 2.25mg/kg or 100mg qd. Take 2 hrs before or at least 1 hr after a meal.	≥6 mo: Pharyngitis/Tonsillitis/Otitis Media: 9mg/kg qd for 10 days. Max: 400mg. ABECB/Otitis Media/ Pharyngitis/Tonsillitis: ≥12 yrs: 400mg qd for 10 days. Max: 400mg/day. CrCl 30-49mL/min: 4.5mg/kg or 200mg qd. CrCl 5-29mL/min: 2.25mg/kg or 100mg qd. Take 2 hrs before or at least 1 hr after a meal.
Cefizox (ceftizoxime)	**Inj:** 1g, 2g, 10g	Treatment of lower respiratory tract, skin and skin structure, intra-abdominal, bone and joint, and urinary tract infections (UTI), pelvic inflammatory disease (PID), gonorrhea, and septicemia.	Uncomplicated UTI: 500mg q12h IM/IV. Other Sites: 1g q8-12h IM/IV. Severe/Refractory Infections: 1-2g IM/IV q8-12h. PID: 2g IV q8h. Life Threatening Infections: 3-4g IV q8h. Uncomplicated Gonorrhea: 1g IM as single dose. Renal Impairment: LD: 500mg-1g IM/IV. Less Severe Infection: Maint: CrCl 50-79mL/min: 500mg q8h. CrCl 5-49mL/min: 250-500mg q12h. CrCl 0-4mL/ min (Dialysis): 500mg q48h or 250mg q24h. Life Threatening Infection: Maint: CrCl 50-79mL/min: 0.75-1.5g q8h. CrCl 5-49mL/min: 0.5-1g q12h. CrCl 0-4mL/min (Dialysis): 0.5-1g q48h or 0.5g q24h.	≥6 mos: 50mg/kg IM/IV q6-8h, up to 200mg/kg/day. Max: 6g/day for serious infections.
Fortaz (ceftazidime)	**Inj:** 500mg, 1g, 1g/50mL, 2g, 2g/50mL, 6g	Treatment of lower respiratory tract (eg, pneumonia), skin and skin structure (SSSI), bone and joint, gynecologic, CNS (eg, meningitis), intra-abdominal, and urinary tract infections (UTI), and septicemia. For use in sepsis.	Usual: 1g IM/IV q8-12h. Uncomplicated UTI: 250 mg IM/IV q12h. Complicated UTI: 500mg IM/IV q8-12h. Bone and Joint Infection: 2g IV q12h. Uncomplicated Pneumonia/SSSI: 500mg-1g IM/IV q8h. Gynecological/Intra-Abdominal/Meningitis/ Severe Life-Threatening Infection: 2g IV q8h. Lung Infection caused by Pseudomonas spp. in Cystic Fibrosis (normal renal function): 30-50mg/kg IV q8h. Max: 6g/day. CrCl 31-50mL/min: 1g q12h. CrCl 16-30mL/min: 1g q24h. CrCl 6-15mL/min: 500mgq24h. CrCl <5mL/min: 500mg q48h. For severe infections (6g/day), increase renal impairment dose by 50% or increase dosing interval. Apply reduced dosage recommendations after initial 1g LD is given. Hemodialysis: Give 1g before then 1g after each hemodialysis. Intra-Peritoneal Dialysis/ Continuous Peritoneal Dialysis: Ambulatory Peritoneal Dialysis: Give 1g followed by 500mg q24h.	≥12 yrs: Usual: 1g IM/IV q8-12h. Uncomplicated UTI: 250mg IM/IV q12h. Complicated UTI: 500mg IM/IV q8-12h. Bone and Joint Infection: 2g IV q12h. Uncomplicated Pneumonia/SSSI: 500mg-1g IM/IV q8h. Gynecological/Intra-Abdominal/Meningitis/ Severe Life-Threatening Infection: 2g IV q8h. Lung Infection caused by Pseudomonas spp. in Cystic Fibrosis (normal renal function): 30-50mg/kg IV q8h Max: 6g/day. CrCl 31-50mL/min: 1g q12h. CrCl 16-30mL/min: 1g q24h. CrCl 6-15mL/min: 500mg q24h. CrCl <5mL/min: 500mg q48h. For severe infections (6g/day), increase renal impairment dose by 50% or increase dosing interval. Apply reduced dosage recommendations after initial 1g LD is given. Hemodialysis: Give 1g before then 1g after each hemodialysis. Intra-Peritoneal Dialysis/Continuous Ambulatory Peritoneal Dialysis: Give 1g followed by 500mg q24h.

(Continued)

BRAND NAME (Generic)	DOSAGE FORM/ STRENGTH	INDICATIONS	ADULT DOSE	PEDIATRIC DOSE
Claforan (cefotaxime sodium)	Inj: 500mg, 1g, 2g, 10g	Treatment of lower respiratory tract, genitourinary, gynecologic, intra-abdominal, skin and skin structure, bone and joint, and CNS infections (eg, meningitis), bacteremia, and septicemia. For surgical prophylaxis.	Gonococcal Urethritis/Cervicitis (Males/Females): 500mg single dose IM. Rectal Gonorrhea: 0.5g (females) or 1g (males) single dose IM. Uncomplicated Infections: 1g IM/IV q12h. Moderate-Severe Infections: 1-2g IM/IV q8h. Septicemia: 2g IV q6-8h. Life-Threatening Infections: 2g IV q4h. Max: 12g/day. Surgical Prophylaxis: 1g IM/IV 30-90 min before surgery. Cesarean Section: 1g IV when umbilical cord is clamped, then 1g IV at 6 and 12 hrs after 1st dose. CrCl <20mL/min/1.73 m²: Give ½ of usual dose.	≥50kg: Use adult dose. Max: 12g/day. 1mo-12 yrs and ≤50kg: 50-180mg/kg/day IM/IV divided in 4-6 doses. 1-4 weeks: 50mg/kg IV q8h. 0-1 week: 50mg/kg IV q12h. CrCl <20mL/min/1.73 m²: Give ½ of usual dose.
Fortaz (ceftazidime)	Inj: 500mg, 1g, 1g/50mL, 2g, 2g/50mL, 6g	Treatment of lower respiratory tract (eg, pneumonia), skin and skin structure (SSSI), bone and joint, gynecologic, CNS (eg, meningitis), intra-abdominal, and urinary tract infections (UTI), and septicemia. For use in sepsis.	Usual: 1g IM/IV q8-12h. Uncomplicated UTI: 250mg IM/IV q12h. Complicated UTI: 500mg IM/IV q8-12h. Bone and Joint Infection: 2g IV q12h. Uncomplicated Pneumonia/SSSI: 500mg-1g IM/IV q8h. Gynecological/Intra-Abdominal/Meningitis/Severe Life-Threatening Infection: 2g IV q8h. Lung Infection Caused by Pseudomonas spp. in Cystic Fibrosis (Normal Renal Function): 30-50mg/kg IV q8h. Max: 6g/day. CrCl 31-50mL/min: 1g q12h. CrCl 16-30mL/min: 1g q24h. CrCl 6-15mL/min: 500mg q24h. CrCl <5mL/min: 500mg q48h. For severe renal impairment dose by 50% or increase dosing interval. Apply reduced dosage recommendations after initial 1g LD is given Hemodialysis: Give 1g before then 1g after each hemodialysis. Intra-Peritoneal Dialysis/Continuous Ambulatory Peritoneal Dialysis: Give 1g followed by 500mg q24h, or add to fluid at 250mg/2L.	1 mo-12 yrs: 30-50mg/kg IV q8h. Max: 6g/day. Neonates (0-4 weeks): 30mg/kg IV q12h. Higher doses for cystic fibrosis or meningitis. CrCl 31-50 mL/min: 1g q12h. CrCl 16-30mL/min: 1g q24h. CrCl 6-15mL/min: 500mg q24h. CrCl <5mL/min: 500mg q48h. For severe infections (6g/day), increase renal impairment dose by 50% or increase dosing interval. Apply reduced dosage recommendations after initial 1g LD is given. Hemodialysis: Give 1g before then 1g after each hemodialysis. Intra-Peritoneal Dialysis/Continuous Ambulatory Peritoneal Dialysis: Give 1g followed by 500mg q24h, or add to fluid at 250mg/2L.

BRAND NAME (Generic)	DOSAGE FORM/ STRENGTH (Continued)	INDICATIONS	ADULT DOSE	PEDIATRIC DOSE
CEPHALOSPORINS, THIRD GENERATION (Continued)				
Omnicef (cefdinir)	Cap: 300mg; Sus: 125mg/5mL, 250mg/5mL [60mL, 100mL]	Community acquired pneumonia (CAP), acute exacerbations of chronic bronchitis (AECB), acute maxillary sinusitis, pharyngitis/tonsillitis, uncomplicated skin and structure infections (SSSI), and acute bacterial otitis media.	(Cap) SSSI/Cap: 300mg q12h for 10 days. AECB/Pharyngitis/Tonsillitis: 300mg q12h for 5-10 days or 600mg q24h for 10 days. Sinusitis: 300mg q12h or 600mg q24h for 10 days. CrCl <30mL/min: 300mg qd.	(Sus) 6 mo-12 yrs: OtitisMedia/Pharyngitis/Tonsillitis: 7mg/kg q12h for 5-10 days or 14mg/kg q24h for 10 days. Sinusitis: 7mg/kg q12h or 14mg/kg q24h for 10 days. SSSI: 7mg/kg q12h for 10 days. (Cap) ≥13 yrs: CAP/SSSI: 300mg q12h for 10 days. AECB/Pharyngitis/Tonsillitis: 300mg q12h for 5-10 days or 600mg q24h for 10 days. Sinusitis: 300mg q12h or 600mg q24h for 10 days. CrCl <30mL/min/1.73m²: 7mg/kg qd. Max: 300mg qd.
Rocephin (ceftriaxone sodium)	Inj: 250mg, 500mg. 1g, 2g, 10g	Treatment of lower respiratory tract infections, skin and skin structure infections, bone and joint infections, intra-abdominal infections, acute otitis media, uncomplicated gonorrhea, pelvic inflammatory disease, UTI, septicemia, and meningitis. For surgical prophylaxis.	Usual: 1-2g/day IV/IM given qd-bid. Max: 4g/day. Gonorrhea: 250mg IM single dose. Surgical Prophylaxis: 1g IV ½-2 hrs before surgery.	Skin Infections: 50-75mg/kg/day IV/IM given qd-bid. Max: 2g/day. Otitis Media: 50mg/kg up to 1g) IM single dose. Serious Infections: 50-75mg/kg/day IM/IV given q12h. Max: 2g/day. Meningitis: Initial: 100mg/kg (up to 4g), then 100mg/kg/day given qd-bid for 7-14 days. Max: 4g/day.
Spectracef (cefditoren pivoxil)	Tab: 200mg	Treatment of acute bacterial exacerbations of chronic bronchitis (ABECB), pharyngitis/tonsillitis, community acquired pneumonia (CAP), and uncomplicated skin and skin-structure infections (SSSI).	ABECB: 400mg bid for 10 days. Pharyngitis/Tonsillitis/SSSI: 200mg bid for 10 days. Cap: 400mg bid for 14 days. CrCl 30-49mL/min: 200mg bid. CrCl<30mL/min: 200mg qd. Take with meals.	≥12 yrs: ABECB: 400mg bid for 10 days. Pharyngitis/Tonsillitis/SSSI: 200mg bid for 10 days. Cap: 400mg bid for 14 days. CrCl 30-49mL/min: 200mg bid. CrCl<30mL/min: 200mg qd. Take with meals.
Suprax (cefixime)	Sus: 100mg/5mL [50mL, 75mL, 100mL]	Otitis media, pharyngitis, tonsillitis, acute bronchitis, acute exacerbation of chronic bronchitis, uncomplicated UTIs, and cervical/urethral gonorrhea caused by susceptible strains.	Usual: 400mg qd. Gonorrhea: 400mg single dose. CrCl 21-60mL/min/Hemodialysis: Give 75% of standard dose. CrCl <20mL/min/CAPD: Give 50% of standard dose.	>12 yrs or >50kg: (Tab/Sus) Usual: 400mg qd. ≥6 mos: (Sus) 8mg/kg qd or 4mg/kg bid. Treat for at least 10 days with S. pyogenes. CrCl 21-60mL/min/Hemodialysis: Give 75% of standard dose. CrCl <20mL/min/CAPD: Give 50% of standard dose.

(Continued)

BRAND NAME (Generic)	DOSAGE FORM/ STRENGTH	INDICATIONS	ADULT DOSE	PEDIATRIC DOSE
Tazicef (ceftazidime)	Inj: 1g, 2g, 6g	Treatment of lower respiratory tract (eg, pneumonia), skin and skin structure (SSSI), bone and joint, gynecologic, CNS (eg, meningitis), intra-abdominal, and urinary tract infections (UTI), and septicemia. For use in sepsis.	Usual: 1g IM/IV q8-12h. Uncomplicated UTI: 250mg IM/IV q12h. Complicated UTI: 500mg IM/IV q8-12h. Bone and Joint Infection: 2g IV q12h. Uncomplicated Pneumonia/SSSI: 500mg-1g IM/IV q8h. Gynecological/Intra-Abdominal/Meningitis/Severe Life-Threatening Infection: 2g IV q8h. Lung Infection caused by Pseudomonas in Cystic Fibrosis (normal renal function): 30-50mg/kg IV q8h. Max: 6g/day. Renal Impairment: CrCl 31-50mL/min: 1g q12h. CrCl 16-30mL/min: 1g q24h. CrCl 6-15mL/min: 500mg q24h. CrCl <5mL/min: 500mg q48h. For severe infections (6g/day), increase renal impairment dose by 50% or increase dosing interval. Apply reduced dosage recommendations after initial 1g LD is given. Hemodialysis: Give 1g before and 1g after each hemodialysis. Intra-Peritoneal Dialysis/Continuous Ambulatory Peritoneal Dialysis: Give 1g followed by 500mg q24h, or add to fluid at 250mg/2L.	Neonates (0-4 weeks): 30mg/kg IV q12h. 1 mo-12 yrs: 30-50mg/kg IV q8h. Max: 6g/day. Higher doses for patients with cystic fibrosis or when treating meningitis. Renal Impairment: CrCl 31-50mL/min: 1g q12h. CrCl 16-30mL/min: 1g q24h. CrCl 6-5mL/min: 500mg q24h. CrCl <5mL/min: 500mg q48h. For severe infections (6g/day), increase renal impairment dose by 50% or increase dosing interval. Apply reduced dosage recommendations after initial 1g LD is given. Hemodialysis: Give 1g before and 1g after each hemodialysis. Intra-Peritoneal Dialysis/ Continuous Ambulatory Peritoneal Dialysis: Give 1g followed by 500mg q24h, or add fluid at 250mg/2L.
Tazidime (ceftazidime)	Inj: 1g, 2g, 6g	Treatment of lower respiratory tract (eg, pneumonia), skin and skin structure (SSSI), bone and joint, gynecologic, CNS (eg, meningitis), intra-abdominal, and urinary tract infections (UTI), and septicemia. For use in sepsis.	Usual: 1g IM/IV q8-12h. Uncomplicated UTI: 250mg IM/IV q12h. Complicated UTI: 500mg IM/IV q8-12h. Bone and Joint Infection: 2g IV q12h. Uncomplicated Pneumonia/Skin and Skin Structure Infection: 500mg-1g IM/IV q8h. Gynecological/Intra-Abdominal/Meningitis/Severe Life-Threatening Infection: 2g IV q8h. Lung Infection caused by Pseudomonas spp. in Cystic Fibrosis (normal renal function): 30-50mg/kg IV q8h. Max: 6g/day. Renal Impairment: CrCl 31-50mL/min: 1g q12h. CrCl 16-30mL/min: 1g q24h. CrCl 6-15mL/min: 500mg q24h. CrCl <5mL/min: 500mg q48h. For severe infections (6g/day), increase renal impairment dose by 50% or increase dosing interval. Apply reduced dosage recommendations after initial 1g LD is given. Hemodialysis: Give 1g before then 1g after each hemodialysis. Intra-Peritoneal Dialysis/Continuous Ambulatory Peritoneal Dialysis: Give 1g followed by 500mg q24h, or add to fluid at 250mg/2L.	Neonates (0-4 weeks): 30mg/kg IV q12h. 1 mo-12 yrs: 30-50mg/kg IV q8h. Max: 6g/day. Higher doses for cystic fibrosis and meningitis. Renal Impairment: CrCl 31-50mL/min: 1g q12h. CrCl 16-30mL/min: 1g q24h. CrCl 6-15mL/min: 500mg q24h. CrCl <5mL/ min: 500mg q48h. For severe infections (6g/day), increase renal impairment dose by 50% or increase dosing interval. Apply reduced dosage recommendations after initial 1g LD is given. Hemodialysis: Give 1g before then 1g after each hemodialysis. Intra-Peritoneal Dialysis/Continuous Ambulatory Peritoneal Dialysis: Give 1g followed by 500mg q24h, or add to fluid at 250mg/2L.

BRAND NAME (Generic)	DOSAGE FORM/ STRENGTH	INDICATIONS	ADULT DOSE	PEDIATRIC DOSE
CEPHALOSPORIN, THIRD GENERATION *(Continued)*				
Vantin (cefpodoxime proxetil)	**Sus:** 50mg/mL [50mL, 100mL], 100mg/5mL [50mL, 75mL, 100mL]; **Tab:** 100mg, 200mg	Acute otitis media, pharyngitis/tonsillitis, community acquired pneumonia (CAP), acute bacterial exacerbation of chronic bronchitis (ABECB), acute uncomplicated urethral and cervical gonorrhea, acute uncomplicated ano-rectal infections in women, uncomplicated skin and skin structure infections (SSSI), acute maxillary sinusitis, uncomplicated urinary tract infections (UTI).	Take tabs with food. Pharyngitis/Tonsillitis: 100mg q12h for 5-10 days. Cap: 200mg q12h for 14 days. ABECB: 200mg q12h for 10 days. Uncomplicated Gonorrhea (Men and Women)/Rectal Gonococcal Infections (women): 200mg single dose. SSSI: 400mg q12h for 7-14 days. Sinusitis: 200mg q12h for 10 days. UTI: 100mg q12h for 7 days. CrCl<30mL/min: Increase interval to q24h. Hemodialysis: Dose 3 times weekly after dialysis.	≥12 yrs: Take tabs with food. Pharyngitis/Tonsillitis: 100mg q12h for 5-10 days. Cap: 200mg q12h for 14 days. ABECB: 200mg q12h for 10 days. Uncomplicated Gonorrhea (men and women)/Rectal Gonococcal Infections (women): 200mg single dose. SSSI: 400mg q12h for 7-14 days. Sinusitis: 200mg q12h for 10 days. UTI: 100mg q12h for 7 days. 2 mos-11 yrs: Otitis Media: 5mg/kg q12h for 5 days. Max: 200mg/dose. Pharyngitis/Tonsillitis: 5mg/kg q12h for 5-10 days. Max: 100mg/dose. Sinusitis: 5mg/kg q12h for 10 days. Max:200mg/dose. CrCl<30mL/min: Increase interval to q24h. Hemodialysis: Dose 3 times weekly after dialysis.
CEPHALOSPORIN, FOURTH GENERATION				
Maxipime (cefepime HCl)	**Inj:** 500mg, 1g, 2g	Treatment of uncomplicated/complicated urinary tract (UTI), uncomplicated skin and skin structure (SSSI), and complicated intra-abdominal infections, and pneumonia. Emperic therapy for febrile neutropenia.	Moderate-Severe Pneumonia: 1-2g IV q12h for 10 days. Febrile Neutropenia Emperic Therapy: 2g IV q8h for 7 days or until neutropenia resolved. Mild-Moderate UTI: 0.5-1g IM/IV q12h for 7-10 days. Severe UTI/Moderate-Severe SSSI: 2g IV q12h for 10 days. Complicated Intra-Abdominal Infections: 2g IV q12h for 7-10 days. CrCl<60mL/min: Initial: Same dose as normal renal function. Maint: Refer to prescribing information for dose-adjustment.	2 months-16 yrs: ≤40kg: UTI/SSSI/Pneumonia: 50mg/kg IV q12h. Febrile Neutropenia: 50mg/kg IV q8h. Max: Do not exceed adult dose. CrCl ≤60mL/min: Initial: Same dose as normal renal function. Maint: Refer to prescribing information for dose adjustment.
FLUOROQUINOLONES				
Avelox (moxifloxacin HCl)	**Inj:** 400mg/250mL; **Tab:** 400mg [ABC pack, 5 tabs]	Acute bacterial sinusitis, acute bacterial exacerbation of chronic bronchitis (ABECB), uncomplicated skin and skin structure infections (SSSI), complicated skin and skin structure infections (cSSSI), complicated intra-abdominal infections (cIAI), and community acquired pneumonia (CAP), including multi-drug resistant *S.pneumoniae*.	≥18 yrs: Sinusitis: 400mg PO/IV q24h for 10 days. ABECB: 400mg PO/IV q24h for 5 days. SSSI: 400mg PO/IV q24h for 7 days. cSSSI: 400mg PO/IV q24h for 7-21 days. cIAI: 400mg IV q24h for 5-14 days. Cap: 400mg PO/IV q24h for 7-14 days.	

(Continued)

BRAND NAME (Generic)	DOSAGE FORM/ STRENGTH	INDICATIONS	ADULT DOSE	PEDIATRIC DOSE
Cipro (ciprofloxacin HCl)	**Sus:** 250mg/5mL, 500mg/5mL [100mL]; **Tab:** 250mg, 500mg, 750mg	Treatment of lower respiratory tract (LRTI), complicated intra-abdominal, skin and skin structure (SSSI), bone and joint, and urinary tract infections (UTI), acute exacerbations of chronic bronchitis, acute sinusitis, acute uncomplicated cystitis in females, chronic bacterial prostatitis, infectious diarrhea, typhoid fever, post-exposure inhalational anthrax, uncomplicated cervical and urethral gonorrhea, complicated UTI and pyelonephritis in pediatrics.	≥18 yrs: Acute Sinusitis/Typhoid Fever: 500mg q12h for 10 days. LRTI/SSSI: Mild-Moderate: 500mg q12h for 7-14 days. Severe/Complicated: 750mg q12h for 7-14 days. Cystitis/Acute Uncomplicated UTI: 250mg q12h for 3 days. Mild-Moderate UTI: 250mg q12h for 7-14 days. Severe/Complicated UTI: 500mg q12h for 7-14 days. Chronic Bacterial Prostatitis: 500mg q12h for 28 days. Intra-Abdominal: 500mg q12h (w/ metronidazole) for 7-14 days. Bone and Joint: Mild-Moderate: 500mg q12h for ≥4-6 weeks. Severe/Complicated: 750mg q12h for ≥4-6 weeks. Infectious Diarrhea: 500mg q12h for 5-7 days. Uncomplicated Urethral/Cervical Gonococcal: 250mg single dose. Inhalational Anthrax: 500mg q12h for 60 days. CrCl 30-50mL/min: 250-500mg q12h. CrCl 5-29mL/min: 250-500mg q18h. Hemodialysis/Peritoneal Dialysis: 250-500mg q24h (after dialysis). Administer at least 2 hrs before or 6 hrs after magnesium or aluminum containing antacids, sucralfate, Videx (didanosine) chewable/buffered tablets or pediatric powder, or other products containing calcium, iron or zinc.	<18 yrs: Inhalational Anthrax: 15mg/kg q12h for 60 days. Max: 500mg/dose. 1-17 yrs: Complicated UTI/Pyelonephritis: 10-20mg/kg q12h for 10-21 days. Max: 750mg/dose.

BRAND NAME (Generic)	DOSAGE FORM/ STRENGTH	INDICATIONS	ADULT DOSE	PEDIATRIC DOSE
FLUOROQUINOLONES (Continued)				
Cipro IV (ciprofloxacin)	**Inj:** 10mg/mL, 200mg/100mL, 400mg/200mL	Treatment of skin and skin structure (SSSI), bone and joint, complicated intra-abdominal infections, lower respiratory (LRTI), and urinary tract infections (UTI), nosocomial pneumonia, acute sinusitis, chronic bacterial prostatitis, post-exposure inhalational anthrax, empirical therapy for febrile neutropenia, complicated UTI and pyelonephritis in pediatrics	≥18 yrs: IV: UTI: Mild-Moderate: 200mg q12h for 7-14 days. Complicated/Severe: 400mg q12h for 7-14 days. LRTI/SSSI: Mild-Moderate: 400mg q12h for 7-14 days. Complicated/Severe: 400mg q8h for 7-14 days. Bone and Joint: Mild-Moderate: 400mg q12h for ≥4-6 weeks. Complicated/Severe: 400mg q8h for ≥4-6 weeks. Nosocomial Pneumonia: 400mg q8h for 10-14 days. Complicated Intra-Abdominal: 400mg q12h (w/metronidazole) for 7-14 days. Acute Sinusitis: 400mg q12h for 10 days. Chronic Bacterial Prostatitis: 400mg q12h for 28 days. Febrile Neutropenia: 400mg q8h (w/piperacillin 50mg/kg q4h) for 7-14 days. Max: 24g/day. Inhalational Anthrax: 400mg q12h for 60 days. Administer over 60 min. CrCl 5-29mL/min: 200-400mg q18-24h.	<18 yrs: Inhalational Anthrax: 10mg/kg q12h for 60 days. Max: 400mg/dose; 800mg/day. 1-17 yrs: Complicated UTI/Pyleonephritis: 6-10mg/kg q8h for 10-21 days. Max: 400mg/dose.
Cipro XR (ciprofloxacin)	**Tab, Extended-Release:** 500mg, 1000mg	Uncomplicated (acute cystitis) and complicated urinary tract infections (UTI), and acute uncomplicated pyelonephritis due to *E.coli*.	≥18 yrs: Uncomplicated UTI: 500mg qd for 3 days. Complicated UTI: 1000mg qd for 7-14 days. Acute Uncomplicated Pyelonephritis: 1000mg qd for 7-14 days. CrCl <30mL/min: 500 mg qd. Acute Uncomplicated Pyelonephritis: 1000mg qd for 7-14 days. CrCl <30mL/min: 500mg qd. Take with fluids. Administer at least 2 hrs before or 6 hrs after magnesium or aluminum containing antacids, sucralfate, Videx (didanosine) chewable/buffered tablets or pediatric powder, metal cations (eg, iron), multivitamins with zinc. Avoid concomitant administration with dairy products alone, or with calcium-fortified products. Space concomitant calcium intake (>800mg) by at least 2 hrs. Do not split, crush, or chew. Swallow tab whole. Dialysis: Give after procedure is completed.	

(Continued)

BRAND NAME (Generic)	DOSAGE FORM/ STRENGTH	INDICATIONS	ADULT DOSE	PEDIATRIC DOSE
Factive (gemifloxacin mesylate)	**Tab:** 320mg	Treatment of community-acquired pneumonia (CAP), including multi-drug resistant *Streptococcus pneumoniae* (MDRSP), and acute bacterial exacerbation of chronic bronchitis (ABECB).	≥18 yrs: ABECB: 320mg qd for 5 days. Cap: 320mg qd for 5 days *S.pneumoniae, H.influenzae, M. pneumoniae,* or *C.pneumoniae* or 7 days (MDRSP, *K.pneumoniae,* or *M.catarrhalis.* Renal Impairment: CrCl ≤40mL/min or Dialysis: 160mg qd. Take with fluids.	
Floxin (ofloxacin)	**Tab:** 200mg, 300mg, 400mg	Treatment of acute urinary tract (UTI) and uncomplicated skin and skin structure infection (SSSI), acute bacterial exacerbation of chronic bronchitis (ABECB), community acquired pneumonia (CAP), acute uncomplicated urethral and cervical gonorrhea, nongonococcal urethritis and cervicitis, mixed infections of the urethra and cervix, acute pelvic inflammatory disease (PID), uncomplicated cystitis, prostatitis.	≥18 yrs: ABECB/CAP/SSSI: 400mg q12h for 10 days. Cervicitis/Urethritis: 300mg q12h for 7 days. Gonorrhea: 400mg single dose. PID: 400mg q12h for 10-14 days. Uncomplicated Cystitis: 200mg q12h for 3 days (*E.coli* or *K.pneumoniae*) or 7 days (other pathogens). Complicated UTI: 200mg q12h for 10 days. Prostatitis: (*E.coli*) 300mg q12h for 6 weeks. CrCl 20-50mL/min: Dose q24h. CrCl <20mL/min: After regular initial dose, give 50% of normal dose q24h. Severe Hepatic Impairment: Max: 400mg/day.	
Floxin IV (ofloxacin)	**Inj:** 4mg/mL, 40mg/mL	Treatment of acute bacterial exacerbation of chronic bronchitis, community-acquired pneumonia, uncomplicated skin and skin structure infections, acute uncomplicated urethral and cervical gonorrhea, nongonococcal urethritis and cervicitis, urethral and cervical infections, acute pelvic inflammatory disease (PID), uncomplicated cystitis, urinary tract infections (UTI), prostatitis.	Lower Respiratory Tract Infection/Skin Structure Infections: 400mg q12h for 10 days. Cervicitis/ Urethritis: 300mg q12h for 7 days. Gonorrhea: 400mg single dose. PID: 400mg q12h for 10-14 days. Uncomplicated Cystitis: 200mg q12h for 3 days. Other Uncomplicated UTIs: 200mg q12h for 7 days. Complicated UTI: 200mg q12h for 10 days. Prostatitis: 300mg q12h for 6 weeks. Renal Impairment: CrCl 20-50mL/min: increase dosing interval to 24 hrs. CrCl<20mL/min: give normal initial dose then 50% of normal dose and increase dosing interval to 24 hrs. Severe Hepatic Impairment: Max: 400mg qdy. Switch to oral form when appropriate. Max: 10 days IV.	

BRAND NAME (Generic)	DOSAGE FORM/ STRENGTH	INDICATIONS	ADULT DOSE	PEDIATRIC DOSE
FLUOROQUINOLONES *(Continued)*				
Levaquin (levofloxacin)	**Inj:** 5mg/mL, 25mg/mL; **Sol:** 25mg/mL; **Tab:** 250mg, 500mg, 750mg [Leva-pak, 5']	Uncomplicated and complicated skin and skin structure (SSSI), and urinary tract infections (UTI), acute bacterial sinusitis, acute bacterial exacerbation of chronic bronchitis (ABECB), community acquired pneumonia (CAP), including multi-drug resistant *Streptococcus pneumoniae*, nosocomial pneumonia, chronic bacterial prostatitis (CBP), and acute pyelonephritis caused by susceptible strains of micro-organisms. Prevention of inhalational anthrax following exposure to *Bacillus anthracis*.	≥18 yrs: IV/PO: ABECB: 500mg qd for 7 days. Cap: 500mg qd for 7-14 days or 750mg qd for 5 days. Sinusitis: 500mg qd for 10-14 days or 750mg qd for 5 days. CBP: 500mg qd for 28 days. Uncomplicated SSSI: 500mg qd for 7-10 days. Complicated SSSI/Nosocomial Pneumonia: 750mg qd for 7-14 days. Inhalational Anthrax: 500mg qd for 60 days.Complicated SSSI/Nosocomial Pneumonia/CAP/Sinusitis: CrCl 20-49mL/min: 750mg, then 750mgq48h. CrCl 10-19mL/min/ Hemodialysis/CAPD: 750mg, then 500mg q48h. ABECB/CAP/Sinusitis/Uncomplicated SSSI/CBP/ Inhalational Anthrax:CrCl 20-49mL/min: 500mg, then 250mg q24h. CrCl 10-19mL/min/Hemodialysis/ CAPD: 500mg,then 250mg q48h. Complicated UTI/ Acute Pyelonephritis: 250mg qd for 10 days. CrCl 10-19mL/min: 250mg, then 250mg q48h. Uncomplicated UTI: 250mg qd for 3 days. Take oral solution 1 hr before or 2 hrs after eating.	
Maxaquin (lomefloxacin HCl)	**Tab:** 400mg	Treatment of acute bacterial exacerbation of chronic bronchitis (ABECB) and uncomplicated/complicated urinary tract infections (UTI). Preoperatively for the prevention of infections from transrectal prostate biopsy (TRPB) and in transurethral surgical procedures (TUSP).	≥18 yrs: ABECB: 400mg qd for 10 days. Uncom- plicated Cystitis: 400mg qd for 3 days *E.coli*. or 10 days *K.pneumoniae, P.mirabilis*, or *S.saprophyticus*. Complicated UTI: 400mg qd for 14 days. Hemodialysis/CrCl≥10 to <40mL/min: LD: 400mg. Maint: 200mg qd. Preoperative Prevention: TRPB: 400mg single dose 1-6 hrs before procedure. TUSP: 400mg single dose 2-6 hrs before procedure.	
Proquin XR (ciprofloxacin HCl)	**Tab, Extended- Release:** 500mg	Treatment of uncomplicated urinary tract infections (acute cystitis) caused by *E.coli* and *K.pneumoniae*.	500mg qd with pm meal for 3 days. Administer at least 4 hrs before or 2 hrs after magnesium or aluminum containing antacids, sucralfate, Videx (didanosine) chewable/buffered tablets of pediatric powder, metal cations (eg, iron), multivitamins with zinc. Do not split, crush, or chew. Swallow tab whole.	

(Continued)

BRAND NAME (Generic)	DOSAGE FORM/ STRENGTH	INDICATIONS	ADULT DOSE	PEDIATRIC DOSE
MACROLIDES				
Biaxin (clarithromycin)	**Sus:** 125mg/5mL, 250mg/5mL [50mL, 100mL]; **Tab:** 250mg, 500mg	Adults: Pharyngitis/tonsillitis, acute maxillary sinusitis, acute bacterial exacerbation of chronic bronchitis (ABECB), community acquired pneumonia (CAP), uncomplicated skin and skin structure infections (SSSI), combination therapy for *H.pylori* infection with duodenal ulcers. MAC prophylaxis in advanced HIV. Pediatrics: Pharyngitis/tonsillitis, CAP, acute maxillary sinusitis, acute otitis media, uncomplicated SSSI, disseminated mycobacterial infections. MAC prophylaxis in advanced HIV.	Pharyngitis/Tonsillitis: 250mg q12h for 10 days, Sinusitis: 500mg q12h for 14 days. ABECB: 250-500mg q12h for 7-14 days. SSSI/Cap: 250mg q12h for 7-14 days. MAC Prophylaxis/Treatment: 500mg bid. *H.pylori:* Triple Therapy: 500mg + amoxicillin 1g + omeprazole 20mg, all q12h for 10 days; or 500mg + amoxicillin 1g + lansoprazole 30mg, all q12h for 10-14 days. Give additional omeprazole 20mg qd for 18 days with active ulcer. Dual Therapy: 500mg q8h + omeprazole 40mg qd for 14 days (give additional omeprazole 20mg qd for 14 days with active ulcer); or 500mg q8h or q12h + ranitidine bismuth citrate 400mg q12h for 14 days (give additional ranitidine bismuth citrate 400mg bid for 14 days with active ulcer). Avoid Biaxin and ranitidine bismuth citrate combination with CrCl<25mL/min.	≥6 mo: Usual: 7.5mg/kg q12h for 10 days. MAC Prophylaxis/Treatment: ≥20 mo: 7.5mg/kg bid, up to 500mg bid. CrCl <30mL/min: Give 50% dose or double interval.
Biaxin XL (clarithromycin)	**Tab, Extended- Release:** 500mg [PAC 14 tabs]	Treatment of acute maxillary sinusitis, community acquired pneumonia (CAP), and acute bacterial exacerbation of chronic bronchitis (ABECB).	Sinusitis: 1000mg qd for 14 days. ABECB/Cap: 1000mg qd for 7 days. CrCl <30mL/min: Give 50% dose or double interval. Take with food.	
E.E.S. (erythromycin ethylsuccinate)	**Sus:** 200mg/5mL, 400mg/5mL [100mL, 480mL]; **Tab:** 400mg	Mild to moderate upper and lower respiratory tract and skin and skin structure infections, listeriosis, pertussis, diphtheria, erythrasma, intestinal amebiasis, acute pelvic inflammatory disease (PID) *N.gonorrhea,* primary syphilis in PCN allergy, Legionnaires' disease, chlamydial infections (eg, newborn conjunctivitis urethral, endocervical, or rectal, etc), and nongonococcal urethritis. Prophylaxis of endocarditis or rheumatic fever.	Usual: 1600mg/day given q6h; q8h or q12h. Max: 4g/day. Treat strep infections for 10 days. Strep-tococcal Infection Prophylaxis with Rheumatic Heart Disease: 400mg bid. Urethritis *C.trachomatis* or *U. urealyticum:* 800mg tid for 7 days. Primary Syphilis: 48-64g in divided doses over 10-15 days. Intestinal Amebiasis: 400mg qid for 10-14 days. Pertussis: 40-50mg/kg/day in divided doses for 5-14 days. Legionnaires' Disease: 1.6-4g/day in divided doses.	Usual: 30-50mg/kg/day in divided doses q6h, q8h or q12h. Double dose for more severe infections. Treat strep infections for 10 days. Intestinal Amebiasis: 30-50mg/kg/day in divided doses for 10-14 days. Pertussis: 40-50mg/kg/day in divided doses for 5-14 days.

BRAND NAME (Generic)	DOSAGE FORM/ STRENGTH	INDICATIONS	ADULT DOSE	PEDIATRIC DOSE
MACROLIDES *(Continued)*				
ERYC (erythromycin)	**Cap, Delayed-Release:** 250mg	Mild to moderate upper and lower respiratory tract and skin and soft tissue infections, pertussis, diphtheria, erythrasma, intestinal amebiasis, acute pelvic inflammatory disease (PID) (*N. gonorrhea*), *Listeria monocytogenes* infections, primary syphilis in PCN allergy, Legionnaires' disease, chlamydial infections (eg, newborn conjunctivitis, urethral, endocervical, or rectal, etc), and nongonococcal urethritis. Prophylaxis of endocarditis or rheumatic fever in PCN allergy.	Usual: 250mg q6h or 500mg q12h. Max: 4g/day. Treat strep infections for 10 days. Chlamydial Urogenital Infection During Pregnancy: 500mg qid for at least 7 days or 250mg qid for 14 days. Urethral/Endocervical/Rectal Chlamydial Infections: 500mg qid for 7 days. Primary Syphilis: 30-40g in divided doses for 10-15 days. Acute PID: 500mg (erythromycin lactobionate) IV q6h for 3 days, then 250mg PO q6h for 7 days. Streptococcal Infection Long-Term Prophylaxis of Rheumatic Fever: 250mg bid. Intestinal Amebiasis: 250mg qid for 10-14 days. Pertussis: 40-50mg/kg/day in divided doses for 5-14 days. Legionnaires' Disease: 1-4g/day in divided doses. Bacterial Endocarditis Prophylaxis: 1g 1 hr before procedure, then 500mg 6 hrs later.	Usual: 30-50mg/kg/day in divided doses without food. Max: 4g/day. Severe Infections: Double dose up to 4g/day. Treat strep infections for 10 days. Intestinal Amebiasis: 30-50mg/kg/day in divided doses for 10-14 days. Bacterial Endocarditis Prophylaxis: 20mg/kg 1 hr before procedure, then 10mg/kg 6 hrs later.
EryPed (erythromycin ethylsuccinate)	**Sus:** 100mg/2.5mL [50mL], 200mg/5mL, 400mg/5mL [5mL, 100mL, 200mL]; **Tab, Chewable:** 200mg	Treatment of mild to moderate upper and lower respiratory tract and skin and skin structure infections, listeriosis, pertussis, diphtheria, erythrasma, intestinal amebiasis, acute pelvic inflammatory disease (PID) *N. gonorrhea*, Legionnaires' disease, chlamydial infections (eg, newborn conjunctivitis, urethral, endocervical, or rectal, etc), and nongonococcal urethritis. Prophylaxis of endocarditis or rheumatic fever.	Usual: 1600mg/day given q6h, q8h or q12h. Max: 4g/day. Treat strep infections for 10 days. Streptococcal Infection Prophylaxis with Rheumatic Heart Disease: 400mg bid. Urethritis *C.trachomatis* or *U. urealyticum*: 800mg tid for 7 days. Primary Syphilis:48-64g in divided doses over 10-15 days. Intestinal Amebiasis: 400mg qid for 10-14 days. Pertussis:40-50mg/kg/day in divided doses for 5-14 days. Legionnaires' Disease: 1.6-4g/day in divided doses.	Usual: 30-50mg/kg/day in divided doses q6h, q8h or q12h. Double dose for more severe infections. Treat strep infections for 10 days. Intestinal Amebiasis: 30-50mg/kg/day in divided doses for 10-14 days. Pertussis: 40-50mg/kg/day in divided doses for 5-14 days.

(Continued)

BRAND NAME (Generic)	DOSAGE FORM/ STRENGTH	INDICATIONS	ADULT DOSE	PEDIATRIC DOSE
Ery-Tab (erythromycin)	**Tab, Delayed-Release:** 250mg, 333mg, 500mg	Mild to moderate upper and lower respiratory tract and skin and skin structure infections, listeriosis, pertussis, diphtheria, erythrasma, intestinal amebiasis, acute pelvic inflammatory disease (PID) (*N.gonorrhoeae*), primary syphilis in PCN allergy, Legionnaires' disease, chlamydial infections (eg, newborn conjunctivitis urethral, endocervical, rectal, etc), and nongonococcal urethritis; Prophylaxis of rheumatic fever.	Usual: 250mg qid, 333mg q8h or 500mg q12h without food. Max: 4g/day. Do not take bid when dose is ≥1g/day. Treat strep infections for 10 days. Chlamydial Urogenital Infection During Pregnancy: 500mg qid or 666mg q8h for 7 days, or 500mg q 12h, 333mg q8h or 250mg qid for 14 days. Urethral/Endocervical/Rectal Chlamydial Infections and Nongonococcal Urethritis: 500mg qid or 666mg q8h for at least 7 days. Primary Syphilis: 30-40g in divided doses for 10-15 days. Acute PID: 500mg (erythromycin lactobionate) IV q6h for 3 days, then 500mg PO q12h or 333mg q8h for 7 days. Streptococcal Infection Long-Term Prophylaxis of Rheumatic Fever: 250mg bid. Intestinal Amebiasis: 500mg q12h, 333mg q8h or 250mg q6h for 10-14 days. Pertussis: 40-50mg/kg/day in divided doses for 5-14 days. Legionnaires' Disease: 1-4g/day in divided doses.	Usual: 30-50mg/kg/day in divided doses without food. Max: 4g/day. Severe Infections: Double dose up to 4g/day. Treat strep infections for 10 days. Chlamydial Conjunctivitis of Newborns and Chlamydial Pneumonia in Infancy: 12.5mg/kg for 2 weeks and 3 weeks, respectively. Intestinal Amebiasis: 30-50mg/kg/day in divided doses for 10-14 days. Long-Term Prophylaxis of Rheumatic Fever: 250mg bid. Intestinal Amebiasis: 30-50mg/kg/day in divided doses for 10-14 days. Pertussis: 40-50mg/kg/day in divided doses for 5-14 days. Legionnaire's Disease: 1-4g/day in divided doses.
Erythrocin (erythromycin stearate)	**Tab:** 250mg, 500mg	Mild to moderate upper and lower respiratory tract, and skin and skin structure infections, listeriosis, pertussis, diphtheria, erythrasma, intestinal amebiasis, acute pelvic inflammatory disease (PID) (gonorrhea), primary syphilis in PCN allergy, Legionnaires' disease, chlamydial infections (eg, newborn conjunctivitis urethral, endocervical, or rectal, etc), and nongonococcal urethritis. Prophylaxis of rheumatic fever.	Usual: 250mg q6h or 500mg q12h without food. Max: 4g/day. Treat strep infections for 10 days. Streptococcal Infection Prophylaxis of Rheumatic Fever: 250mg bid. Chlamydial Urogenital Infection During Pregnancy: 500mg qid for 7 days or 250mg qid for 14 days. Urethral/Endocervical/Rectal Chlamydial Infections and Nongonococcal Urethritis: 500mg qid for at least 7 days. Primary Syphilis: 30-40g in divided doses over 10-15 days. Acute PID: 500mg (erythromycin lactobionate) IV q6h for 3 days, then 500mg PO q12h for 7 days. Intestinal Amebiasis: 250mg qid for 10-14 days. Pertussis: 40-50mg/kg/day in divided doses for 5-14 days. Legionnaires' Disease: 1-4g/day in divided doses.	Usual: 30-50mg/kg/day in divided doses without food. Severe Infections: Double dose up to 4g/day. Streptococcal Infection Prophylaxis of Rheumatic Fever: 250mg bid. Treat strep infections for 10 days. Chlamydial Conjunctivitis of Newborns/Chlamydial Pneumonia in Infancy: 12.5mg/kg for 2 weeks and 3 weeks, respectively. Intestinal Amebiasis: 30-50mg/kg/day in divided doses for 10-14 days. Pertussis: 40-50mg/kg/day in divided doses for 5-14 days.

BRAND NAME (Generic)	DOSAGE FORM/ STRENGTH	INDICATIONS	ADULT DOSE	PEDIATRIC DOSE
MACROLIDES *(Continued)*				
Erythromycin	**Cap, Delayed-Release:** 250mg	Mild to moderate upper and lower respiratory tract and skin and skin structure infections, listeriosis, pertussis, diphtheria, erythrasma, intestinal amebiasis, primary syphilis in PCN allergy, Legionnaires' disease, chlamydial infections (eg, newborn conjunctivitis urethral, endocervical, rectal, etc), and nongonococcal urethritis. Prophylaxis of endocarditis or rheumatic fever.	Usual: 250mg q6h or 500mg q12h without food. Max: 4g/day. Treat strep infections for 10 days. Streptococcal Infection Prophylaxis of Rheumatic Fever: 250mg bid. Chlamydial Urogenital Infection During Pregnancy: 500mg qid for 7 days or 250mg qid for 14 days. Urethral/Endocervical/Rectal Chlamydial Infections: 500mg qid for at least 7 days. Primary Syphilis: Intestinal Amebiasis: 250mg q6h over 10-15 days. Pertussis: 40-50mg/kg/day in divided doses for 5-14 days. Legionnaires' Disease: 1-4g/day in divided doses. Bacterial Endocarditis Prophylaxis: 1g 1 hr before procedure, then 500mg 6 hrs later.	Usual: 30-50mg/kg/day in divided doses without food. Severe Infections: Double dose up to 4g/day. Treat strep infections for 10 days. Streptococcal Infection Prophylaxis of Rheumatic Fever: 250mg bid. Intestinal Amebiasis: 30-50mg/kg/day in divided doses for 10-14 days. Pertussis: 40-50mg/kg/day in divided doses for 5-14 days. Bacterial Endocarditis Prophylaxis: 20mg/kg 1 hr before procedure, then 10mg/kg 6 hrs later.
Erythromycin Base	**Tab:** 250mg	Mild to moderate upper and lower respiratory tract and skin and skin structure infections, listeriosis, pertussis, diphtheria, erythrasma, intestinal amebiasis, acute pelvic inflammatory disease (PID) *(N.gonorrhoeae)*, primary syphilis in PCN allergy, Legionnaires' disease, chlamydial infections (eg, newborn conjunctivitis urethral, endocervical, rectal, etc), and nongonococcal urethritis. Prophylaxis of rheumatic fever.	Usual: 250mg q6h or 500mg q12h without food. Max: 4g/day. Treat strep infections for 10 days. Streptococcal Infection Prophylaxis of Rheumatic Fever: 250mg bid. Chlamydial Urogenital Infection During Pregnancy: 500mg qid for 7 days or 250mg qid for 14 days. Urethral/Endocervical/Rectal Chlamydial Infections and Nongonococcal Urethritis: 500mg qid for at least 7 days. Primary Syphilis: 30-40g in divided doses over 10-15 days. Acute PID: 500mg (erythromycin lactobionate) IV q6h for 3 days, then 500mg PO q12h for 7 days. Intestinal Amebiasis: 250mg qid for 10-14 days. Pertussis: 40-50mg/kg/day in divided doses. Legionnaires' Disease: 1-4g/day in divided doses.	Usual: 30-50mg/kg/day in divided doses without food. Severe Infections: Double dose up to 4g/day. Treat strep infections for 10 days. Streptococcal Infection Prophylaxis of Rheumatic Fever: 250mg bid. Chlamydial Conjunctivitis of Newborns and Chlamydial Pneumonia in Infancy: 12.5mg/kg qid for 2 weeks and 3 weeks, respectively. Intestinal Amebiasis: 30-50mg/kg/day in divided doses for 10-14 days. Pertussis: 40-50mg/kg/day in divided doses for 5-14 days.
Pediazole (sulfisoxazole acetyl-erythromycin ethylsuccinate)	**Sus:** (Erythromycin Ethylsuccinate-Sulfisoxazole Acetyl) 200 mg-600mg/5mL [100 mL, 150mL, 200mL]	Acute otitis media caused by *H.influenzae.*		>2 mos: Dose based on 50mg/kg/day erythromycin or 150mg/kg/day sulfisoxazole given tid-qid for 10 days. Max: 6g/day sulfisoxazole.

(Continued)

BRAND NAME (Generic)	DOSAGE FORM/ STRENGTH	INDICATIONS	ADULT DOSE	PEDIATRIC DOSE
PCE (erythromycin)	Tab, Extended-Release: 333mg, 500mg	Mild to moderate upper and lower respiratory tract and skin and skin structure infections, listeriosis, pertussis, diphtheria, erythrasma, intestinal ame biasis, acute pelvic inflammatory disease (PID) (N.gonorrhoeae), primary syphilis in PCN allergy, Legionnaires' disease, chlamydial infections (eg, newborn conjunctivitis urethral, endocervical, or rectal, etc), and nongonococcal urethritis. Prophylaxis of rheumatic fever.	Usual: 333mg q8h or 500mg q12h without food. Max: 4g/day. Do not take bid when dose is ≥1g/day Treat strep infections for 10 days. Chlamydial Urogenital Infection During Pregnancy: 500mg q8h or 666mg q8h for 7 days, or 500mg q12h, 333mg q8h or 250mg qid for 14 days. Urethral/Endocervical/ Rectal Chlamydial Infections and Nongonococcal Urethritis: 500mg qid or 666mg q8h for at least 7 days. Primary Syphilis: 30-40g in divided doses for 10-15 days. Acute PID: 500mg (erythromycin lactobionate) IV q6h for 3 days, then 500mg PO q12h or 333mg q8h for 7 days. Streptococcal Infection Long-Term Prophylaxis of Rheumatic Fever: 250mg bid. Intestinal Amebiasis: 500mg q12h, or 333mg q8h or 250mg q6h for 10-14 days. Pertussis: 40-50mg/day in divided doses for 5-14 days. Legionnaires' Disease: 1-4g/day in divided doses.	Usual: 30-50mg/kg/day in divided doses without food. Max: 4g/day. Severe Infections: Double dose up to 4g/day. Treat strep infections for 10 days. Chlamydial Conjunctivitis of Newborns and Chlamydial Pneumonia in Infancy: 12.5mg/kg qid for 2 weeks and 3 weeks, respectively. Intestinal Amebiasis: 30-50mg/day in divided doses for 10-14 days. Long-Term Prophylaxis of Rheumatic Fever: 250mg bid. Pertussis: 40-50mg/kg/day in divided doses for 5-14 days. Legionnaires' Disease: 1-4g/day in divided doses.
Zithromax (azithromycin)	Inj: 500mg; Sus: 100mg/5mL [15mL], 200mg/5mL [15mL, 22.5mL, 30mL], 1g/pkt [3⁵ 10⁵]; Tab: 250mg [Z-Pak, 6 tabs], 500mg [Tri-Pak, 3 tabs], 600mg	(PO) Treatment of acute bacterial exacerbations of COPD, community acquired bacterial sinusitis (ABS), community acquired pneumonia (CAP), pharyngitis/tonsillitis, uncomplicated skin and skin structure, urethritis/ cervicitis, genital ulcer disease (men), acute otitis media, prevention of disseminated Mycobacterium avium complex (MAC) disease in advanced HIV infection. (IV) Treatment of CAP and pelvic inflammatory disease (PID).	(PO) COPD/CAP/Pharyngitis/Tonsillitis (second line therapy)/SSSI: ≥16 yrs: 500mg on day 1, then 250 mg qd on days 2-5. COPD: 500mg qd for 3 days. ABS: 500mg qd for 3 days. Genital Ulcer Disease and Non-Gonococcal Urethritis/Cervicitis: 1g single dose. Urethritis/Cervicitis due to gonorrhea: 2g single dose. MAC Prophylaxis: 1200mg once weekly. MAC Treatment: 600mg qd with ethambutol 15mg/ kg/day. (IV) ≥16 yrs: CAP: 500mg qd for at least 2 days; then 500mg PO to complete 7-10 day course. PID: 500mg qd for 1-2 days, then 250mg PO to complete 7-day course.	(Sus) Otitis Media: ≥6 mo: 30mg/kg single dose; 10mg/kg qd for 3 days; or 10mg/kg qd on day 1, then 5mg/kg qd on days 2-5. ABS: ≥6 mo: 10mg/kg qd for 3 days. Cap: ≥6 mo: 10mg/kg qd on day 1, then 5mg/kg qd on days 2-5. (Sus, Tab) Pharyngitis/ Tonsillitis: ≥2 yrs: 12mg/kg qd for 5 days. 1g suspension is not for pediatric use.
Zmax (azithromycin)	Sus, Extended-Release: 2g	Treatment of mild to moderate acute bacterial sinusitis due to Haemophilus influenzae, Moraxella catarrhalis, or Streptococcus pneumoniae. Treatment of community-acquired pneumonia due to Chlamydophila pneumoniae, Haemophilus influenzae, Mycoplasma pneumoniae, or Streptococcus pneumoniae in patients appropriate for oral therapy.	2g single dose. Take on an empty stomach (1 hr before or 2 hrs after a meal).	

BRAND NAME (Generic)	DOSAGE FORM/ STRENGTH	INDICATIONS	ADULT DOSE	PEDIATRIC DOSE
PENICILLINS				
Amoxil (amoxicillin)	**Cap:** 250mg, 500mg; **Sus:** 50mg/mL [15mL, 30mL], 125mg/5mL [80mL, 100mL, 150mL], 200mg/5mL [50mL, 75mL, 100mL], 250mg/5mL [80mL, 100mL, 150mL], 400mg/5mL [5mL, 50mL, 75mL, 100mL]; **Tab:** 500mg, 875mg; **Tab, Chewable:** 200mg, 400mg	Infections of the ear, nose, throat, genitourinary tract, skin and skin structure, lower respiratory tract due to susceptible (beta lactamase negative) organisms; gonorrhea (acute uncomplicated). *H.pylori* eradication to reduce the risk of duodenal ulcer recurrence.	Ear/Nose/Throat/SSSI/GU: (Mild/Moderate): 500mg q12h or 250mg q8h. (Severe): 875mg q12h or 500 mg q8h. LRTI: 875mg q12h or 500mg q8h. Gonorrhea: 3g as single dose. *H.pylori:* (Dual Therapy) 1g + 30mg lansoprazole, both tid for 14 days. (Triple Therapy) 1g + 30mg lansoprazole + 500mg clarithromycin, all q12h X 14 days. CrCl 10-30mL/ min: 250-500mg q12h. <10mL/min: 250-500mg q24h. Hemodialysis: 250-500mg or 250mg q24h, additional dose during and at the end.	**Neonates:** ≤12 weeks: Max: 30mg/kg/day divided q12h. >3 mo: Ear/Nose/Throat/SSSI/GU: (Mild/Moderate): 25mg/kg/day given q12h or 20mg/kg/day given q8h. (Severe): 45mg/kg/day given q12h or 40 mg/kg/day given q8h. LRTI: 45mg/kg/day given q12h or 40mg/kg/day given q8h. Gonorrhea: (Prepubertal) 50mg/kg with 25mg/kg probenecid as single dose. (Not for <2 yrs). >40kg: Dose as adult.
Ampicillin (ampicillin sodium)	**Inj:** 125mg, 250mg, 500mg, 1g, 2g, 10g	Treatment of respiratory tract, urinary tract, and GI infections, bacterial meningitis, septicemia, endocarditis.	IM/IV: Respiratory Tract: ≥40kg: 250-500mg q8h. <40kg: 25-50mg/kg/day given q6-8h. GI/GU Caused by *N.gonorrhea* (Females): ≥40kg: 500mg q6h. <40kg: 50mg/kg/day given q6-8h. Urethritis Caused by *N.gonorrhea* (Males): 500mg q8-12h for 2 doses; may retreat if needed. Bacterial Meningitis: 150-200mg/kg/day IV given q3-4h. Septicemia: 150-200mg/kg/day IV for 3 days, continue with IM q3-4h. Treat for minimum of 10 days and 48-72 hrs after being asymptomatic.	Bacterial Meningitis: 150-200mg/kg/day IV given q3-4h. Septicemia: 150-200mg/kg/day IV given q3-4h for 3 days, continue with IM q3-4h. Treat for minimum of 10 days and 48-72 hrs after being asymptomatic.

(Continued)

BRAND NAME (Generic)	DOSAGE FORM/ STRENGTH	INDICATIONS	ADULT DOSE	PEDIATRIC DOSE
Augmentin (amoxicillin-clavulanate potassium)	(Amoxicillin-Clavulanate) **Sus:** 125-31.25mg/5mL [75mL, 100mL, 150mL] 200-28.5mg/5mL [50mL, 75mL, 100mL], 250-62.5mg/5mL [75mL, 100mL, 150mL], 400-57mg/5mL [50mL, 75mL, 100mL]; **Tab:** 250-125mg, 500-125mg, 875-125mg; Chewable: 200-28.5mg, 250-62.5mg, 400-57/mg	Treatment of lower respiratory tract (LRTI), skin and skin structure (SSSI), and urinary tract infections (UTI), otitis media (OM), sinusitis.	(Dose based on amoxicillin) 500mg q12h or 250mg q8h. Severe Infections/RTI: 875mg q12h or 500mg q8h. May use 125mg/5mL or 250mg/5mL sus in place of 500mg tab and 200mg/5mL sus or 400mg/5mL sus in place of 875mg tab. CrCl <30mL/min: Do not give 875mg tab. CrCl 10-30mL/min: 250-500mg q12h. CrCl <10mL/min: 250-500mg q24h. Hemodialysis: 250-500mg q24h; give additional dose during and at the end of dialysis.	(Dose based on amoxicillin) ≥40kg: Use adult dose. ≥12 weeks: Sinusitis/OM/LRTI/Severe Infections: (Sus/Tab, Chewable) 45mg/kg/day given q12h or 40mg/kg/day given q8h. Less Severe Infections: 25mg/kg/day given q12h or 20mg/kg/day given q8h. <12 weeks:15mg/kg q12h (use 125mg/5mL sus).
Augmentin ES-600 (amoxicillin-clavulanate potassium)	**Sus:** (Amoxicillin-Clavulanate) 600mg-42.9mg/5mL [50mL, 75mL, 100mL, 150mL]	Treatment of recurrent or persistent acute otitis media.		(Dose based on amoxicillin) 3 mo-12 yrs: <40kg: 45mg/kg q12h for 10 days.
Augmentin XR (amoxicillin-clavulanate potassium)	**Tab, Extended-Release:** (Amoxicillin-Clavulanate) 1000 mg-62.5mg	Treatment of community acquired pneumonia (CAP) or acute bacterial sinusitis due to confirmed or suspected β-lactamase producing pathogens.	Sinusitis: 2 tabs q12h for 10 days. Cap: 2 tabs q12h for 7-10 days. Take at the start of a meal.	≥16 yrs: Sinusitis: 2 tabs q12h for 10 days. Cap: 2 tabs q12h for 7-10 days. Take at the start of a meal.
Bicillin C-R (penicillin G benzathine-penicillin G procaine)	**Inj:** (Penicillin G Benzathine-Penicillin G Procaine) 300,000 U/mL, 300,000-300,000 U/mL	Treatment of moderately severe to severe upper-respiratory tract (URTI) and skin and soft-tissue infections (SSTI); scarlet fever and erysipelas due to streptococci. Treatment of moderately severe pneumonia and otitis media due to pneumococci.	Group A Strep: URTI/SSTI/Scarlet Fever/Erysipelas: 2.4 MU IM. Treat at a single session using multiple IM sites, or use an alternative schedule and give ½ of the total dose on Day 1 and ½ on Day 3. Pneumococcal Infections (Except Meningitis): 1.2 MU IM, repeat every 2-3 days until temperature is normal for 48 hrs. Administer IM into upper, outer quadrant of buttock.	Group A Strep: URTI/SSTI/Scarlet Fever/Erysipelas: >60 lbs: 2.4 MU IM. IM. 30-60 lbs: 900,000 U-1.2 MU IM. <30 lbs: 600,000 U IM. Treat at a single session using multiple IM sites, or use an alternative schedule and give ½ of the total dose on Day 1 and ½ on Day 3. Pneumococcal Infections (Except Meningitis): 600,000 U IM, repeat every 2-3 days until temperature is normal for 48 hrs. Administer IM into upper, outer quadrant of buttock. Use the midlateral aspect of thigh in neonates, infants, and small children.

BRAND NAME (Generic)	DOSAGE FORM/ STRENGTH	INDICATIONS	ADULT DOSE	PEDIATRIC DOSE
PENICILLINS *(Continued)*				
Bicillin C-R 900/300 (penicillin G benzathine-penicillin G procaine)	**Inj:** (Penicillin G Benzathine-Penicillin G Procaine) 900,000-300,000 U/2mL	Treatment of moderately severe to severe upper-respiratory tract (URTI) and skin and soft-tissue infections (SSTI), scarlet fever and erysipelas due to streptococci. Treatment of moderately severe pneumonia and otitis media due to pneumococci.		Group A Strep: URTI/SSTI/Scarlet Fever/Erysipelas: 1.2 MU IM single dose. Pneumococcal Infections (Except Meningitis): 1.2 MU IM every 2-3 days until temperature is normal for 48 hrs. Administer IM into upper, outer quadrant of buttock. Use midlateral aspect of thigh in neonates, infants, and small children.
Bicillin L-A (penicillin G benzathine)	**Inj:** 600,000 U/mL	Treatment of mild to moderate upper respiratory tract infections (URTI) due to streptococci and venereal infections (eg, syphilis, yaws, bejel, pinta). Prophylaxis to prevent recurrence of rheumatic fever or chorea.	Group A Strep: URTI: 1.2 MU IM single dose. Primary/Secondary/Latent Syphilis: 2.4 MU IM single dose. Late Syphilis (Tertiary/Neurosyphilis): 2.4 MU IM every 7 days for 3 doses. Yaws/Bejel/Pinta: 1.2 MU IM single dose. Rheumatic Fever/Glomerulonephritis Prophylaxis: 1.2 MU IM once a mo or 600,000 U IM every 2 weeks. Administer IM into upper, outer quadrant of buttock.	Group A Strep: URTI: Older Pediatrics: 900,000 U IM single dose. <60lbs: 300,000-600,000 U IM single dose. Congenital Syphilis: 2-12 yrs: Adjust dose based on adult schedule. <2 yrs: 50,000 U/kg IM single dose. Rheumatic Fever/Glomerulonephritis Prophylaxis: 1.2 MU IM once a mo or 600,000 U IM every 2 weeks. Administer IM into upper, outer quadrant of buttock. Use the midlateral aspect of thigh in neonates, infants, and small children.
Dicloxacillin (dicloxacillin sodium)	**Cap:** 250mg, 500mg; **Sus:** 62.5mg/5mL [100mL]	Infections caused by penicillinase-producing staphylococci.	Mild-Moderate Infection: 125mg q6h. Severe Infection: 250mg q6h for at least 14 days.	<40kg: Mild-Moderate Infection: 12.5mg/kg/day in divided doses q6h. Severe Infection: 25mg/kg/day in divided doses q6h for at least 14 days.
Geocillin (carbenicillin disodium)	**Tab:** 382mg	Treatment of acute and chronic infections of the upper and lower urinary tract (UTI) and asymptomatic bacteriuria.	UTI: *E.coli, Proteus,* and *Enterobacter:* 1-2 tabs qid. *Pseudomonas, Enterococcus:* 2 tabs qid. Prostatitis: *E.coli, Proteus, Enterococcus* and *Enterobacter:* 2 tabs qid. CrCl 10-20mL/min: Adjust dose.	
Penicillin VK, Veetids (penicillin V potassium)	**Sus:** 125mg/5mL, 250mg/5mL [100mL, 200mL]; **Tab:** 250mg, 500mg	Mild to moderately severe bacterial infections including conditions of the respiratory tract, oropharynx, skin and soft tissue. Prevention of recurrence following rheumatic fever and/or chorea.	Usual: Streptococcal Infections (Scarlet Fever, Erysipelas, Upper Respiratory Tract): 125-250mg q6-8h for 10 days. Pneumococcal Infections (Otitis Media, Respiratory Tract): 250-500mg q6h until afebrile for at least 2 days. Staphylococcus Infections (Skin/Soft Tissue): 250-500mg q6-8h. Fusospirochetosis Infections (Oropharynx): 250-500mg q6-8h.	≥12 yrs: Usual: Streptococcal Infections (Scarlet fever, Erysipelas, Upper Respiratory Tract): 125-250mg q6-8h for 10 days. Pneumococcal Infections (Otitis media, Respiratory Tract): 250-500mg q6h until afebrile. Respiratory Tract): 250-500mg q6h until afebrile for at least 2 days. Staphylococcus Infections (Skin/Soft Tissue): 250-500mg q6-8h. Fusospirochetosis Infections (Oropharynx): 250-500mg q6-8h. Rheumatic Fever/Chorea Prevention: 125-250mg bid.

(Continued)

BRAND NAME (Generic)	DOSAGE FORM/ STRENGTH	INDICATIONS	ADULT DOSE	PEDIATRIC DOSE
Pfizerpen (penicillin G potassium)	Inj: 1 MU, 5 MU, 20 MU	For therapy of severe infections when rapid and high blood levels of penicillin required. Management of streptococcal, pneumococcal, staphylococcal, clostridial, fusospirochetal, listeria, and gram negative bacillary, and pasteurella infections. For anthrax, actinomycosis, diphtheria, erysipeloid, meningitis, endocarditis, bacteremia, rat-bite fever, syphilis, and gonorrheal endocarditis and arthritis. With combined oral therapy, prophylaxis against endocarditis in patients with congenital heart disease, rheumatic, or other acquired valvular heart disease undergoing dental procedures or surgical procedures of upper respiratory tract.	Anthrax/Gonorrheal Endocarditis/Severe Infections (Streptococci, Pneumococci, Staphylococci): Minimum of 5 MU/day. Syphilis: Administer in hospital. Determine dose and duration based on age and weight. Meningococcic Meningitis: 1-2 MU IM q2h or 20-30 MU/day continuous IV. Actinomycosis: 1-6 MU/day for cervicofacial cases; 10-20 MU/day for thoracic and abdominal disease. Clostridial Infections: 20 MU/day (adjunct to antitoxin). Fusospirochetal Severe Infections: 5-10 MU/day for oropharynx, lower respiratory tract, and genital area infection. Rat-bite Fever: 12-15 MU/day for 3-4 weeks. Listeria Endocarditis: 15-20 MU/day for 4 weeks. Pasteurella Bacteremia/Meningitis: 4-6 MU/day for 2 weeks. Erysipeloid Endocarditis: 2-20 MU/day for 4-6 weeks. Gram Negative Bacillary Bacteremia: 20-80 MU/day. Diphtheria (carrier state): 0.3-0.4 MU/day in divided doses for 10-12 days. Endocarditis Prophylaxis: 1 MU IM mixed with 0.6 MU procaine penicillin G 0.5-1 hr before procedure. Renal/Cardiac/Vascular Dysfunction: Consider dose reduction. For streptococcal infection, treat for minimum 10 days.	Listeria Infections: Neonates: 0.5-1 MU/day. Congenital Syphilis: Administer in hospital. Determine dose and duration based on age and weight. Endocarditis Prophylaxis: 30,000 U/kg IM mixed with 0.6 MU procaine penicillin G 0.5-1 hr before procedure. For streptococcal infection, treat for minimum 10 days.
Permapen (penicillin G benzathine)	Inj: 600,000 U/mL	Treatment of microorganisms susceptible to low and very prolonged serum levels in upper respiratory tract infections (streptococci group A—without bacteremia), syphilis, yaws, bejel, and pinta. Prophylaxis for rheumatic fever and/or chorea. Follow-up prophylactic therapy for rheumatic heart disease and acute glomerulonephritis.	Streptococcal Infection: 1.2 MU IM single dose. Primary/Secondary/Latent Syphilis: 1 MU IM single dose. Late (Tertiary/Neurosyphilis) Syphilis: 3 MU IM every 7 days for total of 6-9 MU. Yaws/Bejel/Pinta: 1.2 MU IM single dose. Rheumatic Fever/Glomerulonephritis Prophylaxis: 1.2 MU IM once moly or 600,000 U IM twice moly. Use upper outer quadrant of buttock. Rotate injection site.	≤12 yrs: Adjust dose according to age and weight and severity of infection. Streptococcal Infection: 900,000 U IM single dose in older children. Congenital Syphilis: <2 yrs: 50,000 U/kg IM single dose. 2-12 yrs: Adjust dose based on adult schedule. Use midlateral aspect of thigh in infants and small children. May divide dose between 2 buttocks in peds <2 yrs. Rotate injection site.

BRAND NAME (Generic)	DOSAGE FORM/ STRENGTH	INDICATIONS	ADULT DOSE	PEDIATRIC DOSE
PENICILLINS *(Continued)*				
Piperacillin	**Inj:** 2g, 3g, 4g	Treatment of serious intra-abdominal, urinary tract, gynecologic, lower respiratory tract, skin and skin structure, bone and joint, and gonoccocal infections, septicemia, and perioperative surgical prophylaxis.	Usual: 3-4g IM/IV q4-6h. Max: 24g/day. IM: 2g/site. Serious Infections: 200-300mg/kg/day IV divided q4-6h. Complicated UTI: 125-200mg/day IV divided q6-8h. Uncomplicated UTI/Community Acquired Pneumonia: 100-125mg/kg/day IM/IV divided q6-12h. Uncomplicated Gonorrhea: 2g IM single dose with 1g PO probenecid 1/2 hr before injection. Surgical Prophylaxis: 2g IV 20-30 min just prior to anesthesia (See labeling for follow-up dosing). C-Section: 2g IV after cord is clamped, then 2g 4 hrs and 8 hrs after 1st dose. Renal Impairment: Uncomplicated/Complicated UTI: CrCl<20mL/min: 3g q12h. Complicated UTI: CrCl 20-40mL/min: 3g q8h. Serious Infection: CrCl 20-40mL/min: 4g q8h. CrCl<20mL/min: 4g q12h. Hemodialysis: Give 1g additional dose after each dialysis. Max: 2g q8h. Usual treatment is for 7-10 days; treat gynecologic infections for 3-10 days; treat *S.pyogenes* infections for at least 10 days.	≥12 yrs: Usual: 3-4g IM/IV q4-6h. Max: 24g/day. IM: 2g/site. Serious Infections: 200-300mg/kg/day IV divided q4-6h. Complicated UTI: 125-200mg/kg/day IV divided q6-8h. Uncomplicated UTI/Community Acquired Pneumonia: 100-125mg/kg/day IM/IV divided q6-12h. Uncomplicated Gonorrhea: 2g IM single dose with 1g PO probenecid 1/2 hr before injection. Surgical Prophylaxis: 2g IV 20-30 minute just prior to anesthesia (See labeling for follow-up dosing). C-section: 2g IV after cord is clamped, then 2g 4 hrs and 8 hrs after 1st dose. Renal Impairment: Uncomplicated/Complicated UTI: CrCl <20mL/min: 3g q12h. Complicated UTI: CrCl 20-40mL/min: 3g q8h. Serious Infection: CrCl 20-40mL/min: 4g q8h. CrCl <20mL/min: 4g q12h. Hemodialysis: Give 1g additional dose after each dialysis. Max: 2g q8h. Usual treatment is for 7-10 days; treat gynecologic infections for 3-10 days; treat *S.pyogenes* infections for at least 10 days.
Timentin (ticarcillin-clavulanate potassium)	**Inj:** (Ticarcillin-Clavulanate) 3g-100mg, 3g-100mg/100mL, 30g-1g	Treatment of lower respiratory tract, bone and joint, skin and skin structure, urinary tract (UTI), gynecologic, and intra-abdominal infections, and septicemia.	≥60kg: UTI/Systemic Infection: 3g-100mg (3.1g vial) IV given q4-6h. Gynecologic Infections: Moderate: 200mg/kg/day ticarcillin IV given q6h. Severe: 300mg/kg/day ticarcillin IV given q4h.<60kg: Usual: 200-300mg/kg/day ticarcillin IV given q4-6h. UTI: 3g-200mg (3.2g vial) q8h. Renal Impairment (based on ticarcillin): CrCl 60-30mL/min: 2g IV q4h. CrCl 30-10mL/min: 2g IV q8h. CrCl<10mL/min: 2g IV q12h (2g IV q24h with hepatic dysfunction). Peritoneal Dialysis: 3.1g IV q12h. Hemodialysis: 2g IV q12h, and 3.1g after each dialysis. Apply reduced dosage after initial 3.1g LD is given.	≥3 mo: >60kg: Mild to Moderate: 3g-100mg (3.1g vial) IV q6h. Severe: 3g-100mg (3.1g vial) IV q4h. <60kg: Mild to Moderate: 50mg/kg ticarcillin IV q6h. Severe: 50mg/kg ticarcillin IV q4h. Renal Impairment (based on ticarcillin): CrCl 60-30mL/min: 2g IV q4h. CrCl 30-10mL/min: 2g IV q8h. CrCl<10mL/min: 2g IV q12h (2g IV q24h with hepatic dysfunction). Peritoneal Dialysis: 3.1g IV q12h. Hemodialysis: 2g IV q12h, and 3.1g after each dialysis. Apply reduced dosage after initial 3.1g LD is given.

(Continued)

BRAND NAME (Generic)	DOSAGE FORM/ STRENGTH	INDICATIONS	ADULT DOSE	PEDIATRIC DOSE
Unasyn (ampicillin sodium/ sulbactam sodium)	**Inj:** (Ampicillin-Sulbactam) 1g-0.5g, 2g-1g, 10g-5g	Treatment of skin and skin structure (SSSI), intra-abdominal, and gynecological infections caused by susceptible microorganisms.	1.5-3g (ampicillin + sulbactam) IM/IV q6h. Max: 4g/day sulbactam. Renal Impairment: CrCl ≥30mL/min: 1.5-3g q6-8h. CrCl 15-29mL/min: 1.5-3g q12h. CrCl 5-14mL/min: 1.5-3g q24h.	≥1 yr: SSSI: 1.5-3g (ampicillin + sulbactam) IM/IV q6h. Max: 4g/day sulbactam.
Veetids (penicillin V potassium)	**Sus:** 125mg/5mL, 250mg/5mL [100mL, 200mL]; **Tab:** 250mg, 500mg	Mild to moderately severe bacterial infections including conditions of the respiratory tract, oropharynx, skin and soft tissue. Prevention of recurrence following rheumatic fever and/or chorea.	Streptococcal Infections (Scarlet Fever, Erysipelas, Upper Respiratory Tract): 125-250mg q6-8h for 10 days. Pneumococcal Infections (Otitis media, Respiratory Tract): 250-500mg q6h until afebrile for at least 2 days. Staphylococcus Infections (Skin/Soft Tissue): 250-500mg q6-8h. Fusospirochetosis Infections (Oropharynx): 250-500mg q6-8h. Rheumatic Fever/Chorea Prevention: 125-250mg bid.	Streptococcal Infections (Scarlet fever, Erysipelas, Upper Respiratory Tract): 125-250mg q6-8h for 10 days. Pneumococcal Infections (Otitis media, Respiratory Tract): 250-500mg q6h until afebrile for at least 2 days. Staphylococcus Infections (Skin/Soft Tissue): 250-500mg q6-8h. Fusospirochetosis Infections (Oropharynx): 250-500mg q6-8h. Rheumatic Fever/Chorea Prevention: 125-250mg bid.
Zosyn (piperacillin sodium-tazobactam)	**Inj:** (Piperacillin-Tazobactam) 40mg-5mg/mL, 60mg-7.5mg/mL, 2g-0.25g, 3g-0.375g, 4g-0.5g, 4g-0.5g/100mL, 36g-4.5g	Treatment of appendicitis, peritonitis, uncomplicated/complicated skin and skin structure infections, postpartum endometritis, pelvic inflammatory disease, moderate severity of community acquired pneumonia, and moderate to severe nosocomial pneumonia.	Usual: 3.375g q6h for 7-10 days. Nosocomial Pneumonia: 4.5g q6h for 7-14 days plus aminoglycoside. CrCl 20-40mL/min: 2.25g q6h. CrCl <20mL/min: 2.25g q8h. Hemodialysis: Max: 2.25g q12h.Give 1 additional 0.75g dose after each dialysis period.	
STREPTOMYCES DERIVATIVES				
Sumycin (tetracycline HCl)	**Sus:** 125mg/5mL; **Tab:** 250mg, 500mg	Treatment of respiratory tract, urinary tract, and skin and skin structure infections, lymphogranuloma psittacosis, trachoma, uncomplicated urethral/endocervical/rectal infection caused by *Chlamydia*, nongonococcal urethritis, chancroid, plague, cholera, brucellosis, and others. When PCN is contraindicated, treatment of uncomplicated gonorrhea, syphilis, listeriosis, anthrax, *Clostridium* species, and others. Adjunct therapy for amebicides and severe acne.	Mild-Moderate: 250mg qid or 500mg bid. Severe: 500mg qid. Continue for 24-48 hrs after symptoms subside (minimum 10 days with Group A hemolytic streptococci). Severe Acne: Initial: 1g/day in divided doses. Maint: After improvement, 125-500mg/day. Brucellosis: 500mg qid for 3 weeks plus streptomycin 1g IM bid for 1 week, then qd for 1 week. Syphilis: 30-40g equally divided over 10-15 days. Gonorrhea: 500mg q6h for 7 days. Chlamydia: 500mg qid for at least 7 days. Renal Dysfunction: Reduce dose or extend dose interval.	Usual: 25-50mg/kg divided bid-qid. Continue for 24-48 hrs after symptoms subside (minimum 10 days with Group A β-hemolytic streptococci). Severe Acne: Initial: 1g/day in divided doses. Maint: After improvement, 125-500mg/day. Renal Dysfunction: Reduce dose or extend dose interval.

BRAND NAME (Generic)	DOSAGE FORM/ STRENGTH	INDICATIONS	ADULT DOSE	PEDIATRIC DOSE
STREPTOMYCES DERIVATIVES *(Continued)*				
Lincocin (lincomycin HCl)	Inj: 300mg/mL	Treatment of serious infections due to streptococci, pneumococci, and staphylococci. Reserve for PCN allergy or if PCN is inappropriate.	IM: Serious Infection: 600mg q24h. More Severe Infection: 600mg q12h or more often. IV: Dose depends on severity. Serious Infection: 600mg-1g q8-12h. More Severe Infection: Increase dose. Infuse over ≥1 hr. Life-Threatening Situation: Up to 8g/day has been given. Max: 8g/day. Severe Renal Dysfunction: 25-30% of normal dose.	>1 mo: IM: Serious Infection: 10mg/kg q24h. More Severe Infection: 10mg/kg q12h or more often. IV: 10-20mg/kg/day, depending on severity infused in divided doses as described for adults. Severe Renal Dysfunction: 25-30% of normal dose.
TETRACYCLINE DERIVATIVES				
Declomycin (demeclocycline HCl)	Tab: 150mg, 300mg	Treatment of infections due to *rickettsiae*, *Mycoplasma pneumoniae*, *B.recurrentis*, agents of psittacosis, ornithosis, lymphogranuloma venereum or granuloma inguinale. Treatment of gram-negative infections (eg, respiratory, urinary tract), gram-positive infections (eg, respiratory tract, skin and soft tissue), trachoma, inclusion conjunctivitis. When PCN is contraindicated, treatment of gonorrhea, syphilis, listeriosis, anthrax, *Clostridium* species, and others. Adjunct therapy for amebicides.	Usual: 150mg qid or 300mg bid. Gonorrhea: Initial: 600mg, then 300mg q12h for 4 days. Gonorrhea: 600mg followed by 300mg q12h for 4 days to a total of 3g. Renal/Hepatic Impairment: Reduce dose and/or extend dose intervals. Continue therapy for at least 24-48 hrs after symptoms subside. Treat strep infections for at least 10 days. Take at least 1 hr before or 2 hrs after meals with plenty of fluids.	>8 yrs: Usual: 3-6mg/lb/day given bid-qid. Gonorrhea: 600mg followed by 300mg q12h for 4 days to a total of 3g. Renal/Hepatic Impairment: Reduce dose and/or extend dose intervals. Continue therapy for at least 24-48 hrs after symptoms subside. Treat strep infections for at least 10 days. Take at least 1 hr before or 2 hrs after meals with plenty of fluids.
Doryx (doxycycline hyclate)	Cap: 75mg, 100mg	Treatment of susceptible infections including respiratory, urinary, skin and skin structure, lymphogranuloma, psittacosis, trachoma, uncomplicated urethral/endocervical/rectal, nongonococcal urethritis, rickettsiae, chancroid, plague, cholera, brucellosis, anthrax. When penicillin is contraindicated, treatment of syphilis, listeriosis, *Clostridium* species, and others. Adjunct therapy for amebiasis and severe acne.	Usual: 100mg q12h on 1st day, followed by 100mg qd. Severe Infections/Chronic UTI: 100mg q12h. Uncomplicated Gonococcal Infections (Men, except anorectal infections): 100mg bid for 7 days, or 300mg followed in 1 hr by another 300mg dose. Acute Epididymo-Orchitis: 100mg bid for at least 10 days. Primary/Secondary Syphilis: 300mg/day in divided doses for at least 10 days. Nongonococcal Urethritis, Uncomplicated Urethral/Endocervical/Rectal Infection: 100mg bid for at least 7 days. Inhalational Anthrax (post-exposure): 100mg bid for 60 days. Treat Strep infections for 10 days.	>8 yrs: >100 lbs: 100mg q12h on 1st day, followed by 100mg qd. Severe Infections/Chronic UTI: 100mg q12h. ≤100 lbs: 2mg/lb given bid on Day 1, followed by 1mg/lb given qd-bid thereafter. Severe Infections: Up to 2mg/lb. Inhalational Anthrax (post-exposure): <100 lbs: 1mg/lb bid for 60 days. <100 lbs: 100mg bid for 60 days.

(Continued)

A177

BRAND NAME (Generic)	DOSAGE FORM/ STRENGTH	INDICATIONS	ADULT DOSE	PEDIATRIC DOSE
Dynacin (minocycline HCl)	**Cap:** 50mg, 75mg, 100mg; **Tab:** 50mg, 75mg, 100mg	Treatment of inclusion conjunctivitis, nongonococcal urethritis, and other infections (eg, respiratory tract, endocervical, rectal, urinary tract, skin and skin structure) caused by susceptible strains of microorganisms. Alternative treatment in certain other infections (eg, urethritis, gonococcal, syphilis, anthrax). Adjunctive therapy in acute intestinal amebiasis and severe acne. Treatment of *Mycobacterium marinum* and asymptomatic carriers of *Neisseria meningitidis*.	Usual: 200mg initially; then 100mg q12h; alternative is 100-200mg initially, then 50mg qid. Uncomplicated Gonococcal Infection (Men, Other Than Urethritis and Anorectal Infections): 200mg initially, then 100mg q12h for minimum 4 days. Uncomplicated Gonococcal Urethritis (Men): 100mg q12h for 5 days. Syphilis: Administer usual dose for 10-15 days. Meningococcal Carrier State: 100mg q12h for 5 days. *Mycobacterium marinum*: 100mg q12h for 6-8 weeks. Uncomplicated urethral, endocervical, or rectal infection: 100mg q12h for at least 7 days. Renal Dysfunction: Reduce dose and/or extend dose intervals.	>8 yrs: 4mg/kg initially followed by 2mg/kg q12h. Take with plenty of fluids.
Minocin (minocycline HCl)	**Cap:** 50mg, 100mg;	Treatment of inclusion conjunctivitis, nongonococcal urethritis, and other infections (eg, respiratory tract, endocervical, rectal, urinary tract, skin and skin structure) caused by susceptible strains of microorganisms. Alternative treatment in certain other infections (eg, urethritis, gonococcal, syphilis, anthrax). Adjunctive therapy in acute intestinal amebiasis and severe acne. Treatment of *Mycobacterium marinum* and asymptomatic carriers of *Neisseria meningitidis*.	Usual: 200mg initially, then 100mg q12h; alternative is 100-200mg initially, then 50mg qid. Uncomplicated Gonococcal Infection (Men, other than urethritis and anorectal infections): 200mg initially, then 100mg q12h for minimum 4 days. Uncomplicated Gonococcal Urethritis (Men): 100mg q12h for 5 days. Syphilis: Administer usual dose for 10-15 days. Meningococcal Carrier State: 100mg q12h for 5 days. *Mycobacterium marinum*: 100mg q12h for 6-8 weeks. Uncomplicated Urethral, Endocervical, or Rectal Infection Caused by *Chlamydia trachomatis* or *Ureaplasma urealyticum*: 100mg q12h for at least 7 days. Gonorrhea in Patients Sensitive to PCN: 200mg initially, then 100mg q12h for at least 4 days, with post-therapy cultures within 2-3 days. Take with plenty of fluids. Renal Dysfunction: Max: 200mg/24hrs.	>8 yrs: 4mg/kg initially followed by 2mg/kg q12h. Take with plenty of fluids. Renal Dysfunction: Max: 200mg/24 hrs.

BRAND NAME (Generic)	DOSAGE FORM/ STRENGTH	INDICATIONS	ADULT DOSE	PEDIATRIC DOSE
TETRACYCLINE DERIVATIVES *(Continued)*				
Monodox (doxycycline monohydrate)	Cap: 50mg, 100mg	Treatment of respiratory tract, urinary tract, skin and skin structure, uncomplicated urethral/endocervical/rectal infection caused by *C.trachomatis*, nongonococcal urethritis caused by *C.trachomatis* and *U.urealyticum*, lymphogranuloma, psittacosis, trachoma, chancroid, plague, cholera, brucellosis. Treatment of uncomplicated gonorrhea, syphilis, listeriosis, anthrax, *Clostridium* species when PCN is contraindicated. Adjunct therapy for amebicides and severe acne.	Usual: 100mg q12h or 50mg q6h for 1 day, then 100 mg/day. Severe Infection: 100mg q12h. Uncomplicated Gonococcal Infections (except anorectal infections in men): 100mg bid for 7 days or 300mg stat, then repeat in 1 hr. Acute Epididymo-Orchitis caused by *N.gonorrhea* or *C.trachomatis*: 100mg bid for at least 10 days. Primary/Secondary Syphilis: 300mg/day in divided dose for at least 10 days. Uncomplicated Urethral/Endocervical/Rectal Infection caused by *C.trachomatis*: 100mg bid for at least 7 days. Nongonococcal Urethritis caused by *C.trachomatis* and *U.urealyticum*: 100mg bid for at least 7 days. Take with full glass of water. Take with food if GI upset occurs.	>8 yrs: ≤100 lbs: 2mg/lb divided in 2 doses for 1 day, then 1mg/lb daily in single or 2 divided doses. Severe Infection: May use up to 2mg/lb/day. >100 lbs; 100mg q12h or 50mg q6h for 1 day, then 100mg/day. Severe Infection: 100mg q12h. Take with a full glass of water. Take with food if GI upset occurs.
Oracea (doxycycline)	Cap: 40mg	Treatment of only inflammatory lesions (papules and pustules) of rosacea.	40mg qd in am. Take on empty stomach.	
Periostat (doxycycline hyclate)	Tab: 20mg	Adjunct to scaling and root planing to promote attachment level gain and reduces pocket depth in patients with adult periodontitis.	Following scaling and root planing, 20mg bid, 1 hour prior to morning and evening meals for up to 9 mos. Maintain adequate fluid intake with caps to reduce risk of esophageal irritation and ulceration.	
Solodyn (minocycline HCl)	Tab, Extended-Release: 45mg, 90mg, 135mg.	Treatment of inflammatory lesions of non-nodular moderate to severe acne vulgaris in patients ≥12 yrs.	1mg/kg for 12 weeks. Reduce dose with renal impairment.	≥12 yrs: 1mg/kg qd for 12 weeks. Reduce dose with renal impairment.
Vibra-tabs (doxycycline hyclate)	Tab: 100mg	Treatment of susceptible infections including respiratory, urinary, skin and skin structure, lymphogranuloma, psittacosis, trachoma, uncomplicated urethral/endocervical/rectal, nongonococcal urethritis, rickettsiae, chancroid, plague, cholera, brucellosis, anthrax. When penicillin is contraindicated, treatment of uncomplicated gonorrhea, syphilis, listeriosis, *Clostridium* species, and others. Adjunct therapy for amebiasis and severe acne. Prophylaxis of malaria.	Usual: 100mg q12h on day 1, then 100mg qd or 50mg q12h. Severe Infection: 100mg q12h. Treat for 10 days with strep infection. Uncomplicated Gonococcal Infection (Except Anorectal in Men): 100mg bid for 7 days or 300mg followed by 300mg in 1 hr. Uncomplicated Urethral/Endocervical/Rectal Infection and Nongonococcal Urethritis: 100mg bid for 7 days. Syphilis: 100mg bid for 2 weeks. Syphilis for >1 yr: 100mg bid for 4 weeks. Acute Epididymo-orchitis: 100mg bid for at least 10 days. Inhalation Anthrax (Post-Exposure): 100mg bid for 60 days. Malaria Prophylaxis: 100mg qd. Begin 1-2 days before travel and continue for 4 weeks after leaving malarious area.	

(Continued)

BRAND NAME (Generic)	DOSAGE FORM/ STRENGTH	INDICATIONS	ADULT DOSE	PEDIATRIC DOSE
Vibramycin (doxycycline)	**Cap:** (Doxycycline Hyclate) 50mg, 100mg; **Syrup:** (Doxycycline Calcium) 50mg/5mL; **Sus:** (Doxycycline Monohydrate) 25mg/5mL [60mL]	Treatment of susceptible infections including respiratory, urinary, skin and skin structure, lymphogranuloma, psittacosis, trachoma, uncomplicated urethral/endocervical/rectal, nongonococcal urethritis, rickettsiae, chancroid, plague, cholera, brucellosis, anthrax. When penicillin is contraindicated, treatment of uncomplicated gonorrhea, syphilis, listeriosis, *Clostridium species*, and others. Adjunct therapy for amebiasis and severe acne. Prophylaxis of malaria.	Usual: 100mg q12h on day 1, then 100mg qd or 50mg q12h. Severe Infection: 100mg q12h. Treat for 10 days with strep infection. Uncomplicated Gonococcal Infection (Except Anorectal in Men): 100mg bid for 7 days or 300mg followed by 300mg in 1 hr. Uncomplicated Urethral/Endocervical/Rectal Infection and Nongonococcal Urethritis: 100mg bid for 7 days. Syphilis: 100mg bid for 2 weeks. Syphilis for >1 yr: 100mg bid for 4 weeks. Acute Epididymo-orchitis: 100mg bid for at least 10 days. Inhalation Anthrax (Post-Exposure): 100mg bid for 60 days. Malaria Prophylaxis: 100mg qd. Begin 1-2 days before travel and continue for 4 weeks after leaving malarious area.	>8 yrs: ≤100 lbs: 1mg/lb bid on day 1, then 1mg/lb qd or 0.5mg/lb bid. Severe Infections: Maint: 2mg/lb. >100 lbs: Usual: 100mg q12h on day 1, then 100mg qd or 50mg q12h. Severe Infection: 100mg q12h. Treat for 10 days with strep infection. Inhalation Anthrax (Post-Exposure): <100 lbs: 1mg/lb bid for 60 days. ≥100 lbs: 100mg bid for 60 days. Malaria Prophylaxis: 2mg/kg qd. Max: 100mg/day. Begin 1-2 days before travel and continue for 4 weeks after leaving malarious area.
Vibramycin IV (doxycycline hyclate)	**Inj:** 100mg, 200mg	Treatment of *rickettsiae, Mycoplasma pneumoniae, psittacosis,* ornithosis, lymphogranuloma venereum, granuloma inguinale, relapsing fever, chancroid, *Pasteurella pestis, Pasturella tularensis, Bartonella bacilliformis, Bacteroides species, Vibrio comma, Vibrio fetus, Brucella species, E.coli, Enterobacter aerogenes, Shigella species, Mima species, Herellea species, Haemophilus influenzae, Klebsiella species, Streptococcus species, Diplococcus pneumoniae, Staphylococcus aureus,* anthrax, and trachoma. When PCN is contraindicated; treatment of *Neisseria gonorrhea, N.meningitidis;* syphilis, yaws, *Listeria monocytogenes, Clostridium species, Fusobacterium fusiforme* and *Actinomyces species.* Adjunct therapy for amebiasis.	Usual: 200mg IV divided qd-bid on Day 1 then 100-200mg/day IV depending on severity, with 200mg administered in 1 or 2 infusions. Primary/Secondary Syphilis: 300mg/day IV for at least 10 days. Inhalational Anthrax (Post-Exposure): 100mg IV bid. Institute oral therapy as soon as possible and continue therapy for a total of 60 days.	>8 yrs: >100 lbs: Usual: 200mg IV divided qd-bid on Day 1 then 100-200mg/day IV depending on severity, with 200mg administered in 1 or 2 infusions. ≤100 lbs: 2mg/lb IV divided qd-bid on Day 1 then 1-2mg/lb/day IV divided qd-bid depending on severity. Inhalational Anthrax (Post-Exposure): ≤100 lbs: 1mg/lb IV bid. Institute oral therapy as soon as possible and continue therapy for a total of 60 days.

BRAND NAME (Generic)	DOSAGE FORM/ STRENGTH	INDICATIONS	ADULT DOSE	PEDIATRIC DOSE
MISCELLANEOUS				
Bactrim (trimethoprim-sulfamethoxazole)	(Sulfamethoxazole [SMX]-Trimethoprim [TMP]) **Tab:** 400mg-80mg; Tab. **DS:** 800mg-160mg	Treatment of urinary tract infection (UTI), acute otitis media, acute exacerbation of chronic bronchitis (AECB), travelers' diarrhea, Shigellosis, and pneumocystitis carinii pneumonia (PCP).	UTI: 800mg SMX-160mg TMP q12h for 10-14 days. Shigellosis: 800mg SMX-160mg TMP q12h for 5 days. AECB: 800mg SMX-160mg TMP q12h for 14 days. PCP Treatment: 15-20mg/kg TMP and 75-100 mg/kg SMX per 24 hrs given q6h for 14-21 days. PCP Prophylaxis: 800mg SMX-160mg TMP qd. Traveler's Diarrhea: 800mg SMX-160mg TMP q12h for 5 days. CrCl: 15-30mL/min: 50% usual dose. CrCl: <15mL/min: Not recommended.	≥2 mo: UTI/Otitis Media: 4mg/kg TMP and 20mg/kg SMX q12h for 10 days. Shigellosis: 8mg/kg TMP and 40mg/kg SMX per 24 hrs given q12h for 5 days. PCP Treatment: 15-20mg/kg TMP and 75-100mg/kg SMX per 24 hrs given q6h for 14-21 days. PCP Prophylaxis: 150mg/m2/day TMP with 750mg/m2/day SMX given bid, on 3 consecutive days/week. Max: 320mg TMP/1600mg SMX/day. CrCl: 15-30mL/min: 50% usual dose. CrCl: <15mL/min: Not recommended.
Cleocin (clindamycin)	**Cap:** (HCl) 75mg, 150mg, 300mg; **Inj:** (Phosphate) 150mg/ mL, 300mg/50mL, 600mg/50mL, 900mg/50mL; **Sus:** (HCl) 75mg/5mL [100g]	Serious infections caused by anaerobes, streptococci, pneumococci and staphylococci.	Serious Infection: 150-300mg PO q6h or 600-1200 mg/day IM/IV given bid-qid. More Severe Infection: 300-450mg PO q6h or 1200-2700mg/day IM/IV given bid-qid. Life-threatening infections: Up to 4800mg/day IV. Max: 600mg per IM injection. Take oral form with full glass of water. Treat β-hemolytic strep for at least 10 days.	Birth-16 yrs: Serious Infection: 8-16mg/kg/day PO. More Severe Infection: 16-20mg/kg/day PO. 1 mo-16 yrs: 20-40mg/kg/day IM/IV given tid-qid: use higher dose for more severe infection. <1 mo: 15-20mg/kg/day IM/IV given tid-qid. Take oral form with full glass of water. Treat β-hemolytic strep for at least 10 days.
Coly-Mycin M (colistimethate sodium)	**Inj:** 150mg	Treatment of acute or chronic infections due to certain gram-negative bacilli (eg, Pseudomonas aeruginosa, Enterobacter aerogenes, E.coli, Klebsiella pneumoniae).	Usual: 2.5-5mg/kg/day IV/IM in 2-4 divided doses. Max: 5mg/kg/day. SCr 1.3-1.5mg/dL: 2.5-3.8mg/ kg/day IV/IM in 2 divided doses. SCr: 1.6-2.5mg/dL: 2.5mg/kg/day IV/IM in 1-2 divided doses. SCr 2.6-4mg/dL: 1.5mg/kg/day IV/IM q36h. Obesity: Base dose on IBW.	Usual: 2.5-5mg/kg/day IV/IM in 2-4 divided doses. Max: 5mg/kg/day. SCr 1.3-1.5mg/dL: 2.5-3.8mg/kg/day IV/IM in 2 divided doses. SCr 1.6-2.5mg/dL: 2.5mg/kg/day IV/IM in 1-2 divided doses. SCr 2.6-4mg/dL: 1.5mg/kg/day IV/IM q36h. Obesity: Base dose on IBW.
Cubicin (daptomycin)	**Inj:** 500mg	Susceptible complicated skin and skin structure infections (cSSSI). Staphylococcus aureus blood stream infections (bacteremia).	≥18 yrs: Administer as IV infusion over 30 minutes. cSSSI: 4mg/kg once every 24 hrs for 7-14 days. S.aureus Bacteremia: 6mg/kg once every 24 hrs for minimum 2-6 weeks. Renal impairment: CrCl <30 mL/min, Hemodialysis or CAPD: (cSSSI) 4mg/kg or (S.aureus bacteremia) 6mg/kg once every 48 hrs.	
Flagyl IV (metronidazole HCl)	**Inj:** 500mg, 500mg (RTU)	Treatment of anaerobic intra-abdominal, skin and skin structure, gynecologic, bone and joint, CNS, lower respiratory tract infections, endocarditis, and septicemia.	LD: 15mg/kg IV. Maint: 6 hrs later, 7.5mg/kg IV q6h for 7-10 days or more. Max: 4g/24 hrs.	

(Continued)

BRAND NAME (Generic)	DOSAGE FORM/ STRENGTH	INDICATIONS	ADULT DOSE	PEDIATRIC DOSE
Hiprex (methenamine hippurate)	**Tab:** 1g	Prophylaxis or suppression of recurrent urinary tract infections when long-term therapy is necessary. For use only after infection is eradicated by other appropriate antimicrobials.	1g bid.	>12 yrs: 1g bid. 6 to 12 yrs: 0.5g-1g bid.
Ketek (telithromycin)	**Tab:** 300mg [20ˢ], 400mg [60ˢ, Ketek Pak, 100ˢ]	Treatment of mild to moderate community-acquired pneumonia (CAP).	800mg qd for 7-10 days. Severe Renal Impairment (CrCl <30mL/min): 600mg qd. Hemodialysis: Give after dialysis session on dialysis days. Severe Renal Impairment (CrCl <30mL/min) with Hepatic Impairment: 400mg qd.	
Macrobid (nitrofurantoin monohydrate)	**Cap:** 100mg	Treatment of acute uncomplicated urinary tract infections (acute cystitis).	100mg every 12 hrs for 7 days. Take with food.	>12 yrs: 100mg every 12 hrs for 7 days. Take with food.
Macrodantin (nitrofurantoin macrocrystals)	**Cap:** 25mg, 50mg, 100mg	Treatment of urinary tract infection.	50-100mg qid for at least 7 days. Take with food. Long-term Suppressive Use: 50-100mg at bedtime.	≥1 mo: 5-7mg/kg/day given qid for at least 7 days. Take with food. Long-term Suppressive Use: 1mg/kg/day given qd-bid.
Monurol (fosfomycin tromethamine)	**Pow:** 3g/sachet	Uncomplicated urinary tract infection (acute cystitis) in women.	≥18 yrs: 1 single-dose sachet. Mix with 3-4oz of water before ingesting.	
Primsol (trimethoprim HCl)	**Sol:** 50mg/5mL	Treatment of acute otitis media in pediatrics and urinary tract infection (UTI) in adults.	UTI: Usual: 100mg q12h or 200mg q24h for 10 days. CrCl: 15-30mL/min: Give 50% of usual dose.	Otitis Media: ≥6 mos: 5mg/kg q12h for 10 days. CrCl: 15-30mL/min: Give 50% of usual dose.
Rifadin (rifampin)	**Cap:** 150mg; 300mg; **Inj:** 600mg	Treatment of all forms of tuberculosis (TB). Treatment of asymptomatic carriers of *Neisseria meningitidis* to eliminate meningococci from the nasopharynx.	TB: 10mg/kg PO/IV qd. Max: 600mg/day. Meningococcal Carriers: 600mg bid for 2 days. Take 1 hr before or 2 hrs after a meal with a full glass of water.TB: 10-20mg/kg PO/IV qd. Max: 600mg/day.	Meningococcal Carriers: ≥1 mo: 10mg/kg q12h for 2 days. Max: 600mg/dose. <1 mo: 5mg/kg q12h for 2 days. Take 1 hr before or 2 hrs after a meal with a full glass of water.
Rifamate (isoniazid–rifampin)	**Cap:** (Isoniazid–Rifampin) 150mg-300mg	For pulmonary tuberculosis (TB). Not for initial therapy or prevention of TB.	2 caps qd. Take 1 hr before or 2 hrs after meals. Give with pyridoxine in the malnourished, those predisposed to neuropathy (eg, alcoholics, diabetics), and adolescents.	

BRAND NAME (Generic)	DOSAGE FORM/ STRENGTH	INDICATIONS	ADULT DOSE	PEDIATRIC DOSE
MISCELLANEOUS (Continued)				
Rifater (isoniazid-rifampin-pyrazinamide)	**Tab:** (Isoniazid-Pyrazinamide-Rifampin) 50mg-300mg-120mg	For initial phase of pulmonary tuberculosis treatment	≥44kg: 4 tabs single dose qd. 45-54kg: 5 tabs single dose. ≥55kg: 6 tabs single dose. Give pyridoxine in malnourished, if predisposed to neuropathy (eg, alcoholics, diabetics), and adolescents. Take 1 hr before or 2 hrs after meals with full glass of water. Treatment usually lasts 2 months.	≥15 yrs: ≤44kg: 4 tabs single dose qd. 45-54kg: 5 tabs qd single dose. ≥55kg: 6 tabs qd single dose. Give pyridoxine in malnourished, if predisposed to neuropathy (eg, alcoholics, diabetics), and adolescents. Take 1 hr before or 2 hrs after meals with full glass of water. Treatment usually lasts 2 months.
Septra (sulfamethoxazole-trimethoprim)	(Sulfamethoxazole [SMX]-Trimethoprim [TMP]) **Inj:** 80mg-16mg/mL; **Sus:** 200mg-40mg/5mL [100mL, 473mL]; **Tab:** 400mg-80mg; Tab, DS: 800mg-160mg	(Inj, Sus, Tab) Treatment of urinary tract infection (UTI), pneumocystitis carinii pneumonia (PCP) and enteritis caused by *Shigella*. (Sus, Tab). Treatment of acute exacerbation of chronic bronchitis (AECB), travelers' diarrhea, and acute otitis media.	(Sus, Tab) UTI: 800mg-160mg PO q12h for 10-14 days. Shigellosis/Traveler's Diarrhea: 800mg-160mg PO q12h for 5 days. AECB: 800mg-160mg PO q 12h for 14 days. PCP Treatment: 15-20mg/kg TMP and 75-100mg/kg SMX per 24 hrs given PO q6h for 14-21 days PCP Prophylaxis: 800mg-160mg PO qd. (Inj) Severe UTI: 8-10mg/kg TMP IV given in divided doses q6, 8 or 12h for up to 14 days. PCP Treatment: 15-20mg/kg TMP IV given in divided doses q6-8h for up to 14 days. Shigellosis: 8-10mg/kg TMP IV given in divided doses q6, 8 or 12h for 5 days. (Inj, Sus, Tab) Renal Impairment: CrCl 15-30 mL/min: 50% usual dose. CrCl <15mL/min: Not recommended.	(Sus, Tab) ≥2 mo: UTI/Otitis Media: 4mg/kg TMP and 20mg/kg SMX q12h for 10 days. Shigellosis/ Traveler's Diarrhea: 4mg/kg TMP and 20mg/kg SMX q12h for 5 days. PCP Treatment: 15-20mg/kg TMP and 75-100mg/kg SMX/24 hrs given q6h for 14-21 days. PCP Prophylaxis: 150mg/m2/day TMP and 750mg/m2/day SMX PO given bid, on 3 consecutive days per week. Max: 320mg TMP and 1600mg SMX per day. (Inj) Severe UTI: 8-10mg/kg TMP IV given in divided doses q6, 8 or 12h for up to 14 days. PCP Treatment: 15-20mg/kg TMP IV given in divided doses q6-8h for up to 14 days. Shigellosis: 8-10mg/ kg TMP IV given in divided doses q6, 8 or 12h for 5 days. (Inj, Sus, Tab) Renal Impairment: CrCl 15-30mL/ mL/min: 50% usual dose. CrCl <15mL/min: Not recommended.
Synercid (dalfopristin-quinupristin)	**Inj:** (Dalfopristin-Quinupristin) 350mg-150mg per 500mg vial	Treatment of serious or life-threatening infections associated with vancomycin-resistant *Enterococcus faecium* (VREF) bacteremia and complicated skin and skin structure infections (SSSI) caused by *Staphylococcus aureus* (methicillin susceptible) or *Streptococcus pyogenes*.	VREF: 7.5mg/kg IV q8h. Duration depends on site and severity of infection. Complicated SSSI: 7.5mg/ kg IV q12h for at least 7 days. Hepatic Cirrhosis (Child Pugh A or B): May need dose reduction.	≥16 yrs: VREF: 7.5mg/kg IV q8h. Duration depends on site and severity of infection. Complicated SSSI: 7.5mg/kg IV q12h for at least 7 days. Hepatic Cirrhosis (Child Pugh A or B): May need dose reduction.

(Continued)

BRAND NAME (Generic)	DOSAGE FORM/ STRENGTH	INDICATIONS	ADULT DOSE	PEDIATRIC DOSE
Vancocin (vancomycin HCl)	**Inj:** 500mg/100mL, 1g/200mL	Treatment of severe infections caused by susceptible strains of methicillin-resistant staphylococci. Indicated for penicillin-allergic patients, those who cannot receive or have failed to respond to other drugs, and for vancomycin-susceptible organisms that are resistant to other antimicrobials.	Usual: 500mg IV q6h or 1g IV q12h. Mild to Moderate Renal Impairment: Initial: 15mg/kg/day. Maint: 1.9mg/kg/d. Administer 10mg/min or over at least 60 min, whichever is longer. Renal Dysfunction: Initial: 15mg/kg. Dose is about 15x the GFR in mL/min (refer to table in labeling). Elderly: Require greater dose reduction. Functionally Anephric: Initial: 15mg/kg, then 1.9mg/kg/24hrs. Marked Renal Dysfunction: 250-1000mg every several days. Anuria: 1000mg every 7-10 days.	Usual: 10mg/kg IV q6h. Infants/Neonates: Initial: 15mg/kg, then 10mg/kg q12h for neonates in the 1st week of life and q8h thereafter until 1 mo of age. Administer over at least 60 min. Renal Dysfunction: Initial: 15mg/kg. Dose is about 15x the GFR in mL/min (refer to table in labeling). Premature Infants: Require greater dose reduction.
Vancocin Oral (vancomycin HCl)	**Cap:** 125mg, 250mg	Staphylococcal enterocolitis and antibiotic-associated pseudomembranous colitis caused by *C.difficile*.	500mg-2g/day given tid-qid for 7-10 days.	40mg/kg/day given tid-qid for 7-10 days. Max: 2g/day.
Zyvox (linezolid)	**Inj:** 2mg/mL [100mL, 200mL, 300mL]; **Sus:** 100mg/5mL; **Tab:** 400mg, 600mg	Vancomycin resistant *Enterococcus faecium* (VRE) infections, nosocomial pneumonia caused by *Staphylococcus aureus* (methicillin-susceptible and -resistant strains) or *Streptococcus pneumoniae* (including multi-drug resistant strains [MDRSP]), complicated skin and skin structure infections (SSSI) including diabetic foot infections without concomitant osteomyelitis caused by *Staphylococcus aureus* (methicillin-susceptible and -resistant strains), *Streptococcus pyogenes*, or *Streptococcus agalactiae*, uncomplicated SSSI caused by *Staphylococcus aureus* (methicillin-susceptible only) or *Streptococcus pyogenes*, community-acquired pneumonia (CAP) caused by *Streptococcus pneumoniae* (MDRSP), including concurrent bacteremia, or *Staphylococcus aureus* (methicillin-susceptible strains only).	Complicated SSSI/CAP/Nosocomial Pneumonia: 600mg IV/PO q12h for 10-14 days. VRE: 600mg IV/PO q12h for 14-28 days. Uncomplicated SSSI: 400mg PO q12h for 10-14 days.	Complicated SSSI/CAP/Nosocomial Pneumonia: Treat for 10-14 days. ≥12 yrs: 600mg IV/PO q12h. Birth-11 yrs: 10mg/kg IV/PO q8h. VRE: Treat for 14-28 days: 10mg/kg IV/PO q8h. Uncomplicated SSSI: Treat for 10-14 days: ≥12 yrs: 600mg PO q12h. 5-11 yrs: 10mg/kg PO q12h. <5 yrs: 10mg/kg PO q8h. Neonates <7 days should be initiated with dosing regimen of 10mg/kg q12h; may increase to 10mg/kg q8h if suboptimal response. All neonatal patients should receive 10mg/kg q8h by 7 days of life.

HIV/AIDS PHARMACOTHERAPY

DRUG	BRAND	HOW SUPPLIED	USUAL DOSE	FOOD EFFECT
CCR5 ANTAGONISTS				
Maraviroc (MVC)	Selzentry	**Tab:** 150mg, 300mg	**Adults:** >16 yrs: Give in combination with other anti-retroviral medications. With Strong CYP3A Inhibitors (with or without CYP3A inducers) Including PIs (excepts tipranavir/ritonavir), Delavirdine: 150mg bid. With NRTIs, Tipranavir/Ritonavir, Nevirapine, Other Drugs That Are Not Strong CYP3A Inhibitors/Inducers: 300mg bid. With CYP3A Inducers (without strong CYP3A inhibitor): 600mg bid.	Take without regard to meals.
HIV INTEGRASE STRAND TRANSFER INHIBITOR				
Raltegravir	Isentress	**Tab:** 400mg	**Adults:** 400mg bid.	Take without regard to meals.
NUCLEOSIDE REVERSE TRANSCRIPTASE INHIBITORS (NRTIs)				
Abacavir (ABC)	Ziagen	**Sol:** 20mg/mL [240mL]; **Tab:** 300mg	**Adults:** >16 yrs: or 600mg qd. **Pediatrics: 3 months-16 yrs:** 8mg/kg bid. **Max:** 300mg bid.	Take without regard to meals.
Didanosine (ddI)	Videx Powder for Oral Sol; Videx EC	**Powder for Sol:** 2g, 4g; **Cap, Delayed Release:** (Videx EC) 125mg, 200mg, 250mg, 400mg	**Adults:** ≥60kg: **(Cap)** 400mg qd, **(Sol)** 200mg bid or 400mg qd. <60kg: **(Cap)** 250mg qd, **(Sol)** 125mg bid or 250mg qd. **Pediatrics: 2 weeks-8 months: (Sol)** 100mg/m² bid. >8 months: 120mg/m² bid.	Take on empty stomach at least 30 minutes before or 2 hrs after meals. Swallow caps whole.
Emtricitabine (FTC)	Emtriva	**Cap:** 200mg; **Sol:** 10mg/mL	**Adults:** ≥18 yrs: Cap: 200 mg qd. Sol: 240mg (24mL) qd. **Pediatrics: 0-3 mos:** 3mg/kg qd. **3 mos-17 yrs: Cap: >33kg:** 200mg qd. Sol: 6mg/kg qd. **Max:** 240mg (24mL).	Take without regard to meals.
Lamivudine	Epivir	**Sol:** 10mg/mL [240mL]; **Tab:** 150mg, 300mg	**Adults:** 150mg bid or 300mg qd. **Pediatrics: 3 months-16 yrs:** 4mg/kg bid. **Max:** 150mg bid.	Take without regard to meals.
Stavudine (d4T)	Zerit	**Cap:** 15mg, 20mg, 30mg, 40mg; **Sol:** 1mg/mL [200mL]	**Adults:** ≥60kg: 40mg q12h. <60kg: 30mg q12h. **Pediatrics:** ≥60kg: 40mg q12h. 30-59 kg: 30mg q12h. ≥14 days and <30kg: 1mg/kg q12h. **Birth-13 days:** 0.5mg/kg q12h.	Take without regard to meals.
Tenofovir Disoproxil Fumarate (TDF)	Viread	**Tab:** 300mg	**Adults:** 300mg once daily.	Take without regard to meals.
Zalcitabine (ddC)	Hivid	**Tab:** 0.375mg, 0.75mg	**Adults:** 0.75mg q8h. **Pediatrics:** >13 yrs: 0.75mg q8h.	Take without regard to meals.
Zidovudine (AZT, ZDV)	Retrovir	**Cap:** 100mg; **Inj:** 10mg/mL; **Syrup:** 50mg/5mL [240mL]; **Tab:** 300mg	**Adults: (Cap, Tab)** 600mg/day in divided doses. **(Inj)** 1mg/kg IV over 1 hr 5-6 times/day. **Pediatrics: 6 weeks-12 yrs:** 160mg/m² PO q8h. **Max:** 200mg PO q8h.	Take without regard to meals.

(Continued)

DRUG	BRAND	HOW SUPPLIED	USUAL DOSE	FOOD EFFECT
NON-NUCLEOSIDE REVERSE TRANSCRIPTASE INHIBITORS (NNRTIs)				
Delavirdine (DLV)	Rescriptor	**Tab:** 100mg, 200mg	**Adults: Usual:** 400mg tid. **Pediatrics:** ≥**16 yrs: Usual:** 400mg tid.	Take without regard to meals.
Efavirenz (EFV)	Sustiva	**Cap:** 50mg, 100mg, 200mg; **Tab:** 600mg	**Adults: Initial:** 600mg qd at bedtime. **Pediatrics:** ≥**3 yrs: 10 to <15kg:** 200mg qd. **15 to <20kg:** 250mg qd. **20 to <25kg:** 300mg qd. **25 to <32.5kg:** 350mg qd. **32.5 to <40kg:** 400mg qd. ≥**40kg:** 600mg qd at bedtime.	Take on an empty stomach.
Etravirine (ETR)	Intelence	**Tab:** 100mg	**Adults:** 200mg bid.	Take with meals.
Nevirapine (NVP)	Viramune	**Sus:** 50mg/5mL [240mL]; **Tab:** 200mg* *scored	**Adults:** 200mg qd for 14 days (lead-in period), then 200mg bid. **Pediatrics: 2 months-8 yrs:** 4mg/kg qd for 14 days, then 7mg/kg bid. **Max:** 400mg/day. **8 yrs:** 4mg/kg qd for 14 days, then 4mg/kg bid. **Max:** 400mg/day.	Take without regard to meals.
PROTEASE INHIBITORS (PIs)				
Atazanavir (ATV)	Reyataz	**Cap:** 100mg, 150mg, 200mg, 300mg	**Adults:** Therapy-naive: 400mg qd. Therapy Experienced: (ATV 300mg + RTV 100mg) qd.	Take with food; avoid taking with antacids.
Darunavir (DRV)	Prezista	**Tab:** 300mg	**Adults:** (DRV 600mg + RTV 100mg) bid.	Take with food.
Fosamprenavir (fAPV)	Lexiva	**Tab:** 700mg **Sus:** 50mg/1mL [225mL]	**Adults:** Therapy-naive: 1400mg bid OR 1400mg qd + RTV 200mg qd OR 700mg bid + RTV 100mg bid. PI-Experienced: 700mg bid + RTV 100mg bid.	Take without regard to meals.
Indinavir (IDV)	Crixivan	**Cap:** 100mg, 200mg, 333mg, 400mg	**Adults:** 800mg q8h OR (IDV 800mg + RTV 100 or 200mg) q12h.	Take 1 hr before or 2 hr after meals; may take with skim milk or low-fat meal. RTV-boosted, take with or without food.
Nelfinavir (NFV)	Viracept	**Sus:** (powder) 50mg/g [144g] **Tab:** 250mg, 625mg	**Adults:** 1250mg bid or 750mg tid. **Pediatrics: 2-13 yrs:** 45-55mg/kg bid; 25-35mg/kg tid. **Max:** 2500mg/day	Take with meals.
Ritonavir (RTV)	Norvir	**Cap:** 100mg **Sol:** 80mg/mL [240mL]	**Adults: Initial:** 300mg bid. **Titrate:** Increase every 2-3 days by 100mg bid. **Maint:** 600mg bid. **Pediatrics: >1 month: Initial:** 250mg/m² po bid. **Titrate:** Increase by 50mg/m² every 2-3 days. **Maint:** 350-400mg/m² po bid or highest tolerated dose. **Max:** 600mg bid.	Take with food, may improve tolerability.
Saquinavir (SQV)	Invirase	**Hard Gel Cap:** 200mg **Tab:** 500mg	**Adults/Pediatrics: >16 yrs:** 1000mg bid with RTV 100mg bid OR 1000mg bid with LPV/RTV 400/100mg bid (no additional RTV).	Take within 2 hrs after a meal when taken with RTV.

(Continued)

DRUG	BRAND	HOW SUPPLIED	USUAL DOSE	FOOD EFFECT
PROTEASE INHIBITORS (PIs) *(Continued)*				
Tipranavir (TPV)	Aptivus	**Cap:** 250mg	**Adults:** (500mg + RTV 200mg) bid.	Take with food.
FUSION INHIBITORS				
Enfuvirtide (T20)	Fuzeon	**Inj:** 90mg/1ml (60s)	**Adults:** 90mg SQ bid. **Pediatrics: 6-16 yrs:** 2mg/kg SQ bid. **Max:** 90mg bid. 11-15.5kg: 27mg bid. 15.6-20.0kg: 36mg bid. 20.1-24.5kg: 45mg bid. 24.6-29.0kg: 54mg bid. 29.1-33.5kg: 63mg bid. 33.6-38.0kg: 72mg bid. 38.1-42.5kg: 81mg bid. ≥42.6kg: 90mg bid.	
COMBINATIONS				
EFV/FTC/TDF	Atripla	**Tab:** (Efavirenz-Emtricitabine-Tenofovir DF) 600mg-200mg-300mg	**Adults:** ≥18 yrs: 1 tab qd.	Take on empty stomach.
3TC/ZDV	Combivir	**Tab:** (Lamivudine-Zidovudine) 150mg-300mg	**Adults:** 1 tab bid. **Pediatrics:** ≥12 yrs: 1 tab bid. Do not give if CrCl ≥50mL/min.	Take without regard to meals.
ABC/3TC	Epzicom	**Tab:** (Abacavir Sulfate-Lamivudine) 600mg-300mg	**Adults:** ≥18 yrs: CrCl >50 mL/min: 1 tab qd.	Take without regard to meals.
LPV/RTV	Kaletra	**Tab:** (Lopinavir-Ritonavir) 200mg-50mg; 100mg-25mg; **Sol:** (Lopinavir-Ritonavir) 80mg-20mg/mL [160mL]	**Adults: Therapy-Naive:** 400/100mg (2 tabs or 5mL) bid or 800/200mg qd (4 tabs or 10mL). **Therapy Experienced:** 400/100mg bid (2 tabs or 5mL).	Take without regard to meals. **Sol:** Take with meal.
ABC/ZDV/3TC	Trizivir	**Tab:** (Abacavir-Lamivudine-Zidovudine) 300mg-150mg-300mg	**Adults:** >40kg and CrCl >50mL/min: 1 tab bid.	Take without regard to meals.
FTC/TDF	Truvada	**Tab:** (Emtricitabine-Tenofovir Disoproxil Fumarate) 200mg-300mg	**Adults:** ≥18 yrs: CrCl ≥50mL/min: 1 tab qd. CrCl 30-49mL/min: 1 tab q48h.	Take without regard to meals.

Sources: FDA Approved Labeling; Guidelines for the Use of Antiretroviral Agents in HIV-1-Infected Adults and Adolescents - October 10, 2006.

ADHD AGENTS

BRAND (GENERIC)	HOW SUPPLIED	ADULT DOSE	PEDIATRIC DOSE
Adderall (Amphetamine plus dextroamphetamine)	Tab: 5mg*, 7.5mg*, 10mg*, 12.5mg*, 15mg*, 20mg*, 30mg* *scored		**3-5 yrs:** Initial: 2.5mg qd. Titrate: May increase by 2.5mg weekly. **≥6 yrs:** 5mg qd-bid. May increase by 5mg weekly. Max (usual): 40mg/day.
Adderall XR* (Amphetamine salt combo)	Cap: 5mg, 10mg, 15mg, 20mg, 25mg, 30mg	Initial: 20mg qam. Currently Using Adderall: Switch to Adderall XR at the same total daily dose, taken once daily. Titrate at weekly intervals as needed.	**≥6 yrs:** Initial: 10mg qam. Titrate: May increase weekly by 5-10mg/day. Max: 30mg/day. **13-17 yrs:** Initial: 10mg/day. Titrate: May increase to 20mg/day after one week. Currently Using Adderall: Switch to Adderall XR at the same total daily dose, taken once daily. Titrate at weekly intervals as needed.
Concerta** (Methylphenidate HCl)	Tab: Extended-Release: 18mg, 27mg, 36mg, 54mg	Methylphenidate-Naive or Receiving Other Stimulant: Initial: 18mg qam. Titrate: Adjust dose at weekly intervals. Previous Methylphenidate Use: Initial: 18mg qam if previous dose 10-15mg/day; 36mg qam if previous dose 20-30mg/day; 54mg qam if previous dose 30-45mg/day. Initial conversion should not exceed 54mg/day. Titrate: Adjust dose at weekly intervals. Max: 72mg/day. Reduce dose or d/c if paradoxical aggravation of symptoms occurs. D/C if no improvement after appropriate dosage adjustments over 1 month.	**≥6 yrs:** Methylphenidate-Naive or Receiving Other Stimulant: Initial: 18mg qam. Titrate: Adjust dose at weekly intervals. Max: **6-12 yrs:** 54mg/day. **13-17 yrs:** 72mg/day not to exceed 2mg/kg/day. Previous Methylphenidate Use: Initial: 18mg qam if previous dose 10-15mg/day; 36mg qam if previous dose 20-30mg/day; 54mg qam if previous dose 30-45mg/day. Initial conversion should not exceed 54mg/day. Titrate: Adjust dose at weekly intervals. Max: 72mg/day. Reduce dose or d/c if paradoxical aggravation of symptoms occurs. D/C if no improvement after appropriate dosage adjustments over 1 month.
Daytrana (Methylphenidate transdermal system)	Patch: 10mg/9 hrs, 15mg/9 hrs, 20mg/9 hrs, 30mg/9 hrs [10S, 30S]	Individualize dose. Apply to hip area 2 hrs before effect is needed and remove 9 hrs after application. Recommended Titration Schedule: Week 1: 10mg/9 hrs. Week 2: 15mg/9 hrs. Week 3: 20mg/9 hrs. Week 4: 30mg/9 hrs.	**≥6 yrs:** Individualize dose. Apply to hip area 2 hrs before effect is needed and remove 9 hrs after application. Recommended Titration Schedule: Week 1: 10mg/9 hrs. Week 2: 15mg/9 hrs. Week 3: 20mg/9 hrs. Week 4: 30mg/9 hrs.
Desoxyn (Methamphetamine HCl)	Tab: 5mg		**≥6 yrs:** Initial: 5mg qd-bid. Titrate: Increase weekly by 5mg/day until optimum response. Usual: 20-25mg/day given bid.
Dexedrine (Dextroamphetamine sulfate)	Cap: Extended-Release: (Spansules) 5mg, 10mg, 15mg; Tab: 5mg* *scored		**3-5 yrs:** Initial: 2.5mg qd. Titrate: Increase weekly by 2.5mg/day. **≥6 yrs:** 5mg qd-bid. Titrate: Increase weekly by 5mg/day. Max: 40mg/day. For tabs, give 1st dose upon awakening and additional every 4-6 hrs. May give caps once daily.

BRAND (GENERIC)	HOW SUPPLIED	ADULT DOSE	PEDIATRIC DOSE
DextroStat (Dextroamphetamine sulfate)	Tab: 5mg*, 10mg* *scored		**3-5 yrs:** Initial: 2.5mg/day. Titrate: Increase weekly by 2.5mg/day until optimum response. **6-16 yrs:** Initial 5mg qd-bid. Titrate: Increase weekly by 5mg/day until optimum response. Give 1st dose upon awakening, and additional doses q4-6h.
Focalin (Dexmethylphenidate HCl)	Tab: 2.5mg, 5mg, 10mg	Take bid at least 4 hrs apart. Methylphenidate Naive: Initial: 2.5-5mg/day. Titrate: Increase weekly by 2.5-5mg/day. Max: 20mg/day. Currently on Methylphenidate: Initial: Take ½ of methylphenidate dose. Max: 20mg/day. Reduce or d/c if paradoxical aggravation of symptoms. D/C if no improvement after appropriate dosage adjustments over 1 month.	**≥6 yrs:** Take bid at least 4 hrs apart. Methylphenidate Naive: Initial: 2.5mg/day. Titrate: Increase weekly by 2.5-5mg/day. Max: 20mg/day. Currently on Methylphenidate: Initial: Take ½ of methylphenidate dose. Max: 20mg/day. Reduce or d/c if paradoxical aggravation of symptoms. D/C if no improvement after appropriate dosage adjustments over 1 month.
Focalin XR* (Dexmethylphenidate HCl)	Cap, Extended-Release: 5mg, 10mg, 15mg, 20mg	Methylphenidate Naive: Initial: 10mg/day. Titrate: May adjust weekly by 10mg/day. Max: 20mg/day. Currently on Methylphenidate: Initial: Take ½ of methylphenidate dose. Max: 20mg/day. Reduce or d/c if paradoxical aggravation of symptoms. D/C if no improvement after appropriate dosage adjustments over 1 month.	**≥6 yrs:** Methylphenidate Naive: Initial: 5mg/day. Titrate: May adjust weekly by 5mg/day. Max: 20mg/day. Currently on Methylphenidate: Initial: Take ½ of methylphenidate dose. Max: 20mg/day. Reduce or d/c if paradoxical aggravation of symptoms. D/C if no improvement after appropriate dosage adjustments over 1 month.
Metadate CD* (Methylphenidate HCl)	Cap, Extended-Release: 10mg, 20mg, 30mg, 40mg, 50mg, 60mg		**≥6 yrs:** Usual: 20mg qam before breakfast. Titrate: Increase weekly by 10-20mg depending on tolerability/efficacy. Max: 60mg/day. Reduce dose or d/c if paradoxical aggravation of symptoms occur. D/C if no improvement after appropriate dose adjustments over 1 month.
Metadate ER* (Methylphenidate HCl)	Tab, Extended-Release: 10mg, 20mg	(Immediate-Release Methylphenidate) 10-60mg/day given bid-tid 30-45 min ac. If insomnia occurs, take last dose before 6 pm.†	**≥6 yrs:** (Immediate-Release Methylphenidate) Initial: 5mg bid before breakfast and lunch. Titrate: Increase gradually by 5-10mg weekly. Max: 60mg/day. Reduce dose or d/c if paradoxical aggravation of symptoms occur. D/C if no improvement after appropriate dose adjustment over 1 month.†
Methylin* (Methylphenidate HCl)	Sol: 5mg/5mL [500mL], 10mg/5mL [500mL]; Tab: 5mg, 10mg, 20mg; Tab, Chewable: 2.5mg, 5mg, 10mg; Tab, Extended-Release: 10mg, 20mg	(Sol/Tab/Tab, Chewable) 10-60mg/day given bid-tid 30-45 min ac. If insomnia occurs, take last dose before 6 pm.†	**≥6 yrs:** (Sol/Tab/Tab, Chewable) Initial: 5mg bid before breakfast and lunch. Titrate: Increase gradually by 5-10mg weekly. Max: 60mg/day. Reduce dose or d/c if paradoxical aggravation of symptoms occur. D/C if no improvement after appropriate dose adjustment over 1 month.†

(Continued)

BRAND (GENERIC)	HOW SUPPLIED	ADULT DOSE	PEDIATRIC DOSE
Ritalin, Ritalin LA*, Ritalin SR** (Methylphenidate HCl)	Cap, Extended-Release (Ritalin LA): 10mg, 20mg, 30mg, 40mg; Tab (Ritalin): 5mg, 10mg*, 20mg*; Tab, Extended-Release (Ritalin SR): 20mg *scored	(Tab) 10-60mg/day given bid-tid 30-45 min ac. Take last dose before 6 pm if insomnia occurs. **(Cap, ER)** Initial: 20mg qam. Titrate: Adjust weekly by 10mg. Max: 60mg qam.†	**≥6 yrs:** (Tab) Initial: 5mg bid before breakfast and lunch. Titrate: Increase gradually by 5-10mg weekly. Max: 60mg/day. (Cap, ER) Initial: 20mg qam. Titrate: Adjust weekly by 10mg. Max: 60mg qam. Previous Methylphenidate Use: May use as qd in place of IR dosed bid or daily dose of methylphenidate-SR. Reduce dose or d/c if paradoxical aggravation of symptoms occurs: D/C if no improvement after appropriate dose adjustment over 1 month.†
Strattera (Atomoxetine HCl)	Cap: 10mg, 18mg, 25mg, 40mg, 60mg, 80mg, 100mg	Initial: 40mg/day given qam or evenly divided doses in the am and late afternoon/early evening. Titrate: Increase after minimum of 3 days to target dose of about 80mg/day. After 2-4 weeks, may increase to max of 100mg/day. Max: 100mg/day. Dose adjust in hepatic insufficiency and when used with concomitant CYP450 2D6 inhibitors. See PI for detailed dosing information	**≥6 yrs:** ≤70kg: Initial: 0.5mg/kg/day given qam or evenly divided doses in the am and late afternoon or early evening. Titrate: Increase after minimum of 3 days to target dose of about 1.2mg/kg/day. Max: 1.4mg/kg/day or 100mg, whichever is less. >70kg: Initial: 40mg/day given qam or evenly divided doses in the am and late afternoon/ early evening. Titrate: Increase after minimum of 3 days to target dose of about 80mg/day. After 2-4 weeks, may increase to max of 100mg/day. Max: 100mg/day. Dose adjust in hepatic insufficiency and when used with concomitant CYP450 2D6 inhibitors. See PI for detailed dosing information.
Vyvanse (Lisdexamfetamine dimesylate)	Cap: 20mg, 30mg, 40mg, 50mg, 60mg, 70mg	Individualize dose. Usual: 30mg qam. Titrate: If needed, may increase in increments of 10mg or 20mg at weekly intervals. Max: 70mg/day. Swallow caps or dissolve contents in glass of water; do not store once dissolved. Re-evaluate periodically.	Individualize dose. **6-12 yrs:** Usual: 30mg qam. Titrate: If needed, may increase in increments of 10mg or 20mg at weekly intervals. Max: 70mg/day. Swallow caps or dissolve contents in glass of water; do not store once dissolved. Re-evaluate periodically.

ADHD = attention-deficit/hyperactivity disorder.
* Swallow cap whole or open cap and sprinkle contents on applesauce; do not chew beads.
**Swallow whole; do not chew, crush, or divide.
†Tab, Extended-Release: May use in place of immediate-release tabs when the 8-hr dose corresponds to the titrated 8-hr immediate-release dose.

ORAL CONTRACEPTIVES

DRUG	ESTROGEN	PROGESTIN	STRENGTH (ESTROGEN/PROGESTIN)
MONOPHASIC			
Alesse, Levlite	Ethinyl Estradiol	Levonorgestrel	20mcg/0.1mg
Brevicon, Modicon	Ethinyl Estradiol	Norethindrone	35mcg/0.5mg
Demulen 1/35	Ethinyl Estradiol	Ethynodiol Diacetate	35mcg/1mg
Demulen 1/50	Ethinyl Estradiol	Ethynodiol Diacetate	50mcg/1mg
Desogen, Ortho-Cept	Ethinyl Estradiol	Desogestrel	30mcg/0.15mg
Levlen, Nordette-28	Ethinyl Estradiol	Levonorgestrel	30mcg/0.15mg
Loestrin 21 1/20, Loestrin Fe 1/20	Ethinyl Estradiol	Norethindrone Acetate	20mcg/1mg
Loestrin 21 1.5/30, Loestrin Fe 1.5/30	Ethinyl Estradiol	Norethindrone Acetate	30mcg/1.5mg
Lo/Ovral	Ethinyl Estradiol	Norgestrel	30mcg/0.3mg
Lybrel	Ethinyl Estradiol	Levonorgestrel	20mcg/90mcg
Modicon	Ethinyl Estradiol	Norethindrone	0.035mg/0.5mg
Norinyl 1/35, Ortho-Novum 1/35	Ethinyl Estradiol	Norethindrone	35mcg/1mg
Norinyl 1/50, Ortho-Novum 1/50	Mestranol	Norethindrone	50mcg/1mg
Ortho-Cept	Ethinyl Estradiol	Desogestrel	0.03mg/0.15mg
Ortho-Cyclen	Ethinyl Estradiol	Norgestimate	35mcg/0.25mg
Ovcon 35	Ethinyl Estradiol	Norethindrone	35mcg/0.4mg
Ovcon 50	Ethinyl Estradiol	Norethindrone	50mcg/1mg
Seasonale	Ethinyl Estradiol	Levonorgestrel	30mcg/0.15mg
Seasonique	Ethinyl Estradiol	Levonorgestrel	0.01mg, 0.15mg/0.03mg
Yasmin	Ethinyl Estradiol	Drospirenone	30mcg/3mg
YAZ	Ethinyl Estradiol	Drospirenone	0.02mg/3mg
BIPHASIC			
Ortho-Novum 10/11	Ethinyl Estradiol	Norethindrone	**Phase 1:** 35mcg/0.5mg **Phase 2:** 35mcg/1mg
Mircette	Ethinyl Estradiol	Desogestrel	**Phase 1:** 20mcg/0.15mg **Phase 2:** 10mcg/NONE
TRIPHASIC			
Cyclessa	Ethinyl Estradiol	Desogestrel	**Phase 1:** 25mcg/0.1mg **Phase 2:** 25mcg/0.125mg **Phase 3:** 25mcg/0.15mg
Estrostep Fe	Ethinyl Estradiol	Norethindrone Acetate	**Phase 1:** 20mcg/1mg **Phase 2:** 30mcg/1mg **Phase 3:** 35mcg/1mg
Ortho-Novum 7/7/7	Ethinyl Estradiol	Norethindrone	**Phase 1:** 35mcg/0.5mg **Phase 2:** 35mcg/0.75mg **Phase 3:** 35mcg/1mg
Ortho Tri-Cyclen	Ethinyl Estradiol	Norgestimate	**Phase 1:** 35mcg/0.18mg **Phase 2:** 35mcg/0.215mg **Phase 3:** 35mcg/0.25mg
Ortho Tri-Cyclen Lo	Ethinyl Estradiol	Norgestimate	**Phase 1:** 25mcg/0.18mg **Phase 2:** 25mcg/0.215mg **Phase 3:** 25mcg/0.25mg

(Continued)

DRUG	ESTROGEN	PROGESTIN	STRENGTH (ESTROGEN/PROGESTIN)
TRIPHASIC *(Continued)*			
Tri-Levlen, Triphasil, Trivora 28	Ethinyl Estradiol	Levonorgestrel	**Phase 1:** 30mcg/0.05mg **Phase 2:** 40mcg/0.075mg **Phase 3:** 30mcg/0.125mg
Tri-Norinyl	Ethinyl Estradiol	Norethindrone	**Phase 1:** 35mcg/0.5mg **Phase 2:** 35mcg/1mg **Phase 3:** 35mcg/0.5mg
PROGESTIN ONLY			
Nor-Q.D., Ortho-Micronor		Norethindrone	0.35mg

ASTHMA MANAGEMENT

DRUG (BRAND)	DOSAGE FORM	ADULT DOSE	CHILD DOSE*
ANTICHOLINERGIC			
Ipratropium (Atrovent HFA)	**MDI:** 0.017mg/inh [12.9g]	2 inh qid	
Tiotropium (Spiriva)	**Cap, Inhalation:** 18mcg	1 cap qd	
SYSTEMIC CORTICOSTEROIDS			
Methylprednisolone	**Tab:** 2, 4, 8, 16, 32mg	7.5-60mg qd in a single dose or qod prn for control. Short course "burst": 40-60 mg/day as single dose or 2 divided doses for 3-10 days.	0.25-2mg/kg qd in a single dose or qod prn for control. Short course "burst": 1-2mg/kg/day. **Max:** 60mg/day for 3-10 days.
Prednisolone	**Tab:** 5mg; **Liq:** 5mg/5mL, 15mg/5mL		
Prednisone	**Tab:** 1, 2.5, 5, 10, 20, 50mg **Liq:** 5mg/mL, 5mg/5mL		
CROMOLYN & NEDOCROMIL			
Cromolyn (Intal)	**MDI:** 800mcg/puff	2 puffs qid	1-2 puffs tid-qid
Nedocromil (Tilade)	**MDI:** 1.75mg/puff	2-4 puffs bid-qid	1-2 puffs bid-qid
SHORT-ACTING β₂-AGONISTS			
Albuterol	**MDI:** 0.09mg/inh; **Sol (neb):** 0.083%, 0.5%; **Syrup:** 2mg/5mL; **Tab:** 2mg*, 4mg*; **Tab, Extended-Release (Repetabs):** 4mg *scored	2 inh q4-6h or 1 inh q4h. **(Repetabs) Initial:** 4-8mg q12h. **Max:** 32mg/day. **(Sol)** 2.5mg tid-qid by nebulizer. **(Syrup, Tabs)** 2-4mg tid qid. **Max:** 32mg/day (8mg qid).	**(Syrup) Initial:** 2-4mg tid-qid. **Max:** 8mg (Aerosol) 2 inh q4-6h or 1 inh q4h. **(Sol)** 2.5mg tid-qid by nebulizer. **(Tabs) Initial:** 2-4mg tid-qid.
Albuterol Sulfate (ProAir HFA, Proventil HFA, Ventolin HFA)	**MDI:** 90mcg/inh	2 inh q4-6h or 1 inh q4h	2 inh q4-6h or 1 inh q4h
Aformoterol (Brovana)	**Sol, Inhalation:** 15mcg/2mL	5mcg bid	
Levalbuterol (Xopenex, Xopenex HFA)	**Sol:** 0.31mg/3mL, 0.63mg/3mL, 1.25mg/3mL (HFA) 45mcg/inh	0.63mg tid, q6-8h (HFA) 2 inh (90mcg) q4-6h or 1 inh (45mcg) q4h	0.63mg tid, q6-8h (HFA) 2 inh (90mcg) q4-6h or 1 inh (45mcg) q4h
Pirbuterol (Maxair)	**Autohaler:** 0.2mg/inh; **MDI:** 0.2mg/inh [14g]	1-2 inh q4-6h	1-2 inh q4-6h
LONG-ACTING β₂-AGONISTS			
Salmeterol (Serevent)	**DPI:** 50mcg/blister	1 blister q 12 hours	1 blister q 12 hours
Formoterol (Foradil)	**DPI:** 12mcg	1 cap q 12 hours	1 cap q 12 hours
COMBINATION AGENTS			
Ipratropium/Albuterol (Combivent)	**MDI:** (Albuterol-Ipratropium) 0.09mg-0.018mg/inh [14.7g]	2 inh qid.	
Ipratropium/Albuterol (Duoneb)	**Sol, Inhalation:** (Albuterol-Ipratropium) 3mg-0.5mg/3mL	3mL qid via nebulizer	
Fluticasone/ Salmeterol (Advair)	**DPI:** 100, 250, 500mcg/50mcg	1 puff bid	(100mcg/50mcg) 1 puff bid
Fluticasone/ Salmeterol (Advair HFA)	**MDI:** (45/21) 0.045mg-0.021mg/inh, (115/21) 0.115mg-0.021mg/inh, (230/21) 0.230mg-0.021mg/inh	Initial: 2 inh of 45/21 bid or 1 inh of 115/21 bid. **Max:** 2 inh of 230/21 bid.	Initial: 2 inh of 45/21 bid or 1 inh of 115/21 bid. **Max:** 2 inh of 230-21 bid.
Budesonide/Formoterol (Symbicort)	**MDI:** (Budesonide-Formoterol) 80mcg-4.5mcg/inh, 160mcg-4.5mcg/inh [10.2g]	2 puff bid of 80/4.5 or 160/4.5 depending on asthma severity. **Max:** 640mcg/18mcg (2 puff bid of 160/4.5).	2 inh bid of 80/4.5 or 160/4.5 depending on asthma severity. **Max:** 640mcg/18mcg (2 inh of 160/4.5).

(Continued)

DRUG (BRAND)	DOSAGE FORM	ADULT DOSE	CHILD DOSE*
METHYLXANTHINE			
Theophylline	Elixir; Caps & Tabs, Extended-Release	**Initial:** 10mg/kg/day up to 300mg max. **Usual Max:** 800mg/day.	**Initial:** 10mg/kg/day. **Usual Max:** <1 yr: 0.2 x age in weeks + 5 = mg/kg/day. 1 yr: 16mg/kg/day.
LEUKOTRIENE MODIFIERS			
Montelukast (Singulair)	**Tab:** 10mg; **Tab, Chewable:** 4mg, 5mg	10mg qhs	2-5 yrs: 4mg qhs. 6-14 yrs: 5mg qhs. 15 yrs: 10mg qhs.
Zafirlukast (Accolate)	**Tab:** 10mg, 20mg	20mg bid	≥12 yrs: 20mg bid. 5-11 yrs: 10mg bid.
Zileuton (Zyflo)	**Tab:** 600mg	600mg qid	≥12 yr: 600mg qid

ESTIMATED COMPARATIVE DAILY DOSAGES FOR INHALED CORTICOSTEROIDS

DRUG	LOW DAILY DOSE		MEDIUM DAILY DOSE		HIGH DAILY DOSE	
	ADULT	CHILD*	ADULT	CHILD*	ADULT	CHILD*
Beclomethasone HFA 40, 80mcg/puff (QVAR)	80-240mcg	80-160mcg	240-480mcg	160-320mcg	>480mcg	>320mcg
Budesonide DPI 200mcg/inhalation (Pulmicort Turbuhaler)	200-600mcg	200-400mcg	600-1200mcg	400-800mcg	>1200mcg	>800mcg
Budesonide Neb Sol: 0.25, 0.5mg/2mL (Pulmicort Respules)	N/A	0.5mg	N/A	1.0mg	N/A	2mg
Flunisolide 250mcg/puff (Aerobid)	500-1000mcg	500-750mcg	1000-2000mcg	1000-1250mcg	>2000mcg	>1250mcg
Fluticasone MDI 44, 110, or 220mcg/puff (Flovent HFA)	88-264mcg	88-176mcg	264-660mcg	176-440mcg	>660mcg	>440mcg
Mometasone Twisthaler 110mcg/inh, 220mcg/inh (Asmanex)	220-440mcg	220-440mcg	N/A	N/A	>880mcg	>880mcg
Triamcinolone acetonide 100mcg/puff (Azmacort)	400-1000mcg	400-800mcg	1000-2000mcg	800-1200mcg	>2000mcg	>1200mcg

*Children ≤12 yrs unless otherwise noted. MDI: metered-dose inhaler; DPI: dry powder inhaler.
Adopted from: The NAEPP Expert Panel Report: Guidelines for the Diagnosis and Management of Asthma–
Update on Selected Topics 2002. http://www.nhlbi.nih.gov/guidelines/asthma/asthsumm.htm

ASTHMA TREATMENT PLAN

CLASSIFICATION	LUNG FUNCTION	STEPWISE APPROACH TO THERAPY IN PATIENTS >12 YEARS OF AGE
Intermittent • Symptoms ≤2 days a week • Short-acting ß$_2$-agonist use for symptom control ≤2 days a week • Nighttime awakenings ≤2 times/month • Interference with normal activity - none	• Normal FEV$_1$ b/w exacerbations • FEV$_1$ ≥80% predicted • FEV$_1$/FVC - normal	**Step 1** • **Short-acting inhaled ß$_2$-agonists as needed (2-4 puffs prn).** • Severe exacerbations may occur, separated by long periods of normal lung function and no symptoms; a course of systemic corticosteroids is recommended.
Mild persistent • Symptoms >2 days/week but not daily • Short-acting ß$_2$-agonist use for symptom control >2days/wk but not daily, and not more than 1x on any day • Nighttime awakenings 3-4x/month • Interference with normal activity - minor limitation	• FEV$_1$ ≥80% predicted • FEV$_1$/FVC - normal	**Step 2** • **Low-dose inhaled corticosteroids.** • **Short-acting ß$_2$-agonists as needed (2-4 puffs prn).** ALTERNATIVE TREATMENT: • Cromolyn, leukotriene modifier, nedocromil OR theophylline
Moderate persistent • Daily symptoms • Short-acting ß$_2$-agonist use for symptom control daily • Nighttime awakenings >1x/wk but not nightly • Interference with normal activity - some limitation	• FEV$_1$ >60% but <80% predicted • FEV$_1$/FVC reduced 5%	**Step 3** • **Low- to medium-dose inhaled corticosteroids** AND • **Long-acting inhaled ß$_2$-agonists.** • **Short-acting inhaled ß$_2$-agonists as needed (2-4 puffs prn).** ALTERNATIVE TREATMENT: • Low-dose ICS + either LTRA, theophylline, OR Zileuton
Severe persistent • Symptoms throughout the day • Short-acting ß$_2$-agonist use for symptom several times per day • Nighttime awakenings often >7x/week • Interference with normal activity - extreme limitation	• FEV$_1$ ≤60% predicted • FEV$_1$/FVC reduced >5%	**Step 4 or Step 5** • **Medium-dose ICS + LABA OR** • **High-dose ICS + LABA** AND • Consider Omalizumab for patients who have allergies • **Short-acting inhaled ß$_2$-agonists as needed (2-4 puffs prn).** ALTERNATIVE TREATMENT: • Medium-dose ICS + either LTRA, Theophylline, OR Zileuton

Note: Preferred treatments are in bold.

Key Points:

- Stepwise approach presents general guidelines. Review treatment every 1 to 6 months; a gradual stepwise reduction in treatment may be possible. If control is not maintained, consider step up.

- The presence of one of the features of severity is sufficient to place a patient in that category. An individual should be assigned to the most severe grade in which any feature occurs (PEF is % of personal best; FEV is % predicted).

- Intensity of treatment will depend on severity of exacerbation; up to 3 treatments at 20-minute intervals or a single nebulizer treatment as needed. Course of systemic corticosteroids may be needed.

- Use of short-acting beta$_2$-agonists >2 days/week for a symptom relief generally indicates inadequate control and the need to step up treatment

- Airflow obstruction is indicated by reduced FEV$_1$ and FEV$_1$/FVC values relative to reference or predicted values.

- Abnormalities of lung function are categorized as restrictive and obstructive defects. A reduced ratio of FEV$_1$/FVC (eg, <65%) indicates obstruction to the flow of air from the lungs, whereas a reduced FVC with a normal FEV$_1$/FVC ratio suggests a restrictive pattern.

Abbreviations: FEV$_1$: Forced expiratory volume in one second. FVC: Forced vital capacity.

*Adapted from the Full Report 2007 *Guidelines for the Diagnosis and Management of Asthma.* NAEPP Expert Panel Report III.

RECOMMENDED IMMUNIZATION SCHEDULE FOR PERSONS AGED 0-6 YEARS

Vaccine ▼ Age ►	Birth	1 month	2 months	4 months	6 months	12 months	15 months	18 months	19–23 months	2–3 years	4–6 years
Hepatitis B[1]	HepB	HepB		see footnote 1		HepB					
Rotavirus[2]			Rota	Rota	Rota						
Diphtheria, Tetanus, Pertussis[3]			DTaP	DTaP	DTaP	see footnote 3	DTaP				DTaP
Haemophilus influenzae type b[4]			Hib	Hib	Hib	Hib					
Pneumococcal[5]			PCV	PCV	PCV	PCV				PPV	
Inactivated Poliovirus			IPV	IPV		IPV					IPV
Influenza[6]						Influenza (Yearly)					
Measles, Mumps, Rubella[7]						MMR					MMR
Varicella[8]						Varicella					Varicella
Hepatitis A[9]						HepA (2 doses)				HepA Series	
Meningococcal[10]										MCV4	

   ▨ Range of recommended ages   ▨ Certain high-risk groups

This schedule indicates the recommended ages for routine administration of currently licensed childhood vaccines, as of December 1, 2007, for children aged 0 through 6 years. Additional information is available at **www.cdc.gov/vaccines/recs/schedules.** Any dose not administered at the recommended age should be administered at any subsequent visit, when indicated and feasible. Additional vaccines may be licensed and recommended during the year. Licensed combination vaccines may be used whenever any components of the combination are indicated and other components of the vaccine are not contraindicated and if approved by the Food and Drug Administration for that dose of the series. Providers should consult the respective Advisory Committee on Immunization Practices statement for detailed recommendations, including for **high-risk conditions: http://www.cdc.gov/vaccines/pubs/ ACIP-list.htm.** Clinically significant adverse events that follow immunization should be reported to the Vaccine Adverse Event Reporting System (VAERS). Guidance about how to obtain and complete a VAERS form is available at **http://www.vaers.hhs.gov** or by telephone, **800-822-7967.**

1. **Hepatitis B vaccine (HepB).** *(Minimum age: birth)*
   At birth:
   - Administer monovalent HepB to all newborns prior to hospital discharge.
   - If mother is hepatitis B surface antigen (HBsAg) positive, administer HepB and 0.5 mL of hepatitis B immune globulin (HBIG) within 12 hours of birth.
   - If mother's HBsAg status is unknown, administer HepB within 12 hours of birth. Determine the HBsAg status as soon as possible and if HBsAg positive, administer HBIG (no later than age 1 week).
   - If mother is HBsAg negative, the birth dose can be delayed, in rare cases, with a provider's order and a copy of the mother's negative HBsAg laboratory report in the infant's medical record.

   After the birth dose:
   - The HepB series should be completed with either monovalent HepB or a combination vaccine containing HepB. The second dose should be administered at age 1–2 months. The final dose should be administered no earlier than age 24 weeks. Infants born to HBsAg-positive mothers should be tested for HBsAg and antibody to HBsAg after completion of at least 3 doses of a licensed HepB series, at age 9–18 months (generally at the next well-child visit).

   4-month dose:
   - It is permissible to administer 4 doses of HepB when combination vaccines are administered after the birth dose. If monovalent HepB is used for doses after the birth dose, a dose at age 4 months is not needed.

2. **Rotavirus vaccine (Rota).** *(Minimum age: 6 weeks)*
   - Administer the first dose at age 6–12 weeks.
   - Do not start the series later than age 12 weeks.
   - Administer the final dose in the series by age 32 weeks. Do not administer any dose later than age 32 weeks.
   - Data on safety and efficacy outside of these age ranges are insufficient.

3. **Diphtheria and tetanus toxoids and acellular pertussis vaccine (DTaP).** *(Minimum age: 6 weeks)*
   - The fourth dose of DTaP may be administered as early as age 12 months, provided 6 months have elapsed since the third dose.
   - Administer the final dose in the series at age 4–6 years.

4. **Haemophilus influenzae type b conjugate vaccine (Hib).** *(Minimum age: 6 weeks)*
   - If PRP-OMP (PedvaxHIB® or ComVax® [Merck]) is administered at ages 2 and 4 months, a dose at age 6 months is not required.
   - TriHIBit® (DTaP/Hib) combination products should not be used for primary immunization but can be used as boosters following any Hib vaccine in children age 12 months or older.

(Continued)

5. Pneumococcal vaccine. *(Minimum age: 6 weeks for pneumococcal conjugate vaccine [PCV]; 2 years for pneumococcal polysaccharide vaccine [PPV])*

- Administer one dose of PCV to all healthy children aged 24–59 months having any incomplete schedule.
- Administer PPV to children aged 2 years and older with underlying medical conditions.

6. Influenza vaccine. *(Minimum age: 6 months for trivalent inactivated influenza vaccine [TIV]; 2 years for live, attenuated influenza vaccine [LAIV])*

- Administer annually to children aged 6–59 months and to all eligible close contacts of children aged 0–59 months.
- Administer annually to children 5 years of age and older with certain risk factors, to other persons (including household members) in close contact with persons in groups at higher risk, and to any child whose parents request vaccination.
- For healthy persons (those who do not have underlying medical conditions that predispose them to influenza complications) ages 2–49 years, either LAIV or TIV may be used.
- Children receiving TIV should receive 0.25 mL if age 6–35 months or 0.5 mL if age 3 years or older.
- Administer 2 doses (separated by 4 weeks or longer) to children younger than 9 years who are receiving influenza vaccine for the first time or who were vaccinated for the first time last season but only received one dose.

7. Measles, mumps, and rubella vaccine (MMR). *(Minimum age: 12 months)*

- Administer the second dose of MMR at age 4–6 years. MMR may be administered before age 4–6 years, provided 4 weeks or more have elapsed since the first dose.

8. Varicella vaccine. *(Minimum age: 12 months)*

- Administer second dose at age 4–6 years; may be administered 3 months or more after first dose.
- Do not repeat second dose if administered 28 days or more after first dose.

9. Hepatitis A vaccine (HepA). *(Minimum age: 12 months)*

- Administer to all children aged 1 year (i.e., aged 12–23 months). Administer the 2 doses in the series at least 6 months apart.
- Children not fully vaccinated by age 2 years can be vaccinated at subsequent visits.
- HepA is recommended for certain other groups of children, including in areas where vaccination programs target older children.

10. Meningococcal vaccine. *(Minimum age: 2 years for meningococcal conjugate vaccine (MCV4) and for meningococcal polysaccharide vaccine (MPSV4))*

- Administer MCV4 to children aged 2–10 years with terminal complement deficiencies or anatomic or functional asplenia and certain other high-risk groups. MPSV4 is also acceptable.
- Administer MCV4 to persons who received MPSV4 3 or more years previously and remain at increased risk for meningococcal disease.

The Recommended Immunization Schedules for Persons Aged 0–18 Years are approved by the Advisory Committee on Immunization Practices (http://www.cdc.gov/vaccines/recs/acip), the American Academy of Pediatrics (http://www.aap.org), and the American Academy of Family Physicians (http://www.aafp.org).

RECOMMENDED IMMUNIZATION SCHEDULE FOR PERSONS AGED 7-18 YEARS

Vaccine ▼ Age ►	7–10 years	11–12 years	13–18 years
Diphtheria, Tetanus, Pertussis[1]	see footnote 1	Tdap	Tdap
Human Papillomavirus[2]	see footnote 2	HPV (3 doses)	HPV Series
Meningococcal[3]	MCV4	MCV4	MCV4
Pneumococcal[4]	PPV		
Influenza[5]	Influenza (Yearly)		
Hepatitis A[6]	HepA Series		
Hepatitis B[7]	HepB Series		
Inactivated Poliovirus[8]	IPV Series		
Measles, Mumps, Rubella[9]	MMR Series		
Varicella[10]	Varicella Series		

Range of recommended ages	Catch-up immunization	Certain high-risk groups

This schedule indicates the recommended ages for routine administration of currently licensed childhood vaccines, as of December 1, 2007, for children aged 7–18 years. Additional information is available at **www.cdc.gov/vaccines/recs/schedules**. Any dose not administered at the recommended age should be administered at any subsequent visit, when indicated and feasible. Additional vaccines may be licensed and recommended during the year. Licensed combination vaccines may be used whenever any components of the combination are indicated and other components of the vaccine are not contraindicated and if approved by the Food and Drug Administration for that dose of the series. Providers should consult the respective Advisory Committee on Immunization Practices statement for detailed recommendations, including for **high risk conditions: http://www.cdc.gov/vaccines/pubs/ACIP-list.htm**. Clinically significant adverse events that follow immunization should be reported to the Vaccine Adverse Event Reporting System (VAERS). Guidance about how to obtain and complete a VAERS form is available at **www.vaers.hhs.gov** or by telephone, **800-822-7967**.

1. **Tetanus and diphtheria toxoids and acellular pertussis vaccine (Tdap).** *(Minimum age: 10 years for BOOSTRIX® and 11 years for ADACEL™)*

   • Administer at age 11–12 years for those who have completed the recommended childhood DTP/DTaP vaccination series and have not received a tetanus and diphtheria toxoids (Td) booster dose.

   • 13–18-year-olds who missed the 11–12 year Tdap or received Td only are encouraged to receive one dose of Tdap 5 years after the last Td/DTaP dose.

2. **Human papillomavirus vaccine (HPV).** *(Minimum age: 9 years)*

   • Administer the first dose of the HPV vaccine series to females at age 11–12 years.

   • Administer the second dose 2 months after the first dose and the third dose 6 months after the first dose.

   • Administer the HPV vaccine series to females at age 13–18 years if not previously vaccinated.

3. **Meningococcal vaccine.**

   • Administer MCV4 at age 11–12 years and at age 13–18 years if not previously vaccinated. MPSV4 is an acceptable alternative.

   • Administer MCV4 to previously unvaccinated college freshmen living in dormitories.

   • MCV4 is recommended for children aged 2–10 years with terminal complement deficiencies or anatomic or functional asplenia and certain other high-risk groups.

   • Persons who received MPSV4 3 or more years previously and remain at increased risk for meningococcal disease should be vaccinated with MCV4.

4. **Pneumococcal polysaccharide vaccine (PPV).**

   • Administer PPV to certain high-risk groups.

5. **Influenza vaccine.**

   • Administer annually to all close contacts of children aged 0–59 months.

   • Administer annually to persons with certain risk factors, health-care workers, and other persons (including household members) in close contact with persons in groups at higher risk.

   • Administer 2 doses (separated by 4 weeks or longer) to children younger than 9 years who are receiving influenza vaccine for the first time or who were vaccinated for the first time last season but only received one dose.

   • For healthy nonpregnant persons (those who do not have underlying medical conditions that predispose them to influenza complications) ages 2–49 years, either LAIV or TIV may be used.

6. **Hepatitis A vaccine (HepA).**

   • Administer the 2 doses in the series at least 6 months apart.

   • HepA is recommended for certain other groups of children, including in areas where vaccination programs target older children.

(Continued)

7. Hepatitis B vaccine (HepB).

- Administer the 3-dose series to those who were not previously vaccinated.
- A 2-dose series of Recombivax HB® is licensed for children aged 11–15 years.

8. Inactivated poliovirus vaccine (IPV).

- For children who received an all-IPV or all-oral poliovirus (OPV) series, a fourth dose is not necessary if the third dose was administered at age 4 years or older.
- If both OPV and IPV were administered as part of a series, a total of 4 doses should be administered, regardless of the child's current age.

9. Measles, mumps, and rubella vaccine (MMR).

- If not previously vaccinated, administer 2 doses of MMR during any visit, with 4 or more weeks between the doses.

10. Varicella vaccine.

- Administer 2 doses of varicella vaccine to persons younger than 13 years of age at least 3 months apart. Do not repeat the second dose if administered 28 or more days following the first dose.
- Administer 2 doses of varicella vaccine to persons aged 13 years or older at least 4 weeks apart.

The Recommended Immunization Schedules for Persons Aged 0–18 Years are approved by the Advisory Committee on Immunization Practices (**http://www.cdc.gov/**), the American Academy of Pediatrics (**http://www.aap.org**), and the American Academy of Family Physicians (**http://www.aafp.org**).

CATCH-UP IMMUNIZATION SCHEDULE FOR PERSONS AGED 4 MONTHS-18 YEARS WHO START LATE OR WHO ARE MORE THAN 1 MONTH BEHIND

CATCH-UP SCHEDULE FOR PERSONS AGED 4 MONTHS–6 YEARS

Vaccine[1]	Minimum Age for Dose 1	Minimum Interval Between Doses			
		Dose 1 to Dose 2	Dose 2 to Dose 3	Dose 3 to Dose 4	Dose 4 to Dose 5
Hepatitis B[1]	Birth	4 weeks	8 weeks (and 16 weeks after first dose)		
Rotavirus[2]	6 wks	4 weeks	4 weeks		
Diphtheria, Tetanus, Pertussis[3]	6 wks	4 weeks	4 weeks	6 months	6 months[3]
Haemophilus influenzae type b[4]	6 wks	4 weeks if first dose administered at younger than 12 months of age / 8 weeks (as final dose) if first dose administered at age 12-14 months / No further doses needed if first dose administered at 15 months of age or older	4 weeks[a] if current age is younger than 12 months / 8 weeks (as final dose)[b] if current age is 12 months or older and second dose administered at younger than 15 months of age / No further doses needed if previous dose administered at age 15 months or older	8 weeks (as final dose) This dose only necessary for children aged 12 months–5 years who received 3 doses before age 12 months	
Pneumococcal[5]	6 wks	4 weeks if first dose administered at younger than 12 months of age / 8 weeks (as final dose) if first dose administered at age 12 months or older or current age 24–59 months / No further doses needed for healthy children if first dose administered at age 24 months or older	4 weeks if current age is younger than 12 months / 8 weeks (as final dose) if current age is 12 months or older / No further doses needed for healthy children if previous dose administered at age 24 months or older	8 weeks (as final dose) This dose only necessary for children aged 12 months–5 years who received 3 doses before age 12 months	
Inactivated Poliovirus[6]	6 wks	4 weeks	4 weeks	4 weeks[6]	
Measles, Mumps, Rubella[7]	12 mos	4 weeks			
Varicella[8]	12 mos	3 months			
Hepatitis A[9]	12 mos	6 months			

CATCH-UP SCHEDULE FOR PERSONS AGED 7–18 YEARS

Vaccine[1]	Minimum Age for Dose 1	Dose 1 to Dose 2	Dose 2 to Dose 3	Dose 3 to Dose 4	Dose 4 to Dose 5
Tetanus, Diphtheria/ Tetanus, Diphtheria, Pertussis[10]	7 yrs[10]	4 weeks	4 weeks if first dose administered at younger than 12 months of age / 6 months if first dose administered at age 12 months or older	6 months if first dose administered at younger than 12 months of age	
Human Papillomavirus[11]	9 yrs	4 weeks	12 weeks (and 24 weeks after the first dose)		
Hepatitis A[9]	12 mos	6 months			
Hepatitis B[1]	Birth	4 weeks	8 weeks (and 16 weeks after first dose)		
Inactivated Poliovirus[6]	6 wks	4 weeks	4 weeks	4 weeks[6]	
Measles, Mumps, Rubella[7]	12 mos	4 weeks			
Varicella[8]	12 mos	4 weeks if first dose administered at age 13 years or later / 3 months if first dose administered at younger than 13 years of age			

The table above provides catch-up schedules and minimum intervals between doses for children whose vaccinations have been delayed. A vaccine series does not need to be restarted, regardless of the time that has elapsed between doses. Use the section appropriate for the child's age.

1. Hepatitis B vaccine (HepB).

- Administer the 3-dose series to those who were not previously vaccinated.
- A 2-dose series of Recombivax HB® is licensed for children aged 11–15 years.

2. Rotavirus vaccine (Rota).

- Do not start the series later than age 12 weeks.
- Administer the final dose in the series by age 32 weeks.
- Do not administer a dose later than age 32 weeks.
- Data on safety and efficacy outside of these age ranges are insufficient.

3. Diphtheria and tetanus toxoids and acellular pertussis vaccine (DTaP).

- The fifth dose is not necessary if the fourth dose was administered at age 4 years or older.
- DTaP is not indicated for persons aged 7 years or older.

4. Haemophilus influenzae type b conjugate vaccine (Hib).

- Vaccine is not generally recommended for children aged 5 years or older.
- If current age is younger than 12 months and the first 2 doses were PRP-OMP

(PedvaxHIB® or ComVax® [Merck]), the third (and final) dose should be administered at age 12–15 months and at least 8 weeks after the second dose.
- If first dose was administered at age 7–11 months, administer 2 doses separated by 4 weeks plus a booster at age 12–15 months.

5. Pneumococcal conjugate vaccine (PCV).

- Administer one dose of PCV to all healthy children aged 24–59 months having any incomplete schedule.
- For children with underlying medical conditions, administer 2 doses of PCV at least 8 weeks apart if previously received less than 3 doses, or 1 dose of PCV if previously received 3 doses.

(Continued)

6. Inactivated poliovirus vaccine (IPV).

- For children who received an all-IPV or all-oral poliovirus (OPV) series, a fourth dose is not necessary if third dose was administered at age 4 years or older.
- If both OPV and IPV were administered as part of a series, a total of 4 doses should be administered, regardless of the child's current age.
- IPV is not routinely recommended for persons aged 18 years and older.

7. Measles, mumps, and rubella vaccine (MMR).

- The second dose of MMR is recommended routinely at age 4–6 years but may be administered earlier if desired.
- If not previously vaccinated, administer 2 doses of MMR during any visit with 4 or more weeks between the doses.

8. Varicella vaccine.

- The second dose of varicella vaccine is recommended routinely at age 4–6 years but may be administered earlier if desired.
- Do not repeat the second dose in persons younger than 13 years of age if administered 28 or more days after the first dose.

9. Hepatitis A vaccine (HepA).

- HepA is recommended for certain groups of children, including in areas where vaccination programs target older children. See *MMWR* 2006;55 (No. RR-7):1–23.

10. Tetanus and diphtheria toxoids vaccine (Td) and tetanus and diphtheria toxoids and acellular pertussis vaccine (Tdap).

- Tdap should be substituted for a single dose of Td in the primary catch-up series or as a booster if age appropriate; use Td for other doses.
- A 5-year interval from the last Td dose is encouraged when Tdap is used as a booster dose. A booster (fourth) dose is needed if any of the previous doses were administered at younger than 12 months of age. Refer to ACIP recommendations for further information. See *MMWR* 2006;55(No. RR-3).

11. Human papillomavirus vaccine (HPV).

- Administer the HPV vaccine series to females at age 13–18 years if not previously vaccinated.

Information about reporting reactions after immunization is available online at **http://www.vaers.hhs.gov** or by telephone via the 24-hour national toll-free information line 800-822-7967. Suspected cases of vaccine-preventable diseases should be reported to the state or local health department. Additional information, including precautions and contraindications for immunization, is available from the National Center for Immunization and Respiratory Diseases at **http://www.cdc.gov/vaccines** or telephone, **800-CDC-INFO (800-232-4636)**.

RECOMMENDED ADULT IMMUNIZATION SCHEDULE, BY VACCINE AND AGE GROUP

VACCINE ▼ AGE GROUP ▶	19–49 years	50–64 years	≥65 years
Tetanus, diphtheria, pertussis (Td/Tdap)[1,*]	1 dose Td booster every 10 yrs — Substitute 1 dose of Tdap for Td		
Human papillomavirus (HPV)[2,*]	3 doses females (0, 2, 6 mos)		
Measles, mumps, rubella (MMR)[3,*]	1 or 2 doses	1 dose	
Varicella[4,*]	2 doses (0, 4–8 wks)		
Influenza[5,*]		1 dose annually	
Pneumococcal (polysaccharide)[6,7]	1–2 doses		1 dose
Hepatitis A[8,*]	2 doses (0, 6–12 mos or 0, 6–18 mos)		
Hepatitis B[9,*]	3 doses (0, 1–2, 4–6 mos)		
Meningococcal[10,*]	1 or more doses		
Zoster[11]			1 dose

Covered by the Vaccine Injury Compensation Program.

For all persons in this category who meet the age requirements and who lack evidence of immunity (e.g., lack documentation of vaccination or have no evidence of prior infection)

Recommended if some other risk factor is present (e.g., on the basis of medical, occupational, lifestyle, or other indications)

Report all clinically significant postvaccination reactions to the Vaccine Adverse Event Reporting System (VAERS). Reporting forms and instructions on filing a VAERS report are available at **www.vaers.hhs.gov** or by telephone, 800-822-7967.

Information on how to file a Vaccine Injury Compensation Program claim is available at **www.hrsa.gov/vaccine compensation** or by telephone, 800-338-2382. To file a claim for vaccine injury, contact the U.S. Court of Federal Claims, 717 Madison Place, N.W., Washington, D.C. 20005; telephone, 202-357-6400.

Additional information about the vaccines in this schedule, extent of available data, and contraindications for vaccination is also available at **www.cdc.gov/vaccines** or from the CDC-INFO Contact Center at 800-CDC-INFO (800-232-4636) in English and Spanish, 24 hours a day, 7 days a week.

Use of trade names and commercial sources is for identification only and does not imply endorsement by the U.S. Department of Health and Human Services.

This schedule indicates the recommended age groups for which administration of currently licensed vaccines is commonly indicated for adults ages 19 years and older, as of October 1, 2007. Licensed combination vaccines may be used whenever any components of the combination are indicated and when the vaccine's other components are not contraindicated. For detailed recommendations on all vaccines, including those used primarily for travelers or that are issued during the year, consult the manufacturers' package inserts and the complete statements from the Advisory Committee on Immunization Practices **(www.cdc.gov/vaccines/pubs/acip-list.htm)**.

1. **Tetanus, diphtheria, and acellular pertussis (Td/Tdap) vaccination.** Tdap should replace a single dose of Td for adults aged <65 years who have not previously received a dose of Tdap. Only one of two Tdap products (Adacel® [sanofi pasteur]) is licensed for use in adults.
Adults with uncertain histories of a complete primary vaccination series with tetanus and diphtheria toxoid–containing vaccines should begin or complete a primary vaccination series. A primary series for adults is 3 doses of tetanus and diphtheria toxoid–containing vaccines; administer the first 2 doses at least 4 weeks apart and the third dose 6–12 months after the second. However, Tdap can substitute for any one of the doses of Td in the 3-dose primary series. The booster dose of tetanus and diphtheria toxoid–containing vaccine should be administered to adults who have completed a primary series and if the last vaccination was received ≥10 years previously. Tdap or Td vaccine may be used, as indicated.
If the person is pregnant and received the last Td vaccination ≥10 years previously, administer Td during the second or third trimester; if the person

received the last Td vaccination in <10 years, administer Tdap during the immediate postpartum period. A one-time administration of 1 dose of Tdap with an interval as short as 2 years from a previous Td vaccination is recommended for postpartum women, close contacts of infants aged <12 months, and all health-care workers with direct patient contact. In certain situations, Td can be deferred during pregnancy and Tdap substituted in the immediate postpartum period, or Tdap can be administered instead of Td to a pregnant woman after an informed discussion with the woman. Consult the ACIP statement for recommendations for administering Td as prophylaxis in wound management.

2. **Human papillomavirus (HPV) vaccination.** HPV vaccination is recommended for all females aged ≤26 years who have not completed the vaccine series. History of genital warts, abnormal Papanicolaou test, or positive HPV DNA test is not evidence of prior infection with all vaccine HPV types; HPV vaccination is still recommended for these persons.

(Continued)

Ideally, vaccine should be administered before potential exposure to HPV through sexual activity; however, females who are sexually active should still be vaccinated. Sexually active females who have not been infected with any of the HPV vaccine types receive the full benefit of the vaccination. Vaccination is less beneficial for females who have already been infected with one or more of the HPV vaccine types.

A complete series consists of 3 doses. The second dose should be administered 2 months after the first dose; the third dose should be administered 6 months after the first dose.

Although HPV vaccination is not specifically recommended for females with the medical indications described in Figure 2, "Vaccines that might be indicated for adults on medical and other indications," it is not a live-virus vaccine and can be administered. However, immune response and vaccine efficacy might be less than in persons who do not have the medical indications described or who are immunocompetent.

3. **Measles, mumps, rubella (MMR) vaccination.**
Measles component: Adults born before 1957 can be considered immune to measles. Adults born during or after 1957 should receive ≥1 dose of MMR unless they have a medical contraindication, documentation of ≥1 dose, history of measles based on health-care provider diagnosis, or laboratory evidence of immunity.

A second dose of MMR is recommended for adults who 1) have been recently exposed to measles or are in an outbreak setting; 2) have been previously vaccinated with killed measles vaccine; 3) have been vaccinated with an unknown type of measles vaccine during 1963–1967; 4) are students in postsecondary educational institutions; 5) work in a health-care facility; or 6) plan to travel internationally.
Mumps component: Adults born before 1957 can generally be considered immune to mumps. Adults born during or after 1957 should receive 1 dose of MMR unless they have a medical contraindication, history of mumps based on health-care provider diagnosis, or laboratory evidence of immunity.

A second dose of MMR is recommended for adults who 1) are in an age group that is affected during a mumps outbreak; 2) are students in postsecondary educational institutions; 3) work in a health-care facility; or 4) plan to travel internationally. For unvaccinated health-care workers born before 1957 who do not have other evidence of mumps immunity, consider administering 1 dose on a routine basis and strongly consider administering a second dose during an outbreak.
Rubella component: Administer 1 dose of MMR vaccine to women whose rubella vaccination history is unreliable or who lack laboratory evidence of immunity. For women of childbearing age, regardless of birth year, routinely determine rubella immunity and counsel women regarding congenital rubella syndrome. Women who do not have evidence of immunity should receive MMR vaccine upon completion or termination of pregnancy and before discharge from the health-care facility.

4. **Varicella vaccination.** All adults without evidence of immunity to varicella should receive 2 doses of single-antigen varicella vaccine unless they have a medical contraindication. Special consideration should be given to those who 1) have close contact with persons at high risk for severe disease (e.g., health-care personnel and family contacts of immunocompromised persons) or 2) are at high

risk for exposure or transmission (e.g., teachers; child care employees; residents and staff members of institutional settings, including correctional institutions; college students; military personnel; adolescents and adults living in households with children; nonpregnant women of childbearing age; and international travelers).

Evidence of immunity to varicella in adults includes any of the following: 1) documentation of 2 doses of varicella vaccine at least 4 weeks apart; 2) U.S.-born before 1980 (although for health-care personnel and pregnant women birth before 1980 should not be considered evidence of immunity); 3) history of varicella based on diagnosis or verification of varicella by a health-care provider (for a patient reporting a history of or presenting with an atypical case, a mild case, or both, health-care providers should seek either an epidemiologic link with a typical varicella case or to a laboratory-confirmed case or evidence of laboratory confirmation, if it was performed at the time of acute disease); 4) history of herpes zoster based on health-care provider diagnosis; or 5) laboratory evidence of immunity or laboratory confirmation of disease. Assess pregnant women for evidence of varicella immunity. Women who do not have evidence of immunity should receive the first dose of varicella vaccine upon completion or termination of pregnancy and before discharge from the health-care facility. The second dose should be administered 4–8 weeks after the first dose.

5. **Influenza vaccination.** *Medical indications:* Chronic disorders of the cardiovascular or pulmonary systems, including asthma; chronic metabolic diseases, including diabetes mellitus, renal or hepatic dysfunction, hemoglobinopathies, or immunosuppression (including immunosuppression caused by medications or human immunodeficiency virus [HIV]); any condition that compromises respiratory function or the handling of respiratory secretions or that can increase the risk of aspiration (e.g., cognitive dysfunction, spinal cord injury, or seizure disorder or other neuromuscular disorder); and pregnancy during the influenza season. No data exist on the risk for severe or complicated influenza disease among persons with asplenia; however, influenza is a risk factor for secondary bacterial infections that can cause severe disease among persons with asplenia.
Occupational indications: Health-care personnel and employees of long-term care and assisted-living facilities.
Other indications: Residents of nursing homes and other long-term care and assisted-living facilities; persons likely to transmit influenza to persons at high risk (e.g., in-home household contacts and caregivers of children aged 0–59 months, or persons of all ages with high-risk conditions); and anyone who would like to be vaccinated. Healthy, nonpregnant adults aged ≤49 years without high-risk medical conditions who are not contacts of severely immunocompromised persons in special care units can receive either intranasally administered live, attenuated influenza vaccine (FluMist®) or inactivated vaccine. Other persons should receive the inactivated vaccine.

6. **Pneumococcal polysaccharide vaccination.**
Medical indications: Chronic pulmonary disease (excluding asthma); chronic cardiovascular diseases; diabetes mellitus; chronic liver diseases, including liver disease as a result of alcohol abuse (e.g., cirrhosis); chronic alcoholism, chronic renal

(Continued)

failure or nephrotic syndrome; functional or anatomic asplenia (e.g., sickle cell disease or splenectomy [if elective splenectomy is planned, vaccinate at least 2 weeks before surgery]); immunosuppressive conditions; and cochlear implants and cerebrospinal fluid leaks. Vaccinate as close to HIV diagnosis as possible.

Other indications: Alaska Natives and certain American Indian populations and residents of nursing homes or other long-term care facilities.

7. **Revaccination with pneumococcal polysaccharide vaccine.** One-time revaccination after 5 years for persons with chronic renal failure or nephrotic syndrome; functional or anatomic asplenia (e.g., sickle cell disease or splenectomy); or immunosuppressive conditions. For persons aged ≥65 years, one-time revaccination if they were vaccinated ≥5 years previously and were aged <65 years at the time of primary vaccination.

8. **Hepatitis A vaccination.** *Medical indications:* Persons with chronic liver disease and persons who receive clotting factor concentrates.
Behavioral indications: Men who have sex with men and persons who use illegal drugs.
Occupational indications: Persons working with hepatitis A virus (HAV)–infected primates or with HAV in a research laboratory setting.
Other indications: Persons traveling to or working in countries that have high or intermediate endemicity of hepatitis A (a list of countries is available at **wwwn.cdc.gov/travel/contentdiseases.aspx**) and any person seeking protection from HAV infection. Single-antigen vaccine formulations should be administered in a 2-dose schedule at either 0 and 6–12 months (Havrix®), or 0 and 6–18 months (Vaqta®). If the combined hepatitis A and hepatitis B vaccine (Twinrix®) is used, administer 3 doses at 0, 1, and 6 months.

9. **Hepatitis B vaccination.** *Medical indications:* Persons with end-stage renal disease, including patients receiving hemodialysis; persons seeking evaluation or treatment for a sexually transmitted disease (STD); persons with HIV infection; and persons with chronic liver disease.
Occupational indications: Health-care personnel and public-safety workers who are exposed to blood or other potentially infectious body fluids.
Behavioral indications: Sexually active persons who are not in a long-term, mutually monogamous relationship (e.g., persons with more than 1 sex partner during the previous 6 months); current or recent injection-drug users; and men who have sex with men.
Other indications: Household contacts and sex partners of persons with chronic hepatitis B virus (HBV) infection; clients and staff members of institutions for persons with developmental disabilities; international travelers to countries with high or intermediate prevalence of chronic HBV infection (a list of countries is available at **wwwn.cdc.gov/travel/contentdiseases.aspx**); and any adult seeking protection from HBV infection.
Settings where hepatitis B vaccination is recom-

mended for all adults: STD treatment facilities; HIV testing and treatment facilities; facilities providing drug-abuse treatment and prevention services; health-care settings targeting services to injection-drug users or men who have sex with men; correctional facilities; end-stage renal disease programs and facilities for chronic hemodialysis patients; and institutions and nonresidential daycare facilities for persons with developmental disabilities.
Special formulation indications: For adult patients receiving hemodialysis and other immunocompromised adults, 1 dose of 40 μg/mL (Recombivax HB®), or 2 doses of 20 μg/mL (Engerix-B®) administered simultaneously.

10. **Meningococcal vaccination.** *Medical indications:* Adults with anatomic or functional asplenia, or terminal complement component deficiencies.
Other indications: First-year college students living in dormitories; microbiologists who are routinely exposed to isolates of Neisseria meningitidis; military recruits; and persons who travel to or live in countries in which meningococcal disease is hyperendemic or epidemic (e.g., the "meningitis belt" of sub-Saharan Africa during the dry season [December–June]), particularly if their contact with local populations will be prolonged. Vaccination is required by the government of Saudi Arabia for all travelers to Mecca during the annual Hajj. Meningococcal conjugate vaccine is preferred for adults with any of the preceding indications who are aged ≤55 years, although meningococcal polysaccharide vaccine (MPSV4) is an acceptable alternative. Revaccination after 3–5 years might be indicated for adults previously vaccinated with MPSV4 who remain at increased risk for infection (e.g., persons residing in areas in which disease is epidemic).

11. **Herpes zoster vaccination.** A single dose of zoster vaccine is recommended for adults aged ≥60 years regardless of whether they report a prior episode of herpes zoster. Persons with chronic medical conditions may be vaccinated unless a contraindication or precaution exists for their condition.

12. **Selected conditions for which *Haemophilus influenzae* type b (Hib) vaccine may be used.** Hib conjugate vaccines are licensed for children aged 6 weeks–71 months. No efficacy data are available on which to base a recommendation concerning use of Hib vaccine for older children and adults with the chronic conditions associated with an increased risk for Hib disease. However, studies suggest good immunogenicity in patients who have sickle cell disease, leukemia, or HIV infection or who have had splenectomies; administering vaccine to these patients is not contraindicated.

13. **Immunocompromising conditions.** Inactivated vaccines are generally acceptable (e.g., pneumococcal, meningococcal, and influenza [trivalent inactivated influenza vaccine]), and live vaccines generally are avoided in persons with immune deficiencies or immune suppressive conditions. Information on specific conditions is available at **www.cdc.gov/vaccines/pubs/acip-list.htm**.

RECOMMENDED ADULT IMMUNIZATION SCHEDULE, BY VACCINE AND MEDICAL AND OTHER INDICATIONS

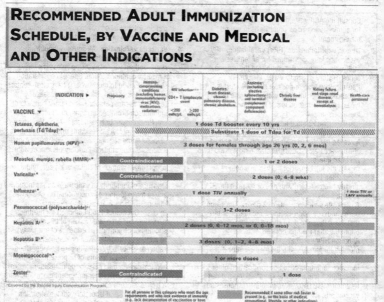

INDICATION ► / VACCINE ▼	Pregnancy	Immuno-compromising conditions (excluding human immunodeficiency virus [HIV], medications, radiation)	HIV infection CD4+ T lymphocyte count <200 cells/µL	HIV infection CD4+ T lymphocyte count ≥200 cells/µL	Diabetes, heart disease, chronic pulmonary disease, chronic alcoholism	Asplenia (including elective splenectomy and terminal complement component deficiencies)	Chronic liver disease	Kidney failure, end-stage renal disease, receipt of hemodialysis	Health-care personnel
Tetanus, diphtheria, pertussis (Td/Tdap)*	1 dose Td booster every 10 yrs · Substitute 1 dose of Tdap for Td								
Human papillomavirus (HPV)*	3 doses for females through age 26 yrs (0, 2, 6 mos)								
Measles, mumps, rubella (MMR)*	Contraindicated		1 or 2 doses						
Varicella*	Contraindicated		2 doses (0, 4–8 wks)						
Influenza*	1 dose TIV annually								1 dose TIV or 1 LAIV annually
Pneumococcal (polysaccharide)*	1–2 doses								
Hepatitis A*	2 doses (0, 6–12 mos, or 0, 6–18 mos)								
Hepatitis B*	3 doses (0, 1–2, 4–6 mos)								
Meningococcal*	1 or more doses								
Zoster	Contraindicated			1 dose					

*Covered by the Vaccine Injury Compensation Program

For all persons in this category who meet the age requirements and who lack evidence of immunity (e.g., lack documentation of vaccination or have no evidence of prior infection)

Recommended if some other risk factor is present (e.g., on the basis of medical, occupational, lifestyle, or other indications)

Report all clinically significant postvaccination reactions to the Vaccine Adverse Event Reporting System (VAERS). Reporting forms and instructions on filing a VAERS report are available at **www.vaers.hhs.gov** or by telephone, 800-822-7967.

Information on how to file a Vaccine Injury Compensation Program claim is available at **www.hrsa.gov/vaccine compensation** or by telephone, 800-338-2382. To file a claim for vaccine injury, contact the U.S. Court of Federal Claims, 717 Madison Place, N.W., Washington, D.C. 20005; telephone, 202-357-6400.

Additional information about the vaccines in this schedule, extent of available data, and contraindications for vaccination is also available at **www.cdc.gov/vaccines** or from the CDC-INFO Contact Center at 800-CDC-INFO (800-232-4636) in English and Spanish, 24 hours a day, 7 days a week.

Use of trade names and commercial sources is for identification only and does not imply endorsement by the U.S. Department of Health and Human Services.

This schedule indicates the recommended medical indications for which administration of currently licensed vaccines is commonly indicated for adults ages 19 years and older, as of October 1, 2007. Licensed combination vaccines may be used whenever any components of the combination are indicated and when the vaccine's other components are not contraindicated. For detailed recommendations on all vaccines, including those used primarily for travelers or that are issued during the year, consult the manufacturers' package inserts and the complete statements from the Advisory Committee on Immunization Practices (**www.cdc.gov/vaccines/pubs/acip-list.htm**).

---

1. **Tetanus, diphtheria, and acellular pertussis (Td/Tdap) vaccination.** Tdap should replace a single dose of Td for adults aged <65 years who have not previously received a dose of Tdap. Only one of two Tdap products (Adacel® [sanofi pasteur]) is licensed for use in adults.

   Adults with uncertain histories of a complete primary vaccination series with tetanus and diphtheria toxoid–containing vaccines should begin or complete a primary vaccination series. A primary series for adults is 3 doses of tetanus and diphtheria toxoid–containing vaccines; administer the first 2 doses at least 4 weeks apart and the third dose 6–12 months after the second. However, Tdap can substitute for any one of the doses of Td in the 3-dose primary series. The booster dose of tetanus and diphtheria toxoid–containing vaccine should be administered to adults who have completed a primary series and if the last vaccination was received ≥10 years previously. Tdap or Td vaccine may be used, as indicated.

   If the person is pregnant and received the last Td vaccination ≥10 years previously, administer Td during the second or third trimester; if the person received the last Td vaccination in <10 years, administer Tdap during the immediate postpartum period. A one-time administration of 1 dose of Tdap with an interval as short as 2 years from a previous Td vaccination is recommended for postpartum women, close contacts of infants aged <12 months, and all health-care workers with direct patient contact. In certain situations, Td can be deferred during pregnancy and Tdap substituted in the immediate postpartum period, or Tdap can be administered instead of Td to a pregnant woman after an informed discussion with the woman.

(Continued)

Consult the ACIP statement for recommendations for administering Td as prophylaxis in wound management.

2. **Human papillomavirus (HPV) vaccination.** HPV vaccination is recommended for all females aged ≤26 years who have not completed the vaccine series. History of genital warts, abnormal Papanicolaou test, or positive HPV DNA test is not evidence of prior infection with all vaccine HPV types; HPV vaccination is still recommended for these persons.

Ideally, vaccine should be administered before potential exposure to HPV through sexual activity; however, females who are sexually active should still be vaccinated. Sexually active females who have not been infected with any of the HPV vaccine types receive the full benefit of the vaccination. Vaccination is less beneficial for females who have already been infected with one or more of the HPV vaccine types.

A complete series consists of 3 doses. The second dose should be administered 2 months after the first dose; the third dose should be administered 6 months after the first dose.

Although HPV vaccination is not specifically recommended for females with the medical indications described in Figure 2, "Vaccines that might be indicated for adults based on medical and other indications," it is not a live-virus vaccine and can be administered. However, immune response and vaccine efficacy might be less than in persons who do not have the medical indications described or who are immunocompetent.

3. **Measles, mumps, rubella (MMR) vaccination.** *Measles component:* Adults born before 1957 can be considered immune to measles. Adults born during or after 1957 should receive ≥1 dose of MMR unless they have a medical contraindication, documentation of ≥1 dose, history of measles based on health-care provider diagnosis, or laboratory evidence of immunity.

A second dose of MMR is recommended for adults who 1) have been recently exposed to measles or are in an outbreak setting; 2) have been previously vaccinated with killed measles vaccine; 3) have been vaccinated with an unknown type of measles vaccine during 1963–1967; 4) are students in postsecondary educational institutions; 5) work in a health-care facility; or 6) plan to travel internationally. *Mumps component:* Adults born before 1957 can generally be considered immune to mumps. Adults born during or after 1957 should receive 1 dose of MMR unless they have a medical contraindication, history of mumps based on health-care provider diagnosis, or laboratory evidence of immunity.

A second dose of MMR is recommended for adults who 1) are in an age group that is affected during a mumps outbreak; 2) are students in postsecondary educational institutions; 3) work in a health-care facility; or 4) plan to travel internationally. For unvaccinated health-care workers born before 1957 who do not have other evidence of mumps immunity, consider administering 1 dose on a routine basis and strongly consider administering a second dose during an outbreak.

Rubella component: Administer 1 dose of MMR vaccine to women whose rubella vaccination history is unreliable or who lack laboratory evidence of immunity. For women of childbearing age, regardless of birth year, routinely determine rubella immunity and counsel women regarding congenital rubella syndrome. Women who do not have evidence of

immunity should receive MMR vaccine upon completion or termination of pregnancy and before discharge from the health-care facility.

4. **Varicella vaccination.** All adults without evidence of immunity to varicella should receive 2 doses of single-antigen varicella vaccine unless they have a medical contraindication. Special consideration should be given to those who 1) have close contact with persons at high risk for severe disease (e.g., health-care personnel and family contacts of immunocompromised persons) or 2) are at high risk for exposure or transmission (e.g., teachers; child care employees; residents and staff members of institutional settings, including correctional institutions; college students; military personnel; adolescents and adults living in households with children; nonpregnant women of childbearing age; and international travelers).

Evidence of immunity to varicella in adults includes any of the following: 1) documentation of 2 doses of varicella vaccine at least 4 weeks apart; 2) U.S.-born before 1980 (although for health-care personnel and pregnant women birth before 1980 should not be considered evidence of immunity); 3) history of varicella based on diagnosis or verification of varicella by a health-care provider (for a patient reporting a history of or presenting with an atypical case, a mild case, or both, health-care providers should seek either an epidemiologic link with a typical varicella case or to a laboratory-confirmed case or evidence of laboratory confirmation, if it was performed at the time of acute disease); 4) history of herpes zoster based on health-care provider diagnosis; or 5) laboratory evidence of immunity or laboratory confirmation of disease. Assess pregnant women for evidence of varicella immunity. Women who do not have evidence of immunity should receive the first dose of varicella vaccine upon completion or termination of pregnancy and before discharge from the health-care facility. The second dose should be administered 4–8 weeks after the first dose.

5. **Influenza vaccination.** *Medical indications:* Chronic disorders of the cardiovascular or pulmonary systems, including asthma; chronic metabolic diseases, including diabetes mellitus, renal or hepatic dysfunction, hemoglobinopathies, or immunosuppression (including immunosuppression caused by medications or human immunodeficiency virus [HIV]); any condition that compromises respiratory function or the handling of respiratory secretions or that can increase the risk of aspiration (e.g., cognitive dysfunction, spinal cord injury, or seizure disorder or other neuromuscular disorder); and pregnancy during the influenza season. No data exist on the risk for severe or complicated influenza disease among persons with asplenia; however, influenza is a risk factor for secondary bacterial infections that can cause severe disease among persons with asplenia.

Occupational indications: Health-care personnel and employees of long-term care and assisted-living facilities.

Other indications: Residents of nursing homes and other long-term care and assisted-living facilities; persons likely to transmit influenza to persons at high risk (e.g., in-home household contacts and caregivers of children aged 0–59 months, or persons of all ages with high-risk conditions); and anyone who would like to be vaccinated. Healthy, nonpregnant adults aged ≤49 years without high-risk medical conditions who are not contacts of

(Continued)

severely immunocompromised persons in special care units can receive either intranasally administered live, attenuated influenza vaccine (FluMist®) or inactivated vaccine. Other persons should receive the inactivated vaccine.

6. **Pneumococcal polysaccharide vaccination.**
   Medical indications: Chronic pulmonary disease (excluding asthma); chronic cardiovascular diseases; diabetes mellitus; chronic liver diseases, including liver disease as a result of alcohol abuse (e.g., cirrhosis); chronic alcoholism, chronic renal failure or nephrotic syndrome; functional or anatomic asplenia (e.g., sickle cell disease or splenectomy [if elective splenectomy is planned, vaccinate at least 2 weeks before surgery]); immunosuppressive conditions; and cochlear implants and cerebrospinal fluid leaks. Vaccinate as close to HIV diagnosis as possible.
   Other indications: Alaska Natives and certain American Indian populations and residents of nursing homes or other long-term care facilities.

7. **Revaccination with pneumococcal polysaccharide vaccine.** One-time revaccination after 5 years for persons with chronic renal failure or nephrotic syndrome; functional or anatomic asplenia (e.g., sickle cell disease or splenectomy); or immunosuppressive conditions. For persons aged ≥65 years, one-time revaccination if they were vaccinated ≥5 years previously and were aged <65 years at the time of primary vaccination.

8. **Hepatitis A vaccination.** *Medical indications:* Persons with chronic liver disease and persons who receive clotting factor concentrates.
   Behavioral indications: Men who have sex with men and persons who use illegal drugs.
   Occupational indications: Persons working with hepatitis A virus (HAV)–infected primates or with HAV in a research laboratory setting.
   Other indications: Persons traveling to or working in countries that have high or intermediate endemicity of hepatitis A (a list of countries is available at **wwwn.cdc.gov/travel/contentdiseases.aspx**) and any person seeking protection from HAV infection. Single-antigen vaccine formulations should be administered in a 2-dose schedule at either 0 and 6–12 months (Havrix®), or 0 and 6–18 months (Vaqta®). If the combined hepatitis A and hepatitis B vaccine (Twinrix®) is used, administer 3 doses at 0, 1, and 6 months.

9. **Hepatitis B vaccination.** *Medical indications:* Persons with end-stage renal disease, including patients receiving hemodialysis; persons seeking evaluation or treatment for a sexually transmitted disease (STD); persons with HIV infection; and persons with chronic liver disease.
   Occupational indications: Health-care personnel and public-safety workers who are exposed to blood or other potentially infectious body fluids.
   Behavioral indications: Sexually active persons who are not in a long-term, mutually monogamous relationship (e.g., persons with more than 1 sex partner during the previous 6 months); current or recent injection-drug users; and men who have sex with men.
   Other indications: Household contacts and sex partners of persons with chronic hepatitis B virus (HBV) infection; clients and staff members of institutions for persons with developmental disabilities; international travelers to countries with high or

intermediate prevalence of chronic HBV infection (a list of countries is available at **wwwn.cdc.gov/travel/contentdiseases.aspx**); and any adult seeking protection from HBV infection.
Settings where hepatitis B vaccination is recommended for all adults: STD treatment facilities; HIV testing and treatment facilities; facilities providing drug-abuse treatment and prevention services; health-care settings targeting services to injection-drug users or men who have sex with men; correctional facilities; end-stage renal disease programs and facilities for chronic hemodialysis patients; and institutions and nonresidential daycare facilities for persons with developmental disabilities.
Special formulation indications: For adult patients receiving hemodialysis and other immunocompromised adults, 1 dose of 40 μg/mL (Recombivax HB®), or 2 doses of 20 μg/mL (Engerix-B®) administered simultaneously.

10. **Meningococcal vaccination.** *Medical indications:* Adults with anatomic or functional asplenia, or terminal complement component deficiencies.
    Other indications: First-year college students living in dormitories; microbiologists who are routinely exposed to isolates of Neisseria meningitidis; military recruits; and persons who travel to or live in countries in which meningococcal disease is hyperendemic or epidemic (e.g., the "meningitis belt" of sub-Saharan Africa during the dry season [December–June]), particularly if their contact with local populations will be prolonged. Vaccination is required by the government of Saudi Arabia for all travelers to Mecca during the annual Hajj. Meningococcal conjugate vaccine is preferred for adults with any of the preceding indications who are aged ≤55 years, although meningococcal polysaccharide vaccine (MPSV4) is an acceptable alternative. Revaccination after 3–5 years might be indicated for adults previously vaccinated with MPSV4 who remain at increased risk for infection (e.g., persons residing in areas in which disease is epidemic).

11. **Herpes zoster vaccination.** A single dose of zoster vaccine is recommended for adults aged ≥60 years regardless of whether they report a prior episode of herpes zoster. Persons with chronic medical conditions may be vaccinated unless a contraindication or precaution exists for their condition.

12. **Selected conditions for which *Haemophilus influenzae* type b (Hib) vaccine may be used.** Hib conjugate vaccines are licensed for children aged 6 weeks–71 months. No efficacy data are available on which to base a recommendation concerning use of Hib vaccine for older children and adults with the chronic conditions associated with an increased risk for Hib disease. However, studies suggest good immunogenicity in patients who have sickle cell disease, leukemia, or HIV infection or who have had splenectomies; administering vaccine to these patients is not contraindicated.

13. **Immunocompromising conditions.** Inactivated vaccines are generally acceptable (e.g., pneumococcal, meningococcal, and influenza [trivalent inactivated influenza vaccine]), and live vaccines generally are avoided in persons with immune deficiencies or immune suppressive conditions. Information on specific conditions is available at **www.cdc.gov/vaccines/pubs/acip-list.htm**.

DRUGS EXCRETED IN BREAST MILK

The following list is not comprehensive; generic forms and alternate brands of some products may be available. When recommending drugs to pregnant or nursing patients, always check product labeling for specific precautions.

Accolate	Cardizem	Diastat	Hydrocortone
Accuretic	Cataflam	Diflucan	HydroDIURIL
Aciphex	Catapres	Digitek	Iberet-Folic
Actiq	Ceclor	Dilacor	Ifex
Activella	Cefizox	Dilantin	Imitrex
Actonel	Cefobid	Dilaudid	Imuran
Actonel with Calcium	Cefotan	Diovan	Inderal
ActoPlus Met	Ceftin	Diprivan	Inderide
Actos	Celebrex	Diuril	Indocin
Adalat	Celexa	Dolobid	INFeD
Adderall	Cerebyx	Dolophine	Inspra
Advicor	Ceredase	Doral	Invanz
Aggrenox	Cipro	Doryx	Inversine
Aldactazide	Ciprodex	Droxia	Isoptin
Aldactone	Claforan	Duraclon	Kadian
Aldomet	Clarinex	Duragesic	Keflex
Aldoril	Claritin	Duramorph	Keppra
Alesse	Claritin-D	Duratuss	Kerlone
Alfenta	Cleocin	Duricef	Ketek
Allegra-D	Climara	Dyazide	Klonopin
Aloprim	Clozaril	Dyrenium	Kronofed-A
Altace	Codeine	E.E.S.	Kutrase
Ambien	CombiPatch	EC-Naprosyn	Lamictal
Anaprox	Combipres	Ecotrin	Lamisil
Androderm	Combivir	Effexor	Lamprene
Antara	Combunox	Elestat	Lanoxicaps
Apresoline	Compazine	EMLA	Lanoxin
Aralen	Cordarone	Enduron	Lariam
Arthrotec	Corgard	Epzicom	Lescol
Asacol	Cortisporin	Equetro	Levbid
Ativan	Corzide	ERYC	Levitra
Augmentin	Cosopt	EryPed	Levlen
Avalide	Coumadin	Ery-Tab	Levlite
Avandia	Covera-HS	Erythrocin	Levora
Avelox	Cozaar	Erythromycin	Levothroid
Axid	Crestor	Esgic-plus	Levoxyl
Axocet	Crinone	Eskalith	Levsin
Azactam	Cyclessa	Estrogel	Levsinex
Azasan	Cymbalta	Estrostep	Lexapro
Azathioprine	Cystospaz	Evista	Lexiva
Azulfidine	Cytomel	FazaClo	Lialda
Bactrim	Cytotec	Felbatol	Lindane
Baraclude	Cytoxan	Feldene	Lioresal
Benadryl	Dapsone	femhrt	Lipitor
Bentyl	Daraprim	Fiorinal	Lithium
Betapace	Darvon	Flagyl	Lithobid
Bextra	Darvon-N	Floxin	Lo/Ovral
Bexxar	Decadron	Foradil	Loestrin
Bicillin	Deconsal II	Fortamet	Lomotil
Blocadren	Demerol	Fortaz	Loniten
Boniva	Demulen	Fosamax Plus D	Lopressor
Brethine	Depacon	Furosemide	Lortab
Brevicon	Depakene	Gabitril	Lotensin
Brontex	Depakote	Galzin	Lotrel
Byetta	DepoDur	Garamycin	Luminal
Caduet	Depo-Provera	Glucophage	Luvox
Cafergot	Desogen	Glyset	Lyrica
Calan	Desoxyn	Guaifed	Macrobid
Campral	Desyrel	Halcion	Macrodantin
Capoten	Dexedrine	Haldol	Marinol
Capozide	DextroStat	Helidac	Maxipime
Captopril	D.H.E. 45	Hycamtin	Maxzide
Carbatrol	Diabinese	Hydrocet	Mefoxin

Menostar
Methergine
Methotrexate
MetroCream/Gel/Lotion
Mexitil
Micronor
Microzide
Migranal
Miltown
Minizide
Minocin
Mirapex
Mircette
M-M-R II
Mobic
Modicon
Moduretic
Monodox
Monopril
Morphine
MS Contin
MSIR
Myambutol
Mycamine
Mysoline
Namenda
Naprelan
Naprosyn
Nascobal
Necon
NegGram
Nembutal
Neoral
Niaspan
Nicotrol
Niravam
Nizoral
Norco
Nor-QD
Nordette
Norinyl
Noritate
Normodyne
Norpace
Norplant
Novantrone
Nubain
Nucofed
Nydrazid
Oramorph
Oretic
Ortho-Cept
Ortho-Cyclen
Ortho-Novum
Ortho Tri-Cyclen
Orudis
Ovcon
Oxistat
OxyContin

OxyFast
OxyIR
Pacerone
Pamelor
Pancrease
Paxil
PCE
Pediapred
Pediazole
Pediotic
Pentasa
Pepcid
Periostat
Persantine
Pfizerpen
Phenergan
Phenobarbital
Phrenilin
Pipracil
Plan B
Ponstel
Pravachol
Premphase
Prempro
Prevacid
Prevacid NapraPAC
PREVPAC
Prinzide
Prograf
Proloprim
Prometrium
Pronestyl
Propofol
Prosed/DS
Protonix
Provera
Prozac
Pseudoephedrine
Pulmicort
Pyrazinamide
Quinidex
Quinine
Raptiva
Reglan
Relpax
Renese
Requip
Reserpine
Restoril
Retrovir
Rifadin
Rifamate
Rifater
Rimactane
Risperdal
Rocaltrol
Rocephin
Roferon A
Roxanol

Rozerem
Sanctura
Sanctura XR
Sandimmune
Sarafem
Seconal
Sectral
Semprex-D
Septra
Seroquel
Seroquel XR
Sinequan
Slo-bid
Soma
Sonata
Spiriva
Sprycel
Stadol
Streptomycin
Stromectol
Symbyax
Symmetrel
Synthroid
Tagamet
Tambocor
Tapazole
Tarka
Tasigna
Tavist
Tazicef
Tazidime
Tegretol
Tenoretic
Tenormin
Tenuate
Testoderm
Thalitone
Theo-24
Theo-Dur
Thorazine
Tiazac
Timolide
Timoptic
Tindamax
Tobi
Tofranil
Tolectin
Toprol-XL
Toradol
Trandate
Tranxene
Trental
Tricor
Triglide
Trilafon
Trileptal
Tri-Levlen
Tri-Norinyl
Triostat

Triphasil
Trivora
Trizivir
Trovan
Truvada
Tygacil
Tylenol
Tylenol with Codeine
Ultane
Ultram
Unasyn
Uniphyl
Uniretic
Unithroid
Urimax
Valium
Valtrex
Vanceril
Vancocin
Vantin
Vascor
Vaseretic
Vasotec
Ventavis
Verelan
Vermox
Versed
Vibramycin
Vibra-Tabs
Vicodin
Vigamox
Viramune
Voltaren
Vytorin
Wellbutrin
Xanax
Xolair
Zantac
Zarontin
Zaroxolyn
Zegerid
Zemplar
Zestoretic
Zetia
Ziac
Zinacef
Zithromax
Zocor
Zomig
Zonalon
Zonegran
Zosyn
Zovia
Zovirax
Zyban
Zydone
Zyloprim
Zyprexa
Zyrtec

DRUGS THAT MAY CAUSE PHOTOSENSITIVITY

The drugs in this table are known to cause photosensitivity in some individuals. Effects can range from itching, scaling, rash, and swelling to skin cancer, premature skin aging, skin and eye burns, cataracts, reduced immunity, blood vessel damage, and allergic reactions. The list is not all-inclusive, and shows only representative brands of each generic. When in doubt, always check specific product labeling. Individuals should be advised to wear protective clothing and to apply sunscreens while taking the medications listed below.

GENERIC	BRAND
Acamprosate	Campral
Acetazolamide	Diamox
Acitretin	Soriatane
Acyclovir	Zovirax
Alendronate	Fosamax
Alitretinoin	Panretin
Almotriptan	Axert
Amiloride/ hydrochlorothiazide	Moduretic
Aminolevulinic acid	Levulan Kerastick
Amiodarone	Cordarone, Pacerone
Amitriptyline	Elavil
Amitriptyline/ chlordiazepoxide	Etrafon, Limbitrol
Amitriptyline/perphenazine	
Amlodipine/atorvastatin	Caduet
Amoxapine	
Amphetamine aspartate/ amphetamine sulfate/ dextroamphetamine saccharate/ dextroamphetamine sulfate	Adderall XR
Anagrelide	Agrylin
Aripiprazole	Abilify
Atazanavir	Reyataz
Atenolol/chlorthalidone	Tenoretic
Atorvastatin	Lipitor
Atovaquone/proguanil	Malarone
Azatadine/ pseudoephedrine	Rynatan, Trinalin
Azithromycin	Zithromax, Zmag
Benazepril	Lotensin
Benazepril/ hydrochlorothiazide	Lotensin HCT
Bendroflumethiazide/ nadolol	Corzide
Bexarotene	Targretin
Bismuth/metronidazole/ tetracycline	Helidac
Bismuth subcitrate potassium/ metronidazole/tetracycline	Pylera
Bisoprolol/ hydrochlorothiazide	Ziac
Brompheniramine/ dextromethorphan/ phenylephrine	Alacol DM, Dimetane DX
Brompheniramine/ dextromethorphan/ pseudoephedrine	Bromfed-DM
Buffered aspirin/ pravastatin	Pravigard PAC
Bupropion	Wellbutrin, Zyban
Candesartan/ hydrochlorothiazide	Atacand HCT
Capecitabine	Xeloda
Captopril	Capoten
Captopril/ hydrochlorothiazide	Capozide
Carbamazepine	Carbatrol, Equetro, Tegretol, Tegretol-XR
Carbinoxamine/ pseudoephedrine	Palgic-D, Palgic-DS, Pediatex-D

GENERIC	BRAND
Carvedilol	Coreg
Carvedilol phosphate	Coreg CR
Celecoxib	Celebrex
Cetirizine	Zyrtec
Cetirizine/pseudoephedrine	Zyrtec-D
Cevimeline	Evoxac
Chlorhexidine gluconate	Hibistat
Chloroquine	Aralen
Chlorothiazide sodium	Diuril I.V.
Chlorpheniramine/ hydrocodone/ pseudoephedrine	Tussend
Chlorpheniramine/ phenylephrine/pyrilamine	Rynatan
Chlorpromazine	Thorazine
Chlorpropamide	Diabinese
Chlorthalidone	Thalitone
Chlorthalidone/clonidine	Clorpres
Cidofovir	Vistide
Ciprofloxacin	Cipro, Cipro XR
Citalopram	Celexa
Clemastine	Tavist
Clindamycin phosphate	Clindagel
Clonidine/chlorthalidone	Clorpres
Clozapine	Clozaril, Fazaclo
Coagulation Factor IX (recombinant)	BeneFIX
Cromolyn sodium	Gastrocrom
Cyclobenzaprine	Flexeril
Cyproheptadine	Cyproheptadine
Dacarbazine	DTIC-Dome
Dantrolene	Dantrium
Demeclocycline	Declomycin
Desipramine	Norpramin
Diclofenac potassium	Cataflam
Diclofenac sodium	Voltaren
Diclofenac sodium/ misoprostol	Arthrotec
Diflunisal	Dolobid
Dihydroergotamine	D.H.E. 45
Diltiazem	Cardizem, Tiazac
Diphenhydramine	Benadryl
Divalproex	Depakote
Doxepin	Sinequan
Doxycycline hyclate	Doryx, Periostat, Vibra-Tabs, Vibramycin
Doxycycline monohydrate	Monodox
Duloxetine	Cymbalta
Efalizumab	Raptiva
Enalapril	Vasotec
Enalapril/felodipine	
Enalapril/ hydrochlorothiazide	Vaseretic
Enalaprilat (injection)	Vasotec I.V.
Epirubicin	Ellence
Eprosartan mesylate/ hydrochlorothiazide	Teveten HCT
Erythromycin/ sulfisoxazole	Pediazole
Escitalopram oxalate	Lexapro
Esomeprazole	Nexium
Estazolam	

GENERIC	BRAND
Estradiol	Gynodiol, Estrogel
Eszopiclone	Lunesta
Ethionamide	Trecator-SC
Etodolac	Lodine
Felbamate	Felbatol
Fenofibrate	Lofibra, Tricor, Triglide
Floxuridine	Sterile FUDR
Flucytosine	Ancobon
Fluorouracil	Efudex
Fluoxetine	Prozac, Sarafem
Fluphenazine	Prolixin
Flutamide	Eulexin
Fluvastatin	Lescol
Fluvoxamine	Luvox
Fosinopril	Monopril
Fosphenytoin	Cerebyx
Furosemide	Lasix
Gabapentin	Neurontin
Gatifloxacin	Tequin
Gemfibrozil	Lopid
Gemifloxacin mesylate	Factive
Gentamicin	Garamycin
Glatiramer acetate	Copaxone
Glimepiride	Amaryl
Glimepiride/pioglitazone hydrochloride	Duetact
Glimepiride/ rosiglitazone maleate	Avandaryl
Glipizide	Glucotrol
Glyburide	DiaBeta, Glynase, Micronase
Glyburide/metformin HCl	Glucovance
Griseofulvin	Fulvicin P/G, Grifulvin, Gris-PEG
Haloperidol	Haldol
Hexachlorophene	pHisoHex
Hydralazine/ hydrochlorothiazide	Hydra-zide
Hydrochlorothiazide	HydroDIURIL, Microzide, Oretic
Hydrochlorothiazide/ fosinopril	Monopril HCT
Hydrochlorothiazide/ irbesartan	Avalide
Hydrochlorothiazide/ lisinopril	Prinzide, Zestoretic
Hydrochlorothiazide/ losartan potassium	Hyzaar
Hydrochlorothiazide/ methyldopa	Aldoril
Hydroclorothiazide/ metoprolol tartrate	Lopressor HCT
Hydrochlorothiazide/ moexipril	Uniretic
Hydrochlorothiazide/ propranolol	Inderide
Hydrochlorothiazide/ quinapril	Accuretic
Hydrochlorothiazide/ spironolactone	Aldactazide
Hydrochlorothiazide/ telmisartan	Micardis HCT
Hydrochlorothiazide/timolol	Timolide
Hydrochlorothiazide/ triamterene	Dyazide, Maxzide
Hydrochlorothiazide/ valsartan	Diovan HCT
Hydroflumethiazide	Hydroflumethiazide

GENERIC	BRAND
Hydroxocobalamin	Cyanokit Antidote
Hydroxychloroquine	Plaquenil
Hypericum	Kira, St. John's wort
Hypericum/vitamin B1/ vitamin C/kava-kava	One-A-Day Tension & Mood
Ibuprofen	Motrin
Imatinib Mesylate	Gleevec
Imipramine	Tofranil
Imiquimod	Aldara
Indapamide	Lozol
Interferon alfa-2b, recombinant	Intron A
Interferon alfa-n3 (human leukocyte derived)	Alferon-N
Interferon beta-1a	Avonex
Interferon beta-1b	Betaseron
Irbesartan/hydrochlorothiazide	Avalide
Isocarboxazid	Marplan
Isoniazid/pyrazinamide/ rifampin	Rifater
Isotretinoin	Accutane, Amnesteem
Itraconazole	Sporanox
Ketoprofen	Orudis, Oruvail
Lamotrigine	Lamictal
Leuprolide acetate	Lupron, Lupron Depot
Levamisole	Levamisole
Levofloxacin	Levaquin
Levofloxacin/5% dextrose	Levaquin Injection
Lisinopril	Zestril
Lisinopril/ hydrochlorothiazide	Prinivil, Zestoretic
Lomefloxacin	Maxaquin
Loratadine	Claritin
Loratadine/ pseudoephedrine	Claritin-D
Losartan	Cozaar
Losartan/ hydrochlorothiazide	Hyzaar
Lovastatin	Altoprev, Mevacor
Lovastatin/niacin	Advicor
Maprotiline	Maprotiline
Mefenamic acid	Ponstel
Meloxicam	Mobic
Mesalamine	Pentasa
Methazolamide	
Methotrexate	Trexall
Methoxsalen	Uvadex, Oxsoralen, 8-MOP
Methyclothiazide	Enduron
Methyldopa/ hydrochlorothiazide	Aldoril
Metolazone	Mykrox, Zaroxolyn
Metoprolol succinate	Toprol-XL
Metoprolol tartrate	Lopressor
Minocycline	Dynacin, Minocin, Solodyn
Mirtazapine	Remeron
Moexipril	Univasc
Moexipril/ hydrochlorothiazide	Uniretic
Moxifloxacin	Avelox
Nabilone	Cesamet
Nabumetone	Relafen
Nadolol/ bendroflumethiazide	Corzide

GENERIC	BRAND
Nalidixic acid	Nalidixic acid
Naproxen	Naprosyn, EC-Naprosyn
Naproxen sodium	Anaprox, Anaprox DS, Naprelan
Naratriptan	Amerge
Nefazodone	Serzone
Nifedipine	Adalat CC, Procardia
Nisoldipine	Sular
Norfloxacin	Noroxin
Nortriptyline	Pamelor
Ofloxacin	Floxin
Olanzapine	Zyprexa
Olanzapine/fluoxetine	Symbyax
Olmesartan medoxomil/ hydrochlorothiazide	Benicar HCT
Olsalazine	Dipentum
Omeprazole/ sodium bicarbonate	Zegerid
Oxaprozin	Daypro
Oxcarbazepine	Trileptal
Oxycodone	Roxicodone
Oxytetracycline	Terramycin
Panitumumab	Vectibix
Pantoprazole	Protonix
Paroxetine hydrochloride	Paxil
Paroxetine mesylate	Pexeva
Pastinaca sativa	Parsnip
Pentosan polysulfate	Elmiron
Pentostatin	Nipent
Perphenazine	Perphenazine
Pilocarpine	Salagen
Piroxicam	Feldene
Polymyxin B sulfate/ trimethopim sulfate	Polytrim
Polythiazide	Renese
Polythiazide/prazosin	Minizide
Porfimer sodium	Photofrin
Pramipexole dihydrochloride	Mirapex
Pravastatin	Pravachol
Pregabalin	Lyrica
Prochlorperazine	Compazine, Compro
Promethazine	Phenergan
Protriptyline	Vivactil
Pyrimethamine/sulfadoxine	Fansidar
Pyrazinamide	Pyrazinamide
Quetiapine	Seroquel
Quinapril	Accupril
Quinapril/ hydrochlorothiazide	Accuretic
Quinidine gluconate	Quinidine
Quinidine sulfate	Quinidex
Rabeprazole sodium	Aciphex
Ramipril	Altace
Rasagiline mesylate	Azilect
Riluzole	Rilutek
Risperidone	Risperdal, Risperdal Consta
Ritonavir	Norvir

GENERIC	BRAND
Rizatriptan	Maxalt, Maxalt-MLT
Ropinirole	Requip
Rosuvastatin	Crestor
Ruta graveolens	Rue
Saquinavir mesylate	Invirase
Selegiline	Eldepryl, Emsam
Sertraline	Zoloft
Sibutramine	Meridia
Sildenafil	Viagra
Simvastatin	Zocor
Simvastatin/ezetimibe	Vytorin
Sirolimus	Rapamune
Somatropin	Serostim
Sotalol	Betapace, Betapace AF
Sulfamethoxazole/ trimethoprim	Bactrim, Septra
Sulfasalazine	Azulfidine
Sulfisoxazole acetyl	Gantrisin Pediatric
Sulindac	Clinoril
Sumatriptan	Imitrex
Tacrolimus	Prograf, Protopic
Tazarotene	Tazorac
Telmisartan/ hydrochlorothiazide	Micardis HCT
Tetracycline	Sumycin
Thalidomide	Thalomid
Thiothixene	Navane
Tiagabine	Gabitril
Tigecycline	Tygacil
Tolazamide	Tolazamide
Tolbutamide	Tolbutamide
Topiramate	Topamax
Tretinoin	Retin-A
Triamcinolone acetonide	Azmacort Inhalation
Triamterene	Dyrenium
Triamterene/ hydrochlorothiazide	Dyazide, Maxzide
Trifluoperazine	Trifluoperazine
Trimipramine	Surmontil
Trovafloxacin	Trovan
Valacyclovir	Valtrex
Valdecoxib	Bextra
Valproate	Depacon
Valproic acid	Depakene
Valsartan/ hydrochlorothiazide	Diovan HCT
Vardenafil	Levitra
Varenicline tartrate	Chantix
Venlafaxine	Effexor
Verteporfin	Visudyne
Vinblastine	Vinblastine
Voriconazole	Vfend
Zalcitabine	Hivid
Zaleplon	Sonata
Ziprasidone	Geodon
Zolmitriptan	Zomig
Zolpidem	Ambien, Ambien CR

DRUGS THAT MAY CAUSE QT PROLONGATION

BRAND NAME	GENERIC NAME	BRAND NAME	GENERIC NAME
Abilify	Aripiprazole	Norpace	Disopyramide phosphate
AcipHex	Rabeprazole sodium	Norpramin	Desipramine
Advair	Fluticasone propionate/ salmeterol xinafoate	Noxafil	Posaconazole
		Orap	Pimozide
Advair HFA	Fluticasone propionate/ salmeterol xinafoate	OsmoPrep	Sodium phosphate mono-basic monohydrate/ sodium phosphate dibasic anhydrous
Aloxi Injection	Palonosetron HCl		
Amerge	Naratriptan HCl		
Amitriptyline	Amitriptyline	Pacerone	Amiodarone HCl
Anzemet	Dolasetron mesylate	PCE	Erythromycin particles
Apokyn	Apomorphine HCl	Perforomist	Formoterol fumarate
Avelox	Moxifloxacin HCl	Plenaxis*	Abarelix
Betapace	Sotalol HCl	Pletal	Cilostazol
Betapace AF	Sotalol HCl	PREVPAC	Lansoprazole/amoxicillin/ clarithromycin
Biaxin	Clarithromycin		
Brovana	Arformoterol tartrate	Procainamide	Procainamide
Celexa	Citalopram HBr	Prograf	Tacrolimus
Cipro	Ciprofloxacin	Prozac	Fluoxetine
Cipro XR	Ciprofloxacin	Quinidine gluconate	Quinidine gluconate
Cordarone	Amiodarone HCl	Quinidine sulfate	Quinidine sulfate
Corvert	Ibutilide fumarate	Ranexa	Ranolazine
Detrol LA	Tolterodine tartrate	Raxar*	Grepafloxacin
Dolophine	Methadone HCl	Razadyne	Galantamine HBr
Doxepin	Doxepin	Risperdal Consta	Risperidone
E.E.S.	Erythromycin ethylsuccinate	Rythmol SR	Propafenone HCl
		Serentil*	Mesoridazine besylate
Effexor XR	Venlafaxine HCl	Serevent	Salmeterol
Eraxis	Anidulafungin	Seroquel	Quetiapine fumarate
ERYC	Erythromycin	Sporanox	Itraconazole
EryPed	Erythromycin ethylsuccinate	Sprycel	Dasatinib
		Strattera	Atomoxetine HCl
Erythrocin stearate	Erythromycin stearate	Sutent	Sunitinib malate
Erythromycin Base Filmtab	Erythromycin	Symbicort	Budesonide/formoterol fumarate dihydrate
Erythromycin Delayed-Release	Erythromycin	Symbyax	Olanzapine/fluoxetine HCl
Exelon Patch	Rivastigmine	Tambocor	Flecainide acetate
Factive	Gemifloxacin mesylate	Tasigna	Nilotinib
Fleet Enema/Enema Extra/ Enema for Children	Monobasic sodium phosphate/dibasic sodium phosphate	Tequin*	Gatifloxacin
		Thioridazine HCl	Thioridazine HCl
		Tikosyn	Dofetilide
Foradil	Formoterol	Tofranil, Tofranil-PM	Imipramine
Geodon	Ziprasidone HCl	Trisenox Injection	Arsenic trioxide
Haldol	Haloperidol	Tykerb	Lapatinib
Halfan*	Halofantrine HCl	Uroxatral	Alfuzosin HCl
Imitrex Injection	Sumatriptan succinate	Vascor*	Bepridil HCl
Inapsine	Droperidol	VFEND	Voriconazole
Invega	Paliperidone	Viracept	Nelfinavir mesylate
Ketek	Telithromycin	Visicol	Sodium phosphate
Levaquin	Levofloxacin	Zagam*	Sparfloxacin
Levitra	Vardenafil HCl	Zanaflex	Tizanidine
Lexapro	Escitalopram oxalate	Zmax	Azithromycin
Maxaquin	Lomefloxacin HCl	Zofran	Ondansetron HCl
Methadose	Methadone HCl	Zolinza	Vorinostat
Namenda	Memantine HCl	Zoloft	Sertraline HCl
Nizoral	Ketoconazole	Zomig	Zolmitriptan
Noroxin	Norfloxacin	Zomig-ZMT	Zolmitriptan

* Drug no longer available in the U.S.
NOTE: This list does not include all of the drugs that may cause QT disturbance. For more information, please refer to the specific product's full Prescribing Information.

DRUGS THAT MAY CAUSE STEVENS-JOHNSON SYNDROME AND TEN*

BRAND NAME	GENERIC NAME	BRAND NAME	GENERIC NAME
ACAM2000	Smallpox vaccine, live	Covera-HS	Verapamil HCl
AcipHex	Rabeprazole sodium	Crixivan	Indinavir sulfate
Adderall XR	Dextroamphetamine sulfate/dextroamphetamine saccharate/amphetamine sulfate/amphetamine aspartate	Cymbalta	Duloxetine HCl
		Daraprim	Pyrimethamine
		Daypro	Oxaprozin
		Depakote ER	Divalproex sodium
Advicor	Niacin/lovastatin	Diamox	Acetazolamide
Agenerase	Amprenavir	Didronel	Etidronate disodium
Aggrenox	Aspirin/dipyridamole	Dilantin	Phenytoin sodium
Albenza	Albendazole	Diovan HCT	Valsartan/ hydrochlorothiazide
Aldoril	Methyldopa/ hydrochlorothiazide	Diuril	Chlorothiazide
		Dolobid	Diflunisal
Aloprim	Allopurinol sodium	Donnatal Extentabs	Phenobarbital
Altace	Ramipril	Duac Topical Gel	Clindamycin, 1%/benzoyl peroxide, 5%
Amoxil	Amoxicillin		
Anaprox	Naproxen	Dynacin	Minocycline HCl
Ancobon	Flucytosine	EC-Naprosyn	Naproxen
Ansaid	Flurbiprofen	E.E.S.	Erythromycin ethylsuccinate
Arava	Leflunomide	Effexor XR	Venlafaxine HCl
Arimidex	Anastrozole	Emend	Aprepitant
Arthrotec	Diclofenac sodium/ misoprostol	Engerix-B Vaccine	Hepatitis B vaccine (recombinant)
Atacand HCT	Candesartan cilexetil/ hydrochlorothiazide	Epzicom	Abacavir sulfate/lamivudine
		Equetro	Carbamazepine
Atripla	Efavirenz/emtricitabine/ tenofovir disoproxil fumarate	EryPed	Erythromycin ethylsuccinate
		Ethyol	Amifostine
		Etodolac	Etodolac
Attenuvax	Measles virus vaccine, live	Exelon	Rivastigmine tartrate
Augmentin	Amoxicillin/clavulanate potassium	Fansidar	Sulfadoxine/pyrimethamine
		Feldene	Piroxicam
Avalide	Irbesartan/ hydrochlorothiazide	Flebogamma 5%	Immune globulin intravenous (human)
Avandamet	Rosiglitazone maleate/ metformin HCl	Flector	Diclofenac epolamine topical patch
Avandia	Rosiglitazone maleate	Fluarix	Influenza virus vaccine
Avelox	Moxifloxacin HCl	Fortaz	Ceftazidime for injection
Azulfidine	Sulfasalazine	Fosamax	Alendronate sodium
Bactrim	Sulfamethoxazole/ trimethoprim	Fosamax Plus D	Alendronate sodium/ cholecalciferol
Betagan	Levobunolol HCl	Furadantin	Nitrofurantoin
Betoptic S	Betaxolol HCl	Gammagard	Immune globulin intravenous (human)
Biaxin	Clarithromycin		
Bleph-10	Sulfacetamide sodium	Gamunex	Immune globulin intravenous (human), 10% caprylate/ chromatography purified
Blephamide	Sulfacetamide sodium/ prednisolone acetate		
Caduet	Amlodipine besylate/ atorvastatin calcium		
		Gantrisin	Acetyl sulfisoxazole
Capoten	Captopril	Gleevec	Imatinib mesylate
Carbatrol	Carbamazepine	Hyzaar	Losartan potassium/ hydrochlorothiazide
Cataflam	Diclofenac potassium		
Ceftin	Cefuroxime axetil	Inderal LA	Propranolol HCl
Celebrex	Celecoxib	Intelence	Etravirine
Cialis	Tadalafil	Intron A	Interferon alfa-2b
Cimzia	Certolizumab pegol	Lozol	Indapamide
Cipro	Ciprofloxacin	Indocin	Indomethacin
Cleocin vaginal ovules	Clindamycin phosphate vaginal suppositories	Lamictal	Lamotrigine
		Lamisil	Terbinafine HCl
Clinoril	Sulindac	Lariam	Mefloquine HCl
Clorpres	Clonidine HCl/chlorthalidone	Lescol	Fluvastatin sodium
Clozaril	Clozapine	Leukeran	Chlorambucil
Combivir	Lamivudine/zidovudine	Leustatin	Cladribine
Combunox	Oxycodone HCl/ibuprofen	Levaquin	Levofloxacin
Comvax	Haemophilus b conjugate (meningococcal protein conjugate)/ hepatitis B (recombinant) vaccine	Lexapro	Escitalopram oxalate
		Lexiva	Fosamprenavir calcium
		Lipitor	Atorvastatin calcium
		Lyrica	Pregabalin

DRUGS THAT MAY CAUSE STEVENS-JOHNSON SYNDROME AND TEN*

BRAND NAME	GENERIC NAME	BRAND NAME	GENERIC NAME
Malarone	Atovaquone/proguanil HCl	Relafen	Nabumetone
Maxalt	Rizatriptan benzoate	Remicade for IV Injection	Infliximab
Mefoxin	Cefoxitin injection		
Merrem	Meropenem for injection	Rescriptor	Delavirdine mesylate
Meruvax II	Rubella virus vaccine, live	Retrovir	Zidovudine
Mevacor	Lovastatin	Reyataz	Atazanavir sulfate
Micardis HCT	Telmisartan/ hydrochlorothiazide	Rituxan	Rituximab
		Rosula NS	Sodium sulfacetamide
Minocin	Minocycline HCl	Septra	Trimethoprim/ sulfamethoxazole
Mintezol	Thiabendazole		
M-M-R II	Measles, mumps, and rubella virus vaccine, live	Seroquel	Quetiapine fumarate
		Solodyn	Minocycline HCl
Mobic	Meloxicam	Stromectol	Ivermectin
Moduretic	Amiloride HCl/ hydrochlorothiazide	Suprax	Cefixime for oral suspension
Motrin	Ibuprofen	Sustiva	Efavirenz
Mumpsvax	Mumps virus vaccine, live	Tamiflu	Oseltamivir phosphate
Nalfon	Fenoprofen calcium	Tarka	Trandolapril/verapamil HCl
Namenda	Memantine HCl	Taxotere	Docetaxel
Naprelan	Naproxen sodium	Tegretol	Carbamazepine
Naprosyn	Naproxen	Teveten HCT	Eprosartan mesylate/ hydrochlorothiazide
Neurontin	Gabapentin		
Nexium	Esomeprazole magnesium	Thalomid	Thalidomide
		Tiazac	Diltiazem HCl
Niravam	Alprazolam orally disintegrating	Ticlid	Ticlopidine HCl
		Timentin	Ticarcillin disodium/ clavulanate potassium
Noroxin	Norfloxacin		
Norvir	Ritonavir	Timolide	Timolol maleate/ hydrochlorothiazide
Nuvigil	Armodafinil		
Nystatin Oral	Nystatin	Tindamax	Tinidazole
Omnicef	Cefdinir	Topamax	Topiramate
Orthoclone OKT3 Sterile Solution	Muromonab-CD3	Tricor	Fenofibrate
		Trileptal	Oxcarbazepine
Ovace	Sodium sulfacetamide	Trizivir	Abacavir sulfate/ lamivudine/zidovudine
Paxil	Paroxetine HCl		
PCE	Erythromycin particles in tablets	Trusopt	Dorzolamide HCl
		Twinrix	Hepatitis A inactivated/ hepatitis B (recombinant) vaccine
PegIntron	Peginterferon alfa-2b		
Pepcid	Famotidine		
Phenytek	Phenytoin sodium	Vancocin	Vancomycin HCl
Plavix	Clopidogrel bisulfate	Varivax	Varicella virus vaccine, live
Pletal	Cilostazol	VFEND	Voriconazole
Ponstel	Mefenamic acid	Viramune	Nevirapine
Prevacid NapraPAC	Lansoprazole/naproxen	Voltaren	Diclofenac sodium
PREVPAC	Lansoprazole/ amoxicillin/clarithromycin	VoSpire ER	Albuterol sulfate
		Vytorin	Ezetimibe/simvastatin
Prezista	Darunavir	Vyvanse	Lisdexamfetamine dimesylate
Primaxin I.M./I.V.	Imipenem/cilastatin		
Prinivil	Lisinopril	Wellbutrin	Bupropion HCl
Prinzide	Lisinopril/ hydrochlorothiazide	Zegerid	Omeprazole/sodium bicarbonate
Prograf	Tacrolimus	Ziagen	Abacavir sulfate
Proleukin	Aldesleukin	Zinacef	Cefuroxime for injection
ProQuad	Measles, mumps, rubella and varicella virus vaccine, live	Zmax	Azithromycin extended release for oral suspension
Protonix	Pantoprazole sodium	Zocor	Simvastatin
Provigil	Modafinil	Zoloft	Sertraline HCl
Prozac	Fluoxetine	Zonegran	Zonisamide
Raniclor	Cefaclor	Zosyn	Piperacillin/tazobactam
Raptiva	Efalizumab	Zovirax	Acyclovir
Recombivax HB	Hepatitis B vaccine (recombinant)	Zyban	Bupropion HCl
		Zyvox	Linezolid

*TEN = toxic epidermal necrolysis.
Note: This list is not comprehensive. For more information, refer to the specific product's full Prescribing Information.

DRUGS THAT SHOULD NOT BE CRUSHED

Listed below are various slow-release as well as enteric-coated products that should not be crushed or chewed. Slow-release (sr) represents products that are controlled-release, extended-release, long-acting, or timed-release. Enteric-coated (ec) represents products that are delayed-release.

In general, capsules containing slow-release or enteric-coated particles may be opened and their contents administered on a spoonful of soft food. Instruct patients not to chew the particles, though. (Patients should, in fact, be discouraged from chewing any medication unless it is specifically formulated for that purpose.)

This list should not be considered all-inclusive. Generic and alternate brands of some products may exist. Tablets intended for sublingual or buccal administration (not included in this list) should also be administered only as intended, in an intact form.

DRUG	FORM	DRUG	FORM	DRUG	FORM
Abletex LA	sr	Ascriptin Enteric	ec	Claritin-D 24 Hour	sr
Aciphex	ec	Atrohist Pediatric	sr	Coldamine	sr
Adalat CC	sr	Augmentin XR	sr	Coldex-A	sr
Adderall XR	sr	Avinza	sr	Concerta	sr
Advicor	sr	Azulfidine Entabs	ec	Contac 12-Hour	sr
Aerohist	sr	Bayer Aspirin Regimen	ec	Correctol	ec
Aerohist Plus	sr	Biaxin XL	sr	Coreg CR	sr
Afeditab CR	sr	Bidex-A	sr	Cotazym-S	ec
Aggrenox	sr	Bidhist	sr	Covera-HS	sr
Ala-Hist	sr	Bidhist-D	sr	CPM 8/PE 20/MSC 1.25	sr
Ala-Hist D	sr	Bisac-Evac	ec	CPM-12	sr
Aleve Cold & Sinus	sr	Biscolax	ec	Creon 5	ec
Aleve Sinus & Headache	sr	Blanex-A	sr	Creon 10	ec
Allegra-D 12 Hour	sr	Bontril Slow-Release	sr	Creon 20	ec
Allegra-D 24 Hour	sr	Bromfed	sr	Cymbalta	ec
Allerx	sr	Bromfed-PD	sr	Dairycare	ec
Allerx-D	sr	Bromfenex	sr	Dallergy	sr
Allfen	sr	Bromfenex PD	sr	Dallergy-Jr	sr
Allfen-DM	sr	Bromfenex PE	sr	Deconamine SR	sr
Alophen	ec	Bromfenex PE Pediatric	sr	Deconex	sr
Altoprev	sr	Budeprion SR	sr	Deconsal II	sr
Ambi 45/800	sr	Budeprion XL	sr	Deconex DM	sr
Ambi 45/800/30	sr	Buproban	sr	Depakote	ec
Ambi 60/580	sr	Calan SR	sr	Depakote ER	sr
Ambi 60/580/30	sr	Campral	ec	Depakote Sprinkles	ec
Ambi 80/700	sr	Carbatrol	sr	Despec SR	sr
Ambi 80/700/40	sr	Cardene SR	sr	Detrol LA	sr
Ambi 1000/55	sr	Cardizem CD	sr	Dexedrine Spansules	sr
Ambien CR	sr	Cardizem LA	sr	D-Feda II	sr
Ambifed-G	sr	Cardura XL	sr	D-Hist D	sr
Ambifed-G DM	sr	Carox Plus	sr	Diabetes Trio	sr
Amdry-C	sr	Cartia XT	sr	Diamox Sequels	sr
Amdry-D	sr	Cemill 500	sr	Dilacor XR	sr
Amibid LA	sr	Cemill 1000	sr	Dilantin	sr
Amrix	sr	Certuss-D	sr	Dilantin Kapseals	sr
Anextuss	sr	Cevi-Bid	sr	Dilatrate-SR	sr
Anti-tussive	sr	Chlorex-A	sr	Diltia XT	sr
Aquabid-DM	sr	Chlor-Phen	sr	Dilt-CD	sr
Aquatab C	sr	Chlor-Trimeton Allergy	sr	Dilt-XR	sr
Aquatab D	sr	Chlor-Trimeton Allergy	sr	Dimetane Extentabs	sr
Aquatab DM	sr	Decongestant		Disophrol Chronotab	sr
Arthrotec	ec	Cipro XR	sr	Ditropan XL	sr
Asacol	ec	Clarinex-D 24 Hour	sr	Donnatal Extentabs	sr
Ascocid-500-D	sr	Claritin-D	sr	Doryx	ec
Ascocid-1000	sr	Claritin-D 12 Hour	sr	D-Phen 1000	sr

Enteric-coated= ec   Slow-release = sr

Drugs That Should Not Be Crushed

DRUG	FORM	DRUG	FORM	DRUG	FORM
Drexophed SR	sr	Fero-Grad-500	sr	Klor-Con 10	sr
Drihist SR	sr	Ferro-Sequels	sr	Klor-Con M10	sr
Drixoral	sr	Ferrous Fumarate DS	sr	Klor-Con M15	sr
Drixoral Plus	sr	Fetrin	sr	Klor-Con M20	sr
Drixoral Sinus	sr	Flagyl ER	sr	Klotrix	sr
Drize-R	sr	Fleet Bisacodyl	ec	K-Tab	sr
Drysec	sr	Focalin XR	sr	K-Tan	sr
D-Tab	sr	Folitab 500	sr	Lescol XL	sr
Dulcolax	ec	Fortamet	sr	Levall G	sr
Duomax	sr	Fumatinic	sr	Levsinex	sr
Durahist	sr	G/P 1200/75	sr	Lexxel	sr
Durahist D	sr	Genacote	ec	Lialda	ec
Durahist PE	sr	GFN 500/DM 30	sr	Lipram 4500	ec
Duratuss	sr	GFN 550/PSE 60	sr	Lipram-PN10	ec
Duratuss CS	sr	GFN 550/PSE 60/DM 30	sr	Lipram-PN16	ec
Duratuss DA	sr	GFN 595/PSE 48	sr	Lipram-PN20	ec
Duratuss GP	sr	GFN 595/PSE 48/DM 32	sr	Liquibid-D	sr
Dynacirc CR	sr	GFN 1000/DM 50	sr	Liquibid-D 1200	sr
Dynahist-ER Pediatric	sr	GFN 1200/DM 60/PSE 60	sr	Liquibid-PD	sr
Dynex LA	sr	GFN 1200/Phenylephrine 40	sr	Lithobid	sr
Dynex VR	sr	GFN 1200/PSE 50	sr	Lodrane-12 Hour	sr
Dytan-CS	sr	Gilphex TR	sr	Lodrane-12D	sr
Easprin	ec	Giltuss TR	sr	Lodrane 24	sr
EC Naprosyn	ec	Glucophage XR	sr	Lodrane 24D	sr
Ecotrin	ec	Glucotrol XL	sr	Lohist-12	sr
Ecotrin Adult Low Strength	ec	Glumetza	sr	Lohist-12D	sr
Ecotrin Maximum Strength	ec	Guaifenex DM	sr	Lusonex	sr
Ecpirin	ec	Guaifenex GP	sr	Mag Delay	ec
Ed A-Hist	sr	Guaifenex PSE 60	sr	Mag64	ec
Effexor-XR	sr	Guaifenex PSE 80	sr	Mag-SR Plus Calcium	sr
Efidac 24 Chlorpheniramine	sr	Guaifenex PSE 120	sr	Mag-Tab SR	sr
Efidac 24 Pseudoephedrine	sr	H 9600 SR	sr	Maxifed	sr
Enablex	sr	Halfprin	ec	Maxifed DM	sr
Endal	sr	Hemax	sr	Maxifed DMX	sr
Entab-DM	sr	Histacol LA	sr	Maxifed-G	sr
Entercote	ec	Hista-Vent DA	sr	Maxiphen DM	sr
Entex LA	sr	Hista-Vent PSE	sr	Medent DM	sr
Entex PSE	sr	Humavent LA	sr	Medent PE	sr
Entocort EC	ec	Humibid	sr	Mega-C	sr
Equetro	sr	Humibid DM	sr	Melfiat	sr
Ery-Tab	ec	Humibid LA	sr	Menopause Trio	sr
Eskalith-CR	sr	Iberet-500	sr	Mestinon Timespan	sr
Execof	sr	Iberet-Folic-500	sr	Metadate CD	sr
Exefen-DM	sr	Icar-C Plus SR	sr	Metadate ER	sr
Exefen-DMX	sr	Imdur	sr	Methylin ER	sr
Exefen-PD	sr	Inderal LA	sr	Micro-K	sr
Extendryl Jr	sr	Indocin SR	sr	Micro-K 10	sr
Extendryl SR	sr	Innopran XL	sr	Mild-C	sr
Extress-30	sr	Invega	sr	Mindal DM	sr
Exetuss-DM	sr	Isochron	sr	Montephen	sr
Extendryl G	sr	Isopro	sr	MS Contin	sr
Extress-60	sr	Isoptin SR	sr	Mucinex	sr
Feen-A-Mint	ec	Kadian	sr	Mucinex D	sr
Femilax	ec	Kaon-Cl 10	sr	Mucinex DM	sr
Fero-Folic-500	sr	Klor-Con 8	sr	Multi-Ferrous Folic	sr

DRUG	FORM	DRUG	FORM	DRUG	FORM
Multiret Folic-500	sr	Paxil CR	sr	Respa-PE	sr
Mydex	sr	PCE Dispertab	sr	Respahist	sr
Mydocs	sr	PCM LA	sr	Respahist-II	sr
Myfortic	ec	Pendex	sr	Respaire-60 SR	sr
Nacon	sr	Pentasa	sr	Respaire-120 SR	sr
Nalex-A	sr	Pentopak	sr	Rhinacon A	sr
Naprelan	sr	Pentoxil	sr	Risperdal Consta	sr
Nasatab LA	sr	Phenabid	sr	Ritalin LA	sr
New Ami-Tex LA	sr	Phenabid DM	sr	Ritalin-SR	sr
Nexium	ec	Phenavent	sr	Rodex Forte	sr
Niaspan	sr	Phenavent D	sr	Rondec-TR	sr
Nicomide\	sr	Phenavent LA	sr	Ru-Tuss	sr
Nifediac CC	sr	Phenavent PED	sr	Ryneze	sr
Nifedical XL	sr	Phendiet-105	sr	Rythmol SR	sr
Nitrocot	sr	Phenytek	sr	SAM-e	ec
Nitro-Time	sr	Phlemex-PE	sr	Sanctura XR	sr
Nohist	sr	Plendil	sr	Scopohist-PE	sr
Nohist-Plus	sr	Poly Hist Forte	sr	Seroquel XR	sr
Nohist-Plus Jr	sr	Poly-Vent	sr	Simuc-GP	sr
Norel SR	sr	Poly-Vent Jr	sr	Sinemet CR	sr
Norpace CR	sr	Prehist D	sr	Sinutuss DM	sr
Obstetrix EC	ec	Prevacid	ec	Sinuvent PE	sr
Omnihist LA	sr	Prilosec	ec	Slo-Niacin	sr
Opana ER	sr	Prilosec OTC	sr	Slow Fe	sr
Oramorph SR	sr	Procanbid	sr	Slow Fe With Folic Acid	sr
Oracea	sr	Procardia XL	sr	Slow-Mag	ec
Oruvail	sr	Prolex PD	sr	Solodyn	sr
Oxycontin	sr	Prolex-D	sr	St. Joseph Pain Reliever	ec
Palcaps 10	ec	Pronestyl-SR	sr	Stahist	sr
Palcaps 20	ec	Proquin XR	sr	Sudafed 12 Hour	sr
Pancrease	ec	Prosed EC	ec	Sudafed 24 Hour	sr
Pancrease MT 10	ec	Proset-D	sr	Sudahist	sr
Pancrease MT 16	ec	Protid	sr	Sudal DM	sr
Pancrease MT 20	ec	Protonix	ec	Sudal SR	sr
Pancrecarb MS-16	ec	Prozac Weekly	ec	Sudatex-DM	sr
Pancrecarb MS-4	ec	Pseubrom	sr	Sudatex-G	sr
Pancrecarb MS-8	ec	Pseubrom-PD	sr	Sudatrate	sr
Pancrelipase 4500	ec	Pseudocot-C	sr	Sudex Tab	sr
Pangestyme CN-10	ec	Pseudocot-G	sr	Sular	sr
Pangestyme CN-20	ec	Pseudovent	sr	Sulfazine EC	ec
Pangestyme EC	ec	Pseudovent 400	sr	Symax Duotab	sr
Pangestyme MT16	ec	Pseudovent DM	sr	Symax-SR	sr
Pangestyme UL12	ec	Pseudovent PED	sr	Tarka	sr
Pangestyme UL18	ec	Quibron-T/SR	sr	Taztia XT	sr
Pangestyme UL20	ec	Quindal	sr	Tegretol-XR	sr
Panmist DM	sr	Ralix	sr	Tenuate Dospan	sr
Panmist Jr	sr	Ranexa	sr	Theo-24	sr
Panmist LA	sr	Razadyne ER	sr	Theochron	sr
Panocaps	ec	Reliable Gentle Laxative	ec	Theo-Time	sr
Panocaps MT 16	ec	Rescon-Jr	sr	Tiazac	sr
Panocaps MT 20	ec	Rescon-MX	sr	Time-Hist	sr
Papacon	sr	Respa-1ST	sr	Toprol XL	sr
Para-Time SR	sr	Respa-AR	sr	Totalday	sr
Paser	sr	Respa-BR	sr	Touro Allergy	sr
Pavacot	sr	Respa-DM	sr	Touro CC	sr

Enteric-coated= ec   Slow-release = sr

DRUGS THAT SHOULD NOT BE CRUSHED

DRUG	FORM	DRUG	FORM	DRUG	FORM
Touro CC-LD	sr	Ultrase	ec	We Mist II LA	sr
Touro DM	sr	Ultrase MT12	ec	Wellbid-D	sr
Touro HC	sr	Ultrase MT18	ec	Wellbid-D 1200	sr
Touro LA	sr	Ultrase MT20	ec	Wellbutrin SR	sr
Touro LA-LD	sr	Uniphyl	sr	Wellbutrin XL	sr
Tranxene-SD	sr	Uni-Tex	sr	Wobenzym N	ec
Trental	sr	Urimax	ec	Woman's Wellbeing	sr
Trikof-D	sr	Uritact-EC	ec	Menopause Relief	
Trinalin Repetabs	sr	Urocit-K 5	sr	Xanax XR	sr
Trituss-ER	sr	Urocit-K 10	sr	Xedec II	sr
Tussafed-LA	sr	Uroxatral	sr	Xiral	sr
Tussall-ER	sr	Utira	sr	Xpect-AT	sr
Tussi-Bid	sr	Veracolate	ec	Xpect-HC	sr
Tussicaps	sr	Verelan	sr	Zephrex LA	sr
Tusso-DM	sr	Verelan PM	sr	Zmax	sr
Tusso-HC	sr	Videx EC	ec	Zorprin	sr
Tylenol Arthritis	sr	Vivotif Berna	ec	Zotex-12D	sr
Ultrabrom	sr	Voltaren	ec	Zyban	sr
Ultrabrom PD	sr	Voltaren-XR	sr	Zymase	ec
Ultracaps MT 20	ec	Vospire	sr	Zyrtec-D	sr
Ultram ER	sr	We Mist LA	sr		

Enteric-coated= ec   **Slow-release = sr**

ADMINISTRATION GUIDELINES FOR EAR DROPS

1. Wash hands thoroughly with soap and water.

2. Carefully wash and dry outside of the ear, taking care not to get water into the ear canal.

3. Warm ear drops to body temperature by holding the container in the palm of your hand for a few minutes.

4. Tilt head to the side, or lie down with the affected ear up. Use gentle restraint for an infant or a young child.

5. Position the dropper tip near, but not inside, the ear canal opening. **NOTE:** To prevent contamination and avoid injuring the ear, do not allow the dropper to touch the ear.

6. Pull ear backward and upward to open the ear canal and place the proper number of drops into the ear canal. Replace the cap on the container.

7. Gently press the small, flat skin flap over the ear canal opening to force out air bubbles and to push the drops down the ear canal.

8. Stay in the same position for the length of time indicated on the product instructions, or gently place a clean piece of cotton into the ear to prevent draining of medication. Do not leave it in the ear longer than one hour.

9. Repeat the procedure in the other ear, if needed.

10. Gently wipe the medication off the outside of the ear, using caution to avoid getting moisture in the ear canal.

11. Do not rinse the dropper after use. Wipe the tip of the dropper with a clean tissue and keep the container tightly closed.

12. Wash hands.

Counseling tips:

- If the drops are a suspension or if the label indicates, shake well before using.

- Do not warm the eardrop container in warm water. Hot ear drops can cause ear pain, nausea, and dizziness.

- Avoid contaminating applicator tip to preserve the sterility of the dropper.

ADMINISTRATION GUIDELINES FOR EYE DROPS & OINTMENT

Administration guidelines for eye drops:

1. Wash hands thoroughly.
2. Tilt head back.
3. Gently pull the lower eyelid away from the eye to create a pocket.
4. Hold the bottle upside down and look up just before applying a single drop. **NOTE:** To prevent contamination, do not let the tip of the eye drop applicator touch any surface (including the eye or eyelid). When not in use, keep the container tightly closed.
5. After applying the drop, look down for several seconds (still holding the eyelid away from the eye).
6. Slowly release the eyelid and close the eyes for 1 to 2 minutes. Do not blink.
7. Gently press on the inside corner of the eye (where the eyelid meets the nose) with a finger.
8. Blot excessive solution from around the eye with a tissue.

Administration guidelines for eye ointment:

1. Wash hands thoroughly.
2. Tilt head back.
3. Gently grasp lower outer eyelid below lashes, and pull eyelid away from the eye.
4. Place ointment tube over eye by directly looking at it. With a sweeping motion, place ¼ to ½-inch of ointment inside the lower eyelid by gently squeezing the tube. **NOTE:** To prevent contamination, do not let the tip of the tube touch any surface (including the eye or eyelid). When not in use, keep the tube tightly closed.
5. Slowly release eyelid and close eyes for 1 to 2 minutes.
6. Blot excessive ointment from around the eye with a tissue.
7. Vision may be temporarily blurred. Until vision clears, avoid activities requiring good visual ability.

Counseling tips:

- If having difficulty determining whether an eye dropper has touched the eye surface, keep the dropper in a refrigerator (not in a freezer).
- If more than one drop is needed, wait at least 5 minutes before instilling the next drop to prevent flushing away or diluting the first drop.
- If both eye drop and ointment therapy are needed, instill the eye drop at least 10 minutes before the ointment.

POISON ANTIDOTE CHART

WARNING: While every effort has been made to ensure the accuracy of this chart, it is not intended to serve as the sole source of information on antidotes. Guidelines may need to be adjusted based on factors such as anticipated usage in the hospital's local area, the nearest alternate sources of antidotes, and distance to tertiary care institutions. Contact your nearest regional poison control center (1-800-222-1222) for treatment information regarding any exposure, including indications for use of antidote therapy. Directions in this chart assume that all basic life support and decontamination measures have been initiated as needed.

ANTIDOTE	POISON/DRUG/TOXIN	SUGGESTED MINIMUM STOCK QUANTITY	COMMENTS
N-Acetylcysteine (Acetadote®, Mucomyst®)	Acetaminophen Carbon tetrachloride Other hepatotoxins	Oral product: 600 mL in 10 mL or 30 mL vials of 20% solution IV product: One carton of four 30 mL vials of 20% solution	Acetaminophen is the most common drug involved in intentional and unintentional poisonings. 600 mL (120 g) of the oral product provides enough antidote to treat an adult for an entire 3-day course of therapy, or enough to treat three adults for 24 h. Several vials may be stocked in the ED to provide a loading dose and the remaining vials in the pharmacy for the q 4 h maintenance doses. The IV product dose of 120 mL (24 g) will treat one adult patient for an entire 20-hour IV protocol.
Amyl nitrite, sodium nitrite, and sodium thiosulfate (Cyanide antidote kit)	Acetonitrile Acrylonitrile Bromates (thiosulfate only) Chlorates (thiosulfate only) Cyanide (e.g., HCN, KCN and NaCN) Cyanogen chloride Cyanogenic glycoside natural sources (e.g., apricot pits and peach pits) Hydrogen sulfide (nitrites only) Laetrile Mustard agents (thiosulfate only) Nitroprusside (thiosulfate only) Smoke inhalation (combustion of synthetic materials)	One to two kits Each kit contains: Twelve 0.3 mL amyl nitrite ampules Two vials 3% sodium nitrite, 10 mL each Two vials 25% sodium thiosulfate, 50 mL each	Stock one kit in the ED. Consider also stocking one kit in the pharmacy. Note: This kit has a short shelf life of 24 months. Note: Stocking this kit may be unnecessary if adequate supply of hydroxocobalamin is available.
Antivenin, *Crotalidae* Polyvalent (equine origin)	Pit viper envenomation (e.g., rattlesnakes, cottonmouths, and timber rattlers	None	As of March 31, 2007, this product is no longer available from the manufacturer. See Antivenin, *Crotalidae* Polyvalent Immune Fab–Ovine in this chart.

(Continued)

This chart is adapted from material furnished by the Illinois Poison Center, a program of the Metropolitan Chicago Healthcare Council (MCHC).

ANTIDOTE	POISON/DRUG/TOXIN	SUGGESTED MINIMUM STOCK QUANTITY	COMMENTS
Antivenin, *Crotalidae* Polyvalent Immune Fab–Ovine (CroFab®)	Pit viper envenomation (e.g., rattlesnakes, cottonmouths, copperheads, and timber rattlers)	Four to six vials	Advised in geographic areas with endemic populations of copperhead, water moccasin, eastern massasauga, or timber rattlesnake. In low-risk areas, know nearest alternate source of antivenin. This product may have a lower risk of hypersensitivity reaction than previously marketed equine product. Average dose in premarketing trials was 12 vials, but more may be needed. Stock in pharmacy. Store in refrigerator. Equine product is no longer available after March 31, 2007.
Antivenin, *Latrodectus mactans* (Black widow spider)	Black widow spider envenomation	Zero to one vial	Serious *Latrodectus* envenomations are rare. This product is only used for severe envenomations. Antivenin must be given in a critical care setting since it is an equine-derived product. Know the nearest source of antidote. Note: Product must be refrigerated at all times.
Atropine sulfate	Alpha$_2$ agonists (e.g., clonidine, guanabenz, and guanfacine) Alzheimer's drugs (e.g., donepezil, galantamine, rivastigmine, tacrine) Antimyesthenic agents (e.g., pyridostigmine) Bradyarrhythmia-producing agents (e.g., beta blockers, calcium channel blockers, and digitalis glycosides) Cholinergic agonists (e.g., bethanechol) Muscarine-containing mushrooms (e.g., Clitocybe and Inocybe) Nerve agents (e.g., sarin, soman, tabun, and VX) Organophosphate and carbamate insecticides	Total 100 mg to 150 mg Available in various formulations: 0.4 mg/mL (1 mL, 0.4 mg ampules) 0.4 mg/mL (20 mL, 8 mg vials) 0.1 mg/mL (10 mL, 1 mg ampules) Atropine sulfate military-style auto-injectors: 2mg/0.7 mL, 1 mg/0.7 mL, 0.5 mg/0.7 mL, 0.25 mg/0.3 mL	The product should be immediately available in the ED. Some may also be stored in the pharmacy or other hospital sites, but should be easily mobilized if a severely poisoned patient needs treatment. Note: Product is necessary for adequate preparedness for a weapon of mass destruction (WMD) incident; the suggested amount may not be sufficient for mass-casualty events. Auto-injectors are available from Bound Tree Medical, Inc. Drug stocked in chempack container is intended only for use in mass-casualty events.
Calcium disodium EDTA (Versenate®)	Lead Zinc salts (e.g., zinc chloride)	One 5 mL amp (200 mg/mL)	Stock in pharmacy. One vial provides one day of therapy for a child. More may be needed in lead-endemic areas. Important note: Edetate disodium (Endrate®) is not the same as calcium disodium EDTA, and is used primarily as an IV chelator for emergent treatment of hypercalcemia, etc.
Calcium chloride and Calcium gluconate	Beta blockers Calcium channel blockers Fluoride salts (e.g., NaF) Hydrofluoric acid (HF) Hyperkalemia (not digoxin-induced) Hypermagnesemia	10% calcium chloride: fifteen 10 mL vials 10% calcium gluconate: five 10 mL vials	Stock in ED. More may be stocked in pharmacy. Many ampules of calcium chloride may be necessary in life-threatening calcium channel blocker or hydrofluoric acid poisoning.

(Continued)

ANTIDOTE	POISON/DRUG/TOXIN	SUGGESTED MINIMUM STOCK QUANTITY	COMMENTS
Deferoxamine mesylate (Desferal®)	Iron	Twelve 500 mg vials	Stock in pharmacy. Note: Per package insert, the maximum daily dose is 6 g (12 vials). However, this dose may be exceeded in serious poisonings.
Digoxin immune Fab (Digibind®, DigiFab®)	Cardiac glycoside-containing plants (e.g., foxglove and oleander) Digitoxin Digoxin	Ten vials	Stock in ED or pharmacy. This amount (ten vials) may be given to a digoxin-poisoned patient in whom the digoxin level is unknown. This amount would effectively neutralize a steady-state digoxin level of 14.2 ng/mL in a 70-kg patient. More may be necessary in severe intoxications. Know nearest source of additional supply.
Dimercaprol (BAL in oil)	Arsenic Copper Gold Lead Lewisite Mercury	Two 3 mL amps (100 mg/mL)	Stock in pharmacy. This amount provides two doses of 3 to 5 mg/kg/dose given q 4 h to treat one seriously poisoned adult or provides enough to treat a 15-kg child for 24 h.
Ethanol	Ethylene glycol Methanol	6 L of 5% alcohol in D_5W 10% alcohol in D_5W was discontinued in 2004; however, it can be prepared from 5% alcohol in D_5W and dehydrated alcohol. Consult Poison Control Center.	Stock in pharmacy. This amount (6 L) provides enough to treat two adults with a loading dose followed by a maintenance infusion for 4 hours each. More alcohol or fomepizole will be needed during dialysis or prolonged treatment. 95% or 40% alcohol diluted in juice may be given po if IV alcohol is unavailable. Note: Ethanol is unnecessary if fomepizole is stocked. See also fomepizole in this chart.
Flumazenil (Romazicon®)	Benzodiazepines Zaleplon Zolpidem	Total 1 mg: two 5 mL vials (0.1 mg/mL)	Suggested minimum is for ED stocking. Due to risk of seizures, use with extreme caution, if at all, in poisoned patients. More may be stocked in the pharmacy for use in reversal of conscious sedation.
Folic acid and Folinic acid (Leucovorin)	Formaldehyde/Formic Acid Methanol Methotrexate, trimetrexate Pyrimethamine Trimethoprim	Folic acid: three 50 mg vials Folinic acid: one 50 mg vial	Stock in pharmacy. For methanol-poisoned patients with an acidosis, give 50 mg folinic acid initially, then 50 mg of folic acid q 4 h for six doses.
Fomepizole (Antizol®)	Ethylene glycol Methanol	Two 1.5 g vial Note: Available in a kit of four 1.5 g vials	Stock in pharmacy. Know where nearest alternate supply is located. One vial will provide at least one initial adult dose. Hospitals with critical care and hemodialysis capabilities should consider stocking one kit of four vials (enough to treat one patient for up to several days). Note: Product has a 2-year shelf life; however, the manufacturer offers a credit for unused, expired product. Ethanol is unnecessary if adequate supply of fomepizole is stocked.

(Continued)

ANTIDOTE	POISON/DRUG/TOXIN	SUGGESTED MINIMUM STOCK QUANTITY	COMMENTS
Glucagon	Beta blockers Calcium channel blockers Hypoglycemia Hypoglycemic agents	Fifty 1 mg vials	Stock 20 mg in ED and remainder in pharmacy. The total amount (50 mg) provides approximately 5 to 10 hours of high-dose therapy in life-threatening beta blocker or calcium channel blocker poisoning. A protocol using high doses of insulin/dextrose also may be considered. Consult regional poison center for guidelines.
Hydroxocobalamin (Cyanokit®)	Acetonitrile Acrylonitrile Cyanide (e.g., HCN, KCN and NaCN) Cyanogen chloride Cyanogenic glycoside natural sources (e.g., apricot pits and peach pits) Laetrile Nitroprusside Smoke inhalation (combustion of synthetic materials	Two to four kits Each kit contains two 2.5 vials Note: Diluent is not included in the kit.	Seriously poisoned cyanide patients may require 5-10 g (1-2 kits). Stock two kits in ED. Consider also stocking two kits in the pharmacy. The product has a shelf-life of 30 months post-manufacture. Due to its favorable safety profile, this product may be used in a pre-hospital setting.
Hyperbaric oxygen (HBO)	Carbon monoxide Carbon tetrachloride Cyanide Hydrogen sulfide Methemoglobinemia	Post the location and phone number of nearest HBO chamber in the ED.	Consult IPC to determine if HBO treatment is indicated.
Methylene blue	Methemoglobin-inducing agents including: Aniline dyes Dapsone Dinitrophenol Local anesthetics (e.g., benzocaine) Metoclopramide Monomethylhydrazine-containing mushrooms (e.g., Gyromitra) Naphthalene Nitrates and nitrites Nitrobenzene Phenazopyridine	Three 10 mL amps (10 mg/mL)	Stock in pharmacy. This amount provides three doses of 1 to 2 mg/kg (0.1 to 0.2 mL/kg) for an adult patient.
Nalmefene (Revex®) and Naloxone (Narcan®)	ACE inhibitors Alpha₂ agonists (e.g., clonidine, guanabenz, and guanfacine) Coma of unknown cause Imidazoline decongestants (e.g., oxymetazoline and tetrahydrozoline) Loperamide Opioids (e.g., codeine, dextromethorphan, diphenoxylate, fentanyl, heroin, meperidine, morphine, and propoxyphene)	Nalmefene: none required Naloxone: total 40 mg, any combination of 0.4 mg 1 mg, and 2 mg ampules	Stock 20 mg naloxone in the ED and 20 mg elsewhere in the institution. Note: Nalmefene has a longer duration of action but it offers no therapeutic advantage over a maloxone infusion.
D-Penicillamine (Cuprimine®)	Arsenic Copper Lead Mercury	None required as an antidote. Available in bottles of 100 capsules (125 mg or 250 mg/capsule)	D-penicillamine is no longer considered the drug of choice for heavy-metal poisonings. It may be stocked in the pharmacy for other indications such as Wilson's disease or rheumatoid arthritis.

(Continued)

ANTIDOTE	POISON/DRUG/TOXIN	SUGGESTED MINIMUM STOCK QUANTITY	COMMENTS
Physostigmine salicylate (Antilirium®)	Anticholinergic alkaloid-containing plants (e.g., deadly nightshade and jimson weed) Antihistamines Atropine and other anticholinergic agents Intrathecal baclofen	Two 2 mL ampules (1 mg/mL)	Stock in ED or pharmacy. Usual adult dose is 1 to 2 mg slow IV push. Note: Duration of effect is 30 to 60 min.
Phytonadione (Vitamin K_1) (AquaMEPHYTON®, Mephyton®)	Indandione derivatives Long-acting anticoagulant rodenticides (e.g., brodifacoum and bromadiolone)	Two 0.5 mL ampules (2 mg/mL) and ten 1 mL ampules (10 mg/mL) 5 mg tablets available in packages of 10, 14, 20, 30, and 100	Stock in pharmacy.
Pralidoxime chloride (2-PAM) (Protopam®)	Antimyesthenic agents (e.g., pyridostigmine) Nerve agents (e.g., sarin, soman, tabun, and VX) Organophosphate insecticides Tacrine	Six 1 g vials Pralidoxime chloride military-style auto-injectors: 600 mg/2 mL	Stock in ED or pharmacy. Note: Serious intoxications may require 500 mg/h (12 g/day). Product is necessary for adequate preparedness for a weapon of mass destruction (WMD) incident; the suggested amount may not be sufficient for mass-casualty events. Auto-injectors are available from Bound Tree Medical, Inc. Drug stocked in chempack container is intended only for use in mass-casualty events.
Protamine sulfate	Enoxaparin Heparin	Variable, consider recommendation of hospital P&T Committee Available as 5 mL ampules (10 mg/mL) and 25 mL vials (250 mg/25 mL)	Stock in pharmacy.
Pyridoxine hydrochloride (Vitamin B_6)	Acrylamide Ethylene glycol Hydrazine Isoniazid (INH) Monomethylhydrazine-containing mushrooms (e.g., Gyromitra)	One hundred 1 mL vials (100 mg/mL vials)	Stock in ED or pharmacy. Usual dose is 1 g pyridoxine HCl for each gram of INH ingested. If amount ingested is unknown, give 5 g of pyridoxine. Repeat dose if seizures are uncontrolled. Know nearest source of additional supply. For ethylene glycol, a dose of 100 mg/day enhances the clearance of toxic metabolite.
Sodium bicarbonate	Chlorine gas Hyperkalemia Serum alkalinization: Agents producing a quinidine-like effect as noted by widened QRS complex on EKG (e.g., amantadine, carbamazepine, chloroquine, cocaine, diphenhydramine, flecainide, propafenone, propoxyphene, tricyclic antidepressants, quinidine, and related agents) Urine alkalinization: Weakly acidic agents (e.g., chlorophenoxy herbicides, chlorpropamide, phenobarbital, and salicylates)	Twenty 50 mEq vials	Stock 10 vials in the ED and 10 vials elsewhere in the hospital.
Succimer (Chemet®)	Arsenic Lead Lewisite Mercury	One bottle of 100 capsules (100 mg/capsule)	Stock in pharmacy. FDA-approved only for pediatric lead poisoning; however, it has shown efficacy for other heavy-metal poisonings.

USE-IN-PREGNANCY RATINGS

The U.S. Food and Drug Administration's Use-in-Pregnancy rating system weighs the degree to which available information has ruled out risk to the fetus against the drug's potential benefit to the patient. Below is a listing of drugs (by generic name) for which ratings are available.

Contraindicated in pregnancy

Studies in animals or humans, or investigational or postmarketing reports, have demonstrated fetal risk which clearly outweighs any possible benefit to the patient.

Acetohydroxamic Acid
Acitretin
Ambrisentan
Amlodipine Besylate/
    Atorvastatin Calcium
Anisindione
Atorvastatin Calcium
Bexarotene
Bicalutamide
Bosentan
Cetrorelix Acetate
Clomiphene Citrate
Desogestrel/Ethinyl Estradiol
Diclofenac Sodium/Misoprostol
Dihydroergotamine Mesylate
Dutasteride
Estazolam
Estradiol
Estradiol Acetate
Estradiol Cypionate/
    Medroxyprogesterone Acetate
Estradiol Valerate
Estradiol/Levonorgestrel
Estradiol/Norethindrone Acetate
Estrogens, Conjugated
Estrogens, Conjugated, Synthetic A
Estrogens, Conjugated/
    Medroxyprogesterone Acetate
Estrogens, Esterified
Estrogens, Esterified/
    Methyltestosterone
Estropipate
Ethinyl Estradiol/Drospirenone
Ethinyl Estradiol/
    Ethynodiol Diacetate
Ethinyl Estradiol/Etonogestrel
Ethinyl Estradiol/Ferrous
    Fumarate/Norethindrone Acetate
Ethinyl Estradiol/
    Levonorgestrel
Ethinyl Estradiol/Norelgestromin
Ethinyl Estradiol/Norethindrone
Ethinyl Estradiol/Norethindrone
    Acetate

Ethinyl Estradiol/
    Norgestimate
Ethinyl Estradiol/Norgestrel
Ezetimibe/Simvastatin
Finasteride
Fluorouracil
Fluoxymesterone
Flurazepam Hydrochloride
Fluvastatin Sodium
Follitropin Alfa
Follitropin Beta
Ganirelix Acetate
Goserelin Acetate
Histrelin Acetate
Hydromorphone Hydrochloride
Interferon Alfa-2B,
    Recombinant/Ribavirin
Iodine I 131 Tositumomab/
    Tositumomab
Isotretinoin
Leflunomide
Leuprolide Acetate
Levonorgestrel
Lovastatin
Lovastatin/Niacin
Medroxyprogesterone Acetate
Megestrol Acetate
Menotropins
Mequinol/Tretinoin
Mestranol/Norethindrone
Methotrexate Sodium
Methyltestosterone
Miglustat
Misoprostol
Nafarelin Acetate
Norethindrone
Norethindrone Acetate
Norgestrel
Oxandrolone
Oxymetholone
Plicamycin
Pravastatin Sodium
Pravastatin Sodium/
    Aspirin Buffered
Raloxifene Hydrochloride
Ribavirin
Rosuvastatin Calcium
Simvastatin
Tazarotene
Testosterone
Testosterone Enanthate
Thalidomide
Tositumomab
Triptorelin Pamoate
Warfarin Sodium

Positive evidence of risk

Investigational or postmarketing data show risk to the fetus. Nevertheless, potential benefits may outweigh the potential risk.

Alitretinoin
Alprazolam
Altretamine
Amiodarone Hydrochloride
Amlodipine Besylate/
    Benazepril Hydrochloride
Amlodipine Besylate/Olmesartan
    Medoxomil
Amlodipine Besylate/Valsartan*
Anastrozole
Arsenic Trioxide
Aspirin Buffered/
    Pravastatin Sodium
Aspirin/Dipyridamole
Atenolol
Azathioprine
Azathioprine Sodium
Benazepril Hydrochloride*
Benazepril Hydrochloride/
    Hydrochlorothiazide*
Bortezomib
Busulfan
Candesartan Cilexetil*
Candesartan Cilexetil/
    Hydrochlorothiazide*
Capecitabine
Captopril*
Carbamazepine
Carboplatin
Carmustine (BiCNU)
Chlorambucil
Cladribine
Clofarabine
Clonazepam
Cytarabine Liposome
Dactinomycin
Daunorubicin Citrate Liposome
Daunorubicin Hydrochloride
Demeclocycline Hydrochloride
Dexrazoxane Hydrochloride
Diazepam
Divalproex Sodium
Docetaxel
Doxorubicin Hydrochloride
Doxorubicin Hydrochloride Liposome
Doxycycline

* Category C or D depending on the trimester the drug is given.

Doxycycline Calcium
Doxycycline Hyclate
Doxycycline Monohydrate
Efavirenz
Enalapril Maleate*
Enalapril Maleate/
    Hydrochlorothiazide*
Epirubicin Hydrochloride
Eprosartan Mesylate
Erlotinib
Exemestane
Floxuridine
Fludarabine Phosphate
Flutamide
Fosinopril Sodium*
Fosinopril Sodium/
    Hydrochlorothiazide*
Fosphenytoin Sodium
Fulvestrant
Gefitinib
Gemcitabine Hydrochloride
Gemtuzumab Ozogamicin
Genistein/Zinc Chelazome/
    Cholecalciferol
Goserelin Acetate
Ibritumomab Tiuxetan
Idarubicin Hydrochloride
Ifosfamide
Imatinib Mesylate
Irbesartan*
Irbesartan/Hydrochlorothiazide*
Irinotecan Hydrochloride
Ixabepilone
Letrozole
Lisinopril*
Lisinopril/Hydrochlorothiazide*
Lithium Carbonate
Losartan Potassium*
Losartan Potassium/
    Hydrochlorothiazide*
Mechlorethamine Hydrochloride
Melphalan
Melphalan Hydrochloride
Mephobarbital
Mercaptopurine
Methimazole
Midazolam Hydrochloride
Minocycline Hydrochloride
Mitoxantrone Hydrochloride
Moexipril Hydrochloride*
Moexipril Hydrochloride/
    Hydrochlorothiazide*
Nelarabine
Neomycin Sulfate/
    Polymyxin B Sulfate
Nicotine
Nilotinib Hydrochloride Monohydrate
Olmesartan Medoxomil
Oxaliplatin
Pamidronate Disodium
Pemetrexed
Penicillamine
Pentobarbital Sodium
Pentostatin

Perindopril Erbumine*
Phenytoin
Procarbazine Hydrochloride
Quinapril Hydrochloride*
Quinapril Hydrochloride/
    Hydrochlorothiazide*
Ramipril*
Sorafenib
Streptomycin Sulfate
Sunitinib
Tamoxifen Citrate
Telmisartan
Telmisartan/
    Hydrochlorothiazide
Temozolomide
Temsirolimus
Thioguanine
Tigecycline
Tobramycin
Topotecan Hydrochloride
Toremifene Citrate
Trandolapril*
Trandolapril/Verapamil
    Hydrochloride*
Tretinoin
Valproate Sodium
Valproic Acid
Valsartan*
Valsartan/Hydrochlorothiazide*
Vinorelbine Tartrate
Voriconazole
Zoledronic Acid

C

Risk cannot be ruled out

Human studies are lacking, and animal studies are either positive for risk or are lacking as well. However, potential benefits may outweigh the potential risk.

Abacavir Sulfate
Abacavir Sulfate/Lamivudine
Abacavir Sulfate/
    Lamivudine/Zidovudine
Abciximab
Acamprosate Calcium
Acetaminophen
Acetaminophen/
    Butalbital/Caffeine
Acetaminophen/Caffeine/
    Chlorpheniramine
    Maleate/Hydrocodone
    Bitartrate/Phenylephrine
    Hydrochloride
Acetazolamide
Acetazolamide Sodium
Acyclovir
Adapalene
Adefovir Dipivoxil

Adenosine
Alatrofloxacin Mesylate
Albendazole
Albumin (Human)
Albuterol
Albuterol Sulfate
Albuterol Sulfate/
    Ipratropium Bromide
Alclometasone Dipropionate
Aldesleukin
Alemtuzumab
Alendronate Sodium
Alendronate Sodium/
    Cholecalciferol
Allopurinol Sodium
Almotriptan Malate
Alpha1-Proteinase Inhibitor (Human)
Alprostadil
Alteplase
Amantadine Hydrochloride
Amifostine
Aminocaproic Acid
Aminohippurate Sodium
Aminolevulinic Acid Hydrochloride
Aminosalicylic Acid
Amlodipine Besylate
Amlodipine Besylate/Benazepril
    Hydrochloride
Amlodipine Besylate/
    Olmesartan Medoxomil*
Amlodipine Besylate/Valsartan*
Amoxicillin/Clarithromycin/
    Lansoprazole
Amphetamine Aspartate/
    Amphetamine Sulfate/
    Dextroamphetamine Saccharate/
    Dextroamphetamine Sulfate
Amprenavir
Anagrelide Hydrochloride
Anthralin
Antihemophilic Factor (Human)
Antihemophilic Factor (Recombinant)
Anti-Inhibitor Coagulant Complex
Anti-Thymocyte Globulin
Apomorphine Hydrochloride
Aripiprazole
Armodafinil
Arnica Montana/Herbals,
    Multiple/Sulfur
Asparaginase
Atomoxetine Hydrochloride
Atovaquone
Atovaquone/Proguanil Hydrochloride
Atropine Sulfate/Benzoic
    Acid/Hyoscyamine
    Sulfate/Methenamine/
    Methylene Blue/Phenyl Salicylate
Atropine Sulfate/Hyoscyamine
    Sulfate/Scopolamine
    Hydrobromide
Azelastine Hydrochloride
Bacitracin Zinc/Neomycin
    Sulfate/Polymyxin B Sulfate
Baclofen

BCG, Live (Intravesical)
Becaplermin
Beclomethasone Dipropionate
Beclomethasone Dipropionate
    Monohydrate
Benazepril Hydrochloride*
Benazepril Hydrochloride/
    Hydrochlorothiazide*
Bendroflumethiazide
Benzocaine
Benzonatate
Benzoyl Peroxide
Benzoyl Peroxide/Clindamycin
Benzoyl Peroxide/Erythromycin
Betamethasone Dipropionate
Betamethasone
    Dipropionate/Clotrimazole
Betamethasone Valerate
Betaxolol Hydrochloride
Bethanechol Chloride
Bevacizumab
Bimatoprost
Bisacodyl/Polyethylene
    Glycol/Potassium Chloride/Sodium
    Bicarbonate/Sodium Chloride
Bisoprolol Fumarate
Bisoprolol Fumarate/
    Hydrochlorothiazide
Bitolterol Mesylate
Black Widow Spider
    Antivenin (Equine)
Botulinum Toxin Type A
Botulinum Toxin Type B
Brimonidine Tartrate/Timolol Maleate
Brinzolamide
Brompheniramine
    Maleate/Dextromethorphan
    Hydrobromide/Phenylephrine
    Hydrochloride
Budesonide
Bupivacaine Hydrochloride
Bupivacaine Hydrochloride/
    Epinephrine Bitartrate
Buprenorphine Hydrochloride
Buprenorphine
    Hydrochloride/Naloxone
    Hydrochloride
Butabarbital/Hyoscyamine
    Hydrobromide/ Phenazopyridine
    Hydrochloride
Butalbital/Acetaminophen
Butenafine Hydrochloride
Butoconazole Nitrate
Butorphanol Tartrate
Caffeine Citrate
Calcipotriene
Calcitonin-Salmon
Calcitriol
Calcium Acetate
Candesartan Cilexetil*
Candesartan Cilexetil/
    Hydrochlorothiazide*
Capreomycin Sulfate

Captopril*
Carbetapentane
    Tannate/Chlorpheniramine Tannate
Carbetapentane
    Tannate/Chlorpheniramine
    Tannate/Ephedrine
    Tannate/Phenylephrine Tannate
Carbidopa/Entacapone/
    Levodopa
Carbidopa/Levodopa
Carbinoxamine Maleate/
    Dextromethorphan Hydrobromide/
    Pseudoephedrine Hydrochloride
Carteolol Hydrochloride
Carvedilol
Caspofungin Acetate
Celecoxib
Cetirizine Hydrochloride
Cetuximab
Cevimeline Hydrochloride
Chloramphenicol
Chloroprocaine Hydrochloride
Chlorothiazide
Chlorothiazide Sodium
Chlorpheniramine Maleate/
    Methscopolamine Nitrate/
    Phenylephrine Hydrochloride
Chlorpheniramine Maleate/
    Pseudoephedrine Hydrochloride
Chlorpheniramine
    Polistirex/Hydrocodone Polistirex
Chlorpheniramine
    Tannate/Phenylephrine Tannate
Chlorpropamide
Chlorthalidone/Clonidine
    Hydrochloride
Choline Magnesium Trisalicylate
Cidofovir
Cilostazol
Cinacalcet Hydrochloride
Ciprofloxacin Hydrochloride
Ciprofloxacin Hydrochloride/
    Hydrocortisone
Ciprofloxacin/Dexamethasone
Citalopram Hydrobromide
Clarithromycin
Clobetasol Propionate
Clonidine
Clonidine Hydrochloride
Codeine Phosphate/
    Acetaminophen
Colistimethate Sodium
Colistin Sulfate/Hydrocortisone
    Acetate/Neomycin Sulfate/
    Thonzonium Bromide
Corticorelin Ovine Triflutate
Cyanocobalamin
Cycloserine
Cyclosporine
Cytomegalovirus Immune Globulin
Dacarbazine
Daclizumab
Dantrolene Sodium

Dapsone
Darbepoetin Alfa
Darifenacin
Deferoxamine Mesylate
Delavirdine Mesylate
Denileukin Diftitox
Desloratadine
Desloratadine/Pseudoephedrine
    Sulfate
Desoximetasone
Dexamethasone
Dexamethasone Sodium Phosphate
Dexmethylphenidate Hydrochloride
Dexrazoxane
Dextroamphetamine Sulfate
Diazoxide
Dichlorphenamide
Diclofenac Potassium
Diclofenac Sodium
Diflorasone Diacetate
Diflunisal
Digoxin
Digoxin Immune Fab (Ovine)
Diltiazem Hydrochloride
Dimethyl Sulfoxide
Dinoprostone
Diphtheria & Tetanus Toxoids and
    Acellular Pertussis Vaccine
    Adsorbed
Diphtheria & Tetanus Toxoids and
    Acellular Pertussis Vaccine
    Adsorbed/Hepatitis B Vaccine,
    Recombinant/Poliovirus Vaccine
    Inactivated
Dirithromycin
Dofetilide
Donepezil Hydrochloride
Dorzolamide Hydrochloride
Dorzolamide Hydrochloride/Timolol
    Maleate
Doxazosin Mesylate
Dronabinol
Drotrecogin Alfa (Activated)
Duloxetine Hydrochloride
Echothiophate Iodide
Econazole Nitrate
Efalizumab
Eflornithine Hydrochloride
Eletriptan Hydrobromide
Enalapril Maleate*
Enalapril Maleate/Felodipine*
Enalapril Maleate/
    Hydrochlorothiazide*
Entacapone
Entecavir
Epinastine Hydrochloride
Epinephrine
Epoetin Alfa
Eprosartan Mesylate
Erythromycin Ethylsuccinate/
    Sulfisoxazole Acetyl
Escitalopram Oxalate
Eszopiclone

* Category C or D depending on the trimester the drug is given.

A237

Ethionamide
Ethotoin
Etidronate Disodium
Exenatide
Ezetimibe
Factor IX Complex
Felodipine
Fenofibrate
Fentanyl
Fentanyl Citrate
Fentanyl Hydrochloride
Ferrous Fumarate/Folic Acid/
    Intrinsic Factor Concentrate/
    Liver Preparations/
    Vitamin B12/Vitamin C/
    Vitamins with Iron
Fexofenadine Hydrochloride
Fexofenadine Hydrochloride/
    Pseudoephedrine Hydrochloride
Filgrastim
Flecainide Acetate
Fluconazole
Flucytosine
Fludrocortisone Acetate
Flumazenil
Flunisolide
Fluocinolone Acetonide
Fluocinolone Acetonide/
    Hydroquinone/Tretinoin
Fluocinonide
Fluorometholone
Fluorometholone/Sulfacetamide
    Sodium
Fluoxetine Hydrochloride
Fluoxetine Hydrochloride/
    Olanzapine
Flurandrenolide
Flurbiprofen Sodium
Fluticasone Furoate
Fluticasone Propionate
Fluticasone Propionate HFA
Fluticasone Propionate/Salmeterol
    Xinafoate
Fomivirsen Sodium
Formoterol Fumarate
Fosamprenavir Calcium
Foscarnet Sodium*
Fosinopril Sodium*
Fosinopril Sodium/
    Hydrochlorothiazide*
Frovatriptan Succinate
Furosemide
Gabapentin
Gallium Nitrate
Ganciclovir
Ganciclovir Sodium
Gatifloxacin
Gemfibrozil
Gemifloxacin Mesylate
Gentamicin Sulfate
Gentamicin Sulfate/
    Prednisolone Acetate
Glimepiride
Glipizide

Glipizide/Metformin Hydrochloride
Globulin, Immune (Human)
Globulin, Immune (Human)/
    Rho (D) Immune Globulin
    (Human)
Glyburide
Gramicidin/Neomycin Sulfate/
    Polymyxin B Sulfate
Guaifenesin/Hydrocodone Bitartrate
Haemophilus B Conjugate Vaccine
Haemophilus B Conjugate
    Vaccine/Hepatitis B Vaccine,
    Recombinant
Halobetasol Propionate
Haloperidol Decanoate
Hemin
Heparin Sodium
Hepatitis A Vaccine, Inactivated
Hepatitis A Vaccine,
    Inactivated/Hepatitis B Vaccine,
    Recombinant
Hepatitis B Immune Globulin
    (Human)
Hepatitis B Vaccine, Recombinant
Homatropine
    Methylbromide/Hydrocodone
    Bitartrate
Homeopathic Formulations
Hydralazine Hydrochloride/Isosorbide
    Dinitrate
Hydrochlorothiazide
Hydrocodone Bitartrate
Hydrocodone
    Bitartrate/Acetaminophen
Hydrocodone Bitartrate/Ibuprofen
Hydrocortisone
Hydrocortisone Acetate
Hydrocortisone Acetate/Neomycin
    Sulfate/Polymyxin B Sulfate
Hydrocortisone Acetate/Pramoxine
    Hydrochloride
Hydrocortisone Butyrate
Hydrocortisone Probutate
Hydrocortisone/Neomycin
    Sulfate/Polymyxin B Sulfate
Hydromorphone Hydrochloride
Hydroquinone
Hyoscyamine Sulfate
Ibandronate Sodium
Ibutilide Fumarate
Iloprost
Imiglucerase
Imipenem/Cilastatin
Imiquimod
Immune Globulin Intravenous
    (Human)
Indinavir Sulfate
Indocyanine Green
Influenza Virus Vaccine
Insulin Aspart
Insulin Aspart Protamine,
    Human/Insulin Aspart, Human
Insulin Glargine
Insulin Glulisine

Interferon Alfa-2B, Recombinant
Interferon Alfacon-1
Interferon Alfa-N3
    (Human Leukocyte Derived)
Interferon Beta-1A
Interferon Beta-1B
Interferon Gamma-1B
Iodoquinol/Hydrocortisone
Irbesartan*
Irbesartan/Hydrochlorothiazide*
Iron Dextran
Isoniazid/
    Pyrazinamide/Rifampin
Isosorbide Mononitrate
Isradipine
Itraconazole
Ivermectin
Ketoconazole
Ketorolac Tromethamine
Ketotifen Fumarate
Labetalol Hydrochloride
Lamivudine
Lamivudine/Zidovudine
Lamotrigine
Lanreotide Acetate
Lanthanum Carbonate
Latanoprost
Levalbuterol Hydrochloride
Levalbuterol Tartrate
Levamisole Hydrochloride
Levetiracetam
Levobunolol Hydrochloride
Levofloxacin
Linezolid
Lisinopril*
Lisinopril/Hydrochlorothiazide*
Lopinavir/Ritonavir
Losartan Potassium*
Losartan Potassium/
    Hydrochlorothiazide*
Loteprednol Etabonate
Mafenide Acetate
Magnesium Salicylate Tetrahydrate
Measles Virus Vaccine, Live
Measles, Mumps & Rubella Virus
    Vaccine, Live
Mebendazole
Mecamylamine Hydrochloride
Mecasermin [rDNA Origin]
Medrysone
Mefenamic Acid
Mefloquine Hydrochloride
Meloxicam
Meningoccal Polysaccharide
    Diphtheria Toxoid Conjugate
    Vaccine
Meningococcal Polysaccharide
    Vaccine
Meperidine Hydrochloride
Mepivacaine Hydrochloride
Metaproterenol Sulfate
Metaraminol Bitartrate
Metformin Hydrochloride/Pioglitazone
    Hydrochloride

Metformin Hydrochloride/
   Rosiglitazone Maleate
Methamphetamine Hydrochloride
Methazolamide
Methenamine Mandelate/
   Sodium Acid Phosphate
Methocarbamol
Methoxsalen
Methoxy Polyethylene Glycol/
   Epoetin Beta
Methscopolamine Nitrate/
   Pseudoephedrine Hydrochloride
Methyldopa/Chlorothiazide
Methyldopa/Hydrochlorothiazide
Methylphenidate Hydrochloride
Metipranolol
Metoprolol Succinate
Metoprolol Tartrate
Metoprolol
   Tartrate/Hydrochlorothiazide
Metyrosine
Mexiletine Hydrochloride
Micafungin Sodium
Midodrine Hydrochloride
Mivacurium Chloride
Modafinil
Moexipril Hydrochloride*
Moexipril Hydrochloride/
   Hydrochlorothiazide*
Mometasone Furoate
Mometasone Furoate Monohydrate
Morphine Sulfate
Morphine Sulfate, Liposomal
Moxifloxacin Hydrochloride
Mumps Virus Vaccine, Live
Muromonab-CD3
Mycophenolate Mofetil
Mycophenolate Mofetil Hydrochloride
Mycophenolic Acid
Nabumetone
Nadolol
Nadolol/Bendroflumethiazide
Naloxone Hydrochloride/
   Pentazocine Hydrochloride
Naltrexone Hydrochloride
Naphazoline Hydrochloride
Naproxen
Naproxen Sodium
Naratriptan Hydrochloride
Natamycin
Nateglinide
Nebivolol
Nefazodone Hydrochloride
Neomycin Sulfate/Dexamethasone
   Sodium Phosphate
Neomycin Sulfate/Polymyxin B
   Sulfate/Prednisolone Acetate
Nesiritide
Nevirapine
Niacin
Nicardipine Hydrochloride
Nifedipine
Nilutamide
Nimodipine

Nisoldipine
Nitroglycerin
Norfloxacin
Ofloxacin
Olanzapine
Olmesartan Medoxomil/
   Hydrochlorothiazide
Olopatadine Hydrochloride
Olsalazine Sodium
Omega-3-Acid Ethyl Esters
Omeprazole
Oprelvekin
Orphenadrine Citrate
Oseltamivir Phosphate
Oxcarbazepine
Oxycodone Hydrochloride/
   Acetaminophen
Oxycodone Hydrochloride/ Ibuprofen
Oxymorphone Hydrochloride
Palifermin
Palivizumab
Pancrelipase
Paricalcitol
Paroxetine Hydrochloride
Paroxetine Mesylate
Peg-3350/Potassium Chloride/
   Sodium Bicarbonate/
   Sodium Chloride
Pegademase Bovine
Pegaspargase
Pegfilgrastim
Peginterferon Alfa-2A
Peginterferon Alfa-2B
Pemirolast Potassium
Pentazocine Hydrochloride/
   Acetaminophen
Pentoxifylline
Perindopril Erbumine*
Phenoxybenzamine Hydrochloride
Phentermine Hydrochloride
Pilocarpine Hydrochloride
Pimecrolimus
Pimozide
Pioglitazone Hydrochloride
Pirbuterol Acetate
Piroxicam
Plasma Fractions, Human/
   Rabies Immune Globulin (Human)
Plasma Protein Fraction (Human)
Pneumococcal Vaccine, Diphtheria
   Conjugate
Pneumococcal Vaccine, Polyvalent
Podofilox
Polyethylene Glycol
Polyethylene Glycol/
   Potassium Chloride/Sodium
   Bicarbonate/Sodium Chloride
Polyethylene Glycol/Potassium
   Chloride/Sodium
   Bicarbonate/Sodium
   Chloride/Sodium Sulfate
Polymyxin B Sulfate/
   Trimethoprim Sulfate
Polythiazide/Prazosin Hydrochloride

Porfimer Sodium
Potassium Acid Phosphate
Potassium Chloride
Potassium Citrate
Potassium Phosphate/
   Sodium Phosphate
Pralidoxime Chloride
Pramipexole Dihydrochloride
Pramlintide Acetate
Pramoxine Hydrochloride/
   Hydrocortisone Acetate
Prazosin Hydrochloride
Prednisolone Acetate
Prednisolone Acetate/
   Sulfacetamide Sodium
Prednisolone Sodium Phosphate
Pregabalin
Promethazine Hydrochloride
Propafenone Hydrochloride
Proparacaine Hydrochloride
Propranolol Hydrochloride
Pseudoephedrine Hydrochloride
Pyrimethamine
Quetiapine Fumarate
Quinapril Hydrochloride*
Quinidine Sulfate
Rabies Vaccine
Raltegravir Potassium
Ramelteon
Ramipril*
Rasburicase
Remifentanil Hydrochloride
Repaglinide
Reteplase
Rho (D) Immune Globulin (Human)
Rifampin
Rifapentine
Rifaximin
Riluzole
Rimantadine Hydrochloride
Risedronate Sodium
Risedronate Sodium/
   Calcium Carbonate
Risperidone
Rituximab
Rizatriptan Benzoate
Rocuronium Bromide
Rofecoxib
Ropinirole Hydrochloride
Rosiglitazone Maleate
Rotigotine
Rubella Virus Vaccine, Live
Salmeterol Xinafoate
Sapropterin Dihydrochloride
Sargramostim
Scopolamine
Selegiline Hydrochloride
Selenium Sulfide
Sertaconazole Nitrate
Sertraline Hydrochloride
Sevelamer Carbonate
Sevelamer Hydrochloride
Sibutramine Hydrochloride
   Monohydrate

* Category C or D depending on the trimester the drug is given.

Sirolimus
Sodium Benzoate/
    Sodium Phenylacelate
Sodium Phenylbutyrate
Sodium Polysterene Sulfonate
Sodium Sulfacetamide/Sulfur
Solifenacin Succinate
Somatropin
Somatropin (rDNA Origin)
Stavudine
Streptokinase
Succimer
Sulfacetamide Sodium
Sulfamethoxazole/Trimethoprim
Sulfanilamide
Sumatriptan
Sumatriptan Succinate
Tacrine Hydrochloride
Tacrolimus
Telithromycin
Telmisartan*
Telmisartan/
    Hydrochlorothiazide*
Tenecteplase
Terazosin Hydrochloride
Teriparatide
Tetanus & Diphtheria Toxoids
    Adsorbed
Tetanus Immune Globulin (Human)
Theophylline
Theophylline Anhydrous
Thiabendazole
Thrombin
Thyrotropin Alfa
Tiagabine Hydrochloride
Tiludronate Disodium
Timolol Hemihydrate
Timolol Maleate
Timolol Maleate/
    Hydrochlorothiazide
Tinidazole
Tiotropium Bromide
Tipranavir
Tizanidine Hydrochloride
Tobramycin/Dexamethasone
Tobramycin/Loteprednol Etabonate
Tolcapone
Tolterodine Tartrate
Topiramate
Tramadol Hydrochloride
Tramadol Hydrochloride/
    Acetaminophen
Trandolapril*
Trandolapril/Verapamil
    Hydrochloride*
Travoprost
Tretinoin
Triamcinolone Acetonide
Triamterene
Triamterene/Hydrochlorothiazide
Trientine Hydrochloride
Triethanolamine Polypeptide Oleate-
    Condensate

Trifluridine
Trimethoprim Hydrochloride
Trimipramine Maleate
Tropicamide/
    Hydroxyamphetamine
    Hydrobromide
Trospium Chloride
Trovafloxacin Mesylate
Tuberculin Purified Protein
    Derivative, Diluted
Typhoid Vaccine Live Oral Ty21a
Unoprostone Isopropyl
Urea
Valdecoxib
Valganciclovir Hydrochloride
Valsartan*
Valsartan/Hydrochlorothiazide*
Varicella Virus Vaccine, Live
Venlafaxine Hydrochloride
Verapamil Hydrochloride
Verteporfin
Vitamin K₁
Yellow Fever Vaccine
Zalcitabine
Zaleplon
Zanamivir
Zidovudine
Ziprasidone Mesylate
Zolmitriptan
Zolpidem Tartrate
Zonisamide

No evidence of risk in humans

*Either animal findings show risk
while human findings do not, or, if no
adequate human studies have been
done, animal findings are negative.*

Acarbose
Acrivastine
Acyclovir
Acyclovir Sodium
Adalimumab
Agalsidase Beta
Alefacept
Alfuzosin Hydrochloride
Alosetron Hydrochloride
Amiloride Hydrochloride
Amiloride Hydrochloride/
    Hydrochlorothiazide
Amoxicillin
Amoxicillin/Clavulanate Potassium
Amphotericin B
Amphotericin B Lipid Complex
Amphotericin B, Liposomal
Amphotericin B/Cholesteryl Sulfate
    Complex
Ampicillin Sodium/
    Sulbactam Sodium

Anakinra
Antithrombin III
Aprepitant
Aprotinin
Argatroban
Arginine Hydrochloride
Atazanavir Sulfate
Azelaic Acid
Azithromycin
Azithromycin Dihydrate
Aztreonam
Balsalazide Disodium
Basiliximab
Bivalirudin
Brimonidine Tartrate
Budesonide
Bupropion Hydrochloride
Cabergoline
Carbenicillin Indanyl Sodium
Cefaclor
Cefazolin Sodium
Cefdinir
Cefditoren Pivoxil
Cefepime Hydrochloride
Cefixime
Cefoperazone Sodium
Cefotaxime Sodium
Cefotetan Disodium
Cefoxitin Sodium
Cefpodoxime Proxetil
Cefprozil
Ceftazidime Sodium
Ceftibuten Dihydrate
Ceftizoxime Sodium
Ceftriaxone Sodium
Cefuroxime
Cefuroxime Axetil
Cephalexin
Cetirizine Hydrochloride
Ciclopirox
Ciclopirox Olamine
Cimetidine
Cimetidine Hydrochloride
Cisatracurium Besylate
Clindamycin
    Hydrochloride/Clindamycin
    Phosphate
Clindamycin Palmitate Hydrochloride
Clindamycin Phosphate
Clopidogrel Bisulfate
Clotrimazole
Clozapine
Colesevelam Hydrochloride
Cromolyn Sodium
Cyclobenzaprine Hydrochloride
Cyproheptadine Hydrochloride
Dalfopristin/Quinupristin
Dalteparin Sodium
Dapiprazole Hydrochloride
Daptomycin
Desflurane
Desmopressin Acetate
Dicyclomine Hydrochloride

Didanosine
Diphenhydramine Hydrochloride
Dipivefrin Hydrochloride
Dipyridamole
Dolasetron Mesylate
Doripenem
Dornase Alfa
Doxapram Hydrochloride
Doxepin Hydrochloride
Doxercalciferol
Edetate Calcium Disodium
Emtricitabine
Emtricitabine/Tenofovir Disoproxil
    Fumarate
Enfuvirtide
Enoxaparin Sodium
Eplerenone
Epoprostenol Sodium
Ertapenem
Erythromycin
Erythromycin Ethylsuccinate
Erythromycin Stearate
Esomeprazole Magnesium
Esomeprazole Sodium
Etanercept
Ethacrynate Sodium
Ethacrynic Acid
Famciclovir
Famotidine
Fenoldopam Mesylate
Fondaparinux Sodium
Galantamine Hydrobromide
Glatiramer Acetate
Glucagon
Glyburide/Metformin Hydrochloride
Granisetron Hydrochloride
Hydrochlorothiazide
Ibuprofen
Indapamide
Infliximab
Insulin Lispro Protamine,
    Human/Insulin Lispro, Human
Insulin Lispro, Human
Ipratropium Bromide
Iron Sucrose
Isosorbide Mononitrate
Lactulose
Lansoprazole
Lansoprazole/Naproxen
Laronidase
Lepirudin
Levocarnitine
Levocetirizine Dihydrochloride
Lidocaine
Lidocaine Hydrochloride
Lidocaine/Prilocaine

Lindane
Loperamide Hydrochloride
Loracarbef
Loratadine
Malathion
Meclizine Hydrochloride
Memantine Hydrochloride
Meropenem
Mesalamine
Metformin Hydrochloride
Metformin Hydrochloride/
    Sitagliptin Phosphate
Methohexital Sodium
Methyldopa
Metolazone
Metronidazole
Miglitol
Montelukast Sodium
Mupirocin
Mupirocin Calcium
Naftifine Hydrochloride
Nalbuphine Hydrochloride
Nalmefene Hydrochloride
Naloxone Hydrochloride
Naproxen Sodium
Nedocromil Sodium
Nelfinavir Mesylate
Nitazoxanide
Nitrofurantoin Macrocrystals
Nitrofurantoin Macrocrystals/
    Nitrofurantoin Monohydrate
Nizatidine
Octreotide Acetate
Omalizumab
Ondansetron
Ondansetron Hydrochloride
Orlistat
Oxiconazole Nitrate
Oxybutynin
Oxybutynin Chloride
Oxycodone Hydrochloride
Palonosetron Hydrochloride
Pancrelipase
Pantoprazole Sodium
Pegvisomant
Pemoline
Penciclovir
Penicillin G Benzathine
Penicillin G Benzathine/
    Penicillin G Procaine
Penicillin G Potassium
Pentosan Polysulfate Sodium
Permethrin
Piperacillin Sodium
Piperacillin Sodium/
    Tazobactam Sodium

Praziquantel
Progesterone
Propofol
Pseudoephedrine Hydrochloride
Pseudoephedrine Sulfate
Psyllium Preparations
Rabeprazole Sodium
Ranitidine Hydrochloride
Retapamulin
Rifabutin
Ritonavir
Rivastigmine Tartrate
Ropivacaine Hydrochloride
Saquinavir Mesylate
Sevoflurane
Sildenafil Citrate
Silver Sulfadiazine
Sodium Ferric Gluconate
Somatropin
Sotalol Hydrochloride
Sucralfate
Sulfasalazine
Tadalafil
Tamsulosin Hydrochloride
Tenofovir Disoproxil Fumarate
Terbinafine Hydrochloride
Ticarcillin Disodium/
    Clavulanate Potassium
Ticlopidine Hydrochloride
Tirofiban Hydrochloride
Torsemide
Trastuzumab
Treprostinil Sodium
Urokinase
Ursodiol
Valacyclovir Hydrochloride
Vancomycin Hydrochloride
Vardenafil Hydrochloride
Zafirlukast

Controlled studies show no risk

*Adequate, well-controlled studies in
pregnant women have failed to
demonstrate risk to the fetus.*

Liothyronine Sodium
Liotrix
Nystatin

---

* Category C or D depending on the trimester the drug is given.

BOYS LENGTH-FOR-AGE AND WEIGHT-FOR-AGE BIRTH TO 36 MONTHS (5TH-95TH PERCENTILE)

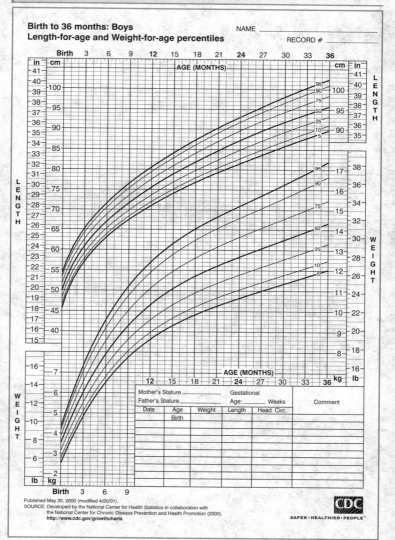

Birth to 36 months: Boys
Length-for-age and Weight-for-age percentiles

NAME _____

RECORD # _____

Published May 30, 2000 (modified 4/20/01).
SOURCE: Developed by the National Center for Health Statistics in collaboration with
the National Center for Chronic Disease Prevention and Health Promotion (2000).
http://www.cdc.gov/growthcharts

CDC

SAFER · HEALTHIER · PEOPLE™

A243

BOYS HEAD CIRCUMFERENCE-FOR-AGE AND WEIGHT-FOR-LENGTH
BIRTH TO 36 MONTHS (5TH-95TH PERCENTILE)

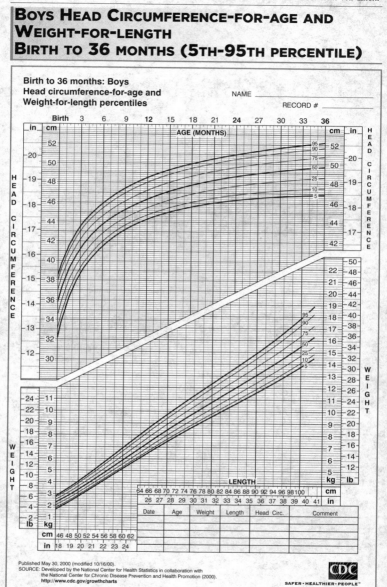

Birth to 36 months: Boys
Head circumference-for-age and
Weight-for-length percentiles

NAME _____

RECORD # _____

Published May 30, 2000 (modified 10/16/00).
SOURCE: Developed by the National Center for Health Statistics in collaboration with
the National Center for Chronic Disease Prevention and Health Promotion (2000).
http://www.cdc.gov/growthcharts

CDC

SAFER · HEALTHIER · PEOPLE™

A245

GIRLS LENGTH-FOR-AGE AND WEIGHT-FOR-AGE
BIRTH TO 36 MONTHS (5TH-95TH PERCENTILE)

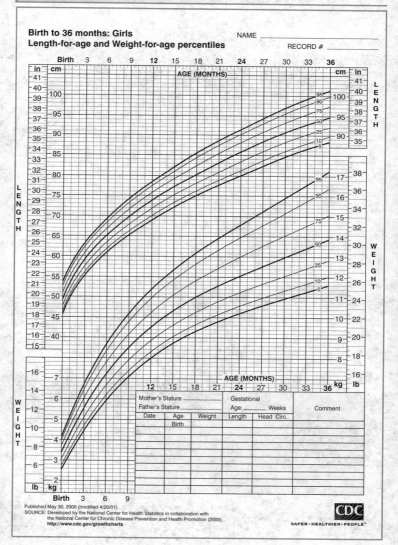

Birth to 36 months: Girls
Length-for-age and Weight-for-age percentiles

NAME _____

RECORD # _____

Published May 30, 2000 (modified 4/20/01).
SOURCE: Developed by the National Center for Health Statistics in collaboration with
the National Center for Chronic Disease Prevention and Health Promotion (2000).
http://www.cdc.gov/growthcharts

CDC
SAFER · HEALTHIER · PEOPLE™

GIRLS HEAD CIRCUMFERENCE-FOR-AGE AND WEIGHT-FOR-LENGTH
BIRTH TO 36 MONTHS (5TH-95TH PERCENTILE)

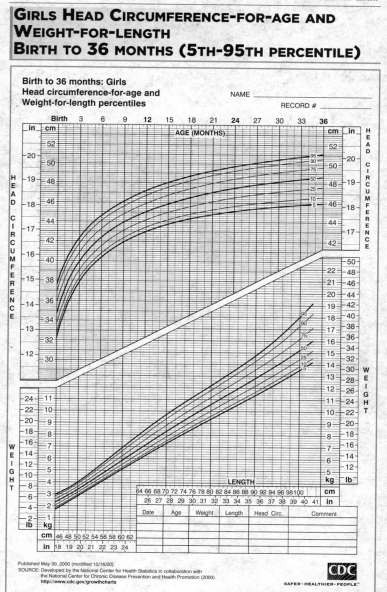

Birth to 36 months: Girls
Head circumference-for-age and
Weight-for-length percentiles

NAME _____

RECORD # _____

Published May 30, 2000 (modified 10/16/00).
SOURCE: Developed by the National Center for Health Statistics in collaboration with
the National Center for Chronic Disease Prevention and Health Promotion (2000).
http://www.cdc.gov/growthcharts

CDC

SAFER·HEALTHIER·PEOPLE™

BOYS STATURE-FOR-AGE AND WEIGHT-FOR-AGE CHILDREN 2 TO 20 YEARS (5TH-95TH PERCENTILE)

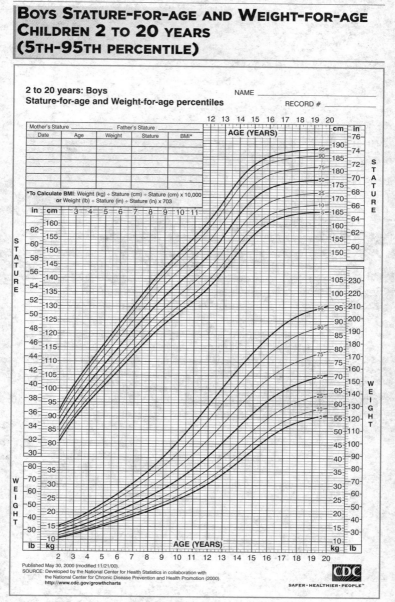

2 to 20 years: Boys
Stature-for-age and Weight-for-age percentiles

NAME

RECORD #

Published May 30, 2000 (modified 11/21/00).
SOURCE: Developed by the National Center for Health Statistics in collaboration with
the National Center for Chronic Disease Prevention and Health Promotion (2000).
http://www.cdc.gov/growthcharts

BOYS BMI-FOR-AGE
CHILDREN 2 TO 20 YEARS (5TH-95TH PERCENTILE)

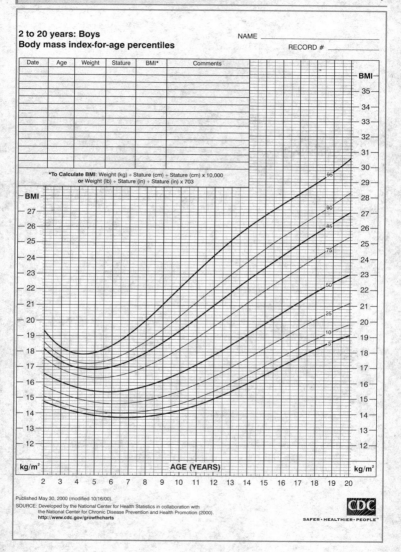

2 to 20 years: Boys
Body mass index-for-age percentiles

NAME _____

RECORD # _____

Date	Age	Weight	Stature	BMI*	Comments

*To Calculate BMI: Weight (kg) ÷ Stature (cm) ÷ Stature (cm) x 10,000
or Weight (lb) ÷ Stature (in) ÷ Stature (in) x 703

AGE (YEARS)

kg/m²

Published May 30, 2000 (modified 10/16/00).
SOURCE: Developed by the National Center for Health Statistics in collaboration with
the National Center for Chronic Disease Prevention and Health Promotion (2000).
http://www.cdc.gov/growthcharts

CDC
SAFER • HEALTHIER • PEOPLE™

A253

GIRLS STATURE-FOR-AGE AND WEIGHT-FOR-AGE CHILDREN 2 TO 20 YEARS (5TH-95TH PERCENTILE)

2 to 20 years: Girls
Stature-for-age and Weight-for-age percentiles

NAME _____

RECORD # _____

Mother's Stature _____ Father's Stature _____

Date	Age	Weight	Stature	BMI*

*To Calculate BMI: Weight (kg) ÷ Stature (cm) ÷ Stature (cm) x 10,000
or Weight (lb) ÷ Stature (in) ÷ Stature (in) x 703

AGE (YEARS)

STATURE

WEIGHT

Published May 30, 2000 (modified 11/21/00).
SOURCE: Developed by the National Center for Health Statistics in collaboration with
the National Center for Chronic Disease Prevention and Health Promotion (2000).
http://www.cdc.gov/growthcharts

CDC

SAFER · HEALTHIER · PEOPLE™

A255

GIRLS BMI-FOR-AGE
CHILDREN 2 TO 20 YEARS (5TH-95TH PERCENTILE)

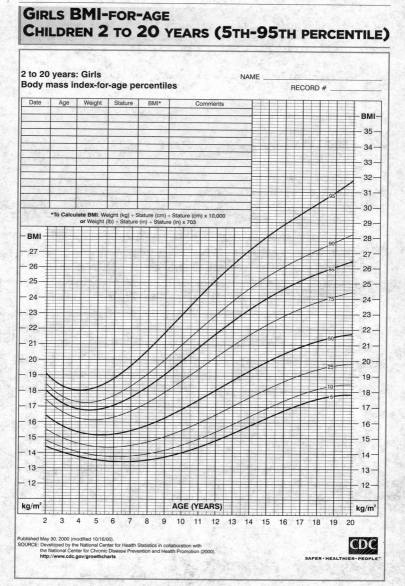

2 to 20 years: Girls
Body mass index-for-age percentiles

NAME _____

RECORD # _____

Date	Age	Weight	Stature	BMI*	Comments

*To Calculate BMI: Weight (kg) ÷ Stature (cm) ÷ Stature (cm) x 10,000
or Weight (lb) ÷ Stature (in) ÷ Stature (in) x 703

AGE (YEARS)

Published May 30, 2000 (modified 10/16/00).
SOURCE: Developed by the National Center for Health Statistics in collaboration with
the National Center for Chronic Disease Prevention and Health Promotion (2000).
http://www.cdc.gov/growthcharts

CDC
SAFER · HEALTHIER · PEOPLE™

BOYS WEIGHT-FOR-STATURE
(5TH-95TH PERCENTILE)

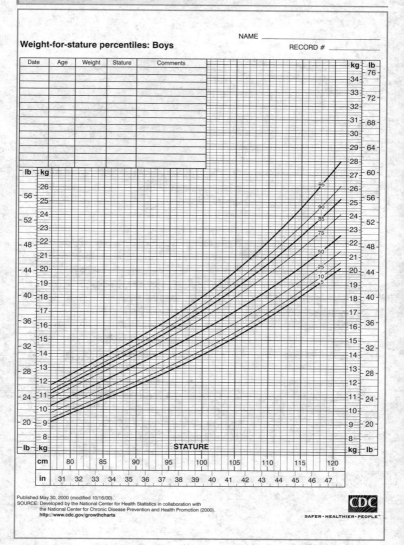

Weight-for-stature percentiles: Boys

NAME _____

RECORD # _____

Published May 30, 2000 (modified 10/16/00).
SOURCE: Developed by the National Center for Health Statistics in collaboration with
the National Center for Chronic Disease Prevention and Health Promotion (2000).
http://www.cdc.gov/growthcharts

CDC
SAFER · HEALTHIER · PEOPLE™

A259

GIRLS WEIGHT-FOR-STATURE
(5TH-95TH PERCENTILE)

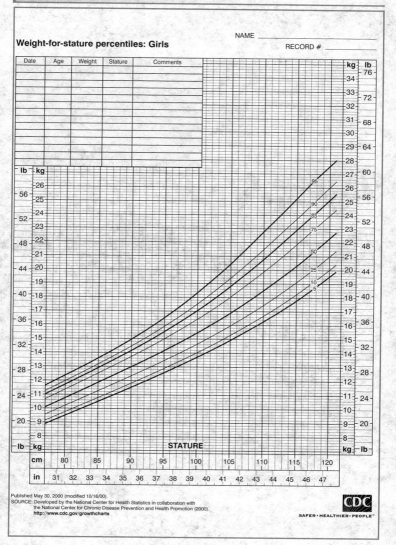

Weight-for-stature percentiles: Girls

NAME _____

RECORD # _____

Date	Age	Weight	Stature	Comments

STATURE

Published May 30, 2000 (modified 10/16/00).
SOURCE: Developed by the National Center for Health Statistics in collaboration with
the National Center for Chronic Disease Prevention and Health Promotion (2000).
http://www.cdc.gov/growthcharts

CDC
SAFER·HEALTHIER·PEOPLE™

A261

BOYS LENGTH-FOR-AGE AND WEIGHT-FOR-AGE BIRTH TO 36 MONTHS (3RD-97TH PERCENTILE)

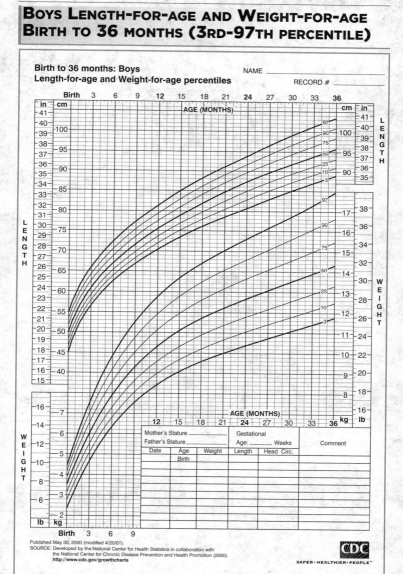

Birth to 36 months: Boys
Length-for-age and Weight-for-age percentiles

NAME

RECORD #

Published May 30, 2000 (modified 4/20/01).
SOURCE: Developed by the National Center for Health Statistics in collaboration with
the National Center for Chronic Disease Prevention and Health Promotion (2000).
http://www.cdc.gov/growthcharts

CDC

SAFER · HEALTHIER · PEOPLE

BOYS HEAD CIRCUMFERENCE-FOR-AGE AND WEIGHT-FOR-LENGTH
BIRTH TO 36 MONTHS (3RD-97TH PERCENTILE)

Birth to 36 months: Boys
Head circumference-for-age and
Weight-for-length percentiles

NAME _____

RECORD # _____

Published May 30, 2000 (modified 10/16/00).
SOURCE: Developed by the National Center for Health Statistics in collaboration with
the National Center for Chronic Disease Prevention and Health Promotion (2000).
http://www.cdc.gov/growthcharts

CDC
SAFER · HEALTHIER · PEOPLE™

GIRLS LENGTH-FOR-AGE AND WEIGHT-FOR-AGE BIRTH TO 36 MONTHS (3RD-97TH PERCENTILE)

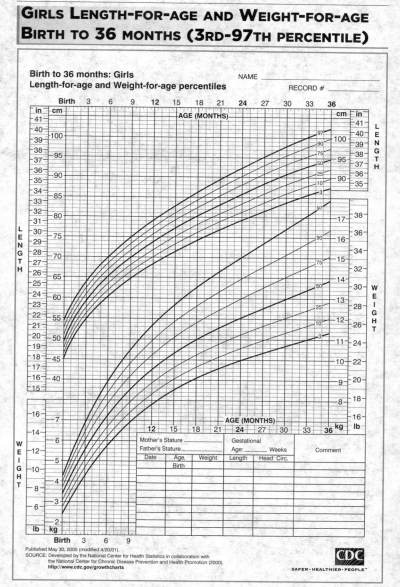

Birth to 36 months: Girls
Length-for-age and Weight-for-age percentiles

NAME _____

RECORD # _____

Published May 30, 2000 (modified 4/20/01).
SOURCE: Developed by the National Center for Health Statistics in collaboration with
the National Center for Chronic Disease Prevention and Health Promotion (2000).
http://www.cdc.gov/growthcharts

SAFER · HEALTHIER · PEOPLE™

A267

GIRLS HEAD CIRCUMFERENCE-FOR-AGE AND WEIGHT-FOR-LENGTH
BIRTH TO 36 MONTHS (3RD-97TH PERCENTILE)

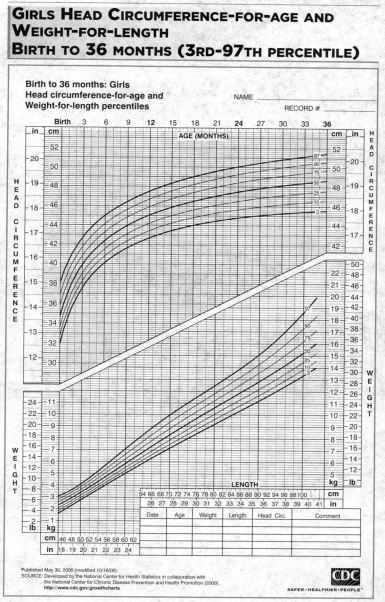

Birth to 36 months: Girls
Head circumference-for-age and
Weight-for-length percentiles

NAME _____

RECORD # _____

Published May 30, 2000 (modified 10/16/00).
SOURCE: Developed by the National Center for Health Statistics in collaboration with
the National Center for Chronic Disease Prevention and Health Promotion (2000).
http://www.cdc.gov/growthcharts

CDC
SAFER · HEALTHIER · PEOPLE™

BOYS STATURE-FOR-AGE AND WEIGHT-FOR-AGE
CHILDREN 2 TO 20 YEARS (3RD-97TH PERCENTILE)

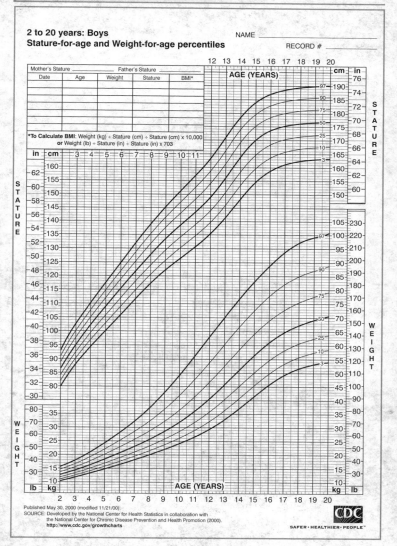

2 to 20 years: Boys
Stature-for-age and Weight-for-age percentiles

NAME _____

RECORD # _____

Mother's Stature _____ Father's Stature _____

Date	Age	Weight	Stature	BMI*

*To Calculate BMI: Weight (kg) ÷ Stature (cm) ÷ Stature (cm) x 10,000
or Weight (lb) ÷ Stature (in) ÷ Stature (in) x 703

AGE (YEARS)

Published May 30, 2000 (modified 11/21/00).
SOURCE: Developed by the National Center for Health Statistics in collaboration with
the National Center for Chronic Disease Prevention and Health Promotion (2000).
http://www.cdc.gov/growthcharts

CDC

SAFER • HEALTHIER • PEOPLE™

BOYS BMI-FOR-AGE
CHILDREN 2 TO 20 YEARS (3RD-97TH PERCENTILE)

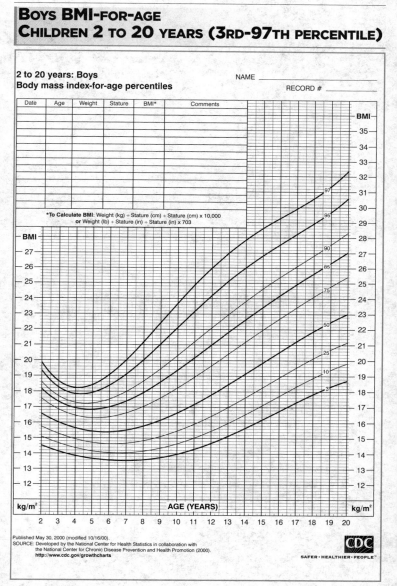

2 to 20 years: Boys
Body mass index-for-age percentiles

NAME _____

RECORD # _____

Date	Age	Weight	Stature	BMI*	Comments

*To Calculate BMI: Weight (kg) ÷ Stature (cm) ÷ Stature (cm) x 10,000
or Weight (lb) ÷ Stature (in) ÷ Stature (in) x 703

AGE (YEARS)

Published May 30, 2000 (modified 10/16/00).
SOURCE: Developed by the National Center for Health Statistics in collaboration with
the National Center for Chronic Disease Prevention and Health Promotion (2000).
http://www.cdc.gov/growthcharts

CDC
SAFER · HEALTHIER · PEOPLE™

A273

GIRLS STATURE-FOR-AGE AND WEIGHT-FOR-AGE
CHILDREN 2 TO 20 YEARS (3RD-97TH PERCENTILE)

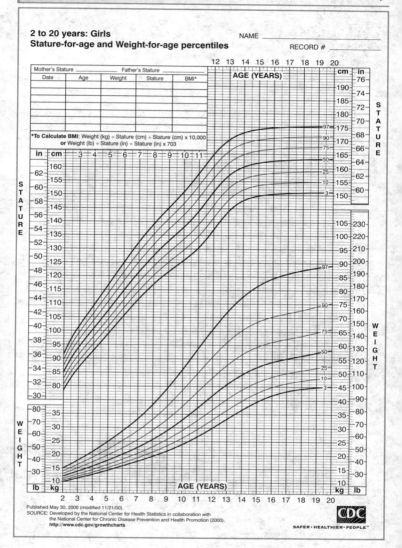

2 to 20 years: Girls
Stature-for-age and Weight-for-age percentiles

NAME _____

RECORD # _____

*To Calculate BMI: Weight (kg) ÷ Stature (cm) ÷ Stature (cm) x 10,000
or Weight (lb) ÷ Stature (in) ÷ Stature (in) x 703

Published May 30, 2000 (modified 11/21/00).
SOURCE: Developed by the National Center for Health Statistics in collaboration with
the National Center for Chronic Disease Prevention and Health Promotion (2000).
http://www.cdc.gov/growthcharts

CDC
SAFER · HEALTHIER · PEOPLE™

GIRLS BMI-FOR-AGE
CHILDREN 2 TO 20 YEARS (3RD-97TH PERCENTILE)

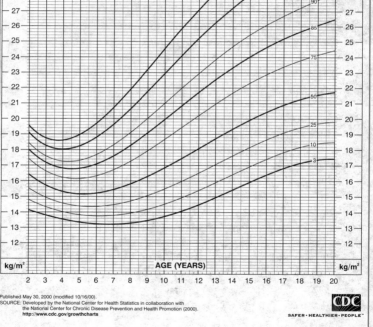

2 to 20 years: Girls
Body mass index-for-age percentiles

NAME _____

RECORD # _____

*To Calculate BMI: Weight (kg) ÷ Stature (cm) ÷ Stature (cm) x 10,000
or Weight (lb) ÷ Stature (in) ÷ Stature (in) x 703

Date	Age	Weight	Stature	BMI*	Comments

AGE (YEARS)

kg/m²

kg/m²

Published May 30, 2000 (modified 10/16/00).
SOURCE: Developed by the National Center for Health Statistics in collaboration with
the National Center for Chronic Disease Prevention and Health Promotion (2000).
http://www.cdc.gov/growthcharts

CDC
SAFER · HEALTHIER · PEOPLE™

BOYS WEIGHT-FOR-STATURE (3RD-97TH PERCENTILE)

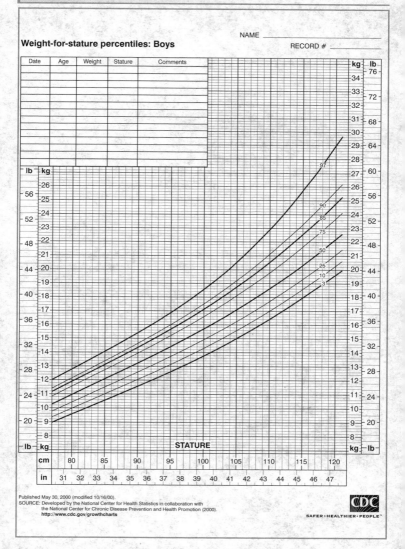

Weight-for-stature percentiles: Boys

NAME _____

RECORD # _____

Date	Age	Weight	Stature	Comments

STATURE

Published May 30, 2000 (modified 10/16/00).
SOURCE: Developed by the National Center for Health Statistics in collaboration with
the National Center for Chronic Disease Prevention and Health Promotion (2000).
http://www.cdc.gov/growthcharts

CDC

SAFER·HEALTHIER·PEOPLE™

A279

GIRLS WEIGHT-FOR-STATURE
(3RD–97TH PERCENTILE)

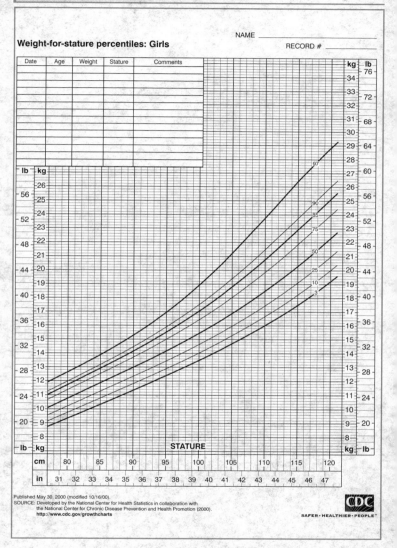

Weight-for-stature percentiles: Girls

NAME _____

RECORD # _____

Date	Age	Weight	Stature	Comments

STATURE

Published May 30, 2000 (modified 10/16/00).
SOURCE: Developed by the National Center for Health Statistics in collaboration with
the National Center for Chronic Disease Prevention and Health Promotion (2000).
http://www.cdc.gov/growthcharts

CDC
SAFER·HEALTHIER·PEOPLE™

A281